Biomarkers in Disease: Methods, Discoveries and Applications

Series Editor

Victor R. Preedy
Department of Nutrition and Dietetics
Division of Diabetes and Nutritional Sciences
Faculty of Life Sciences and Medicine
King's College London
London, UK

In the past decade there has been a sea change in the way disease is diagnosed and investigated due to the advent of high throughput technologies, such as microarrays, lab on a chip, proteomics, genomics, lipomics, metabolomics, etc. These advances have enabled the discovery of new and novel markers of disease relating to autoimmune disorders, cancers, endocrine diseases, genetic disorders, sensory damage, intestinal diseases etc. In many instances these developments have gone hand in hand with the discovery of biomarkers elucidated via traditional or conventional methods, such as histopathology or clinical biochemistry. Together with microprocessor-based data analysis, advanced statistics and bioinformatics these markers have been used to identify individuals with active disease or pathology as well as those who are refractory or have distinguishing pathologies. Unfortunately techniques and methods have not been readily transferable to other disease states and sometimes diagnosis still relies on single analytes rather than a cohort of markers. Furthermore, the discovery of many new markers have not been put into clinical practice, partly because of their cost and partly because some scientists are unaware of their existence or the evidence is still at the preclinical stage. In some cases the work needs further scientific scrutiny. There is thus a demand for a comprehensive and focused evidenced-based text and scientific literature that addresses these issues. Hence the formulation of *Biomarkers in Disease: Methods, Discoveries and Applications*. The series covers a wide number of areas including for example, nutrition, cancer, endocrinology, cardiology, addictions, immunology, birth defects, genetics and so on. The chapters are written by national or international experts and specialists.

Series Titles

1. General Methods in Biomarker Research and Their Applications
2. Biomarkers in Cancer
3. Biomarkers in Cardiovascular Disease
4. Biomarkers in Kidney Disease
5. Biomarkers in Bone Disease
6. Biomarkers in Liver Disease

More information about this series at http://www.springer.com/series/13842

Victor R. Preedy • Vinood B. Patel
Editors

Biomarkers in Cancer

With 176 Figures and 88 Tables

Springer Reference

Editors
Victor R. Preedy
Department of Nutrition and Dietetics
Division of Diabetes and Nutritional Sciences
Faculty of Life Sciences and Medicine
King's College London
London, UK

Vinood B. Patel
Department of Biomedical Sciences
Faculty of Science and Technology
University of Westminster
London, UK

ISBN 978-94-007-7680-7 ISBN 978-94-007-7681-4 (eBook)
ISBN 978-94-007-7682-1 (print and electronic bundle)
DOI 10.1007/978-94-007-7681-4

Library of Congress Control Number: 2015941735

Springer Dordrecht Heidelberg New York London

Printed on acid-free paper

Springer Science+Business Media B.V. Dordrecht is part of Springer Science+Business Media (www.springer.com)

Preface

In the present volume, ***Biomarkers in Cancer***, we have over 40 chapters covering a wide range of conditions, body locations, and cancer types. Their allocations to a traditional grouping presents some difficulty as this may mean having only one chapter in a particular section. Instead, we have adopted a pragmatic approach for ease of navigation and so have the following sections:

- General Aspects: Techniques and Overviews
- Bladder, Kidney, Liver, and Lung
- Brain
- Breast and Prostate
- Cervix and Uterus
- Colorectum
- Head and Neck
- Leukemia and Hodgkin Lymphoma
- Further Knowledge

While the Editors recognize the difficulties in assigning particular chapters to particular sections, the book has enormously wide coverage and includes the following areas, analytes, and platforms: omics, circulating tumor cells, oncoproteomics, cardiotoxicity, DNA methylation, kallikreins, MAP17, CA 19-9, PTTG (Securin), small nuclear RNA, centrosome amplification, cytological specimens, microarrays, cell death markers, epigenetics, molecular markers, maspin, LGR5, 2D-DIGE-MS, imaging, TPS, CD133, mitosis targets, HER2, immunohistochemistry, visceral adipocytes, expression profiling, telomerase, carcinoembryonic antigen family cell adhesion molecules, human papillomavirus (HPV), the NeoMark European project, matrix metalloproteinases, tissue microarrays, FGFR4, whole blood transcriptome, nuclear BMI-1, immunophenotyping, and CD163 and TARC. Tissues and conditions include cancers in general, cancers of the bladder, renal cell, liver, lung, brain, breast, prostate, cervix, endometrium, colorectum, head and neck cancers including the oral cavity, salivary gland, oropharynx, nasopharynx, larynx, leukemia, and Hodgkin lymphoma. Finally, the last chapter is devoted to locating resource material for biomarker discovery and applications. The chapters are written by national or international experts and specialists.

This book is specifically designed for clinical biochemists, oncologists, scientists, epidemiologists, doctors, and nurses, from students to practitioners at the higher level. It is also designed to be suitable for lecturers and teachers in health care and libraries as a reference guide.

April 2015 Victor R. Preedy
London Vinood B. Patel

Series Preface

In the past decade, there has been a sea change in the way disease is diagnosed and investigated due to the advent of high-throughput technologies and advances in chemistry and physics, leading to the development of microarrays, lab on a chip, proteomics, genomics, lipomics, metabolomics, etc. These advances have enabled the discovery of new and novel markers of disease relating to autoimmune disorders, cancers, endocrine diseases, genetic disorders, sensory damage, intestinal diseases, and many other conditions too numerous to list here. In many instances, these developments have gone hand in hand with the discovery of biomarkers elucidated via traditional or conventional methods, such as histopathology, immunoassays, or clinical biochemistry. Together with microprocessor-based data analysis, advanced statistics, and bioinformatics, these markers have been used to identify individuals with active disease as well as those who are refractory or have distinguishing pathologies.

Unfortunately, techniques and methods have not been readily transferable to other disease states, and sometimes, diagnosis still relies on a single analyte rather than a cohort of markers. Furthermore, the discovery of many new markers has not been put into clinical practice partly because of their cost and partly because some scientists are unaware of their existence or the evidence is still at the preclinical stage. There is thus a demand for a comprehensive and focused evidence-based text and scientific literature that addresses these issues. Hence, the book series ***Biomarkers in Disease: Methods, Discoveries and Applications***. It imparts holistic information on the scientific basis of health and biomarkers and covers the latest knowledge, trends, and treatments. It links conventional approaches with new platforms. The ability to transcend the intellectual divide is aided by the fact that each chapter has

- *Key Facts* (areas of focus explained for the lay person)
- *Definitions of Words and Terms*
- *Potential Applications to Prognosis, Other Diseases, or Conditions*
- *Summary Points*

The material in ***Potential Applications to Prognosis, Other Diseases, or Conditions*** pertains to speculative or proposed areas of research, cross-transference to other diseases or stages of the disease, translational issues, and other areas of wide applicability.

The series is expected to prove useful for clinicians, scientists, epidemiologists, doctors and nurses, and also academicians and students at an advanced level.

April 2015
London

Victor R. Preedy

Contents

About the Editors

Victor R. Preedy is a senior member of King's College London (Professor of Nutritional Biochemistry) and King's College Hospital (Professor of Clinical Biochemistry, Honorary). He is attached to both the Diabetes and Nutritional Sciences Division and the Department of Nutrition and Dietetics. He is also founding and current Director of the Genomics Centre and a member of the School of Medicine. Professor Preedy graduated in 1974 with an Honors Degree in Biology and Physiology with Pharmacology. He gained his University of London Ph.D. in 1981. In 1992, he received his Membership of the Royal College of Pathologists, and in 1993, he gained his second Doctoral degree for his contribution to the science of protein metabolism in health and disease. Professor Preedy was elected as a Fellow of the Institute of Biology in 1995 and to the Royal College of Pathologists in 2000. Since then, he has been elected as a Fellow to the Royal Society for the Promotion of Health (2004) and the Royal Institute of Public Health and Hygiene (2004). In 2009, Professor Preedy became a Fellow of the Royal Society for Public Health and in 2012 a Fellow of the Royal Society of Chemistry. In his career, Professor Preedy worked at the National Heart Hospital (part of Imperial College London) and the MRC Centre at Northwick Park Hospital. He has collaborated with research groups in Finland, Japan, Australia, USA, and Germany. He is a leading expert on biomedical sciences and has a long-standing interest in analytical methods and their applications to the study of health and disease. He has lectured nationally and internationally. To his credit, Professor Preedy has published over 500 articles, which includes peer-reviewed manuscripts based on original research, reviews, abstracts, and numerous books and volumes.

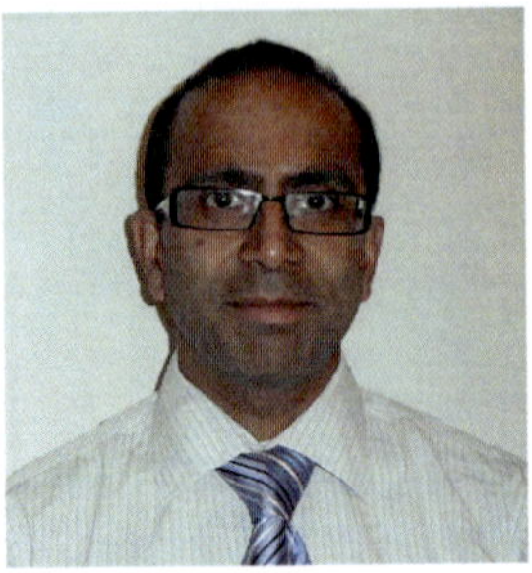

Vinood B. Patel is currently a Senior Lecturer in Clinical Biochemistry at the University of Westminster and honorary fellow at King's College London. He presently directs studies on metabolic pathways involved in liver disease, particularly related to mitochondrial energy regulation and cell death. Research is being undertaken to study the role of nutrients, antioxidants, phytochemicals, iron, alcohol, and fatty acids in the pathophysiology of liver disease. Other areas of interest are identifying new biomarkers that can be used for diagnosis and prognosis of liver disease, understanding mitochondrial oxidative stress in Alzheimer's disease, and gastrointestinal dysfunction in autism. Dr. Patel graduated from the University of Portsmouth with a degree in Pharmacology and completed his Ph.D. in protein metabolism from King's College London in 1997. His postdoctoral work was carried out at Wake Forest University Baptist Medical School studying structural–functional alterations to mitochondrial ribosomes, where he developed novel techniques to characterize their biophysical properties. Dr. Patel is a nationally and internationally recognized liver researcher and was involved in several NIH-funded biomedical grants related to alcoholic liver disease. He has edited biomedical books in the area of nutrition and health prevention, autism, and biomarkers and has published over 150 articles. In 2014, he was elected as a Fellow to The Royal Society of Chemistry.

Editorial Advisors

Caroline J. Hollins Martin School of Nursing, Midwifery and Social Work, College of Health and Social Care, University of Salford, Salford, Greater Manchester, UK

Ross J. Hunter Department of Cardiology, St. Bartholomew's Hospital, Barts Health NHS Trust and Queen Mary, University of London, London, UK

Colin R. Martin Faculty of Society and Health, Buckinghamshire New University, Uxbridge, Middlesex, UK

Rajkumar Rajendram Royal Free London Hospitals, Barnet General Hospital, London, UK

Division of Diabetes and Nutritional Sciences, Faculty of Life Sciences and Medicine, King's College London, London, UK

King Khalid University Hospital, King Saud University Medical City, Riyadh, Saudi Arabia

Contributors

Panagiotis G. Adamopoulos Department of Biochemistry and Molecular Biology, Faculty of Biology, School of Science, University of Athens, Athens, Greece

Soo Kyung Ahn Division of Breast and Endocrine, Department of Surgery, College of Medicine, University of Ulsan, Asan Medical Center, Sonpa-gu, Seoul, South Korea

Robert W. Allan Department of Pathology, Immunology and Laboratory Medicine, University of Florida, Gainesville, FL, USA

Eugenia Allegra Otolaryngology-Head and Neck Surgery, Department of Medical and Surgical Sciences, University Magna Graecia of Catanzaro, Catanzaro, Italy

Samer Z. Al-Quran Department of Pathology, Immunology and Laboratory Medicine, University of Florida, Gainesville, FL, USA

Arunkumar Anandharaj Department of Otolaryngology, Head and Neck Surgery, LSU Health Shreveport, Shreveport, LA, USA

Diego Ardigò MultiMed s.r.l., Cremona, Italy

Andrew J. Armstrong Duke Cancer Institute, Duke Prostate Center, Divisions of Medical Oncology and Urology, Duke University School of Medicine, Durham, NC, USA

Min-Hyun Baek Department of Obstetrics and Gynecology, University of Ulsan College of Medicine, Asan Medical Center, Seoul, South Korea

Ioanna Balkouranidou Analysis of Circulating Tumor Cells Lab, Laboratory of Analytical Chemistry, Department of Chemistry, University of Athens, Athens, Greece

Hirendra Nath Banerjee Department of Biological Sciences and Pharmaceutical Sciences, Elizabeth City State University/University of North Carolina, Elizabeth City, NC, USA

Ancha Baranova Center for the Study of Chronic Metabolic Diseases, School of System Biology, George Mason University, Fairfax, VA, USA

Research Centre for Medical Genetics, Russian Academy of Medical Sciences, Moscow, Russia

Rodrigo Barderas Biochemistry and Molecular Biology I Department, Facultad de Ciencias Químicas, Universidad Complutense de Madrid, Madrid, Spain

Tanios Bekaii-Saab Division of Medical Oncology, The Ohio State University Wexner Medical Center, James Cancer Hospital, Columbus, OH, USA

Manfred Beleut Qlaym Healthcare AG, Goettingen, Germany

Rossana Berardi Medical Oncology Unit, Università Politecnica delle Marche, Azienda Ospedaliero-Universitaria, Ospedali Riuniti Umberto I – GM Lancisi – G Salesi, Ancona, Italy

Roberta Bertorelle Immunology and Molecular Oncology Unit, Istituto Oncologico Veneto, IOV-IRCCS, Padova, Italy

Jaime Berumen Departamento de Medicina Experimental, Facultad de Medicina, Universidad Nacional Autonoma de Mexico, Mexico city, Mexico

Unidad de Medicina Genomica, Hospital General de Mexico, Mexico city, Mexico

Natalia Buza Department of Pathology, Yale University School of Medicine, New Haven, CT, USA

Daniela Cardinale Unit of Cardioncology, Division of Cardiology, European Institute of Oncology, Milan, Italy

Amancio Carnero Instituto de Biomedicina de Sevilla (IBIS), Hospital Universitario Virgen del Rocio, Consejo Superior de Investigaciones Cientificas, Universidad de Sevilla, Sevilla, Spain

Christopher M. Carter Department of Pathology, Immunology and Laboratory Medicine, University of Florida, Gainesville, FL, USA

J. Ignacio Casal Department of Cellular and Molecular Medicine, Functional Proteomics Laboratory, Centro de Investigaciones Biológicas (CSIC), Madrid, Spain

Stefano Cascinu Medical Oncology Unit, Università Politecnica delle Marche, Azienda Ospedaliero-Universitaria, Ospedali Riuniti Umberto I – GM Lancisi – G Salesi, Ancona, Italy

Jimmy Yu-Wai Chan Department of Surgery, Queen Mary Hospital, The University of Hong Kong, Hong Kong, Hong Kong

Samuel Chao GeneNews Limited, Markham, ON, Canada

Kellie A. Charles School of Medical Sciences (Pharmacology), Sydney Medical School, University of Sydney, St Leonards, NSW, Australia

Wei Chua Department of Medical Oncology, Liverpool Hospital, Liverpool, NSW, Australia

Caroline Chung Department of Radiation Oncology, University of Toronto/ University Health Network-Princess Margaret Cancer Centre, Toronto, ON, Canada

Stephen J. Clarke Kolling Institute of Medical Research, Royal North Shore Hospital, University of Sydney, St Leonards, NSW, Australia

Alessandro Colombo Unit of Cardioncology, Division of Cardiology, European Institute of Oncology, Milan, Italy

Ana Conesa Genomics of Gene Expression Laboratory, Centro de Investigación Príncipe Felipe (CIPF), Valencia, Spain

Chiara Copelli Maxillofacial Surgery, University-Hospital of Parma, Parma, Italy

Claudia Corbo CEINGE-Biotecnologie avanzate, s.c.a r.l, Naples, Italy

Manuel José Rolo da Fonseca Link Consulting – Tecnologias De Informaçao S.A., Lisbon, Portugal

Adriana Madeira Álvares da Silva Conforti Department of Biology, Federal University of Espirito Santo – Center of Agrarian Sciences (CCA/UFES), Alegre, ES, Brazil

Oslei Paes de Almeida Piracicaba Dental School, Department of Oral Diagnosis (Pathology), State University of Campinas, Areão, Piracicaba, São Paulo, Brazil

Marco De Fazio STMicroelectronics, Agrate Brianza (MI), Italy

Anita De Rossi Department of Surgery, Oncology and Gastroenterology, Section of Oncology and Immunology, University of Padova, and Istituto Oncologico Veneto, IOV-IRCCS, Padova, Italy

Istituto Oncologico Veneto, Padova, Italy

Luigi Del Vecchio CEINGE-Biotecnologie avanzate, s.c.a r.l, Naples, Italy

Dipartimento di Medicina Molecolare e Biotecnologie Mediche, Università di Napoli "Federico II", Naples, Italy

Connie I. Diakos Kolling Institute of Medical Research, Royal North Shore Hospital, University of Sydney, St Leonards, NSW, Australia

Roberta Lelis Dutra Department of Pathology, University of Sao Paulo, Laboratório de Citogenômica, LIM 03, São Paulo, SP, Brazil

Oleksandr Ekshyyan Department of Otolaryngology, Head and Neck Surgery, LSU Health Shreveport, Shreveport, LA, USA

Diana P. English Department of Obstetrics, Gynecology and Reproductive Sciences, Yale University School of Medicine, New Haven, CT, USA

Ana María Espinosa Unidad de Medicina Genomica, Hospital General de Mexico, Mexico city, Mexico

Konstantinos Exarchos University of Ioannina, Ioannina, Greece

Felipe Paiva Fonseca Piracicaba Dental School, Department of Oral Diagnosis (Pathology), State University of Campinas, Areão, Piracicaba, São Paulo, Brazil

School of Clinical Dentistry, Department of Oral and Maxillofacial Pathology, The University of Sheffield, Claremont Crescent, Sheffield, UK

James Freeman School of Medical Sciences, Edith Cowan University, Perth, WA, Australia

Shinichi Fukushige Department of Molecular Pathology, Center for Regulatory Epigenome and Diseases, Tohoku University School of Medicine, Sendai, Miyagi, Japan

Maher K. Gandhi University of Queensland Diamantina Institute, Translational Research Institute, Brisbane, QLD, Australia

Wei Gao Department of Surgery, Queen Mary Hospital, The University of Hong Kong, Pokfulam, Hong Kong

Miguel Pérez-Guillermo García Department of Pathology, Hospital General Universitario Santa Lucia (HGUSL), Cartagena, Spain

Marica Gemei CEINGE-Biotecnologie avanzate, s.c.a r.l, Naples, Italy

Violaine Goidts Division of Molecular Genetics (B060), German Cancer Research Center (DKFZ), Heidelberg, Germany

Elin S. Gray School of Medical Sciences, Edith Cowan University, Perth, WA, Australia

Mariano Guardado Unidad de Medicina Genomica, Hospital General de Mexico, Mexico city, Mexico

Stephan A. Hahn Department of Molecular Gastrointestinal Oncology, Ruhr-University Bochum, Molecular GI-Oncology (MGO), Bochum, Germany

Ji-Hyun Han Department of Obstetrics and Gynecology, University of Ulsan College of Medicine, Asan Medical Center, Seoul, South Korea

Liz Y. Han Division of Gynecologic Oncology, Kaiser Permanente Northern California, Oakland, CA, USA

Wonshik Han Division of Breast and Endocrine, Department of Surgery, College of Medicine, University of Ulsan, Asan Medical Center, Sonpa-gu, Seoul, South Korea

Woo-Suk Han Department of Obstetrics and Gynecology, University of Ulsan College of Medicine, Asan Medical Center, Seoul, South Korea

Stefan Holdenrieder Institute of Clinical Chemistry and Clinical Pharmacology, University Hospital Bonn, Bonn, Germany

Akira Horii Department of Molecular Pathology, Tohoku University School of Medicine, Sendai, Miyagi, Japan

Viive M. Howell Kolling Institute of Medical Research, Royal North Shore Hospital, University of Sydney, St Leonards, NSW, Australia

Kimberley Jones University of Queensland Diamantina Institute, Translational Research Institute, Brisbane, QLD, Australia

Dimitrios N. Kanakis Department of Pathology, Medical Faculty, Democritus University of Thrace, Alexandroupolis, Greece

Jisun Kim Division of Breast and Endocrine, Department of Surgery, College of Medicine, University of Ulsan, Asan Medical Center, Sonpa-gu, Seoul, South Korea

Elmar Kirches Department of Neuropathology, Medical Faculty, Otto-von-Guericke University, Magdeburg, Germany

Athina Kladi-Skandali Department of Biochemistry and Molecular Biology, University of Athens, Athens, Greece

A-Ra Ko Department of Obstetrics and Gynecology, University of Ulsan College of Medicine, Asan Medical Center, Seoul, South Korea

Nikolaus Kohles Department of Otorhinolaryngology, Helios-Klinikum Erfurt, Erfurt, Germany

Christos K. Kontos Department of Biochemistry and Molecular Biology, Faculty of Biology, School of Science, University of Athens, Athens, Greece

Kavya Krishna Department of Hematology and Oncology, The Ohio State University Wexner Medical Center, James Cancer Hospital, Columbus, OH, USA

Feryel Ksiâa Department of Pathology, University Hospital Farhat Hached, Sousse, Tunisia

Davide Lanfranco Maxillofacial Surgery, University-Hospital of Parma, Parma, Italy

Michelle Mei Lin Lee GeneNews (Malaysia) Limited, Georgetown, Penang, Malaysia

Jing Li Duke University and Cancer Institute, Durham, NC, USA

Ying Li Department of Pathology, Immunology and Laboratory Medicine, University of Florida, Gainesville, FL, USA

Zeng-Hong Li Department of Surgery, The University of Hong Kong, Pokfulam, Hong Kong

Evi S. Lianidou Analysis of Circulating Tumor Cells Lab, Laboratory of Analytical Chemistry, Department of Chemistry, University of Athens, Athens, Greece

Choong Chin Liew GeneNews Diagnostics, Kuala Lumpur, Malaysia

Chun Ren Lim GeneNews (Malaysia) Limited, Georgetown, Penang, Malaysia

Yvonne G. Lin Division of Gynecologic Oncology, Department of Obstetrics-Gynecology, Norris Comprehensive Cancer Center, University of Southern California, Los Angeles, CA, USA

Petr Lokhov Department of Proteomics and Mass-Spectrometry, Orekhovich Institute of Biomedical Chemistry, Russian Academy of Medical Sciences, Moscow, Russia

Iúri Drumond Louro Department of Biology, Federal University of Espirito Santo (UFES), Human and Molecular Genetics Center, Vitória, ES, Brazil

Abdelouahid Maghnouj Department of Molecular Gastrointestinal Oncology, Ruhr-University Bochum, Molecular GI-Oncology (MGO), Bochum, Germany

Athina Markou Analysis of Circulating Tumor Cells Lab, Laboratory of Analytical Chemistry, Department of Chemistry, University of Athens, Athens, Greece

Elena Martinelli Maxillofacial Surgery, University-Hospital of Parma, Parma, Italy

Tasuku Matsuoka Department of Surgical Oncology, Osaka City University Graduate School of Medicine, Osaka, Japan

Hideyasu Matsuyama Department of Urology, Graduate School of Medicine, Yamaguchi University, Ube, Japan

Ingrid Medina Unidad de Medicina Genomica, Hospital General de Mexico, Mexico city, Mexico

Vikas Mehta Department of Otolaryngology, Head and Neck Surgery, LSU Health Shreveport, Shreveport, LA, USA

Suzanny Oliveira Mendes Programa de Pós-graduação em Biotecnologia, Núcleo de Genética Humana e Molecular, Federal University of Espirito Santo (UFES), Vitória, ES, Brazil

Kleita Michaelidou Department of Biochemistry and Molecular Biology, University of Athens, Athens, Greece

Hyeong-Gon Moon Division of Breast and Endocrine, Department of Surgery, College of Medicine, University of Ulsan, Asan Medical Center, Sonpa-gu, Seoul, South Korea

Tara Moore-Medlin Department of Otolaryngology, Head and Neck Surgery, LSU Health Shreveport, Shreveport, LA, USA

Francesca Morgese Medical Oncology Unit, Università Politecnica delle Marche, Azienda Ospedaliero-Universitaria, Ospedali Riuniti Umberto I – GM Lancisi – G Salesi, Ancona, Italy

Sergei Moshkovskii Department of Personalized Medicine, Orekhovich Institute of Biomedical Chemistry, Russian Academy of Medical Sciences, Moscow, Russia

Medico-Biological Faculty, Pirogov Russian National Research Medical University, Moscow, Russia

Susumu Nakata Division of Oncological Pathology, Aichi Cancer Center Research Institute, Nagoya, Japan

Joo-Hyun Nam Department of Obstetrics and Gynecology, University of Ulsan College of Medicine, Asan Medical Center, Seoul, South Korea

Cherie-Ann O. Nathan Department of Otolaryngology, Head and Neck Surgery, LSU Health Shreveport, Shreveport, LA, USA

Claudio Navarre Genomics of Gene Expression Laboratory, Centro de Investigación Príncipe Felipe (CIPF), Valencia, Spain

Dong-Young Noh Division of Breast and Endocrine, Department of Surgery, College of Medicine, University of Ulsan, Asan Medical Center, Sonpa-gu, Seoul, South Korea

Azzurra Onofri Medical Oncology Unit, Università Politecnica delle Marche, Azienda Ospedaliero-Universitaria, Ospedali Riuniti Umberto I – GM Lancisi – G Salesi, Ancona, Italy

Jeong-Yeol Park Department of Obstetrics and Gynecology, University of Ulsan College of Medicine, Asan Medical Center, Seoul, South Korea

Vinood B. Patel Department of Biomedical Sciences, Faculty of Science and Technology, University of Westminster, London, UK

Gabriela Tonini Peterle Programa de Pós-graduação em Biotecnologia, Núcleo de Genética Humana e Molecular, Federal University of Espirito Santo (UFES), Vitória, ES, Brazil

Emma Phillips Division of Molecular Genetics (B060), German Cancer Research Center (DKFZ), Heidelberg, Germany

Marco Picone Department of Information Engineering, University of Parma, MultiMed s.r.l., Cremona, Italy

Tito Poli Maxillofacial Surgery, University-Hospital of Parma, Parma, Italy

Victor R. Preedy Department of Nutrition and Dietetics, Division of Diabetes and Nutritional Sciences, Faculty of Life Sciences and Medicine, King's College London, London, UK

Mikhail Pyatnitsky Department of Bioinformatics, Orekhovich Institute of Biomedical Chemistry, Russian Academy of Medical Sciences, Moscow, Russia

Rajkumar Rajendram Department of General Medicine and Intensive Care, John Radcliffe Hospital, Oxford, UK

Diabetes and Nutritional Sciences Research Division, School of Medicine, King's College London, London, UK

Roshanna Rajendram School of Medicine, University of Birmingham, Edgbaston, Birmingham, UK

Dana Marie Roque Division of Gynecologic Oncology, Greenebaum Cancer Center, University of Maryland-Baltimore, Baltimore, MD, USA

Michela Salvatici Division of Laboratory Medicine, European Institute of Oncology, Milan, Italy

Francesco Salvatore CEINGE-Biotecnologie avanzate, s.c.a r.l, Naples, Italy

Dipartimento di Medicina Molecolare e Biotecnologie Mediche, Università di Napoli "Federico II", Naples, Italy

IRCCS-SDN, Naples, Italy

Dario Salvi Life Supporting Technologies, ETSI Telecomunicación, Universidad Politécnica de Madrid, Madrid, Spain

Maria Teresa Sandri Division of Laboratory Medicine, European Institute of Oncology, Milan, Italy

Alessandro D. Santin Department of Obstetrics, Gynecology and Reproductive Sciences, Yale University School of Medicine, New Haven, CT, USA

Marcelo dos Santos Department of Medicine, Federal University of Rio Grande do Norte (UFRN) – Campus Caicó, Caicó, RN, Brazil

Shinobu Sato Department of Applied Chemistry, Research Center for Biomicrosensing Technology, Kyushu Institute of Technology, Kitakyushu, Fukuoka, Japan

Agnese Savini Medical Oncology Unit, Università Politecnica delle Marche, Azienda Ospedaliero-Universitaria, Ospedali Riuniti Umberto I – GM Lancisi – G Salesi, Ancona, Italy

Peter Schraml Institute of Surgical Pathology, University Hospital Zurich, Zurich, Switzerland

Andreas Scorilas Department of Biochemistry and Molecular Biology, Faculty of Biology, School of Science, University of Athens, Athens, Greece

Enrico Sesenna Maxillofacial Surgery, University-Hospital of Parma, Parma, Italy

Mari Carmen Turpín Sevilla Department of Pathology (HGUSL) Cartagena, Spain; University Francisco of Vitoria, Madrid, Spain

Louise Seymour University of Queensland Diamantina Institute, Translational Research Institute, Brisbane, QLD, Australia

José García Solano Department of Pathology, Hospital General Universitario Santa Lucia (HGUSL), Cartagena, Spain

Facultad de Ciencias de la Salud, Catholic University of Murcia (UCAM), Murcia, Spain

Ioanna Sourvinou Analysis of Circulating Tumor Cells Lab, Laboratory of Analytical Chemistry, Department of Chemistry, University of Athens, Athens, Greece

Paul M. Speight School of Clinical Dentistry, Department of Oral and Maxillofacial Pathology, The University of Sheffield, Claremont Crescent, Sheffield, UK

Sebastian Steger Fraunhofer Institute for Computer Graphics (IGD) Cognitive Computing and Medical Imaging (A7), Darmstadt, Germany

Shigeori Takenaka Department of Applied Chemistry, Research Center for Biomicrosensing Technology, Kyushu Institute of Technology, Kitakyushu, Fukuoka, Japan

Serena Trapasso Otolaryngology-Head and Neck Surgery, Department of Medical and Surgical Sciences, University Magna Graecia of Catanzaro, Catanzaro, Italy

Mounir Trimeche Department of Pathology, University Hospital Farhat Hached, Sousse, Tunisia

Deepak B. Vangala Department of Medicine and Department of Molecular Gastrointestinal Oncology, Ruhr-University Bochum, Knappschaftskrankenhaus, Bochum, Germany

Pablo Agustin Vargas Piracicaba Dental School, Department of Oral Diagnosis (Pathology), State University of Campinas, Areão, Piracicaba, São Paulo, Brazil

Department of Oral Pathology and Oral Biology, School of Dentistry, Faculty of Health Sciences, University of Pretoria, Pretoria, South Africa

Mukesh Verma Methods and Technologies Branch, Epidemiology and Genetics Research Program, Division of Cancer Control and Population Sciences, National Cancer Institute (NCI), National Institutes of Health (NIH), Rockville, MD, USA

Roi Villar-Vázquez Department of Cellular and Molecular Medicine, Functional Proteomics Laboratory, Centro de Investigaciones Biológicas (CSIC), Madrid, Spain

Thian-Sze Wong Department of Surgery, Queen Mary Hospital, The University of Hong Kong, Pokfulam, Hong Kong

Masakazu Yashiro Department of Surgical Oncology, Osaka City University Graduate School of Medicine, Osaka, Japan

Adel Zaatar Gleneagles Medical Centre, Penang, Malaysia

Pablo Conesa Zamora Department of Pathology, Hospital General Universitario Santa Lucia (HGUSL), Cartagena, Spain

Facultad de Ciencias de la Salud, Catholic University of Murcia (UCAM), Murcia, Spain

Mel Ziman School of Medical Sciences, Edith Cowan University, Perth, WA, Australia

Hannah Zoellner Department of Molecular Gastrointestinal Oncology, Ruhr-University Bochum, Molecular GI-Oncology (MGO), Bochum, Germany

Part I

General Aspects: Techniques and Overviews

OMICS for Tumor Biomarker Research

1

Sergei Moshkovskii, Mikhail Pyatnitsky, Petr Lokhov, and Ancha Baranova

Contents

S. Moshkovskii (✉)
Department of Personalized Medicine, Orekhovich Institute of Biomedical Chemistry, Russian Academy of Medical Sciences, Moscow, Russia

Medico-Biological Faculty, Pirogov Russian National Research Medical University, Moscow, Russia
e-mail: smosh@mail.ru; sergei.moshkovskii@ibmc.msk.ru

M. Pyatnitsky
Department of Bioinformatics, Orekhovich Institute of Biomedical Chemistry, Russian Academy of Medical Sciences, Moscow, Russia
e-mail: mpyat@mail.ru

P. Lokhov
Department of Proteomics and Mass-Spectrometry, Orekhovich Institute of Biomedical Chemistry, Russian Academy of Medical Sciences, Moscow, Russia
e-mail: lokhovpg@rambler.ru

A. Baranova
Center for the Study of Chronic Metabolic Diseases, School of System Biology, George Mason University, Fairfax, VA, USA

Research Centre for Medical Genetics, Russian Academy of Medical Sciences, Moscow, Russia
e-mail: abaranov@gmu.edu; aancha@gmail.com

V.R. Preedy, V.B. Patel (eds.), *Biomarkers in Cancer, Biomarkers in Disease: Methods, Discoveries and Applications*,
DOI 10.1007/978-94-007-7681-4_14

Abstract

OMICS generally refers to a study of some gene expression products, either direct, such as RNA and proteins, or indirect, such as metabolites, and is usually based on genome information. Main sections of OMICS sciences include transcriptomics, proteomics, and metabolomics, powerful research instruments capable of high-throughput detection of biomolecules differentially expressed between tumor and non-tumor samples, including excised tissues or biopsies, blood plasma, saliva, and urine. Consequently, thousands of species of RNAs, proteins, and metabolites were suggested as candidate tumor biomarkers alone or as constituents of multiplex signatures. Despite many difficulties encountered by OMICS panels with an intended use in population screening programs, some of the multiplex panels already have found their applications in the field of theranostics. If the patient is already diagnosed with a certain cancer, RNA or protein biomarker signatures may help to select a specific therapy or to predict the probability of a relapse. A number of clinically relevant, validated, and approved signatures of RNA and protein analytes successfully emerged from OMICS pipelines. It is important to remember that an implementation of these clinical tests took the safety of reliable laboratory techniques, such as polymerase chain reaction and immunoassay.

List of Abbreviations

AUC	Area Under the Curve
DNA	Deoxyribonucleic Acid
ENCODE	Encyclopedia of DNA Elements
ESI	Electrospray Ionization
FDA	US Food and Drug Administration
HPLC	High-Performance Liquid Chromatography
IVDMIA	In Vitro Diagnostic Multivariate Index Assay
LC-MS/MS	Liquid Chromatography-Tandem Mass Spectrometry
LDT	Laboratory-Developed Tests
LOOCV	Leave-One-Out Cross Validation
MALDI-TOF	Matrix-Assisted Laser Desorption/Ionization Time-of-Flight Mass Spectrometry
MRM	Multiple Reaction Monitoring
MS	Mass Spectrometry
MS/MS	Tandem Mass Spectrometry
m/z	Molecular Mass/Charge Ratio
mRNA	Matrix Ribonucleic Acid
miRNA	Micro-Ribonucleic Acid
NMR	Nuclear Magnetic Resonance
PCR	Polymerase Chain Reaction
PPV	Positive Predictive Value
qRT-PCR	Quantitative Real-Time Polymerase Chain Reaction
RNA	Ribonucleic Acid

RNAseq	High-Throughput Sequencing of Ribonucleic Acid
ROC	Receiver Operator Characteristics
SELDI	Surface-Enhanced Laser Desorption/Ionization
SRM	Selected Reaction Monitoring

Key Facts of OMICS Sciences

OMICS sciences are focused on the inventory of multiple molecular species in living organisms or their parts.

Each OMICS discipline is designated using the name of molecular species studied plus the "-omics" suffix, such as proteomics for proteins, lipidomics for lipids, glycomics for glycans, etc.

OMICS sciences for medicine have become possible after human genome sequencing.

Some OMICS sciences, such as transcriptomics and proteomics, are directly based on genome sequence, whereas others are indirectly related to genome, e.g., metabolomics.

OMICS sciences are used to compare levels of multiple molecular species between diseased and healthy control tissues or cells to discover differential molecules, i.e., biomarkers.

Today, transcriptomics, proteomics, and metabolomics are most widely used for biomarker discovery.

Transcriptomics uses nucleic acid microarrays and high-throughput nucleic acid sequencing to catalog RNA molecules.

Proteomics uses mass spectrometry and affinity reagents, such as antibodies, on protein microarrays, for protein inventory.

Metabolomics detects low-molecular metabolites by mass spectrometry or nucleic magnetic resonance spectroscopy.

Definitions of Words and Terms

Transcriptome Transcriptome is a whole of genome transcripts, i.e., RNAs, which are contained in a cell, tissue, or organism. The high-throughput detection and quantitation of multiple RNAs based on genome sequence information is transcriptomics.

Proteome Proteome is a whole of proteins, which are contained in a cell, tissue, or organism. High-throughput detection and quantitation of multiple proteins based on gene sequence information is proteomics.

Metabolome Metabolome is a whole of low-molecular substances, i.e., metabolites, which are contained in a cell, tissue, or organism. High-throughput detection and quantitation of multiple metabolites based on their physical and chemical properties is metabolomics.

Liquid Chromatography-Tandem Mass-Spectrometry (LC-MS/MS) LC-MS/MS is an analytical method, where molecules of interest are separated by high-performance liquid chromatography which is coupled with mass spectrometer with electrospray ionization. Such mass spectrometer performs tandem mass spectrometry. It measures the molecular mass/charge ratio (m/z) of original ions which may be further fragmented in mass spectrometer and analyzed for more structural information. LC-MS/MS is widely used in shotgun and targeted proteomics and metabolomics. Detectors used for tandem mass spectrometry include, but not limited to, ion trap, quadrupole time of flight (Q-TOF), triple quadrupole (QQQ), Orbitrap, etc.

Electrospray Ionization (ESI) ESI is a method for ionization of molecules based on the application of electrical field to the molecules which are sprayed in small drops of liquid. It is a mild method of ionization which preserves the structure of biomolecules for detection by mass spectrometry. ESI is widely used in proteomics.

Matrix-Assisted Laser Desorption/Ionization Time-of-Flight Mass Spectrometry (MALDI-TOF MS) MALDI-TOF MS is a specific method of mass spectrometry. It uses ionization of solid substances co-crystallized with a laser-sensitive "matrix" compound. After laser shot, a molecule analyzed is ionized and desorbed from the crystal state and then analyzed by time-of-flight detector. MALDI-TOF MS is a fast and easy method to analyze proteins and peptides.

Multiple Reaction Monitoring (MRM) Multiple reaction monitoring or selected reaction monitoring (SRM) is a method of targeted tandem mass spectrometry. In the MRM mode, a mass spectrometer can detect only molecules with expected narrow range of m/z and its expected fragments. ESI and a triple quadrupole detector are widely used for MRM. This method was originally used for quantitation of small molecules, such as drugs and chemicals. Since 2005, it was suggested for use to quantify peptides in proteomics. An isotope synthetic standard is required for proper measurement quality.

Introduction: A Role of OMICS in Cancer Biomarker Research

OMICS is a recently generated word that was coined by molecular biologists that figured how to analyze molecular entities in a high-throughput manner. In the late 1990s, the genomics became the very first "OMICS" field assessed in this manner. Respectively, the term "genomics" was derived from "genome," yet another recent addition to the dictionaries (Winkler 1920).

Each "OMICS" discipline is focused on its own "-ome." After the genome, a proteome concept was suggested (Wilkins et al. 1996) to represent a sum of proteins within the cell, tissue, or organism of interest. Simultaneously, many other classes of biomolecules got their own "-omes" and "OMICS" – transcriptomics for RNAs, metabolomics for metabolites, and lipidomics for lipids. In addition to "OMICS"-based inventories of various molecular entities, some "OMICS" disciplines are focused on the inventories of events, such as interactomics that systematically analyze interactions between various macromolecules (Cesareni et al. 2005).

It is important to note that the genomics stands apart from other OMICS disciplines as it serves as a background for others. In this context, transcriptomics and proteomics are usually referred to as postgenome technologies. Indeed, deciphering the genome of given species makes it possible for other OMICS sciences to emerge. In this chapter, we will not focus on cancer genomics due to the heaps of information already available. Here, OMICS will generally refer to a study of some gene expression products, either direct, such as RNA and proteins, or indirect, such as metabolites.

A majority of sporadic cancers are due to random somatic mutagenesis by way of environmental exposures and endogenous stress that lead to epigenetic deregulation of expression patterns within the cell (Amin et al. 2009). That is why high-throughput versions of mRNA expression analysis are widely used as means for cancer biomarker discovery. An accumulation of somatic or germ line mutations in chromosomal DNA is recognized as major reason for the proliferative features of cancer phenotype. These crucial genomic events are usually designated as driver mutations (Bignell et al. 2010) that may be caused by viral genome insertions, radiation, chemical mutagens, and other environmental carcinogens. How many driver mutations are exactly necessary and/or sufficient to make a viable cancer cell is a topic of hot discussion. As evident from the studies of transgenic and knockout mice, in most cases these numbers are minimal. However, naturally developed tumors are represented by a mix of competing clones varying in their malignant potential and genomic structure. Hence, the DNA extracted from a piece of tumor tissue may harbor thousands of mutations. Indeed, recent efforts in tumor exome sequencing confirmed these findings (Cancer Genome Atlas Research Network 2012; Stephens et al. 2009) and created solid grounds for generation of cancer-type specific genome atlases that provide a knowledge base for modern biomarker discovery.

The primary difficulty with the biomarker-guided detection of the tumors in general population is due to the multiclonal composition of individual tumors and the resultant variation in the levels and the spectrum of biological molecules expressed by tumors that originated within the same tissue. That is why, with a few notable exceptions, single molecular biomarkers, such as mRNA, miRNA, protein, or metabolite, are rarely successful as population screening tools. Hence, a molecular signature concept was developed for both diagnostic and theranostic applications (Subramanian and Simon 2010; Zimmer et al. 2006). These molecular signatures are often derived from OMICS data. In case of tumor detection, the prevalence of the somatic component makes the OMICS-based approaches especially suitable (Fig. 1). The cancers located within the same organ display substantially different proteome profiles that accurately reflect morphological subtype of the tumor (Kobel et al. 2008). Profiling-based studies may focus on any type of molecular biomarkers and may include somatic cancer mutations within coding

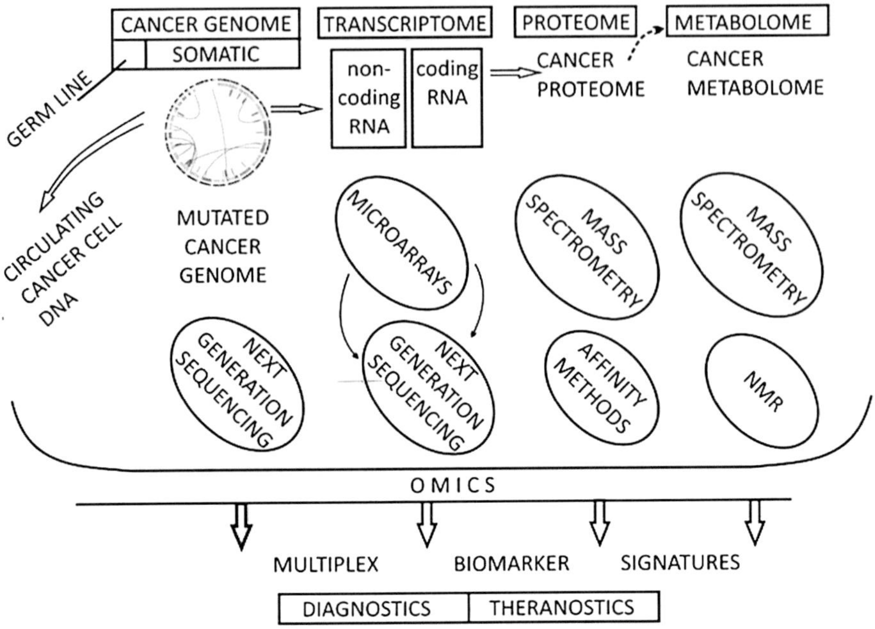

Fig. 1 Outline of main OMICS technologies used for tumor biomarker discovery: from cancer genome to diagnostic and theranostic signature

transcripts (Hawkins et al. 2010), miRNAs (Ferracin et al. 2010), proteins (Kim et al. 2009), or metabolites (Aboud and Weiss 2013).

Measured together, molecular variables of the signature ensure higher diagnostic accuracy or more efficient risk prediction as compared to single biomarkers (Yurkovetsky et al. 2010). The techniques for discerning diagnostic molecular signatures depend on the type of the molecules to be detected. For protein signatures, immunoassays (Edgell et al. 2010) or mass spectrometry (Rodriguez et al. 2010) may be used, while for the detection of mRNA levels, one may use a qRT-PCR, microarrays, or RNAseq. However, the use of "mixed" panels, for example, ones that include both mRNA and protein biomarkers, is limited by substantial increase in costs of performing an assay. The conversion of a series of experimentally quantified values into clinically relevant test is a long journey. The multiplexed signatures require application of the complex statistical techniques, including pattern recognition approaches (Alonzo and Pepe 2007; Hamacher et al. 2009).

An Analysis Pathway for Multiplex Biomarker Panels

A typical clinical classification and risk prediction framework is implemented as follows. Experimental data are collected for samples representing two classes, for example, healthy individuals versus patients with a disease, or two cohorts of

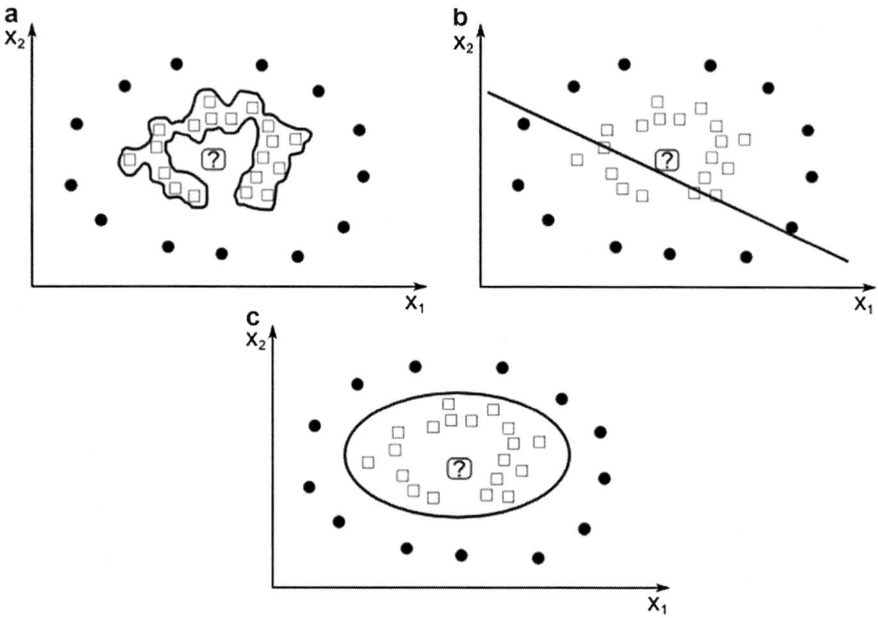

Fig. 2 **Illustration of model overfitting and generalization.** (**a**) Model with many adjustable parameters is capable of error-free classification of training set but performs poorly on novel data. (**b**) Too simple model does not allow discrimination of training data. (**c**) The model with optimum balance between overfitting and generalization

patients, one with poor and one with good prognosis as measured post hoc, by disease outcomes. Variables may represent gene expression, peak intensities from proteomic or metabolomic spectra, results of genotyping, blood biochemistry values, or demographics. These variables require intensive preprocessing, including imputation of missing values, normalization, smoothing out of the noise, and removing of outliers. A distinctive feature of OMICS data is that the number of samples (N) is orders of magnitude smaller than the available number of variables (P). In this context, a variable is often called a feature and refers to a specific gene or protein among the many thousands of molecules assayed in parallel. This "small n, large p" issue greatly complicates the statistical analysis of OMICS experiments and has many consequences. When the volume of the data grows exponentially, the information needed to describe the feature space with the same sampling density also should grow exponentially (so-called curse of dimensionality). In practical sense, this situation described as sparseness of the data may substantially complicate the building of classification models; good separation of the classes may be achieved even for sets of classifiers chosen randomly (Venet et al. 2011) (Fig. 2).

The obvious solution to "dimensionality curse" is to remove a majority of variables, i.e., perform feature selection (Saeys et al. 2007). Indeed, elimination of the features that carry no association with the disease or its outcome aids the discrimination of the sample classes and increases the classification power.

Additionally, it makes sense to eliminate variables that are highly correlated with each other, for example, co-regulated genes, or mass spectrometry peaks that represent modified forms of the same protein (Pyatnitskiy et al. 2010). Leaving only one “best-in-class” feature for every co-correlated group also aids in the interpretation of the results, as these features are more likely to represent highly interacting genes that correspond to the hubs in regulatory networks. Another possible way to attack dimensionality is identify and interpret a pattern within the data. For that, a number of visualization approaches were developed, for example, principal components analysis, clustering, or multidimensional scaling. It is important to note that the visualization of the data is not a required component of multiplexed biomarker test; rather, it serves as a foothold that helps a researcher to gain confidence with massive dataset.

The Holy Grail of biomarker discovery is the building of a decent classification model. This process includes two major steps: the learning step that extracts information contained in training dataset and model evaluation using validation dataset. The ultimate goal is to develop a model that withstands validation step, i.e., shows required accuracy when tested on independent set of samples set and, thus, deemed suitable for real-world applications. To develop the model that is more likely to pass validation, the model’s parameters are fine-tuned to optimize its performance on the training set. An accurate guess whether the model will survive validation is impossible. Perfect classification of training samples does not guarantee good performance in independently collected samples; when good-looking model does perform, we call this model “overfitted” to the training set. When high-dimensional data are inputted in models with many adjustable parameters, the “overfitting” is commonplace. On the other hand, an oversimplified model may not be able to discriminate the samples at all. Thus, the development of the biomarker panel is always a trade-off between overfitting and over simplification.

A great number of classification algorithms have been utilized in the analysis of OMICS data. The most frequently used classifiers include support vector machines (SVM), artificial neural networks, decision trees and random forests, logistic regression, and many others. Comparative studies of various approaches to improve discrimination power of the multidimensional models in terms of prediction accuracy, specificity, and sensitivity had been performed and published earlier. The results of comparisons contradict to each other – in certain cases more sophisticated algorithms like support vector machines outperform others, while in some cases relatively simple techniques show comparable classification accuracy.

It is also important to note that the importance of standard performance metrics is often overestimated (such as area under ROC curve or AUC). As we already mentioned above, overfitted models are unlikely to survive validation in independent cohorts, while underperforming models that rely on solid biological knowledge may actually improve their sensitivity and specificity when validated in larger cohorts. For example, the models generated by neural networks often show superior performance, but, in essence, they remain “black boxes” unavailable for meaningful interpretation. On the other side, the decision trees or the logistic regression models allow easy derivation of relationships between feature values and prediction outcomes, thus contributing to the understanding of the molecular mechanisms underlying a disease or condition. Furthermore, one should keep in mind that the model cannot perform better than the benchmark comparison test. In practical terms, that means that we have to be absolutely sure in the absolute accuracy of the clinician-assisted diagnosis in order to use it as sensitivity and specificity measure for novel test, which creates a self-perpetuating problem.

From statistics viewpoint, the most important limitation of OMICS-based biomarker discovery is a relatively small number of available samples that impose difficulties in assessing the performance of the model. In ideal world, the training and the validation sets of sample must not overlap. Additionally, both of these sets should be as large as possible. In practice, the size of the sets is limited by the availability of the samples, the factor especially important for relatively rare cancers, and the cost of OMICS profiling per sample. The standard way to solve this problem is to use cross validation, a partitioning of the whole dataset into two parts, where one part is used for model training and another is used to test the trained model. For example, leave-one-out cross validation (LOOCV) involves using a single sample from the original set for the validation of the model obtained by using the remaining samples that comprise the training set. This procedure is repeated until each sample is utilized for the validation. The prediction errors obtained at each run are averaged to estimate the final prediction error of the classification model. Other more powerful methods of cross validation are also available.

Both feature selection and cross validation are vital for building the proper model. The selection of features occurs at each step of the cross validation. Since training set is resampled at each step of cross validation, iterations of this process would yield different feature sets. However, in many studies, the feature selection is performed using the whole dataset, upstream of the cross-validation cycle. This simplified procedure may lead to serious underestimation of the prediction error (Ambroise and McLachlan 2002). Additionally, there are ways to learn from cross-validation procedure that should not be discarded. For example, some samples may be misclassified more often than others; they might be outliers, or genuinely misclassified samples, or other interesting cases that do not fit the typical two-bin output of the model. Studying specific properties of these samples may give additional clues on how to improve the classification model.

The main expected outcome of the OMICS data analysis is the development of multivariate biomarker panels that can be integrated in clinical practice for screening, diagnostic, and prognostic purposes. Hence, final validation of multivariate biomarker panel must be performed on samples that were not previously used during classifier learning or cross validation. In fact, to field test the model, these samples shall be collected independently, in some other medical center, and tested in a different lab. However, the large proportion of multivariate biomarkers developed from OMICS data have not been confirmed in independently collected sets of samples (Gerszten et al. 2008; Sung et al. 2012).

Transcriptome Profiling Approaches and Multiplexed Panels Based on mRNA Levels

Transcriptomics was the first non-DNA-based OMICS. In more than two decades of its development, a plethora of transcriptomics studies were done with a purpose of cancer biomarker discovery. In the early 1990s, when the microarray technique evolved from Southern blotting, first attempts of high-throughput expression profiling were done on colon carcinoma samples (Augenlicht et al. 1991). Since that, much technical advancements were made, but key limitation of expression profiling remained firm – the gene expression profiling methods have to deal with either cell and tissue material. This condition restricts application of expression profiling to biofluids except the assaying of circulating cancer cells. Thus, analysis of expression by microarrays has been mostly used to predict cancer outcome from biopsy tissue specimens (Pusztai et al. 2003) or to post hoc analysis of archived tissue blocks (Waldron et al. 2012). Typically, data from microarrays containing thousands of nucleic acid probes were used to select mRNA candidates with an advent of bioinformatics tools and gimmicks, and the reduced set of candidates was further tested on larger specimen cohort using quantitative real-time PCR or a different platform which was more easy to use than the genome-wide microarray. However, in most cases, the number of profiled specimens was not more than 100, and the resultant predictive models rarely survived validation (Ntzani and Ioannidis 2003).

Nowadays, the transcriptomics drastically changed its technological approach toward RNAseq, the "next-generation" sequencing-based estimation of transcript levels (Ding et al. 2010). In a nutshell, the RNAseq approach provides a global survey of transcriptome activity through en masse generation of short sequence reads from random locations along each of profiled RNAs followed by their mapping to appropriate reference genome. A number of reads that map to a particular gene are proportional to the level of its mRNA level. The RNAseq technique requires lesser amount of RNA than typical microarray (Mutz et al. 2013). However, similar to other high-throughput OMICS analyses, RNAseq results should be validated by qRT-PCR.

Another novel hot field within transcriptomics is an analysis of noncoding RNAs. The results of ENCODE project removed all the doubts about the widespread expression of eukaryotic genomes, with current estimates that more than 62 % of human genome participates in transcription events (Bernstein et al. 2012), in drastic contrast to mere 2 % occupied by protein-coding RNAs. So far, in human genome, ENCODE annotated more that 8,800 small RNAs and 9,600 long noncoding RNA, most of which do not have any attributed function but capable of RNA interference. Abundance of these RNAs, especially small RNAs, stimulated attempts to their potential utility as biomarkers. Recent studies showed that small RNAs, especially microRNAs (miRNAs), remain stable in circulation (Weiland et al. 2012). Vast majority of these circulating miRNA molecules originate from the blood and endothelial cells; however, some tissue-specific miRNAs, for example, from the liver and gut, are represented as well, indicating a broad source of tissue contribution to the total circulating miRNAs (Williams et al. 2013). Hence, miRNA profile "fingerprints" were suggested as possible biomarkers of developing tumors. A flood of papers and patents about miRNA in cancer increases exponentially and cannot be reviewed in this chapter.

Herein, we will omit gene expression studies as such and further discuss only examples of successful translation of mRNA-based multi-analyte profiles to clinical practice. To evaluate these tests, the US Food and Drug Administration (FDA) designated a novel group identifier IVDMIA (in vitro diagnostic multivariate index assay). In 2004, before IVDMIA, in frame of broader category of laboratory-developed tests (LDTs), the RNA-based prognostic test Oncotype Dx for breast cancer was approved. Later, this test was reclassified as IVDMIA. Other tests already approved through IVDMIA procedure include MammaPrint (2007), Tissue of Origin (2008), as well as Oncotype Dx for colon cancer (2010) and prostate cancer (2013).

Both Oncotype Dx for breast cancer and the MammaPrint determine the risk of breast cancer metastasis, i.e., its relapse after surgery. Based on the assay result, as well as on other clinical features, a medical practitioner would whether assign to the patient a course of adjuvant chemotherapy or not. Both assays quantify the levels of multiple mRNAs in a biopsy sample of excised primary tumor.

MammaPrint assay (Agendia Inc., Netherlands) includes quantitative measurements of expression for 70 genes in mRNA samples extracted from frozen breast carcinoma biopsies. The test intends to estimate the probability of metastatic progression of previously nonmetastatic breast cancer less than 5 cm in size, in women younger than 61. Technically, the assay is based on custom oligonucleotide hybridization microchip (Agilent Technologies) that includes the probes to the set of mRNAs that corresponds to the signature discovered in the microarray study of 112 relatively young breast cancer patients with known outcomes (Van't Veer et al. 2002). The test assigns each patient to the high-risk or low-risk groups. In the first group, chemotherapy would be of benefit. However, some technology problems were identified after the test approval, including 15 % risk overstatement. As a result, the test was retracted from the US markets but remains available in Europe.

Oncotype Dx breast cancer assay (Genomic Health, USA) intends to identify patients with previously diagnosed estrogen receptor (ER)-positive breast carcinoma who should receive adjuvant chemotherapy on top of conventional treatment with tamoxifen. Substantial technical advantage of this assay is its applicability to paraffinized blocks of fixed tissue. Oncotype Dx breast cancer assay is based on 21-gene signature (Dowsett et al. 2010), 16 of which being cancer biomarkers and 5 serve as reference transcripts. This test is based on quantitative real-time PCR. Expression levels for each of these mRNAs are inputted into proprietary algorithm which calculates so-called Recurrence Score (RS), a predictor of chemotherapy benefit that reflects the probabilistic estimate of possible cancer recurrence in 10 years after diagnosis. Recurrence Score is a number between 0 and 100. This value itself does not provide clinically useful information but denotes a risk category for the given patient. RS values less than 11 correspond to a low risk, while RS values between 11 and 25 and more than 25 are recognized as intermediate and high risk, respectively. Along with other biomarkers, the Recurrence Score guides the decision whether the adjuvant chemotherapy should be administered. Interestingly, low versus high RS patients are significantly more likely to follow the chemotherapy-related recommendation of the test, suggesting a tendency toward less aggressive treatment in high RS that decreases utility of the test (Carlson and Roth 2013).

Both MammaPrint and Oncotype Dx breast cancer assays test for the relative risk of breast carcinoma relapse. Surprisingly, there is only one gene that is common for both signatures, 70-plex in MammaPrint and 21-plex for Oncotype Dx for breast cancer. In one study, both tests were compared side by side using a cohort of 295 patients (Fan et al. 2006). In these settings, the concordance of tests results was at about 80 %. However, 15 of 33 patients classified as intermediate risk by Oncotype Dx were assigned to high-risk group by 70-plex assay. Hence, the intermediate-risk group was the most vulnerable to misclassification. Importantly, OMICS-based molecular tests are especially in demand for this group, as either high- or low-risk patients may be as well ascertained by conventional clinical approach.

A certain contributor to the relative success of the Oncotype Dx is its technological solution to substitute gene expression microarrays by the multiplexed qRT-PCR. Similar platforms are used in Oncotype Dx tests for the colon and prostate cancer. Twelve-plex Oncotype Dx colon cancer assay aims to predict the recurrence for stage II or III of the disease (Venook et al. 2013), while the 17-plex Oncotype Dx prostate cancer assay is developed to provide an opportunity for low-risk patients to avoid invasive treatments such as radical prostatectomy or radiation (Cooperberg et al. 2013). Importantly, only 7 out of 12 colon cancer and 12 out of 17 prostatic carcinoma genes that comprise Oncotype Dx classifiers are target genes; the rest of them are normalization references.

We do not intend to discuss here clinical aspects of the Oncotype Dx test performance, because they are widely described elsewhere (Azim et al. 2013). However, for the biomarker development standpoint, it is important to note that three sets of genes used as signatures for three different cancers do overlap. There are two common transcripts between the colon and the breast tests, one for putative cell cycle protein MKI67 and cell cycle-related transcription factor MYBL2. Additionally, glutathione S-transferase Mu 1 (GSTM1) transcript of breast cancer signature could be paired up with its close homologue and chromosomal locus neighbor GSTM2 in prostate cancer signature. Finally, the colon cancer and the prostate cancer signatures also share one gene, X-chromosome-encoded biglycan (BGN). Moreover, protein-coding genes that comprise Oncotype Dx signatures are closely tied to each other by their functions assessed as protein interaction map (Fig. 3). Note that the hubs of this network are represented by other well-known cancer-associated proteins, such as ERBB2 (HER2) receptor protein kinase that serves as a target for breast cancer drug rituximab and BCL2 proto-oncogene. Oncotype Dx gene sets are also enriched in cluster of neighboring genes co-localized within the same chromosome segments (Table 1). More than one third of the segments share two signature hits. This fact may indicate that the

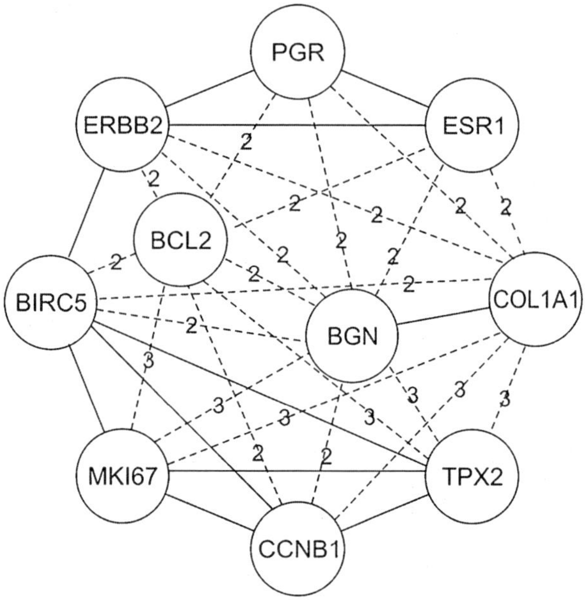

Fig. 3 Functional interactions of Oncomine Dx signature genes. Interaction map of proteins encoded by genes contained in Oncomine Dx breast, colon, and prostate cancer signatures (gene names are shown). The knowledge about protein-protein interactions for bait proteins was received from STRING database (Szklarczyk et al. 2011) with interaction score >0.7 being considered reliable for interaction. Top 10 hub interactors are shown in the network using CytoHubba plug-in (Lin et al. 2008) for Cytoscape software (Shannon et al. 2003). Top hub proteins were specified by Maximal Clique Centrality method. Predicted direct interactions are shown by *solid line*, and indirect connections are shown by *dotted line* with a number of intermediators indicated. Note the well-known cancer-associated proteins, such as ERBB2 (HER2) receptor protein kinase, a target of rituximab drug, and BCL2 proto-oncogene among network hubs

recurrence of human tumors may be associated with specific epigenetic events that require further functional dissection.

The Affymetrix-based transcriptome profiling microchips yielded a practical embodiment in a clinic that is known as a Tissue of Origin test (Pathwork Diagnostics, USA). This test is intended for the determination of tissue type for unassigned metastatic tumors with no lost clear differentiation signs. Tissue of Origin evaluates expression levels for 1,668 genes; these numbers are plugged in the algorithm that assigns the origin of metastatic tumor to one of 15 tissue types. The accuracy of the Tissue of Origin is estimated to be in range of 72–88.5 % for gastric cancer and up to 96.5 % for breast adenocarcinoma. Some modified versions of Tissue of Origin tests are available, such as a 316-plex test for ovary and uterine cancer classification (Lal et al. 2012).

In summary, the main output of gene expression-based signatures is in the field of cancer theranostics, i.e., the personalized management of cancer, rather in its diagnostics.

Table 1 Protein-coding human genes contained in Oncomine Dx breast, colon, and prostate cancer signatures used to determine the recurrence score of these cancers (Cooperberg et al. 2013; Dowsett et al. 2010; Venook et al. 2013) and the genome location of the genes. Gene names are used according to the NextProt knowledge base (www.nextprot.org). Chromosome locations are filled and shown by italic where more than one signature gene is situated. Genes which are contained in more than one cancer signature are highlighted in the same manner

	Type of cancer		
Genome location	Breast (16 genes)	Colon (7 genes)	Prostate (12 genes)
1p13	*GSTM1*	–	*GSTM2*
2p23-24	–	FAP	SRD5A2
5q13	CCNB1	–	–
6q25	ESR1	–	–
7p14	–	INHBA	SFRP4
9p13	BAG1	–	TPM2
9q22	CTSL2	–	–
9q32-33	–	–	ORM1, GSN
10q21	–	–	FAM13C
10q26	*MKI67*	*MKI67*	–
11p15	SCUBE2	–	–
11q22	PGR, MMP11	–	–
15q22	–	DENND4A (C-MYC)	–
17p13	CD68	–	–
17q12	GRB1, ERBB2 (HER2)	–	–
17q21	–	–	COL1A1
17q25	BIRC5	–	–
18q21	BCL2		
19p13	–	GADD45B	KLK2
20q11	–	–	TPX2
20q13	*MYBL2*, AURKA	*MYBL2*	–
Xq28	–	*BGN*	*BGN*

Proteomics: From MALDI-TOF Through Shotgun Techniques to Targeted Approach

The proteomics is technology-driven field that aims at high-throughput inventory of individual proteomes. The basics of protein separation, such as two-dimensional gel electrophoresis, which could visualize whole proteomes or at least their subsets were developed in the 1970s (O'Farrell 1975). At that time, proteome studies were limited by difficulties of identification of proteins within the bands or spots on electrophoretic gels. Availability of genome sequence made possible an identification of proteins by mass spectrometry that deduces the identities of proteins and peptide fragments from mass-to-charge ratios (m/z) being compared to all possible m/z predicted by comparison to the genome parsed into open reading frames (Aebersold 2003).

This process allows one to calculate a probability that theoretically predicted peptide of protein actually exists in the given sample. It is important to note that mass spectrometry provides probabilistic identification of the given protein or peptide but does not sequence this protein de novo. An introduction of the protein sequencing into the routine of the lab would be welcomed, but these techniques are not gaining any traction yet (Hughes et al. 2010).

In mass spectrometry, the accuracy of m/z and, correspondingly, molecular weight quantification is inversely related to the size of analyzed molecule. That is why many proteomics studies start with whole proteome digestion by trypsin and the analysis of resultant mixture. This approach is known as *bottom-up* or *shotgun* proteomics (Washburn et al. 2001). Its main advantage is in ease of separation and identification of short peptides, and its main drawback is the significant loss of information due to the destruction of protein integrity. Conventional pipelines of bottom-up LC-MS/MS proteomics workflow include (i) digestion by isolated protein fraction by trypsin, (ii) separation of resultant peptides by nanoflow HPLC, (iii) electrospray ionization (ESI) of peptides in the flux from HPLC column and tandem mass spectrometry (MS/MS) of peptides and their fragments generated in the mass spectrometer, and (iv) probabilistic identification of peptides from tandem mass spectra by various search algorithms based on genome sequence (Chalkley 2010). Modern bottom-up proteomics pipelines may identify from 1,000 to 10,000 proteins in one sample depending on the workflow and the specimen nature (Zubarev 2013).

Alternative proteomics approach is a "top down," where proteins are analyzed by mass spectrometry in their intact form. Due to their large molecular weights, native protein identification remains far from being routine. The pioneering modifications to tandem mass spectrometry recently demonstrated its power to correctly discern hundreds of proteins in one sample (Tran et al. 2011). However, the complicated, time-consuming procedure of intact proteomics cannot be yet adapted for biomarker discovery. Luckily, in the early 2000s, a relatively simple top-down approach was developed specifically for that purpose, a time-of-flight mass spectrometry with matrix-assisted laser desorption ionization (MALDI-TOF) that could be used for direct profiling of biological fluids, for example, plasma or urine. In this technique, the sample is subjected to fast separation or desalting and applied to the metallic chip (Karpova et al. 2010). In this approach, small proteins and peptides are registered in its intact form but remain unidentified unless downstream experiments are performed.

General experiment design for the MALDI-TOF profiling of the body fluid samples includes the following steps: (i) diseased and control sample preparation with fast separation, (ii) mass-spectra acquisition, (iii) mass-spectra processing to ascertain the intensities for each m/z peak as set of features present in each sample, and (iv) selection of m/z peaks capable of discriminating samples collected from patients with tumors from matched controls and development of multi-peak diagnostic model. Many early papers reported high levels of diagnostic accuracy of MALDI-TOF spectra, some in range of above 90 % (Petricoin et al. 2002). Unfortunately, the MALDI profiles strongly depend on the choice of suitable solvents and the methods of sample preparation. This is a major limitation of MALDI-TOF, as the variation in purity and amounts of buffer components, as well as nontarget lipids and carbohydrates, prevents efficient ionization of the proteins, contributes to the technical variation in test outputs, and precludes efficient reproduction of the profiles in independent lab settings. The most disturbing observation coming from the study of Hu and coauthors demonstrated that changes in the protocol result in the reproducible shift in protein profiles masking more subtle changes corresponding to different histological subtypes of cancer (Hu et al. 2005). Because of that, a hope that the MALDI-TOF peak profiles itself would become a backbone of future diagnostics failed to translate into clinically approved test products. Nevertheless, the efforts in the field of MALDI-TOF plasma profiling continue until now (McLerran et al. 2008). Recent attempts to improve reproducibility (Mann et al. 2013) may inspire further clinical studies.

Today, many peptide and protein peaks capable of discriminating plasma samples of patients with malignancies from healthy controls are already identified as either gel electrophoresis (Tolson et al. 2004) or HPLC (Zhang et al. 2004), followed by trypsin digestion and tandem mass spectrometry (Karpova et al. 2010). Candidate protein biomarkers are often validated by independent assay, such as immunoassay (Moshkovskii et al. 2007; Zhang et al. 2004). Most, if not all, peptide and protein candidates identified by MALDI-TOF plasma profiling represent highly abundant products, such as inflammatory acute-phase proteins (complement fragments, serum amyloid A), lipoproteins, and protease inhibitors (inter-alpha-trypsin inhibitor). It is believed that the levels of these molecules in plasma change are due to the reaction of the body to the presence of tumor, rather than being specific products expressed by tumor cells. This understanding casts a doubt at the utility of these molecules as biomarkers suitable for the screening of general populations (Diamandis 2003). To overcome the shortfalls of MALDI-TOF-based profiling, the shotgun proteomics by LC-MS/MS was proposed as the next contender for high-throughput biomarker discovery in cancer. However, a complexity of its data files, not much improved reproducibility, and highly variable quantitative outputs curtailed its raise.

A tremendous proportion of studies that involve complex processing of data are accompanied by statistical flows and subsequent lack of reproducibility. A plethora of proteins were pinpointed as differentially expressed in cancer and considered candidate cancer biomarkers; however, practical outputs of these studies were close to nil (Polanski and Anderson 2007). In general, the most important challenge of proteome profiling in cancer is the selection of proper candidates for validation. Recent meta-analysis of the proteomics profiling in colorectal cancer (Luo et al. 2013) vividly highlights the statement above. Between 2008 and 2012, 28 attempts to profile-excised colorectal cancer and control tissue specimens by proteomics were made. On average, each study involved 27 human subjects, while average number of differentially expressed proteins was 96, with one paper reporting as many as 555 (Table 2; see the arguments above in data analysis sections). Obviously, the "dimensionality curse" was ignored by a majority of scientists. As partial excuse, we shall point that some peaks were identified and

Table 2 Overview of the methodology, cohort sizes, and numbers of differential proteins used for colorectal cancer biomarker discovery by proteomics based on recent review by Luo et al. (2013)

Specimen type	Methodology: MALDI-TOF vs. LC-MS/MS, number of papers	Cohort size, average ± standard deviation (min, max)	Number of differentially expressed proteins/biomarkers, average ± standard deviation (min, max)	Ratio between the number of biomarkers found and cohort size in each paper, average ± standard deviation (min, max)
Tissue	MALDI-TOF: LC-MS/MS	27.3 ± 21.4 (8, 118)	95.8 ± 146.3 (5, 555)	4.8 ± 9.3 (0.2, 45.9)
	16:10, total 26			
Blood derivatives	MALDI-TOF: LC-MS/MS	57.7 ± 28.7 (20, 92)	10.9 ± 8.2 (3, 28)	0.3 ± 0.3 (0.1, 0.9)
	4:3, total 7			

validated by immunoassays. Note that the majority of the studies employed less laborious MALDI-TOF profiling rather than more complicated LC-MS/MS workflow (16 vs. 10). In the studies that aimed at discovery of biomarkers in plasma, the cohort sizes were larger (average $N = 58$), and a number of peaks identified as biomarkers was threefold to tenfold smaller than the cohort size (Table 2).

However, the studies of plasma provide extra challenge for assay sensitivity; plasma is filled with highly abundant proteins that interfere with mass-spectrometry-based detection of less abundant but possibly tumor-derived protein species (Archakov et al. 2012). Subsequently, many proteomics studies of plasma samples include the sample processing step that depletes the most abundant protein species. However, many potential serum biomarkers are bound to carrier proteins that are usually depleted during sample preparation. Accumulation on circulating protein carriers or specially designed hydrogel nanoparticles amplifies the total serum/plasma concentration of the measurable biomarkers (Longo et al. 2009). Examination of the carrier-bound molecules represents an important future avenue in tumor marker discovery.

Despite all these challenges, MALDI (SELDI)-TOF plasma profiling efforts yielded one clinical innovation, albeit not in diagnostics but in theranostics of ovarian cancer (Fung 2010). OVA1 is a 5-biomarker panel for ovarian cancer management. When a woman is diagnosed by ultrasound study to have the ovarian adnexal mass and scheduled to surgery, OVA1 helps to assess the risk of malignancy in this pelvic mass and to select the postsurgical therapy (Bristow et al. 2013). The list of the proteins comprising the OVA1 panel was compiled by rigorous analysis of MALDI-TOF profiles collected from the plasma of ovarian cancer patients (Zhang et al. 2004). Selected proteins then were developed as immunoassay-based test. In the marketed test, OvaCalc® algorithm combines abundancy values for these proteins and returns the risk value. Two proteins of OVA1 which are upregulated in cancer include beta-2 microglobulin and mucin-16 (cancer antigen 125; CA 125 II), whereas three other members of the panel are downregulated in cancer and include apolipoprotein A1, transthyretin (prealbumin), and transferrin proteins. Importantly, one of the panel components, CA 125, is an established ovarian cancer biomarker, although its specificity is far from being perfect when this biomarker is used alone. Thus, OVA1 panel augments this biomarker with four other molecules. Interestingly, another recently introduced biomarker of ovarian carcinoma, a human epididymis protein 4 (HE4), is not included in the OVA1, most likely due to intellectual property-related issues. Marketed multiplexed ovarian carcinoma tests include one more assay, the "risk of ovarian malignancy algorithm" (ROMA) that includes both CA-125 and HE-4 (Simmons et al. 2013). However, the ROMA has not been derived from OMICS studies.

Since 2005, a new technological avenue of proteomics has been developed. In this so-called "targeted proteomics" approach, the candidate protein-derived peptides are selected beforehand, at the stage of experimental design. Since the 1980s, the multiple reaction monitoring (or selected reaction monitoring; MRM or SRM) has been used to detect known chemicals in biofluids (Anderson and Hunter 2006). In its proteomics reincarnation, this method relies on rational selection of the peptides likely to be derived from proteins of interests, their synthesis and use as a set of standards (Vizcaíno et al. 2010). Any triple quadrupole mass spectrometer, or one of its more powerful analogs, may be adjusted to detect only the m/z of the desired peptides in its first filter, while the second MS in the triplet would dissociate the peptide ions of interest, and the third part would detect the fragments. Thus, in MRM approach, the mass spectrometer is requested to analyze complex mixture in such a way that would allow exclusive detection of selected features, thus simultaneously dealing with "dimensionality curse" and improving sensitivity and reproducibility (Picotti and Aebersold 2012). For absolute protein quantifying, two unique synthetic peptides are labeled by stable isotopes and used for internal calibration.

In general, the MRM approach is comparable to immunoassays (Aebersold et al. 2013) in its analytical characteristics, such as coefficient of variation, and it may be multiplexed to analyze 30–50 proteins per 1 h LC-MS/MS run. Many attempts to develop absolute quantification MRM assays for conventional biomarkers are reported (Fortin et al. 2009). In order to increase sensitivity, some methods preface MRM with an enrichment for specific analytes by cognizant antibodies (Kuhn et al. 2012); however, this step contributes to the substantial increase in the costs of assay.

Just recently, a use of 13-plex MRM assay was reported to predict the benign nature of the node found in the lung by imaging (Li et al. 2013). This test is thought to help in lung cancer management. It measures levels of 13 blood proteins in major protein-depleted plasma.

In conclusion, three main mass-spectrometry-based proteomics solutions are currently employed for biomarker discovery and validation (Fig. 4). Of them, MALDI-TOF already brought some fruit as it served as the tool to select candidates that augment theranostics performance of ovarian cancer biomarker CA125 in OVA1 biomarker panel. So far, the shotgun approach is mostly used for biomarker discovery, but its results rarely withstand rigorous validation. Targeted proteomics is comparable to affinity methods and is a promising tool for translation of mass-spectrometry to clinics as it is already done in the field of therapeutic drug monitoring.

Apart from mass-spectrometry methods, affinity reagents for protein detection are widely developed for the purpose of tumor biomarker discovery. Arrays containing such reagents, including antibodies, may be immobilized on various kinds of solid supports or beads; protein arraying approaches are widely known and reviewed elsewhere (Lee et al. 2013). In reverse phase arrays for tumor marker identification, multiple analytes represented by tested sample are immobilized within the same spot, but the spot array is probed with one detection molecule at a time, thus detecting a single protein analyte in a number of samples under the same conditions (Espina et al. 2003). An advantage of reverse protein arrays is its ability to detect analytes in very small volume of sample, e.g., in 30–60 μl of whole cell lysate or in core needle biopsies obtained with a 16 or 18 gauge needle (Espina et al. 2003).

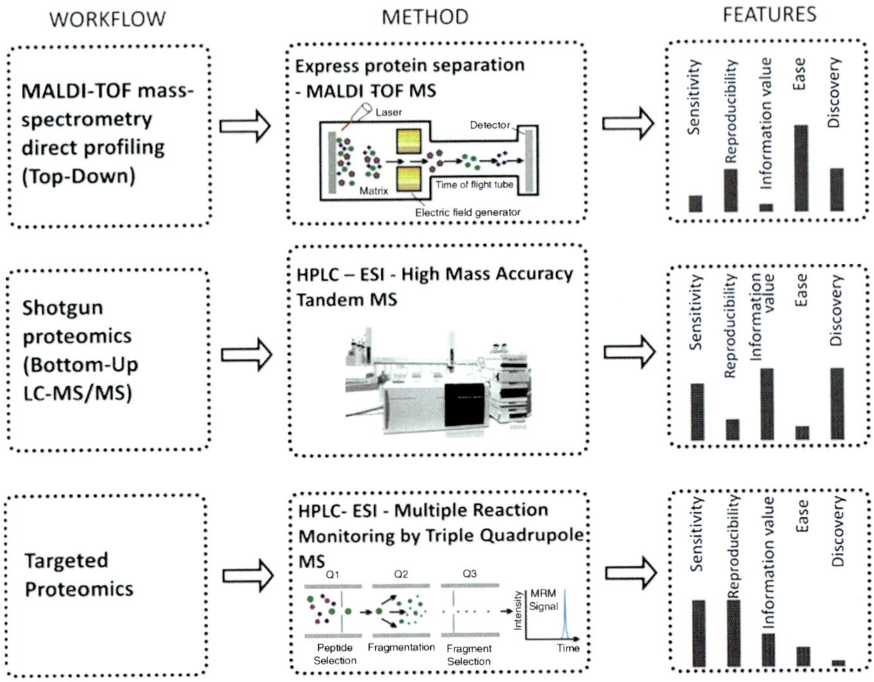

Fig. 4 Mass-spectrometry-based proteomics workflows employed for tumor biomarker discovery and validation. Features of the workflows shown in the *right panel* are ranked by the authors based on their expert opinion

To quantitatively match the antibody and the analyte concentrations, sample dilutions are printed on same array. This helps to expand the linear range of detection and improves the sensitivity and specificity of this technique. A major limiting factor of reverse phase arrays is the unavailability of specific and high-affinity antibodies for a range of interesting targets (Espina et al. 2003). Unlike DNA probes that allow for affinity customization, affinity probes for protein arrays usually represent a "black box," so multiple probes need to be pretested in order to find the most reliable molecule that allows high-fidelity analyte quantification. Reverse protein arrays allow to rapidly screen for autoantibodies and phosphorylated or otherwise modified forms of human proteins (Liu et al. 2012).

A relatively novel class of affinity reagents, aptamers, is especially suitable for multiplexed quantification of the proteins in biofluids. Aptamers are oligonucleotide products of combinatorial chemical synthesis selected for their ability of high-affinity binding to target proteins (Ulrich and Wrenger 2009). As aptamers originate from natural protein-binding motifs within RNA or DNA, they commonly attach to the positively charged proteins and their fragments. The most advanced kind of aptamers is known as somamers (slow off-rate modified aptamers) that have advantageous kinetic features of ligand binding. Recently, an array of somamers with specific affinity to about 800 human proteins was employed in a search for biomarkers of lung cancer in blood plasma with promising results (Kraemer et al. 2011).

Metabolomics: A Promising New Direction for Biomarker Discovery

The recent decade was marked by explosive increase in a number of publications on high-throughput analysis of metabolites, so-called metabolomics. In sensu stricto, metabolomics cannot be considered postgenome research field; however, a set of metabolites produced in the human body and in the tumor cells may be viewed as an ultimate phenotypic expression of the genome. Moreover, metabolomics is especially relevant to the context of tumor biomarkers, as cancer cells are known to modulate their metabolism to assist their uncontrolled proliferation and survival in hypoxic conditions. For example, they prefer anaerobic energy supply instead of normal mitochondrial work, the phenomenon called Warburg effect (Schulze and Harris 2012). Consequently, a variety of tumor-specific metabolites were discovered, such as 2-hydroxyglutarate produced by mutant enzyme (Dang et al. 2010).

High-throughput metabolite profiling is an attractive method to look for novel cancer biomarkers and signatures, which was made possible by recent developments in the analytical detection of low-molecular-weight organic compounds (Trifonova et al. 2013). However, this technology is not free from pitfalls. As metabolite levels vary according to circadian cycle, diet, physical exercises, etc., an interpretation of the signatures and an extraction of disease-specific features are far from being trivial.

As in other OMICS sciences, metabolite profiling is performed either in biological fluids or in tissue samples. Two types of analytical platforms are used, namely, nuclear magnetic resonance (NMR) spectroscopy and mass spectrometry (MS). The profiling based on NMR spectroscopy is often discussed as "metabonomics," whereas the term "metabolomics" is reserved for MS-based metabolite profiling. In other edition, metabonomics relates to the drug and other xenobiotic studies, whereas metabolomics is alternatively used for profiling of naturally occurring metabolites. NMR spectroscopy is a workhorse of metabolic profiling as it in use for more than 20 years. It is quantitative, is highly reproducible, and does not require an extensive sample preparation; the technique can be used even with intact blood plasma. However, the sensitivity of NMR is relatively low as it detects only several dozens of metabolites in plasma by NMR (Kirschenlohr et al. 2006).

Metabolomics by mass spectrometry is similar to an approach of shotgun proteomics (see previous section of this chapter). Briefly, metabolites are extracted from the sample, then separated by gas or liquid chromatography or by capillary electrophoresis, and analyzed by mass spectrometer with ESI or other ionization types and high-accuracy detector. A separation stage is sometimes omitted (Lokhov et al. 2013). After data acquisition, metabolites are identified and/or selected for diagnostic signatures by a bunch of data analysis techniques described above. Typical metabolomics study is designed similarly to its proteomics counterparts that compare tumor and control cohorts using either the profiling mode that monitors all detectable metabolites or the targeted approach with a focus on a couple of dozens or low hundreds of predetermined metabolites, reviewed in Aboud and Weiss (2013). An example of a typical output of a large metabolomics study is a finding that glycine derivative sarcosine concentrations are increased in all types of samples collected from prostate carcinoma patients, including urine (Sreekumar et al. 2009). Discriminatory metabolic profiles of not yet identified metabolites were described for various cancers (Lokhov et al. 2010; Huang et al. 2013).

It is important to note that metabolomics profiling is still in its diapers. No clinical applications of metabolomics are approved up to date. However, there is a lot of promise in these kinds of studies. Mass-spectrometry-based metabolite profiling has an important advantage over LC-MS/MS proteomics: it deals with the intact metabolites which can be measured directly with high mass accuracy, whereas proteins in proteomics should be digested before analyzing. This remarkable detail enables scalability of metabolite analysis and gives us hope that its analytical parameters, such as coefficient of variance, would be soon enough fine-tuned for practical application.

Potential Applications to Prognosis, Other Diseases, or Conditions

A lot of papers have described various uses of OMICS for cancer diagnostics, but cancer prognosis still remains in the area of genomics and epigenomics due to their context nature. Approved tests for theranostics based on molecular signatures as described above are not prognostic but predict patient's response to therapies. In turn, other diseases and conditions also are in focus of OMICS profiling. Substantially any condition which is difficult to diagnose by conventional laboratory methods has been studied extensively by transcriptomics, proteomics, or other profiling methods.

Conclusion

Main sections of OMICS sciences include transcriptomics, proteomics, and metabolomics, a set of powerful research instruments capable of high-throughput detection of differentially expressed biomolecules between tumor and non-tumor samples, including excised tissues or biopsies, blood plasma, saliva, and urine. Consequently, thousands species of RNAs, proteins, and metabolites were suggested as candidate tumor biomarkers alone or as constituents of multiplex signatures. However, only a handful of OMICS-derived biomarkers entered the clinical practice for theranostics purposes, and none are used as stand-alone diagnostics. The reasons for that are multiple, and some of them are beyond the realm of science.

To understand it better, we would have to have a closer look at a positive predictive value (PPV) of candidate diagnostic test, something that is very important for real-life applicability of the test, besides its accuracy. PPV is defined as a ratio of true diagnoses among all positively diagnosed subjects and is influenced by the frequency of the disease in general populations. Most types of the malignant tumors occur relatively rarely. For example, about 40 ovarian cancer cases could be found by a screening of 100,000 postmenopausal women. Thus, if a biomarker or a panel of biomarkers has sensitivity as high as 99.6 %, the screening of general population would miss about 0.16 cases. However, for the same test, the specificity of 99.6 % would yield 440 cancer diagnoses, per same population of 100,000 women, and 400 of them would be false positives. With that, a PPV of our test will be not more than 10 %. Yes, all 40 cancers would be diagnosed, but 400 patients would be assigned false-positive cancer diagnosis, thus producing unnecessary worries in these women.

The stress mentioned above has a substantial economical and social impact. Due to extremely polymorphic molecular etiology of each cancer type, OMICS-based tests hardly approach 90 % overall accuracy even when tested in small, homogenous cohorts. Hence, even after an extension of cohorts and test validation, the economically appropriate performance of these tests is not anticipated.

Despite all these limitations, OMICS-based tests are being seriously considered. Recently, mock submissions of multiplexed protein mass spectrometry peak-based assay and glycoprotein immunological array-based tests to US Food and Drug Administration were performed (Regnier et al. 2010). The reason for this mock study was to deliver to the community a preliminary report on main regulatory challenges facing biomarker assay developers. The chief shortage of targeted mass-spectrometry platform was seen in the need to digest the proteins before their quantitative assessment, and the digestion step is difficult to standardize; hence, it will likely contribute to overall inter-assay variation. For glycan microarrays that contain hundreds of different antibodies, the analytical bottleneck is in the variation in the affinity of individual antibodies to their antigens. Additionally, it is likely that both types of assays may run into the problem with unacceptably low positive predictive values that were mentioned above.

Despite so far insurmountable difficulties encountered by OMICS panels with an intended use in population screening programs, some of the multiplex panels already have found their applications in the field of theranostics. If the patient is already diagnosed with a certain cancer, RNA or protein biomarker signatures may help to select a specific therapy or to predict the probability of a relapse. A number of clinically relevant, validated, and approved signatures of RNA (Oncomine Dx, MammaPrint) and protein (OVA1) analytes successfully emerged from OMICS pipelines. However, it is important to remember that an implementation of these clinical tests took the safety of reliable laboratory techniques, such as qRT-PCR and immunoassay.

Summary Points

This chapter describes the use of postgenome research disciplines widely designated as OMICS sciences for malignant tumor biomarker discovery and validation.

The general challenge in cancer biomarker discovery is that various molecular pathways may be involved in one cancer type with common set of clinical signs.

Molecular variables included in OMICS diagnostic signature have to be selected to avoid overfitting-based result mutilation, and the diagnostic signature has to be adequately validated.

Transcriptomics, the RNA inventory, was developed based on microarrays and, more recently, genome-wide RNA sequencing.

Proteomics is a way to detect and quantify proteins, and it is based on mass-spectrometry protein and peptide identification or on the protein profiling with affinity reagents, such as antibodies and aptamers.

Metabolomics is used to catalog the metabolites in the tissue and blood, and both mass spectrometry and nucleic magnetic resonance spectroscopy are used to detect and quantify these low-molecular species.

In recent decade, transcriptomics, proteomics, and metabolomics have reported thousands of molecular species, both distinctively and in signatures, as potential tumor biomarkers, but very few entered more extensive clinical trials.

Based on transcriptomics results, some molecular tests are approved for practice in breast, colon, and prostate cancer theranostics, i.e., for correct selection of therapy in diseased person (e.g., Oncotype Dx tests).

One molecular test is approved for ovarian cancer theranostics based on results of proteomics (OVA1 test).

Acknowledgments This work was supported by the Human Proteome Program of the Russian Academy of Medical Sciences, by the grant # 12-04-33109 of the Russian Fund for Basic Research and by the contracts # 14.512.11.0090 (27th June 2013) under the call # 2013-1.2-14-512-0042 and # 8273 (27th August 2012) under the call # 2012-1.1-12-000-2008-067 of the Ministry of Education and Science of Russia.

References

Aboud OA, Weiss RH. New opportunities from the cancer metabolome. Clin Chem. 2013;59(1):138–46.

Aebersold R. A mass spectrometric journey into protein and proteome research. J Am Soc Mass Spectrom. 2003;14(7):685–95.

Aebersold R, Burlingame AL, Bradshaw RA. Western blots vs. SRM assays: time to turn the tables? Mol Cell Proteomics. 2013;12(9):2381–2.

Alonzo TA, Pepe MS. Development and evaluation of classifiers. Methods Mol Biol. 2007;404:89–116.

Ambroise C, McLachlan GJ. Selection bias in gene extraction on the basis of microarray gene-expression data. Proc Natl Acad Sci U S A. 2002;99(10):6562–6.

Amin ARMR, Kucuk O, Khuri FR, Shin DM. Perspectives for cancer prevention with natural compounds. J Clin Oncol. 2009;27(16):2712–25.

Anderson L, Hunter CL. Quantitative mass spectrometric multiple reaction monitoring assays for major plasma proteins. Mol Cell Proteomics. 2006;5(4):573–88.
Archakov A, Zgoda V, Kopylov A, et al. Chromosome-centric approach to overcoming bottlenecks in the Human Proteome Project. Expert Rev Proteomics. 2012;9(6):667–76.
Augenlicht LH, Taylor J, Anderson L, Lipkin M. Patterns of gene expression that characterize the colonic mucosa in patients at genetic risk for colonic cancer. Proc Natl Acad Sci U S A. 1991;88(8):3286–9.
Azim HA, Michiels S, Zagouri F, et al. Utility of prognostic genomic tests in breast cancer practice: the IMPAKT 2012 Working Group Consensus Statement. Ann Oncol. 2013;24(3):647–54.
Bernstein BE, Birney E, Dunham I, Green ED, Gunter C, Snyder M. An integrated encyclopedia of DNA elements in the human genome. Nature. 2012;489(7414):57–74.
Bignell GR, Greenman CD, Davies H, et al. Signatures of mutation and selection in the cancer genome. Nature. 2010;463(7283):893–8.
Bristow RE, Smith A, Zhang Z, et al. Ovarian malignancy risk stratification of the adnexal mass using a multivariate index assay. Gynecol Oncol. 2013;128(2):252–9.
Cancer Genome Atlas Research Network. Comprehensive molecular characterization of human colon and rectal cancer. Nature. 2012;487(7407):330–7.
Carlson JJ, Roth JA. The impact of the Oncotype Dx breast cancer assay in clinical practice: a systematic review and meta-analysis. Breast Cancer Res Treat. 2013;141(1):13–22.
Cesareni G, Ceol A, Gavrila C, Palazzi LM, Persico M, Schneider MV. Comparative interactomics. FEBS Lett. 2005;579(8):1828–33.
Chalkley R. Instrumentation for LC-MS/MS in proteomics. Methods Mol Biol. 2010;658:47–60.
Cooperberg M, Simko J, Falzarano S, et al. Development and validation of the biopsy-based genomic prostate score (GPS) as a predictor of high grade or extracapsular prostate cancer to improve patient selection for active surveillance. American Urological Association Meeting, San Diego, CA, USA. 2013; Abstract 2131.
Dang L, White DW, Gross S, et al. Cancer-associated IDH1 mutations produce 2-hydroxyglutarate. Nature. 2010;465(7300):966.
Diamandis EP. Point: proteomic patterns in biological fluids: do they represent the future of cancer diagnostics? Clin Chem. 2003;49(8):1272–5.
Ding L, Wendl MC, Koboldt DC, Mardis ER. Analysis of next-generation genomic data in cancer: accomplishments and challenges. Hum Mol Genet. 2010;19(R2):R188–96.
Dowsett M, Cuzick J, Wale C, et al. Prediction of risk of distant recurrence using the 21-gene recurrence score in node-negative and node-positive postmenopausal patients with breast cancer treated with anastrozole or tamoxifen: a TransATAC study. J Clin Oncol. 2010;28(11):1829–34.
Edgell T, Martin-Roussety G, Barker G, et al. Phase II biomarker trial of a multimarker diagnostic for ovarian cancer. J Cancer Res Clin Oncol. 2010;136(7):1079–88.
Espina V, Mehta AI, Winters ME, et al. Protein microarrays: molecular profiling technologies for clinical specimens. Proteomics. 2003;3(11):2091–100.
Fan C, Oh DS, Wessels L, et al. Concordance among gene-expression-based predictors for breast cancer. N Engl J Med. 2006;355(6):560–9.
Ferracin M, Veronese A, Negrini M. Micromarkers: miRNAs in cancer diagnosis and prognosis. Expert Rev Mol Diagn. 2010;10(3):297–308.
Fortin T, Salvador A, Charrier JP, et al. Clinical quantitation of prostate-specific antigen biomarker in the low nanogram/milliliter range by conventional bore liquid chromatography-tandem mass spectrometry (multiple reaction monitoring) coupling and correlation with ELISA tests. Mol Cell Proteomics. 2009;8(5):1006–15.
Fung ET. A recipe for proteomics diagnostic test development: the OVA1 test, from biomarker discovery to FDA clearance. Clin Chem. 2010;56(2):327–9.
Gerszten RE, Accurso F, Bernard GR, et al. Challenges in translating plasma proteomics from bench to bedside: update from the NHLBI Clinical Proteomics Programs. Am J Physiol Lung Cell Mol Physiol. 2008;295(1):L16–22.

Hamacher M, Stephan C, Meyer HE, Eisenacher M. Data handling and processing in proteomics. Expert Rev Proteomics. 2009;6(3):217–9.

Hawkins RD, Hon GC, Ren B. Next-generation genomics: an integrative approach. Nat Rev Genet. 2010;11(7):476–86.

Hu J, Coombes KR, Morris JS, Baggerly KA. The importance of experimental design in proteomic mass spectrometry experiments: some cautionary tales. Brief Funct Genomic Proteomic. 2005;3(4):322–31.

Huang Q, Tan Y, Yin P, et al. Metabolic characterization of hepatocellular carcinoma using nontargeted tissue metabolomics. Cancer Res. 2013;73(16):4992–5002.

Hughes C, Ma B, Lajoie GA. De novo sequencing methods in proteomics. Methods Mol Biol. 2010;604:105–21.

Karpova MA, Moshkovskii SA, Toropygin IY, Archakov AI. Cancer-specific MALDI-TOF profiles of blood serum and plasma: biological meaning and perspectives. J Proteomics. 2010;73(3):537–51.

Kim K, Visintin I, Alvero AB, Mor G. Development and validation of a protein-based signature for the detection of ovarian cancer. Clin Lab Med. 2009;29(1):47–55.

Kirschenlohr HL, Griffin JL, Clarke SC, et al. Proton NMR analysis of plasma is a weak predictor of coronary artery disease. Nat Med. 2006;12(6):705–10.

Kobel M, Kalloger SE, Boyd N, et al. Ovarian carcinoma subtypes are different diseases: implications for biomarker studies. PLoS Med. 2008;5(12):e232.

Kraemer S, Vaught JD, Bock C, et al. From SOMAmer-based biomarker discovery to diagnostic and clinical applications: a SOMAmer-based, streamlined multiplex proteomic assay. PLoS One. 2011;6(10):e26332.

Kuhn E, Whiteaker JR, Mani DR, et al. Interlaboratory evaluation of automated, multiplexed peptide immunoaffinity enrichment coupled to multiple reaction monitoring mass spectrometry for quantifying proteins in plasma. Mol Cell Proteomics. 2012;11(6): M111.013854.

Lal A, Panos R, Marjanovic M, et al. A gene expression profile test for the differential diagnosis of ovarian versus endometrial cancers. Oncotarget. 2012;3(2):212–23.

Lee J-R, Magee DM, Gaster RS, LaBaer J, Wang SX. Emerging protein array technologies for proteomics. Expert Rev Proteomics. 2013;10(1):65–75.

Li XJ, Hayward C, Fong PY, et al. A blood-based proteomic classifier for the molecular characterization of pulmonary nodules. Sci Transl Med. 2013;5(207):207ra142.

Lin C-Y, Chin C-H, Wu H-H, Chen S-H, Ho C-W, Ko M-T. Hubba: hub objects analyzer – a framework of interactome hubs identification for network biology. Nucleic Acids Res. 2008;36 (Web Server issue):W438–43.

Liu BC-S, Dijohnson DA, O'Rourke DJ. Antibody profiling with protein antigen microarrays in early stage cancer. Expert Opin Med Diagn. 2012;6(3):187–96.

Lokhov PG, Dashtiev MI, Moshkovskii SA, Archakov AI. Metabolite profiling of blood plasma of patients with prostate cancer. Metabolomics. 2010;6(1):156–63.

Lokhov PG, Trifonova OP, Maslov DL, Archakov AI. Blood plasma metabolites and the risk of developing lung cancer in Russia. Eur J Cancer Prev. 2013;22(4):335–41.

Longo C, Patanarut A, George T, et al. Core-shell hydrogel particles harvest, concentrate and preserve labile low abundance biomarkers. PLoS One. 2009;4(3):e4763.

Luo Y, Wang L, Wang J. Developing proteomics-based biomarkers for colorectal neoplasms for clinical practice: opportunities and challenges. Proteomics Clin Appl. 2013;7(1–2):30–41.

Mann M, Kulak NA, Nagaraj N, Cox J. The coming age of complete, accurate, and ubiquitous proteomes. Mol Cell. 2013;49(4):583–90.

McLerran D, Grizzle WE, Feng Z, et al. SELDI-TOF MS whole serum proteomic profiling with IMAC surface does not reliably detect prostate cancer. Clin Chem. 2008;54(1):53–60.

Moshkovskii S, Vlasova M, Pyatnitskiy M, et al. Acute phase serum amyloid A in ovarian cancer as an important component of proteome diagnostic profiling. Proteomics Clin Appl. 2007;1(1):107–17.

Mutz K-O, Heilkenbrinker A, Lönne M, Walter J-G, Stahl F. Transcriptome analysis using next-generation sequencing. Curr Opin Biotechnol. 2013;24(1):22–30.
Ntzani EE, Ioannidis JPA. Predictive ability of DNA microarrays for cancer outcomes and correlates: an empirical assessment. Lancet. 2003;362(9394):1439–44.
O'Farrell PH. High resolution two-dimensional electrophoresis of proteins. J Biol Chem. 1975;250(10):4007–21.
Petricoin EF, Ardekani AM, Hitt BA, et al. Use of proteomic patterns in serum to identify ovarian cancer. Lancet. 2002;359(9306):572–7.
Picotti P, Aebersold R. Selected reaction monitoring-based proteomics: workflows, potential, pitfalls and future directions. Nat Methods. 2012;9(6):555–66.
Polanski M, Anderson NL. A list of candidate cancer biomarkers for targeted proteomics. Biomark Insights. 2007;1:1–48.
Pusztai L, Ayers M, Stec J, Hortobágyi GN. Clinical application of cDNA microarrays in oncology. Oncologist. 2003;8(3):252–8.
Pyatnitskiy M, Karpova M, Moshkovskii S, Lisitsa A, Archakov A. Clustering mass spectral peaks increases recognition accuracy and stability of SVM-based feature selection. J Proteomics Bioinform. 2010;3:048–54.
Regnier FE, Skates SJ, Mesri M, et al. Protein-based multiplex assays: mock presubmissions to the US Food and Drug Administration. Clin Chem. 2010;56(2):165–71.
Rodriguez H, Tezak Z, Mesri M, et al. Analytical validation of protein-based multiplex assays: a workshop report by the NCI-FDA interagency oncology task force on molecular diagnostics. Clin Chem. 2010;56(2):237–43.
Saeys Y, Inza I, Larrañaga P. A review of feature selection techniques in bioinformatics. Bioinformatics. 2007;23(19):2507–17.
Schulze A, Harris AL. How cancer metabolism is tuned for proliferation and vulnerable to disruption. Nature. 2012;491(7424):364–73.
Shannon P, Markiel A, Ozier O, et al. Cytoscape: a software environment for integrated models of biomolecular interaction networks. Genome Res. 2003;13(11):2498–504.
Simmons AR, Baggerly K, Bast RC. The emerging role of HE4 in the evaluation of epithelial ovarian and endometrial carcinomas. Oncology. 2013;27(6):548–56.
Sreekumar A, Poisson LM, Rajendiran TM, et al. Metabolomic profiles delineate potential role for sarcosine in prostate cancer progression. Nature. 2009;457(7231):910–4.
Stephens PJ, McBride DJ, Lin ML, et al. Complex landscapes of somatic rearrangement in human breast cancer genomes. Nature. 2009;462(7276):1005–10.
Subramanian J, Simon R. Gene expression-based prognostic signatures in lung cancer: ready for clinical use? J Natl Cancer Inst. 2010;102(7):464–74.
Sung J, Wang Y, Chandrasekaran S, Witten DM, Price ND. Molecular signatures from omics data: from chaos to consensus. Biotechnol J. 2012;7(8):946–57.
Szklarczyk D, Franceschini A, Kuhn M, et al. The STRING database in 2011: functional interaction networks of proteins, globally integrated and scored. Nucleic Acids Res. 2011;39 (Database issue):D561–8.
Tolson J, Bogumil R, Brunst E, et al. Serum protein profiling by SELDI mass spectrometry: detection of multiple variants of serum amyloid alpha in renal cancer patients. Lab Investig. 2004;84(7):845–56.
Tran JC, Zamdborg L, Ahlf DR, et al. Mapping intact protein isoforms in discovery mode using top-down proteomics. Nature. 2011;480(7376):254–8.
Trifonova O, Lokhov P, Archakov A. Postgenomics diagnostics: metabolomics approaches to human blood profiling. OMICS. 2013;17(11):550–9.
Ulrich H, Wrenger C. Disease-specific biomarker discovery by aptamers. Cytometry A. 2009;75(9):727–33.
Van't Veer LJ, Dai H, van de Vijver MJ, et al. Gene expression profiling predicts clinical outcome of breast cancer. Nature. 2002;415(6871):530–6.

Venet D, Dumont JE, Detours V. Most random gene expression signatures are significantly associated with breast cancer outcome. PLoS Comput Biol. 2011;7(10):e1002240.
Venook AP, Niedzwiecki D, Lopatin M, et al. Biologic determinants of tumor recurrence in stage II colon cancer: validation study of the 12-gene recurrence score in cancer and leukemia group B (CALGB) 9581. J Clin Oncol. 2013;31(14):1775–81.
Vizcaíno JA, Foster JM, Martens L. Proteomics data repositories: providing a safe haven for your data and acting as a springboard for further research. J Proteomics. 2010;73(11):2136–46.
Waldron L, Ogino S, Hoshida Y, et al. Expression profiling of archival tumors for long-term health studies. Clin Cancer Res. 2012;18(22):6136–46.
Washburn MP, Wolters D, Yates JR. Large-scale analysis of the yeast proteome by multidimensional protein identification technology. Nat Biotechnol. 2001;19(3):242–7.
Weiland M, Gao X-H, Zhou L, Mi Q-S. Small RNAs have a large impact: circulating microRNAs as biomarkers for human diseases. RNA Biol. 2012;9(6):850–9.
Wilkins MR, Pasquali C, Appel RD, et al. From proteins to proteomes: large scale protein identification by two-dimensional electrophoresis and amino acid analysis. Biotechnology. 1996;14(1):61–5.
Williams Z, Ben-Dov IZ, Elias R, et al. Comprehensive profiling of circulating microRNA via small RNA sequencing of cDNA libraries reveals biomarker potential and limitations. Proc Natl Acad Sci U S A. 2013;110(11):4255–60.
Winkler H. Verbreitung und Ursache der Parthenogenesis im Pflanzen – und Tierreiche. Jena: Verlag Fischer; 1920. p. 165.
Yurkovetsky Z, Skates S, Lomakin A, et al. Development of a multimarker assay for early detection of ovarian cancer. J Clin Oncol. 2010;28(13):2159–66.
Zhang Z, Bast RC, Yu Y, et al. Three biomarkers identified from serum proteomic analysis for the detection of early stage ovarian cancer. Cancer Res. 2004;64(16):5882–90.
Zimmer JS, Monroe ME, Qian WJ, et al. Advances in proteomics data analysis and display using an accurate mass and time tag approach. Mass Spectrom Rev. 2006;25(3):450–82.
Zubarev RA. The challenge of the proteome dynamic range and its implications for in-depth proteomics. Proteomics. 2013;13(5):723–6.

Circulating Tumor Cells as Biomarkers in Cancer

2

James Freeman, Elin S. Gray, and Mel Ziman

Contents

Abstract

Circulating tumor cells (CTCs) can be found in the peripheral blood of metastatic cancer patients. Recently, with the development of technologies sufficiently sensitive to detect very rare cells, there has been a considerable increase in research to improve detection of CTCs. Here we discuss the current technologies employed for the enumeration and characterization of CTCs. The implementation of such technologies has enabled research into determining the clinical significance of CTCs and has shown that the concentration of CTCs in patient blood correlates with prognosis and is a clinically relevant prognostic biomarker for patients with metastatic breast, prostate, and colorectal cancers.

J. Freeman • E.S. Gray • M. Ziman (✉)
School of Medical Sciences, Edith Cowan University, Perth, WA, Australia
e-mail: james.freeman@ecu.edu.au; e.gray@ecu.edu.au; m.ziman@ecu.edu.au

V.R. Preedy, V.B. Patel (eds.), *Biomarkers in Cancer, Biomarkers in Disease: Methods, Discoveries and Applications*,
DOI 10.1007/978-94-007-7681-4_21

Additionally, CTCs may be a useful marker for more accurately staging patients as well as to identify early-stage patients at risk of developing metastatic disease who are likely to benefit from a more aggressive adjuvant therapy. Furthermore, various studies have shown that temporal monitoring of CTCs can be used to evaluate patient responses to therapy and to detect genetic and phenotypic changes to tumors in real time, allowing more effective treatment guidance.

List of Abbreviations

CTC	Circulating Tumor Cell
EMT	Epithelial to Mesenchymal Transition
EpCAM	Epithelial Cell Adhesion Molecule
FISH	Fluorescence in Situ Hybridization
ISET	Isolation by Size of Epithelial Tumor Cells
MET	Mesenchymal to Epithelial Transition
qRT-PCR	Quantitative Reverse Transcription Polymerase Chain Reaction
RT-PCR	Reverse Transcription Polymerase Chain Reaction

Key Facts About Circulating Tumor Cells (CTCs)

- CTCs are cancer cells which have broken away from the primary tumor and circulate in peripheral blood.
- CTCs are responsible for invading and proliferating within tissues and organs distant to the primary tumor, leading to the formation of secondary tumors.
- CTCs differ from other cells in the blood in terms of size and the genes they express.
- Technologies which have been developed to isolate CTCs from blood take advantage of their increased size or specifically target proteins on the cell surface which are absent on other cells in the blood.
- Studies have shown that an increased concentration of CTCs in the blood is associated with poor prognosis.
- Some studies have shown that monitoring the number of CTCs before, during, and after therapy is useful for predicting patient outcomes.
- Monitoring CTC numbers may be useful for evaluating treatment efficacy and more effectively guiding treatment programs.
- Research is being undertaken to characterize CTCs in different cancers to determine if there are subpopulations of CTCs more able to form secondary tumors.
- Characterization of CTCs offers potential to develop new targeted therapies.

Definition of Words and Terms

Circulating Tumor Cells (CTCs) Cells derived from solid tumors which circulate in the blood of metastatic cancer patients.

Epithelial to Mesenchymal Transition (EMT) The transformation of epithelial cancer cells in response to expression of transcription factors resulting in adoption of a mesenchymal phenotype with enhanced metastatic capability.

Mesenchymal to Epithelial Transition (MET) Reversal of the EMT process.

CTC Enrichment The process of separating CTCs from whole blood for downstream analysis.

The CELLSEARCH® System A method for enriching CTCs from patient blood using EpCAM antibody-coated immunomagnetic beads and identifying CK-positive, CD45-negative cells by automated fluorescence microscopy.

Isolation by Size of Epithelial Tumor Cells (ISET) A method for enriching CTCs by passing whole blood through a filter (8 μm pore size) allowing capture of large CTCs and elimination of small leukocytes and erythrocytes.

Microemboli Clusters of CTCs which are thought to have greater metastatic potential than single CTCs.

Tumor-Initiating Cells Subpopulations of cancer cells which exhibit greater tumorigenic capacity than the bulk cancer cell population. Tumor-initiating capability is associated with an undifferentiated, stem cell like phenotype.

Introduction to Circulating Tumor Cells

The vast majority of cancer-related deaths occur as a consequence of metastasis, the process of cells shedding from a primary tumor, entering circulation, and subsequently invading and proliferating within the distant tissues. The ability to identify circulating tumor cells (CTCs) before the development of clinically detectable metastases offers promise as a prognostic measure, allowing both identification of residual disease following primary tumor resection and identification of patients at risk of disease progression who may benefit from adjuvant therapy. Furthermore, CTC detection offers the potential to monitor patient responses to therapy and thus evaluate treatment efficacy in cancers which are notoriously difficult to treat.

The process which allows tumor cells to enter the circulation and subsequently invade and proliferate at distant sites, giving rise to metastases, remains poorly understood. In short, metastasis begins when cells within the primary tumor invade the surrounding tissue and enter the vasculature of the circulatory or lymphatic systems, a process known as intravasation. The early stages of metastasis can often be detected by biopsy of the sentinel lymph nodes, the first nodes into which the primary tumor drains (Das and Skobe 2008). However, it seems the vast majority of metastatic dissemination occurs via the circulatory system (Chambers et al. 2002). Subsequently, for the development of metastases, CTCs must exit the vasculature

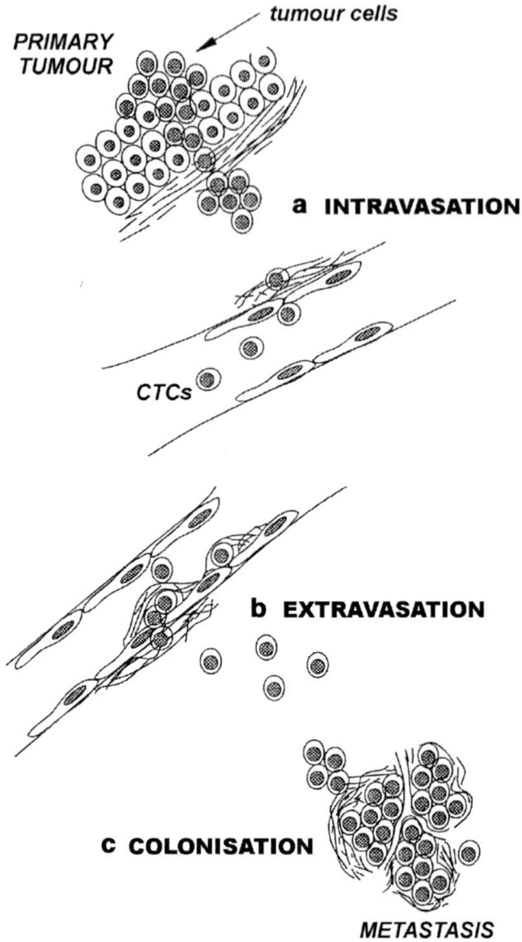

Fig. 1 The metastatic process. Cells within the primary tumor intravasate (**a**) and circulate in the blood as CTCs. CTCs subsequently extravasate at distant sites (**b**) and adapt to and colonize their new environment leading to metastasis formation (**c**) (Adapted with permission from Pantel et al. 1999)

and invade adjacent tissue in a process termed extravasation. CTCs must then adapt to their new environment and begin to proliferate, a process known as colonization (Fig. 1). It is uncertain what proportion of viable CTCs are able to undergo this process; however, it has been suggested that only a small subpopulation of CTCs with a highly metastatic phenotype, known as tumor-initiating cells, give rise to metastases (Ishizawa et al. 2010; Chaffer and Weinberg 2011).

In order to escape the primary tumor, cells undergo an epithelial to mesenchymal transition (EMT), a process that is vital in early embryogenesis for cell migration. EMT is initiated by expression of a number of transcription factors that are activated in response to signaling between tumor cells and the surrounding stroma (Yang et al. 2008; Chaffer and Weinberg 2011). Cells which adopt a mesenchymal phenotype are invasive, migratory, and resistant to apoptosis, so they more readily enter circulation and invade distant tissues, increasing their metastatic potential (Kalluri and Weinberg 2009). Following tissue invasion, cells revert to an epithelial phenotype by undergoing mesenchymal to epithelial transition (MET), allowing them to proliferate (Yang et al. 2008).

Detection of tumor cells in the circulation as an indication of tumor progression is the subject of a plethora of studies leading to the generation of new technologies; however, the rarity of CTCs makes reliable detection a considerable challenge. Although CTC concentrations appear to vary significantly between patients and tumor types, they are estimated to circulate in the blood of metastatic cancer patients at a concentration of one cell in a billion blood cells (Yu et al. 2011). Although many technologies allowing enrichment of CTCs from whole blood have emerged in recent years, there is as yet no standardized method of CTC detection suitable for clinical use across a number of metastatic cancers. Techniques allowing reliable, sensitive detection of CTCs are required for accurate downstream analysis in order to evaluate their clinical utility. This chapter provides an overview of the current methodologies available for CTC detection and discusses enumeration and characterization of CTCs resulting from implementation of these technologies.

Detection of CTCs by RT-PCR

Circulating tumor cell mRNA can be detected in the blood of cancer patients by reverse transcription polymerase chain reaction (RT-PCR). This technique is able to detect the expression of tumor-associated markers in patient peripheral blood, suggesting the presence of CTCs. Studies have shown that detection of tumor markers in the blood of patients correlates with prognosis and predicts disease outcome (Reynolds et al. 2003; Ignatiadis et al. 2008; Helo et al. 2009).

Although this method has improved with the use of multi-marker quantitative RT-PCR (qRT-PCR) (Xi et al. 2007; Reid et al. 2013), there are many disadvantages to the use of RT-PCR for CTC detection in whole blood. Low specificity of this method has been reported, resulting in a large number of false positives (Paterlini-Brechot and Benali 2007). This technique may also detect free mRNA transcripts circulating in the blood rather than intact CTCs with metastatic capability (Chen et al. 2000; Silva et al. 2002). Additionally, as cell lysis is required, CTCs are unable to be enumerated or characterized further. The use of PCR for detection of CTCs in whole blood is now rarely used, with more recent research adopting methods to enrich intact CTCs.

CTC Enrichment Technologies

Enriching intact, viable CTCs from whole blood enables enumeration of CTCs. Further analysis of the enriched fraction allows characterization of CTCs in regard to their genetic and morphological characteristics. There are a number of properties which distinguish CTCs from other cells in the circulatory system. Technologies developed to enrich CTCs from whole blood take advantage of their physical properties, such as their increased size compared to leukocytes or the expression of tumor-associated markers.

Enrichment by Physical Properties

Physical properties, such as differences in size and density, can distinguish the majority of CTCs from other cells in the blood and can therefore be useful for isolation of CTCs. Density gradient centrifugation, as used by the OncoQuick® system (Greiner Bio-One), can be used to enrich mononuclear cells, including CTCs, from whole blood (Rosenberg et al. 2002). However, samples processed by density gradient centrifugation have significant leukocyte contamination; thus, this method is usually used as a precursor to other CTC detection procedures such as RT-PCR-based techniques.

Methods enriching CTCs based on their physical properties usually take advantage of their increased size. Isolation by size of epithelial tumor cells (ISET) (Rarecells Diagnostics) involves enrichment of CTCs from whole blood by filtration through a membrane with a pore size of 8 μm; thus, large CTCs are captured, while smaller leukocytes and erythrocytes pass through (Vona et al. 2000). The benefit of this method is that there is no discrimination applied to the type of CTCs enriched, as cells do not have to sufficiently express a particular marker to be detected. This is especially useful for highly heterogeneous tumors, since many subtypes of CTCs, marked by a variety of gene expression profiles, can be enriched, providing they are of sufficient size. Another advantage of this technique is that, due to minimal disturbance of cells passing through the filter, clusters of CTCs, or microemboli, which may have increased metastatic capability (Paterlini-Brechot and Benali 2007), remain intact and can be visualized (Fig. 2) (Farace et al. 2011). Enriching intact cells also allows for further characterization by immunocytochemistry or molecular biology. The downside of the ISET filtration technique is its low specificity, which results in the isolated CTCs being contaminated by a large number of leukocytes (Paterlini-Brechot and Benali 2007). Also, although the majority of CTCs are relatively large and are therefore captured by the membrane, it has been observed that CTCs are heterogeneous in size, as well as gene expression, and thus smaller CTCs will be lost with this method (Marrinucci et al. 2007).

Recently, another filtration device, ScreenCell®, like the ISET system, has become commercially available. The ScreenCell method comes in three formats allowing immunocytochemistry, molecular biology, or culture of enriched CTCs for further characterization. This technology demonstrates high sensitivity and specificity of enrichment, based on spiking experiments with cancer cell lines, and like other size-filtration methods is not biased in terms of preferentially selecting CTCs which express a particular marker (Desitter et al. 2011).

Cell Surface Marker-Based Enrichment

Most commonly, CTCs are enriched from whole blood by targeting markers expressed on the surface of tumor cells. Epithelial markers, such as EpCAM, are useful targets for methods that enrich CTCs derived from epithelial tumors of the breast, prostate, colon, and lung, among others. However, other cancers such as

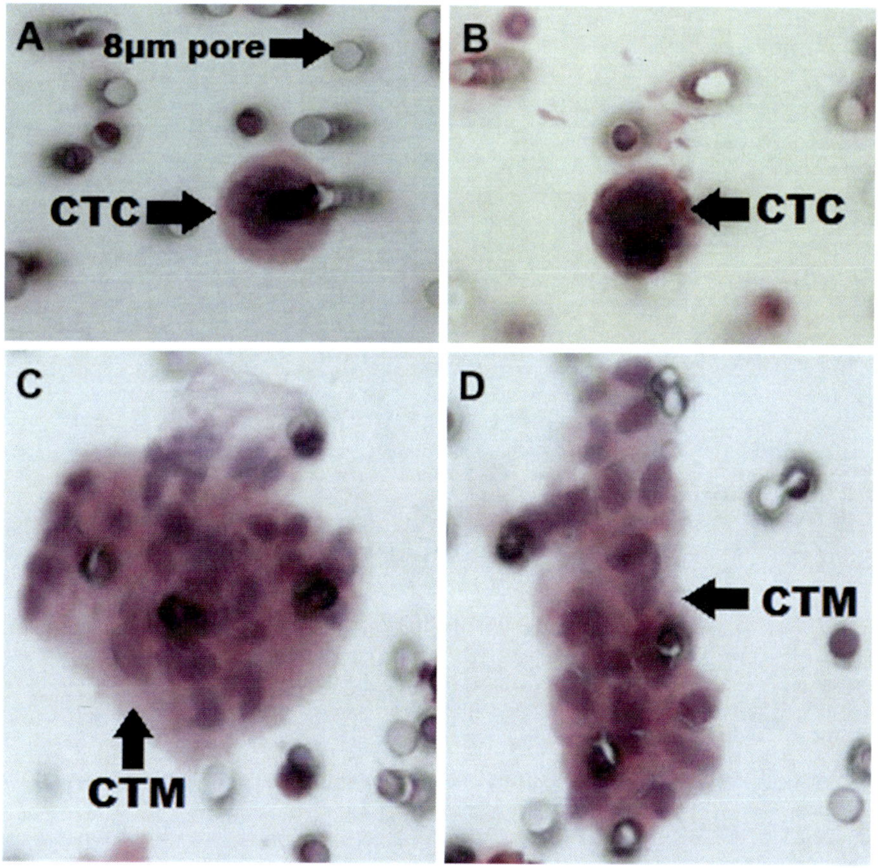

Fig. 2 Isolation by size of epithelial tumor cells (ISET). CTCs enriched by ISET from a patient with prostate cancer (**a** and **b**) and circulating tumor microemboli (*CTM*) from a patient with kidney cancer (**c** and **d**). Cells were enriched by the ISET method and stained with hematoxylin and eosin. CTCs are characterized by high nuclear/cytoplasmic ratio, irregular nuclei, and nonhomogeneous texture (Adapted with permission from Paterlini-Brechot and Benali 2007)

sarcomas and malignant melanoma do not express EpCAM and need to be detected by targeting other surface markers.

The CELLSEARCH® System (Veridex) is a semiautomated method which enriches epithelial tumor cells from the blood using EpCAM antibody-coated immunomagnetic beads. Isolated cells are immunocytochemically labeled with antibodies for CD45 and cytokeratins (CK) 8, 18, and 19, as well as DAPI for nuclear staining. Epithelial-derived CTCs (DAPI positive, CK positive, CD45 negative) can then be distinguished from contaminating leukocytes (CD45 positive) by semiautomated fluorescence microscopy (Fig. 3) (Cristofanilli et al. 2004). The CELLSEARCH® System has been FDA (Food and Drug Administration) approved for clinical use in metastatic breast, prostate, and colorectal cancer, although more

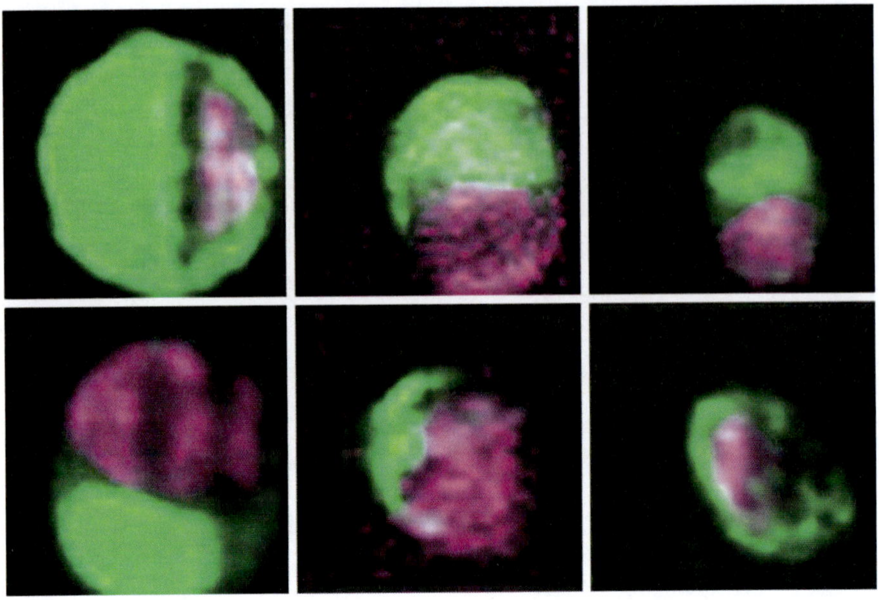

Fig. 3 CTCs isolated by the CELLSEARCH® System. Images of 6 CTC candidates enriched by the CELLSEARCH® System and identified by the CellTracks® Analyzer II. The images show an overlay of DAPI (*purple*) and cytokeratin (*green*). All cells were CD45 negative and classified as CTCs by 6 of 6 trained operators (Adapted with permission from Miller et al. 2010)

recent studies have also demonstrated the prognostic significance of CTCs in both small cell (Hou et al. 2009) and non-small cell lung cancer (Krebs et al. 2011) using this method.

As CTCs must sufficiently express EpCAM to be enriched, there are a number of drawbacks to this method. As epithelial cancers tend to be heterogeneous, enriching CTCs by EpCAM expression may allow detection of only a specific subtype of CTCs, not necessarily representative of the total CTC population. Also, CTCs which have undergone EMT during the metastatic process may not be detected due to loss of expression of epithelial markers (Kalluri and Weinberg 2009). This could be a problem when quantifying CTCs or when characterizing CTCs with metastatic capability.

For non-epithelial malignancies, where EpCAM is not a useful target marker, alternate kits are available for enriching CTCs; for example, Veridex has recently released the CELLTRACKS® Circulating Melanoma Cell Kit, for enriching melanoma CTCs. Instead of targeting EpCAM and staining for cytokeratins, this kit targets CD146, a marker expressed on the surface of melanoma cells, and stains for high molecular weight-melanoma-associated antigen (HMW-MAA) in addition to CD45 and CD34 for exclusion of leukocytes and endothelial cells, respectively (Rao et al. 2011).

There are also commercially available kits which allow magnetic beads to be conjugated to antibodies of the researcher's choice for enrichment of rare cells, including CTCs. For example, the CELLection Pan Mouse IgG Kit (Invitrogen) includes immunomagnetic beads conjugated to anti-mouse antibody which are able to enrich CTCs pre-labeled with any mouse antibody (Sakaizawa et al. 2012). Alternatively, commercially available and chemically activated magnetic beads can be directly labeled with a variety of antibodies to tumor-associated markers. Targeting multiple-cell surface markers has been shown to increase the proportion of total CTCs captured (Freeman et al. 2012).

The AdnaTest (AdnaGen) utilizes immunomagnetic beads conjugated to antibodies targeting EpCAM and MUC1 to capture CTCs, in combination with a multiplex RT-PCR to determine the presence of cancer-derived transcripts (Fehm et al. 2007; Lankiewicz et al. 2008). The AdnaTest allows the detection of CTCs with dedifferentiated characteristics such as mesenchymal and stem cell phenotypes (Barriere et al. 2012). However, this method does not determine whether these markers are co-expressed or if they are derived from different CTCs.

The MagSweeper is an automated immunomagnetic separation device allowing efficient enrichment of epithelial tumor cells from whole blood with limited sample manipulation. Whole blood is first incubated with magnetic beads coated with EpCAM antibody. Bead-bound cells are subsequently enriched by a sweeping magnetic device which creates shear force removing nonspecifically bound blood cells (Talasaz et al. 2009). Captured cells can subsequently be released from the magnet and visualized by microscopy. An advantage of the MagSweeper technology is that it allows single viable CTCs to be aspirated for downstream applications allowing characterization of individual CTCs (Talasaz et al. 2009; Powell et al. 2012).

Emerging Technologies

Microfluidic Devices

More recently, a number of technologies have emerged which promise improved CTC enrichment with increased sensitivity and specificity. Many of these use microfluidic technology, usually within a chip-like device. The CTC-Chip relies on laminar flow to pass whole blood through a chip containing 78,000 microposts coated with EpCAM antibody. The microposts bind and isolate epithelial tumor cells from the blood, for subsequent quantification and characterization (Nagrath et al. 2007). This technology offers improved sensitivity and specificity of CTC enrichment, demonstrating positive CTC detection in the majority of patients with metastatic carcinoma, as well as in early-stage patients with no clinical evidence of metastasis (Nagrath et al. 2007; Stott et al. 2010b). This technology was further improved with the development of the Herringbone-Chip, which passively mixes cells through the generation of microvortices, maximizing the interaction of cells with the antibody-coated walls of the chip (Stott et al. 2010a). In addition to improved sensitivity and specificity of enrichment, microfluidic devices, like filtering methods, are gentle on processed cells and allow detection of intact tumor cell clusters (Fig. 4) (Stott et al. 2010a). Serial CTC monitoring using the

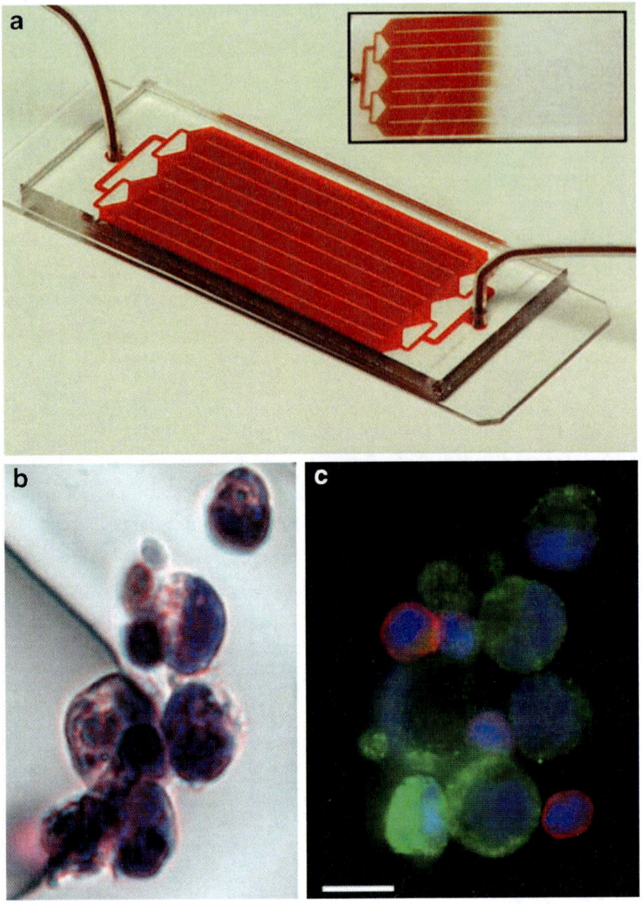

Fig. 4 **The Herringbone-Chip.** (**a**) The Herringbone-Chip is a device which allows passage of whole blood through microfluidic channels enabling capture of CTCs by the EpCAM antibody-coated chip surface. Gentle processing of blood allows capture of CTC clusters or microemboli. (**b**) and (**c**) show a CTC cluster isolated from a metastatic prostate cancer patient stained with hematoxylin and eosin (**b**) and fluorescently labeled with DAPI (*blue*), prostate-specific antigen (*green*), and CD45 (*red*); scale bar represents 10 μm (**c**) (Adapted with permission from Stott et al. 2010a)

Herringbone-Chip combined with RNA fluorescence in situ hybridization (RNA-FISH) detection of EMT markers shows an association of mesenchymal CTCs with disease progression (Yu et al. 2013). The Herringbone-Chip capture, however, allows only limited characterization of the isolated CTCs, as they remain fixed within the chip.

Further refinements to the CTC-Chip have resulted in an integrated microfluidic system (CTC-iChip) that combines three sequential separation steps: removal of red blood cells, inertial focusing of nucleated cells, and deflection of magnetic tagged

CTCs (Ozkumur et al. 2013). The CTC-iChip allows the isolation of CTCs in suspension, and it is compatible with downstream single-cell molecular analysis as well as standard cytopathology.

The OncoCEE™ (Cell Enrichment and Extraction) platform (Biocept Laboratories) also consists of a microfluidic device to efficiently capture and detect CTCs (Pecot et al. 2011). This system enables sequential recovery of both CK-positive and CK-negative CTCs for subsequent testing by fluorescence in situ hybridization (FISH). Its efficacy is attributed to its use of a cocktail containing antibodies directed toward a variety of epithelial cell surface antigens (EpCAM, HER2, MUC1, EGFR, folate-binding protein receptor and TROP2) and mesenchymal or stem cell antigens (c-MET, N-Cadherin, CD318, and mesenchymal stem cell antigen). However, this method does not allow the recovery of CTCs for further molecular characterization.

High-Definition CTC

The high-definition (HD)-CTC assay (EPIC Sciences) identifies CTCs in whole blood. Following erythrocyte lysis, cells are attached as a monolayer to custom-made glass slides. Using automated digital microscopy, CTCs are defined as CK-positive, CD45-negative cells with intact, non-apoptotic, DAPI-stained nuclei. CTCs must also be morphologically distinct from surrounding WBCs, by displaying characteristics used in standard diagnostic pathology for identification of malignant cells (Cho et al. 2012; Marrinucci et al. 2012). There is minimal sample processing required, due to the absence of enrichment, which results in high sensitivity of CTC detection. The EPIC system demonstrates significantly higher sensitivity of detection in comparison to the CELLSEARCH® System while maintaining high specificity, with very few CTC like cells detected in blood samples from healthy donors (Marrinucci et al. 2012). Minimal processing also enables detection of CTC clusters, which are observed in a high proportion of patients. The drawback of this method is that it only allows CTC quantification and analysis of morphology; it is not designed for downstream characterization of CTCs.

DEParray

The DEParray™ (Silicon Biosystems) is an instrument allowing selection of pure single CTCs for downstream single-cell analysis. Following enrichment and fluorescent labeling of CTCs by a compatible methodology, such as the CELLSEARCH® CTC kit, cells are loaded into a silicon chip and positioned on the instrument. Microelectrodes within the chip trap individual cells in electromagnetic cages generated by a nonuniform electrical field (Fuchs et al. 2006; Fabbri et al. 2013; Peeters et al. 2013). Identified cells of interest are subsequently maneuvered and recovered by activation and deactivation of the electrodes, automatically controlled through software manipulation. The advantage of this technology is that it enables isolation of pure single cells for downstream applications not possible with an impure enriched cell fraction (Fabbri et al. 2013; Peeters et al. 2013). The ability to characterize individual CTCs is extremely useful for investigating CTC heterogeneity and for monitoring changes in CTC profiles as a consequence of therapy, which may influence patient outcomes. The downside of this method, however, is that the chip only processes approximately two thirds of the loaded sample in order to avoid the uptake of air, resulting in significant cell loss (Peeters et al. 2013). Taken together with CTC losses during the initial enrichment step, this is a considerable drawback for samples with very few CTCs.

Positive Versus Negative Enrichment of CTCs

Positive enrichment of CTCs, for example, by size or expression of particular tumor-associated antigens, inevitably introduces discrimination into CTC selection. As CTC phenotype remains largely unknown, targeting particular markers or properties of CTCs may inadvertently exclude various subpopulations of CTCs from the enriched fraction. For this reason, there is some thought that negative enrichment of CTCs, by removal of all hematologic cells and other circulating non-tumor cells, offers improved enrichment of all CTCs, including rare subtypes (Yang et al. 2009). There are, however, advantages and disadvantages associated with both positive and negative enrichment of CTCs. Typically, positive enrichment generates a higher purity of CTCs, whereas negative enrichment results in a greater number of contaminating leukocytes (Liu et al. 2011). While negative enrichment of CTCs may allow the detection of rare CTC subpopulations, which may not express common tumor-associated antigens, lower purity of enriched CTCs limits the potential for further characterization as CTC concentration may be below the detection limit of many downstream assays. However, although positive selection of CTCs may be more suitable for downstream applications due to increased purity, the discrimination applied to the selection process may diminish the significance of the results.

Quantification of CTCs as a Predictor of Survival and a Marker of Therapy Response

Research has shown that detection of CTCs in patient blood correlates with poor prognosis and shorter overall survival (Fig. 5). Studies using the CELLSEARCH® System have shown that a cutoff of five CTCs per 7.5 ml of blood can be used to sort metastatic breast and prostate cancer patients into favorable and unfavorable prognostic groups (Cristofanilli et al. 2004; Danila et al. 2007; de Bono et al. 2008). On the other hand, a cutoff of three CTCs per 7.5 ml of blood has been shown to discriminate metastatic colorectal cancer patients with poorer prognosis (Cohen et al. 2008).

Metastatic breast cancer patients with five or more CTCs per 7.5 ml of blood at baseline were shown to have both shorter progression-free survival (median 2.7 months vs. 7 months) and shorter overall survival (median 10.1 months vs. >18 months) than patients with fewer than five CTCs (Cristofanilli et al. 2004).

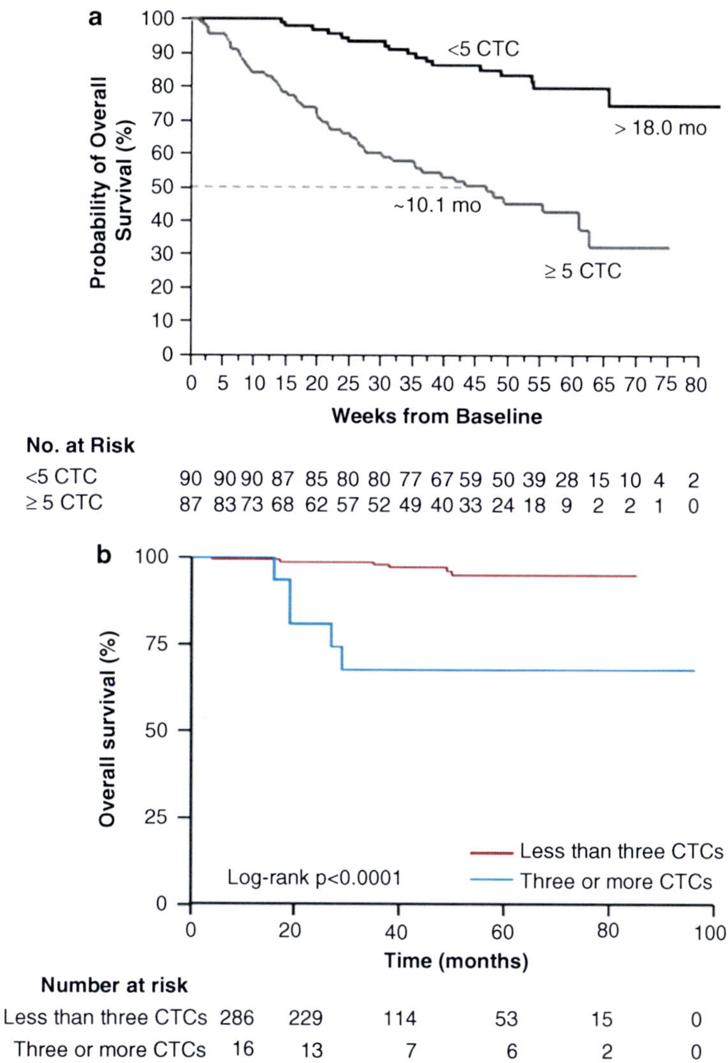

Fig. 5 Prognostic value of CTC enumeration by the CELLSEARCH® System. Kaplan-Meier curves demonstrating the relationship between CTC number and overall survival in metastatic breast cancer (**a**) and early-stage, non-metastatic breast cancer (**b**) (Adapted with permission from Cristofanilli et al. 2004; Lucci et al. 2012)

Follow-up of these patients during therapy determined that CTC numbers were a strong predictor of disease progression and mortality at any given time point (Hayes et al. 2006). Interestingly, it was observed that patients with five or more CTCs at baseline who had a reduction in CTCs (<5) following initiation of therapy had improved overall survival (median 19.8 months), while patients with less than five

CTCs at baseline who had an increase in CTCs ($\geq$5) following initiation of therapy had shorter overall survival (10.6 months).

In castration-resistant prostate cancer patients, five or more CTCs per 7.5 ml of blood are also associated with shorter overall survival (median 6.8 months) compared with fewer than five CTCs (median >26 months) (de Bono et al. 2008). CTC enumeration before and after therapy demonstrated that patients with five or more CTCs at baseline, who had a reduction in CTCs (<5) following treatment, had improved overall survival (median 21.3 months), while patients with fewer than five CTCs, who had an increase in CTCs ($\geq$5) following treatment, had shorter overall survival (median 9.3 months).

Similarly, CTCs have been shown to be a useful marker for evaluating treatment effectiveness in studies utilizing different methods of CTC detection. Serial monitoring of CTCs with the CTC-Chip has demonstrated that while CTC numbers are independent of tumor burden, CTCs respond to therapy in a manner similar to that of solid tumors and are therefore a useful marker of treatment efficacy (Nagrath et al. 2007; Maheswaran et al. 2008). These results suggest that monitoring CTCs before, during, and after therapy is a useful measure of patient response and could be used to test the effectiveness of multiple treatments on individual patients, resulting in improved treatment outcomes.

Although the CELLSEARCH® System is currently only approved for clinical use in patients with metastatic disease, some recent studies have applied the method to early-stage, non-metastatic patients in order to determine if CTCs are a predictor of disease progression. A study in non-metastatic breast cancer detected CTCs in 24 % of patients and demonstrated that those patients with detectable CTCs had shorter progression-free survival and overall survival (Lucci et al. 2012). With improvements in technology, efficient CTC detection would allow improved staging and disease management in early-stage patients.

CTC Characterization and Monitoring Therapy Responses

In addition to CTC enumeration, further characterization of these cells can provide information about the tumor from which they are derived and indicate changes that take place during therapy. Evaluating the presence of a variety of markers may also be useful for identifying subpopulations in the CTC fraction, such as metastasis-initiating cells (Baccelli et al. 2013), stemness, and mesenchymal phenotype (Gazzaniga et al. 2010; Gradilone et al. 2011a; Wang et al. 2012) or CTCs with treatment-resistant markers (Maheswaran et al. 2008).

In breast cancer, hormone replacement therapy and trastuzumab (Herceptin) treatment are determined according to the HER2 status and hormone receptor expression of the initial tumor. Various studies have demonstrated a discrepancy between the primary tumor and the CTCs in regard to their expression of HER2 (Fehm et al. 2010; Munzone et al. 2010; Hayashi et al. 2012), estrogen receptor alpha (Aktas et al. 2011; Gradilone et al. 2011b), and progesterone receptor (Aktas et al. 2011). A study of patients with metastatic breast cancer, starting a new

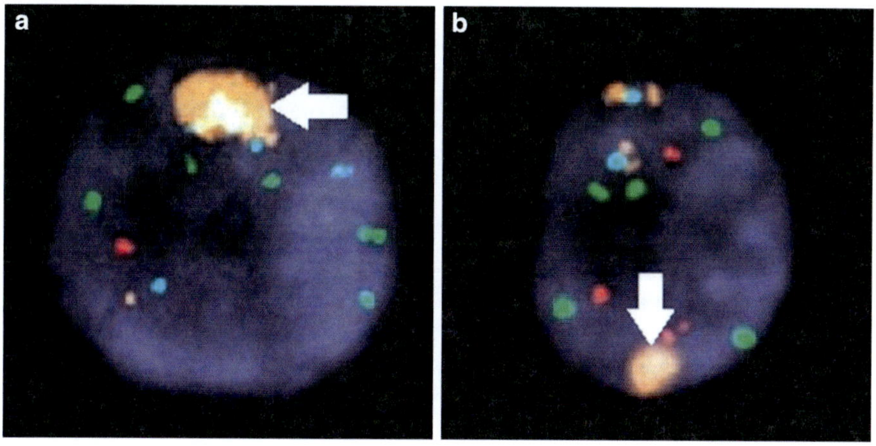

Fig. 6 Androgen receptor (AR) gene amplification in CTCs observed by FISH. CTCs were enriched by the CELLSEARCH® System and subsequently hybridized with probes for AR (*orange*) among other genes. AR amplification can be seen in both (**a**) and (**b**), as indicated by the *arrows* (Adapted with permission from Leversha et al. 2009)

systemic therapy, demonstrated that HE2-positive CTCs, not present at baseline but at first follow-up, were associated with shorter progression-free survival (Hayashi et al. 2012). Despite being a low-powered study that requires further confirmation, these results suggest that HER2-positive CTCs at first follow-up predict resistance to treatment, and therefore these patients might benefit from a change of therapy.

Flow cytometry can be used for characterization of CTCs, following staining for tumor-associated markers and other phenotypic markers of EMT and stemness (Liu et al. 2011; Fusi et al. 2012; Wang et al. 2012). Flow cytometry allows rapid enumeration of a large number of cells and multiple markers; however, it does not allow cells to be visualized, and therefore CTC morphology cannot be analyzed. Moreover, given the low frequency of CTCs in the blood of most patients, flow cytometric analysis is at the limit of reliable detection.

Fluorescence in situ hybridization (FISH) can be used for confirmation and further characterization of enriched CTCs by detection of chromosomal aberrations, such as gene amplification and translocations, associated with various malignancies. Following enrichment of CTCs, gene-specific fluorescently labeled probes are hybridized to denatured DNA allowing visualization of specific chromosomal regions by microscopy. CTCs can be identified by detection of known chromosomal aberrations, for example, amplification of the androgen receptor (AR) gene in metastatic prostate cancer CTCs (Fig. 6) (Shaffer et al. 2007; Leversha et al. 2009), and further characterization can be performed by identification of novel abnormalities. Chromosomal amplification of AR, rearrangement of ERG gene, PTEN deletion, and MYC amplification were detected in CTCs from patients with metastatic prostate cancer by FISH (Attard et al. 2009; Leversha et al. 2009). Significant heterogeneity of AR copy number gain and PTEN loss was observed in CTCs, illustrating the heterogeneity of the tumors and the representation of this diversity in CTCs.

Rearrangement in the ALK gene can be detected in CTCs from patients with lung cancer and strongly correlated with contemporaneous tumor biopsies (Ilie et al. 2012). Given that crizotinib (Xalkori) treatment is restricted to patients with ALK rearrangements (Ou et al. 2012), molecular profiling of CTCs may allow screening for patients who will benefit from this treatment without the need to undergo an invasive tumor biopsy.

Allele-specific PCR amplification revealed mutations in the epidermal growth factor receptor (EGFR) in DNA recovered from CTCs and from matched tumor biopsy specimens (Maheswaran et al. 2008). Moreover, the drug-resistant mutation T790M was detected in CTCs isolated from patients with EGFR mutations that had received tyrosine kinase inhibitors gefitinib (Iressa®) or erlotinib (Tarceva®). The presence of the T790M mutation correlated with reduced progression-free survival. This result supports the idea of monitoring changes in tumor genotypes during the course of treatment, by genotyping CTCs.

Similarly, another study describes the detection of the KRAS mutation in CTCs from colorectal cancer patients (Yang et al. 2010). The presence of KRAS mutations in EGFR-positive colorectal cancer is used to identify patients likely to not respond to anti-EGFR mAb cetuximab (Erbitux). This study suggested that blood might be a better sample to assess the tumor genotype for treatment decisions.

The BRAF V600E/K mutation is present in around 50 % of melanoma cases, and two targeted therapies are now available for the treatment of this subtype of metastatic melanoma. The detection of the BRAFV600E mutation in isolated CTCs has been previously reported (Kitago et al. 2009; Freeman et al. 2012) with a 91 % (19/21) correspondence with the matched tumor tissue (Liu et al. 2011). Moreover, in one of those individuals, CTCs were shown to bear the BRAFV600E mutation while this was not at detectable levels at the tissue level (Liu et al. 2011). This is consistent with the previous observations of intra- and inter-tumor heterogeneity of BRAF mutation status in melanoma (Sensi et al. 2006; Yancovitz et al. 2012). A recent report by Sakaizawa and colleagues successfully identified BRAF- and KIT-activating mutations at a single-cell level in CTCs from patients with melanoma (Sakaizawa et al. 2012).

A recent study described comprehensive genomic profiling of CTCs using array comparative genomic hybridization (CGH) and next-generation sequencing (Heitzer et al. 2013). The authors identified multiple colorectal cancer-associated copy number changes, many of which were also present in the respective primary tumors. Mutations in known driver genes [e.g., APC, KRAS, or PIK3CA] found in the primary tumor and metastasis were also detected in corresponding CTCs. However, some mutations initially found only in CTCs were also present at subclonal levels in the primary tumors and metastases from the same patient (Heitzer et al. 2013). This study constitutes the beginning of a new era in the CTC field by integrating single-cell genomics for comprehensive analysis of these cells.

Concluding Remarks

Altogether, these studies support CTCs as a superior sample with which to examine the genetic profile of the sum of the patient's tumors and may therefore be useful for monitoring the development of escape mutations during treatment. Nevertheless, it is a limitation in some studies that the isolation and analysis of CTCs is based on only one or two surface proteins, gene deletions, amplifications, or point mutations. More comprehensive studies are required that determine the extent to which CTCs represent the parental tumors. The rapid progress in next-generation sequencing and onco-proteomics will enable better characterization of CTCs in the near future. Hopefully this will uncover more informative biomarkers with which to select CTCs and thus provide more specific information about patients who will benefit from targeted treatments as well as improve evaluation of therapeutic responses.

In parallel, improvements in the methodologies used to isolate and quantify CTCs are needed. Different methodologies that bias toward different tumor cell subsets might not reflect overall tumor heterogeneity. Issues such as the impact on disease outcome of collective migration (microemboli detection), presence of EMT, and cancer stem cell markers need to be addressed in the context of well-designed clinical studies. Moreover, there is little evidence of the metastatic potential of CTCs (Kupas et al. 2011; Baccelli et al. 2013), and it is yet to be confirmed that CTCs are indeed the source of metastasis. The use of CTCs as an independent marker of treatment response is a valuable tool that should be evaluated as part of clinical trials to facilitate a swift implementation into clinical practice. However, it is likely that this will be different for different cancer types and therapeutic interventions.

Summary Points

- CTCs circulate in patient blood at very low frequency, and therefore, reliable detection is a significant technical challenge.
- Recent technological advances have improved our capacity to detect and isolate CTCs for quantification and molecular characterization.
- CTC isolation technologies are based on the physical and biological properties that differentiate CTCs from other cells in circulation.
- The concentration of CTCs in peripheral blood has been shown to be prognostic of overall survival in colon, breast, and prostate cancers, non-small and small cell lung cancers, and melanoma patients.
- Gene expression in CTCs is highly heterogeneous; thus, targeting a single marker for CTC isolation is not ideal for efficient detection.
- Research has shown that cancer cells are able to undergo epithelial to mesenchymal transition (EMT) which is associated with an invasive phenotype and may give rise to CTCs with high metastatic potential.

- Some research has shown that CTC concentration is a useful marker of treatment efficacy and may be an effective predictor of disease relapse or progression.
- Temporal monitoring of CTCs has shown potential for detecting genetic changes in CTCs which can lead to treatment resistance.

References

Aktas B, Muller V, Tewes M, et al. Comparison of estrogen and progesterone receptor status of circulating tumor cells and the primary tumor in metastatic breast cancer patients. Gynecol Oncol. 2011;122:356–60.

Attard G, Swennenhuis JF, Olmos D, et al. Characterization of ERG, AR and PTEN gene status in circulating tumor cells from patients with castration-resistant prostate cancer. Cancer Res. 2009;69:2912–8.

Baccelli I, Schneeweiss A, Riethdorf S, et al. Identification of a population of blood circulating tumor cells from breast cancer patients that initiates metastasis in a xenograft assay. Nat Biotechnol. 2013;31:539–44.

Barriere G, Riouallon A, Renaudie J, et al. Mesenchymal characterization: alternative to simple CTC detection in two clinical trials. Anticancer Res. 2012;32:3363–9.

Chaffer CL, Weinberg RA. A perspective on cancer cell metastasis. Science. 2011;331:1559–64.

Chambers AF, Groom AC, MacDonald IC. Dissemination and growth of cancer cells in metastatic sites. Nat Rev Cancer. 2002;2:563–72.

Chen XQ, Bonnefoi H, Pelte MF, et al. Telomerase RNA as a detection marker in the serum of breast cancer patients. Clin Cancer Res. 2000;6:3823–6.

Cho EH, Wendel M, Luttgen M, et al. Characterization of circulating tumor cell aggregates identified in patients with epithelial tumors. Phys Biol. 2012;9:016001.

Cohen SJ, Punt CJ, Iannotti N, et al. Relationship of circulating tumor cells to tumor response, progression-free survival, and overall survival in patients with metastatic colorectal cancer. J Clin Oncol. 2008;26:3213–21.

Cristofanilli M, Budd GT, Ellis MJ, et al. Circulating tumor cells, disease progression, and survival in metastatic breast cancer. N Engl J Med. 2004;351:781–91.

Danila DC, Heller G, Gignac GA, et al. Circulating tumor cell number and prognosis in progressive castration-resistant prostate cancer. Clin Cancer Res. 2007;13:7053–8.

Das S, Skobe M. Lymphatic vessel activation in cancer. Ann N Y Acad Sci. 2008;1131:235–41.

de Bono JS, Scher HI, Montgomery RB, et al. Circulating tumor cells predict survival benefit from treatment in metastatic castration-resistant prostate cancer. Clin Cancer Res. 2008;14:6302–9.

Desitter I, Guerrouahen BS, Benali-Furet N, et al. A new device for rapid isolation by size and characterization of rare circulating tumor cells. Anticancer Res. 2011;31:427–41.

Fabbri F, Carloni S, Zoli W, et al. Detection and recovery of circulating colon cancer cells using a dielectrophoresis-based device: KRAS mutation status in pure CTCs. Cancer Lett. 2013;335:225–31.

Farace F, Massard C, Vimond N, et al. A direct comparison of CellSearch and ISET for circulating tumour-cell detection in patients with metastatic carcinomas. Br J Cancer. 2011;105:847–53.

Fehm T, Becker S, Duerr-Stoerzer S, et al. Determination of HER2 status using both serum HER2 levels and circulating tumor cells in patients with recurrent breast cancer whose primary tumor was HER2 negative or of unknown HER2 status. Breast Cancer Res. 2007;9:R74.

Fehm T, Muller V, Aktas B, et al. HER2 status of circulating tumor cells in patients with metastatic breast cancer: a prospective, multicenter trial. Breast Cancer Res Treat. 2010;124:403–12.

Freeman JB, Gray ES, Millward M, et al. Evaluation of a multi-marker immunomagnetic enrichment assay for the quantification of circulating melanoma cells. J Transl Med. 2012;10:192.

Fuchs AB, Romani A, Freida D, et al. Electronic sorting and recovery of single live cells from microlitre sized samples. Lab Chip. 2006;6:121–6.

Fusi A, Liu Z, Kummerlen V, et al. Expression of chemokine receptors on circulating tumor cells in patients with solid tumors. J Transl Med. 2012;10:52.

Gazzaniga P, Gradilone A, Petracca A, et al. Molecular markers in circulating tumour cells from metastatic colorectal cancer patients. J Cell Mol Med. 2010;14:2073–7.

Gradilone A, Iacovelli R, Cortesi E, et al. Circulating tumor cells and "suspicious objects" evaluated through CellSearch(R) in metastatic renal cell carcinoma. Anticancer Res. 2011a;31:4219–21.

Gradilone A, Naso G, Raimondi C, et al. Circulating tumor cells (CTCs) in metastatic breast cancer (MBC): prognosis, drug resistance and phenotypic characterization. Ann Oncol. 2011b;22:86–92.

Hayashi N, Nakamura S, Tokuda Y, et al. Prognostic value of HER2-positive circulating tumor cells in patients with metastatic breast cancer. Int J Clin Oncol. 2012;17:96–104.

Hayes DF, Cristofanilli M, Budd GT, et al. Circulating tumor cells at each follow-up time point during therapy of metastatic breast cancer patients predict progression-free and overall survival. Clin Cancer Res. 2006;12:4218–24.

Heitzer E, Auer M, Gasch C, et al. Complex tumor genomes inferred from single circulating tumor cells by array-CGH and next-generation sequencing. Cancer Res. 2013;73:2965–75.

Helo P, Cronin AM, Danila DC, et al. Circulating prostate tumor cells detected by reverse transcription-PCR in men with localized or castration-refractory prostate cancer: concordance with CellSearch assay and association with bone metastases and with survival. Clin Chem. 2009;55:765–73.

Hou JM, Greystoke A, Lancashire L, et al. Evaluation of circulating tumor cells and serological cell death biomarkers in small cell lung cancer patients undergoing chemotherapy. Am J Pathol. 2009;175:808–16.

Ignatiadis M, Kallergi G, Ntoulia M, et al. Prognostic value of the molecular detection of circulating tumor cells using a multimarker reverse transcription-PCR assay for cytokeratin 19, mammaglobin A, and HER2 in early breast cancer. Clin Cancer Res. 2008;14:2593–600.

Ilie M, Long E, Butori C, et al. ALK-gene rearrangement: a comparative analysis on circulating tumour cells and tumour tissue from patients with lung adenocarcinoma. Ann Oncol. 2012;23:2907–13.

Ishizawa K, Rasheed ZA, Karisch R, et al. Tumor-initiating cells are rare in many human tumors. Cell Stem Cell. 2010;7:279–82.

Kalluri R, Weinberg RA. The basics of epithelial-mesenchymal transition. J Clin Invest. 2009;119:1420–8.

Kitago M, Koyanagi K, Nakamura T, et al. mRNA expression and BRAF mutation in circulating melanoma cells isolated from peripheral blood with high molecular weight melanoma-associated antigen-specific monoclonal antibody beads. Clin Chem. 2009;55:757–64.

Krebs MG, Sloane R, Priest L, et al. Evaluation and prognostic significance of circulating tumor cells in patients with non-small-cell lung cancer. J Clin Oncol. 2011;29:1556–63.

Kupas V, Weishaupt C, Siepmann D, et al. RANK is expressed in metastatic melanoma and highly upregulated on melanoma-initiating cells. J Invest Dermatol. 2011;131:944–55.

Lankiewicz S, Zimmermann S, Hollmann C, et al. Circulating tumour cells as a predictive factor for response to systemic chemotherapy in patients with advanced colorectal cancer. Mol Oncol. 2008;2:349–55.

Leversha MA, Han J, Asgari Z, et al. Fluorescence in situ hybridization analysis of circulating tumor cells in metastatic prostate cancer. Clin Cancer Res. 2009;15:2091–7.

Liu Z, Fusi A, Klopocki E, et al. Negative enrichment by immunomagnetic nanobeads for unbiased characterization of circulating tumor cells from peripheral blood of cancer patients. J Transl Med. 2011;9:70.

Lucci A, Hall CS, Lodhi AK, et al. Circulating tumour cells in non-metastatic breast cancer: a prospective study. Lancet Oncol. 2012;13:688–95.

Maheswaran S, Sequist LV, Nagrath S, et al. Detection of mutations in EGFR in circulating lung-cancer cells. N Engl J Med. 2008;359:366–77.

Marrinucci D, Bethel K, Bruce RH, et al. Case study of the morphologic variation of circulating tumor cells. Hum Pathol. 2007;38:514–9.

Marrinucci D, Bethel K, Kolatkar A, et al. Fluid biopsy in patients with metastatic prostate, pancreatic and breast cancers. Phys Biol. 2012;9:016003.

Miller MC, Doyle GV, Terstappen LW. Significance of circulating tumor cells detected by the CellSearch system in patients with metastatic breast colorectal and prostate cancer. J Oncol. 2010;2010:617421.

Munzone E, Nole F, Goldhirsch A, et al. Changes of HER2 status in circulating tumor cells compared with the primary tumor during treatment for advanced breast cancer. Clin Breast Cancer. 2010;10:392–7.

Nagrath S, Sequist LV, Maheswaran S, et al. Isolation of rare circulating tumour cells in cancer patients by microchip technology. Nature. 2007;450:1235–9.

Ou SH, Bartlett CH, Mino-Kenudson M, et al. Crizotinib for the treatment of ALK-rearranged non-small cell lung cancer: a success story to usher in the second decade of molecular targeted therapy in oncology. Oncologist. 2012;17:1351–1375.

Ozkumur E, Shah AM, Ciciliano JC, et al. Inertial focusing for tumor antigen-dependent and -independent sorting of rare circulating tumor cells. Sci Transl Med. 2013;5:179ra147.

Pantel K, Cote RJ, Fodstad O. Detection and clinical importance of micrometastatic disease. J Natl Cancer Inst. 1999;91:1113–24.

Paterlini-Brechot P, Benali NL. Circulating tumor cells (CTC) detection: clinical impact and future directions. Cancer Lett. 2007;253:180–204.

Pecot CV, Bischoff FZ, Mayer JA, et al. A novel platform for detection of CK+ and CK- CTCs. Cancer Discov. 2011;1:580–6.

Peeters DJ, De Laere B, Van den Eynden GG, et al. Semiautomated isolation and molecular characterisation of single or highly purified tumour cells from CellSearch enriched blood samples using dielectrophoretic cell sorting. Br J Cancer. 2013;108:1358–67.

Powell AA, Talasaz AH, Zhang H, et al. Single cell profiling of circulating tumor cells: transcriptional heterogeneity and diversity from breast cancer cell lines. PLoS One. 2012;7: e33788.

Rao C, Bui T, Connelly M, et al. Circulating melanoma cells and survival in metastatic melanoma. Int J Oncol. 2011;38:755–60.

Reid AL, Millward M, Pearce R, et al. Markers of circulating tumour cells in the peripheral blood of patients with melanoma correlate with disease recurrence and progression. Br J Dermatol. 2013;168:85–92.

Reynolds SR, Albrecht J, Shapiro RL, et al. Changes in the presence of multiple markers of circulating melanoma cells correlate with clinical outcome in patients with melanoma. Clin Cancer Res. 2003;9:1497–502.

Rosenberg R, Gertler R, Friederichs J, et al. Comparison of two density gradient centrifugation systems for the enrichment of disseminated tumor cells in blood. Cytometry. 2002;49:150–8.

Sakaizawa K, Goto Y, Kiniwa Y, et al. Mutation analysis of BRAF and KIT in circulating melanoma cells at the single cell level. Br J Cancer. 2012;106:939–46.

Sensi M, Nicolini G, Petti C, et al. Mutually exclusive NRASQ61R and BRAFV600E mutations at the single-cell level in the same human melanoma. Oncogene. 2006;25:3357–64.

Shaffer DR, Leversha MA, Danila DC, et al. Circulating tumor cell analysis in patients with progressive castration-resistant prostate cancer. Clin Cancer Res. 2007;13:2023–9.

Silva JM, Rodriguez R, Garcia JM, et al. Detection of epithelial tumour RNA in the plasma of colon cancer patients is associated with advanced stages and circulating tumour cells. Gut. 2002;50:530–4.

Stott SL, Hsu CH, Tsukrov DI, et al. Isolation of circulating tumor cells using a microvortex-generating herringbone-chip. Proc Natl Acad Sci U S A. 2010a;107:18392–7.

Stott SL, Lee RJ, Nagrath S, et al. Isolation and characterization of circulating tumor cells from patients with localized and metastatic prostate cancer. Sci Transl Med. 2010b;2:25ra23.

Talasaz AH, Powell AA, Huber DE, et al. Isolating highly enriched populations of circulating epithelial cells and other rare cells from blood using a magnetic sweeper device. Proc Natl Acad Sci U S A. 2009;106:3970–5.

Vona G, Sabile A, Louha M, et al. Isolation by size of epithelial tumor cells: a new method for the immunomorphological and molecular characterization of circulating tumor cells. Am J Pathol. 2000;156:57–63.

Wang N, Shi L, Li H, et al. Detection of circulating tumor cells and tumor stem cells in patients with breast cancer by using flow cytometry: a valuable tool for diagnosis and prognosis evaluation. Tumour Biol. 2012;33:561–9.

Xi L, Nicastri DG, El-Hefnawy T, et al. Optimal markers for real-time quantitative reverse transcription PCR detection of circulating tumor cells from melanoma, breast, colon, esophageal, head and neck, and lung cancers. Clin Chem. 2007;53:1206–15.

Yancovitz M, Litterman A, Yoon J, et al. Intra- and inter-tumor heterogeneity of BRAF(V600E) mutations in primary and metastatic melanoma. PLoS One. 2012;7:e29336.

Yang G, Li Y, Nishimura EK, et al. Inhibition of PAX3 by TGF-beta modulates melanocyte viability. Mol Cell. 2008;32:554–63.

Yang L, Lang JC, Balasubramanian P, et al. Optimization of an enrichment process for circulating tumor cells from the blood of head and neck cancer patients through depletion of normal cells. Biotechnol Bioeng. 2009;102:521–34.

Yang MJ, Chiu HH, Wang HM, et al. Enhancing detection of circulating tumor cells with activating KRAS oncogene in patients with colorectal cancer by weighted chemiluminescent membrane array method. Ann Surg Oncol. 2010;17:624–33.

Yu M, Stott S, Toner M, et al. Circulating tumor cells: approaches to isolation and characterization. J Cell Biol. 2011;192:373–82.

Yu M, Bardia A, Wittner BS, et al. Circulating breast tumor cells exhibit dynamic changes in epithelial and mesenchymal composition. Science. 2013;339:580–4.

Oncoproteomic Approaches to Cancer Marker Discovery: The Case of Colorectal Cancer

3

Francesco Salvatore, Claudia Corbo, Marica Gemei, and Luigi Del Vecchio

Contents

F. Salvatore (✉)
CEINGE-Biotecnologie avanzate, s.c.a r.l, Naples, Italy

Dipartimento di Medicina Molecolare e Biotecnologie Mediche, Università di Napoli "Federico II", Naples, Italy

IRCCS-SDN, Naples, Italy
e-mail: salvator@unina.it

C. Corbo • M. Gemei
CEINGE-Biotecnologie avanzate, s.c.a r.l, Naples, Italy
e-mail: corbo@ceinge.unina.it; gemei@ceinge.unina.it

L. Del Vecchio
CEINGE-Biotecnologie avanzate, s.c.a r.l, Naples, Italy

Dipartimento di Medicina Molecolare e Biotecnologie Mediche, Università di Napoli "Federico II", Naples, Italy
e-mail: luigi.delvecchio@unina.it

V.R. Preedy, V.B. Patel (eds.), *Biomarkers in Cancer, Biomarkers in Disease: Methods, Discoveries and Applications*,
DOI 10.1007/978-94-007-7681-4_16

Abstract

Colorectal cancer (CRC) is one of the most common types of cancer; it is diagnosed in more than one million people each year and causes the death of about half of them. Early detection can help to decrease CRC-related mortality. In fact, the 5-year survival rate exceeds 90 % when the disease is localized and is only 10 % in case of metastases. Consequently, it is imperative to improve methods for the early detection of the disease. In this context, genomic approaches have resulted in new CRC biomarkers and have helped to shed light on the genetic basis of cancer as a whole. However, the proteome provides a more dynamic and faithful image of the genetic program of a cell. Hence, given the importance of proteins as effectors of cellular behavior, proteomic analysis has the potential to identify biomarkers that can help to classify and predict CRC. Several proteomic technique, such as matrix-assisted laser desorption ionization-time of flight mass spectrometry (MALDI-TOF MS), quantitative isotopic protein labeling (SILAC, ICAT, and iTRAQ), and two-dimensional gel electrophoresis (2D-PAGE and 2D-DIGE), are being used in cancer research and can improve the diagnosis of patients; they are also helping to optimize personalized therapy.

In this chapter, the main proteomic approaches used in biomarker research will be discussed, together with their impact and potential in the clinical setting. The proteomic biomarkers currently used for CRC diagnosis and/or therapy monitoring will be also described.

List of Abbreviations

2D-DIGE	Two-Dimensional Differential In-gel Electrophoresis
2D-PAGE	Two-Dimensional Polyacrylamide Gel Electrophoresis
APC	Adenomatous Polyposis Coli
CEA	Carcinoembryonic Antigen
CRC	Colorectal Cancer
Cy2	Cyanine 2 Fluorescent Dye
Cy3	Cyanine 3 Fluorescent Dye
Cy5	Cyanine 5 Fluorescent Dye
DCBE	Double-Contrast Barium Enema
ESI	Electrospray Ionization
FIT	Fecal Immunological Test
FOBT	Fecal Occult Blood Test
ICAT	Isotope-Coded Affinity Tag
IMAC	Immobilized Metal Affinity Chromatography
iTRAQ	Isobaric Tags for Relative and Absolute Quantitation
LC-MS	Liquid Chromatography Mass Spectrometry

MALDI	Matrix-Assisted Laser Desorption Ionization
MOAC	Metal Oxide Affinity Chromatography
MS	Mass Spectrometry
MW	Molecular Weight
pI	Isoelectric Point
PTM	Post-translational Modification
SCX	Strong Cation Exchange Chromatography
SILAC	Stable Isotope Labeling with Amino Acids in Cell Culture
TOF	Time of Flight

Key Facts

- Approximately one million people each year are diagnosed with colorectal cancer.
- About 50 % of diagnosed people die each year.
- To improve therapy efficacy, it is important to screen for early detection biomarkers.
- Due to the poor specificity of the biomarkers currently used, efforts are being made to discover new more efficient colorectal cancer biomarkers.
- Proteomic approaches have had great impact in this field and have great potential.

Definition of Words and Terms

Adenocarcinoma A carcinoma originated from the glandular tissue or a carcinoma in which the cells form glandular structures.

Biomarker It is an indicator of a biological state; it should be objectively measured and it is used to indicate a normal or a pathological biological process or a response to pharmacologic therapy.

Biopsy It is the removal of tissue from the living body; it is usually evaluated by microscopic analysis. It is performed when a precise diagnosis is required.

Cell Line A population of cells from a multicellular organism that keeps undergoing division. The cells can therefore be grown for prolonged periods *in vitro* and are thus widely used in biotechnology.

Colorectal Cancer A cancer from uncontrolled cell growth in the colon or rectum.

Early Detection In medicine, "early detection" means discovering a disorder or disease during the early stage of its progression.

Glycosylation This post-translational modification consists in the attachment of sugar moieties to proteins; several kinds of glycosidic linkages exist: *N*-, *O*-, and *C*-linked glycosylation, the glycosylphosphatidylinositol anchor attachment to the plasma membrane called glypiation, and phosphoglycosylation. This post-translational modification is involved in several cellular processes, including cell-to-cell adhesion and protein-ligand interactions in the cell. A branch of proteomics called "glycoproteomics" is devoted to the characterization of glycoproteins, and it is focused on different types of strategies of enrichment of this class of proteins.

Mass Spectrometry An analytical method that detects ions and measures their mass-to-charge (m/z) ratio. Each mass spectrometer is constituted by three elements: a source, an analyzer, and a detector. The first step in an MS analysis is to generate charged molecules or molecule fragments; hence, the sample (solid, liquid, or gas) is charged by an ion source. Then the generated ions are separated by an analyzer according to their typical m/z ratio. Finally, the ion signals are processed by a detector into the spectra of the relative abundance of ions as a function of the m/z. The atoms or molecules being analyzed are identified using molecular masses (obtained from the m/z ratio) or through a characteristic fragmentation pattern.

Phosphorylation A post-translational modification of proteins in which a serine, a threonine, or a tyrosine is modified by a kinase that adds a covalently bound phosphate group. Phosphorylation of a protein acts as a molecular switch that turns the protein activity on or off.

Proteome The term "proteome," coined in 1994 by Marc Wilkins, arose as a combination of the words *prote*in and gen*ome*. The proteome is the entire set of proteins expressed in an organism or tissue or cell or biological system. Proteomics is the study on a large scale of all the proteins with particular focus on their structures and functions.

Introduction

Colorectal Cancer

Cancer is a devastating public health problem worldwide, irrespective of a country's level of development. Approximately one million people per year worldwide get colorectal cancer (CRC), which accounts for 30 % of all tumors. Despite recent improvements in the treatment of CRC, nearly 50 % of treated cases relapse and are expected to die within 5 years of diagnosis (Newton et al. 2012).

Genetic mechanisms have an important impact on CRC. In fact, more than 25 % of diagnosed patients have a family history of the disease (Gala and Chung 2011). According to the genetic model of tumorigenesis, a tumor is the result of the accumulation of mutations in genes, i.e., tumor suppressor genes and oncogenes (Fearon and Vogelstein 1990).

A number of genes play a role in colorectal carcinogenesis: adenomatous polyposis coli (APC), rat sarcoma oncogene K-ras, tumor suppressor TP53, the DNA glycosylase gene MUTYH, and the murine sarcoma oncogene BRAF (Ettarh 2012). However, the most frequently mutated gene in CRC patients is APC which results in the constitutive activation of the Wnt-signaling pathway, which is a critical event in the development of CRC (Corbo et al. 2012).

The development of CRC is a long process; it originates from the epithelial cells lining the interior of the large intestine. In fact, due to accumulation of mutations and the consequent change in gene function, these cells lose their normal biological behavior and acquire the characteristics of tumor cells. There are three ways to interfere in the progression of CRC depending on the stage of disease. The first concerns early-stage cancer or adenoma. Early detection of CRC is the most effective way to reduce cancer mortality. The fecal occult blood test (FOBT), colonoscopy, sigmoidoscopy, and the immunological FOBT (FIT) can identify CRC in time to manage the disease successfully. Secondly, in the case of stage II and III CRC, the first issue is to establish if patients need to be treated with adjuvant chemotherapy after surgical resection. The second issue is to choose the most appropriate regimen for each patient according to the specific biologic characteristics of their disease. Thirdly, in the case of stage IV/metastatic CRC, curative options are no longer available, and patients are treated with systemic therapy, which is a mix of the conventional chemotherapeutic approach and the more innovative approach based on the use of biological drugs. In these cases, even more than in stage II/III CRC, it is vital to select the combination of drugs that best meets the needs of patients, rather than applying the same strategy regardless of the specificity of patient's conditions.

The last 5 years have seen surge in research to identify biomarkers that can improve the current diagnostic and prognostic scenario for CRC screening and management. Proteomics is a promising area of research in CRC biomarker identification.

Biomarkers in Cancer

A biomarker, also called a "signature molecule," is defined as a biological molecule objectively measurable in body fluids (e.g., blood, urine) or tissues that may be used as an indicator of a normal/abnormal biological process or of a pathological condition. A biomarker can be employed in the detection of a disease and in the prediction of prognosis or to forecast the pharmacologic responses to a therapeutic intervention. Usually, a given biomarker has to ameliorate life expectancy or the quality of life in order to be considered in clinical practice (Newton et al. 2012). There are three main types of biomarkers depending on the purpose for which they are employed (Table 1). **Diagnostic biomarkers** are used to determine the disease from which the patient is suffering. These kinds of biomarkers can support the conventional imaging techniques. They are probably the most important biomarkers and are also useful to reveal recurring diseases. **Prognostic biomarkers** serve to predict the probable course of a disease; they can reflect the ability to metastasize, tumor aggressiveness, or the probable growth rate. These biomarkers

Table 1 **Biomarker classification**. Summary of the differences in the use of biomarkers based on clinical needs

Type of biomarkers	Use	Clinical applications
Diagnostic	To help diagnose a cancer and to reveal the possibility of relapse	Screening
Prognostic	To forecast the aggressiveness of the disease process and/or how a patient can expect to fare in the absence of therapy	Predict recurrence
Predictive	Used to identify which patients will respond to a specific pharmacological treatment. It also means to show predisposition (increase of risk) to have the disease (genetic marker)	Personalized therapy

can be used to evaluate the disease outcome and to inform treatment and care decisions. **Predictive biomarkers** can help to predict a subpopulation of patients that may benefit from a specific therapy. A predictive biomarker can forecast the possible effects of treatment and can also be used as a treatment target. It can also indicate "predisposition", namely an increased risk of acquiring a given disease (Biomarkers in cancer: an introductory guide for advocates. Research advocacy network 2010).

Any measurable molecular alteration at DNA, RNA, protein, or metabolite level in a cancer cell is a putative cancer biomarker. This chapter deals with protein biomarkers and the approach currently used to discover protein biomarkers. Biomarker discovery starts with an investigation of putative biomarkers, which can be performed either in a hypothesis-driven or in a hypothesis-free manner. In the former case, researchers follow updates in the knowledge of the specific pathology condition, while in the latter case, i.e., the "fishing exercise," researchers investigate differentially expressed markers in patients versus healthy individuals without any starting hypothesis (Newton et al. 2012). In recent years, biomarker discovery has become a major focus of cancer research, as shown by the number of scientific publications on the topic over the past decade. Between the years 2003 to 2012, the number of articles published in peer-reviewed journals indexed on PubMed – the main biomedical publication database in the United States – has increased year by year. In 2012 alone, more than 42,000 articles related to biomarkers were published in the scientific and medical literature (Fig. 1), a number twice that of 2002. Another indicator of the topicality of biomarkers is the increase in the number of biomedical journals devoted entirely to the topic like *Journal of Biomarkers*, *Biomarkers*, *The Open Biomarkers Journal*, *Biomarkers in Medicine-Future Medicine*, *Journal of Biomarkers in Cancer*, and *Journal of Molecular Biomarkers & Diagnosis*, to name just a few.

Why Proteomics?

Cancer results from the accumulation of genetic changes that lead to an alteration of several cellular processes including angiogenesis, proliferation, apoptosis, and senescence. As a consequence, markers were initially searched for using genomics

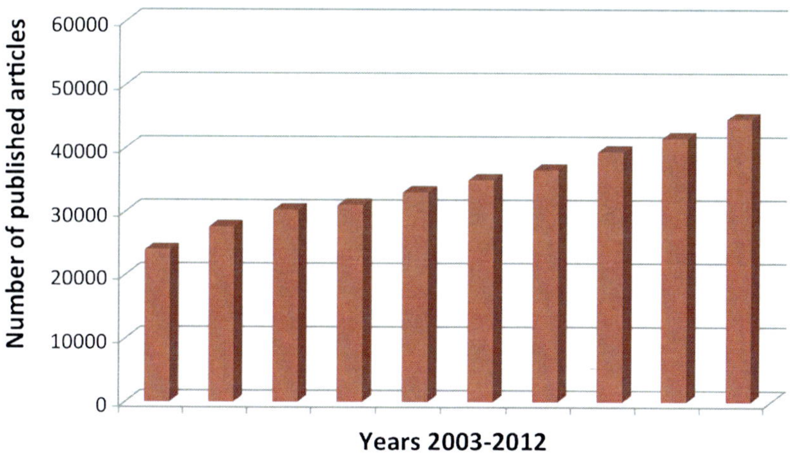

Fig. 1 Number of scientific or medical articles related to biomarkers. A graphical representation of the published scientific or medical articles related to biomarkers (Source: PubMed database, keyword "biomarker" limited to the years stated)

and transcriptomic approaches, which increased our understanding of the molecular basis of cancer. However, progressive knowledge revealed the need to obtain a more complete landscape of the cell. In fact, it soon became clear that genetic analysis alone does not tell the whole story.

Through alternative splicing of mRNA in combination with numerous post-translational modifications (e.g., phosphorylation, acetylation, and glycosylation), one gene codes for different kinds of proteins with different sequences and, as a consequence, different activities. The proteome harbors more information than the genome; it is more dynamic and hence it is a more accurate mirror of the genetic information of a cell. Therefore, proteomics can fill in the gap between the genome and cell behavior.

Since proteins are the main effectors of cell behavior, interrogation of the functional proteome has great potential in such medical settings as neurodegenerative diseases, infectious diseases, and cardiovascular diseases (Engwegen 2006). The potential of proteomics in oncology is not surprising: cancer originates in mutated genes and causes aberrant protein expression. Oncoproteomics allows one to investigate the identity and function of thousands of proteins that derive from cancer cells and that are consequently involved in the mechanisms underlying cancer (Cho and Chen 2007). This in turn opens the possibility of using some of these proteins as therapeutic targets and markers for the early detection, therapy, and prognostic evaluation of patients. Furthermore, protein markers can be readily measured on routinely available body fluids such as serum rather than on fresh or frozen tissue biopsies. Thus, oncoproteomic approaches are widely applicable in the clinical setting and could have an important impact on cancer diagnosis and treatment monitoring (Chan and Lee 2013; van der Merwe 2007).

Proteomic Technologies

The term "proteomics" refers to the set of analytical tools used to depict the protein compartment of a cell. It is the natural continuation of genomics, and it moves away from classical protein chemistry while drawing on the heritage of knowledge and methods developed in the latter field. The great innovation of proteomics is, in fact, the concept that one must study the entire proteome as a single analyte in order to study cellular molecular mechanisms in which proteins play a key role (Anderson and Anderson 1998). This means that the proteins being analyzed are no longer purified and isolated from their highly complex context in living systems. Indeed, they are analyzed together within their context so providing a true picture of the proteome in a given cell state. However, proteome analysis is hindered by several analytical problems. First is the wide range of protein concentrations present in samples. For example, in human serum, the most abundant proteins represent almost 100 % of the total protein mass but are only less than 0.1 % in number (Guerrier et al. 2006). Another important challenge is the detection of post-translational modifications (PTMs). In fact, only a minor part of the proteins of interest are post-translationally modified. The high sample complexity in terms of number of analytes is another feature that must be taken in account in proteomic analysis. Consequently, proteomic analysis needs a pool of methodologies and technologies that are high throughput, sensitive, and selective toward the proteins that are the target of the analysis and that have a large dynamic range effectiveness. Many chromatographic and electrophoresis tools are available to fractionate analytes. However, although the separation techniques differ, the various strategies have a common final step: mass spectrometry (MS) analysis, which gives a name to each protein. Several of the most widely used technologies in colorectal cancer research are detailed below.

Two-Dimensional Gel Electrophoresis

Mammalian cells contain thousands of different proteins and only a small number of them change under circumstances such as in response to stress or in pathological conditions. The primary goal of expression proteomics is to reveal differences in protein expression profiles between samples in two different conditions. Proteome analysis is based on two essential components: protein separation and protein identification. Historically, the tool of choice for maximal separation of proteins was two-dimensional electrophoresis (2D-PAGE) that separates proteins according to their isoelectric point (pI) and molecular weight (MW).

Based on their specific amino acidic sequence, post-translational modifications (e.g., phosphorylation, glycosylation, and nitrosylation), and the pH of the environment, the net charge of proteins varies and can be positive, negative, or zero. The pI of a protein is the pH at which the number of positive charges is equal to the number of negative charges, so the protein has no net charge. When a mixture of proteins is loaded on a pH gradient, they will be separated on the basis of their specific pI. In a region with a pH greater than its pI, a given protein is charged negatively and moves toward the cathode (+). While in a region with a pH below its pI, a given protein is charged positively and migrates toward the anode (−). Moreover, the charge decreases during migration and becomes null when the proteins reach the pH equal to their pI, at which point proteins cease to migrate. In the original 2DE method devised by O'Farrell (1975), carrier ampholytes in tube gels are used to generate a pH gradient. However, this method had drawbacks in the resolving power and in the pH gradient stability. Commercial immobilized pH gradient strips, in which the carrier ampholytes are copolymerized into the gel matrix, improved the reproducibility and performance of isoelectrofocusing (IEF) in 2D-PAGE. The second dimension uses the traditional SDS-PAGE technique in which proteins are separated in a sort of molecular sieve constituted by polyacrylamide gel. Traditional 2D gel electrophoresis is a well-established technique, but it is labor intensive and time consuming; moreover, it does not satisfactorily separate low-abundant proteins, proteins with an extreme pI, or membrane proteins. In addition, various sources of variability in 2DE can distort the difference in protein expression, for instance, (a) analytical variations due to treatment of the sample, to procedures for staining, or to image acquisition and (b) biological variations due to the environment in which the sample was produced, processed, and preserved. These variations can be minimized by working with multiple biological and analytical replicates, but this increases the difficulty of analysis.

The introduction of 2D differential in-gel electrophoresis (2D-DIGE) in 1997 overcame this limitation because it allows three samples to be compared in a single 2D-PAGE gel (Unlu et al. 1997). In fact, typically, during a 2D-DIGE experiment, the proteomes of three different samples, e.g., healthy, diseased, and internal control, are labeled with fluorescent dyes (Cy3, Cy5, and Cy2), each with a specific excitation and emission wavelength. Thus, the same experimental procedure is applied to different samples, and a protein labeled with the three different dyes will migrate to the same position on the 2D gel and on the overlay. This overcomes issues due to experimental variation and ensures accurate within-gel matching, reproducibility, and quantization. 2D-DIGE is widely used in the clinical setting especially in laboratories involved in disease biomarker discovery. The 2D-PAGE and 2D-DIGE experimental workflows are shown in Fig. 2.

Gel-Free Proteomics: Isotopic Labeling

As mentioned above, traditionally, quantitative analysis was carried out using a 2D-PAGE or 2D-DIGE approach whereby the comparison of the spot sizes reveals differences in the protein amount and MS identifies the protein (Neilson et al. 2011). Recently, quantitative proteomics has moved beyond the 2D gel electrophoresis approach. Now gel-free isotopic procedures are available that, through a chemical reaction, add isotope-enriched tags to proteins using isotope-coded affinity tags (ICATs), isobaric tags for relative and absolute quantitation

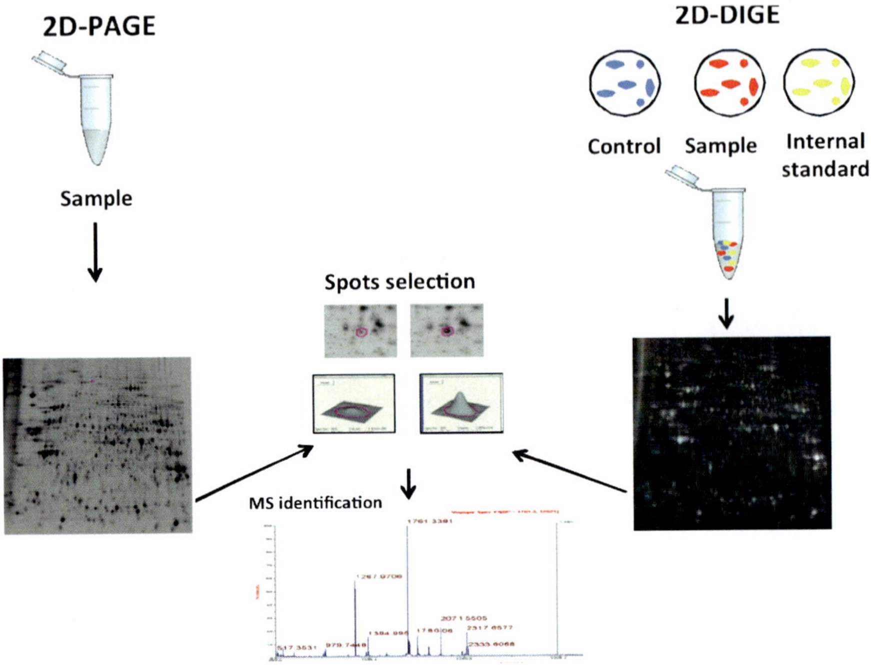

Fig. 2 **Basic workflow of gel-based proteomic approaches**. The 2D-PAGE separates proteins according to their pI and MW, giving rise to a gel representing a protein map. Two or more samples are compared by analyzing their specific protein map on two or more different gels (inter-gel comparison). The 2D-DIGE implies the labeling of three different protein samples with fluorescent dyes and then the mixed samples are submitted to 2D gel separation. This procedure reveals differences in spots and in expression between samples analyzed on the same gel (intra-gel comparison). In both techniques, protein spots of interest are then submitted to in situ digestion protocol and analyzed by MS

(iTRAQ), or stable isotope labeling with amino acids in cell culture (SILAC). These high-throughput techniques can provide results complementary to the traditional gel-based proteomic approaches.

The ICAT (Han et al. 2001) reagent is marketed in two different isotopic forms with a different distribution of the 12C/13C atoms thereby allowing the relative quantitative estimation between two samples in MS mode. It is generally used to compare a sample in two different conditions. Its reactivity is at the level of cysteine residues; therefore, the disadvantage of this approach is that proteins without cysteines cannot be detected.

The iTRAQ (Ross et al. 2004) strategy, by a combination of C, N, and O isotopes, enables peptide isobaric labeling, and peptide abundances are measured during MS/MS fragmentation thereby overcoming the need to interpret MS spectra. The iTRAQ kit is available as a set of four or eight isobaric labeling molecules so that eight samples can be multiplexed simultaneously. Its reactivity is at the level of the primary amino group so that all proteins will be tagged by iTRAQ.

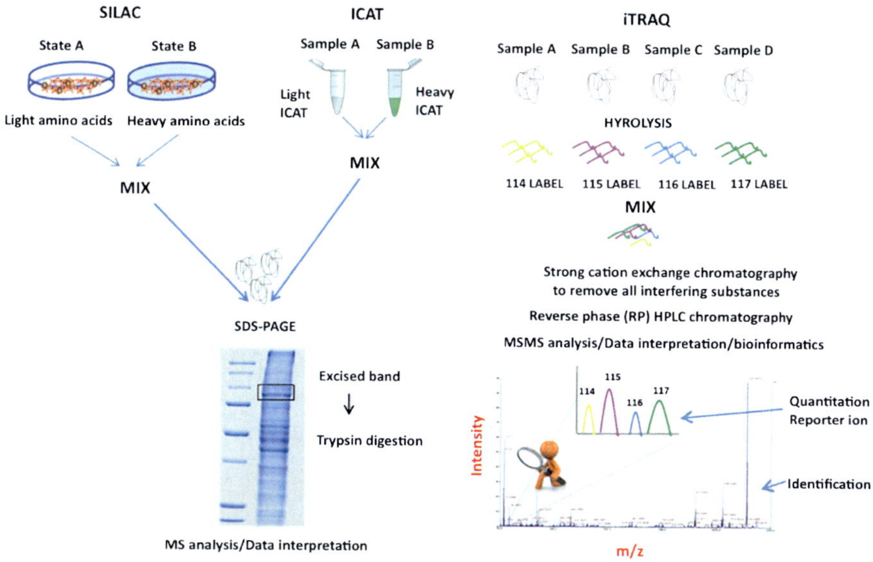

Fig. 3 Representative workflows for SILAC, ICAT, and iTRAQ. The main differences among labeling techniques are (i) SILAC and ICAT labeling are applied on intact proteins, while iTRAQ labeling is performed on peptides, and (ii) in the case of SILAC and ICAT, peptides are quantified during MS analysis, while in the case of iTRAQ, quantitation occurs during fragmentation, i.e., MS/MS analysis

The SILAC (Ong et al. 2002) strategy is based on cell growth in isotope-enriched amino acid medium, thus allowing the incorporation of the isotopic and non-isotopic form of amino acids in the proteins. In a typical experiment, heavy arginine or lysine (13C or 15 N) is added to the cell culture medium of the sample of interest, while the cell culture medium of the control sample consists of normal amino acids.

The above strategies are widely used in protein quantitation because of their accuracy; unfortunately, they entail the use of expensive molecules and of specific software to analyze data. Moreover, the number of samples that can be simultaneously analyzed is limited by the number of available labels, and not all strategies can be applied to all types of samples (Neilson et al. 2011). Representative workflows for the SILAC, ICAT, and iTRAQ technologies are shown in Fig. 3.

Label-Free Mass Spectrometry

Thanks to the development of novel instrumentation and progresses in bioinformatics, a promising label-free LC-MS approach is emerging. By definition, label-free LC-MS shotgun screening is done without isotope labeling. There are two categories of label-free-based measurements: peak area (or ion intensity) and spectral counting. These two methods are mostly used for relative quantification.

The peak area method measures analyte quantity based on the integrated peak area obtained from the extracted ion chromatogram. The principle is that the detected ion signal is positively proportional to the analyte concentration. The practical constraints of this type of label-free method are related to the LC-MS method, which must be highly reproducible. Any drifts in retention time and m/z will complicate the peak alignment process. Second, high-resolution MS instruments must be used because it is difficult to distinguish the overlapping peaks that are obtained with low-resolution instruments.

The spectral counting label-free method is a much simpler procedure. Spectral counts are the number of MS/MS spectra assigned to one protein. Thus, this method measures how many times the MS/MS events are performed for each peptide belonging to one protein. The principle is that in a given LC-MS/MS analysis, the total number of MS/MS spectra derived from the fragmentation of a peptide belonging to a protein is linearly correlated with the abundance of that protein in the sample. It is important to underline that it is not possible to detect all peptides using spectral counting because of competition among ions, dynamic range, and sensitivity limitations (Zhang et al. 2006). Thanks to attempts to improve these issues, label-free MS may become widely used for biomarker discovery and validation (Pastor et al. 2013).

Detection of Post-Translational Modifications

Post-translational modifications are chemical or enzymatic modifications of a protein after its synthesis. The analysis of protein PTMs is one of the reasons why proteomics is so challenging. Amino acids can be modified by hundreds of modifications that change their molecular weights and charge, which are the fundamental physical properties measured by MS. PTMs extend the range of functions of proteins by linking proteins to chemical functional groups that modify the chemical nature of amino acids or by making structural changes. PTMs are attracting attention because they play a critical role in cellular machinery and they vary in response to external stimuli and to diseases. They include phosphorylation, glycosylation, acetylation, proteolytic cleavage, oxidation, methylation, nitration, nitrosylation, and many other processes.

Phosphorylation and glycosylation are two PTMs that have a major impact on the cell, and their role in the progression of many types of cancer is growing day by day. Phosphorylation is the addition of a phosphate group to specific amino acid residues. Phosphorylation of proteins and peptides is one of the most frequent PTMs and is a biochemical process of biological relevance; in fact, kinases and phosphatases, the enzymes that promote protein phosphorylation and dephosphorylation, account for 2–4 % of eukaryotic proteomes (Moorhead et al. 2009). Phosphorylation cycles are very dynamic and rapid in order to satisfy the cell's need for highly dynamic regulation processes. Phosphorylation acts as a molecular switch, in a reversible manner, to turn the activity of a protein or of a cellular signaling pathway "on" or "off" and to regulate a protein's enzymatic activities, substrate specificities, folding and function, localization, formation of complexes, and degradation. Cellular processes such as cell cycling, differentiation, development, hormone response, and signal transduction are regulated by protein phosphorylation. It is estimated that almost one-third of eukaryotic proteins are phosphorylated (Sefton and Shenolikar 2001). Protein phosphorylation is a sub-stoichiometric modification; in fact, phosphoproteins represent about 1–2 % of the total proteins in a cell. Consequently, the detection of phosphorylation, in terms of definition of sites and abundance, is a challenging task for proteomics.

Various enrichment strategies have been devised for the immunoaffinity or immunoprecipitation identification of phosphorylated proteins. The most frequently used enrichment strategies are affinity based, namely, immobilized metal affinity chromatography, metal oxide affinity chromatography, and strong cation exchange chromatography (Pastor et al. 2013; Schmidt et al. 2007; Engholm-Keller and Larsen 2013). Separation methods include electrophoresis, 2D-PAGE or 2D-DIGE, associated to staining specific for phosphoprotein (Pro-Q Diamond) or isotope labeling (ICAT or SILAC). The methods used to analyze and identify phosphoproteins are based on MS (e.g., MALDI-TOF MS, LC-ESI-MS, and LC-ESI-MS/MS). In fact, because a phosphate group increases the protein mass by 80 Da, MS enables one to determine the average number of phosphorylation sites just by comparing the increment of the protein mass versus control. Given the key role of kinases and phosphatases as regulators of signaling cascades, the analysis of the phosphoproteome of colon cancer may help to unveil the link between the phosphorylation status of cells and the mechanisms of cancer.

Alteration of the glycosylation state is a characteristic of cancer cells, and several kinds of glycans have been shown to be markers of tumor progression (Varki et al. 1999). The glycosylation profile of cells continuously changes during embryonic development and cellular activation in vertebrates. Thus, the role of glycans as markers of malignant transformation and tumor progression is not surprising. Their marker potential was first recognized consequent to the observation that plant lectins bind to animal tumor cells. Subsequently, *in vitro* experiments showed that the transformation of cells was associated to an increased size of metabolically labeled glycopeptides (Hakomori et al. 1986). Moreover, after the advent of monoclonal antibody technology, researchers searching for the "right" molecule against cancer cells revealed that many of the antibodies directed against cancer recognize sugars (Feizi 1985). Hence, the characterization of the glycosidic portion of the glycoproteins, the so-called "glycoproteome analysis," may help to improve the diagnosis, prognosis, and immunotherapy of tumors (Lowe 2001).

Typically, the workflow for a glycoproteomic experiment starts with the chemical or enzymatic digestion of the protein sample in a mixture of peptides and glycopeptides. Then, enrichment procedures (lectin affinity chromatography) are applied to select glycosylated peptides. Mapping experiments are generally carried out by online nano-LC–ES-MS/MS or by MALDI-TOF/TOF. Glycoprotein enrichment can be done before digestion; in this case, it is followed by 2D-PAGE and 2D-DIGE coupled with staining specific for glycoproteins (e.g., Pro-Q Emerald) and MS for identification.

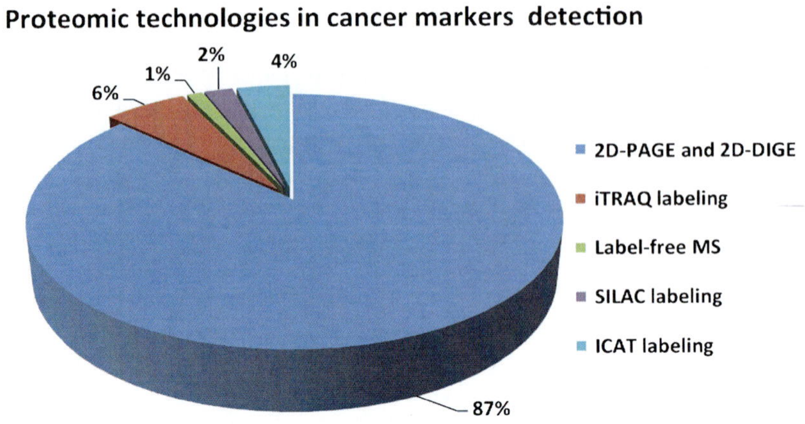

Fig. 4 **Proteomic technologies used in the detection of cancer markers**. Percent of the proteomic approaches used based on the number of published scientific or medical articles related to the application of the specific technology in biomarker discovery (Source: PubMed database, keyword "biomarker and cancer and the selected proteomic approach"). 2D gel-based methods are clearly the procedure of choice in biomarker research

Figure 4 shows the described proteomic technologies used in biomarker cancer research. Despite the progress made in label-based and free-label methods, 2D-gel-based approaches remain the methods of choice in biomarker research.

Early Detection Screening Technologies and Samples for CRC Biomarker Research

Prevention of CRC mortality is closely related to early detection. Greater use of screening methods, i.e., fecal occult blood test, sigmoidoscopy, colonoscopy, and barium enema (see Table 2) may decrease the number of deaths from CRC. However, people tend to avoid these tests because of the discomfort involved. Consequently, blood- and stool-based *in vitro* molecular tests and novel targets for noninvasive molecular screening are required.

As mentioned above, proteins are good biomarkers in a diagnostic scenario because they can be revealed by antibody-based methods. The CRC cell lines are widely used in research laboratories as a model of cancer tissues since they can be easily reproduced when necessary in huge amounts. Various human CRC cell lines are available for research purposes, each with specific molecular properties. They are easy to handle in an experimental procedure; moreover, they are particularly suitable when the goal is to isolate by biochemical fractionation different proteome subpopulations, e.g., nuclear matrix, secretome, plasma membrane, exosomes, etc. Biochemical fractionation is one of the strategies used to reduce sample complexity, thereby enabling the investigator to probe deeper into the cell proteome and to identify low-abundant proteins. Despite these advantages, all the available CRC

Table 2 Current early detection screening technologies for colorectal cancer. A brief description of the principles of widely used early detection screening methods

Early detection tests for colorectal cancer
One or more of these tests are indicated for CRC screening, particularly, in people older than 50 with a CRC case in the family history
A fecal occult blood test (FOBT) detects hidden blood in the stool, which is one of the first CRC alarm bells. This test should be performed every 1–2 years in people between 50 and 80 years old; it decreases the number of CRC deaths by 30 %
A sigmoidoscopy is an inspection of the rectum and of the sigmoid colon (final portion of the bowel) using an instrument called a "sigmoidoscope" which is a small tube with a small light attached. Sigmoidoscopy can reveal precancerous or cancerous growths
A colonoscopy is an inspection of the rectum and entire colon using an instrument called "colonoscope." Colonoscopy can reveal precancerous or cancerous conditions in the whole colon, unlike sigmoidoscopy. Moreover, during colonoscopy, it is possible to remove suspicious growths, and thus, it is a screening and a therapeutic method
In double-contrast barium enema, the colon and rectum undergo a series of x-rays. The first step in this test is the introduction of a barium solution into the colon, and then air is also added to delineate the colon and rectum on the x-ray. This procedure may not detect small polyps

cell lines derive from malignant tumors, i.e., adenocarcinomas, so they are not suitable for studies of premalignant adenomas. Furthermore, comparative studies conducted with CRC cell lines are complicated by the absence of normal epithelial cells, i.e., controls (Jimenez et al. 2010).

Biomarkers for blood-based CRC detection can be identified by comparing the proteins in the serum of cancer patients with those of healthy control serum. Thus, biomarkers can be detected directly in a biological fluid (serum or plasma) that would be employed for cancer screening. However, the discovery of new biomarkers is hindered by the complexity of these samples (Jimenez et al. 2010). In fact, current high-resolution MS methods are able to detect proteins at concentrations up to four orders of magnitude, and the dynamic concentration range of blood proteins is 11 orders of magnitude, so typically they identify only the most abundant proteins in a biological sample. For an in-depth analysis of the proteome and to detect low-abundant proteins, cell components must be fractionated. Tumor-associated proteins are highly diluted in the bloodstream, and therefore, the concentration of most potential protein biomarkers in the blood is below detection limits.

Protein Biomarkers of Colon Cancer

Carcinoembryonic antigen (CEA) and fecal hemoglobin are the only approved, soluble protein biomarkers of CRC.

Carcinoembryonic Antigen

Carcinoembryonic antigen is an immunoglobulin involved in cell adhesion, whose carboxy-terminal region is anchored to the cell membrane by covalent attachment to the glycosylphosphatidylinositol moiety, and this protein, which has been identified in serum, has long been used as a biomarker of CRC and of other types of cancers. The progression of CRC is associated to high CEA expression and usually decreases after surgery. However, CEA expression is also high in serum of heavy smokers, in conditions of inflammation, in colitis, in liver cirrhosis, and in pancreatitis (Tanaka et al. 2010). Consequently, it is not considered sensitive and reliable for the early detection of CRC. However, it is reliable in predicting prognosis and is useful in monitoring the disease course, the response to treatment, and the recurrence posttreatment. In CRC patients, the higher the CEA level, the poorer the prognosis. In fact, the higher the CEA level at the time of CRC diagnosis, the greater the possibility that the cancer is in an advanced stage (Tanaka et al. 2010). As mentioned above, the CEA level is expected to decrease after surgery; in fact, this antigen is the standard marker with which to monitor CRC patients during and after treatment to evaluate if the cancer is responding to treatment or if it has recurred after treatment (Newton et al. 2012). In conclusion, CEA should be interpreted with caution but can be useful on a case-by-case basis.

Fecal Hemoglobin

The detection of CRC based on stool analysis is a completely noninvasive screening method and is easy to perform and inexpensive. The most widely used CRC screening test is the FOBT (see Table 2) that detects hemoglobin enzymatically or immunologically. Enzymatic FOBT is an assay that measures the peroxidase-like activity of hemoglobin. This method does not distinguish the origin of the hemoglobin; hence, this assay identifies hemorrhage from the colorectal and upper gastrointestinal tracts. A false-positive result can occur if the patient has ingested red meat, vegetables, or anti-inflammatory drugs. Immunological FOBT is based on antibodies that specifically recognize human hemoglobin and is not affected by plant peroxidases in the diet (Tumor Markers Fact Sheet American Cancer Society 2013). The major drawback of the FOBT is its low ability to detect early-stage lesions. In fact, this screening method reduces CRC mortality by only 30 %; thus, it must be associated to other kinds of screening (Tanaka et al. 2010).

Potential Application of Proteomics to Prognosis, Other Diseases, or Conditions

Recent progresses in proteomics have led to progress in cancer-related biomarker discovery. The new proteomic technologies and improved tools for data handling and interpretation have opened new avenues in the search for biomarkers able to predict the outcome of cancer treatment. In recent years, a substantial set of CRC-related proteins has been identified thanks to proteomic-based methods (Corbo et al. 2012, 2013; Gemei et al. 2013; Van Houdt et al. 2011; de Wit et al. 2012). These proteins may have the potential to be CRC biomarkers. Hopefully, studies devoted to these and other putative protein biomarkers will result in a panel of markers with sufficient sensitivity and specificity for CRC in the clinical setting.

It is expected that in the next few years, many proteins associated to CRC will be discovered by proteomic studies, and most of them could be candidate biomarkers of CRC. This is especially due to the heterogeneity of the disease and to the need for multiple markers to characterize accurately each specific CRC subtype. Finally, the biomarker potential of novel CRC-associated proteins should be validated in body fluids; this is a challenging task that could be overcome by progresses in new targeted MS methods (Anderson et al. 2009; Rifai et al. 2006; Jimenez et al. 2010).

Summary Points

- Early detection of colorectal cancer is critically important.
- The 5-year survival rate after surgical removal of a localized tumor exceeds 90 % versus 10 % in the case of a tumor with metastasis.
- The protein biomarkers accepted for clinical use in colorectal cancer are carcinoembryonic antigen and fecal hemoglobin; however, they lack specificity.
- There is a need to discover new protein biomarker candidates.
- Proteomics is widely used in cancer research.
- Proteomic platforms used for cancer biomarker discovery include gel-based and gel-free methods.
- 2D-DIGE is the most widely used and rigorous gel-based method.
- ICAT and iTRAQ are chemical labeling gel-free methods, and SILAC is a metabolic labeling method.
- Posttranslational modifications are often associated with cancer; understanding the role of phosphorylation in signaling pathways could pave the way to the identification of targets for future clinical research.
- Colorectal cancer proteomics can help the search for new biomarkers.

Acknowledgments The original experiments by the authors cited in this paper were supported by grants L.502/94 2006 from the Ministero della Salute and L.5/95 (to L.D.V.), grant POR Campania FSE 2007/2013 (C.RE.ME) from the Regione Campania (to F.S.), and grant RF-2010-2318372 from the Ministry of Health (to F.S.).

References

Anderson NL, Anderson NG. Proteome and proteomics: new technologies, new concepts, and new words. Electrophoresis. 1998;19:1853–61.

Anderson NL, Anderson NG, Pearson TW, Borchers CH, Paulovich AG, Patterson SD, et al. A human proteome detection and quantitation project. Mol Cell Proteomics. 2009;8:883–6.

Biomarkers in cancer: an introductory guide for advocates. Research advocacy network. 2010. http://researchadvocacy.org/images/uploads/downloads/BiomarkerinCancer_WebDownloadVersion.pdf. Retrieved 26 Apr 2013.

Chan D, Lee SC. Serial changes in expression of proteins in response to neoadjuvant chemotherapy in breast cancer. In: Yahwardiah S, editor. Oncogene and cancer – from bench to clinic. InTech; 2013. p. 3–38.

Cho WC, Cheng CH. Oncoproteomics: current trends and future perspectives. Expert Rev Proteomics. 2007;4(3):401–10.

Corbo C, Orrù S, Gemei M, Noto RD, et al. Protein cross-talk in CD133+ colon cancer cells indicates activation of the Wnt pathway and upregulation of SRp20 that is potentially involved in tumorigenicity. Proteomics. 2012;12(12):2045–59.

Corbo C, Orrù S, Salvatore F. SRp20: an overview of its role in human diseases. Biochem Biophys Res Commun. 2013;436(1):1–5.

de Wit M, Jimenez CR, Carvalho B, et al. Cell surface proteomics identifies glucose transporter type 1 and prion protein as candidate biomarkers for colorectal adenoma-to-carcinoma progression. Gut. 2012;61(6):855–64.

Engholm-Keller K, Larsen MR. Technologies and challenges in large-scale phosphoproteomics. Proteomics. 2013;13(6):910–31.

Engwegen J.Y.M.N, Gast M.C.W, Schellens J.H.M, Beijnen J.H. Clinical proteomics: searching for better tumour markers with SELDI-TOF mass spectrometry. Trends Pharmacol Sci 2006;27(5):2517–259.

Ettarh R. Colorectal cancer: it starts and it runs. In: Ettarh R, editor. Colorectal cancer biology – from genes to tumor. 2012. p. 1–8. http://www.intechopen.com/books/colorectal-cancer-biology-from-genes-to-tumor/colorectal-cancer-it-startsand-it-runs.

Fearon ER, Vogelstein B. A genetic model for colorectal tumorigenesis. Cell. 1990;61:759–67.

Feizi T. Demonstration by monoclonal antibodies that carbohydrate structures of glycoproteins and glycolipids are onco-developmental antigens. Nature. 1985;314:53–7.

Gala M, Chung DC. Hereditary colon cancer syndromes. Semin Oncol. 2011;38(4):490–9.

Gemei M, Mirabelli P, Di Noto R, et al. CD66c is a novel marker for colorectal cancer stem cell isolation, and its silencing halts tumor growth in vivo. Cancer. 2013;119(4):729–38.

Guerrier L, Thulasiraman V, Castagna A, et al. Reducing protein concentration range of biological samples using solid-phase ligand libraries. J Chromatogr B Analyt Technol Biomed Life Sci. 2006;833(1):33–40.

Hakomori S. Tumor-associated glycolipid antigens, their metabolism and organization. Chem Phys Lipids. 1986;42:209–33.

Han DK, Eng J, Zhou H, Aebersold R. Quantitative profiling of differentiation-induced microsomal proteins using isotope-coded affinity tags and mass spectrometry. Nat. Biotechnol. 2001;19:946–51

Jimenez CR, Knola JC, Meijerb GA, Fijnemanb RJA. Proteomics of colorectal cancer: overview of discovery studies and identification of commonly identified cancer-associated proteins and candidate CRC serum markers. J Proteomics. 2010;73:1873–95.

Lowe JB. Glycosylation, immunity, and autoimmunity. Cell. 2001;104(6):809–12.

Moorhead GB, De Wever V, Templeton G, Kerk D. Evolution of protein phosphatases in plants and animals. Biochem J. 2009;417:401–9.

Neilson KA, Ali NA, Muralidharan S, Mirzaei M, Mariani M, Assadourian G, Lee A, van Sluyter SC, Haynes PA. Less label, more free: approaches in label-free quantitative mass spectrometry. Proteomics. 2011;11(4):535–53.

Newton KF, Newman W, Hill J. Review of biomarkers in colorectal cancer. Colorectal Dis. 2012;14(1):3–17.

O'Farell PH. High resolution two-dimensional electrophoresis of proteins. J Biol Chem. 1975;250:4007–21.

Ong SE, Blagoev B, Kratchmarova I, Kristensen DB, Steen H, Pandey A, and Mann M. Stable isotope labeling by amino acids in cell culture, SILAC, as a simple and accurate approach to expression proteomics. Mol. Cell Proteomics. 2002;1(5):376–386.

Pastor MD, Nogal A, Molina-Pinelo S, Paz-Ares L, Carnero A. Oncoproteomic approaches in lung cancer research. In: López-Camarillo C, Aréchaga-Ocampo E, editors. Oncogenomics and cancer proteomics – novel approaches in biomarkers discovery and therapeutic targets in cancer. 2013. Chapter 7. http://www.intechopen.com/books/oncogenomics-and-cancer-proteomics-novel-approaches-in-biomarkers-discovery-and-therapeutic-targets-in-cancer/oncoproteomic-approaches-in-lung-cancer-research.

Rifai N, Gillette MA, Carr SA. Protein biomarker discovery and validation: the long and uncertain path to clinical utility. Nat Biotechnol. 2006;24:971–83.

Ross PL, Huang YN, Marchese JN, et al. Multiplexed protein quantitation in Saccharomyces cerevisiae using aminereactive isobaric tagging reagents. Molecular and Cellular Proteomics. 2004;3:1154–1169.

Schmidt SR, Schweikart F, Andersson ME. Current methods for phosphoprotein isolation and enrichment. J Chromatogr B Analyt Technol Biomed Life Sci. 2007;849(1–2):154–62.

Sefton BM, Shenolikar S. Overview of protein phosphorylation. Curr Protoc Mol Biol. 2001;11:3–4, Chapter 18 (Unit 18).

Tanaka T, Tanaka M, Takahiro T, Ishigamori R. Biomarkers for colorectal cancer. Int J Mol Sci. 2010;11:3209–25.

Tumor markers fact sheet. American Cancer Society 2013. www.cancer.org/tumor-markers-pdf

Unlu M, Morgan ME, Minden JS. Difference gel electrophoresis: a single gel method for detecting changes in protein extracts. Electrophoresis. 1997;18:2071–7.

van der Merwe DE, Oikonomopoulou K, Marshall J, Diamandis EP. Mass spectrometry: uncovering the cancer proteome for diagnostics. Adv Cancer Res. 2007;96:23–50.

Van Houdt WJ, Emmink BL, Pham TV, et al. Comparative proteomics of colon cancer stem cells and differentiated tumor cells identifies BIRC6 as a potential therapeutic target. Mol Cell Proteomics. 2011;10(12):M111.011353.

Varki A. Glycosylation changes in cancer. In: Varki A, Cummings R, Esko J, et al., editors. Essentials of glycobiology. 1999. Chapter. http://www.ncbi.nlm.nih.gov/books/NBK20710/.

Zhang B, VerBerkmoes NC, Langston MA, et al. Detecting differential and correlated protein expression in label-free shotgun proteomics. J Proteome Res. 2006;5(11):2909–18.

Cancer Cardiotoxicity and Cardiac Biomarkers

4

Michela Salvatici, Daniela Cardinale, Alessandro Colombo, and Maria Teresa Sandri

Contents

M. Salvatici • M.T. Sandri (✉)
Division of Laboratory Medicine, European Institute of Oncology, Milan, Italy
e-mail: michela.salvatici@ieo.it; maria.sandri@ieo.it

D. Cardinale • A. Colombo
Unit of Cardioncology, Division of Cardiology, European Institute of Oncology, Milan, Italy
e-mail: daniela.cardinale@ieo.it; alessandro.colombo@ieo.it

V.R. Preedy, V.B. Patel (eds.), *Biomarkers in Cancer, Biomarkers in Disease: Methods, Discoveries and Applications*,
DOI 10.1007/978-94-007-7681-4_20

Abstract

Modern cancer therapies are highly effective in the treatment of malignancy; however, they are associated with the possible development of side effects, in particular involving heart function. This particular form of cardiotoxicity is related to many factors: age, cumulative dose of the drug administered, drug combination, smoking, prior radiotherapy, and prior cardiovascular disease. Different types of events may manifest: the more important and difficult to manage is a progressive LV dysfunction, which may lead to the development of cardiac failure. Other side effects are represented by acute coronary syndromes, hypertension, thromboembolic events, and arrhythmias. Anthracyclines are one of the anticancer drugs more studied, and they are known to cause CTX through different molecular mechanisms; the damage induced by AC is dose dependent and usually irreversible. Also newer therapies like targeted therapy (i.e., trastuzumab) or angiogenesis inhibitors are all associated with some form of cardiac toxicity: while targeted drugs may induce a reversible damage, angiogenesis inhibitors have a prothrombotic activity, which leads to a high incidence of thromboembolic events.

Patients were followed up with serial cardiological visits and evaluation of the LVEF, which however detects the damage already installed. In the last 20 years, a new appealing approach has been proposed: it is based on the evaluation of circulating troponin and/or natriuretic peptides. Especially for troponin, many studies underlined the predictive value of this marker, which can detect minimal cardiac damage, well before the onset of cardiac dysfunction, allowing for a personalized follow-up and cardiological preventive treatment.

In this light, many studies have recently evaluated the protective effect of different drugs, such as dexrazoxane, beta blockers, and ACE inhibitors, with in some cases very promising results.

List of Abbreviations

AC	Anthracycline
ACEIs	Angiotensin-Converting Enzyme Inhibitors
ANP	Atrial Natriuretic Peptide
ASCO	American Society of Clinical Oncology
BB	β-blockers
BNP	Brain Natriuretic Peptide
CHF	Congestive Heart Failure
CNP	C-Type Natriuretic Peptide
cTn	Cardiac Troponin
CT	Chemotherapy
CTX	Cardiotoxicity
ESMO	European Society for Medical Oncology
ECG	Electrocardiogram
FDA	Food and Drug Administration
HDC	High-Dose Chemotherapy

HER2, ErB2	Epidermal Growth Factor Receptor-2
hs-cTn	High-Sensitivity Troponin
LV	Left Ventricular
LVEF	Left Ventricular Ejection Fraction
MUGA	Multi-Gated Radionuclide Angiography
MRI	Magnetic Resonance Imaging
NPs	Natriuretic Peptide
ROS	Reactive Oxygen Species
RT	Radiotherapy
TnC	Troponin C
TnI	Troponin I
TnT	Troponin T
TKI	Tyrosine Kinase Inhibitor
VEGF	Vascular Endothelial Growth Factor

Definition of Words and Terms

Anthracyclines Anthracycline antibiotics are natural products derived from the actinobacteria *Streptomyces peucetius* about more than 40 years ago. They are commonly used in the treatment of a number of diverse tumor types but are among the best characterized chemotherapeutic drugs leading to a myocardial cell loss.

Antiangiogenic targeted therapies The production of a network of blood vessels is a condition necessary to tumor survival. Angiogenesis inhibitors interfere with the development of blood vessels making the cancer unable to receive the oxygen and nutrients it needs to survive.

Biomarkers A biomarker is a molecule which may be used as an indicator of some biological state or condition. The measurement of biomarkers is often used to examine normal biological processes, pathogenic processes, or pharmacologic responses to a therapeutic intervention.

E:A ratio The ratio of peak early to late diastolic filling velocity is an index to characterize patterns of impaired diastolic filling. Abnormalities in the E:A ratio, determined on echocardiography, suggest that the left ventricle, which pumps blood into the circulation, cannot fill with blood properly in the period between contractions.

Free radicals A free radical is a molecule that contains one or more unpaired electrons. A molecule containing an unpaired electron will be more reactive and once produced can interact with other nearby molecules in an attempt to regain the paired electron state.

High-dose chemotherapy (HDC) With this treatment, high doses of chemotherapy are given in order to destroy cancer cells than would be possible with conventional (standard dose) chemotherapy. However, HDC also destroys hematopoietic stem cells, which are responsible for the production of blood cells. In order to restore blood cell production after high-dose chemotherapy, stem cells must be replaced. The procedure that restores the stem cells is called stem cell transplantation. Historically, high-dose chemotherapy and hematopoietic stem cell transplantation have been considered to provide patients with a better chance for longer survival than other therapies. However, the newer agents are providing high response rates, with significantly prolonged survival as well. Thus, the role of high-dose chemotherapy and stem cell transplantation in the treatment of cancer is currently limited.

Immunoassay detection methodology The immunoassays are used to quantify molecules of biological interest based on the specificity and selectivity of antibody to recognize and bind a specific molecule. The molecule bound by an antibody is referred to as an antigen, and the area on an antigen to which the antibody binds is called an epitope.

Interobserver variability Interobserver variability is a systematic difference which arises when the measurement is not performed by a single observer but by two or more observers. In clinical practice, especially in cases of qualitative assessment, the variability that exists between two or more observers could produce different values of the same measurement.

Left ventricular ejection fraction (LVEF) LVEF represents the measurement of how much blood is being pumped out of the left ventricle with each heartbeat or cardiac cycle.

Natriuretic effect It is the excretion of a large amount of sodium in the urine as a result from direct inhibition of sodium absorption in the collecting duct, increased glomerular filtration, and inhibition of aldosterone production and secretion.

Radiotherapy (RT) It is the use of high-energy rays, usually x-rays and similar rays (such as electrons), to treat or control cancer; it is a very common cancer treatment worldwide. It works by destroying the cells in the treated area. However, if the normal cells can usually repair themselves from the damages of radiation therapy, the cancer cell cannot.

Reactive oxygen species (ROS) Oxygen can be converted to different reactive oxygen species depending on the number of electrons and protons it accepts into its stable structure, from the other molecules. They can either exert beneficial physiological effects (control of gene expression and mitogenesis) or damage cell structures, including lipids and membranes, proteins, and nucleic acids, leading to cell death.

Targeted therapy It is the use of drugs that interfere with specific target pathways in neoplastic tissue to destroy cancer cells. They work by changing the way that cells interact with or signal to each other, modifying essential pathways involved in the proliferation, angiogenesis, and differentiation of the neoplasm.

Introduction

Anticancer therapies have greatly improved the survival of cancer patients. However, both due to the longer expectancy of life and to the higher knowledge of cardiac toxicity of antineoplastic agents, a great amount of studies underlined the importance of chemotherapy-induced cardiotoxicity. The most common adverse event is heart failure, which can appear months to years after the end of anticancer treatment (Yeh and Bickford 2009). Patients are usually followed by means of regular cardiologic follow-up and with the evaluation of left ventricular ejection fraction, which declines progressively before CHF appearance (Wouters et al. 2005).

In the last two decades, efforts have been made to find tools that are useful not only in detecting a decline in LVEF but also able to stratify patients at risk. Troponins and natriuretic peptides have progressively emerged as useful biomarkers, which may increase during or after chemotherapy administration and identify with high-sensitivity subjects at risk for future cardiac impairment (Cardinale and Sandri 2010).

Thanks to this new approach, patients can be offered preventive cardiologic therapies, which may significantly lower their risk of developing a cardiac disease.

Cardiotoxicity of Cancer Therapy

CTX is one of the most severe complications of cancer treatment. Recent advances in early detection and in antitumoral therapies led to a remarkable improvement in longevity after cancer diagnosis in spite of a higher risk to develop cardiovascular disease. CTX represents an adverse event difficult to manage by the oncologists: in fact even minor cardiac damages may lead to a review of the anticancer therapy, sometimes with dose reduction or with a change in the type of the administered drug, possibly with a less aggressive one. This may impact on the outcome of the patients, who need to be adequately cured for the malignancy. The most frequent and recurrent cardiac complication of cardiotoxicity is the development of a late/dilated hypokinetic cardiomyopathy, generally beginning with asymptomatic diastolic or systolic dysfunction, which may progress until overt CHF, which may lead to death (Yeh and Bickford 2009). A number of risk factors for the development of CTX have been identified (Cardinale et al. 2013; Jones et al. 2007). Cumulative dose and delivery schedule of the drug administered, patient's age at the time of therapy, treatment with a combination of chemotherapeutic agents, smoking, current or prior radiation therapy, preexisting cardiovascular disease (including coronary artery disease, hypertension, peripheral vascular disease, and dyslipidemia), and comorbidities (diabetes, obesity, renal dysfunction, sepsis, endocrinopathies, etc.) are well-recognized risk factors. A large body of data have demonstrated the relationship between AC exposure and CTX. For example, in a study conducted on 3,941 patients treated with anthracyclines, 88 developed symptomatic heart failure during follow-up with an incidence ranging from 0.14 % in patients receiving <400 mg/m^2, to 7 % and 18 % in patients who received 550 and 700 mg/m^2, respectively (Bristow et al. 1981). Another report on 630 oncological patients treated with doxorubicin found that 26 % of the patients receiving a cumulative dose of 550 mg/m^2 developed heart failure (Swain et al. 2003). According to these evidences, it has been recommended to limit the cumulative doses of doxorubicin to 450–500 mg/m^2 in adults. Although limiting the cumulative dose of anthracyclines is an important approach to prevent CTX, the surveillance of myocardial function during and after therapy, with early detection of adverse cardiac effects, remains the cornerstone in preventing CTX.

Young patients, with a longer life expectancy, are more exposed to the risk of developing CTX (Hershman et al. 2008), and on the other hand, the older age itself is a notable risk, especially for cancer patients who receive anthracyclines and for old women with breast cancer who receive trastuzumab in the adjuvant setting (Tarantini et al. 2012; Du et al. 2009). An additional risk factor for CTX development is prior or concomitant irradiation. RT may amplify and accelerate the development of cardiovascular injury inducing endothelial cell damage and compromising coronary artery blood flow (Shapiro et al. 1998). Moreover, the concomitant administration of different agents may further increase the susceptibility to CTX, resulting in a synergistic toxicity.

This phenomenon is expected to rise as a consequence of the increasing number of patients undergoing cancer chemotherapy, the improved efficacy of anticancer therapies, and therefore the prolonged survival of patients (Meinardi et al. 1999). Data from the National Cancer Institute, the Centers for Disease Control and Prevention, and the Eurocare studies estimate that in the developed countries, there are currently more than 11 million cancer survivors, and many of them should be considered to be at potential risk of long-term cardiovascular toxicity (American Cancer Society 2010).

To date, there is still no single definition of drug-induced cardiotoxicity because the development of adverse cardiac events, such as acute coronary syndromes, hypertension, arrhythmias, decreased cardiac contractile function, episodes of ECG changes, and thromboembolic events, is all regarded as an expression of CTX (Hull et al. 2003). Even the time of onset of CTX induced by chemotherapy can be highly variable: from the onset during or in the days immediately following the administration of anticancer therapy to few weeks until several years after the end of the entire chemotherapy treatment. The early form is rare, usually dose independent, and reversible. It may present as asymptomatic electrocardiographic changes, arrhythmias, heart block, or more rarely as an acute myocarditis and in the majority of cases resolves after discontinuation of the therapy. The late-onset cardiotoxicity may present months or years after the end of the treatment and may evolve toward an irreversible cardiomyopathy (Barrett-Lee et al. 2009; Lipshultz et al. 1995).

Currently, both American and European scientific societies define the CTX as a decline of the LVEF greater than 10 % points with a final LVEF <50 % or as an LVEF reduction greater than 15 % points with a final LVEF >50 % (Bird and Swain 2008).

Although many aspects of cardiotoxicity need to be better investigated, the severity and the incidence of cardiovascular toxicities demand a more accurate prediction of the risk in a preclinical and early clinical stage. This approach would allow to avoid restrictions in prescription practice (indications and dose levels) and drug withdrawal that are recommended when the cardiac damage is already clinically evident and moreover to plan closer monitoring.

Summary Points

- This chapter focuses on CTX that represents a serious adverse effect of antitumoral drugs.
- CTX can impact the quality of life and overall survival of cancer patients limiting their therapeutic opportunities.
- The typical example of CTX from cancer treatment is the development of a late/dilated hypokinetic cardiomyopathy, but different cardiovascular diseases (from arrhythmias to thromboembolic events) can be an expression of CTX.
- The incidence of cardiotoxic event is expected to rise.
- A number of risk factors (age, smoking, prior or concomitant RT, etc.) can increase the risk to develop cardiovascular toxicity.
- Although the term "cardiotoxicity" has been used to describe an adverse cardiac event, now the definition of CTX is generally referred to an LVEF decline greater than 10 % with a final LVEF <50 % or reduction greater than 15 % with a final LVEF >50 %.
- Cardiovascular complications may be observed acutely or subacutely (anytime from the initiation of the therapy) till several years after treatment.
- The early identification, prevention, and treatment of CTX induced by anticancer agents remain an important strategy to reduce morbidity and mortality of cancer patients.

Key Facts of Cardiotoxicity

- If the event of acute toxicity has become rare as a consequence of improved dosing practices, the risk to experience a chronic dilated cardiomyopathy remains considerable (Gianni et al. 2008).
- It is not clear, in the older patients, if the increase in the susceptibility to anthracycline-induced damage is due to a preexisting heart disease or whether it is due to a less functional reserve which is unable to tolerate additional myocardial damage.
- A cumulative mediastinal radiation >30 Gy is a clear risk factor for CTX.

Chemotherapeutic Agents

There is an extensive list of chemotherapeutic agents that have the potential to induce CHF or predispose patients to CTX (Table 1). Traditional chemotherapeutic agents, such as AC, have been known to cause cardiovascular morbidities months to years after administration; however, new targeted drugs such as monoclonal antibodies, TKI, and several others have been recently evaluated in the context of their impact on clinical presentation of cardiovascular disease.

Anthracycline

Anthracycline antibiotics, such as doxorubicin, daunorubicin, and epirubicin, are one of the most effective and widespread chemotherapeutic agents used for the treatment of both hematological and solid malignancies (i.e., breast carcinomas and sarcomas). Isolated in the 1960s from the *Streptomyces* bacterium, this class of drugs acts preventing DNA and RNA synthesis by insertion into the DNA of the replicating cells and inhibition of topoisomerase II enzyme. Their introduction in the clinical practice consistently improved the management of certain malignancies, but unfortunately, their toxic effects were soon revealed. In particular, it was evident that chronic treatment with anthracyclines could often be associated with the development of an irreversible form of dilated cardiomyopathy and dose-dependent CTX (Yeh and Bickford 2009). Even if the exact mechanism by which these agents cause cardiac injury is not still well understood, data from extensive myocardial biopsy and observations of elevated troponin levels after anthracycline administration have established that anthracyclines destroy myocytes causing a permanent damage. The therapeutic activity of anthracycline is mediated by their insertion into the DNA of replicating cells, causing DNA fragmentation, inhibition of polymerases, and decreased DNA, RNA, and protein synthesis. However, the pathophysiological mechanism implicated in the myocardial damage involves probably different pathways, since myocytes are not actively replicating. Myocardial changes following anthracycline treatment include (i) vacuolar degeneration of the sarcoplasmic reticulum, (ii) swelling and disruption of the mitochondria, (iii) myofilament degeneration, and (iv) myocardial cell loss by necrosis or apoptosis. The molecular mechanisms of myocyte injury are likely to be multifactorial. A commonly mentioned pathway involves anthracycline-induced production of ROS with an increase in oxidative stress, which causes irreversible damage in multiple cellular components including lipids of the cell membranes, proteins, and nucleic acids. The myocytes, more susceptible to ROS activity since terminally differentiated, are not able to replace damaged cells, and this leads to myocyte cell death and myocardial replacements by fibrous tissue (Kalyanaraman et al. 2002; Barry et al. 2007). Although the ROS model, leading to direct oxidative damage to cellular components, remains a common postulated mechanism for anthracycline cardiotoxicity, it is not sufficient to fully explain the development of cardiac dysfunction. Other potentially cardiotoxic actions of the anthracyclines include the production of toxic metabolites, inhibition of

Table 1 Systemic cancer drugs with important cardiovascular side effects, selected indications

	Class/drug	Selected indications	Important CV side effects
Cytostatic chemotherapeutics	Anthracyclines/analogs		
	Doxorubicin	Lymphoma	Cardiac dysfunction/ heart failure
	Daunorubicin	Leukemia	
	Epirubicin	Breast cancer	
		Ovarian cancer	
		Sarcoma	
	Mitoxantrone	Leukemia	
		Multiple sclerosis	
	Pyrimidine analogs		
	Fluorouracil (5-FU)	Colorectal cancer	Coronary spasms/ ischemia
	Capecitabine	Breast cancer	
	Alkylating agents		
	Cyclophosphamide	Breast cancer	Myocarditis (rare)
	Cisplatin	Genitourinary cancer	Thrombosis
	Anti-microtubule agents		
	Paditaxel	Breast cancer	Bradycardia
		Colorectal cancer	
Signalling inhibitors	Anti-HER2		
	Trastuzumab	Breast cancer	Cardiac dysfunction
	Lapatinib	Gastric cancer	
	Angiogenesis inhibitors/ anti-VEGF		
	Bevacizumab	Gastrointestinal cancer	Hypertension
	Sunitinib	Renal cell carcinoma	Endovascular damage
	Sorafenib	Hepatocellular carcinoma	
	BCR-ABL inhibitors		
	Imatinib	Leukemia	Edema, cardiac dysfunction (rare)
	Dasatinib	Gastric cancer	QTc prolongation
	Nilotinib		

Data from Suter and Ewer (2013), with the permission from the publishers

nucleic acid and protein synthesis, release of vasoactive amines, decreased expression of specific genes, impairment of mitochondrial membrane binding, and disturbance in intracellular calcium homeostasis. Separate effects mediated by cardiomyocyte topoisomerases and disruption of sarcomere preservation may also be important (Fig. 1) (Zhang et al. 2012).

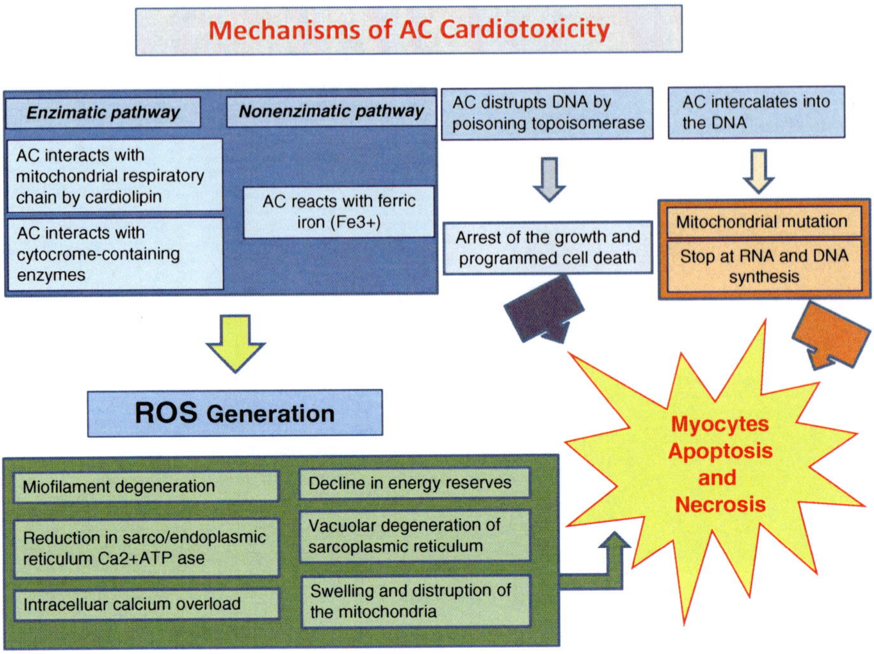

Fig. 1 Mechanisms of anthracycline cardiotoxicity: overview

Targeted Therapy

Trastuzumab

Trastuzumab is a humanized monoclonal antibody directed against the human epidermal growth factor receptor-2 (ErB2, also called EGFR2 or HER2) approved by the FDA for the treatment of positive HER2 breast cancer. Approximately 20–25 % of breast cancer patients have tumors that overexpress the HER2 receptors or with amplification of the *HER2/neu* gene, a maker that identifies aggressive tumor with a worse prognosis. Trastuzumab therapy is important in the treatment of early and advanced breast cancer overexpressing HER2: in monotherapy, trastuzumab has been shown to induce a clinical response in 12–26 % of patients, and if used concurrently with anthracycline (Vogel et al. 2002), it enhances the effect of traditional chemotherapy leading to an increase of the response to the therapy and an improvement in overall survival (Salmon et al. 2001). Its use, however, results in a small to modest and initially unexpected risk for CTX, often manifested by an asymptomatic decrease in LVEF and less often by clinical heart failure. The reported incidence of cardiotoxicity varies due to differences in definition of cardiac dysfunction, chemotherapy schedules, and eligibility criteria for trial entry. In a phase 3 trastuzumab clinical trial in metastatic breast cancer patients, the incidence of cardiac dysfunction raised among patients who received trastuzumab plus anthracycline or trastuzumab plus paclitaxel (27 % and 13 % of adverse cardiac events, respectively) (Salmon et al. 2001). This would confirm the hypothesis that trastuzumab favors the onset of cardiomyopathy supported by anthracycline, although it seems that some cardiac dysfunction can also occur when trastuzumab is used alone with incidence rates of around 3–7 % (Seidman et al. 2002).

In contrast to anthracycline-induced cardiotoxicity, the cardiac injury due to trastuzumab is not related to the cumulative dose, is not associated with severe ultrastructural changes on myocardial biopsy, is often reversible after treatment discontinuation, and can be administered once again, if indicated, after recovery (Ewer and Lippman 2005). However if the anthracycline cardiomyopathy has been reasonably characterized, the features of trastuzumab CTX, such as the precise pathophysiological mechanism, capacity of recovery, long-term implications, and overall clinical importance, are not fully understood. Some of the uncertainties are due to the fact that HER2-positive breast cancer patients are concomitantly treated with both trastuzumab and anthracycline, making difficult the identification of the effects of each agent from a synergistic interaction between them. Evidences from both in vivo and in vitro studies indicate the importance of epidermal growth signal pathway (HER2) also in the heart, suggesting that trastuzumab's CTX is related to HER2 blockade which causes a subsequent impairment of cell-protective, growth-promoting, antiapoptotic pathways in the myocardium (Hayes and Picard 2006).

Inhibitors of Angiogenesis

The VEGF inhibitors are a group of targeted therapies used to treat a variety of solid organ malignancies, including renal cell cancer, hepatocellular carcinoma, and gastrointestinal stromal tumor. This class of angiogenesis inhibitors are monoclonal antibodies against VEGF receptor (bevacizumab) and "multi-targeted" tyrosine kinase inhibitors (sunitinib and sorafenib), which block downstream signalling in VEGF and other tumor growth pathways. Extensive data indicate that these drugs are associated with cardiovascular adverse events, such as hypertension, thromboembolic episode, myocardial ischemia, asymptomatic LV dysfunction, and CHF (Criscitello et al. 2012). The mechanism of LV dysfunction is likely related to both hypertensive cardiomyopathy and direct myocardial toxicity. Different studies have been performed looking at the cardiac adverse events during or after the administration of these drugs (Richards et al. 2011; Choueiri et al. 2010, 2011). One review focusing on thromboembolic events indicated that incidence of these events associated with sorafenib and sunitinib treatment was 1.4 % with a relative risk 3.03 compared with control patients (Choueiri et al. 2010). As far as CHF is concerned, a large analysis of 6,935 patients, with a variety of malignancies, treated with sunitinib found that the incidence of high-grade CHF in the sunitinib arm versus placebo was 2.6 %, with a relative risk of 3.3 (Richards et al. 2011). A meta-analysis of five randomized trials of bevacizumab in patients with metastatic breast cancer demonstrated an overall incidence of 1.6 % of high-grade CHF and a relative risk of 4.74 versus control/placebo group (Choueiri et al. 2011).

Summary Points

- This chapter focuses on the description of the pathophysiological mechanisms through which anthracycline, the most cardiotoxic drug commonly used in the conventional therapy, and the new targeted therapies (monoclonal antibodies and tyrosine kinase inhibitors) induce myocardial dysfunction.
- The therapeutic activity of anthracycline is mediated by their insertion into the DNA of replicating cells, inhibition of polymerases, and decrease of DNA, RNA, and protein synthesis.
- The mechanism of anthracycline-induced cardiotoxicity is not fully understood but it is probably multifactorial. The leading pathway is the increase of ROS within the cardiac myocyte mitochondria; adult myocytes are more susceptible to ROS activity because they are terminally differentiated and cannot replace cells damage during treatment.
- Trastuzumab is a monoclonal antibody approved for the treatment of HER2-overexpressing breast cancer. The early trials of evaluating trastuzumab in metastatic breast cancer point out an unexpected CTX, most evident when trastuzumab was coadministered with doxorubicin.
- The mechanism of trastuzumab-induced cardiotoxicity is probably due to the blockade of HER2 receptor on myocyte.
- Contrary to the irreversible cardiomyocyte damage caused by anthracyclines, trastuzumab-mediated toxicity seems to be reversible.
- An increasing number of antiangiogenesis therapies is broadening the therapeutic opportunities for cancer patients. Nevertheless, these agents are associated with cardiovascular adverse events, such as hypertension, thromboembolic episode, myocardial ischemia, asymptomatic LV dysfunction, and CHF.

Key Facts of Chemotherapeutic Agents

- Anthracyclines disrupt DNA by poisoning topoisomerase, a critical enzyme for unwinding of the DNA for replication and synthesis, causing thereby growth arrest and programmed cell death.
- Anthracycline can induce the generation of oxygen-derived free radicals through two main pathways: a nonenzymatic pathway that utilizes iron and an enzymatic one that use the mitochondrial respiratory chain through a link between anthracycline and cardiolipin.
- The difference between cardiotoxicity from anthracycline and trastuzumab led to the terms "type I" and "type II" chemotherapy-related cardiac dysfunction. Type I is associated with the anthracyclines and results in myocyte destruction and clinical heart failure; it is dose related and in most cases may trigger an irreversible cardiac damage. Type II is a form of CTX that is not unique to trastuzumab, more often associated with a loss of contractility without severe

ultrastructural damage of heart tissue. It is not dose dependent and in most cases reversible after drug withdrawal (Ewer and Lippman 2005).

- ErB2 function seems to be necessary for the repair of the oxidative damage caused by AC and its inactivation increases heart vulnerability. In ErB2 knockout mice, trastuzumab causes ventricular swelling, cardiac wall thinning, and a decline in the muscle contractility
- Overlapping mechanisms have been proposed to explain the high incidence of thromboembolic events in patients treated with antiangiogenic targeted therapies. VEGF inhibition causes endothelial dysfunction blocking the capability of endothelial cells to regenerate, decreases the production of vasodilator and triggers the procoagulant pathways, and increases hematocrit and blood viscosity. The prothrombotic activity mediated by the antiangiogenic therapy combined with the oncological patient's predisposition to thrombosis explains the increased incidence in these patients.

Monitoring of Drug-Induced Cardiotoxicity

The potential cardiotoxicity of chemotherapeutic agents is becoming increasingly manifest and prevalent thanks to a close clinical monitoring by the use of serological makers and cardiac imaging techniques, which include echocardiograms, MUGA, and MRI. This approach as part of routine evaluation of patients receiving cardiotoxic therapies allows the identification of both patients at risk, prior to becoming symptomatic, and of subjects which may develop cardiotoxicity that may limit the use of potentially lifesaving chemotherapy agents. Early identification of patients who are at risk for chemotherapy-induced CTX should be a primary goal to plan and to develop individualized therapeutic strategies and intervention in cancer patients (Wouters et al. 2005).

Cardiac Imaging

Given that many anticancer compounds induce some degree of CTX, a proper management of subsequent cardiac dysfunction after the oncological therapy is becoming increasingly important, especially as the number of patients at risk continues to grow. However, even if cardiac function after the chemotherapeutic treatment can be monitored in several ways, evidence-based guidelines have yet to be established. At present, the most recommended modality for detecting CTX is a regular monitoring of cardiac function by means of LVEF measurements through either echocardiography or MUGA (Jones et al. 2009; Bovelli et al. 2010; Eschenhagen et al. 2011). However, the current standard for monitoring cardiac function, based on periodic assessment of LVEF, detects CTX only when a functional impairment has already occurred, precluding any chance of preventing its

Table 2 Cardiac imaging modalities in the detection of CTX: advantages and drawbacks

	Echocardiography	MUGA	MRI	Endomyocardial biopsy
Advantages	Noninvasive	Noninvasive	Noninvasive	No radiation
	No radiation	Lack of the need for geometric remodeling	No radiation	Histological evidence of CTX
	Complete cardiac assessment (including valvular, diastolic, and pericardial assessment and chamber size)	Low interobserver variability	Accurate and reproducible assessment of LVEF	
			Gold standard for the evaluation of LV volumes, mass, and function	
Disadvantages	Low reproducibility	Exposure to radioactivity	Low availability	Invasive
	High interobserver variability	Incomplete cardiac assessment (focusing only on LVEF value)	Expensive	Low availability
			Long processing time	Less sensitive
			Not applicable in patients with metal devices and renal dysfunction	High variability in interpretation

development. This approach, in fact, represents a relatively insensitive tool for identifying CTX at an early stage because no considerable change in LVEF occurs until a severe myocardial damage is present. Furthermore, the conventional two-dimensional transthoracic echocardiography has a low reproducibility, and the image quality is related to the assumption of LV geometry, dependency on acoustic windows, and expertise (Table 2).

Serological Markers

Due to the relative low sensitivity of imaging techniques in the prediction of myocardial dysfunction, recently, there has been a significant interest in looking for alternative diagnostic tools that are noninvasive, sensitive, specific, and reproducible as well as low cost. In this light, assessment of biochemical markers of myocardial injury and ventricular dysfunction (troponin and natriuretic peptide) has emerged as probably a very useful strategy.

Summary Points

- This chapter focuses on the most recognized methods used in clinical practice for detecting and monitoring CTX.
- Even if no consensus guidelines exist for the monitoring of cardiac function in adults undergoing chemotherapy, cardiac assessment by periodic evaluation of LVEF function is recommended.
- CTX is traditionally monitored serially during the treatment by echocardiography or radionuclide angiography. Although both methods detect significant changes in LV function, they show a low diagnostic accuracy and a poor predictive power.
- Many studies have investigated the utility of cardiac biomarkers that may predict and monitor cardiac injury (troponin) or volume changes (natriuretic peptide) during anticancer therapy cycles.
- Biomarker assessment seems a cost-effective diagnostic tool for an early and real-time identification, assessment, and monitoring of cancer CTX.

Key Facts of Monitoring of Drug-Induced Cardiotoxicity

- To date, there are no evidence-based guidelines for CTX monitoring during and after anticancer therapies in adult, and guidelines in pediatric oncology are subject to debate. Although several guidelines are available, none specify how often, by what means, or how long cardiac function should be monitored during and after cancer treatment (Eschenhagen et al. 2011).
- However, the American Heart Association recommends in both pediatric and adult patients receiving potentially cardiotoxic chemotherapy several evaluations of LVEF (Cheitlin et al. 2003).
- MUGA scan could reduce interobserver variability with the disadvantages of including the exposure to radioactivity.
- MRI is considered the gold standard for the evaluation of LV volumes, mass, and function. However, its lack of availability and high cost limit its routine use.
- On the other hand, endomyocardial biopsy, which provides histological evidence of cardiotoxicity, is not routinely used in clinical practice and has not gained clinical acceptance due to its invasiveness and for the considerable expertise requests to interpret biopsy samples.

Troponins

Troponins constitute a regulatory complex composed of three protein subunits, troponin C (TnC), troponin T (TnT), and troponin I (TnI), localized in all types of

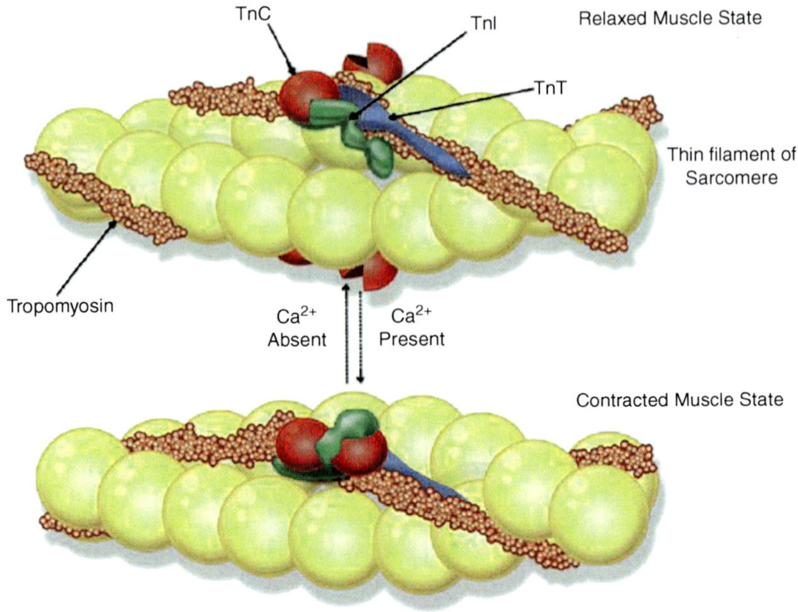

Fig. 2 Schematic of cardiac muscle showing location of cardiac troponin I (*TnI*), cardiac troponin T (*TnT*), and cardiac troponin C (*TnC*) in relation to actin and tropomyosin. Figure illustration by Craig Skaggs (Data from Shave et al. (2010), with the permission from the publishers)

striated (cardiac and skeletal) muscle. Each unit performs a specific function in the process of contraction by mediating actin-myosin interaction. TnC binds Ca^{2+} released from the sarcoplasmic reticulum, TnI inhibits the ATPase activity of actomyosin, and TnT provides for the binding of the troponin complex to tropomyosin. Whereas TnC is common to all muscle types, rendering this protein unsuitable for diagnostic use, three human isoforms have been described for TnT and TnI: one of the cardiac muscle and one of the fast- and the slow-twitch skeletal muscle, respectively (Fig. 2). Cardiac troponin (cTn) is complexed with actin in cardiac myofibrils with an incompletely clarified fraction (about 3–8 %) soluble in the cytoplasm. When ischemia occurs, a modification of myocyte membrane integrity happens, causing rapid depletion of the soluble cytoplasmic pool, followed by larger and more sustained release of troponin into the circulation as the contractile apparatus breaks down. Useful markers for diagnosing myocardial injury and acute coronary syndromes, troponins have been also evaluated in the oncological setting for the early detection and monitoring of the cardiac damage induced by chemotherapy (Lipshultz et al. 1997, 2004; Cardinale et al. 2000, 2002, 2004; Auner et al. 2003; Sandri et al. 2003; Kilickap et al. 2005). In an animal model, troponin T was released from doxorubicin-damaged myocytes, and the serum concentrations of cTnT correlated with the dose of drug received as well as the degree of myocardial damage (Herman et al. 1999). A fairly large number of studies suggest that elevations of cTnT and/or cTnI may be useful in the assessment of cardiac function degree in patients receiving potentially cardiotoxic therapy. The first information that emerges from these studies is that in about one-third of patients undergoing chemotherapy, an increase in the plasma concentration of troponin occurs, confirming the presence of a myocardial damage due to chemotherapy treatment in cancer patients. Different studies pointed out that the troponin measurements would be able to predict an LV dysfunction, months before its development (Lipshultz et al. 1997, 2004). In a population of children with acute lymphoblastic leukemia treated with doxorubicin, cTnT increases in about 30 % of cases predicting a myocardial injury manifested by an LV dilatation and wall thickening. This increase, sometimes persisting for months, was evocative of a cardiac damage educed by AC that may last for a long time (Lipshultz et al. 1997). Longer monitoring of the cardiac outcome, on the same population followed up for 5 years after treatment, showed that the presence of at least one increase in cTnT during CT identified children who would later manifest cardiac abnormalities at echocardiography (Lipshultz et al. 2004). Similarly, in 41 adults with various hematological malignancies in whom serum troponin T and LVEF were serially measured after AC-containing chemotherapy, patients with an elevated cTnT level had a significantly greater posttreatment decrease in LVEF than those without an elevation in the marker (10 % vs. 2 %; $P = 0.17$) (Auner et al. 2003). Further studies employing cTnI measurements have found results comparable to cTnT (Cardinale et al. 2000, 2002; Sandri et al. 2003). In patients undergoing high-dose chemotherapy (HDC) for a variety of malignancies, a raise of cTnI plasma levels during chemotherapy predicts a significantly lower LVEF at 7 months as compared to baseline and also provides information on the severity of the dysfunction. In contrast for patients who did not have elevated cTnI levels, LVEF returned to baseline at 7 months following a transient reduction at 3 months (Cardinale et al. 2000). Therefore cTnI gave both qualitative and quantitative information, identifying patients at greater risk of developing cardiac dysfunction over time and suggesting an estimate of the future functional impairment (Cardinale et al. 2000, 2002). A correlation between persistently elevated levels of post-chemotherapy TnI and CTX was demonstrated in a large study on 703 patients with cancer undergoing high-dose chemotherapy (Cardinale et al. 2004). TnI was measured before treatment, during 3 days after the end of chemotherapy infusion (early evaluation), and after 1 month (late evaluation). Patients without TnI elevation after HDC had a good cardiac prognosis: no significant reduction in LVEF was observed and a low incidence (1 %) of cardiac events occurred during the follow-up. In contrast, the presence of persistently elevated TnI levels 1 month after the last administration of the chemotherapy infusion was correlated with a worst prognosis identified as the occurrence of major adverse cardiac events in the first year of follow-up. The result of this study highlighted the high negative predictive value of TnI (99 %) and its capability to identify patients at low risk of experiencing cardiac complications after chemotherapy, who do not require very close cardiac monitoring, directing clinicians to implement a more stringent surveillance in patients showing a persistent TnI increase. In addition, these data emphasize the need to collect blood sample at several time periods to document a potential increase of this marker.

Troponin measurements have proved to be useful not only for the early identification of CTX induced by high-dose chemotherapy but also its determination gave important information on the prediction and monitoring of cardiac dysfunction in patients treated with standard dose of chemotherapy (Auner et al. 2003; Specchia et al. 2005; Kilickap et al. 2005) and newer targeted cancer drugs (Cardinale et al. 2010). In 78 hematological patients receiving standard doses of AC, cTnT serially measured revealed a delayed subclinical myocardial damage even after minor anthracycline exposure and identified patients at risk for subsequent myocardial dysfunction (Auner et al. 2003). Follow-up echocardiography showed a greater absolute decrease in LVEF in cTnT-positive patients compared to the cTnT-negative ones (10 % vs. 7 %, $P = 0.017$). This result has also confirmed that a prolonged monitoring by troponin measurements allows to disclose delayed decrease in LVEF. In addition, increased serum cTnT level detected in patients treated with standard doses of AC, in the first 3–5 days following the administration of chemotherapy, was associated with diastolic dysfunction of the left ventricle (Kilickap et al. 2005). Although the measurement of the different isoforms of troponin has proven to be able to detect the early cardiac damage produced by anthracyclines, much less is known about the usefulness of biomarkers in the setting of the newer targeted therapy. In 251 breast cancer patients treated with trastuzumab, the elevation in serum cTnI identified a subgroup of patients that were more likely to develop trastuzumab-induced cardiotoxicity and less likely to recover, even when treated for cardiac dysfunction (Cardinale et al. 2010). Furthermore, patients showing an increase of TnI during the treatment had a 25-fold increase in risk for major adverse cardiac events. An important indication emerges from this study: the elevation of troponin I in addition to its prognostic capability allows to distinguish between reversible and irreversible cardiac injury. In an observational study on 86 patients with metastatic renal cancer treated with either sunitinib or sorafenib, cTnT assessed serially (at baseline, bimonthly, and at the occurrence of clinical symptoms) was found elevated in 10 % of patients (Schmidinger et al. 2008). Ninety percent of them experienced a decrease of LVEF or regional contraction abnormalities following the increase in TnT. These data confirm that troponin measurement may be a useful marker designed for CTX testing in patients under both conventional and newer cancer therapy. It seems that a release of troponins reflects a final common event for multiple cardiotoxic mechanisms. Following all these evidences, the ESMO Clinical Practice Guidelines, published a clinical practice guideline in which the determination of troponin I at baseline and periodically during therapy may help in the identification of patients who may need a strict cardiologic follow-up (level of evidence III, grade of recommendation B) (Curigliano et al. 2012).

It must be said that, contrary to the previous findings, others have failed to detect any change in cTn during or after antineoplastic treatments (Soker and Kervancioglu 2005; Kismet et al. 2004). This discrepancy may be due to many factors: (i) the cumulative dose of CT and treatment protocols employed; (ii) different time of sampling for troponin measurement relative to the CT

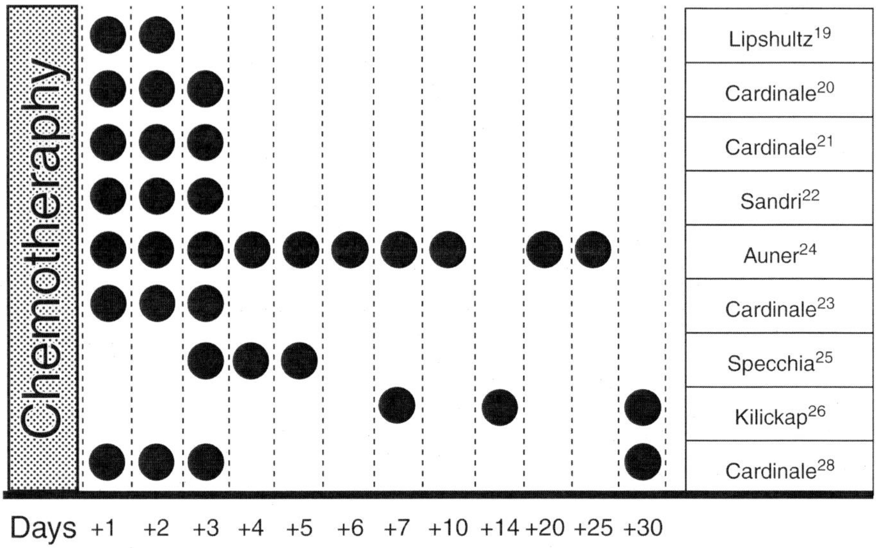

Fig. 3 Timing for sampling troponins in different studies (Data are from Cardinale and Sandri (2010), with the permission from the publishers)

administration (Fig. 3); (iii) the poor harmonization and the lack of standardization of the immunoassays currently used that present different formulation and cutoff levels, compromising the interchangeability of troponin measurements; (iv) the cardiologic end point and follow-up considered; and (v) the imprecision in LVEF estimates. A new generation of highly sensitive troponin assay, able to detect a very low amount of troponin, has been recently released on different platforms. These tests could be of particular relevance and could offer some advantages in a context of cardiotoxicity compared to previous assays, as often troponin concentrations found in cancer patients are just slightly above the cutoff. In a multicenter study, 32 breast cancer patients treated with anthracyclines and trastuzumab were studied prior to in addition to 3 and 6 months post-CT in order to assess whether early increases in biomarkers could predict the development of chemotherapy-induced cardiotoxicity (Sawaya et al. 2011). Elevation of hs-cTnI at 3 months posttreatment was able to detect a decrease in LVEF in six of the nine patients who met the criteria for cardiotoxicity. Decreases in peak longitudinal strain and increases in hs-cTnI concentrations at the completion of the chemotherapy were also observed in a similar study on 81 women with newly diagnosed human epidermal growth factor receptor-2-positive breast cancer treated with anthracyclines followed by trastuzumab and taxane. Changes in hs-TnI levels were predictive of subsequent cardiac side effects (Sawaya et al. 2012). This confirms the evidence that even a small increase in troponin is an independent risk factor for the development of CTX in the follow-up.

Summary Points

- This chapter focuses on structure, physiologic function, and applications of troponin in the oncological setting.
- Cardiac troponin I and T are structural proteins of the heart, involved in the heart muscle contraction and relaxation. These proteins are found mostly in the sarcomere of myocardial cells and in smaller quantities in the cytoplasm of the same cells. Accordingly, their measurements in peripheral blood indicate cardiomyocyte necrosis.
- Troponins have an absolute cardiac tissue specificity and a high sensitivity for detecting small amounts of myocardial necrosis.
- These markers are useful in the cardiac risk stratification as their elevation correlates with clinical severity of the disease and cardiac outcome.
- Recent data have revealed that the evaluation of troponin serum levels could be an efficient and alternative tool for the early cardiotoxic detection.
- Troponin elevation during chemotherapy treatment allows:
  (i) Detection of myocardial damage and the identification of patients at risk of cardiac event in an early preclinical phase
  (ii) Prediction of the severity of cardiac dysfunction and the stratification of the cardiac risk after CT (since its maximal elevation and the number of positive cTn are tightly correlated with LVEF reduction)
  (iii) Opportunity to schedule a strength surveillance monitoring of cardiac function in selected high-risk patients for whom preventive therapy can be planned
- More recently, increases in troponin levels have been also observed in patients who received newer antitumor agents.
- Guidelines exist suggesting the use of troponins for the early detection/prediction of cardiac dysfunction.

Key Facts of Troponin

- The dominant forms of cTnI detectable in serum following the ischemic insult are non-covalent ternary complexed cTnT-I-C (TIC complex) and binary complexed cTnI-C (IC complex) although complexed cTnI-T (IT complex) and free forms are also present.
- There is only one cTnT assay (available from Roche Diagnostics); a number of cTnI assays are available.
- In the last decade, cardiac troponins have become the biomarkers of choice for the diagnosis of acute myocardial infarction. In addition to acute coronary syndromes, the employment of cTn has been extended to a wide range of cardiac pathological conditions such as LV hypertrophy, CHF, stroke, pulmonary embolism, sepsis, chronic kidney disease, and cardiotoxicity (Mahajan and Jarolim 2011).

- A recent expert consensus document about the clinical use of cTn recognizes the utility of this biomarker in detecting cardiotoxicity and stratifying risk of the severity of left ventricular dysfunction (Newby et al. 2012).
- Comparison between cTnI platforms is difficult due to a lack of common standard, variability in antibodies in the commercial assays, and choice of epitopes.
- However, differences on cTnI manufactures exist, and there are those due to a variation in immunoassay detection methodology as well as to various cTnI forms which may alter epitope-binding sites when cTnI is phosphorylated or posttranslationally modified (oxidized, reduced, or partially digested by proteases).
- Since different antibodies used in the commercial assays may have different sensitivities to the modified forms of cTnI, these methods do not produce numerically similar results.
- The high negative predictive value of cTn allows to safely identify patients at low risk of cardiotoxicity and to reserve resources necessary for a tight cardiac monitoring of cTn-positive patients. The exclusion of troponin-negative subjects from the programs of long-term cardiac monitoring with the use of expensive imaging methods would result in an improvement in the cost-effectiveness of the management of cancer patients.

Natriuretic Peptides

Natriuretic peptides (NPs) are hormones produced by the myocardium and released into the circulation in response to wall strain and pressure overload. The more widely investigated members of the NP family (Fig. 4) are ANP and BNP and their co-secreted and biologically inactive N-terminal amino acid fragment (NT-proANP and NT-proBNP). The recognition that CHF and left ventricular systolic dysfunction are pathophysiologically related to profound changes in a variety of neurohormonal substances led to the hypothesis that such mediators could act as biomarkers of systolic dysfunction, hemodynamic upset, and myocyte injury. In effect, several studies have assessed the potential clinical utility of ANP, BNP, and their related fragment measurement, as biomarkers in diagnosis and risk stratification of patients with CHF. In particular, BNP has become a very valuable tool for the diagnosis, estimation of prognosis, and treatment efficacy of CHF, so that it has been incorporated in guidelines for diagnosis and management of CHF (Clerico and Emdin 2006). In the last decade, a great interest has grown about the use of BNP and NT-proBNP in patients with chemotherapy-induced cardiac impairment. In a very early study (Suzuki et al. 1998) on 27 patients with hematological malignancy treated with AC, persistent elevations of BNP were associated with reduced cardiac tolerance to cardiotoxic agents. After this report, multiple articles were published (Soker and Kervancioglu 2005; Ekstein et al. 2007; Dodos et al. 2008; Dolci et al. 2008; Roziakova et al. 2012) and some of these have evaluated the possible

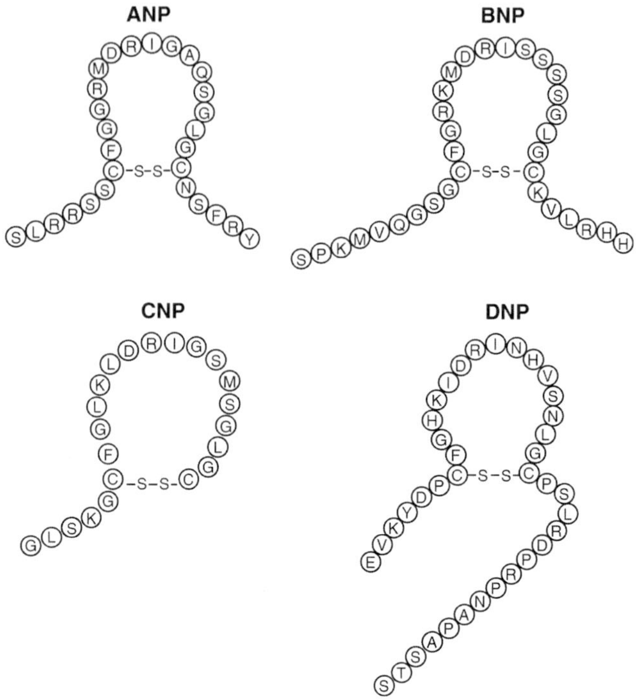

Fig. 4 Peptide chain of natriuretic peptide hormones *ANP*, *BNP*, *CNP*, and *DNP*. The CNH shares the same structure characterized by a cysteine bridge (Data are from Clerico and Emdin (2006), with the permission from the publishers)

employment of NP in the prediction of late CTX and in the early stratification of patients at high risk of cardiac dysfunction (Sandri et al. 2005; Romano et al. 2011). With few exceptions (Dodos et al. 2008; Ekstein et al. 2007), persistently elevated levels of posttreatment BNP and/or NT-proBNP correlate with echocardiographic indexes of myocardial dysfunction in most studies (Soker and Kervancioglu 2005; Sandri et al. 2005; Romano et al. 2011; Roziakova et al. 2012). Data from a retrospective study on 52 patients treated with HDC for aggressive malignancies, in whom a regularly monitoring of diastolic and systolic function was performed, showed the possible predictive role of NT-proBNP (Sandri et al. 2005). Cardiac function was assessed by echo at baseline and at 4 and 12 months after the end of the treatment, while NT-proBNP concentrations were measured in six different times of sampling during and after the CT administration (at baseline, at the end of the infusion, and 12, 24, 36, and 72 h after the end of each CT cycle). According to the changes of NT-proBNP levels, patients were divided into three groups: (i) group A, 32 % of the patients, in which NT-proBNP increased significantly immediately after the end of the infusion, with high concentrations still present at 72 h; (ii) group B, 36 % of the patients, in which NT-proBNP transiently increased after 12–36 h from the end of the treatment but decreased from the baseline to 72 h;

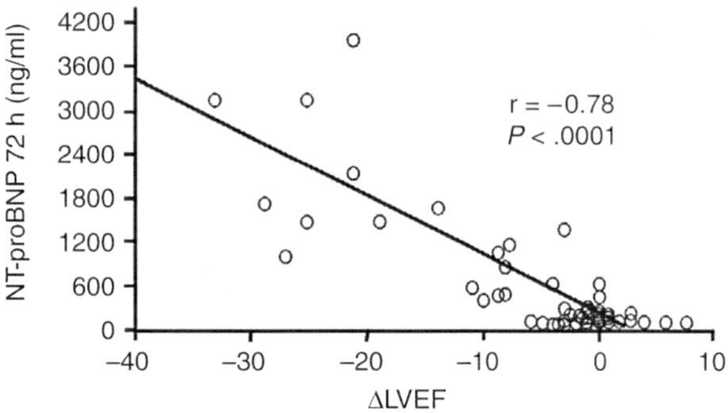

Fig. 5 Scatterplot of NT-proBNP value at 72 h against LVEF changes at 12 months versus baseline (Data are from Cardinale and Sandri (2010), with the permission from the publishers)

and (iii) group C, 32 % of the patients, in which low levels of NT-proBNP were maintained in all the samplings. Patients of group A and of group B did not manifest significant echocardiographic changes during the following months of observation. On the contrary, both diastolic (mitral deceleration time, isovolumetric relaxation time, and mitral E:A ratio) and systolic (LVEF) indexes decreased significantly over time in patients with persistently elevated level of NT-proBNP. In particular, in this group, LVEF was significantly decreased reaching a mean value below 50 % after 12 months. A strong relationship was also found between NT-proBNP value at 72 h and LVEF changes at 12 months versus baseline evaluation (Fig. 5) (Cardinale and Sandri 2010). Another study evaluated the role of NT-proBNP determination in women with breast cancer treated with standard dose of AC (Romano et al. 2011). These patients were followed for 1 year, and in 38 % of them, persistently elevated levels of the marker were found. This finding was associated with a significant decrease of LVEF at 1 year. On the other hand, in a study of 100 adults receiving AC-based chemotherapy and monitored over a period of 1 years (Dodos et al. 2008), 15 patients develop a cardiac event, but among these, none exhibited an alteration of NT-proBNP. Moreover, none of the patients with early NT-proBNP increase developed a systolic dysfunction, and only four patients presented a reduction of E:A ratio during follow-up.

The role of NPs in the patients treated with new targeted agents is less understood. Few studies on small populations, mainly breast cancer patients treated with trastuzumab, have analyzed the information of NP assay in the setting, leading to conflicting results (Perik et al. 2006; Knobloch et al. 2008; Sawaya et al. 2011, 2012; Onitilo et al. 2012). In fact, if some studies have defined NT-proBNP measurement as a promising tool in the management of the patients treated with new therapy (Perik et al. 2006; Knobloch et al. 2008), others have failed to reveal any predictive role of the NT-proBNP (Sawaya et al. 2012; Onitilo et al. 2012). Therefore, further investigation and prospective studies on larger populations are needed to better understand if BNP determination may be a useful approach in the prediction and detection of new treatment-related CTX (Perik et al. 2006; Knobloch et al. 2008). Data available in the literature do not allow to propose a definite conclusion on the possible information provided by natriuretic peptide in the assessment of CT-induced CTX. Different timing of biomarker assessment and specimen collection, insufficient sample size, heterogeneity of the studied population, variability of the treatments and schedules adopted, and different cardiological outcome measured make the comparison of the results of the different study quite difficult. Moreover, important methodological aspects, linked to the diagnostic assays available, need to be clarified too. Although BNP and NT-proBNP originate from a common precursor protein (proBNP), these two molecules show completely different biochemical structure, molecular weight, biological activity, and degradation pathways, making impossible the commutability of the clinical information provided. Furthermore, among BNP methods, there are systematic and wide differences in both analytical performances and the methods are not interchangeable. This highlights that caution must be adopted when NPs are determined with different assays during patient follow-up.

Summary Points

- This chapter focuses on structure, physiologic function, and applications of natriuretic peptides in the oncological setting.
- Natriuretic peptides are hormones secreted from the heart in response to a wall stretch and pressure overload and involved in the maintenance of cardiovascular homeostasis.
- ANP and BNP and their N-terminal counterparts (NT-proANP and NT-proBNP) constitute the system of the cardiac natriuretic peptides.
- The recognition that heart failure and left ventricular dysfunction are pathophysiologically related to changes in a variety of neurohormonal substances led to the hypothesis that NPs evaluation may be useful in the detection of many conditions related to cardiovascular diseases.
- The measurement of circulating BNP and its related peptides is now considered to be a useful marker of myocardial function. Recent international guidelines recommend its use for the diagnosis, risk stratification, and follow-up of patients with chronic or acute heart failure.
- In the last decade, several studies have focused on the survey of the information provided to the measurement of NPs in the detection and, less frequently, in the prediction of cardiotoxicity induced by anticancer drugs.
- With few exceptions, changes in plasma BNP and/or NT-proBNP levels were associated with echocardiographic indices of myocardial dysfunction in most studies.
- To date, few studies are available on the role of NPs in the setting of the targeted therapies; therefore, consistent information on their employment is not possible.
- The development of common definitions of cardiac outcomes, larger sample size with longer follow-up time, and standardization both of sampling time for biomarker measurements and of the commercial diagnostic assays need to be reached to validate the use of NPs in cardioncology.

Key Facts of Natriuretic Peptide

- The natriuretic peptide family includes four principal peptides: ANP, BNP, CNP, and urodilatin. Even though structurally related to the ANP/BNP family, CNP and urodilatin are produced and secreted not by a cardiomyocyte but by other tissues and do not have natriuretic proprieties (Clerico and Emdin 2006).
- Cardiac natriuretic hormones (ANP and BNP) constitute a complex of related peptide with similar peptide chains and analogous degradation pathways as well as physiological effects (Clerico and Emdin 2006).
- Cardiac natriuretic peptides carry out several and important physiological actions. They play an important role in the regulation of electrolytes and water balance through their diuretic and natriuretic effects. They also inhibit the renin-angiotensin-aldosterone system and regulate the permeability of systemic vasculature. In addition, they inhibit the activity of the sympathetic nervous system (Clerico and Emdin 2006).
- The prohormones (proANP and proBNP) produced by cardiomyocytes are split into a biologically active peptide (ANP and BNP) and a longer amino-terminal fragment (NT-proANP and NT-proBNP), which are secreted in the blood in equimolar amounts. However, owing to their longer half-lives, the inactive forms are more stable in the blood and consequently have higher plasma concentrations than the respective free hormones (Clerico and Emdin 2006).
- Recent studies have found significant differences in the analytical characteristics and measured values among the commercially available immonoassays for BNP and NT-proBNP, especially among the immunoassays for BNP measurement. These differences are probably due to (i) cross-reactions against the precursor proBNP and other related peptide share by the immunoassay and (ii) different analytical characteristics and material used by most used commercial platforms.

Potential Application to Prognosis and Other Disease Conditions

Although the evolution of cancer treatments and the prophylactic therapy has changed the prevalence and spectrum of manifesting an adverse event after CT in cancer patients, the prognosis of these patients still remains critical. Cardiopulmonary diseases are the third leading cause of death in children cancer survivors, next only to the development of recurrence and second malignancies, with a death rate of cardiac causes eight to ten times higher than those of age-matched control (Mertens et al. 2001). In adult patients previously treated with CT and RT, the rates of cardiovascular disease and mortality are respectively 15-fold and 7-fold higher than the general population (Cardinale et al. 2002).

In patients with CT-induced cardiotoxicity, the prevention of cardiac damage is strategically more important than any therapeutic interventions aimed at counteracting an already existing damage, which can be frequently progressive and irreversible (Yeh and Bickford 2009; Bird and Swain 2008). According to the

American College of Cardiology and American Heart Association Guidelines, patients receiving CT may be considered a stage A CHF group, namely, those with an increased risk of developing cardiac dysfunction (Bonow et al. 2005).

Therefore, a proper management of the patient undergoing a potentially cardiotoxic chemotherapy treatment should include before starting CT a careful cardiological evaluation by (i) a comprehensive medical history and physical examination to find current signs or history of cardiac CHF, hypertension, diabetes, hyperlipidemia, smoking, obesity, coronary artery disease, valvular heart disease, and prior exposure to AC and to mediastinal radiation and (ii) a standard 12-lead ECG and assessment of LVEF. Cardiovascular risk reduction interventions, treatment optimization of preexistent heart disease, and lifestyle modifications (i.e., smoking cessation, regular exercise, and weight loss) are recommended. If appropriate, treatment of hypertension, diabetes, and hyperlipidemia, by the use of BB and ACEIs, should be started. Optimization of medical therapy for patients with coronary artery disease is essential, and in selected cases, a coronary revascularization could be taken into account. The evaluation of baseline cardiological status may influence the choice of cytotoxic regimen; therefore, a multidisciplinary consultation (oncologist/cardiologist) is always recommended before starting CT (Jones et al. 2009).

Several approaches to reduce the risk of cardiac event due to cardiotoxicity have been proposed, and these include limiting the lifetime cumulative dose, slowing down CT administration, using infusional rather than bolus administration schedule, and using less cardiotoxic structural analogs such as liposomal formulation. However, the use of adjunctive cardioprotective agents and detection of early signs of cardiotoxicity by biomarkers remain the two most promising strategies (Wouters et al. 2005; Cardinale et al. 2008). The benefit of the addition of cardioprotectants (e.g., beta blockers such as carvedilol) to AC treatment was confirmed first in an in vitro study (Spallarossa et al. 2004) and then in a randomized study in which its prophylactic use prevented LV dysfunction and reduced mortality in a small population of patients treated with AC (Kalay et al. 2006). Also the protective effect of nebivolol has been recently demonstrated (Kaya et al. 2013); in 27 patients receiving nebivolol during AC therapy, LVEF and NT-proBNP remained unchanged after 6 months from baseline, conversely, in the placebo group, and significantly lower LVEF and higher NT-proBNP values were observed. Dexrazoxane is an iron-chelating agent that significantly reduces AC-related cardiotoxicity in adults with different solid tumors and in children with acute lymphoblastic leukemia and Ewing's sarcoma (Jones et al. 2007; Lipshultz et al. 2004; Huh et al. 2010). Nevertheless, dexrazoxane is not routinely used in clinical practice, and according to the ASCO guidelines, its use, as a cardioprotectant, is recommended only in patients with metastatic breast cancer who have already received more than 300 mg/m^2 of doxorubicin, because of concerns about potential impact on antitumor efficacy. However, the results of a meta-analysis found no significant difference, in terms of antitumor efficacy or occurrence of secondary malignancies, between patients who were treated with and without dexrazoxane (Wouters et al. 2005; Van Dalen et al. 2011; Tebbi et al. 2007).

A pharmacological preventive approach extended to all cancer patients treated with cardiotoxic chemotherapy has a high cost/benefit ratio and exposes patients to possible adverse effects, including a potential antagonist effect to antitumor activity.

Biomarkers used in cardiology are clearly an important adjunct also in oncology. In a study looking at BNP-guided therapy over the course of treatment for heart failure, cardiologists were assessing the patients so they should be able to figure out symptoms or physical findings (Troughton et al. 2000). Even with this knowledge, the group that had BNP-guided treatment had fewer cardiac events and a better reduction in either heart failure or death during the course of the study.

The employment of cardiac biomarkers as rationale for identifying patients at high risk of developing cardiotoxicity and also the development of tailored preventive strategies directed at reducing the clinical impact of cardiotoxicity are of great interest.

Increasing knowledge about the trend of serum levels of biomarkers during the therapy and in the follow-up could also increase opportunities to begin or to guide a cardioprotective treatment and to improve the prognosis of these patients. Several evidences (Lipshultz et al. 2012; Cardinale et al. 2006; Ederhy et al. 2012) have supported the utility of an associated biomarker-guided clinical decision in patients receiving potentially cardiotoxic therapy.

Specific cardiological treatments could be performed according to two different approaches: (i) in selected cancer patients identified by an increase in these markers during the treatment and (ii) at same time of the CT administration to prevent or blunt the rise of these markers or interfere with their persistence after first increase.

A larger randomized placebo-controlled study compared patients who received doxorubicin alone versus children who receive doxorubicin in association with dexrazoxane (Lipshultz et al. 2004). Serial measurements of cTnT have showed, in the dexrazoxane group, fewer elevation of the marker compared with the control group (50 % vs. 21 %, respectively; $P < 0.001$), even if no difference in cardiac function by means of echocardiography at time of therapy completion was registered. In a small randomized study including 49 patients free of cardiovascular diseases and affected by a variety of solid cancers, the possible role of telmisartan in preventing myocardial damage induced by epirubicin was investigated (Cadeddu et al. 2010). The 25 patients treated with telmisartan 1 week before CT compared to the 24 patients receiving only epirubicin showed no significant reductions in myocardial deformation parameters (peak strain rate) as evaluated by using tissue Doppler echocardiogram or any significant increase in reactive oxygen species or in interleukin-6.

The usefulness of biomarkers in the screening setting for the selection of patients requiring prophylactic cardioprotective therapy was investigated in a randomized, controlled trial on 473 patients treated with HDC (Cardinale et al. 2006). The cardioprotective effects of enalapril were evaluated. In 58 of 114 patients with an early TnI increase, enalapril was initiated 1 month after the completion of CT, titrated at the maximal tolerated dose, and continued for 1 year. In the enalapril-treated group, significant reduction in cardiotoxicity was observed without any change of LVEF during the follow-up period. Conversely, 25 of 58 patients in the placebo control group had a progressive reduction in LVEF and an increase in end-diastolic and end-systolic volumes. Moreover, a significantly lower incidence of adverse cardiac events at a 1-year follow-up was found in enalapril-treated patients than in controls (2 % vs. 52 %; $P < 0.001$).

Although the use of ACEIs and BB have proven to be effective in the managing of CTX and in the prevention of the LVEF reduction and late cardiac event, the limited data and the concern in using these medications in cancer patients influence their employment as first-line therapy only in symptomatic patients.

Summary Points

- This chapter focuses on approaches to reduce the risk of a CT-induced cardiac damage.
- The best treatment of CTX is prevention. A proper management of cancer patients receiving cardiotoxic therapy should provide before starting CT a careful cardiological evaluation and the treatment of existing comorbidities.
- A cooperative working group (between cardiologists and oncologists) should be recommended.
- Limiting the lifetime cumulative dose, administering CT via infusion rather than as a bolus dose, and using structural analogs are all possible strategies to maximize the beneficial effects of CT decreasing or preventing their cardiotoxic effects.
- Another approach is the use of cardioprotective agents in conjunction with cancer treatment. A number of different classes of agents have been evaluated for their cardioprotective activity with varying degrees of success.
- The most promising and commonly used agents are ACE inhibitors, beta blockers, and dexrazoxane. However, owing to the fear of interference with the antitumor efficacy of AC and facilitation of the occurrence of secondary malignancies (as well as by its possible myelosuppressive effect), the ASCO recommends the use dexrazoxane only in patients treated from metastatic disease who have received a cumulative dose of doxorubicin ≥ 300 mg/m^2.
- Extending a pharmacological preventive approach to all cancer patients treated with cardiotoxic CT has a high cost/benefit ratio. There are growing evidences that support the employment of cardiac biomarkers as rationale for the beginning of a preventive strategy and for reducing the clinical impact of CTX.
- A cardioprotectant treatment could be performed (a) in addition to the CT administration to prevent or blunt the rise of these markers or interfere with their persistence after first increase (b) only in selected patients identified by an increase of the marker during CT.

Key Facts of Potential Application to Prognosis and Other Disease Conditions

- Although restraining the dose has been one primary strategy to decrease cardiotoxic effects, this approach is limited by the eventual reduction in treatment efficacy. In addition, this strategy does not consider patients still at risk after receiving limiting doses or patients at increased risk as a result of their cardiac history.
- Carvedilol is a beta blocker with α1-blocking vasodilatory properties. It has also shown strong antioxidant activity that gives it a cardioprotective effect against doxorubicin (Wouters et al. 2005).
- Other chemical agents, such as coenzyme Q10, carnitine, *N*-acetylcysteine, the antioxidant vitamins E and C, erythropoietin, the endothelin-1 receptor antagonist bosentan, the lipid-lowering agents probucol and statins, and iron-chelating agents (deferoxamine and ethylenediaminetetraacetic acid), have been evaluated as cardioprotectants with promising results. However, although preliminary findings found that all these agents may have cardioprotective effects, their utility in preventing CTX needs to be confirmed by further investigation (Wouters et al. 2005; Van Dalen et al. 2011).

References

American Cancer Society. Cancer facts & figures 2010. www.cancerfactsfigures/cancerfactsfigures/cancerfacts-and-figures-2010

Auner HW, Tinchon C, Linkesch W, et al. Prolonged monitoring of troponin T for the detection of anthracycline cardiotoxicity in adults with hematological malignancies. Ann Hematol. 2003;82:218–22.

Barrett-Lee PJ, Dixon JM, Farrell C, et al. Expert opinion on the use of anthracyclines in patients with advanced breast cancer at cardiac risk. Ann Oncol. 2009;20:816–27.

Barry E, Alvarez JA, Scully RE, et al. Anthracycline-induced cardiotoxicity: course, pathophysiology, prevention and management. Expert Opin Pharmacother. 2007;8:1039–58.

Bird BR, Swain SM. Cardiac toxicity in breast cancer survivors: review of potential cardiac problems. Clin Cancer Res. 2008;14:14–24.

Bonow RO, Bennett S, Casey Jr DE, American College of Cardiology, American Heart Association Task Force on Performance Measures, Heart Failure Society of America, et al. ACC/AHA clinical performance measures for adults with chronic heart failure: a report of the American College of Cardiology/American Heart Association Task Force on Performance Measures (Writing Committee to Develop Heart Failure Clinical Performance Measures): endorsed by the Heart Failure Society of America. Circulation. 2005;112:1853–87.

Bovelli D, Plataniotis G, Roila F, ESMO Guidelines Working Group. Cardiotoxicity of chemotherapeutic agents and radiotherapy-related heart disease: ESMO Clinical Practice Guidelines. Ann Oncol. 2010;21 Suppl 5:277–82.

Bristow MR, Mason JW, Billingham ME, et al. Dose-effect and structure-function relationship in doxorubicin cardiomyopathy. Am Heart J. 1981;102:709–18.

Cadeddu C, Piras A, Mantovani G, et al. Protective effects of the angiotensin II receptor blocker telmisartan on epirubicin-induced inflammation, oxidative stress, and early ventricular impairment. Am Heart J. 2010;160:487.e1–7.

Cardinale D, Sandri MT. Role of biomarkers in chemotherapy-induced cardiotoxicity. Prog Cardiovasc Dis. 2010;53:121–9.

Cardinale D, Sandri MT, Martinoni A, et al. Left ventricular dysfunction predicted by early troponin I release after high-dose chemotherapy. J Am Coll Cardiol. 2000;36:517–22.

Cardinale D, Sandri MT, Martinoni A, et al. Myocardial injury revealed by plasma troponin I in breast cancer treated with high-dose chemotherapy. Ann Oncol. 2002;13:710–5.

Cardinale D, Sandri MT, Colombo A, et al. Prognostic value of Troponin I in cardiac risk stratification of cancer patients undergoing high-dose chemotherapy. Circulation. 2004;109:2749–54.

Cardinale D, Colombo A, Sandri MT, et al. Prevention of high-dose chemotherapy- induced cardiotoxicity in high-risk patients by angiotensin-converting enzyme inhibition. Circulation. 2006;114:2474–81.

Cardinale D, Colombo A, Cipolla CM. Prevention and treatment of cardiomyopathy and heart failure in patients receiving cancer chemotherapy. Curr Treat Options Cardiovasc Med. 2008;10:486–95.

Cardinale D, Colombo A, Torrisi R, et al. Trastuzumab-induced cardiotoxicity: clinical and prognostic implications of troponin I evaluation. J Clin Oncol. 2010;28:3910–6.

Cardinale D, Bacchiani G, Beggiato M, et al. Strategies to prevent and treat cardiovascular risk in cancer patients. Semin Oncol. 2013;40:186–98.

Cheitlin MD, Armstrong WF, Aurigemma GP, et al. ACC/AHA/ASE 2003 guideline update for the clinical application of echocardiography: summary article: a report of the American College of Cardiology/American Heart Association Task Force on Practice Guidelines (ACC/AHA/ASE Committee to Update the 1997 Guidelines for the Clinical Application of Echocardiography). Circulation. 2003;108:1146–62.

Choueiri TK, Schutz FA, Je Y, et al. Risk of arterial thromboembolic events with sunitinib and sorafenib: a systematic review and meta-analysis of clinical trials. J Clin Oncol. 2010;28:2280–5.

Choueiri TK, Mayer EL, Je Y, et al. Congestive heart failure risk in patients with breast cancer treated with bevacizumab. J Clin Oncol. 2011;29:632–8.

Clerico A, Emdin M. Natriuretic peptides. The hormones of the heart. Berlin: Springer; 2006.

Criscitello C, Metzger-Filho O, Saini KS, et al. Targeted therapies in breast cancer: are heart and vessels also being targeted? Breast Cancer Res. 2012;14:209.

Curigliano G, Cardinale D, Suter T, et al. Cardiovascular toxicity induced by chemotherapy, targeted agents and radiotherapy: ESMO Clinical Practice Guidelines. Ann Oncol. 2012;23 Suppl 7:155–66.

Dodos F, Halbsguth T, Erdmann E, et al. Usefulness of myocardial performance index and biochemical markers for early detection of anthracycline-induced cardiotoxicity in adults. Clin Res Cardiol. 2008;97:318–26.

Dolci A, Dominici R, Cardinale D, et al. Biochemical markers for prediction of chemotherapy-induced cardiotoxicity: systematic review of the literature and recommendations for use. Am J Clin Pathol. 2008;130:688–95.

Du XL, Xia R, Liu CC, et al. Cardiac toxicity associated with anthracycline-containing chemotherapy in older women with breast cancer. Cancer. 2009;115:5296–308.

Ederhy S, Massard C, Dufaitre G, et al. Frequency and management of troponin I elevation in patients treated with molecular targeted therapies in phase I trials. Invest New Drugs. 2012;30:611–5.

Ekstein S, Nir A, Rein AJ, et al. N-terminal-proB-type natriuretic peptide as a marker for acute anthracycline cardiotoxicity in children. J Pediatr Hematol Oncol. 2007;29:440–4.

Eschenhagen T, Force T, Ewer MS, et al. Cardiovascular side effects of cancer therapies: a position statement from the Heart Failure Association of the European Society of Cardiology. Eur J Heart Fail. 2011;13:1–10.

Ewer MS, Lippman SM. Type II chemotherapy-related cardiac dysfunction: time to recognize a new entity. J Clin Oncol. 2005;23:2900–2.

Gianni L, Herman EH, Lipshultz SE, et al. Anthracycline cardiotoxicity: from bench to bedside. J Clin Oncol. 2008;26:3777–84.

Hayes DF, Picard MH. Heart of darkness: the downside of trastuzumab. J Clin Oncol. 2006;24:4056–8.

Herman EH, Zhang J, Lipshultz SE, et al. Correlation between serum levels of cardiac troponin-T and the severity of the chronic cardiomyopathy induced by doxorubicin. J Clin Oncol. 1999;17:2237–43.

Hershman DL, McBride RB, Eisenberger A, et al. Doxorubicin, cardiac risk factors, and cardiac toxicity in elderly patients with diffuse B-cell non-Hodgkin's lymphoma. J Clin Oncol. 2008;26:3159–65.

Huh WW, Jaffe N, Durand JB, et al. Comparison of doxorubicin cardiotoxicity in pediatric sarcoma patients when given with dexrazoxane versus continuous infusion. Pediatr Hematol Oncol. 2010;27:546–57.

Hull MC, Morris CG, Pepine CJ, et al. Valvular dysfunction and carotid, subclavian, and coronary artery disease in survivors of Hodgkin lymphoma treated with radiation therapy. JAMA. 2003;290:2831–7.

Jones LW, Haykowsky MJ, Swartz JJ, et al. Early breast cancer therapy and cardiovascular injury. J Am Coll Cardiol. 2007;50:1435–41.

Jones AL, Barlow M, Barrett-Lee PJ, et al. Management of cardiac health in trastuzumab-treated patients with breast cancer: updated United Kingdom National Cancer Research Institute recommendations for monitoring. Br J Cancer. 2009;100:684–92.

Kalay N, Basar E, Ozdogru I, et al. Protective effects of carvedilol against anthracyclines induced cardiomyopathy. J Am Coll Cardiol. 2006;48:2258–62.

Kalyanaraman B, Joseph J, Kalivendi S, et al. Doxorubicin-induced apoptosis: implications in cardiotoxicity. Mol Cell Biochem. 2002;234–235:119–24.

Kaya MG, Ozkan M, Gunebakmaz O, et al. Protective effects of nebivolol against anthracycline-induced cardiomyopathy: a randomized control study. Int J Cardiol. 2013;167:2306–10.

Kilickap S, Barista I, Akgul E, et al. cTnT can be a useful marker for early detection of anthracycline cardiotoxicity. Ann Oncol. 2005;16:798–804.

Kismet E, Varan A, Ayabakan C, et al. Serum troponin T levels and echocardiographic evaluation in children treated with doxorubicin. Pediatr Blood Cancer. 2004;42:220–4.

Knobloch K, Tepe J, Lichtinghagen R, et al. Simultaneous hemodynamic and serological cardiotoxicity monitoring during immunotherapy with trastuzumab. Int J Cardiol. 2008;125:113–5.

Lipshultz SE, Lipsitz SR, Mone SR, et al. Female sex and drug dose as risk factors for late cardiotoxic effects of doxorubicin therapy for childhood cancer. N Engl J Med. 1995;332:1738–43.

Lipshultz SE, Rifai N, Sallan SE, et al. Predictive value of cardiac troponin T in pediatric patients at risk for myocardial injury. Circulation. 1997;96:2641–8.

Lipshultz SE, Rifai N, Dalton VM, et al. The effects of dexrazoxane on myocardial injury in doxorubicin-treated children with acute lymphoblastic leukemia. N Engl J Med. 2004;351:1451–2.

Lipshultz SE, Miller TL, Scully RE, et al. Changes in cardiac biomarkers during doxorubicin treatment of pediatric patients with high-risk acute lymphoblastic leukemia: associations with long-term echocardiographic outcomes. J Clin Oncol. 2012;30:1042–9.

Mahajan VS, Jarolim P. How to interpret elevated cardiac troponin levels. Circulation. 2011;124:2350–4.

Meinardi MT, van der Graaf WT, van Veldhuisen DJ, et al. Detection of anthracycline-induced cardiotoxicity. Cancer Treat Rev. 1999;25:237–47.

Mertens AC, Yasui Y, Neglia JP, et al. Late mortality experience in five-year survivors of childhood and adolescent cancer: the Childhood Cancer Survivor Study. J Clin Oncol. 2001;19:3163–72.

Newby LK, Jesse RL, Babb JD, et al. ACCF 2012 expert consensus document on practical clinical considerations in the interpretation of troponin elevations: a report of the American College of Cardiology Foundation Task Force on Clinical Expert Consensus Documents. J Am Coll Cardiol. 2012;60:2427–63.

Onitilo AA, Engel JM, Stankowski RV, et al. High-sensitivity C-reactive protein (hs-CRP) as a biomarker for trastuzumab-induced cardiotoxicity in HER2-positive early-stage breast cancer: a pilot study. Breast Cancer Res Treat. 2012;134:291–8.

Perik PJ, Lub-De Hooge MN, Gietema JA, et al. Indium-111-labeled trastuzumab scintigraphy in patients with human epidermal growth factor receptor 2-positive metastatic breast cancer. J Clin Oncol. 2006;24:2276–82.

Richards CJ, Je Y, Schutz FA, et al. Incidence and risk of congestive heart failure in patients with renal and nonrenal cell carcinoma treated with sunitinib. J Clin Oncol. 2011;29:3450–6.

Romano S, Fratini S, Ricevuto E, et al. Serial measurements of NT-proBNP are predictive of not-high-dose anthracycline cardiotoxicity in breast cancer patients. Br J Cancer. 2011;105:1663–8.

Roziakova L, Bojtarova E, Mistrik M, et al. Serial measurements of cardiac biomarkers in patients after allogeneic hematopoietic stem cell transplantation. J Exp Clin Cancer Res. 2012;31:13.

Salmon DJ, Leyland-Jones B, Shak S, et al. Use of chemotherapy plus monoclonal antibody against HER2 for metastatic breast cancer that overexpresses HER2. N Engl J Med. 2001;344:783–92.

Sandri MT, Cardinale D, Zorzino L, et al. Minor increases in plasma troponin I predict decreased left ventricular ejection fraction after high-dose chemotherapy. Clin Chem. 2003;49:248–52.

Sandri MT, Salvatici M, Cardinale D, et al. N-terminal pro-B-type natriuretic peptide after high-dose chemotherapy: a marker predictive of cardiac dysfunction? Clin Chem. 2005;51:1405–10.

Sawaya H, Sebag IA, Plana JC, et al. Early detection and predictor of cardiotoxicity in chemotherapy-treated patients. Am J Cardiol. 2011;9:1375–80.

Sawaya H, Sebag IA, Plana JC, et al. Assessment of echocardiography and biomarkers for the extended prediction of cardiotoxicity in patients treated with anthracyclines, taxanes, and trastuzumab. Circ Cardiovasc Imaging. 2012;5:596–603.

Schmidinger M, Zielinski CC, Vogl UM, et al. Cardiac toxicity of sunitinib and sorafenib in patients with metastatic renal cell carcinoma. J Clin Oncol. 2008;26:5204–12.

Seidman A, Hudis C, Pierri MK, et al. Cardiac dysfunction in the trastuzumab clinical trial experience. J Clin Oncol. 2002;20:1215–21.

Shapiro CL, Haedenbergh PH, Gelman R, et al. Cardiac effects of adjuvant doxorubicin and radiation therapy in breast cancer patients. J Clin Oncol. 1998;16:3493–501.

Shave R, Baggish A, George K, et al. Exercise-induced cardiac troponin elevation: evidence, mechanisms, and implications. J Am Coll Cardiol. 2010;56:169–176.

Soker M, Kervancioglu M. Plasma concentrations of NT-pro-BNP and cardiac troponin-I in relation to doxorubicin-induced cardiomyopathy and cardiac function in childhood malignancy. Saudi Med J. 2005;26:1197–202.

Spallarossa P, Garibaldi S, Altieri P, et al. Carvedilol prevents doxorubicin-induced free radical release and apoptosis in cardiomyocytes in vitro. J Mol Cell Cardiol. 2004;37:837–46.

Specchia G, Buquicchio C, Pansini N, et al. Monitoring of cardiac function on the basis of serum troponin I levels in patients with acute leukemia treated with anthracyclines. J Lab Clin Med. 2005;145:212–20.

Suter TM, Ewer MS. Cancer drugs and the heart: importance and management. Eur Heart J. 2013;34:1102–1111.

Suzuki T, Hayashi D, Yamazaki T, et al. Elevated B-type natriuretic peptide levels after anthracycline administration. Am Heart J. 1998;136:362–3.

Swain SM, Whaley FS, Ewer MS. Congestive heart failure in patients treated with doxorubicin: a retrospective analysis of three trials. Cancer. 2003;97:2869–79.

Tarantini L, Cioffi G, Gori S, et al. Trastuzumab adjuvant chemotherapy and cardiotoxicity in real-world women with breast cancer. J Card Fail. 2012;18:113–9.

Tebbi CK, London WB, Friedman D, et al. Dexrazoxane-associated risk for acute myeloid leukemia/myelodysplastic syndrome and other secondary malignancies in pediatric Hodgkin's disease. J Clin Oncol. 2007;25:493–500.

Troughton RW, Frampton CM, Yandle T, et al. Treatment of heart failure guided by plasma aminoterminal brain natriuretic peptide (N-BNP) concentrations. Lancet. 2000;355:1126–30.

Van Dalen EC, Caron HN, Dickinson HO, et al. Cardioprotective interventions for cancer patients receiving anthracyclines. Cochrane Database Syst Rev. 2011;6:CD003917.

Vogel CL, Cobleigh MA, Tripathy D, et al. Efficacy and safety of trastuzumab as a single agent in first-line treatment of HER2-overexpressing metastatic breast cancer. J Clin Oncol. 2002;20:719–26.

Wouters KA, Kremer LCM, Miller TL, et al. Protecting against anthracycline-induced myocardial damage: a review of the most promising strategies. Br J Haematol. 2005;131:561–78.

Yeh ET, Bickford CL. Cardiovascular complications of cancer therapy: incidence, pathogenesis, diagnosis, and management. J Am Coll Cardiol. 2009;53:2231–47.

Zhang S, Liu X, Bawa-Khalfe T, et al. Identification of the molecular basis of doxorubicin-induced cardiotoxicity. Nat Med. 2012;18:1639–42.

DNA Methylation as a Biomarker in Cancer

5

Shinichi Fukushige and Akira Horii

Contents

S. Fukushige (✉)
Department of Molecular Pathology, Center for Regulatory Epigenome and Diseases, Tohoku University School of Medicine, Sendai, Miyagi, Japan
e-mail: fukushige@med.tohoku.ac.jp

A. Horii
Department of Molecular Pathology, Tohoku University School of Medicine, Sendai, Miyagi, Japan
e-mail: horii@med.tohoku.ac.jp

V.R. Preedy, V.B. Patel (eds.), *Biomarkers in Cancer, Biomarkers in Disease: Methods, Discoveries and Applications*,
DOI 10.1007/978-94-007-7681-4_45

Abstract

DNA methylation alteration is one of the most prominent epigenetic changes in cancer. Because DNA originated from cancer cells is a stable molecule that is easily detectable in clinical specimens such as blood, sputum, urine, and stool, DNA methylation alterations in tumorigeneses have become one of the promising candidate biomarkers for early detection, prognosis, therapeutic response prediction, and recurrence monitoring in cancer patients. Recent development of technologies has allowed global genome-wide DNA methylation analysis in normal as well as in cancer cells and has provided extensive information for candidate biomarkers. Herein we summarize the features of DNA methylation in cancer, their suitability as DNA methylation biomarkers in comparison with others, and their status in applications of DNA methylation biomarkers in cancer. The research field of DNA methylation biomarking is evolving rapidly with promising results that have the potential to confer enormous benefits for cancer patients in the future.

List of Abbreviations

5-Aza-CdR	5-Aza-2′-Deoxycytidine
5-Aza-CR	5-Azacytidine
5caC	5-Carboxylcytosine
5fC	5-Formylcytosine
5-FU	5-Fluorouracil
5hmC	5-Hydroxymethylcytosine
5mC	5-Methylcytosine
ACF	Aberrant Crypt Foci
ALX1	ALX Homeobox 1
APC	Adenomatous Polyposis Coli
BRCA1	Breast Cancer 1
C-CIMP	Colorectal Cancer CIMP
CDKN2A	Cyclin-Dependent Kinase Inhibitor 2A
CGI	CpG Island
CIMP	CpG Island Methylator Phenotype
CIMP-H	CIMP-High
CIMP-L	CIMP-Low
CK1α	Casein Kinase 1α
DKO	Double Knockout
DNMT	DNA Methyltransferase
G-CIMP	Glioblastoma CIMP
GSK3	Glycogen Synthase Kinase 3
GSTP1	Glutathione S-Transferase Pi 1
HIST1H4F	Histone Cluster 1 H4f
HOXA9	Homeobox A9
HR	Hazard Ratio
HRAS	Harvey Rat Sarcoma Viral Oncogene Homologue
IDH	Isocitrate Dehydrogenase

IGF2	Insulin-like Growth Factor 2
IHEC	International Human Epigenome Consortium
LAD	Lamin-Associated Domain
LEF	Lymphoid Enhancer-Binding Factor
LINE-1	Long Interspersed Nuclear Element-1
LOCK	Large Organized Chromatin Lysine Modification
LOI	Loss of Imprinting
LRES	Long-Range Epigenetic Silencing
MAGE	Melanoma-Associated Antigen
MAP	Methyl-Binding Domain Affinity Purification
MBD	Methyl-CpG-Binding Domain
MeDIP	Methyl-DNA Immunoprecipitation
MeTA	Methyl-CpG Targeted Transcriptional Activation
MGMT	O^6-Methylguanine-DNA Methyltransferase
MLH1	MutL Homologue 1
MSP	Methylation-Specific PCR
NPBWR1	Neuropeptides B/W Receptor 1
NSCLC	Non-small Cell Lung Cancer
oxBS-seq	Oxidative Bisulfite Sequencing
PCDHGB6	Protocadherin Gamma Subfamily B, 6
PcG	Polycomb Group Protein
PCR	Polymerase Chain Reaction
PSA	Prostate-Specific Antigen
RB1	Retinoblastoma 1
RFS	Relapse-Free Survival
ROS	Reactive Oxygen Species
SAM	*S*-Adenosylmethionine
$SCF^{\beta\text{-TrCP}}$	SKP1-Cullin 1-F-Box
SFRP	Secreted Frizzled-Related Protein
SMRT-seq	Single-Molecule Real-Time Sequencing
TAB-seq	TET-Assisted Bisulfite Sequencing
TCF	T-Cell Factor
tDMR	Tissue-Specific Differentially Methylated Region
TET	Ten Eleven Translocation
α-KG	α-Ketoglutarate

Key Facts

Key Facts of DNMT: DNA Methyltransferase

- About 70 % of the CpG dinucleotides in the human genome are chemically modified by the covalent attachment of a methyl group to the C5 position of the cytosine ring.

- DNMTs are responsible for DNA methylation reaction.
- The *de novo* methyltransferases DNMT3A and DNMT3B are mainly responsible for introducing cytosine methylation at previously unmethylated CpG dinucleotides.
- On the other hand, the maintenance methyltransferase DNMT1 copies the parental-strand methylation patterns onto the progeny DNA strand.
- DNA methylation is essential for normal mouse development, because targeted disruption of Dnmt1 or Dnmt3b results in embryonic lethality in mice, and homozygous Dnmt3a knockout mice die at about 4 weeks of age.
- Mutations of human *DNMT3B* gene cause immunodeficiency, centromeric instability, and facial anomalies (ICF) syndrome.

Key Facts of CGIs: CpG Islands

- The human genome is punctuated by non-methylated DNA sequences that contain a high density of CpG dinucleotides termed CpG islands (CGIs).
- CGIs are approximately 1-kb in length and overlap the promoter regions of 60–70 % of human genes.
- CGIs were first identified by digestion of genomic DNA using the methyl-CpG-sensitive restriction enzyme *Hpa*II, and thus it was called HTF (*Hpa*II tiny fragment) islands.
- CGI was initially defined as a region with greater than 50 % G + C content, a length of greater than 200-bp, and greater than 0.6 CpG frequency (observed/expected).
- Then the stringency has been increased to 55 % or more of the G + C content, a length of 500 bp or more, and 0.65 or higher CpG frequency to exclude the vast majority of contaminating *Alu* elements.
- Hypermethylation of CGIs is a common event in carcinogenesis, and the transcriptional silencing of tumor-suppressor genes by promoter CGI hypermethylation can contribute to oncogenesis.

Key Facts of MBD Proteins: Methyl-CpG-Binding-Domain Proteins

- MBD proteins specifically recognize methyl-CpG sequences through the methyl-CpG-binding domain (MBD) consisting of about 80 amino acid residues.
- The mammalian MBD proteins consist of five members named MBD1, MBD2, MBD3, MBD4, and MeCP2.
- MBD proteins recruit transcriptional corepressors through transcriptional repression domain (TRD) to silence transcription.
- MBD2 and MeCP2 are involved in histone deacetylase-dependent repression, whereas MBD1 interacts with the histone H3 lysine 9 (H3K9) methyltransferase SETDB1 and provides a link between DNA methylation and chromatin remodeling and modification.

- Mutations in the human *MECP2* gene cause Rett syndrome, a debilitating neurological disease that affects ~1 in 10,000 female live births.
- MBD4 contains a C-terminal DNA glycosylase catalytic domain in addition to an N-terminal MBD, and thus, it has been thought to be involved in DNA repair.

Definitions of Words and Terms

CpG Islands (CGIs) A region that contains a high density of CpG dinucleotides in the genome and is located at the promoters of many genes.

CpG Island Methylator Phenotype (CIMP) A distinct trait exhibiting concordant tumor-specific DNA methylation.

CpG Island Shore (CGI Shore) The region up to 2 kb from the CpG island and the location of most cancer-specific and tissue-specific differentially methylated regions.

DNA Demethylating Agents Drugs that induce DNA demethylation by inhibiting DNA methyltransferases. Cytidine analogs such as 5-azacytidine and 5-aza-2-′-deoxycytidine are the most commonly used demethylating agents. They are used in the treatment of myelodysplastic syndrome (MDS).

DNA Hypermethylation An increased level of DNA methylation in a DNA sample relative to a reference DNA sample.

DNA Hypomethylation A decreased level of DNA methylation in a DNA sample relative to a reference DNA sample.

DNA Methylation Biomarker A molecular target that undergoes DNA methylation changes in tumorigenesis. It is useful for early detection, prognosis, therapeutic response prediction, and recurrence monitoring in cancer patients.

Driver Gene Mutation A mutation that confers a selective growth advantage to the cell.

Epigenetic Alteration Changes in gene expression or cellular phenotype caused by mechanisms other than changes in the DNA sequence.

Lamin-Associated Domains (LADs) Large genomic regions that specifically associate with lamina, an inner nuclear membrane-associated protein. They are often positioned at the nuclear periphery and are usually linked to transcriptional repression.

Large Organized Chromatin Lysine Modifications (LOCKs) Large genomic regions that are enriched for heterochromatin posttranslational modifications, such as histone H3 lysine 9 dimethylation (H3K9me2). They expand during differentiation and are lost in cancer.

Long-Range Epigenetic Silencing (LRES) Transcriptional lockdown spanning large chromosomal domains and resulting in the coordinate silencing of numerous genes.

Loss of Imprinting (LOI) Loss of the parental allele-specific expression in cancer of imprinted genes, first observed for insulin-like growth factor 2 (*IGF2*) in embryonal tumors of childhood, such as Wilms' tumor.

Methyl-CpG-Binding Domain (MBD) A conserved domain consisting of about 80 amino acid residues that recognizes and binds to methylated DNAs.

Methylation-Specific PCR (MSP) A method for analysis of DNA methylation status in CpG islands. The assay requires initial DNA modification by sodium bisulfite, converting unmethylated, but not methylated, cytosines to uracil, and subsequent amplification with primers specific for methylated versus unmethylated DNA.

Tissue-Specific Differentially Methylated Regions (tDMRs) Differentially methylated regions that distinguish normal tissues from each other.

Introduction

Cancer is caused by the accumulation of a series of alterations of relevant genes that drive a selective growth advantage. Driver genes can be classified into 12 signaling pathways that regulate three core cellular processes: cell fate, cell survival, and genome maintenance (Vogelstein et al. 2013). Genomic alterations that include single-base substitution, insertion, deletion, amplification, and translocation are particularly well suited to be vehicles of persistent phenotypic change. For this reason, cancer has traditionally been viewed as a set of diseases based principally on genetics (Hanahan and Weinberg 2011). For example, colorectal cancers have been thought to evolve from normal cells to premalignant foci, to localized lesions, to invasive tumors, and to metastatic lesions by acquiring a series of mutations over time. The indirect support for the requirement of multiple mutations for clinically detectable cancers is the age dependency of most adult human cancers. Notably, the incidence of some adult cancers increases with the sixth power of age, suggesting that human cancers require six sequential rate-limiting events to produce a clinically apparent tumor (Armitage and Doll 1954). Recent comprehensive sequencing efforts have revealed that the number of mutated driver genes is often three to six in common adult tumors such as pancreatic, colorectal, breast, and brain cancers, although some tumors have only one or two driver gene mutations (Vogelstein et al. 2013). This obvious difference in numbers of driver gene mutations may be explained by epigenetic alterations, including DNA methylation and histone modification. In fact, loss of proper gene function in human cancer can occur through both genetic and epigenetic mechanisms (Herman and Baylin 2003). A recent study of colorectal cancers showed that more than 10 % of the protein-coding genes were differentially methylated when compared with normal colorectal epithelial cells (Beggs et al. 2013). Some of these epigenetic changes in driver genes are likely to provide a selective growth advantage (Feinberg and Tycko 2004). For example, DNA methylation in gene promoter regions of cyclin-dependent kinase inhibitor 2A (*CDKN2A*, also known as *p16*) and mutL homologue 1 (*MLH1*) is much more common than mutational inactivation of either of these two driver genes (Beggs et al. 2013).

In addition to the above information, we now know that it takes decades to develop cancer and that the incurable stage, metastasis, occurs only a few years before death (Jones et al. 2008). That means that the vast majority of cancer patients would not die if their cancers were detected in the first 90 % of the cancers' lifetimes and were removed by proper surgical therapies. This knowledge encourages us to detect genetic and epigenetic changes as early as possible in relevant body fluids such as urine for genitourinary cancers, sputum for lung cancers, stool for gastrointestinal cancers, and plasma/serum for all types of cancers. Of these genetic and epigenetic changes, DNA methylation changes in cancer have great potential for early detection and prevention, as well as for prediction in prognosis and drug sensitivity to therapy (Fukushige and Horii 2013). We believe that cancer deaths can be extensively reduced if greater efforts are made in DNA methylation biomarker research. Thus, we introduce DNA methylation biomarkers in this chapter.

DNA Methylation in Normal Cells

DNA methylation in the mammalian genome occurs after DNA synthesis by enzymatic transfer of a methyl group from the universal methyl donor, *S*-adenosylmethionine (SAM), to the 5 position of cytosine residues (Fig. 1). This modification is imposed only on cytosines that precede a guanosine in the DNA sequence (CpG dinucleotide). DNA methyltransferases (DNMTs) are responsible for this enzymatic reaction and are essential for mammalian development. DNA methylation is established by the activity of the *de novo* DNMTs, DNMT3A and DNMT3B, and is subsequently inherited after DNA replication and primarily owing to the activity of the maintenance DNMT, DNMT1, with the help of both DNMT3A and DNMT3B (Jones and Liang 2009). The CpG dinucleotide varies greatly in methylation status throughout the genome, but little is known about the mechanisms that underlie this methylation pattern. A recent study indicated that DNA methylation patterns are guided in part by primary DNA sequence context and that transcription factors play important roles in this process (Lienert et al. 2011). In the human genome, 70–80 %

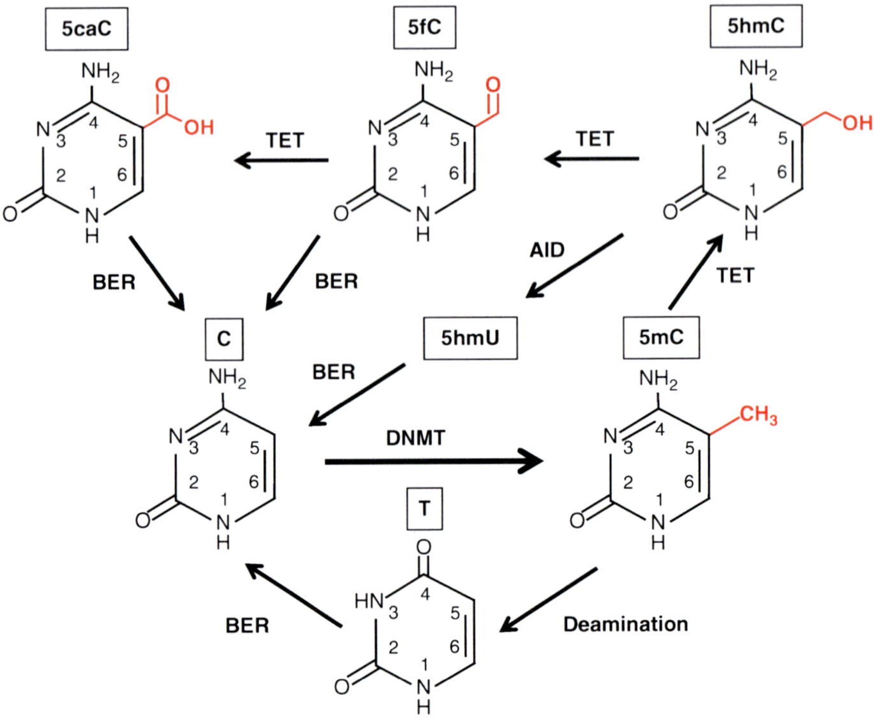

Fig. 1 DNA methylation and demethylation. The process of DNA methylation is carried out by DNA methyltransferases (DNMTs). These enzymes catalyze the covalent addition of a methyl group from a donor *S*-adenosylmethionine to the 5′ position of the cytosine ring, predominantly within the CpG dinucleotide. TET family proteins catalyze 5mC oxidation to 5hmC. 5hmC can be further oxidized by TET proteins to produce 5fC and 5caC, and the latter may be recognized and excised by thymine DNA glycosylase (TDG) to generate cytosine. Alternatively, 5hmC may be further deaminated to become 5hmU by activation-induced cytidine deaminase (AID). 5hmU in turn can be converted to cytosine following base excision repair (BER) pathway-mediated demethylation. It remains unknown whether there are decarboxylases or deformylases that can remove the modification directly. 5mC and its oxidative derivatives may undergo passive demethylation during DNA replication. 5mC is also spontaneously deaminated to thymine (T), resulting in a G/T mismatch which, in turn, is processed by the BER pathway. If this mismatch is not repaired, a C to T change remains.

of all CpG dinucleotides are heavily methylated. As a result, the overall frequency of CpGs is substantially less than what would be expected, because spontaneous hydrolytic deamination of 5-methylcytosine (5mC) residues gives rise to T residues (Fig. 1) (Bird 2002). The globally methylated, CpG-poor genomic landscape is punctuated, however, by short regions with unmethylated CpGs occurring at higher density, forming distinct islands in the genome (Fig. 2) (Bird et al. 1985). These so-called CpG islands (CGIs) are protected from DNA methylation in part by guanine-cytosine (GC) strand asymmetry and accompanying R-loop formation and possibly by active demethylation mediated by the ten-eleven translocation

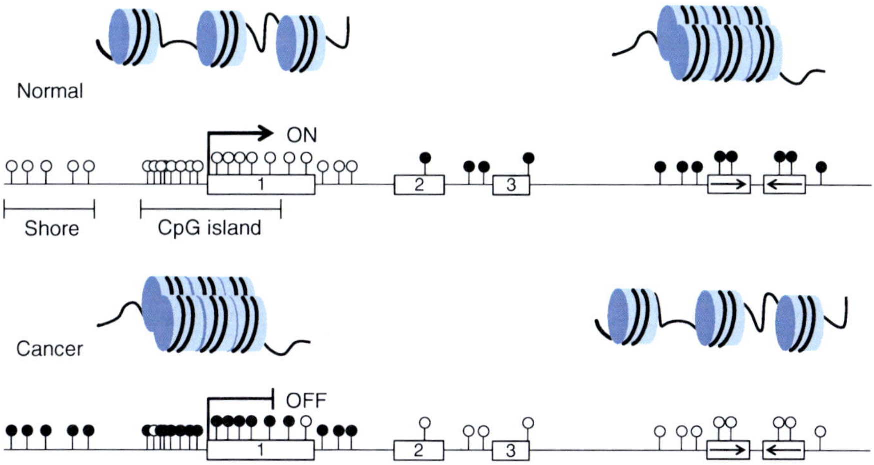

Fig. 2 Normal versus cancer epigenomes. Boxes with a number indicate exons and lines indicate introns as well as the regions outside the genes. Short stretches of CpG-rich sequences, usually around 1 kb in size, are termed CpG islands (CGIs). CpG island shores are regions of comparatively low CpG density located approximately 2 kb from CGIs. In normal cells, most CpG sites outside of CGIs and shores, including gene bodies, repeat elements (indicated by *boxes* with *arrows*), and pericentromeric regions, are methylated and are packaged as closed chromatin (the inset above methylated CpGs shows multiple nucleosomes with higher-order, tight compaction) unfavorable for transcription, whereas most CGIs and shores are unmethylated and reside in regions of open chromatin (inset, upstream of transcription start site shows three nucleosomes with wide spacing), or euchromatic states, favorable for gene transcription (*arrow in upper panel*). In cancer cells, on the other hand, many CpG sites outside of CGIs and shores are unmethylated, but most CGIs and shores are methylated. Aberrant promoter methylation serves to turn off the gene (*lower panel*). Filled and open circles represent methylated and unmethylated CpG sites, respectively.

(TET) family enzymes. Many CGIs are approximately 1 kb in length and reside at the 5′ ends of genes, where they function as promoter elements (Illingworth and Bird 2009). Approximately 70 % of annotated gene promoters are associated with a CGI, making this the most common promoter type in the vertebrate genome. On the other hand, most tissue-specific differentially methylated regions (tDMRs) do not occur in promoters or in CpG islands; they are instead found in regions located within 2 kb of islands with comparatively low CpG densities, termed "CpG island shores" (Fig. 2; Irizarry et al. 2009). The functional role of these tDMRs has been proposed to regulate alternative transcription during differentiation.

Relationship Between CGI DNA Methylation and Transcriptional Repression

Methylated DNA is recognized by proteins containing a methyl-CpG-binding domain (MBD) or a C_2H_2 zinc finger. The mammalian MBD proteins consist of five members: MBD1, MBD2, MBD3, MBD4, and MeCP2 (Hendrich and Bird 1998).

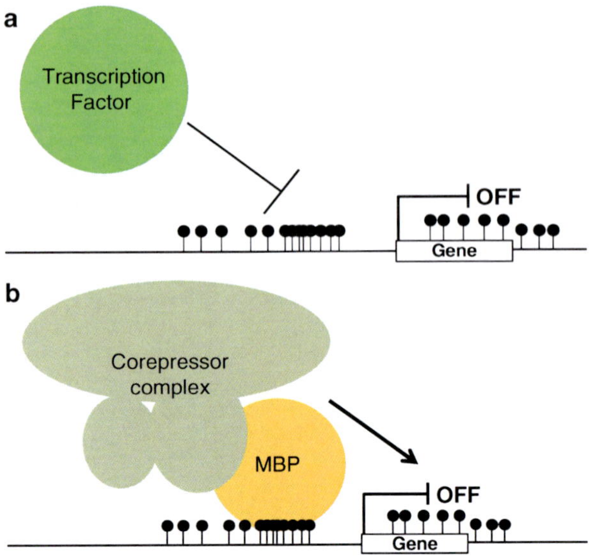

Fig. 3 **Two mechanisms of transcriptional repression by DNA methylation**. (**a**) A transcription factor (*green circle*) is unable to bind to its recognition site when DNA is methylated. Filled circles represent methylated CpGs. (**b**) DNA methylation can attract a protein complex including the methyl-CpG-binding protein (MBP, *orange circle*) and the corepressor complex (*gray ovals*).

Among these, MBD1, MBD2, MBD4, and MeCP2 all specifically recognize methyl-CpG sequences: MBD3 contains amino acid substitutions that prevent binding to methylated DNA. On the other hand, Kaiso (ZBTB33), ZBTB4, and ZBTB38 proteins use zinc finger domains to bind methylated DNA (Prokhortchouk et al. 2001).

MBD proteins and Kaiso are believed to participate in DNA methylation-mediated transcriptional repression of tumor-suppressor genes (Fig. 3). DNA methylation is thought to cause CGI promoter silencing principally by the following two mechanisms: First, DNA methylation inhibits the binding of transcription factors to their cognate DNA sequences. Second, transcriptional silencing is mediated by MBD proteins that recruit chromatin-modifying activities to methylated DNA (Klose and Bird 2006). It seems that CGI methylation is not the initiating event in gene silencing; it is seen as a stabilizing permanent mark important for long-term maintenance of the silent state. For example, during X chromosome inactivation in the female, X-linked CGIs do not become methylated until after gene silencing and the acquisition of several silencing chromatin modifications such as H3K27me3 (Payer and Lee 2008). DNA methylation is, however, required for stable maintenance of X chromosome inactivation, because inhibition of DNA methylation leads to gene reactivation in a fraction of cells (Sado et al. 2000).

DNA Methylation in Cancer Cells

Most studies of cancer epigenetics have focused on DNA methylation as the epigenetic mark, because this modification is able to survive various forms of sample processing, including DNA extraction, formalin fixation, and paraffin embedding (Laird 2010). There are two seemingly contradictory findings in the altered DNA methylation pattern seen in cancer: global hypomethylation and promoter hypermethylation (Fig. 2). Genome-wide DNA hypomethylation was first reported in HeLa cells (Diala and Hoffman 1982), and reduced levels of DNA methylation were found in specific genes of primary human tumors compared to adjacent normal tissues (Feinberg and Vogelstein 1983a). Many laboratories have identified cancer-related genes activated by DNA hypomethylation, including oncogenes, such as the Harvey rat sarcoma viral oncogene homologue (*HRAS*) (Feinberg and Vogelstein 1983b), and the family of genes expressed normally in testis and aberrantly activated in tumors, such as the melanoma-associated antigen (MAGE) family in melanoma (De Smet et al. 1996). DNA hypomethylation involves unwanted transcription of transposable elements, abnormal activation of cancer-related genes, and predisposition to genomic instability through disruption of chromosome replication control. In addition to DNA hypomethylation, promoter DNA hypermethylation is another major altered DNA methylation pattern observed in cancer. Aberrant silencing of genes by promoter hypermethylation was first identified in a CGI upstream of the retinoblastoma 1 (*RB1*) gene (Greger et al. 1989) and is important in the initiation and progression of tumors. Many tumor-suppressor genes have since been associated with hypermethylated CGIs (Baylin and Jones 2011).

The causal relevance of epigenetic changes in cancer was initially questioned, but it is now apparent that cancer is also driven by epigenetic changes that are mediated by mechanisms that do not affect the primary DNA sequence. Many tumor-suppressor genes have been shown to be silenced by promoter CGI hypermethylation. Importantly, these silencing events are mutually exclusive to structural or mutational inactivation of the same gene, such as the case for breast cancer 1 (*BRCA1*) in ovarian cancer (The Cancer Genome Atlas Research Network 2011) and for *CDKN2A* in squamous cell lung cancer (The Cancer Genome Atlas Research Network 2012). These observations reinforce the concept that epigenetic silencing can serve as an alternative mechanism in Knudson's two-hit hypothesis (Jones and Laird 1999). Furthermore, DNA methylation contributes substantially to tumor development in mouse models of cancer (Laird et al. 1995). Finally, a recent study indicated that some DNA methylation changes appear to be essential for the survival of cancer cells, suggesting an acquired addiction to epigenetic alterations (De Carvalho et al. 2012).

5-Hydroxymethylcytosine and Its Derivatives in Cancer

The variety of epigenetic modifications in mammalian DNA has recently increased further with the discovery of 5-hydroxymethylcytosine (5hmC) in mammalian neurons and embryonic stem cells (Tahiliani et al. 2009). Ten-eleven translocation (TET) proteins are Fe(II)- and α-ketoglutarate (α-KG)-dependent dioxygenases that successively oxidize 5-methylcytosine (5mC) to 5hmC, 5-formylcytosine (5fC), and 5-carboxylcytosine (5caC) (Fig. 1). These oxidized methylcytosines are believed to be intermediates in the process of 5mC demethylation (Pastor et al. 2013). TET proteins play an important role in regulating DNA methylation fidelity, and their inactivation contributes to the CpG island methylator phenotype (CIMP) in cancer. Due to their structural similarity, 5mC and 5hmC are experimentally indistinguishable using established 5mC mapping techniques such as differential enzymatic digestion and bisulfite sequencing (Nestor et al. 2010). Therefore, the existing 5mC data sets will require careful re-evaluation in the context of the possible presence of 5hmC. Single-molecule real-time sequencing (SMRT-seq), as well as the oxidative bisulfite sequencing (oxBS-seq) and TET-assisted bisulfite sequencing (TAB-seq) methods, has been developed for quantitative mapping of 5hmC in genomic DNA at single-nucleotide resolution (Pastor et al. 2013). 5hmC has been found in nearly all mouse embryonic tissues, but, with the exception of brain tissue and bone marrow, only very low levels (0.05–0.2 % of all cytosines) are detectable in adult tissue (Ruzov et al. 2011). Given that 5hmC is most abundant in brain tissue, it is important to unravel the function of this modified base in the brain.

The levels of 5hmC in cancer are strongly reduced relative to the corresponding normal tissue surrounding the tumor (Jin et al. 2011). Furthermore, Lian et al. reported that the reintroduction of TET2 restored 5hmC levels and decreased metastatic potential of melanoma cells (Lian et al. 2012). The immunostaining of tissue sections with antibodies against 5hmC and against the Ki67 antigen indicated that 5hmC and Ki67 are almost never present simultaneously in a single cell, suggesting that the combined analysis of 5hmC and Ki67 may become a potential biomarker for cancer diagnosis (Jin et al. 2011). In addition, mutations in the *TET2* gene are commonly observed in human myeloid malignancies and are associated with decreased 5hmC levels (Delhommeau et al. 2009). The TET family is directly responsible for the generation of 5hmC, and the catalytic reaction requires cofactor α-KG (Tahiliani et al. 2009), which is mainly controlled by isocitrate dehydrogenases (IDHs) (Xu et al. 2011). Heterozygous mutations in catalytic arginine residues of *IDH1* or *IDH2* are also common in glioma, acute myeloid leukemia, chondrosarcoma, cholangiocarcinoma, and angioimmunoblastic T-cell lymphomas (Cairns and Mak 2013). These studies suggest the important roles of 5hmC, TET, and IDH in cancer; however, it is still unclear how this epigenetic marker and these related enzymes are associated with cancer initiation and progression and whether they are suitable for use as biomarkers.

Long-Range Coordinated Disruptions in DNA Methylation

Although alterations in nuclear shape are often used for cancer diagnosis, we are now beginning to understand the molecular basis of these altered structures. The human genome is partitioned into both euchromatic and heterochromatic domains. The euchromatic domain is more open to transcription due to posttranslational histone modifications and lower nucleosome density, whereas the heterochromatic domain is not. Large organized chromatin lysine modifications (LOCKs) and

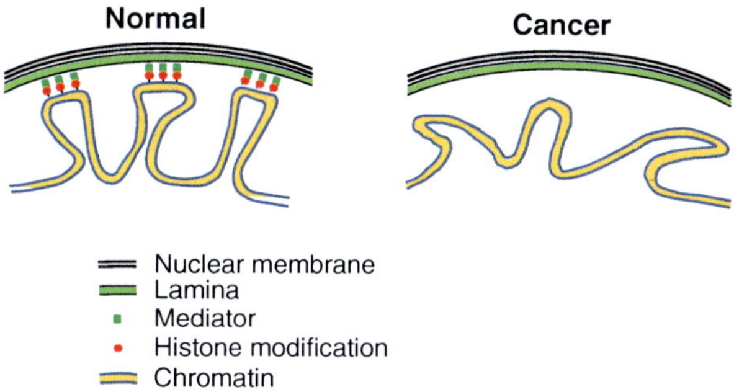

Fig. 4 **Model of a higher-order chromatin structure mediated by LOCKs and LADs.** In normal cells, large organized lysine modifications (LOCKs) and lamin-associated domains (LADs) are associated with the nuclear membrane and are generally heterochromatic, with a high level of DNA methylation. In cancer cells, there are reductions of LOCKs and LADs, as well as general disorganization of the nuclear membrane and hypomethylation of large blocks of DNA corresponding approximately to the LOCKs and LADs.

lamin-associated domains (LADs) are associated with the nuclear membrane and are generally heterochromatic, with a high level of DNA methylation (Fig. 4: Wen et al. 2009; Zullo et al. 2012). In cancer, there is a reduction of LOCKs and general disorganization of the nuclear membrane. Furthermore, large blocks of hypomethylated DNA ranging from 28 to 10 Mb in size have been identified in cancer by comparing colorectal cancer to matched normal mucosa from same patients, and these hypomethylated blocks mostly correspond to LOCKs and LADs (Hansen et al. 2011). CGI hypermethylation is enriched in the hypomethylated blocks, suggesting that these two events may be mechanistically linked but confined to distinct areas of the genome near the nuclear periphery (Berman et al. 2012). These large blocks of DNA hypomethylation and inactive histone modifications, along with promoter CGI methylation, are also consistent with a phenomenon called long-range epigenetic silencing (LRES) (Coolen et al. 2010). In addition, abnormal hypomethylation in the genomic regions in cancer often coordinates with DNA breakpoint hotspots and may therefore contribute to copy number alterations (De and Michor 2011).

CpG Island Methylator Phenotype

Aberrant DNA methylation was initially viewed as a rare and random process that is selected for in neoplastic cells. However, the discovery of colorectal cancers with concordant tumor-specific DNA methylation throughout the genome suggested the existence of a systemic methylation defect in the cell. This phenomenon was referred to as a "CpG island methylator phenotype" (CIMP) (Toyota et al. 1999), analogous to the mutator phenotypes in cancer, mostly resulting from defects in DNA mismatch repair. The concept of CIMP was initially met with considerable argument, but it has since been adopted owing to the substantial accumulated supporting evidence, including more recent genome-scale DNA methylation analyses in colorectal cancer (Hinoue et al. 2012) and glioblastoma (Noushmehr et al. 2010). As an example, colorectal cancer was classified into four distinct subtypes, and each subtype showed characteristic genetic and clinical features. A CIMP-high (CIMP-H) subtype, which exhibits an exceptionally high frequency of cancer-specific DNA hypermethylation, is tightly associated with *MLH1* hypermethylation and the activating mutation of *BRAF* oncogene (*BRAF*^{V600E}). A CIMP-low (CIMP-L) subtype is enriched for *KRAS* mutations. Non-CIMP tumors can be separated into two distinct subsets. One non-CIMP subtype is distinguished by a significantly high frequency of *TP53* mutations and frequent occurrence in the distal colon, whereas the other non-CIMP subtype exhibits a low frequency of both cancer-specific DNA hypermethylation and gene mutations and is significantly enriched for rectal tumors. In the case of glioblastoma CIMP (G-CIMP), the *IDH1* mutation appears to be a causal contributor to the phenotype (Turcan et al. 2012), but the *BRAF* mutation does not appear to be directly implicated in colorectal cancer CIMP (C-CIMP) (Hinoue et al. 2009). Although there are some overlaps with respect to genes targeted by C-CIMP and G-CIMP, and although *IDH1* and genes that affect the same metabolic pathway, such as *IDH2* and *TET2*, have been shown to be causally involved in the generation of CIMP in glioma and leukemia, cancer-specific differences still exist, and the cause of CIMP in the majority of cancer types remains to be identified. In addition, CIMP is associated with a favorable prognosis for colorectal cancer and gliomas. Extensive research has been conducted in these two cancer types with respect to identifying genes that are associated with clinical and molecular features of the tumors. These findings suggest that the hypermethylation of specific gene panels associated with the CIMP phenotype in a specific tumor type could be of potential prognostic or predictive value.

Methods of Isolating DNA Methylation Biomarkers in Cancer

A number of techniques have been used to identify aberrant DNA methylation in cancer. DNA methylation analysis previously restricted to specific loci can now be performed on a genome scale. The most direct method is whole-genome bisulfite sequencing, which allows for an unbiased assessment of the profile of DNA methylomes. This method utilizes bisulfite-induced modification of genomic DNA under conditions whereby cytosine is converted into uracil, but 5mC remains unchanged (Fig. 5; Frommer et al. 1992). After bisulfite conversion, next-generation sequencing technology is used to obtain a complete overview of CpG methylation level at a single-base resolution. Although whole-genome bisulfite sequencing has been successfully employed, more indirect methods have been preferentially utilized. In one such indirect method, methylated DNA fragments are first purified and then coupled with microarrays to map them at specific genomic loci or to sequence them extensively. Two approaches have been used to purify

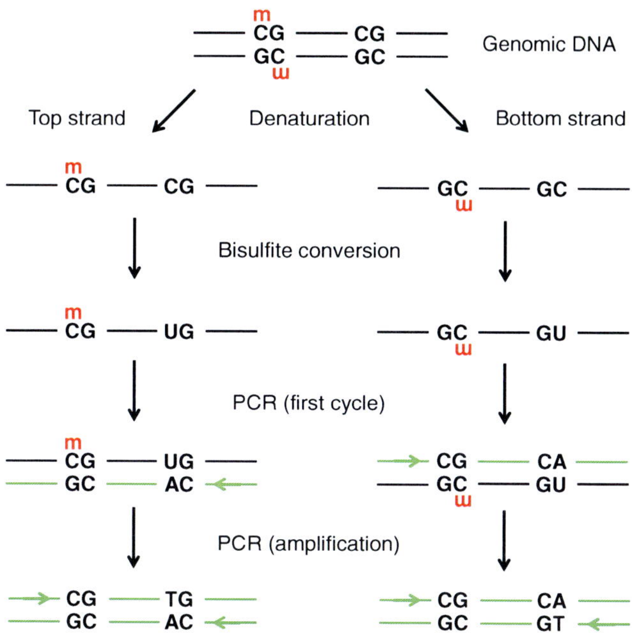

Fig. 5 **Bisulfite treatment of DNA**. DNA is denatured and then treated with sodium bisulfite to convert unmethylated cytosine to uracil, which is then converted to thymine by PCR. Bisulfite conversion of genomic DNA and subsequent PCR amplification give rise to two PCR products for any given locus. PCR primers are designed to assay the methylation status of a specific strand by bisulfite sequencing or methylation-specific PCR (MSP).

methylated DNA fragments. In one approach, unmethylated and methylated DNA fractions are enriched using a series of methylation-sensitive restriction enzymes (Fig. 6a; Irizarry et al. 2008). In the other approach, strategies based on the use of either a monoclonal antibody raised against 5mC (methyl-DNA immunoprecipitation; MeDIP) (Weber et al. 2007) or an MBD domain (methyl-binding domain affinity purification; MAP) (Cross et al. 1994) are exploited to purify methylated DNA (Fig. 6b). CpG-specific array technology is an alternative option for determining a genome-wide DNA methylation profile. Multiplexed methylation-specific primer extension of bisulfite-converted DNA at different CpG sites is performed using primers that are specific for methylated and unmethylated sequences at each site (Fig. 6c). The primers for the two different methylation states are labeled with different fluorescent dyes, and the products are hybridized to bead arrays. The Infinium HumanMethylation 450 K BeadChip Kit (Illumina Inc., CA) allows the high-resolution, genome-wide DNA methylation profiling of human samples, covering 99 % of all RefSeq genes and more than 480,000 CpGs. All of these methods have proven to be useful for identifying hypermethylated CGI sites, but we still do not know which methylated CGIs are involved in transcriptional repression. Therefore, global changes in the gene expression profiles of cancer cell lines have been

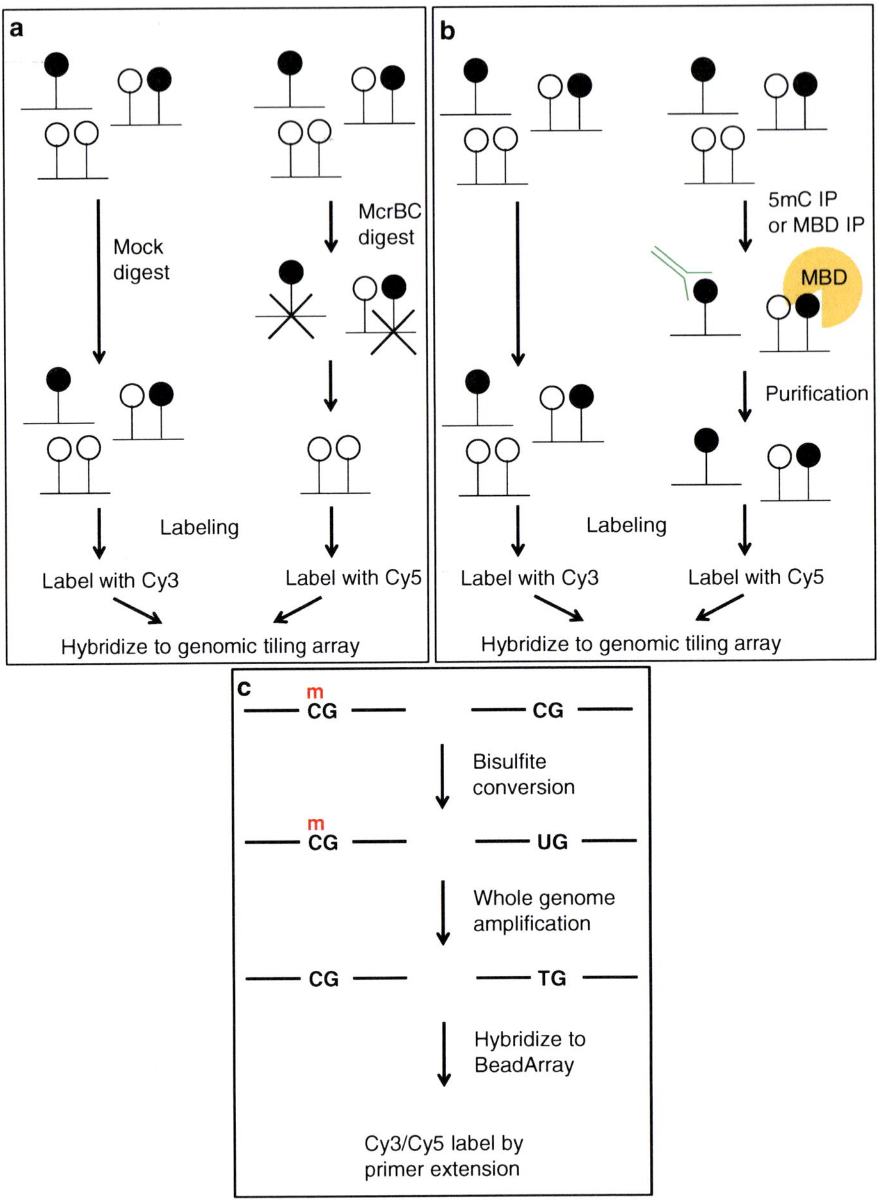

Fig. 6 **Three approaches to DNA methylation microarray analysis**. (**a**) Detection of methylated DNA fragments with methylation-sensitive restriction digestion using McrBC. *Filled circles* denote methylated CpGs, and *open circles* denote unmethylated CpGs. A methylated region of genomic DNA is digested with McrBC, and unmethylated DNA fragments are then enriched in the McrBC-treated samples. (**b**) Affinity enrichment of methylated DNA. Genomic DNA is denatured and then affinity purified with either an anti-5mC antibody (*green*, methylated DNA immunoprecipitation; MeDIP) or a methyl-CpG-binding domain (*orange*, methyl-binding domain affinity

analyzed after treatment with DNA demethylating agents such as 5-aza-2′-deoxycytidine (5-Aza-CdR; decitabine) or 5-azacytidine (5-Aza-CR; azacitidine) (Suzuki et al. 2002). Candidate genes targeted for aberrant DNA methylation in cancer cells are identified, and then a number of clinical samples are examined for DNA methylation and gene expression. Although this strategy is useful for identifying a substantial number of candidate genes, it also identifies genes whose promoters seem to be unmethylated (Suzuki et al. 2002), thus leading to the development of more specific and sensitive methods.

As mentioned before, MBD proteins directly bind to hypermethylated promoters of human genes and are associated with transcriptional silencing through histone modifications. That means that it would be very easy to detect hypermethylated genes if the genes occupied by MBD proteins were specifically reactivated. Therefore, a method termed "methyl-CpG targeted transcriptional activation (MeTA)," which uses a fusion gene comprised of the MBD from MBD2 protein and the NFκB transcriptional activation domain, has been developed (Fukushige et al. 2008). Microarray coupled with MeTA (MeTA-array) has successfully identified tumor-specific methylated genes (Shimizu et al. 2011). These results suggest that it is more advantageous to use this technique to identify methylated genes involved in transcriptional repression than to use strategies such as MeDIP, MAP, or DNA demethylating agents coupled with microarray.

DNA Methylation Changes in Early Tumorigenesis

A number of studies have shown that although the abnormal epigenetic silencing of genes associated with DNA hypermethylation may arise at any time during tumor progression, it is increasingly apparent that it occurs well before invasive cancer, sometimes during the early stages of tumor development and possibly during the abnormal expansion of stem and progenitor cells (Baylin and Ohm 2006). This silencing event may predispose the stem cells to abnormal clonal expansion. This information offered us a new point of view: all tumors can begin not only with genetic mutations but also with epigenetic alterations. The silenced genes may allow cells to abnormally survive the hostile environments that are risk factors for cancer development: for example, chronic inflammation with the concomitant

Fig. 6 (continued) purification; MAP) that can be attached to a column. (**c**) Illumina's bisulfite treatment-based approach. Genomic DNA is treated with sodium bisulfite to convert the unmethylated cytosine into uracil. The bisulfite-treated DNA is subjected to whole-genome amplification, and the products are then applied to the chip. Hybridization is followed by single-nucleotide primer extension with labeled dideoxynucleotides. The Infinium Human Methylation 450 K BeadChip allows the simultaneous quantitative monitoring of more than 480,000 CpG positions.

generation of DNA damaging agents such as reactive oxygen species (ROS). Cells involved in injury repair might normally undergo apoptosis from such DNA damage, but if they are able to survive and expand, they may select for gene mutations and/or epigenetic alterations, which may favor subsequent tumor progression.

There are several key examples of an early role for DNA hypermethylation and gene silencing in tumor progression. One of the most common tumor-suppressor genes affected in many tumor types is *CDKN2A*, whose loss of function leads to cell cycle abnormalities and uncontrolled growth. *CDKN2A* mutations in most cancer types are rare, but the hypermethylation of this gene is observed during progression of tumors such as breast cancer and non-small cell lung cancer (NSCLC) as early as in preneoplastic lesions (Belinsky et al. 1998). A role for this loss of function in early tumorigenesis can be predicted from the data from *CDKN2A* knockout mice indicating that germ line loss of this gene can increase the stem cell life span (Janzen et al. 2006). Experimental loss of *CDKN2A* appears to facilitate early tumorigenesis by permitting subsequent emergence of genomic instability and may cause a sequential process, polycomb group protein (PcG)-mediated silencing, and DNA hypermethylation, in other genes.

Another excellent example for early epigenetic abnormalities involves the Wnt developmental pathway, which is essential for stem/progenitor cell function, expansion, and maintenance in the normal intestine and elsewhere during embryogenesis and adult cell renewal (Fig. 7). The risk of colon cancer can begin with the appearance of aberrant crypt foci (ACF) in the colon epithelium; these harbor preadenomatous, premalignant hyperplastic cells that are derived from individual colon epithelial villi. The evolution of colon cancer is highly dependent on abnormal activation of the Wnt pathway, which is driven by mutations in downstream pathway genes such as adenomatous polyposis coli (*APC*) and *β-catenin*. Most ACF cells do not contain such mutations; instead they have frequent promoter hypermethylation and gene silencing of the genes encoding secreted frizzled-related proteins (*SFRPs*) that antagonize Wnt activation at the cell membrane (Suzuki et al. 2004). This hypermethylation of *SFRPs* occurs in early tumorigenesis, persists throughout colon tumor progression, and can later collaborate with downstream mutations in driving the Wnt pathway (Baylin and Ohm 2006; Suzuki et al. 2004). There are two pieces of evidence that loss of *SFRP* expression is required for clonal expansion of colon cancer cells by using one extensively studied human colon cancer cell line, HCT116, which originally has *SFRP* hypermethylation (Suzuki et al. 2004). First, the *DNMT1* and *DNMT3B* double knockout (DKO) cells derived from HCT116 show *SFRP* promoter demethylation and re-expression, resulting in the downregulation of Wnt signaling and induction of apoptosis, despite the fact that these cells express activated forms of β-catenin. Second, exogenous re-expression of *SFRP* genes in HCT116 cells and in another cell line, SW480 with *APC* mutation, similarly blocks Wnt signaling and results in induction of apoptosis. These examples highlight the importance of epigenetic events in driving tumorigenesis; reversal of these events may have prevention or therapeutic potential.

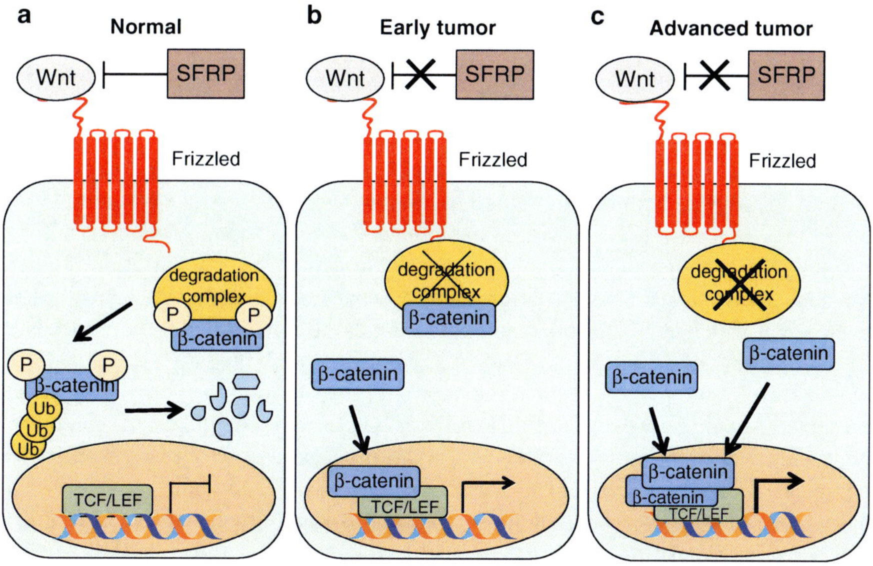

Fig. 7 Epigenetic inactivation of SFRPs occurs in the early stages of colon tumorigenesis. (**a**) In normal colon epithelial cells, secreted frizzled-related proteins (SFRPs) function as antagonists of Wnt signaling by competing with the Frizzled receptors to bind Wnt ligands. When Wnt signaling is inactive, a degradation complex that comprises glycogen synthase kinase 3 (GSK3), casein kinase 1α (CK1α), Axin, and adenomatous polyposis coli (APC) promotes the phosphorylation of β-catenin, which leads to its ubiquitylation by SKP1-cullin 1-F-box ($SCF^{\beta\text{-TrCP}}$) E3 ligase and to its degradation by the 26S proteasome. This prevents the accumulation of nuclear β-catenin and its ability to engage its transcription factor partners, which results in the differentiation and homeostasis of colon epithelial cells. (**b**) When epigenetic silencing of the *SFRP* genes occurs, Wnt signaling becomes activated through the Frizzled receptors. This Wnt signaling inhibits the degradation complex, thereby blocking the degradation of β-catenin. β-catenin then accumulates in the nucleus, binds to lymphoid enhancer-binding factor (LEF) and T-cell factor (TCF) proteins, and acts as a transcriptional co-activator to modulate the expression of target genes such as *MYC*, *cyclin D*, and other genes whose products promote cell proliferation and survival. This sequence results in the expansion of the colon epithelial stem and progenitor cells and formation of atypical crypt foci (ACF). (**c**) Persistent activation of the Wnt pathway allows mutations to occur in other pathway components, such as those that permanently disable the degradation complex and promote nuclear accumulation of β-catenin. These cells are selected for because of their survival and proliferative advantages. This combination of epigenetic and genetic events fully activates the Wnt pathway to promote tumor progression.

The Suitability of DNA Methylation Changes as Biomarkers

The use of promoter-hypermethylation sequences as a molecular signature is providing one of the most promising biomarker strategies for cancer (Herman and Baylin 2003; Laird 2003). One of the most striking features of DNA methylation biomarkers is the relative stability of DNA as compared with many proteins and RNA; methylated sequences can be detected even in paraffin-embedded clinical samples.

Using sensitive polymerase chain reaction (PCR)-based assays such as methylation-specific PCR (MSP), abnormally methylated genes have been detected in sources as diverse as DNA extracted from tumors, lymph nodes, serum, sputum, bronchial lavage fluid, ductal lavage fluid, and urine from patients with all varieties of cancer types (Herman and Baylin 2003; Laird 2003). In comparison with genetic approaches such as mutational analysis, DNA methylation-based approaches have several advantages with regard to their clinical application. First, DNA methylation alterations generally occur at higher percentages of tumors than genetic variations, resulting in a higher sensitivity, even in single-gene DNA methylation studies. Second, aberrant DNA methylation can be sensitively detected in cancer cells, even when it is embedded in substantial amounts of contaminating normal DNA. Third, detection of aberrant DNA methylation is technically simple. DNA hypermethylation only occurs at a rather small promoter region called CGIs; it can be detected using only one set of PCR primers. On the other hand, genetic mutations occur throughout the length of the gene, and it is necessary to use many primers for complete analysis of the gene. Fourth, aberrant DNA methylation can occur in early-stage tumors, as described above, causing loss and/or gain of function of key processes and signaling properties. Although DNA methylation biomarkers have several advantages over genetic markers as previously noted, most importantly, a combination of DNA methylation and genetic analyses could exploit the advantages of both techniques, as has been shown for the diagnosis of colorectal cancers (Ahlquist et al. 2012).

Although DNA hypomethylation is also another major epigenetic alteration in cancer and has been proposed as a valid biomarker for cancer, its diagnostic use is limited, because it is technically more difficult and challenging to detect a loss of DNA methylation than a gain of DNA methylation. However, it has been suggested that DNA hypomethylation of the repetitive element, long interspersed nuclear element-1 (LINE-1), has frequently been observed and is a potential biomarker for the prediction of a response to oral fluoropyrimidines in colorectal cancer patients (Kawakami et al. 2011). Furthermore, loss of imprinting (LOI) at the insulin-like growth factor 2 (*IGF2*) gene, which results in the activation of the normally silent allele of the *IGF2* gene, is associated with various types of cancer and has diagnostic potential for colon cancer (Cui et al. 2002).

DNA Methylation as Early Detection Biomarkers

DNA methylation alterations have been reported to occur early in tumorigenesis; they are therefore potentially good early indicators of existing cancer. Early detection of cancer using DNA methylation biomarkers can result in an improved clinical outcome. Using minimally invasive methods such as the analysis of blood, stool, sputum, or urine samples has clear advantages over invasive ones such as the analysis of biopsy specimens. Tumors release a substantial amount of genomic DNA into biological fluids. Tumor cells can directly be released from the tissue of origin, whereas necrotic and apoptotic tumor cells are engulfed by phagocytes and subsequently the free tumor DNA directly reaches the fluids by cell lysis. Analysis of epigenetic alterations can then be carried out by examining these noninvasive samples. The most promising candidate for a biomarker for noninvasive diagnosis is *GSTP1* hypermethylation in prostate cancer. *GSTP1* encodes the only member of the human pi class of glutathione S-transferase superfamily and is involved in cellular detoxification of xenobiotics and carcinogens. The *GSTP1* promoter is unmethylated in all normal human cells and tissues, but it has frequently been found to be hypermethylated in prostate cancer (Lee et al. 1994). *GSTP1* hypermethylation was consistently validated in more than 30 independent studies, and a meta-analysis pooling almost 3,500 subjects, composed of 2,389 prostate cancer patients and 1,082 normal controls, established *GSTP1* as a promising biomarker of prostate cancer with a sensitivity of 82 % and a specificity of 95 % (Van Neste et al. 2011). *GSTP1* hypermethylation has also been investigated in different stages of prostatic carcinogenesis using 27 laser-capture microdissected samples (Nakayama et al. 2003). Normal prostate epithelium, benign prostatic hyperplasia, proliferative inflammatory atrophy, high-grade prostatic intraepithelial neoplasia, and prostate cancer show *GSTP1* hypermethylation frequencies of 0 %, 0 %, 6.3 %, 68.8 %, and 90.9 % respectively. These results indicate that *GSTP1* hypermethylation is an early event in tumorigenesis, underlining its importance for diagnosis. Meta-analysis of 22 studies that analyzed the value of *GSTP1* as a biomarker for prostate cancer in biological fluids, including plasma, serum, and urine, revealed a high specificity of 89 % but a modest sensitivity of 52 % (Wu et al. 2011). Measuring *GSTP1* hypermethylation in biological fluids presents a promising alternative to conventional methods of detection of prostate cancer. In particular, the combination of *GSTP1* with additional biomarker genes and prostate-specific antigen (PSA) testing could highly improve the sensitivity of diagnosis.

DNA Methylation Biomarkers for Prediction of Drug Sensitivity

One of the most promising uses for DNA methylation biomarkers is for prediction of drug sensitivity. Hypermethylation of the promoter of O^6-methylguanine-DNA methyltransferase (*MGMT*) is one of the very few DNA methylation biomarkers that is already in widespread clinical use, especially for the prediction of chemosensitivity to temozolomide in gliomas. *MGMT* encodes for a protein that removes alkylation adducts from the O^6 position of guanines in DNA, and the absence of *MGMT* can thus promote tumorigenesis through an increased mutation rate (Herman and Baylin 2003). Epigenetic silencing of *MGMT* due to promoter hypermethylation frequently occurs in many types of tumor, including gliomas, and the constituent cells have a diminished capacity to repair alkylation damage, rendering them sensitive to alkylating agents such as temozolomide (Hegi et al. 2005). Thus, multiple studies have revealed that determination of *MGMT* promoter methylation status may allow the selection of patients most likely to benefit from temozolomide treatment. Recently, Ebert et al. published the specific association of a particular promoter methylation status with therapy response in colorectal cancer (Ebert et al. 2012). Hypermethylation of transcription factor AP-2 epsilon (*TFAP2E*) in primary as well as metastatic colorectal cancers was shown to be associated with decreased expression of this gene and with nonresponsiveness to 5-fluorouracil (5-FU). The fact that hypermethylation of *TFAP2E* was observed in 51 % of the patients in this cohort indicates the possible impact this knowledge could have on future colorectal cancer treatment. In addition, if this gene was not methylated, it would result in a six times higher response rate than in the total colorectal cancer population (Ebert et al. 2012).

Future Perspectives

Although we now know that DNA methylation is one of the biomarkers with a great potential for assessing cancer risk, early detection, prognosis, and predicting therapeutic responses (see Table 1), their use in clinical settings is still very limited, partly due to the insufficient sensitivity and specificity in noninvasively obtained clinical samples. For example, genes that are specifically methylated in cancer cells but not in the normal epithelial cells might be excellent biomarkers in biopsies but may not be as promising in noninvasive clinical specimens, if they are found to be methylated in normal lymphocytes. In order to discover biomarkers with high sensitivity and high specificity, reference DNA methylation data sets obtained from the profiles of different healthy individuals and tissue types are used to estimate the variance of a particular CpG site or of regions such as promoters. Using high-resolution technologies, these reference data sets have been created in consortia such as Blueprint, the International Human Epigenome Consortium (IHEC), and Roadmap. Genomic loci that are unstable in DNA methylation

Table 1 **A selected list of potential DNA-based biomarkers in cancer**. A selected list of DNA biomarkers described in this chapter are shown in this table:

Gene name	Gene function	Application	Cancer type	Tissue examined
SFRP	Wnt pathway	Early detection	Colon	ACF
CDKN2A	Cell cycle control	Early detection Prognosis	NSCLC, breast	Tumor, mediastinal lymph node biopsy
MGMT	DNA repair	Predicting drug sensitivity	Glioma, colon, lung, lymphoma	Tumor
GSTP1	Detoxification	Predicting drug sensitivity	Prostate, breast, kidney	Tumor, urine
PYCARD	Apoptosis	Prognosis	NSCLC	Sputum
TFAP2E	Transcription factor	Predicting drug sensitivity	Colon	Tumor
LINE-1	Transposition	Predicting drug sensitivity	Colon	Tumor
IGF2	Cell growth	Prognosis	Colon	Tumor

between individuals are excluded as unsuitable CpG sites before biomarker candidate selection starts. Further reference cancer genomes and DNA methylomes are required to increase the sensitivity and specificity of DNA methylation biomarkers; consortia such as the 1,000 Genomes Project for genome sequencing and the Blueprint, IHEC, and Roadmap projects for methylome mapping currently aim to generate such reference data sets. The data obtained from genomics, transcriptomics, and epigenomics are combined and integrated to determine profiles predicting disease outcome in terms of patient prognosis and treatment response. All of these efforts will contribute to finding useful DNA methylation biomarkers for cancer patients, and these specific and sensitive DNA methylation biomarkers will allow diagnosis and prediction of disease prognosis to be more accurate than is possible at present.

Potential Applications to Prognosis, Other Diseases, or Conditions

The presence of tumor-specific methylation markers in biological fluids such as serum, plasma, sputum, or urine of patients has also been reported to be of prognostic significance. For example, the concomitant methylation of three or more of six genes (*CDKN2A*, *MGMT*, *DAPK*, *RASSF1A*, *PAX5β*, and *GATA5*) in sputum collected within 18 months of diagnosis was associated with a 6.5-fold increase in the risk for lung cancer (Belinsky et al. 2006). In addition, hypermethylation of the proapoptotic gene *PYCARD* (also known as *ASC/TMS1*) in sputum may be useful for predicting which patients with surgically resected early-stage lung cancers may recur (Machida et al. 2006). NSCLC accounts for 80 % of all lung cancer, and the absence of validated prognostic biomarkers could be relevant; even patients with stage I NSCLC who undergo potentially curative surgical resection are at high risk of dying from recurrent disease, with a 5-year relapse rate of 35–50 %. A DNA methylation microarray that analyzes 450,000 CpG sites was applied to study tumor DNA obtained from 444 patients with NSCLC that included 237 stage I tumors (Sandoval et al. 2013). Unsupervised clustering of the 10,000 most variable DNA methylation sites in the discovery cohort identified patients with high-risk stage I NSCLC who had shorter relapse-free survival (RFS; hazard ratio [HR], 2.35; 95 % CI, 1.29–4.28; $P = 0.004$). The study in the validation cohort of the significant methylated sites from the discovery cohort found that hypermethylation of five genes, including histone cluster 1, H4f (*HIST1H4F*), protocadherin gamma subfamily B, 6 (*PCDHGB6*), neuropeptides B/W receptor 1 (*NPBWR1*), ALX homeobox 1 (*ALX1*), and homeobox A9 (*HOXA9*), was significantly associated with shorter RFS in stage I NSCLC (Sandoval et al. 2013). A signature based on the number of hypermethylated events distinguished patients with high- and low-risk stage I NSCLC (HR, 3.24; 95 % CI, 1.61–6.54; $P = 0.001$). These DNA methylation biomarkers indicate which patients should receive adjuvant chemotherapy and could be useful for generating treatment guidelines for early-stage NSCLC.

Summary Points

1. Aberrant DNA methylation is the most well-defined epigenetic change in cancer.
2. DNA methylation profiles represent a more stable source of molecular diagnostic information than RNA or most proteins.
3. DNA methylation can occur during the early stages of human tumor progression and involves disruption or over-activation of key developmental pathways and cell-signaling properties.
4. Recent genome-wide DNA methylation analysis in normal as well as cancer cells has provided extensive information for candidate biomarkers.
5. Tumor-specific DNA methylation can be detected in noninvasive biological fluids such as blood, stool, sputum, or urine and offers a promising approach to the early detection of cancer.

References

Ahlquist DA, Zou H, Domanico M, et al. Next-generation stool DNA test accurately detects colorectal cancer and large adenomas. Gastroenterology. 2012;142:248–56.

Armitage P, Doll R. The age distribution of cancer and a multi-stage theory of carcinogenesis. Br J Cancer. 1954;8:1–12.

Baylin SB, Jones PA. A decade of exploring the cancer epigenome – biological and translational implications. Nat Rev Cancer. 2011;11:726–34.

Baylin SB, Ohm JE. Epigenetic gene silencing in cancer – a mechanism for early oncogenic pathway addiction? Nat Rev Cancer. 2006;6:107–16.

Beggs AD, Jones A, El-Bahwary M, et al. Whole-genome methylation analysis of benign and malignant colorectal tumours. J Pathol. 2013;229:697–704.

Belinsky SA, Nikula KJ, Palmisano WA, et al. Aberrant methylation of $p16^{INK4a}$ is an early event in lung cancer and a potential biomarker for early diagnosis. Proc Natl Acad Sci U S A. 1998;95:11891–6.

Belinsky SA, Liechty KC, Gentry FD, et al. Promoter hypermethylation of multiple genes in sputum precedes lung cancer incidence in a high-risk cohort. Cancer Res. 2006;66:3338–44.

Berman BP, Weisenberger DJ, Aman JF, et al. Regions of focal DNA hypermethylation and long-range hypomethylation in colorectal cancer coincide with nuclear lamina-associated domains. Nat Genet. 2012;44:40–6.

Bird A. DNA methylation patterns and epigenetic memory. Genes Dev. 2002;16:6–21.

Bird A, Taggart M, Frommer M, et al. A fraction of the mouse genome that is derived from islands of nonmethylated, CpG-rich DNA. Cell. 1985;40:91–9.

Cairns RA, Mak TW. Oncogenic isocitrate dehydrogenase mutations: mechanisms, models, and clinical opportunities. Cancer Discov. 2013;3:730–41.

Coolen MW, Stirzaker C, Song JZ, et al. Consolidation of the cancer genome into domains of repressive chromatin by long-range epigenetic silencing (LRES) reduces transcriptional plasticity. Nat Cell Biol. 2010;12:235–46.

Cross SH, Charlton JA, Nan X, et al. Purification of CpG islands using a methylated DNA binding column. Nat Genet. 1994;6:236–44.

Cui H, Onyango P, Brandenburg S, et al. Loss of imprinting in colorectal cancer linked to hypomethylation of *H19* and *IGF2*. Cancer Res. 2002;62:6442–6.

De Carvalho DD, Sharma S, You JS, et al. DNA methylation screening identifies driver epigenetic events of cancer cell survival. Cancer Cell. 2012;21:655–67.

De Smet C, De Backer O, Faraoni I, et al. The activation of human gene *MAGE-1* in tumor cells is correlated with genome-wide demethylation. Proc Natl Acad Sci U S A. 1996;93:7149–53.

De S, Michor F. DNA secondary structures and epigenetic determinants of cancer genome evolution. Nat Struct Mol Biol. 2011;18:950–5.

Delhommeau F, Dupont S, Valle VD, et al. Mutations in *TET2* in myeloid cancers. N Engl J Med. 2009;360:2289–301.

Diala ES, Hoffman RM. Hypomethylation of HeLa cell DNA and the absence of 5-methylcytosine in SV40 and adenovirus (type 2) DNA: analysis by HPLC. Biochem Biophys Res Commun. 1982;107:19–26.

Ebert MP, Tänzer M, Balluff B, et al. *TFAP2E-DKK4* and chemoresistance in colorectal cancer. N Engl J Med. 2012;366:44–53.

Feinberg AP, Tycko B. The history of cancer epigenetics. Nat Rev Cancer. 2004;4:143–53.

Feinberg AP, Vogelstein B. Hypomethylation distinguishes genes of some human cancers from their normal counterparts. Nature. 1983a;301:89–92.

Feinberg AP, Vogelstein B. Hypomethylation of ras oncogenes in primary human cancers. Biochem Biophys Res Commun. 1983b;111:47–54.

Frommer M, McDonald LE, Millar DS, et al. A genomic sequencing protocol that yields a positive display of 5-methylcytosine residues in individual DNA strands. Proc Natl Acad Sci U S A. 1992;89:1827–31.

Fukushige S, Horii A. DNA methylation in cancer: a gene silencing mechanism and the clinical potential of its biomarkers. Tohoku J Exp Med. 2013;229:173–85.

Fukushige S, Kondo E, Horii A. Methyl-CpG targeted transcriptional activation allows re-expression of tumor suppressor genes in human cancer cells. Biochem Biophys Res Commun. 2008;377:600–5.

Greger V, Passarge E, Höpping W, et al. Epigenetic changes may contribute to the formation and spontaneous regression of retinoblastoma. Hum Genet. 1989;83:155–8.

Hanahan D, Weinberg RA. Hallmarks of cancer: the next generation. Cell. 2011;144:646–74.

Hansen KD, Timp W, Bravo HC, et al. Increased methylation variation in epigenetic domains across cancer types. Nat Genet. 2011;43:768–75.

Hegi ME, Diserens A-C, Gorlia T, et al. *MGMT* gene silencing and benefit from temozolomide in glioblastoma. N Engl J Med. 2005;352:997–1003.

Hendrich B, Bird A. Identification and characterization of a family of mammalian methyl-CpG binding proteins. Mol Cell Biol. 1998;18:6538–47.

Herman JG, Baylin SB. Gene silencing in cancer in association with promoter hypermethylation. N Engl J Med. 2003;349:2042–54.

Hinoue T, Weisenberger DJ, Pan F, et al. Analysis of the association between CIMP and $BRAF^{V600E}$ in colorectal cancer by DNA methylation profiling. PLoS One. 2009;4:e8357.

Hinoue T, Weisenberger DJ, Lange CP, et al. Genome-scale analysis of aberrant DNA methylation in colorectal cancer. Genome Res. 2012;22:271–82.

Illingworth RS, Bird AP. CpG islands-'A rough guide'. FEBS Lett. 2009;583:1713–20.

Irizarry RA, Ladd-Acosta C, Carvalho B, et al. Comprehensive high-throughput arrays for relative methylation (CHARM). Genome Res. 2008;18:780–90.

Irizarry RA, Ladd-Acosta C, Wen B, et al. The human colon cancer methylome shows similar hypo- and hypermethylation at conserved tissue-specific CpG island shores. Nat Genet. 2009;41:178–86.

Janzen V, Forkert R, Fleming HE, et al. Stem-cell ageing modified by the cyclin-dependent kinase inhibitor $p16^{INK4a}$. Nature. 2006;443:421–6.

Jin S-G, Jiang Y, Qiu R, et al. 5-hydroxymethylcytosine is strongly depleted in human cancers but its levels do not correlate with *IDH1* mutations. Cancer Res. 2011;71:7360–5.

Jones PA, Laird PW. Cancer epigenetics comes of age. Nat Genet. 1999;21:163–7.

Jones PA, Liang G. Rethinking how DNA methylation patterns are maintained. Nat Rev Genet. 2009;10:805–11.

Jones S, Chen W-D, Parmigiani G, et al. Comparative lesion sequencing provides insights into tumor evolution. Proc Natl Acad Sci U S A. 2008;105:4283–8.

Kawakami K, Matsunoki A, Kaneko M, et al. Long interspersed nuclear element-1 hypomethylation is a potential biomarker for the prediction of response to oral fluoropyrimidines in microsatellite stable and CpG island methylator phenotype-negative colorectal cancer. Cancer Sci. 2011;102:166–74.

Klose RJ, Bird AP. Genomic DNA methylation: the mark and its mediators. Trends Biochem Sci. 2006;31:89–97.

Laird PW. The power and the promise of DNA methylation markers. Nat Rev Cancer. 2003;3:253–66.

Laird PW. Principles and challenges of genome-wide DNA methylation analysis. Nat Rev Genet. 2010;11:191–203.

Laird PW, Jackson-Grusby L, Fazeli A, et al. Suppression of intestinal neoplasia by DNA hypomethylation. Cell. 1995;81:197–205.

Lee W-H, Morton RA, Epstein JI, et al. Cytidine methylation of regulatory sequences near the π-class glutathione *S*-transferase gene accompanies human prostatic carcinogenesis. Proc Natl Acad Sci U S A. 1994;91:11733–7.

Lian CG, Xu Y, Ceol C, et al. Loss of 5-hydroxymethylcytosine is an epigenetic hallmark of melanoma. Cell. 2012;150:1135–46.

Lienert F, Wirbelauer C, Som I, et al. Identification of genetic elements that autonomously determine DNA methylation states. Nat Genet. 2011;43:1091–7.

Machida EO, Brock MV, Hooker CM, et al. Hypermethylation of *ASC/TMS1* is a sputum marker for late-stage lung cancer. Cancer Res. 2006;66:6210–8.

Nakayama M, Bennett CJ, Hicks JL, et al. Hypermethylation of the human glutathione *S*-transferase-π gene (*GSTP1*) CpG island is present in a subset of proliferative inflammatory atrophy lesions but not in normal or hyperplastic epithelium of the prostate. Am J Pathol. 2003;163:923–33.

Nestor C, Ruzov A, Meehan RR, et al. Enzymatic approaches and bisulfite sequencing cannot distinguish between 5-methylcytosine and 5-hydroxymethylcytosine in DNA. Biotechniques. 2010;48:317–9.

Noushmehr H, Weisenberger DJ, Diefes K, et al. Identification of a CpG island methylator phenotype that defines a distinct subgroup of glioma. Cancer Cell. 2010;17:510–22.

Pastor WA, Aravind L, Rao A. TETonic shift: biological roles of TET proteins in DNA demethylation and transcription. Nat Rev Mol Cell Biol. 2013;14:341–56.

Payer B, Lee JT. X chromosome dosage compensation: how mammals keep the balance. Annu Rev Genet. 2008;42:733–72.

Prokhortchouk A, Hendrich B, Jørgensen H, et al. The p120 catenin partner Kaiso is a DNA methylation-dependent transcriptional repressor. Genes Dev. 2001;15:1613–8.

Ruzov A, Tsenkina Y, Serio A, et al. Lineage-specific distribution of high levels of genomic 5-hydroxymethylcytosine in mammalian development. Cell Res. 2011;21:1332–42.

Sado T, Fenner MH, Tan S-S, et al. X inactivation in the mouse embryo deficient for *Dnmt1*: distinct effect of hypomethylation on imprinted and random X inactivation. Dev Biol. 2000;225:294–303.

Sandoval J, Mendez-Gonzalez J, Nadal E, et al. A prognostic DNA methylation signature for stage I non-small-cell lung cancer. J Clin Oncol. 2013;31:4140–7.

Shimizu H, Horii A, Sunamura M, et al. Identification of epigenetically silenced genes in human pancreatic cancer by a novel method "microarray coupled with methyl-CpG targeted transcriptional activation" (MeTA-array). Biochem Biophys Res Commun. 2011;411:162–7.

Suzuki H, Gabrielson E, Chen W, et al. A genomic screen for genes upregulated by demethylation and histone deacetylase inhibition in human colorectal cancer. Nat Genet. 2002;31:141–9.

Suzuki H, Watkins DN, Jair K-W, et al. Epigenetic inactivation of *SFRP* genes allows constitutive WNT signaling in colorectal cancer. Nat Genet. 2004;36:417–22.

Tahiliani M, Koh KP, Shen Y, et al. Conversion of 5-methylcytosine to 5-hydroxymethylcytosine in mammalian DNA by MLL partner TET1. Science. 2009;324:930–5.

The Cancer Genome Atlas Research Network. Integrated genomic analyses of ovarian carcinoma. Nature. 2011;474:609–15.

The Cancer Genome Atlas Research Network. Comprehensive genomic characterization of squamous cell lung cancers. Nature. 2012;489:519–25.

Toyota M, Ahuja N, Ohe-Toyota M, et al. CpG island methylator phenotype in colorectal cancer. Proc Natl Acad Sci U S A. 1999;96:8681–6.

Turcan S, Rohle D, Goenka A, et al. IDH1 mutation is sufficient to establish the glioma hypermethylator phenotype. Nature. 2012;483:479–83.

Van Neste L, Herman JG, Otto G, et al. The epigenetic promise for prostate cancer diagnosis. Prostate. 2011;72:1248–61.

Vogelstein B, Papadopoulos N, Velculescu VE, et al. Cancer genome landscapes. Science. 2013;339:1546–58.

Weber M, Hellmann I, Stadler MB, et al. Distribution, silencing potential and evolutionary impact of promoter DNA methylation in the human genome. Nat Genet. 2007;39:457–66.

Wen B, Wu H, Shinkai Y, et al. Large histone H3 lysine 9 dimethylated chromatin blocks distinguish differentiated from embryonic stem cells. Nat Genet. 2009;41:246–50.

Wu T, Giovannucci E, Welge J, et al. Measurement of GSTP1 promoter methylation in body fluids may complement PSA screening: a meta-analysis. Br J Cancer. 2011;105:65–73.

Xu W, Yang H, Liu Y, et al. Oncometabolite 2-hydroxyglutarate is a competitive inhibitor of α-ketoglutarate-dependent dioxygenases. Cancer Cell. 2011;19:17–30.

Zullo JM, Demarco IA, Piqué-Regi R, et al. DNA sequence-dependent compartmentalization and silencing of chromatin at the nuclear lamina. Cell. 2012;149:1474–87.

Kallikreins as Biomarkers in Human Malignancies

6

Kleita Michaelidou, Athina Kladi-Skandali, and Andreas Scorilas

Contents

K. Michaelidou • A. Kladi-Skandali
Department of Biochemistry and Molecular Biology, University of Athens, Athens, Greece
e-mail: mkleita@gmail.com; kladi_athina@yahoo.gr

A. Scorilas (✉)
Department of Biochemistry and Molecular Biology, Faculty of Biology, School of Science, University of Athens, Athens, Greece
e-mail: ascorilas@biol.uoa.gr

V.R. Preedy, V.B. Patel (eds.), *Biomarkers in Cancer, Biomarkers in Disease: Methods, Discoveries and Applications*,
DOI 10.1007/978-94-007-7681-4_18

Abstract

The human tissue kallikrein and kallikrein-related peptidases are secreted serine proteases, which are expressed in a broad spectrum of tissues, fulfilling a plethora of physiological functions. During the past few years, the KLK family members have drawn a constantly increasing attention regarding their biomarker capabilities. The frequently observed deregulated KLK expression patterns in human malignancies, along with their active involvement in cancer pathobiology and the successful utilization of PSA/KLK3 in routine clinical practice, prompted researchers to evaluate the clinical significance of KLKs. KLK members have been proposed as tissue and/or serological biomarkers for early diagnosis, effective prognosis, and treatment monitoring of cancer patients. This chapter presents an overview of the current knowledge concerning the immense potential of KLKs as biomarkers in human malignancies.

List of Abbreviations

%fPSA	Ratio of fPSA to Total PSA
AD	Alzheimer's Disease
ALL	Acute Lymphoblastic Leukemia
BC	Breast Cancer
BPH	Benign Prostate Hyperplasia
CA125	Cancer Antigen 125
CaP	Prostate Cancer
CAP18	Cationic Antimicrobial Protein 18
CC	Cervical Cancer
CNS	Central Nervous System
CRC	Colorectal Cancer
DFS	Disease-Free Survival
ECM	Extracellular Matrix
EMT	Epithelial-to-Mesenchymal Transition
ER	Estrogen Receptor
fPSA	Free PSA
GC	Gastric Cancer
IGFBPs	Insulin-like Growth Factor-Binding Proteins
IGFs	Insulin-like Growth Factors
IHC	Immunohistochemistry
KLKs	Kallikreins
LEKTI	Lymphoepithelial Kazal-Type-Related Inhibitor
MMPs	Matrix Metalloproteinases
MS	Multiple Sclerosis
NAF	Nipple Aspirate Fluid
NS	Netherton Syndrome
NSCLC	Non-small Cell Lung Cancer
OC	Ovarian Cancer
OS	Overall Survival

PARs	Proteinase-Activated Receptors
PCR	Polymerase Chain Reaction
PD	Parkinson's Disease
PR	Progesterone Receptor
PSA/KLK3	Prostate-Specific Antigen
RCC	Renal Cell Carcinoma
REG4	Regenerating Islet-Derived Family, Member 4
SNPs	Single-Nucleotide Polymorphisms
SPINK5	Serine Peptidase Inhibitor Kazal-Type 5
TC	Testicular Cancer
tPSA	Total PSA
uPA-uPAR	Urokinase-Type Plasminogen Activator and Its Receptor
UPSC	Uterine Papillary Serous Carcinoma
UTR	Untranslated Region
VTCN1	V-Set Domain-Containing T-Cell Activation Inhibitor 1

Key Facts on Kallikrein Family

- The first member of the kallikrein family (KLK1) was identified in the 1930s, by Kraut, Frey, and Werle, as a proteolytic enzyme with high concentrations in the pancreas (kallikreas in Greek).
- The group of "classical" members, namely, *KLK1*, *KLK2*, and *KLK3*, were discovered during the late 1980s, while the "novel" members, *KLK4–KLK15*, were subsequently identified in mid- to late 1990s.
- KLKs are characterized by several common features, in terms of structure and function. For example, *KLK* genes are composed of five coding exons and have the same exon/intron organization, while KLKs are synthesized as pre-proenzymes that require sequential cleavage, in order to produce mature and active enzyme forms.
- KLKs exert their actions in highly regulated proteolytic networks, with other KLKs and/or proteases.
- The two most well-studied interaction networks between several KLK members are the semen liquefaction (KLK2, KLK3, KLK5, and KLK14) and skin desquamation (KLK5, KLK7, and KLK14) cascades.
- Aberrations of KLK gene expression, as well as synthesis, secretion, and activation, have been linked with disease development.
- Notably, KLK expression is associated with clinicopathological characteristics of cancer patients, as well as with disease outcome, and therefore, these family members represent promising molecular tumor markers.
- Prostate-specific antigen (PSA/KLK3), the most well-known kallikrein, was approved by the FDA for prostate cancer patients' treatment monitoring and screening, in 1986 and 1994, respectively.

Definitions of Words and Terms

Serine Proteases Serine proteases represent one of the five main mechanistic classes of proteases and are named after the active serine residue in the catalytic site of the molecule. The other known classes of proteolytic enzymes are metalloproteinases, aspartic proteases, cysteine proteases, and threonine proteases.

KLK Activome The term "KLK activome" describes the activation of pro-KLKs, (inactive zymogens) by other mature KLKs.

A Cancer Biomarker A cancer biomarker can be a biological molecule (e.g., DNA, mRNA, miRNA, protein) or even a process (e.g., apoptosis) that are either produced by cancer cells or by the body as a response to the presence of the tumor. An ideal molecular marker should be cancer specific, easily and reliably measured, and able to provide diagnostic, prognostic, and predictive information.

Types of biomarkers: (a) screening biomarkers can detect and identify a certain type of cancer in asymptomatic population. **(b) Prognostic markers** are used to evaluate the course of disease and patients' outcome and therefore provide valuable information for disease surveillance. **(c) A predictive marker** can be used to segregate patients according to their ability to respond to a certain anticancer treatment and thereby guides treatment choice.

Specificity and Sensitivity The terms specificity and sensitivity are used to describe the accuracy of a diagnostic test. Specificity describes the capacity of a marker to correctly recognize healthy individuals [i.e., true-negative/(true-negative + false-positive)]. Sensitivity refers to the ability of a marker to identify patients [i.e., true-positive/(true-positive + false-negative)].

Total PSA (tPSA) In blood circulation, PSA/KLK3 occurs in two forms: complexed with endogenous protease inhibitors (~80 %) and free PSA/KLK3 (~5–40 %). The ratio of fPSA to tPSA improves the diagnostic specificity of PSA/KLK3 testing.

DNA Methylation DNA methylation is a common epigenetic event that refers to the addition of a methyl group at 5′ position of the cytosine ring within CpG dinucleotides. In cancer, aberrant DNA hypermethylation is involved in transcriptional silencing of tumor suppressor genes.

Multiparametric In multiparametric panels, cancer-related molecules, including KLKs, are combined in order to achieve superior sensitivity and specificity compared to each biomarker alone.

IGFs IGFs are mitogenic peptides that regulate cell proliferation, differentiation, and apoptosis, by their attachment to the transmembrane receptor (IGFR).

The bioavailability of IGFs and their interaction with the corresponding receptor is regulated by a family of six IGF-binding proteins (IGFBPs).

Proteinase-Activated Receptors (PAR1–4) Proteinase-activated receptors (PAR1–4) are members of the G-protein-coupled receptor superfamily, and through signaling, they can regulate several processes such as inflammation and cell proliferation.

Extracellular Matrix (ECM) The extracellular matrix (ECM) is composed by a well-organized network of macromolecules and is a physical barrier against cell migration. In terms of cancer, abnormal ECM degradation contributes in tumor progression, angiogenesis, and metastasis.

Epithelial-to-Mesenchymal Transition (EMT) Epithelial-to-mesenchymal transition (EMT) confers morphological changes in cancer cells toward a mesenchymal phenotype, loss of cell polarity, and detachment from the basement membrane, inducing in this way the migratory capacity and invasiveness of tumor cells.

Introduction

The human tissue kallikrein (*KLK1*) and kallikrein-related peptidase (*KLK2–15*) genes encode for a subfamily of 15 homologous, secreted trypsin- and chymotrypsin-like serine endopeptidases, which belong to the S1 protease family of clan PA. All 15 *KLK* genes are tightly and uninterruptedly clustered on human chromosomal region 19q13.3–19q13.4, forming the largest contiguous family of protease genes. Notably, KLK family members share multiple common structural and functional features, at the gene and protein levels (Yousef et al. 2000, 2005). For instance, all *KLKs* are subjected to alternative splicing, and multiple mRNA transcript variants for the same gene have been detected so far. The expression of *KLK* genes is controlled by steroid hormones such as androgens and estrogens. Additionally, *KLK*s encode for single-chain pre-proenzymes, which are activated by sequential proteolytic cleavage by KLKs ("KLK activome") or other proteases (Lawrence et al. 2010; Paliouras and Diamandis 2006; Sotiropoulou et al. 2009).

KLKs are predominantly expressed by glandular epithelial cells of the prostate, breast, skin, salivary glands, brain, colon, and pancreas and are subsequently secreted directly into biofluids such as serum, seminal plasma, and cerebrospinal fluid. Several members of the KLK family are often co-expressed within a specific tissue, a fact that militates in favor of their functional collaboration and/or participation in proteolytic cascades (Shaw and Diamandis 2007; Sotiropoulou et al. 2009). The normal functional properties of KLKs are extremely broad and include, among others, blood pressure control (e.g., KLK1), skin desquamation (e.g., KLK5, KLK7, KLK14), semen liquefaction (e.g., PSA/KLK3), regulation of neural plasticity (e.g., KLK6, KLK8), innate immunity (e.g., KLK5, KLK7), and inflammatory responses (e.g., KLK14) (Fig. 1a) (Emami and Diamandis 2007;

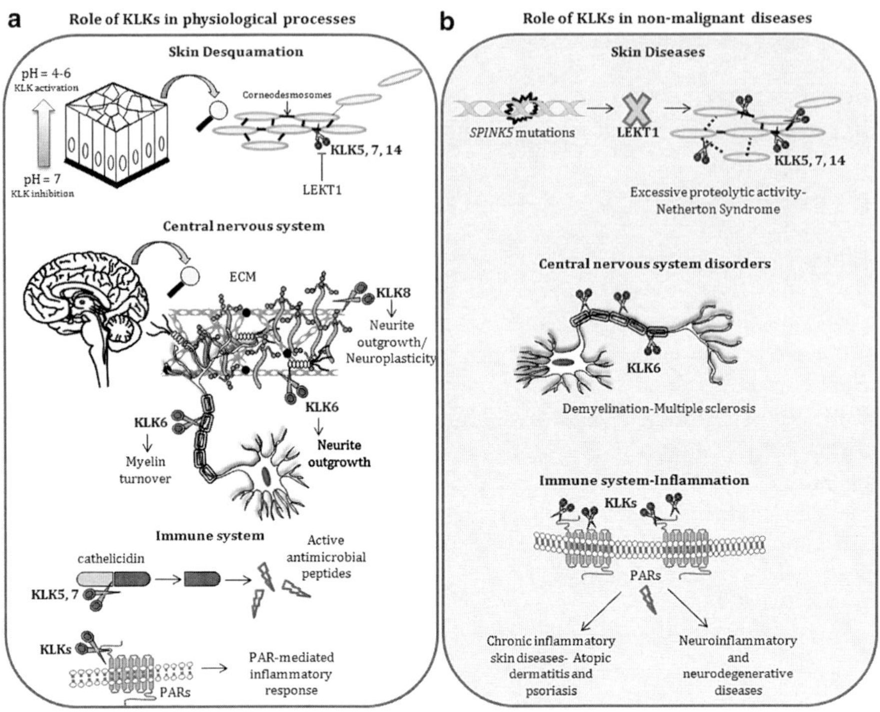

Fig. 1 The diverse roles of KLKs in multiple physiological processes and pathological conditions. (**a**) KLKs participate in *skin desquamation* through cleavage of adhesive proteins of the extracellular part of corneodesmosomes at the epidermis surface. This procedure is mediated by LEKT1-KLK interaction which is regulated by pH gradient through the epidermis. In *brain physiology*, both KLK8 and KLK6 regulate neurite outgrowth by cleavage of distinct ECM molecules. KLK6 is also involved in de- and remyelination processes of neurite axons. In *innate immunity*, KLKs have major functions, through the generation of antimicrobial peptides and in *inflammatory responses* via activation of PAR-signaling pathways. (**b**) In *Netherton syndrome*, mutations of the *SPINK5* gene which result in LEKT1 deficiency and thus in excessive KLK proteolytic activity in stratum corneum. Increased KLK6 expression and activation contributes in demyelination events in *multiple sclerosis*. KLK activation of PAR-signaling pathways plays a prominent role in diverse *inflammatory disorders* in the CNS and skin. *SPINK5* serine peptidase inhibitor Kazal-type 5, *LEKTI* lymphoepithelial Kazal-type-related inhibitor, *PARs* proteinase-activated receptors

Oikonomopoulou et al. 2010; Sotiropoulou et al. 2009; Pampalakis and Sotiropoulou 2007). It is currently apparent that the regulation of KLK gene expression, as well as synthesis, secretion, and activity, requires a robust and fine-tuned control system of many levels, including transcriptional (e.g., steroid hormones, epigenetic modifications), posttranscriptional (e.g., miRNAs), and post-translational (e.g., internal auto-fragmentation) modifications (Emami and Diamandis 2007; Lawrence et al. 2010; Yousef 2008).

Nonetheless, a variety of abnormalities in KLK regulation machinery are documented to be strongly linked with disease development, including cancer.

Indeed, abnormal KLK-mediated activities facilitate several hallmarks of cancer, such as tumor cell growth, angiogenesis, invasion, and metastasis (Avgeris et al. 2012; Borgono and Diamandis 2004; Borgono et al. 2004; Pampalakis and Sotiropoulou 2007). In particular, several KLKs are involved in early events of neoplastic progression by regulating tumor cell proliferation, mainly through cleavage of IGF-binding proteins (IGFBPs) and/or via proteolytic activation of proteinase-activated receptors (PARs). Several data indicate that KLKs are able to provoke invasion and angiogenesis directly through cleavage of extracellular matrix (ECM) proteins, e.g., fibronectin, laminin, collagens, and proteoglycans, and/or indirectly via activation of signaling pathways that involve matrix metalloproteinases (MMPs), urokinase-type plasminogen activator and its receptor (uPA-uPAR), plasminogen, and kinin (Fig. 2). KLKs also induce epithelial-to-mesenchymal transition (EMT)-like changes in cancer cells enhancing in this way their migratory capacity. Finally, the role of KLKs in the establishment of metastatic tumors has been documented, in particular regarding bone metastasis of prostate cancer cells. Contrariwise, KLKs may exhibit inhibitory effects during carcinogenesis, depending upon cancer type and tumor microenvironment. For instance, PSA/KLK3 activity upon several ECM proteins can lead into generation of products with antiangiogenic properties (Avgeris et al. 2012; Blaber et al. 2010; Borgono and Diamandis 2004; Emami and Diamandis 2007; Mavridis et al. 2014; Kryza et al. 2013).

KLK Family: A Rich Source of Cancer Biomarkers

An emerging field of contemporary cancer research is the identification of novel biomarkers. The exploitation of reliable tumor markers, alone or in combinational panels with other biomarkers in clinical practice, will facilitate early diagnosis, effective prognosis, and treatment management of cancer patients.

There are many good reasons to search for such cancer biomarkers in the KLK family. Firstly, PSA/KLK3 is an already established tumor marker, extensively used in prostate cancer screening, prognosis, and treatment monitoring. Secondly, the vast majority of human malignancies display aberrant *KLK* gene expression, as well as KLK synthesis, secretion, and/or activity, which is often associated with patients' prognosis. In addition, the fact that KLKs are secreted molecules makes them ideal biomarker candidates since they can be easily detected in serum and other bodily fluids. Not surprisingly, *KLKs* have been suggested as potential tumor markers for at least one type of malignancy (Avgeris et al. 2010; Borgono et al. 2004; Emami and Diamandis 2008; Kontos and Scorilas 2012; Mavridis and Scorilas 2010).

Among the vast number of studies that highlight the diagnostic, prognostic, and predictive value of KLKs, we have made an effort to summarize the most prominent results regarding the role of this family in several human malignancies (Fig. 3).

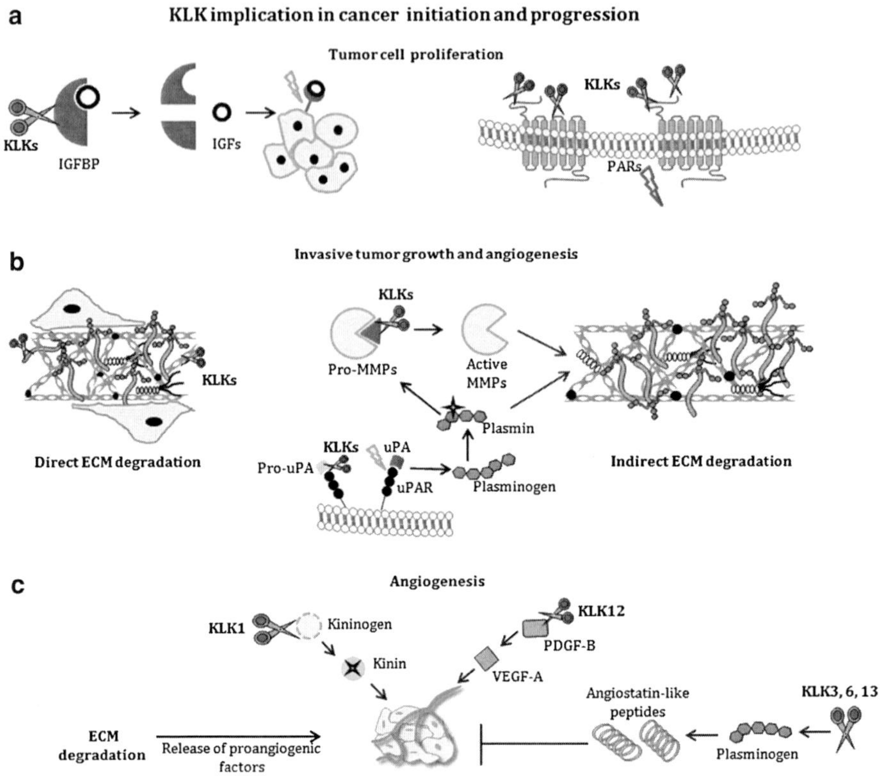

Fig. 2 KLK implication in cancer initiation and progression. KLKs are involved in: (**a**) tumor cell proliferation by proteolytic cleavage of IGFBPs and sequential release of IGFs as well as via activation of PAR-signaling pathways and (**b**) invasive tumor growth through direct and/or indirect ECM degradation. In the latter, KLKs are able to cleave pro-uPA to liberate uPA that binds to its receptor uPAR, resulting in plasmin formation from plasminogen. Plasmin activates MMP proteolytic pathways and both participate in cleavage of ECM components. (**c**) Angiogenesis through degradation of many ECM proteins and activation of growth factors (e.g., VEGF-A). In addition, KLK1 releases active kinin peptides with angiogenic role, whereas plasminogen fragmentation by KLK3, KLK6, and KLK13 produces angiostatin-like peptides that act as inhibitors of angiogenesis. *IGFBPs* insulin-like growth factor-binding proteins, *IGFs* insulin-like growth factors, *PARs* proteinase-activated receptors, *ECM* extracellular matrix, *MMPs* matrix metalloproteinases, *uPA-uPAR* urokinase-type plasminogen activator and its receptor, *VEGF-A* vascular endothelial growth factor, *PDGF-B* platelet-derived growth factor B

Prostate Cancer

Prostate cancer (CaP) is the second most frequently diagnosed cancer in the male population globally (Jemal et al. 2011). The principal clinical aim is the detection of this disease at an early curable stage. Undoubtedly, PSA/KLK3 testing has drastically improved the detection and management of patients with prostatic carcinomas and until to date, is the most broadly used cancer biomarker (Lilja et al. 2008; Ulmert et al. 2009).

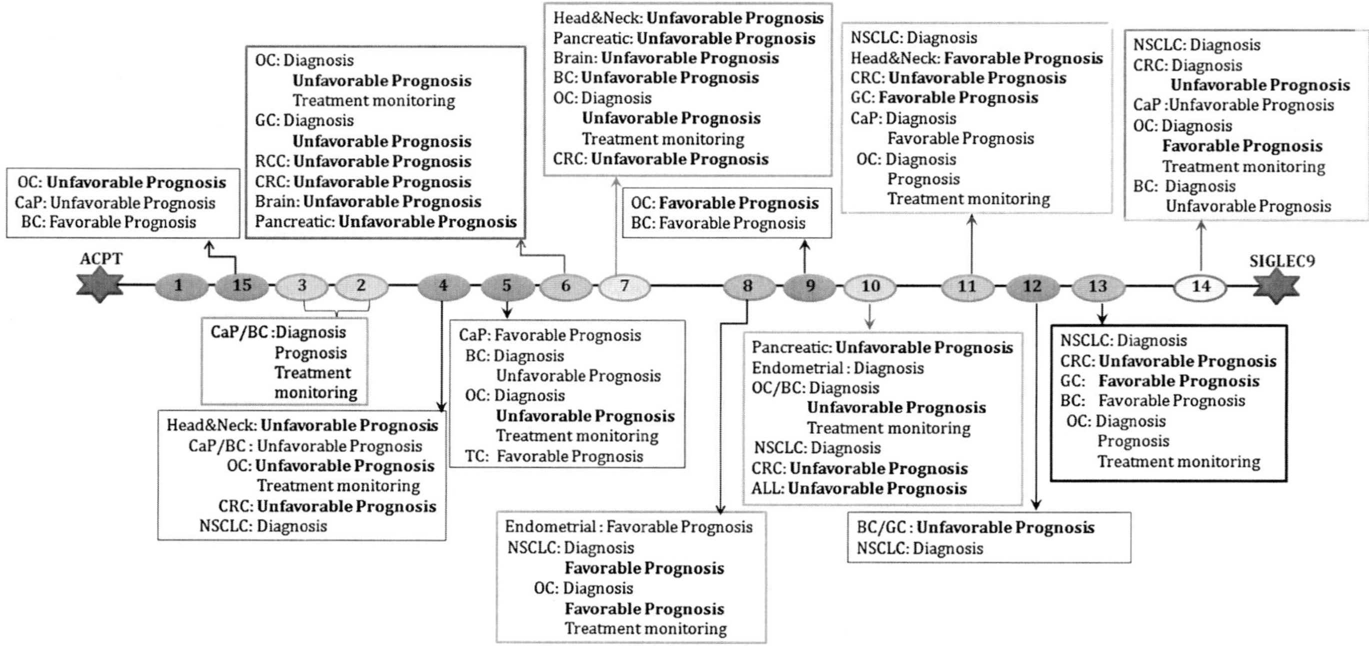

Fig. 3 **Schematic representation of the human kallikrein gene locus and the possible clinical implications of family members in human malignancies.** Prognosis in terms of disease-free and overall survival is indicated in bold font. *ALL* acute lymphoblastic leukemia, *BC* breast cancer, *CaP* prostate cancer, *CRC* colorectal cancer, *GC* gastric cancer, *NSCLC* non-small cell lung cancer, *OC* ovarian cancer, *RCC* renal cell carcinoma, *TC* testicular cancer

Prostate-Specific Antigen (PSA/KLK3): A Long-Used yet Disputed Biomarker for CaP Screening and Diagnosis

The prostate-specific antigen (PSA), encoded by the *KLK3* gene, is the most abundant *KLK* expressed in the prostate gland. Despite the fact that PSA/KLK3 levels are higher in normal compared to neoplastic prostate tissues (Magklara et al. 2000), the cancer-related perturbation of prostate tissue architecture enables its leakage into circulation, resulting in increased amounts of PSA/KLK3 in the blood of CaP patients (Lilja et al. 2008). In 1994, the Food and Drug Administration (FDA) approved serum PSA/KLK3 testing for asymptomatic male population screening, and since then, it has been established as a valuable tool for CaP detection at a preclinical stage. PSA/KLK3 serum concentrations usually increase 5–10 years before other CaP-related clinical symptoms appear, enabling physicians to detect slow-growing and not palpable tumors that might otherwise have escaped diagnosis (Stenman et al. 2005).

Nonetheless, the use of PSA/KLK3 test for screening remains debatable. The foremost limitations of its use are its relatively low diagnostic specificity and its inability to distinguish indolent from aggressive prostate tumors. PSA/KLK3 serum levels increase during other noncancerous prostate disease conditions, including benign prostate hyperplasia (BPH), and are significantly influenced by many factors such as patients' age. These variations may lead into false-positive results, which in turn increase the risk for unnecessary biopsies. In order to improve PSA/KLK3 diagnostic accuracy, several approaches have been introduced, such as the measurement of free PSA (fPSA), PSA velocity (rate of PSA increase), and PSA density (incorporating prostate volume). The ratio of fPSA to total PSA (tPSA), generally expressed as "%fPSA," is lower in CaP patients compared to those with BPH. Therefore, %fPSA adds significant information and improves tPSA diagnostic specificity for men with elevated serum PSA/KLK3, especially for those who fall within the so-called tPSA gray zone (2.5–10 ng/ml) (Avgeris et al. 2012; Lilja et al. 2008; Mavridis and Scorilas 2010; Ulmert et al. 2009).

PSA/KLK3: Applications in CaP Patients' Treatment Monitoring and Prediction of Clinical Outcome

Initially, PSA/KLK3 serum concentration measurement has been approved by the FDA, for CaP patients' treatment monitoring. Increased preoperative serum PSA/KLK3 levels positively correlate with advanced clinical stages of disease and high risk of recurrence after radical prostatectomy (Lilja et al. 2008). Posttreatment PSA/KLK3 serum levels constitute an exceptional marker for the effectiveness of the therapy given, either local or systemic. In this way, the clinicians become aware early of any residual tumors, before other clinical manifestations of recurrence appear, resulting in early initiation of adjuvant treatment. In particular, postoperatively, PSA/KLK3 serum concentration rapidly decreases to reach undetectable levels. As a result, any subsequent increase above a certain level, known as biochemical recurrence, is the first sign of treatment failure. After radiation therapy, PSA levels decrease progressively, and lower nadir PSA levels and a longer time to reach it are both favorable predictors of disease-free survival.

In patients treated with androgen deprivation therapy, the percentage of PSA/KLK3 decrease and the time needed to reach PSA nadir are significant predictors of patients' outcome. Posttreatment increase of PSA/KLK3 nadir levels indicates poor patient clinical outcome due to progression of hormonally resistant disease. Finally, PSA/KLK3 changes are useful for the evaluation of the effectiveness of chemotherapy in patients with metastatic CaP. However, a decline of PSA/KLK3 serum concentration may not always reflect clinical benefit for patients, since several drug-based treatments may influence PSA/KLK3 levels (Avgeris et al. 2012; Lilja et al. 2008; Shariat et al. 2011; Stephan et al. 2007).

Emerging Biomarkers in Prostate Cancer from the Kallikrein Family: Can They Follow and/or Enrich the Success of PSA/KLK3?

Diagnostic Significance

In addition to PSA/KLK3, both KLK2 and KLK11 have been proposed as prospective diagnostic biomarkers in CaP. In fact, KLK2 has attracted researchers' attention, mainly because of its high expression in CaP and its significant sequence similarity to PSA/KLK3. Several reports have documented that when used in conjunction with PSA/KLK3, KLK2 could enhance diagnostic specificity for CaP detection. The ratio of KLK2 to fPSA serum levels exhibits high specificity and effectively discerns CaP cases among individuals with tPSA serum levels within the PSA gray zone. Recently, a four-kallikrein panel consisting of KLK2 and distinct molecular forms of PSA (tPSA, fPSA, and intact PSA) has been shown to be a powerful predictor of prostate biopsy results, in men with elevated PSA/KLK3 serum levels. The application of this panel could result in significant reduction of CaP overdiagnosis, thereby decreasing the number of unnecessary biopsies (Carlsson et al. 2013; Emami and Diamandis 2008; Mavridis and Scorilas 2010; Romero Otero et al. 2014; Shariat et al. 2011).

Regarding KLK11, clinical research studies suggest that the KLK11/tPSA ratio is decreased in men with CaP, compared to those with BPH. In addition, the assessment of the KLK11/tPSA ratio in combination with %fPSA can also be useful in the diagnosis of CaP (Table 1), and thus, rational clinical decisions could be made in order to prevent unneeded biopsies (Mavridis and Scorilas 2010; Nakamura et al. 2003; Stephan et al. 2007). At the tissue level, *KLK4* and *KLK15* mRNA expression is upregulated in CaP compared to BPH specimens, a fact that unravels their diagnostic potential (Avgeris et al. 2012; Romero Otero et al. 2014).

Prostate Cancer Prognosis and Patients' Treatment Monitoring

KLK2 serum levels and *KLK4*, *KLK5*, *KLK11*, *KLK14*, and *KLK15* tissue expression have been demonstrated to possess prognostic and/or predictive value for CaP (Avgeris et al. 2010; Dorn et al. 2013). Specifically, increased KLK2 serum levels combined with low % fPSA are associated with an adverse clinical outcome and are predictors of biochemical relapse in treated CaP patients (Mavridis and Scorilas 2010). Moreover, increased *KLK4* and *KLK14* mRNA levels indicate unfavorable

Table 1 An overview of combinational panels of KLKs and other biomarkers in prostate, ovarian, and lung cancer. Biomarker panels that include KLK members, as well as other cancer-related molecules or established markers, exhibit improved diagnostic, prognostic, and predictive value and therefore can provide additional insights for optimal cancer patients' management. *CA125* cancer antigen 125, *VTCN1* V-set domain-containing T-cell activation inhibitor 1

Type of malignancy	KLK panel or multiparametric model	Expression level studied	Tissue/fluid	Clinical utility	Reference
Prostate cancer	Ratio KLK2/fPSA, %fPSA	Protein	Serum	Diagnosis of prostate cancer Enhanced diagnostic specificity within PSA ranges of 2–10 ng/ml	(Carlsson et al. 2013; Stephan et al. 2007)
	KLK2, tPSA, fPSA, and intact PSA	Protein	Blood		
	Ratio KLK11/tPSA, %fPSA	Protein	Serum		
Ovarian cancer	KLK5–8, KLK10, KLK11, KLK13, KLK14	Protein	Ascites/pleural effusion fluids	Diagnosis of ovarian cancer Discrimination of OC from benign conditions	(Avgeris et al. 2012; Emami and Diamandis 2008)
	KLK 6–8, KLK10	Protein	Ascites/pleural effusion fluids		
	KLK6, CA125	Protein	Serum	Diagnosis of ovarian cancer Improves diagnostic sensitivity of CA125 testing Predictor of shorter overall survival	(Avgeris et al. 2012)
	KLK10, CA125	Protein	Serum	Diagnosis of ovarian cancer Improves diagnostic specificity of CA125 testing	(Avgeris et al. 2012)
	KLK6, KLK13, CA125	mRNA	Tissue	Diagnosis of ovarian cancer Enhanced diagnostic sensitivity and predictive value of CA125 testing	(White et al. 2009)
	KLK7, KLK10, VTCN1, and spondin 2	Protein	Serum	Predictor of patients' 1-year survival after chemotherapy	(Oikonomopoulou et al. 2008b)
	KLK5–7 and VTCN1	Protein	Serum	Predictor of patients' response to chemotherapy	
	CA125, KLK7, KLK8, and spondin 2	Protein	Serum	Predictor of disease progression in treated patients	
Lung cancer	KLK4, KLK8, and KLK10–14	Protein	Serum	Diagnosis of non-small cell lung cancer	(Planque et al. 2008)

outcome, since they are associated with several established clinicopathological parameters of poor prognosis in CaP, such as advanced stage and high Gleason score. Additionally, elevated KLK14 tissue expression is associated with high risk of relapse and disease progression in patients treated with radical prostatectomy, and KLK14 protein expression was found to be an independent prognostic factor in CaP (Avgeris et al. 2012; Rabien et al. 2008). Increased KLK15 protein expression levels are associated with poor patients' outcome, and similarly, *KLK15* overexpression is associated with more aggressive features of prostate tumors (Avgeris et al. 2010). Furthermore, according to a recent study, high *KLK15* classical variant expression levels can independently predict an increased risk of biochemical relapse in CaP patients (Mavridis et al. 2013). On the other hand, higher *KLK5* and *KLK11* expression levels are found in less aggressive CaP and thus are both considered as prognostic markers of favorable patients' outcome (Dorn et al. 2013).

Ovarian Cancer

Ovarian cancer (OC) is the most lethal of all common gynecologic neoplasms worldwide. This is mostly owing to the absence of early detectable symptoms and the lack of highly sensitive and effective screening and diagnostic methods for this malignancy. Apart from that, the drug-resistant nature of OC hampers the effectiveness of the available therapeutic strategies, enhancing disease lethality. Unfortunately, serum cancer antigen 125 (CA125) measurements in combination with imaging methods are deemed insufficient for optimal patients' management, making the identification of novel and more reliable blood-borne or tissue-based tumor markers mandatory (Dorn et al. 2012, 2013).

KLK6, KLK10, and Other KLK Family Members as Promising Markers in Ovarian Cancer Diagnosis

The expression profiles of a vast majority of KLK family members are abnormally altered in OC. In fact, several *KLKs* (*KLK3–KLK11*, *KLK13–KLK15*) are found to be overexpressed in OC tissues, compared to noncancerous controls. At the protein level, KLK3–11, KLK13, and KLK14 are demonstrated to be increased in cancerous versus normal ovarian tissues or other nonmalignant conditions (Schmitt et al. 2013). More importantly, the levels of KLK5–8, KLK10, KLK11, KLK13, and KLK14 are augmented in pleural effusion or ascites fluids of women with OC, in comparison to patients with benign ovarian conditions, and KLK6–8 and KLK10 exhibit significant combinatorial diagnostic value. The above findings underline the role of several KLKs as valuable biomarkers for OC diagnosis (Shih Ie et al. 2007).

Among the aforementioned family members, KLK6 and KLK10 exhibit the most promising competence as serum biomarkers for OC diagnosis at an early stage. Increased KLK6 and KLK10 levels are found in serum of OC patients compared to healthy women. As far as KLK6 is concerned, KLK6 overexpression appears to be an early event in neoplastic transformation in OC, highlighting its diagnostic value. Moreover, the combination of KLK6 serum measurements with CA125 testing improves the sensitivity (21 % increase at 90 % specificity) and enhances the diagnostic potential of CA125 (Diamandis et al. 2003; Rosen et al. 2005). The assessment of *KLK6*, *CA125*, and *KLK13* gene expression in a combinational panel exhibits enhanced diagnostic sensitivity compared to the determination of serum CA125 alone (White et al. 2009). In addition, the unique KLK6 N-glycosylation pattern, identified in ascites fluid of patients with OC, strengthens the diagnostic value of KLK6 for this malignancy (Kuzmanov et al. 2009).

Similar results have been reported for KLK10, underscoring its potential use as a novel serological diagnostic biomarker of OC. KLK10 serum measurements can successfully improve the diagnostic sensitivity of CA125 in OC. Interestingly, KLK10 exhibits the highest diagnostic specificity compared to KLK6 and/or CA125. Increased KLK10 serum levels are also found in a number of patients that lack CA125 expression. This observation prompted the use of KLK10 (along with KLK6) in a combinational panel with other serological biomarkers, in order to improve diagnosis of those OC patients with no or low CA125 expression (Avgeris et al. 2012; Dorn et al. 2012; Kontos and Scorilas 2012).

KLK5 can represent a promising marker for differential diagnosis, since KLK5 concentration is significantly higher in serum samples from OC patients, relatively to those with nonmalignant or borderline ovarian tumors. A similar upward expression trend for KLK5 was observed in ascites fluids of OC patients compared to those harboring benign lesions or other cancer types (Avgeris et al. 2012; Dorn et al. 2013).

KLKs with Potential Prognostic and/or Predictive Value in Ovarian Cancer

A number of studies suggest that *KLK 4–7*, *KLK10*, and *KLK15* are indicators of poor prognosis in OC patients, whereas *KLK8–9* and *KLK14* can effectively predict a favorable disease outcome. Particularly, *KLK4* and *KLK15* mRNA expression and *KLK5* and *KLK7* mRNA and protein levels are independent markers of unfavorable prognosis in OC, since their expression positively correlates with advanced-stage and higher-grade tumors as well as with limited DFS and OS. Interestingly, the expression of alternative splice variants of both *KLK5* and *KLK7* is related to aggressive phenotypes of the disease, suggesting the need for further evaluation of their prognostic potential in OC (Dong et al. 2003). According to a recent study, increased KLK5 serum and ascites fluid levels are associated with shorter progression-free survival and thus poor patients' outcome (Dorn et al. 2011b).

KLK6 and KLK10 are the two of the most extensively studied members of the KLK family in OC, which apart from their significant diagnostic potential, exhibit substantial prognostic capabilities. Elevated KLK6 protein expression in OC tumors was associated with aggressive disease phenotype as well as with limited progression-free survival and OS periods. In addition, increased KLK6 serum concentration correlates with late-stage tumors and along with CA125 are strong predictors of short survival intervals of the patients. Similarly, KLK10 protein expression in tissues and serum samples obtained from patients with OC is associated with advanced stage, inadequate patients' response to chemotherapy, and adverse outcome (in terms of shorter DFS and OS). Besides, *KLK6* and *KLK13* mRNA levels can predict disease recurrence in epithelial OC (Avgeris et al. 2012).

As opposed to the KLKs discussed above, *KLK8*, *KLK9*, and *KLK14* are markers of favorable prognosis, as the increased transcription of these genes is associated with less aggressive disease phenotypes, minimal residual tumor volume, and better DFS and OS. In addition, *KLK14* mRNA levels are negatively correlated with preoperative CA125 serum levels, reinforcing its value as a marker of favorable prognosis (Kontos and Scorilas 2012). KLK8 expression has been studied in OC tissues, as well as in cytosolic extracts, effusion specimens, and the serum, leading in opposite results. Specifically, KLK8 expression in OC tissues is associated with unfavorable disease outcome, whereas its protein concentration in cytosolic extracts, effusion specimens, and the serum was found to be a predictor of favorable prognosis (Avgeris et al. 2012). Recent data report that expression differences of KLK8, KLK5–7, KLK10–11, KLK13, and uPA and its inhibitor, between primary and metastatic tumors, are significantly associated with disease progression and OC patients' outcome (Dorn et al. 2011a). Finally, elevated *KLK11* and *KLK13* mRNA levels in OC tissues are indicative of aggressive disease, whereas increased KLK11 and KLK13 protein concentrations are favorable markers in terms of DFS and OS (Dorn et al. 2013).

Apart from their prognostic value, many members of the KLK family have been evaluated for their potential use as novel predictive tumor markers in OC. For instance, KLK4 gene and protein expression can distinguish paclitaxel-resistant patients from the responder ones. Furthermore, measurement of KLK5, KLK7, and CA125 serum concentrations at baseline or after first chemotherapy cycle can effectively predict response to carboplatin and/or paclitaxel, whereas KLK7 protein overexpression in OC tissues is associated with resistance to carboplatin and/or paclitaxel. High KLK6 protein content in serum is indicative of reduced response to platinum-based therapy. KLK6, in conjunction with KLK8 and KLK13 protein levels, cancer stage, and debulking status, can assist in recognizing OC patients who will potentially benefit of platinum-based antineoplastic drugs. Moreover, the comparison of pre- and posttreatment KLK6 serum levels revealed a significant decline in KLK6 expression after tumor surgical removal. This observation is of particular interest, since KLK6 serum levels in combination with CA125 can be exploited not only for diagnostic purposes but for patients' treatment monitoring as well. Furthermore, KLK8 seems to be a promising predictive biomarker in a proportion of OC patients with low or absent CA125 levels. Finally, higher KLK11 and KLK13 protein levels and *KLK14* mRNA expression, in OC tissues, are associated with better response to chemotherapy, whereas an increase of KLK10 concentration in sera reflects platinum-based therapy resistance (Dorn et al. 2012).

Currently, intensive research efforts focus on the design of multiparametric models for identifying panels of biomarkers with greater diagnostic, prognostic, and predictive potential (Table 1). Plenty of KLKs have been incorporated in biomarker panels along with other cancer-related molecules such as regenerating islet-derived family, member 4 (REG4), V-set domain-containing T-cell activation inhibitor 1 (VTCN1, also known as B7-H4), spondin 2, and CA125, with very promising results. For example, a panel which includes KLK7, KLK10, VTCN1, and spondin 2 constitutes a predictor of posttreatment patients' survival. Additionally, baseline values of KLK5–7, along with VTCN1, can predict patients' response to chemotherapy. Finally, assessment of CA125, KLK7, KLK8, and spondin 2 revealed their combinatorial prognostic value (Oikonomopoulou et al. 2008b).

Breast Cancer

Breast cancer (BC) is the most frequently diagnosed neoplasm and the leading cause of cancer-related deaths in the female population worldwide. BC is an extremely heterogeneous disease entity and remains until now a significant scientific and clinical challenge in terms of disease management (Jemal et al. 2011). The successful identification and use of BC-specific biomarkers is essential for diagnosis, prognosis, and treatment monitoring of patients.

KLKs with Diagnostic Significance for Breast Cancer

Several *KLKs* exhibit aberrant expression patterns in BC, and the majority of *KLKs* are reported to be downregulated in BC, at mRNA and/or protein levels, compared to noncancerous breast tissues. On the contrary, *KLK4* and *KLK15* mRNA expression levels appear to be elevated in BC specimens compared to benign or normal ones (Schmitt et al. 2013). KLK5, KLK10, and KLK14 have been reported to possess diagnostic value for BC. More precisely, serum KLK5, KLK10, and KLK14 protein levels appear to be elevated in subset of patients with BC, compared to healthy individuals (Avgeris et al. 2012). Recently, the quantification of *KLK5* mRNA levels in breast tumors revealed its potential application in differential diagnosis between BC and benign breast diseases (Avgeris et al. 2011). Furthermore, PSA/KLK3 may also have diagnostic application in BC, since fPSA is accumulated in higher concentrations in the serum of BC, compared to healthy women. However, its low diagnostic sensitivity is the major difficulty for its use in BC diagnosis (Black and Diamandis 2000; Black et al. 2000).

Prognosis and Treatment Monitoring

Emerging evidence highlights the promising prognostic capabilities of *KLK* family members in BC. Firstly, the increased mRNA expression of *KLK4*, *KLK5*, *KLK7*, *KLK10*, *KLK12*, and *KLK14*, is correlated with unfavorable clinical outcome for BC patients (Kontos and Scorilas 2012). In particular, *KLK4* overexpression seems to be associated with advanced-stage and high-grade tumors, and thus, *KLK4* may be regarded as a potential marker of poor prognosis in BC. *KLK5* and *KLK7* are both downregulated in BC; however, high *KLK5* or *KLK7* expression levels are significantly associated with shorter DFS and OS periods, pointing to their value as biomarkers of unfavorable prognosis in BC (Avgeris et al. 2012). Regarding

KLK10, this member of the family has been thoroughly studied in BC and is considered to function as a tumor suppressor gene. More specifically, expression analysis of *KLK10* by an in situ hybridization assay demonstrated the tumor-specific loss of *KLK10* expression during BC progression, which in the preponderance of breast carcinomas is attributed to the hypermethylation of the third exon of the gene. On the basis of these findings, a different study explored and uncovered the prognostic value of *KLK10* methylation status in BC patients, as it was found to be associated with limited DFS and OS survival periods (Kioulafa et al. 2009). Additionally, high KLK10 tissue protein levels are associated with shorter progression-free survival after the start of tamoxifen-based treatment and therefore, constitute important predictors of patients' response to treatment (Luo et al. 2002). *KLK12* transcript variant expression levels are correlated with an adverse BC patient outcome in terms of shorter DFS and OS. *KLK14* positivity was more frequently found in advanced-stage mammary gland tumors and in patients with decreased DFS and OS periods. The observation that higher KLK14 protein expression is associated with dedifferentiated tumors and positive nodal status strengthens its value as a biomarker of adverse prognosis in BC (Mavridis and Scorilas 2010; Obiezu and Diamandis 2005).

On the other hand, several other *KLKs* such as *PSA/KLK3*, *KLK9*, *KLK13*, and *KLK15* may hold clinical value as biomarkers of favorable prognosis for BC patients' outcome. PSA/KLK3 may be a valuable biomarker for BC, by the virtue of its potential to indicate patients' outcome and response to treatment. Several studies measuring PSA/KLK3 levels in BC tissue extracts provide evidence that PSA/KLK3 expression levels correlate with less aggressive tumors and with significantly lower risk for relapse and death compared to patients with PSA/KLK3-negative ones. Another important finding is that PSA/KLK3 levels are lower in NAF obtained from patients with large-size and advanced-stage breast tumors plus in patients with metastasis (Sauter et al. 2004). PSA/KLK3 may serve as an important predictor of patients' response to endocrine therapy, since increased PSA/KLK3 tissue levels in patients with recurrent disease are related to inadequate clinical response to tamoxifen. Similarly, increased KLK10 levels are significantly associated with poor response to tamoxifen, and therefore, KLK10 along with PSA/KLK3 can be taken into consideration for the selection of those patients who will benefit from the antiestrogen treatment. Finally, mRNA expression analyses of *KLK9*, *KLK13*, and *KLK15* in BC, using quantitative real-time PCR, have revealed their capabilities as independent biomarkers of favorable prognosis, since they are associated with superior DFS and OS intervals of BC patients (Avgeris et al. 2012; Luo et al. 2002).

Endometrial and Cervical Cancer

Carcinomas of the uterine cervix and corpus are significant causes of mortality, with high prevalence, especially in developing countries. Despite the widespread use of the Pap smear test and improvements in early diagnosis, many unmet clinical needs still persist for the management of these patients, and alternative approaches of cytology screening are required, particularly in developing countries (Jemal et al. 2011).

KLKs with Potential Clinical Utility in Endometrial Carcinomas

KLK4, KLK6, KLK8, and KLK10 are aberrantly expressed in endometrial cancer; however, their potential clinical value has not been fully elucidated yet. In particular, the expression of KLK4, as detected by immunohistochemistry (IHC), was reported to be higher in cancerous compared to hyperplastic and/or normal endometrial tissues. Likewise, increased KLK8 expression was more frequently found in endometrial carcinomas, at both the mRNA and protein levels. Elevated KLK8 protein expression was observed in early stage and low-grade tumors, indicating its potential as biomarker of favorable prognosis in endometrial cancer. Patients suffering from uterine papillary serous carcinoma (UPSC), a more aggressive type of endometrial cancer, exhibit both upregulated *KLK6* mRNA expression and elevated KLK6 serum concentrations. Finally, KLK10 protein is also significantly elevated in the serum of patients with UPSC (Dorn et al. 2013).

KLKs with Potential Clinical Utility in Cervical Cancer

In the case of cervical cancer (CC), only KLK7 holds a significant value for patients suffering from this type of malignancy. In fact, the IHC staining of KLK7 exhibits an increasing trend with cervical disease severity, and thus, it could potentially be used as a biomarker for the classification of different disease stages. Additionally, a significant percentage of cervical adenocarcinomas were found with intense KLK7 IHC staining, suggesting that KLK7 could be a potential adjunct marker in Pap test screening. Furthermore, KLK8 is highly expressed in CC, whereas its prognostic relevance has not been demonstrated yet (Dorn et al. 2013).

Renal Cell Carcinoma and Urinary Bladder Cancer

Renal cell carcinoma (RCC) represents the most common type of kidney neoplasms, whereas bladder cancer exhibits high rates of tumor recurrence after treatment (Jemal et al. 2011). Hence, the identification of novel biomarkers is essential for improving patients' prognosis and quality of life.

KLKs with Potential Clinical Utility in RCC and Bladder Cancer

In the view of the fact that until to date there are no clinically established diagnostic markers for RCC triggered the study of several KLK family members, in order to unravel their capabilities as biomarkers for this malignancy. In particular, the expression of KLK5, KLK6, KLK10, and KLK11, as detected by IHC, is significantly decreased in RCC compared to normal kidney tissues. The same study showed that a higher percentage of more aggressive tumors expressed KLK6 and KLK10, compared to less aggressive ones, while KLK6 and KLK11 expression was positively correlated with disease stage. Additionally, KLK6 expression was found to be a predictor of shorter DFS, supporting its value as prognosticator of unfavorable outcome (Petraki et al. 2006). According to a different study, KLK7 expression may have a potential use in distinguishing between oncocytoma (benign) and chromophobe RCC (malignant), which are histologically similar and difficult to differentiate. KLK6 and KLK7 exhibited strong IHC staining in low-grade tumors compared to high-grade kidney ones, whereas KLK1 expression was found to be increased in high-grade clear cell RCC (Gabril et al. 2010). Finally, *KLK1*, *KLK3*, *KLK6*, and *KLK7* mRNA expression is downregulated in RCC, compared to normal kidney tissues, revealing a potential diagnostic utility for these *KLKs* (White et al. 2010).

In the case of urinary bladder cancer, an increase in *KLK5*, *KLK6*, *KLK8*, and *KLK9* mRNA expression and KLK5, KLK6, KLK10, and KLK11 protein expression was observed in cancerous compared to normal bladder tissues. However, the expression profiles of KLKs and their potential clinical applications have not been fully elucidated yet in bladder cancer (Dorn et al. 2013).

Gastric and Colon Cancer

Gastric cancer (GC) represents one of the most lethal malignancies globally, mainly due to the asymptomatic nature of the disease which leads to late-stage diagnosis. Colorectal cancer (CRC) remains one of the three most frequently diagnosed malignancies in both genders, despite the recent achievements in resection procedures and chemotherapy (Kontos et al. 2013). As a consequence, the identification and establishment of novel biomarkers for GC and CRC is necessary for optimal clinical management of these patients.

KLKs with Potential Clinical Utility in Gastric Cancer

Several recent findings suggest that certain KLK family members are capable of providing prognostic information for patients suffering from GC. In particular, *KLK6* and *KLK10* mRNA as well as KLK6 and KLK12 protein expression is associated with unfavorable prognosis, whereas KLK11 and *KLK13* seem to be prognosticators of favorable patients' outcome. KLK6 protein expression is an independent prognostic indicator of tumor recurrence and decreased OS intervals in GC patients. Elevated KLK6 serum levels have been observed in GC patients compared to healthy controls, highlighting its potential use as a serological marker for this malignancy. Moreover, increased *KLK6* and *KLK10* mRNA expression is positively correlated with lymphatic invasion and more advanced clinical stages. In addition to this, the *KLK6* mRNA expression status appears to be a significant prognostic marker of shorter OS. Likewise, KLK12 is overexpressed in GC and is associated with aggressive disease phenotypes and shorter OS periods (Kontos et al. 2013).

On the other hand, *KLK11* and *KLK13* possess a potential clinical value as predictors of favorable GC patients' outcome. KLK11 is significantly downregulated at both mRNA and protein levels in GC tissues and appears to be an independent marker of superior DFS and OS (Unal et al. 2013). Regarding *KLK13*, is downregulated in GC tissues compared to their normal counterparts and its expression is associated with less GC aggressive features and improved DFS and OS (Kontos et al. 2013). Recent results revealed that *KLK13* expression is modulated in cultivated GC cell lines, after their exposure to different antineoplastic agents, suggesting that *KLK13* may be employed as a treatment-response predictor for GC (Florou et al. 2012).

KLKs with Potential Clinical Utility in Colon Cancer

In the case of CRC, KLK4, KLK6, KLK7, KLK8, KLK10, KLK11, KLK13, and KLK15 are found to be overexpressed in cancerous tissue parts compared to adjacent normal mucosa. Moreover, KLK5–7, KLK11, KLK13, and KLK14 protein content was associated with inferior OS, revealing their potential as markers of unfavorable patients' prognosis. In low rectal cancer, increased KLK11 expression is associated with late-stage disease and shorter OS (Kontos et al. 2013). At mRNA level, *KLK4* is upregulated in advanced-stage and/or poorly differentiated tumors and correlates with tumor size. *KLK4* overexpression is an independent marker of increased risk of relapse (Kontos et al. 2012). *KLK6* and *KLK10* mRNA expression is correlated with disease aggressiveness and limited survival intervals, supporting their role as predictors of unfavorable outcome in CRC patients (Alexopoulou et al. 2013; Ogawa et al. 2005). *KLK7* and *KLK14* have not only prognostic but also discriminatory value. Their prognostic potential stems from the fact that *KLK7* and *KLK14* mRNA expression is indicative of shorter DFS, while *KLK14* is also associated with limited OS. Additionally, the significant increase in *KLK7* and *KLK14* transcripts in cancer tissues compared to adenoma specimens can be exploited for the discrimination between these conditions (Kontos et al. 2013).

Other Types of Human Cancer

Although KLKs are long known for their biomarker capabilities in CaP, OC, and BC, a steadily increasing number of studies suggest that members of the family are of clinical value for other types of human cancer as well, such as those of the brain, pancreas, head and neck, and blood. The research is still ongoing and is expected to uncover the clinical relevance of KLKs in these malignancies in the near future.

Intracranial tumors**:** in brain malignancies, a promising prognostic value has been suggested only for *KLK6* and *KLK7*. A recent study demonstrated that *KLK6* expression is more frequently found in histological types of high malignancy, compared to low malignancy ones, and patients harboring *KLK6*-positive tumors displayed shorter DFS and high risk for relapse (Talieri et al. 2012). Regarding *KLK7*, its expression was found to be associated with shorter OS in patients and with increased invasive potential in cultivated brain tumor cells, highlighting its value in predicting adverse clinical outcome (Prezas et al. 2006).

Pancreatic cancer**:** co-expression of KLK6 and KLK10 in pancreatic ductal adenocarcinoma is significantly associated with shorter OS intervals and unfavorable patient prognosis, suggesting a potential interaction between these two KLKs that contributes to cancer progression. Additionally, KLK7 constitutes an indicator of unfavorable prognosis for patients with unresectable pancreatic ductal adenocarcinoma, given that KLK7 positivity is significantly associated with reduced OS intervals. Finally, three members of the family, namely, *KLK6*, *KLK8*, and *KLK10*, are upregulated in pancreatic cancer compared to normal tissues, whereas *KLK1* is downregulated at mRNA level, as revealed by an in silico analysis (Avgeris et al. 2010; Kontos et al. 2013).

Head and neck cancers: *KLK4*, *KLK7*, and *KLK11* seem to have diagnostic and/or prognostic potential in head and neck cancers. In particular, IHC staining of primary oral cancers revealed a strongest staining intensity for both KLK4 and KLK7 in poor differentiated tumors; the corresponding patients exhibited significantly shorter OS. These observations suggest that these KLKs may be used as markers of unfavorable prognosis in the disease. Regarding laryngeal squamous cell carcinoma, *KLK11* mRNA expression analysis could contribute to both differential diagnosis and disease prognosis. *KLK11* expression was significantly lower in cancerous specimens compared to nonmalignant ones, while *KLK11* positivity was related to prolonged OS intervals, disclosing its value as a biomarker of favorable patients' prognosis (Kontos and Scorilas 2012).

Lymphoblastic leukemia: in a manner similar to BC, a significant downregulation of *KLK10* mRNA expression via epigenetic mechanisms has been demonstrated in acute lymphoblastic leukemia (ALL) patients as well. In particular, *KLK10* gene silencing in ALL occurs through hypermethylation of either the gene promoter, 5′-UTR, or the coding region. Notably, the methylation status of the *KLK10* gene provides important prognostic information in ALL patients and is significantly associated with shorter DFS intervals and inferior patients' prognosis (Paliouras et al. 2007; Roman-Gomez et al. 2004).

Lung cancer: a serum-based panel of KLKs, namely, KLK4, KLK8, and KLK10–14, appears to have a relatively good accuracy for the differential diagnosis of non-small cell lung cancer (NSCLC) from healthy individuals (Table 1). Furthermore, the serum levels of KLK5, KLK7, KLK8, KLK10, and KLK12 are significantly decreased, whereas KLK11, KLK13, and KLK14 are increased in NSCLC patients in relation to healthy individuals. *KLK6*, *KLK8*, and *KLK12* mRNA levels are upregulated in NSCLC tissues compared to nonmalignant counterparts, whereas both *KLK7* and *KLK10* expression is significantly downregulated, suggesting a possible clinical value for these KLKs in diagnosis (Planque et al. 2008). In terms of prognostic significance, increased KLK8 mRNA and protein expression is associated with longer DFS, and thus, KLK8 may constitute a potential indicator of favorable patients' outcome. On the other hand, elevated protein and mRNA levels of *KLK6* and *KLK8* type 4 splice variant appear to be independent markers of poor disease outcome (Heuzé-Vourc'H and Courty 2012). Similarly, *KLK11* is upregulated in a subgroup of neuroendocrine tumors with adverse outcome. A strong correlation has been reported for KLK11 and KLK12 with disease stage, while *KLK5* and *KLK10* overexpression is associated with lung cancer histotype. Finally, *KLK13* expression is an indicator of poor outcome as it is related to lower OS probabilities (Mavridis and Scorilas 2010).

Testicular cancer: According to preliminary data, *KLK5*, *KLK10*, *KLK13*, and *KLK14* are downregulated at the mRNA level in TC compared to normal tissues. Moreover, IHC staining of KLK10 protein in testicular tissues confirmed that malignant germ cells lack KLK10 expression. Additionally, expression analysis of *KLK13* transcript variants revealed that all alternative transcripts, except the classical form, are restricted in normal testicular tissues compared to adjacent tumors, suggesting their plausible use as biomarkers in TC. Finally, quantification of *KLK5* mRNA expression in TC tissues revealed that late-stage (II/III) tumors exhibited significantly lower *KLK5* expression compared to early stage ones, suggesting a clinical value as a biomarker of favorable prognosis (Dorn et al. 2013; Emami and Diamandis 2008; Paliouras et al. 2007).

KLK-Targeting MicroRNAs: A New Era in Cancer Research Has Just Begun

The discovery of microRNAs (miRNAs), a class of small, noncoding RNA molecules, has attracted great attention in scientific communities, while the observation that miRNA expression is deregulated in human malignancies has opened up new horizons in cancer research.

Accumulating evidence supports that miRNAs act as posttranscriptional regulators of *KLK* gene expression (Pasic et al. 2012; Yousef 2008). Interestingly, a study using a bioinformatics approach reported that 96 miRNAs are predicted to target one or more KLKs (Chow et al. 2008). Several KLK-targeting miRNAs have been experimentally validated. For instance, a more recent study demonstrated that transfection of CaP cell lines, with miR-99a, miR-99b, or miR-100, resulted in both decreased expression of PSA/KLK3 and significant inhibition of cancer cell growth, suggesting a possible mechanism for regulating PSA/KLK3 in vivo (Sun et al. 2011). Other experimentally validated miRNA regulators of KLK expression include miR-224 for KLK1 and KLK10, let-7f for KLK6 and KLK10, miR-516a for KLK10, miR-143 for KLK10, and miR-331-3p for KLK4 (Pasic et al. 2012; White et al. 2012). Nonetheless, further understanding of the miRNA-KLK axis of interaction will provide new insights into the mechanisms that control KLK deregulation in cancer and will ultimately lay the foundation for the development of novel anticancer therapeutic strategies.

Single-Nucleotide Polymorphisms (SNPs) in the Human KLK Locus

SNPs represent the most common type of sequence variation in the human genome, and numerous SNPs have been identified within the *KLK* family locus until to date. Interestingly, certain SNPs in *KLK2*, *KLK3*, and *KLK15* are found to be associated with an elevated risk for CaP, BC, or OC and thereby may represent valuable tools for individualized risk stratification and treatment planning. In particular, an SNP located at exon 5 of *KLK2* is found to be associated with CaP risk, whereas SNPs located in *KLK2* may also be useful in BC risk prediction. Additionally, certain SNPs at *KLK2*, when used in combinatorial models with other clinicopathological variables, can significantly improve the prediction of biochemical recurrence after primary cancer treatment in CaP patients. Regarding *KLK3*, two SNPs located within the gene and the *KLK2–KLK3* intergenic region are strongly associated with CaP patients' survival; also, a functional SNP located at one of the androgen response elements of *KLK3* was found to be associated with increased serum PSA levels. Finally, two individual SNPs at *KLK3* and *KLK15* are strongly related to poorer OC patients' survival (Batra et al. 2013; Kontos and Scorilas 2012; Mavridis et al. 2012).

Methodologies and Analytical Techniques

So far, several techniques have been developed and employed for the detection and quantification of KLK expression levels in different biological sources. In particular, real-time PCR (qPCR) is used for the quantification of *KLK* mRNA levels in different tissues or conditions. ELISA immunoassays, radioimmunoassay (RIA), and immunofluorescence-based methods are usually employed for evaluating KLK expression in several biofluids such as serum, CFS, and ascites fluid, as well as in tissue extracts. For instance, sandwich-type ELISA was employed in order to study the protein levels of KLK5–8, KLK10, and KLK11, as well as CA125, VTCN1, and spondin 2, in OC patients' serum. Immunofluorometric methods are used for the determination of tPSA and fPSA in serum samples of CaP and BPH patients. In order to monitor the proportion of enzymatically active KLKs, in biological fluids or supernatants of cell cultures, a serine proteinase-targeted activity-based probe (ABP) coupled to antibody capture assay can be employed. Interestingly, a recent study developed and used this method in order to quantify the proportion of enzymatically active KLK6 in ascites fluid and OC cancer cell culture supernatant. The findings revealed that KLK6 exists in these fluids, mainly in its inactive form. Furthermore, IHC confirms the cellular and subcellular localization of the KLK proteins, providing a clue about their potential function in various tissues (Kontos and Scorilas 2012; Oikonomopoulou et al. 2008a; Paliouras and Diamandis 2006).

Potential Applications of KLK Family Members to Prognosis, Nonmalignant Diseases, or Conditions

A considerable amount of studies have focused on the elucidation of the putative roles of KLKs in a number of human diseases, apart from cancer, in order to unravel their clinical value and therapeutic potential. Many experimental data implicate the aberrations of KLK expression and proteolytic activity in the pathogenesis of nonmalignant disease states in the central nervous system (CNS) and skin (Fig. 1b). Notably, altered KLK levels are found in CNS lesions, serum, and/or cerebrospinal fluid (CSF) of patients with neurological disorders such as multiple sclerosis (MS), Alzheimer's disease (AD), and Parkinson's disease (PD). In addition, KLKs play important roles in inflammatory skin diseases such as psoriasis, Netherton syndrome, and atopic dermatitis. Finally, KLK1 is involved in hypertension, inflammation, renal nephritis, and diabetic renal disease (Bayani and Diamandis 2011; Emami and Diamandis 2007; Goettig et al. 2010; Sotiropoulou and Pampalakis 2012).

KLKs and CNS Disorders

Several KLK family members are expressed and are essential in numerous physiological and pathological processes in the human brain. Among the KLKs expressed in CNS, KLK6 and KLK8 are the two most widely studied members of the family. The former appears to be involved in demyelination events and hence in CNS diseases, in which the myelin sheath is damaged, such as MS. The expression of numerous KLKs, including KLK6, is upregulated in activated immune cells, and recently, it has been postulated that KLKs may contribute to neurodegenerative disorders, through PAR activation which in turn triggers inflammation. KLK6 is also implicated in AD through its amyloidogenic activity which results in accumulation of amyloid plaques in patients' brain, while it is also involved in α-synuclein cleavage and thereby prevents its polymerization in Lewy bodies that represent a typical characteristic of PD (Bayani and Diamandis 2011; Oikonomopoulou et al. 2010; Scarisbrick et al. 2008; Sotiropoulou and Pampalakis 2012). Focusing on KLK8, its expression is induced in CNS by injury processes and it is believed that it regulates pathogenic procedures in the hippocampus/CNS (Sotiropoulou and Pampalakis 2012).

***Multiple sclerosis*:** MS is a common demyelinating disorder, in which KLKs may have an important clinical value. In particular, increased KLK6 expression is reported in CSF of MS patients with advanced disease compared to controls, as well as in demyelinating MS lesions. A recent study revealed that KLK1 and KLK6 serum levels are significantly elevated in MS patients and are found to be associated with secondary progressive disease, suggesting that these KLKs may serve as serological markers for patients. Elevated KLK1 was also correlated with concurrent disability and KLK6 with future disease worsening (Bayani and Diamandis 2011; Scarisbrick et al. 2008).

***Alzheimer's and Parkinson's disease*:** AD is a neurodegenerative disease and the main cause of dementia in the elderly. KLK6 expression is significantly reduced in AD plaques compared to controls. Similarly, decreased KLK6 expression levels were found in serum as well as in CSF and brain extracts of AD patients over controls. Ashby et al. determined KLK6 protein and mRNA levels in patients suffering from AD and vascular dementia and normal controls and found anomalous expression in both diseases. The authors suggested that altered KLK6 expression may play a role in vascular abnormalities in these disorders. A different study using plasma samples from AD patients and healthy individuals reported that KLK6 levels decrease with age in AD. KLK6 plasmatic levels differed significantly between AD, vascular dementia, and pseudodementia patients and the control group and therefore may be useful for the discrimination of AD patients from subjects without neurodegenerative dementia. Notably, measurement of KLK6 plasma concentration in patients with mild cognitive impairment can be a valuable test to predict disease progression and the risk of developing AD and dementia with vascular component (Ashby et al. 2010; Bayani and Diamandis 2011). Furthermore, KLK10 CSF concentration is significantly elevated, whereas KLK7 CFS levels are lower in AD patients compared to controls. Lower levels of KLK7 in CSF were associated with the possession of ApoE4 alleles, which in turn are associated with risk of AD. Finally, an increase of *KLK8* mRNA expression was reported in hippocampal tissues from AD patients compared to normal tissues. In the case of PD, KLK6 expression is found to be decreased and is localized in Lewy bodies in the brain (Bayani and Diamandis 2011; Diamandis et al. 2004).

KLKs in Skin Disorders

In skin physiology, KLK5, KLK7, and KLK14 facilitate cell shedding at late stages of epidermal turnover through cleavage of corneodesmosomal adhesive proteins (DSG1, DSC1, and CDSN). Additionally, several KLKs play a critical role in skin permeability and antimicrobial defense. KLK5 and KLK7 can cleave human cathelicidin inactive protein CAP18 (which is implicated in innate immunity) into the major mature and active peptide as well as into other smaller peptides, with enhanced antimicrobial activity. Recent experimental data suggest the implication of KLK-PAR axis in inflammation and itching phenotype of skin disorders (Fig. 1). Briot et al. reported that KLK5 activates PAR2, which in turn results to upregulation of molecules which are crucial mediators of inflammation, suggesting an activator role of KLK5-PAR2 signaling cascade in innate immunity (Emami and Diamandis 2007; Oikonomopoulou et al. 2010; Sotiropoulou and Pampalakis 2012).

***Netherton syndrome*:** the crucial role of KLKs in skin homeostasis has been mainly elucidated by studies of Netherton syndrome (NS), a rare autosomal recessive disease caused by mutations in *SPINK5* (serine peptidase inhibitor, Kazal-type 5), which encodes for the inhibitor LEKTI (lymphoepithelial Kazal-type-related inhibitor). Recent data suggest a possible pH-dependent inhibitory effect of LEKTI on KLK5, KLK7, and KLK14, which regulates cell shedding. These data are confirmed by studies in knockout mouse models of *SPINK5* where the absence of LEKTI leads into excessive proteolytic activity of KLK5, KLK7, and KLK14 in the skin, resulting in the severe symptoms of NS. Apart from the abovementioned mechanism, KLKs are involved in NS through proteolytic cascades which include PARs and another subgroup of proteases known as matriptases (Deperthes and Kündig 2012; Sotiropoulou and Pampalakis 2012).

***Atopic dermatitis*:** this skin disorder is a chronic inflammatory disease, characterized by increased KLK expression in stratum corneum and serum.

Patients suffering from atopic dermatitis share common symptoms with NS individuals. The disturbance of LEKTI-KLK7 interaction plays crucial role in deregulated skin desquamation. Moreover, atopic dermatitis patients exhibit upregulation of PAR2 and co-localization with members of the KLK family. An insertion in 3′UTR of *KLK7* has been associated with atopic dermatitis, while KLK8 expression is significantly elevated in serum samples from patients (Deperthes and Kündig 2012).

***Psoriasis*:** patients with psoriasis demonstrate aberrant KLK expression in the stratum corneum and serum. In particular, KLK6, KLK10, KLK13, and KLK14 are significantly elevated in the stratum corneum of psoriatic patients compared to normal tissues. In untreated patients, KLK6, KLK8, KLK10, and KLK13 serum levels are correlated with disease severity. After therapy, serum KLK5 and KLK11 levels decrease, whereas those of KLK14 increase in patients with psoriasis. Moreover, high KLK8 levels were found in serum of patients with psoriatic disease, as well as in skin lesions and synovial fluid of patients with psoriatic arthritis. Additionally, serum KLK8 levels were independently associated with cutaneous psoriasis severity (Deperthes and Kündig 2012; Eissa et al. 2013).

Conclusions

This chapter outlines the enormous potential of KLKs as tissue and/or serological biomarkers in early diagnosis, effective prognosis, and treatment monitoring of cancer patients. The successful utilization of PSA/KLK3, along with the deregulated expression patterns of KLKs, in malignant tissues and the circulatory system of cancer patients, as well as the active involvement of KLKs in cancer pathobiology, underline their clinical importance as biomarkers. Enhanced understanding of the molecular mechanisms that lead in deregulated expression of KLKs in cancer, as well as the identification of KLK substrates and functional properties, may ultimately contribute to the development of innovative therapeutic agents. Finally, the designation of multiparametric KLK panels will provide new insights to the improved prediction of patients' clinical outcome and selection of the optimal therapeutic strategy.

Summary Points

- Kallikreins are found to be involved in hallmark processes of cancer progression, such as tumor cell proliferation, angiogenesis, invasion, and metastasis.
- KLK aberrant expression is a common event in human neoplasias and is often associated with various clinicopathological parameters of cancer patients.
- The KLK family members have drawn much research attention, by the virtue of their potential as cancer biomarkers, with KLK5, KLK6, KLK7, KLK11, and KLK14 being the most encouraging members concerning cancer patients' prognosis.

- PSA/KLK3, which is the most well-known KLK family member, is currently used in routine clinical practice, for prostate cancer screening, diagnosis, and patients' treatment monitoring, despite ongoing debates.
- In ovarian cancer, the assessment of KLK6 and KLK10 serum levels holds great promises in diagnosis, prognosis, and therapeutic stratification.
- KLK5, KLK10, and KLK14 are regarded as plausible serum biomarkers for breast cancer diagnosis and prediction of unfavorable disease outcome.
- KLKs expression has been studied and evaluated in terms of diagnostic and prognostic significance in many other cancer types (e.g., gastrointestinal cancer, lung cancer, bladder cancer, and lymphoblastic leukemia) with auspicious results.
- A current trend in KLK-related research is the integration of KLKs in multiparametric models with markers from other cancer-related families resulting in the identification of combined panels with improved diagnostic, prognostic, and/or predictive value.
- KLKs represent attractive molecular targets for the development of innovative targeted strategies for cancer, skin diseases, and other human pathologies.

References

Alexopoulou DK, Papadopoulos IN, Scorilas A. Clinical significance of kallikrein-related peptidase (KLK10) mRNA expression in colorectal cancer. Clin Biochem. 2013;46:1453–61.

Ashby EL, Kehoe PG, Love S. Kallikrein-related peptidase 6 in Alzheimer's disease and vascular dementia. Brain Res. 2010;1363:1–10.

Avgeris M, Mavridis K, Scorilas A. Kallikrein-related peptidase genes as promising biomarkers for prognosis and monitoring of human malignancies. Biol Chem. 2010;391:505–11.

Avgeris M, Papachristopoulou G, Polychronis A, Scorilas A. Down-regulation of kallikrein-related peptidase 5 (KLK5) expression in breast cancer patients: a biomarker for the differential diagnosis of breast lesions. Clin Proteomics. 2011;8:5.

Avgeris M, Mavridis K, Scorilas A. Kallikrein-related peptidases in prostate, breast, and ovarian cancers: from pathobiology to clinical relevance. Biol Chem. 2012;393:301–17.

Batra J, O'Mara T, Patnala R, Lose F, Clements JA. Genetic polymorphisms in the human tissue kallikrein (KLK) locus and their implication in various malignant and non-malignant diseases. Biol Chem. 2013;393:1365–90.

Bayani J, Diamandis EP. The physiology and pathobiology of human kallikrein-related peptidase 6 (KLK6). Clin Chem Lab Med. 2011;50:211–33.

Blaber M, Yoon H, Juliano MA, Scarisbrick IA, Blaber SI. Functional intersection of the kallikrein-related peptidases (KLKs) and thrombostasis axis. Biol Chem. 2010;391:311–20.

Black MH, Diamandis EP. The diagnostic and prognostic utility of prostate-specific antigen for diseases of the breast. Breast Cancer Res Treat. 2000;59:1–14.

Black MH, Giai M, Ponzone R, Sismondi P, Yu H, Diamandis EP. Serum total and free prostate-specific antigen for breast cancer diagnosis in women. Clin Cancer Res. 2000;6:467–73.

Borgono CA, Diamandis EP. The emerging roles of human tissue kallikreins in cancer. Nat Rev Cancer. 2004;4:876–90.

Borgono CA, Michael IP, Diamandis EP. Human tissue kallikreins: physiologic roles and applications in cancer. Mol Cancer Res. 2004;2:257–80.

Carlsson S, Maschino A, Schroder F, et al. Predictive value of four kallikrein markers for pathologically insignificant compared with aggressive prostate cancer in radical prostatectomy specimens: results from the European Randomized Study of Screening for Prostate Cancer section Rotterdam. Eur Urol. 2013;64:693–9.

Chow TF, Crow M, Earle T, El-Said H, Diamandis EP, Yousef GM. Kallikreins as microRNA targets: an in silico and experimental-based analysis. Biol Chem. 2008;389:731–8.

Deperthes D, Kündig C. Kallikrein-related peptidases as pharmaceutical targets. In: Magdolen V, Sommerhoff CP, Fritz H, Schmitt M, editors. Kallikrein-related peptidases: characterization, regulation, and interactions within the protease web, vol. 1. Berlin/Boston: De Gruyter; 2012. p. 161–86.

Diamandis EP, Scorilas A, Fracchioli S, et al. Human kallikrein 6 (hK6): a new potential serum biomarker for diagnosis and prognosis of ovarian carcinoma. J Clin Oncol. 2003;21:1035–43.

Diamandis EP, Scorilas A, Kishi T, et al. Altered kallikrein 7 and 10 concentrations in cerebrospinal fluid of patients with Alzheimer's disease and frontotemporal dementia. Clin Biochem. 2004;37:230–7.

Dong Y, Kaushal A, Brattsand M, Nicklin J, Clements JA. Differential splicing of KLK5 and KLK7 in epithelial ovarian cancer produces novel variants with potential as cancer biomarkers. Clin Cancer Res. 2003;9:1710–20.

Dorn J, Harbeck N, Kates R, et al. Impact of expression differences of kallikrein-related peptidases and of uPA and PAI-1 between primary tumor and omentum metastasis in advanced ovarian cancer. Ann Oncol. 2011a;22:877–83.

Dorn J, Magdolen V, Gkazepis A, et al. Circulating biomarker tissue kallikrein-related peptidase KLK5 impacts ovarian cancer patients' survival. Ann Oncol. 2011b;22:1783–90.

Dorn J, Milou V, Kulasingam V, Schmalfeldt B, Diamandis EP, Schmitt M. Clinical relevance of kallikrein-related peptidases in ovarian cancer. In: Magdolen V, Sommerhoff CP, Fritz H, Schmitt M, editors. Kallikrein-related peptidases: novel cancer-related biomarkers, vol. 2. Berlin/Boston: De Gruyter; 2012. p. 145–66.

Dorn J, Bayani J, Yousef GM, et al. Clinical utility of kallikrein-related peptidases (KLK) in urogenital malignancies. Thromb Haemost. 2013;110:408–22.

Eissa A, Cretu D, Soosaipillai A, et al. Serum kallikrein-8 correlates with skin activity, but not psoriatic arthritis, in patients with psoriatic disease. Clin Chem Lab Med. 2013;51:317–25.

Emami N, Diamandis EP. New insights into the functional mechanisms and clinical applications of the kallikrein-related peptidase family. Mol Oncol. 2007;1:269–87.

Emami N, Diamandis EP. Utility of kallikrein-related peptidases (KLKs) as cancer biomarkers. Clin Chem. 2008;54:1600–7.

Florou D, Mavridis K, Scorilas A. The kallikrein-related peptidase 13 (KLK13) gene is substantially up-regulated after exposure of gastric cancer cells to antineoplastic agents. Tumour Biol. 2012;33:2069–78.

Gabril M, White NM, Moussa M, et al. Immunohistochemical analysis of kallikrein-related peptidases in the normal kidney and renal tumors: potential clinical implications. Biol Chem. 2010;391:403–9.

Goettig P, Magdolen V, Brandstetter H. Natural and synthetic inhibitors of kallikrein-related peptidases (KLKs). Biochimie. 2010;92:1546–67.

Heuzé-Vourc'H N, Courty Y. Pathophysiology of kallikrein-related peptidases in lung cancer. In: Magdolen V, Sommerhoff CP, Fritz H, Schmitt M, editors. Kallikrein-related peptidases: novel cancer-related biomarkers, vol. 2. Berlin/Boston: De Gruyter; 2012. p. 3–26.

Jemal A, Bray F, Center MM, Ferlay J, Ward E, Forman D. Global cancer statistics. CA Cancer J Clin. 2011;61:69–90.

Kioulafa M, Kaklamanis L, Stathopoulos E, Mavroudis D, Georgoulias V, Lianidou ES. Kallikrein 10 (KLK10) methylation as a novel prognostic biomarker in early breast cancer. Ann Oncol. 2009;20:1020–5.

Kontos CK, Scorilas A. Kallikrein-related peptidases (KLKs): a gene family of novel cancer biomarkers. Clin Chem Lab Med. 2012;50:1877–91.

Kontos CK, Chantzis D, Papadopoulos IN, Scorilas A. Kallikrein-related peptidase 4 (KLK4) mRNA predicts short-term relapse in colorectal adenocarcinoma patients. Cancer Lett. 2012;330:106–12.

Kontos CK, Mavridis K, Talieri M, Scorilas A. Kallikrein-related peptidases (KLKs) in gastrointestinal cancer: mechanistic and clinical aspects. Thromb Haemost. 2013;110:450–7.

Kryza T, Achard C, Parent C, et al. Angiogenesis stimulated by human kallikrein-related peptidase 12 acting via a platelet-derived growth factor B-dependent paracrine pathway. FASEB J. 2013;28:740–51.

Kuzmanov U, Jiang N, Smith CR, Soosaipillai A, Diamandis EP. Differential *N*-glycosylation of kallikrein 6 derived from ovarian cancer cells or the central nervous system. Mol Cell Proteomics. 2009;8:791–8.

Lawrence MG, Lai J, Clements JA. Kallikreins on steroids: structure, function, and hormonal regulation of prostate-specific antigen and the extended kallikrein locus. Endocr Rev. 2010;31:407–46.

Lilja H, Ulmert D, Vickers AJ. Prostate-specific antigen and prostate cancer: prediction, detection and monitoring. Nat Rev Cancer. 2008;8:268–78.

Luo LY, Diamandis EP, Look MP, Soosaipillai AP, Foekens JA. Higher expression of human kallikrein 10 in breast cancer tissue predicts tamoxifen resistance. Br J Cancer. 2002;86:1790–6.

Magklara A, Scorilas A, Stephan C, et al. Decreased concentrations of prostate-specific antigen and human glandular kallikrein 2 in malignant versus nonmalignant prostatic tissue. Urology. 2000;56:527–32.

Mavridis K, Scorilas A. Prognostic value and biological role of the kallikrein-related peptidases in human malignancies. Future Oncol. 2010;6:269–85.

Mavridis K, Schmitt M, Scorilas A. Kallikrein-related peptidases as biomarkers in personalized cancer medicine. In: Magdolen V, Sommerhoff CP, Fritz H, Schmitt M, editors. Kallikrein-related peptidases: novel cancer-related biomarkers, vol. 2. Berlin/Boston: De Gruyter; 2012. p. 201–18.

Mavridis K, Stravodimos K, Scorilas A. Quantified KLK15 gene expression levels discriminate prostate cancer from benign tumors and constitute a novel independent predictor of disease progression. Prostate. 2013;73:1191–201.

Mavridis K, Avgeris M, Scorilas A. Targeting kallikrein-related peptidases in prostate cancer. Expert Opin Ther Targets. 2014;18:365–83.

Nakamura T, Scorilas A, Stephan C, Jung K, Soosaipillai AR, Diamandis EP. The usefulness of serum human kallikrein 11 for discriminating between prostate cancer and benign prostatic hyperplasia. Cancer Res. 2003;63:6543–6.

Obiezu CV, Diamandis EP. Human tissue kallikrein gene family: applications in cancer. Cancer Lett. 2005;224:1–22.

Ogawa K, Utsunomiya T, Mimori K, et al. Clinical significance of human kallikrein gene 6 messenger RNA expression in colorectal cancer. Clin Cancer Res. 2005;11:2889–93.

Oikonomopoulou K, Hansen KK, Baruch A, Hollenberg MD, Diamandis EP. Immunofluorometric activity-based probe analysis of active KLK6 in biological fluids. Biol Chem. 2008a;389:747–56.

Oikonomopoulou K, Li L, Zheng Y, et al. Prediction of ovarian cancer prognosis and response to chemotherapy by a serum-based multiparametric biomarker panel. Br J Cancer. 2008b;99:1103–13.

Oikonomopoulou K, Diamandis EP, Hollenberg MD. Kallikrein-related peptidases: proteolysis and signaling in cancer, the new frontier. Biol Chem. 2010;391:299–310.

Paliouras M, Diamandis EP. The kallikrein world: an update on the human tissue kallikreins. Biol Chem. 2006;387:643–52.

Paliouras M, Borgono C, Diamandis EP. Human tissue kallikreins: the cancer biomarker family. Cancer Lett. 2007;249:61–79.

Pampalakis G, Sotiropoulou G. Tissue kallikrein proteolytic cascade pathways in normal physiology and cancer. Biochim Biophys Acta. 2007;1776:22–31.

Pasic MD, Olkhov E, Bapat B, Yousef GM. Epigenetic regulation of kallikrein-related peptidases: there is a whole new world out there. Biol Chem. 2012;393:319–30.

Petraki CD, Gregorakis AK, Vaslamatzis MM, et al. Prognostic implications of the immunohistochemical expression of human kallikreins 5, 6, 10 and 11 in renal cell carcinoma. Tumour Biol. 2006;27:1–7.

Planque C, Li L, Zheng Y, et al. A multiparametric serum kallikrein panel for diagnosis of non-small cell lung carcinoma. Clin Cancer Res. 2008;14:1355–62.

Prezas P, Scorilas A, Yfanti C, et al. The role of human tissue kallikreins 7 and 8 in intracranial malignancies. Biol Chem. 2006;387:1607–12.

Rabien A, Fritzsche F, Jung M, et al. High expression of KLK14 in prostatic adenocarcinoma is associated with elevated risk of prostate-specific antigen relapse. Tumour Biol. 2008;29:1–8.

Roman-Gomez J, Jimenez-Velasco A, Agirre X, et al. The normal epithelial cell-specific 1 (NES1) gene, a candidate tumor suppressor gene on chromosome 19q13.3-4, is downregulated by hypermethylation in acute lymphoblastic leukemia. Leukemia. 2004;18:362–5.

Romero Otero J, Garcia Gomez B, Campos Juanatey F, Touijer KA. Prostate cancer biomarkers: an update. Urol Oncol. 2014;32:252–60.

Rosen DG, Wang L, Atkinson JN, et al. Potential markers that complement expression of CA125 in epithelial ovarian cancer. Gynecol Oncol. 2005;99:267–77.

Sauter ER, Klein G, Wagner-Mann C, Diamandis EP. Prostate-specific antigen expression in nipple aspirate fluid is associated with advanced breast cancer. Cancer Detect Prev. 2004;28:27–31.

Scarisbrick IA, Linbo R, Vandell AG, et al. Kallikreins are associated with secondary progressive multiple sclerosis and promote neurodegeneration. Biol Chem. 2008;389:739–45.

Schmitt M, Magdolen V, Yang F, et al. Emerging clinical importance of the cancer biomarkers kallikrein-related peptidases (KLK) in female and male reproductive organ malignancies. Radiol Oncol. 2013;47:319–29.

Shariat SF, Semjonow A, Lilja H, Savage C, Vickers AJ, Bjartell A. Tumor markers in prostate cancer I: blood-based markers. Acta Oncol. 2011;50 Suppl 1:61–75.

Shaw JL, Diamandis EP. Distribution of 15 human kallikreins in tissues and biological fluids. Clin Chem. 2007;53:1423–32.

Shih Ie M, Salani R, Fiegl M, et al. Ovarian cancer specific kallikrein profile in effusions. Gynecol Oncol. 2007;105:501–7.

Sotiropoulou G, Pampalakis G. Targeting the kallikrein-related peptidases for drug development. Trends Pharmacol Sci. 2012;33:623–34.

Sotiropoulou G, Pampalakis G, Diamandis EP. Functional roles of human kallikrein-related peptidases. J Biol Chem. 2009;284:32989–94.

Stenman UH, Abrahamsson PA, Aus G, et al. Prognostic value of serum markers for prostate cancer. Scand J Urol Nephrol Suppl. 2005;216:64–81.

Stephan C, Jung K, Lein M, Diamandis EP. PSA and other tissue kallikreins for prostate cancer detection. Eur J Cancer. 2007;43:1918–26.

Sun D, Lee YS, Malhotra A, et al. miR-99 family of MicroRNAs suppresses the expression of prostate-specific antigen and prostate cancer cell proliferation. Cancer Res. 2011;71:1313–24.

Talieri M, Zoma M, Devetzi M, Scorilas A, Ardavanis A. Kallikrein-related peptidase 6 (KLK6) gene expression in intracranial tumors. Tumour Biol. 2012;33:1375–83.

Ulmert D, O'Brien MF, Bjartell AS, Lilja H. Prostate kallikrein markers in diagnosis, risk stratification and prognosis. Nat Rev Urol. 2009;6:384–91.

Unal D, Tasdemir A, Oguz A, et al. Is human kallikrein-11 in gastric cancer treated with surgery and adjuvant chemoradiotherapy associated with survival? Pathol Res Pract. 2013;209:779–83.

White NM, Mathews M, Yousef GM, Prizada A, Popadiuk C, Dore JJ. KLK6 and KLK13 predict tumor recurrence in epithelial ovarian carcinoma. Br J Cancer. 2009;101:1107–13.

White NM, Bui A, Mejia-Guerrero S, et al. Dysregulation of kallikrein-related peptidases in renal cell carcinoma: potential targets of miRNAs. Biol Chem. 2010;391:411–23.

White NM, Youssef YM, Fendler A, Stephan C, Jung K, Yousef GM. The miRNA-kallikrein axis of interaction: a new dimension in the pathogenesis of prostate cancer. Biol Chem. 2012;393:379–89.

Yousef GM. microRNAs: a new frontier in kallikrein research. Biol Chem. 2008;389:689–94.

Yousef GM, Chang A, Scorilas A, Diamandis EP. Genomic organization of the human kallikrein gene family on chromosome 19q13.3-q13.4. Biochem Biophys Res Commun. 2000;276:125–33.

Yousef GM, Obiezu CV, Luo LY, et al. Human tissue kallikreins: from gene structure to function and clinical applications. Adv Clin Chem. 2005;39:11–79.

MAP17 as Biomarker for Cancer Treatment 7

Amancio Carnero

Contents

Abstract

MAP17 is a small 17 kDa membrane-associated protein present in a high proportion of tumors, not only carcinoma. It has been found that it is not present in adenoma and benign tumors and highly expressed in metastatic carcinoma. Therefore, the expression correlates with tumor stage and malignant status of the tumor. The expression is mainly driven at transcriptional level either by promoter activation or demethylation. Expression of MAP17 in primary cells triggers senescence through p38, but in already tumoral cells, it enhances the tumoral capabilities of these cells increasing proliferation, migration, resistance to apoptosis, etc. MAP17 expression increases the levels of oxidative species, ROS, in cells which may account for some of the increased tumoral properties. In turn, a further increase of ROS might switch the balance toward apoptosis. Thus, MAP17 may increase the efficacy of therapies increasing ROS and

A. Carnero (✉)
Instituto de Biomedicina de Sevilla (IBIS), Hospital Universitario Virgen del Rocio, Consejo Superior de Investigaciones Cientificas, Universidad de Sevilla, Sevilla, Spain
e-mail: acarnero-ibis@us.es; acarnero@ibis-sevilla.es; acarnero@us.es

V.R. Preedy, V.B. Patel (eds.), *Biomarkers in Cancer, Biomarkers in Disease: Methods, Discoveries and Applications*,
DOI 10.1007/978-94-007-7681-4_27

therefore constitute a biomarker for better prognosis of these tumors. In cervix tumors, currently treated with cisplatin and radiotherapy, the presence of MAP17 is a marker for good response to therapy and good survival of the patients. Therefore, MAP17 is not only a marker for stage and malignant status but also of a better response to drugs involving oxidative stress.

Key Facts

- Biomarkers are necessary to couple the cancer patient to the most suitable therapy.
- MAP17 is an oncogene capable to enhance the tumorigenic capability of melanoma, breast, and cervix tumor cells.
- MAP17 is overexpressed in a large proportion in human carcinomas, and its levels correlate with malignant status and advanced stages of tumors.
- MAP17 increases reactive oxygen species, ROS, and these seem to be necessary for the tumorigenic activity of MAP17.
- Study of cohorts of cervix tumors treated with cisplatin and radiotherapy indicates that the expression of MAP17 correlates with better response to these therapies.

Definitions of Words and Terms

Biomarker Marker of biological origin (DNA, RNA, protein, lipid, etc.) that helps classify the patient for diagnosis, prognosis, or response to therapy. It is the basis of personalized medicine since the markers will define the specific treatment that a patient should receive.

MAP17 Membrane-associated protein of 17 kDa, also called DD96 and PDZK1IP1

Tumoral phenotype Tumoral cells have an altered physiology that confers them some tumoral properties, sustained growth, resistance to apoptosis, immortality, ability to invade the surrounding tissue, etc., which differentiate them from non-tumoral cells. These properties can be easily measured experimentally.

ROS Reactive oxygen species are chemical products of the metabolism involving oxygen; they are highly reactive with other structures (DNA, proteins, etc.) providing chemical modifications.

Immunohistochemistry Technique commonly used to study a tumor sample. Consists in the processing of the tumor sample to identify either the structure or the expression of one specific protein. It is routinely used in hospitals for diagnosis.

Diagnosis Identification of the nature and cause of illness

Prognosis Evaluation of the evolution of the illness to predict the possible outcome

Predictive response to therapy Evaluate and predict the possible outcome of a disease in the presence of one specific therapy.

Chemotherapy Therapy given through the use of chemical compounds, to differentiate from surgery or radiotherapy, for example. In cancer, it is commonly used for drugs acting no specifically on targets, such as cisplatin, taxanes, 5FU, doxorubicin, etc.

Gene overexpression Genes are regulated inside the cells, and their levels are determined. Naturally occurring or artificially induced high increase of the levels of the gene in the cells is considered overexpression.

Introduction

Initial cancer treatments were based on medical experience. Empirically tested drugs were applied to tumors grouped by location, clinical features, or size. As the understanding of the disease was increasing, anatomopathological analysis and fine clinical phenotype were included as the initial markers for tumor treatment selection. Different treatments were given to different tumor types, and both were evolving together along with the discovery of new drugs. Nowadays, more than 200 types of tumors with many more subtypes can be identified, many more drugs either cytotoxic or targeted have been developed, and a treatment is given to a patient according to a combination of clinical features, pathological analysis, and molecular markers. However, this assignment is far from clear. From some time is known the complexity of assigning an adequate treatment or to predict the individual response to a specific one, even if it is the indicated to that type of tumor.

There is a clear need to predict the response of an individual tumor to any given drug in order to select the more adequate therapy among the possible ones. There is also a need to identify the response of the patient to predict the degree of toxicity associated to the treatment proposed in order to adapt the dosage and obtain the best benefit/quality of life ratio for the patient. Given the molecular variability among the tumors of the different individuals discovered by recent whole genome sequentiation projects, it seems that every tumor became a unique entity with its unique treatment challenges. This is what has been called for some time as personalized medicine.

Beyond anatomopathological analysis, which still provides important information about diagnosis, every aspect of the biology has been used to provide putative biomarkers, generating also large subfields highly specialized. Biomarkers have been searched in the genome (or its variations with nonstructural modifications, epigenome), proteins, RNA, and metabolic products. Most of the markers usually come from large data collections and exhaustive statistical analysis of whole genome/cell/tissue information collection(s). Going from the general to the particular has been the more recurrent path to find differentiating profiles and, in some cases, unique entities to diagnose or predict the behavior of one specific tumor. Using genome-wide retroviral gain or loss of function screenings, new genes with causal relevance in cancer have been identified, and therefore new possibilities of find biomarkers for diagnosis, prognosis, or predictive of response in cancer therapy (Vergel and Carnero 2010; Leal et al. 2007; Guijarro et al. 2007a; Bordogna et al. 2005; Castro et al. 2008; Ferrer et al. 2011).

MAP17 (PDZK1IP1)

Tumorigenesis occurs when the mechanisms involved in the control of tissue homeostasis are disrupted and cells stop responding to physiological signals. Therefore, genes capable of desensitizing tumoral cells to physiological signals may provide a selective advantage within the tumoral mass and influence the outcome of the disease. We undertook a large-scale genetic screen to identify genes capable of altering the cellular response to physiological signals that resulted in a selective advantage during tumorigenesis (Carnero et al. 2000; Hannon et al. 1999; Vergel and Carnero 2010). Out of this screen, MAP17 was identified (Guijarro et al. 2007a), a small non-glycosylated membrane-associated protein that localizes to the plasma membrane and the Golgi apparatus (Blasco et al. 2003). The MAP17 protein sequence contains two transmembrane regions and a hydrophobic amino-terminus encoding a PDZ-binding domain (Jaeger et al 2000; Fig. 1). MAP17 binds several PDZ domain-containing proteins, including NHeRF proteins, NaPi-IIa, and NHe3 (Carnero 2012). Overexpression of MAP17 in opossum kidney cells participates in NaPi-IIa internalization to the trans-Golgi network (Lanaspa et al. 2007). MAP17 acts as an atypical anchoring site for PDZK1 and other NHeRF proteins and interacts with the NaPi-IIa/PDZK1 protein complex in renal proximal tubular cells (Pribanic et al. 2003). The physiological role of MAP17 in proximal tubules is not fully understood, but it does stimulate specific Na-dependent transport of mannose and glucose in *Xenopus* oocytes (Blasco et al. 2003) and some human cells (Guijarro et al. 2007a).

MAP17 in Human Tumors

MAP17 overexpression in carcinomas was first detected by using the technique of differential display (Kocher et al. 1995). MAP17 overexpression in carcinomas occurs mostly through mRNA amplification, but promoter activation has also been observed by some oncogenes (Guijarro et al. 2007c; Kocher et al. 1995). Immunohistochemical analysis of MAP17 during cancer progression shows that

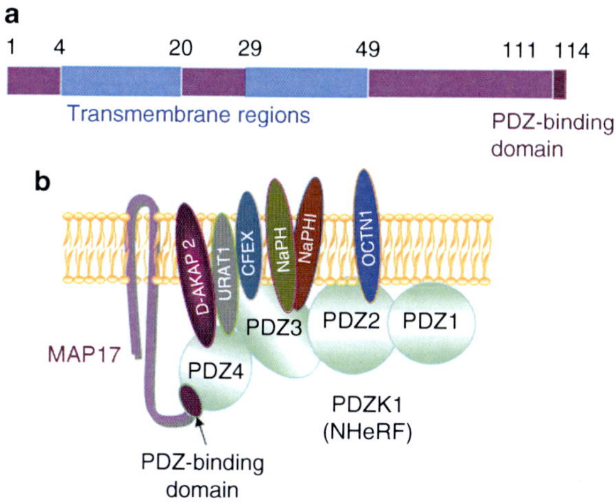

Fig. 1 Schematic representation of structure and binding of MAP17 protein. (**a**) 2D representation of domains in MAP17 protein. (**b**) Cartoon representing the possible structure of MAP17 in the membrane and binding to PDZK1 and transporters

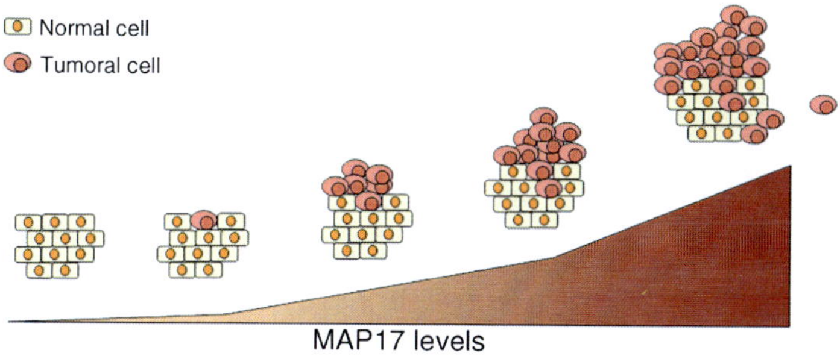

Fig. 2 Representative scheme indicating the relation between tumor stage and MAP17 expression. Normal cells and benign tumors usually do not show MAP17 protein. However, levels of MAP17 increase along with the stage and malignant status of the tumor

overexpression of the protein strongly correlates with tumoral progression (Fig. 2). Generalized MAP17 overexpression in human carcinomas indicates that MAP17 can be a good marker for tumorigenesis and especially for malignant progression. In-depth analysis of MAP17 overexpression in carcinomas by immunohistochemistry showed that the MAP17 protein is overexpressed in a large percentage of the tumors analyzed and is significantly correlated with the tumor grade in ovarian, breast, and prostate carcinomas (Guijarro et al. 2007c, 2012). The analysis of mRNA levels by Q-PCR or by hybridization comparing tumoral versus non-tumoral tissues of the same patient demonstrated an even higher percentage of tumor samples with MAP17 overexpression. In tumors such as ovary, colon, stomach, cervix, and thyroid gland, the percentage of overexpression in tumor samples is higher than 70 %, while in the lung, uterus, and rectum it is approximately 50 %. Although more samples need to be analyzed to confirm these high

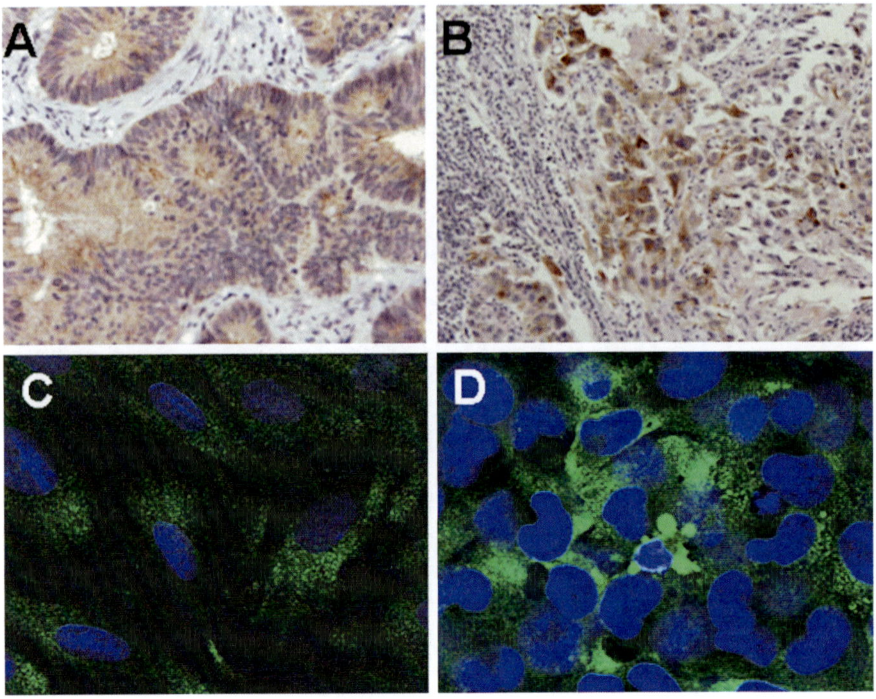

Fig. 3 Representative pictures of MAP17-positive tumors by immunohistochemistry and cells by immunofluorescence. The figures show pictures of immunostained tumors using antibodies anti-MAP17. (**a**) Colorectal adenocarcinoma. (**b**) Cervix tumor. (**c**, **d**) Show pictures of relative levels and distribution of MAP17 in different cell lines (**c** REF52; **d** HBL100). MAP17 proteins are represented in *green* by immunofluorescence

rates, the data suggest that MAP17 overexpression is the most common marker of tumorigenesis in carcinomas. The relevance of MAP17 as a general marker for the malignant stages of human tumors still needs to be confirmed in additional tumor types and larger cohorts. However, all tissues explored thus far have shown similar patterns of MAP17 expression (Fig. 3). Furthermore, MAP17 expression seems to correlate with AKT phosphorylation at Ser473. These expression patterns provide a mechanistic insight and a possible target for future therapies.

In a meta-analysis of public microarray databases for different skin diseases, it was discovered (Noh et al. 2010) that MAP17 is commonly upregulated, suggesting that it may be associated with abnormal keratinocyte differentiation. MAP17 was significantly upregulated in response to interferon gamma, interleukin 4 (IL-4), IL-6, IL-17A, or IL-22 in normal human epidermal keratinocytes. The Th cell cytokine-induced upregulation of MAP17 expression may be linked to the abnormal epidermal differentiation observed in the dermatological diseases through the downregulation of filaggrin (Noh et al. 2010).

Human MAP17 maps to chromosome 1p33, a locus commonly found to be involved in cancer; however, it is not the only interesting gene in this region.

Genes coding for members of the cytochrome P450 family (CYP4B1, CYP4A11), putative oncogenes (SCL/Tal1), MCPH7, CMPK1, and members of the fork head family (FOXE3, FOXD2) are its neighbors.

MAP17 overexpression in carcinomas occurs mostly through mRNA amplification. MAP17 overexpression could be due to the ability of the MAP17 promoter to be activated by oncogenes (Guijarro et al. 2007c; Kocher et al. 1995). Tumorigenic progression involves progressive genetic alterations triggering oncogenic cascades (Vogelstein and Kinzler 2004). In advanced stages, tumors might accumulate oncogenic alterations that result in a high probability of MAP17 promoter activation and increased transcription. This hypothesis could explain the correlation between the MAP17 overexpression and advanced tumor stages observed in many tumor types. In a recent work, it was observed that upon tumor progression there was some degree of demethylation of DNA promoters, resulting in expression of other ways silenced genes. MAP17 was strongly induced by DNA demethylation is these tumors (Rodriguez-Rodero et al. 2013).

Oncogenic Activity of MAP17

Tumor cells that overexpress MAP17 show an increased tumoral phenotype with enhanced proliferative capabilities both in the presence or the absence of contact inhibition, decreased apoptotic sensitivity, and increased migration (Guijarro et al. 2007b, d; Perez et al. 2013). MAP17-expressing clones also grow better in nude mice. The increased malignant cell behavior induced by MAP17 is associated with an increase in reactive oxygen species, ROS, production (Fig. 4), and the treatment of MAP17-expressing cells with antioxidants results in a reduction in the tumorigenic properties of these cells. The MAP17-dependent increase in ROS and tumorigenesis relies on its PDZ-binding domain because disruption of this sequence by point mutations abolishes the ability of MAP17 to enhance ROS production and tumorigenesis (Guijarro et al. 2012).

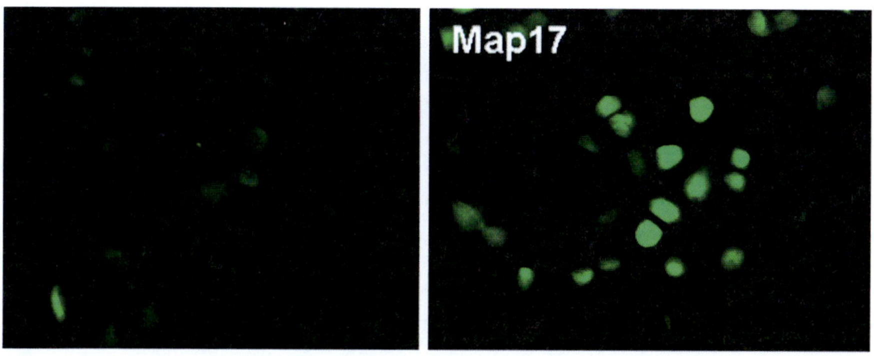

Fig. 4 Expression of ectopic MAP17 results in an increase of reactive oxygen species, ROS, as measured by a ROS probe (*green*)

Potential Applications to Prognosis, Diagnosis, or Response to Therapy

Because the expression of MAP17 increases reactive oxygen species (ROS) generation in cancer cells, we investigated whether MAP17 might be a marker for the activity of treatments involving oxidative stress, such as cisplatin or radiotherapy, and treatments given in many tumors such as in cervix or larynx. First, the transcriptional alterations in genes involved in the oxidative stress induced by MAP17 expression in HeLa cervical tumor cells were confirmed, and it was found that HeLa cells expressing MAP17 were more sensitive to therapies that induce ROS than parental cells. MAP17 was expressed in approximately 70 % of cervical tumors of different types, but they were not expressed in benign adenoma tumors. High levels of MAP17 correlated with improved patient survival after treatment. Furthermore, the patients with high levels of MAP17 present higher survival rates. Therefore, high levels of MAP17 are a marker for good prognosis in patients with cervical tumors after cisplatin plus radiotherapy treatment. These results also suggest that the use of MAP17 as marker may identify patients who are likely to exhibit a better response to treatments that boost oxidative stress in other cancer types.

ROS may promote either proliferation or cell death depending on the intensity and location of the oxidative burst and the activity of the antioxidant system (Haulica et al. 2001; Manda et al. 2009). Considering the proliferative signals delivered by ROS to cancer cells and the consequent resistance of cancer cells to proapoptotic signals, ROS-induced tumor cell death is more likely to be induced by ROS-generating antineoplastic therapies that increase the constitutive status above the critical threshold required for cell death.

In experimental models, ROS generation in tumors and subsequent oxidative stress are at sublethal levels; further ROS increases might lead tumor cells to death (Behrend et al. 2003; Burdon et al. 1990; Guijarro et al. 2007b, 2012; Manda et al. 2009). We hypothesized that MAP17 enhances the oxidative stress in tumor cells close to the threshold separating growth from death and, therefore, might be markers for tumors with high oxidative stress. Therapies increasing ROS might help cells cross this threshold and be beneficial to patients whose tumors exhibit increased levels of MAP17.

ROS are beneficially involved in many signaling pathways that control development and maintain cellular homeostasis (Manda et al. 2009). Under physiological conditions, a tightly regulated redox balance protects cells from injurious ROS activity. However, if altered, ROS promote various pathological conditions including cancer (Bae et al. 1999; Behrend et al. 2003; Burdon 1996; Droge 2002; Irani et al. 1997; Klaunig et al. 1998; Sundaresan et al. 1995). Understanding the duality of ROS as cytotoxic molecules and key mediators in signaling cascades may provide novel opportunities to improve cancer therapeutic interventions.

MAP17 is overexpressed, primarily through increased mRNA levels, in a variety of tumors. Because MAP17 expression increases ROS in cancer cells, we hypothesized that MAP17 might be a marker for tumors with high oxidative stress, and therefore, a further increase in ROS might elevate the levels beyond the apoptotic threshold.

The increased tumorigenic properties induced by MAP17 are associated with an increase in ROS because MAP17 greatly alters the mRNA levels of genes involved in oxidative stress and increases endogenous ROS, and the antioxidant treatment of MAP17-expressing cells entails a reduction in the tumorigenic properties of these cells (Guijarro et al. 2007b, d). Therefore, ROS is generated in a MAP17-dependent manner as an intracellular signal and induces a growth-related genetic program.

A low level of ROS is indispensable for several physiologic cell processes including proliferation, apoptosis, and cell death (Storz 2005). A mild increase in ROS has been shown to activate signaling cascades that can strongly influence the regulation of cell growth and tumorigenic processes (Bae et al. 1999; Burdon 1996; Droge 2002; Finkel and Holbrook 2000; Guijarro et al. 2012; Irani et al. 1997; Klaunig et al. 1998; Marra et al. 2011; Sundaresan et al. 1995). However, a further increase in ROS levels raises oxidative stress and creates a potentially toxic cellular environment. Under normal physiological conditions, a balance between ROS generation and oxidative defenses exists in the cell. In these defenses, endogenous antioxidant enzymes play a significant role. Enzymes such as superoxide dismutase (SOD) and catalase (CAT), which act on O_2^- and H_2O_2, respectively; glutaredoxins; glutathione peroxidases (GPXs), which use glutathione as a co-substrate; peroxiredoxins; and thioredoxins are in a delicate balance with oxidative inputs (Marra et al. 2011). Although many cells can tolerate limited doses of ROS, when the balance tips further in favor of ROS, programmed cell death is initiated (Fruehauf and Meyskens 2007). Excessive ROS accumulates that cellular detox enzymes cannot neutralize in the chemical cellular environment, especially within the mitochondria, initiating the cell death program.

Therefore, it was hypothesized that tumors, not just cervical, expressing high levels of ROS producing MAP17 protein can benefit from therapies that increase oxidative stress, not only cisplatin and radiotherapy, even if they are not the first therapeutic option. Various chemotherapeutic agents including platinum derivatives, doxorubicin, or camptothecin have redox-mediated activity on tumor cells (Simizu et al 1998a, b) without effects on healthy tissues (Yoshikawa et al. 1995). Furthermore, patients could also benefit from combined therapies in which, along with the cytotoxic chemotherapy that induces ROS (i.e., cisplatin and doxorubicin), if boosting of the oxidative stress is induced by a specific pro-oxidative agent (not necessarily the antitumor drug). These combinations of ROS-inducing chemotherapy plus pro-oxidant therapies could result in good antitumor activity. The first attempt to employ pro-oxidant agents in vivo was reported by Nathan and Cohn in 1981 using glucose oxidase as an H_2O_2 precursor, obtaining a significant decrease in tumor growth (Nathan and Cohn 1981).

Because cells can develop adaptive responses to ROS, mostly through increases in detoxifying enzymes (Benhar et al. 2002), it was also hypothesized that the inhibition of classic oxidative stress detoxification enzymes may increase the efficacy of certain antitumor therapies that increase ROS (Nathan et al. 1981), at least in tumors overexpressing MAP17. However, the delicate balance between oxidative stress, cancer, and cell death makes new experimental tests necessary to acquire a deep understanding of these processes.

Summary Points

- There is an urgent need for new biomarkers on cancer, especially on markers predictive of response to treatments.
- This chapter focuses on the identification of MAP17 as a predictive marker for cancer treatment.
- MAP17 is an oncogene capable to enhance the tumorigenic capability of tumor cells.
- MAP17 is overexpressed in a large proportion in human carcinomas, and its levels correlate with malignant status and advanced stages of tumors.
- MAP17 increases reactive oxygen species, ROS, therefore suggesting that treatment which increases ROS might also be more active in cells overexpressing MAP17.
- Study of human tumors treated with cisplatin and radiotherapy indicates that the expression of MAP17 correlates with better response to these therapies.

Acknowledgments This work was supported by grants from the Spanish Ministry of Economy and Competitivity, ISCIII (Fis: PI12/00137, RTICC: RD12/0036/0028), Consejeria de Ciencia e Innovacion, and Consejeria de Salud of the Junta de Andalucia (CTS-6844 and PI-0306-2012).

References

Bae GU, Seo DW, Kwon HK, Lee HY, Hong S, Lee ZW, et al. Hydrogen peroxide activates p70 (S6k) signaling pathway. J Biol Chem. 1999;274:32596–602.

Behrend L, Henderson G, Zwacka RM. Reactive oxygen species in oncogenic transformation. Biochem Soc Trans. 2003;31:1441–4.

Benhar M, Engelberg D, Levitzki A. ROS, stress-activated kinases and stress signaling in cancer. EMBO Rep. 2002;3:420–5.

Blasco T, Aramayona J, Alcalde A, Catalan J, Sarasa M, Sorribas V. Rat kidney MAP17 induces cotransport of Na-mannose and Na-glucose in Xenopus laevis oocytes. Am J Physiol Renal Physiol. 2003;285:F799–810.

Bordogna W, Hudson JD, Buddle J, Bennett DC, Beach DH, Carnero A. EMX homeobox genes regulate microphthalmia and alter melanocyte biology. Exp Cell Res. 2005;311:27–38.

Burdon RH, Gill V, Rice-Evans C. Oxidative stress and tumour cell proliferation. Free Radic Res Commun. 1990;11:65–76.

Burdon RH. Control of cell proliferation by reactive oxygen species. Biochem Soc Trans. 1996;24:1028–32.

Carnero A, Hudson JD, Hannon GJ, Beach DH. Loss-of-function genetics in mammalian cells: the p53 tumor suppressor model. Nucleic Acids Res. 2000;28:2234–41.

Carnero A. MAP17 and the double-edged sword of ROS. Biochim Biophys Acta. 2012;1826:44–52.

Castro ME, Ferrer I, Cascon A, Guijarro MV, Lleonart M, Ramon y Cajal S, et al. PPP1CA contributes to the senescence program induced by oncogenic Ras. Carcinogenesis. 2008;29:491–9.

Droge W. Free radicals in the physiological control of cell function. Physiol Rev. 2002;82:47–95.

Ferrer I, Blanco-Aparicio C, Peregrina S, Canamero M, Fominaya J, Cecilia Y, et al. Spinophilin acts as a tumor suppressor by regulating Rb phosphorylation. Cell Cycle. 2011;10:2751–62.

Finkel T, Holbrook NJ. Oxidants, oxidative stress and the biology of ageing. Nature. 2000;408:239–47.

Fruehauf JP, Meyskens Jr FL. Reactive oxygen species: a breath of life or death? Clin Cancer Res. 2007;13:789–94.

Guijarro MV, Castro ME, Romero L, Moneo V, Carnero A. Large scale genetic screen identifies MAP17 as protein bypassing TNF-induced growth arrest. J Cell Biochem. 2007a;101:112–21.

Guijarro MV, Leal JF, Blanco-Aparicio C, Alonso S, Fominaya J, Lleonart M, et al. MAP17 enhances the malignant behavior of tumor cells through ROS increase. Carcinogenesis. 2007b;28:2096–104.

Guijarro MV, Leal JF, Fominaya J, Blanco-Aparicio C, Alonso S, Lleonart M, et al. MAP17 overexpression is a common characteristic of carcinomas. Carcinogenesis. 2007c;28:1646–52.

Guijarro MV, Link W, Rosado A, Leal JF, Carnero A. MAP17 inhibits Myc-induced apoptosis through PI3K/AKT pathway activation. Carcinogenesis. 2007d;28:2443–50.

Guijarro MV, Vergel M, Marin JJ, Munoz-Galvan S, Ferrer I, Cajal SR, et al. p38alpha limits the contribution of MAP17 to cancer progression in breast tumors. Oncogene. 2012;31:4447.

Hannon GJ, Sun P, Carnero A, Xie LY, Maestro R, Conklin DS, et al. MaRX: an approach to genetics in mammalian cells. Science. 1999;283:1129–30.

Haulica I, Boisteanu D, Neagu B. The role of oxidative stress in normal and pathological adaptive reactions. Rev Med Chir Soc Med Nat Iasi. 2001;105:11–8.

Irani K, Xia Y, Zweier JL, Sollott SJ, Der CJ, Fearon ER, et al. Mitogenic signaling mediated by oxidants in Ras-transformed fibroblasts. Science. 1997;275:1649–52.

Jaeger C, Schaefer B, Wallich R, Kramer M. The membrane-associated protein pKe#192/MAP17 in human keratinocytes. J Invest Dermatol. 2000;115:375–80.

Klaunig JE, Xu Y, Isenberg JS, Bachowski S, Kolaja KL, Jiang J, et al. The role of oxidative stress in chemical carcinogenesis. Environ Health Perspect. 1998;106 Suppl 1:289–95.

Kocher O, Cheresh P, Brown LF, Lee SW. Identification of a novel gene, selectively up-regulated in human carcinomas, using the differential display technique. Clin Cancer Res. 1995;1:1209–15.

Lanaspa MA, Giral H, Breusegem SY, Halaihel N, Baile G, Catalan J, et al. Interaction of MAP17 with NHERF3/4 induces translocation of the renal Na/Pi IIa transporter to the trans-Golgi. Am J Physiol Renal Physiol. 2007;292:F230–42.

Leal JF, Fominaya J, Cascon A, Guijarro MV, Blanco-Aparicio C, Lleonart M, et al. Cellular senescence bypass screen identifies new putative tumor suppressor genes. Oncogene. 2007;27:1961.

Manda G, Nechifor MT, Neagu TM. Reactive oxygen species, cancer and anticancer therapies. Curr Chem Biol. 2009;3:342–66.

Marra M, Sordelli IM, Lombardi A, Lamberti M, Tarantino L, Giudice A, et al. Molecular targets and oxidative stress biomarkers in hepatocellular carcinoma: an overview. J Transl Med. 2011;9:171.

Nathan CF, Arrick BA, Murray HW, DeSantis NM, Cohn ZA. Tumor cell anti-oxidant defenses. Inhibition of the glutathione redox cycle enhances macrophage-mediated cytolysis. J Exp Med. 1981;153:766–82.

Nathan CF, Cohn ZA. Antitumor effects of hydrogen peroxide in vivo. J Exp Med. 1981;154:1539–53.

Noh M, Yeo H, Ko J, Kim HK, Lee CH. MAP17 is associated with the T-helper cell cytokine-induced down-regulation of filaggrin transcription in human keratinocytes. Exp Dermatol. 2010;19:355–62.

Perez M, Praena-Fernandez JM, Felipe-Abrio B, Lopez-Garcia MA, Lucena-Cacace A, Garcia A, et al. MAP17 and SGLT1 protein expression levels as prognostic markers for cervical tumor patient survival. PLoS One. 2013;8:e56169.

Pribanic S, Gisler S, Bacic D, Madjdpour C, Hernando N, Sorribas V, et al. Interactions of MAP17 with the NaPi-IIa/PDZK1 protein complex in renal proximal tubular cells. Am J Physiol Renal Physiol. 2003;285:F784–91.

Rodriguez-Rodero S, Fernandez AF, Fernandez-Morera JL, Castro-Santos P, Bayon GF, Ferrero C, et al. DNA methylation signatures identify biologically distinct thyroid cancer subtypes. J Clin Endocrinol Metab. 2013;98:2811–21.

Simizu S, Takada M, Umezawa K, Imoto M. Requirement of caspase-3(−like) protease-mediated hydrogen peroxide production for apoptosis induced by various anticancer drugs. J Biol Chem. 1998a;273:26900–7.

Simizu S, Umezawa K, Takada M, Arber N, Imoto M. Induction of hydrogen peroxide production and Bax expression by caspase-3(−like) proteases in tyrosine kinase inhibitor-induced apoptosis in human small cell lung carcinoma cells. Exp Cell Res. 1998b;238:197–203.

Storz P. Reactive oxygen species in tumor progression. Front Biosci. 2005;10:1881–96.

Sundaresan M, Yu ZX, Ferrans VJ, Irani K, Finkel T. Requirement for generation of H_2O_2 for platelet-derived growth factor signal transduction. Science. 1995;270:296–9.

Vergel M, Carnero A. Bypassing cellular senescence by genetic screening tools. Clin Transl Oncol. 2010;12:410–7.

Vogelstein B, Kinzler KW. Cancer genes and the pathways they control. Nat Med. 2004;10:789–99.

Yoshikawa T, Kokura S, Tainaka K, Naito Y, Kondo M. A novel cancer therapy based on oxygen radicals. Cancer Res. 1995;55:1617–20.

CA 19-9 as a Serum Biomarker in Cancer

8

Kavya Krishna and Tanios Bekaii-Saab

Contents

K. Krishna
Department of Hematology and Oncology, The Ohio State University Wexner Medical Center, James Cancer Hospital, Columbus, OH, USA
e-mail: Kavya.krishna@osumc.edu

T. Bekaii-Saab (✉)
Division of Medical Oncology, The Ohio State University Wexner Medical Center, James Cancer Hospital, Columbus, OH, USA
e-mail: Tanios.Saab@osumc.edu

V.R. Preedy, V.B. Patel (eds.), *Biomarkers in Cancer, Biomarkers in Disease: Methods, Discoveries and Applications*,
DOI 10.1007/978-94-007-7681-4_17

Abstract

Serum biomarkers in cancer diagnosis or prognosis continue to be part of an evolving field and have been a promising noninvasive tool that may aid in the diagnosis and monitoring of disease in a number of different cancers. Serum carbohydrate antigen 19-9 (CA 19-9) is a biomarker that found utility mainly in biliary tract and pancreatic malignancies as a prognostic marker in monitoring response to treatment and as an indication of disease recurrence. Unfortunately, CA 19-9 levels may lack specificity given that other cancers originating from the ovaries, stomach, colon, and lung may be associated with elevated levels. There are also many benign conditions that are associated with higher levels of CA 19-9. The antigen was discovered in the 1970s and has been studied extensively in various malignancies to validate its utility as a screening, prognostic, or diagnostic tool. CA 19-9 has been used most commonly as a biomarker in pancreatic cancer as a prognostic and predictive tool and less commonly in other malignancies. This chapter will focus mainly on utility of CA 19-9 in pancreatic cancer and biliary tract cancers.

List of Abbreviations

AJCC	American Joint Committee on Cancer
CA 19-9	Carbohydrate Antigen 19-9
CEA	Carcinoembryonic Antigen
CI	Confidence Interval
CRC	Colorectal Cancer
CRT	Chemoradiation
DFS	Disease Free Survival
FIGO	International Federation of Gynecology and Obstetrics
IPMN	Intrapancreatic Mucosal Neoplasm
IU/mL	International Units/Milliliter
Le antigen	Lewis Antigen
mOS	Median Overall Survival
mTTP	Median Time to Progression
NCCN	National Comprehensive Cancer Network
ng/mL	Nanogram/Milliliter
NSCLC	Non-small Cell Lung Cancer
PD	Pancreaticoduodenectomy
RCT	Randomized Controlled Trial
TNM	Tumor Node Metastases
vs	Versus

Definitions of Words and Terms

Prognostic Marker It is a marker or factor which, based on the patient or disease characteristics, provides information on the likely outcome of the disease without treatment. Prognostic markers are reflective of tumor or patient characteristics.

Predictive Marker It is a marker or factor which, based on the patient or disease characteristics, provides information on the likelihood of response to a particular treatment.

Pancreatic Cancer This is a malignancy of the pancreas which typically has adenocarcinoma histology and generally is considered to be very aggressive, and incidence has been increasing over time. It is the fourth leading cause of cancer-related death in the United States and Europe. Primary mode of treatment is resection when the cancer is limited, followed by chemotherapy or chemoradiotherapy based on well-studied guidelines for the benefit of adjuvant therapy. When the disease is locally advanced or unresectable and metastatic, primary treatment is systemic chemotherapy.

TNM Staging in Pancreatic Cancer

T1: tumor size $\leq$2 cm and limited to the pancreas

T2: tumor size is >2 cm and limited to the pancreas

T3: tumor extends beyond the pancreas but without involvement of celiac axis or superior mesenteric artery

T4: tumor involves the celiac axis and or the superior mesenteric artery (unresectable primary tumor)

N: Nodal Stage

N0: no lymph node involvement

N1: regional lymph nodes involved

M: Metastasis

M0: no distant metastases

M1: presence of distant metastases

Staging in Pancreatic Cancer Resectable There is no evidence of distant metastases and no radiographic evidence of superior mesenteric vein (SMV) or portal vein (PV) distortion, and there are clear fat planes around the major blood vessels – including the celiac axis, superior mesenteric artery (SMA), and hepatic artery.

Borderline Resectable There is no evidence of distant metastases and tumor abutment of the SMA not to exceed 180° of circumference of the vessel wall. There is venous involvement of the SMV or PV but with safe resection and replacement being surgically plausible.

Locally Advanced There is no evidence of distant metastases and there is greater than 180° SMA encasement, celiac abutment, IVC, or unreconstructible SMV/PV occlusion or aortic invasion or metastases to lymph nodes beyond the field of resection.

Metastatic There is presence of distant metastases.

Resection Margins
R0: negative for tumor involvement at the margins
R1: positive for microscopic tumor involvement at the margins
R2: positive for macroscopic tumor involvement at the margins or incomplete resection

Neoadjuvant Chemotherapy or Chemoradiotherapy Chemotherapy with or without radiation therapy administered prior to surgical resection of the primary tumor.

Intraductal Papillary Mucinous Neoplasm This is a recently recognized entity and is a tumor arising from the larger ducts in the pancreas and could involve either the main pancreatic duct or side branches or have a mixed pattern. Subsets of IPMN are considered to be premalignant lesions leading to the development of pancreatic cancer.

Biliary Tract Cancers This group consists of intrahepatic and extrahepatic cholangiocarcinoma as well as gall bladder cancer.

Occult Primary This is a relatively common entity and account for nearly 5 % of invasive cancers. Patients usually present with metastatic disease and extensive evaluation for the primary site could be suggestive but not diagnostic. They can present with different histologies including adenocarcinoma, squamous cell carcinoma, poorly differentiated carcinomas, and neuroendocrine carcinoma.

Introduction

CA 19-9 is a sialylated Lewis (Le) A group antigen and is secreted by exocrine epithelial cells. Only patients with the Le ($a - B+$) or Le ($a + B-$) blood groups will express the CA 19-9 antigen. Individuals with genetic absence of Le enzyme (Le $a{-}B$), which would include about 5–10 % of the general population (Tempero et al. 1987), cannot test positive for CA 19-9 irrespective of the tumor burden. It was first discovered in the 1970s when various hybridoma-secreted monoclonal anti-colorectal antibodies that bind to cells of various gastrointestinal malignancies in tissue culture were identified (Herlyn et al. 1982; Koprowski et al. 1979). CA 19-9 can be elevated in several conditions other than pancreatic cancer including, but not limited to, benign neoplasms of the pancreas, acute and chronic pancreatitis, pseudocyst, cystic neoplasms of the pancreas especially in the presence of jaundice (Duraker et al. 2007) as well as tumors of upper gastrointestinal tract, biliary tract cancers, ovarian tumors, hepatocellular carcinoma, and colorectal cancer. It may be elevated in inflammatory conditions of the hepatobiliary system, in many benign conditions such as thyroid disease as well as benign and malignant causes of biliary obstruction.

CA 19-9 Measurement Methodology

Quantification of CA 19-9 is performed using a solid-phase radioimmunometric assay for the monoclonal antibody defined sialylated Lewis A group antigen (Del Villano et al. 1983). In patients with malignancy, CA 19-9 is frequently bound to high-molecular-weight mucin proteins.

CA 19-9 and Its Utility in Pancreatic Cancer

Epidemiology of Pancreas Cancer

Incidence of pancreatic cancer is increasing in the United States with an estimated 45,220 people to be diagnosed in 2013 and with approximately 38,460 people to die of the disease (Siegel et al. 2013). It is the fourth leading cause of cancer-associated mortality in the United States. Surgical resection is the only curative option for patients with pancreas cancer. Unfortunately, only 10–15 % of all patients present with early-stage disease and the majority present at a more advanced stage.

CA 19-9 Level as a Diagnostic Marker/Screening Tool in Pancreatic Cancer

In the last few decades, CA 19-9 serum levels have been evaluated as a potential screening tool for pancreatic cancer. The most notable was a large cross-sectional study which performed mass screening of patients between 1984–1985 and 1987–1988 where 4,506 and 4,250 symptomatic patients were screened and found to have elevated CA 19-9 levels with evidence of pancreatic cancer in 1.9 % and 1.3 % of the patients, respectively. Among the diagnosed patients, 28 out of 85 (32.9 %) and 19 out of 56 (33 %) patients underwent resection for T1/T2 tumors in the two groups, respectively. Among the asymptomatic patients, 10,162 patients in the 1984–1985 group and 2,678 in the 1987–1988 group combined, a total of 4 cases of pancreatic cancer were identified and 3 of the 4 patients did not have resectable disease (Satake et al. 1994). Another mass screening study evaluated 70,940 asymptomatic subjects and found CA 19-9 levels to be elevated in 1,063 (1.5 %) individuals, and malignancy was diagnosed in only 15 of the 1,063 subjects. The various malignancies were pancreatic cancer (4), lung cancer (4), colon cancer (3), gastric cancer (2), hepatocellular cancer (1), and ovarian carcinoma (1). The positive predictive value of CA 19-9 in detecting pancreatic cancer in this study was a dismal 0.9 % (Kim et al. 2004). In a combined analysis of multiple studies, 57 studies with 3,285 pancreatic cancer diagnoses, the combined sensitivity of CA 19-9 was 78.2 %, and in 37 studies with 1,882 cases with benign pancreatic disease, the specificity of CA 19-9 was 82.8 % (Poruk et al. 2013).

Given all this data, it can be concluded that CA 19-9 is not a reliable screening tool for the early detection of pancreatic cancer in the general population given its low positive predictive value (Locker et al. 2006). In high-risk patients such as those with a positive family history or genetic predisposition, the positive predictive value may be higher but the utility of CA 19-9 as the only screening tool for the detection and/or diagnosis of pancreatic cancer is not justifiable (Table 1).

CA 19-9 Level as a Prognostic Marker in Resectable Pancreatic Adenocarcinoma

CA 19-9 appears to have a role as a prognostic marker in pancreatic cancer. It is recommended to obtain a baseline CA 19-9 level as part of the initial diagnostic workup in all patients diagnosed with pancreatic cancer. A number of studies established a correlation between CA 19-9 levels and stage at diagnosis (Table 2). CA 19-9 levels may prove useful to help determine resectability of tumors, especially when combined with other data obtained at diagnosis, including imaging, interventional staging, and tissue biopsy. Higher CA 19-9 levels have been shown to be associated with a higher AJCC stage and lower survival. Several studies have evaluated the relationship between perioperative CA 19-9 levels, resectability rates, and survival outcomes. In one study, 1,543 patients with a diagnosis of pancreatic adenocarcinoma had their preoperative serum levels of CA 19-9, resectability data, and overall survival collected. Additionally, the study included a control cohort of 706 patients with chronic pancreatitis to help assess the predictability of malignancy by CA 19-9 levels as well as to study the effects of hyperbilirubinemia on CA 19-9 level measurements. The resectability and 5-year survival ranged from 38 % to 80 % and 0 % to 27 % in patients with CA 19-9 levels ≥4,000 U/mL versus <37 U/mL, respectively. In the same study, the R0 resection rate in patients with CA 19-9 ≥1,000 U/mL was as low as 15 % (Hartwig et al. 2013) (Figs. 1 and 2).

Additionally, preoperative CA 19-9 levels are strongly associated with pathological stage with lower median CA 19-9 levels noted in patients with negative lymph nodes when compared to those with positive nodes (90 v 164 U/mL) and lower T stage (T1/T2 vs. T3 disease being 41 vs. 162 U/mL, respectively). In the same study, lower preoperative CA 19-9 (<37 U/mL) was associated with a median survival of 2.3 years versus 1.1 years in higher levels (≥2,000 U/mL) (Ferrone et al. 2006). In a retrospective study of 72 patients who had definitive surgery, the presence of R0 resections was associated with significantly lower CA 19-9 values when compared with that of R1/R2 resections (Kim et al. 2009). Hence preoperative CA 19-9 levels may provide prognostic information regarding stage and

Table 1 Various conditions with CA 19-9 elevation

Organ system	Condition	Degree of CA 19-9 elevation	Utility
Pancreas	Pancreatic cancer	Varies depending on stage- higher levels associated with higher stage Resectable disease, median $\leq$352 IU/mL Unresectable disease, median $\geq$ 353 IU/mL (Kim et al. 2009; Zhang et al. 2008)	Prognostic marker Monitoring disease recurrence Response to treatment
	Chronic pancreatitis	Varies, generally mildly elevated (Paganuzzi et al. 1988; Safi et al. 1987)	
	IPMN	Varies, higher levels in higher stage (Alexander et al. 2011)	Prognostic marker
Biliary tract	Cholangiocarcinoma = –0	Varies, higher levels ($\geq$55 IU/mL) associated with increased recurrence (Chung et al. 2011)	Prognostic marker Monitoring disease recurrence Response to treatment
	Gallbladder cancer	Varies depending on stage (D'Hondt et al. 2013; Pais-Costa et al. 2012)	Prognostic marker
	Cholangitis and obstructive jaundice	Varies depending on hyperbilirubinemia and etiology, especially important in PSC- higher levels in PSC predicting higher risk of cancer (Barr Fritcher et al. 2013; Sinakos et al. 2011; Venkatesh et al. 2013)	Differential diagnosis Prognostic marker
Colon/ rectum	Colorectal cancer	Varies, higher levels could be seen in higher TNM stage (Zhang et al. 2013)	Could be prognostic
Stomach	Gastric cancer	Varies, higher levels could be seen in higher TNM stage (Kochi et al. 2000; Ucar et al. 2008)	
Lung	NSCLC	Uncommonly elevated in NSCLC (Li et al. 2012)	
Ovary	Ovarian cancer	Higher levels in mucinous tumors (Dong et al. 2008)	Prognostic marker
	Borderline ovarian tumors	Higher levels in mucinous tumors (Ayhan et al. 2007)	Prognostic marker
	Cystic teratoma of ovary	Higher levels associated with higher rates of bilaterality (Dede et al. 2006)	
Others	Pseudomyxoma peritonei	Varies, higher levels worse survival (Chua et al. 2012; Koh et al. 2013)	Prognostic marker
	Occult primary	Varies, depending on site of primary	

Table 2 Range of CA 19-9 elevation by stage of pancreatic cancer at diagnosis

	Median Range of CA 19-9 by stage (IU/mL) – normal ≤ 37 IU/mL					
Study	Stage 1a	1b	2a	2b	3	4
Ferrone et al. (2006)	20.5	86	105	164		182
Kim et al. (2009)	40.05	2005.28	41.46	87.77	135.83	600.00
Kondo et al. (2010)	96 (stage 1a, 1b)		160 (stage 2–4)			

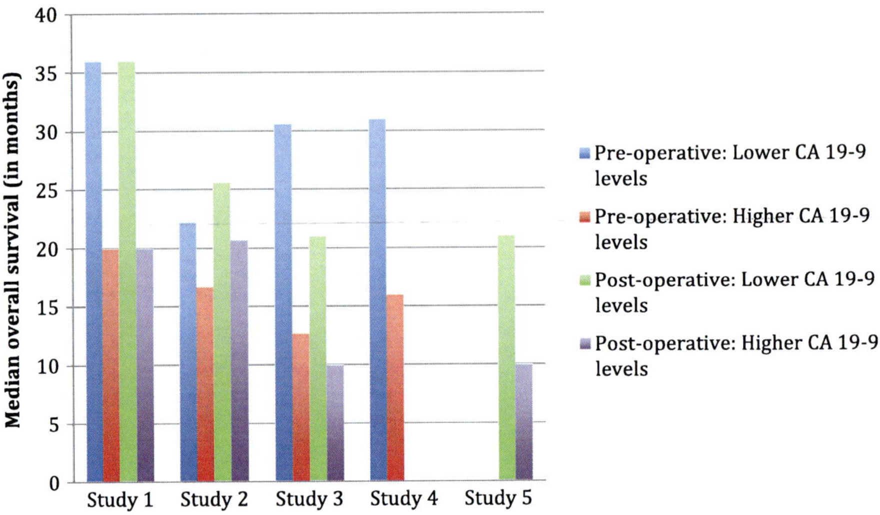

1: (Martin, et al., 2012) 2: (Humphris, et al., 2012) 3: (Waraya, et al., 2009)
4: (Sugiura, et al., 2012) 5: (Berger, et al., 2012)

Fig. 1 Survival in months comparing preoperative and postoperative CA 19-9 levels summarized from studies in resectable pancreas cancer

survival of patients with pancreatic adenocarcinoma (Ferrone et al. 2006; Hartwig et al. 2013; Kau et al. 1999; Kim et al. 2009; Kondo et al. 2010; Lundin et al. 1994).

Postoperative CA 19-9 levels have also been found to be lower in the presence of R0 resections compared to that of R1/R2 resections or in patients with nodal disease (Ferrone et al. 2006; Kondo et al. 2010). In patients undergoing resection, serial drop in CA 19-9 levels postoperatively are favorably associated with improved survival (Berger et al. 2008; Berger et al. 2012; Montgomery et al. 1997). Given that the half-life of CA 19-9 is approximately 14 h, CA 19–9 should not be measured before 4–6 weeks following the operation. CA 19-9 velocity has also been shown to predict overall survival as well as disease progression in addition to baseline CA 19-9 levels (Hernandez et al. 2009; Montgomery et al. 1997; Nishida et al. 1999).

It has been consistently shown that lower stage and the presence of resectable disease are associated with improved survival in patients with pancreatic cancer. However, resectability should not be determined based solely on CA 19-9 levels

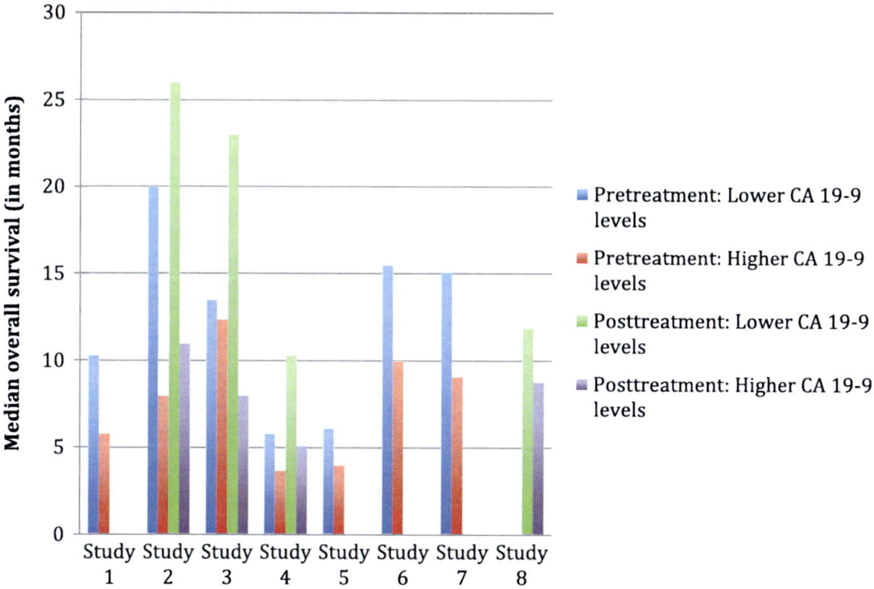

1: (Hess, et al., 2008) 2: (Katz, et al., 1998) 3: (Lee, et al., 2013), (Katz, et al., 1998)
4: (Bauer, et al., 2013) 5: (Haas, et al., 2013) 6: (Reni, et al., 2009) 7: (Yoo, et al., 2011)
8: (Haas, et al., 2013)

Fig. 2 Survival in months comparing pretreatment CA 19-9 levels and survival based on treatment response in CA 19-9 levels summarized from studies in advanced pancreatic cancer

(Locker et al. 2006) but used in conjunction with other investigations and could provide useful prognostic CA 19-9 levels along with other staging workup in pancreatic cancer that may provide useful prognostic information (Table 3).

CA 19-9 Level as a Prognostic Marker in Advanced and Metastatic Pancreatic Adenocarcinoma

Pretreatment CA 19-9 levels were shown to be independent prognostic markers that help predict survival in patients with advanced pancreatic cancer (Hess et al. 2008) and may correlate with tumor burden in patients with advanced pancreatic cancer. Higher levels are typically found to be associated with a decreased overall survival and progression free survival.

A decline in CA 19-9 levels following treatment is a favorable prognostic indicator in terms of survival. It serves as a predictive and prognostic biomarker in patients receiving gemcitabine-based chemotherapy (Bauer et al. 2013). In patients receiving chemotherapy with radiation in the neoadjuvant setting, the decline in serum CA 19-9 is a favorable indicator of response to treatment and negative predictor for progression or development of metastatic disease. An increase in CA 19-9 levels could indicate tumor progression, and these patients

Table 3 Summary of studies of CA 19-9 in resectable pancreas cancer

Paper/year	Description	CA 19-9 range U/mL[a]	Results	Conclusions in papers
Abdel-Misih et al. (2011)	Retrospective review, $N = 93$	≤35 >35	Persistent elevation of CA 19-9 (>35 U/mL) after 6 months following resection – worse survival – similar to unresected or metastatic disease. HR 2.20, p value of 0.002	Post operative CA 19-9 levels are prognostic
Ferrone et al. (2006)	Retrospective review, $N = 424$	Preoperative, median: 41 162 9 164	T1/T2 lesions T3 lesions N0 disease N1 disease	Preoperative CA 19-9 correlates with stage of disease Postoperative CA 19-9 decrease and CA 19-9 value of < 200 U/mL are independent predictors of survival even after adjusting for stage
Hernandez et al. (2009)	Analysis of patients on the control arm of randomized trial and did not receive adjuvant therapy following surgery, $N = 96$	CA 19-9 velocity/4 weeks 131 1	Disease progression No disease progression	Rate of CA 19-9 change is predictive of disease progression
Humphris et al. (2012)	Retrospective review, $N = 260$	Preoperative ≤120 vs. >120 Post resection: <37 vs. 37–120 Normalization of CA 19-9 within 6 months after surgery CA 19-9 did not normalize	Median overall survival in months: 22.2 vs. 16.7 25.6 vs. 20.7 29.9 14.8	Preoperative CA 19-9 levels and normalization of CA 19-9 within 6 months of resection are prognostic markers for survival
Berger et al. (2008)	Phase III randomized trial, patients treated with adjuvant CRT, $N = 385$	Baseline <180 >180	72 % reduction in risk of death More commonly associated with larger tumors, positive lymph nodes	CA 19-9 levels are prognostic for survival and predictive for stage

(*continued*)

Table 3 (continued)

Paper/year	Description	CA 19-9 range U/mL[a]	Results	Conclusions in papers
Kinsella et al. (2008)	Retrospective data, patients treated with surgery followed by radiation therapy, $N = 75$	Post operative: ≤70 and R0 resection ≤70 and R1/R2 resection >70 and R0/R1/R2 resection	Survival 2 years – 80 % 5 years – 65 % 2 years – 40 % 5 years – 10 % 2 years – 10 % 5 years – 0	CA 19-9 levels are prognostic for survival High CA 19-9 levels and positive margins were predictive of early distant metastases
Kondo et al. (2010)	Retrospective review, $N = 109$	Preoperative: <37 ≥37 <100 ≥100 <200 ≥200 <500 ≥500	3 years survival 49 % 10 % 43 % 0 38 % 0 38 % 0	Preoperative CA 19-9 is prognostic for survival
Barton et al. (2009)	Retrospective review, $N = 143$	Preoperative: ≤120 >120	Survival: % 1 year, 3 years, 5 years 76, 41, 31 64, 17, 10	Preoperative CA 19-9 prognostic for survival, not predictive of lymph node status, margin status
Waraya et al. (2009)	Retrospective review, $N = 117$	Preoperative: ≤37 vs. >37	Disease specific survival (months) 30.6 vs. 12.7	Preoperative CA 19-9 is prognostic for survival
Berger et al. (2012)	Analysis of survival data from a large randomized trial to use adjuvant CRT in patients with resected pancreas cancer, $N = 385$	Post resection: <90 vs. ≥90	mOS (months): 21 vs. 10	Post resection CA 19-9 levels is prognostic
Sugiura et al. (2012)	Retrospective review, $N = 154$	Preoperative: <100 ≥100	Early recurrence %[b], 3 years, 5 years % and mOS (months): 11, 47.3, 40.1, 31 53, 21.2, 9.4, 16	Preoperative CA 19-9 are prognostic for early recurrence as well as survival

[a]CA 19-9 in U/mL unless otherwise specified
[b]Early recurrence – within 6 months of surgery

may not be amenable to a successful resection of the tumor (Katz et al. 2010; Willett et al. 1996). Following surgery, CA 19-9 levels could predict the likelihood of a successful completion of margin-negative pancreatic resection (Katz et al. 2010).

Chemotherapy response has been assessed using serial CA 19-9 levels in several studies and it has been found that treatment-related decline in the biomarker is associated with better overall survival in some studies. There are several definitions for assessing the degree of decline such as $\geq$20 % decline as well $\geq$50–75 % decline from pretreatment values in the first 6–8 weeks of treatment. The pretreatment levels have clearly been shown to be prognostic; however, the degree of decline in CA 19-9 and its correlation with survival has shown mixed results (Halm et al. 2000; Hess et al. 2008; Ishii et al. 1997; Maisey et al. 2005; Reni et al. 2009; Saad et al. 2002; Ziske et al. 2003) (Table 4).

Similarly, CA 19-9 levels can be followed serially to monitor response to chemotherapy in metastatic disease. Increasing levels along with imaging studies could indicate disease progression and discontinuation of current therapy. High pretreatment CA 19-9 levels are associated with worse prognosis and could indicate increased tumor burden (Table 4).

CA 19-9 in Intraductal Papillary Mucinous Neoplasms of the Pancreas

Elevated CA 19-9 serves as an adverse risk factor associated with postoperative recurrence of intraductal papillary mucinous neoplasms of the pancreas (Park et al. 2011). Higher CA 19-9 levels are also associated with worse survival (Alexander et al. 2011).

CA 19-9 in Gastric Cancer

Gastric cancer is the second most common cause of worldwide cancer-related death. It is the most common cancer in men in Japan and the highest incidence of gastric cancer is in China. By some estimates, it is the fourth most common cancer worldwide (Kamangar et al. 2006), but its overall incidence has been decreasing worldwide over the last several decades. Several types of gastric cancer (proximal type, diffuse type) have however been increasing in incidence. Gastric cancer is most commonly diagnosed at an advanced stage except in Japan, Korea, and few other countries where screening with endoscopy is prevalent. The incidence and outcomes in patients diagnosed with gastric cancer have significantly improved in Japan, mainly owing to earlier diagnosis, but the overall survival continues to be poor in North America and Europe. In gastric cancer, CA 19-9 can be elevated in up to 20–35 % of patients (Hou et al. 2011; Kochi et al. 2000; Lukaszewicz-Zajac et al. 2011). CA 19-9 measurement alone is not routinely recommended in gastric cancer but in combination with other tumor markers such as CEA and other proinflammatory markers, and it may provide prognostic information. Higher CA 19-9 levels are associated with higher tumor stage, presence of lymph nodes metastases or distant metastases, and decreased overall survival (Kochi et al. 2000; Liu et al. 2012a; Ucar et al. 2008).

Table 4 Summary of studies of CA 19-9 in advanced/ advanced with resectable/metastatic pancreatic cancer

Paper/year	Description	CA 19-9 range U/mL[a]	Results	Conclusions in papers
Hammad et al. (2010)	Analysis of 3 consecutive gemcitabine containing phase 2 trials, $N = 111$		Lower baseline CA 19-9 associated with better OS and TTP	Baseline CA 19-9 values have prognostic value Change in CA 19-9 within 1 month of treatment is not predictive or prognostic
Kim et al. (2009)	Retrospective review, $N = 114$	<92.77 ≥92.77 (along with lower CEA < 2.47 ng/mL and tumor size < 11.85 cm3	R0 resection 90.6 % accuracy R1/R2 resection with 88.6 % accuracy	Lower baseline or preoperative CA 19-9 is predictive of resectability
Tsavaris et al. (2009)	Retrospective study, $N = 215$	>30 x upper limit of normal (37)	Higher levels associated with worse survival	CA 19-9 has prognostic value
Hess et al. (2008)	RCT with patients undergoing treatment with gemcitabine alone or with capecitabine, $N =$ 247 had baseline CA 19-9 levels	Baseline CA 19-9: (ULN: varies from 20 to 37) ≥59 x ULN <59 x ULN	Survival 5.8 months 10.3 months	Pretreatment CA 19-9 is prognostic Decrease in CA 19-9 with treatment is not associated with improved survival
Katz et al. (1998)	Retrospective review of patients treated with radiotherapy, $N =$ 104	Pretreatment median: >680 ≤680 Post treatment: >162.5 ≤162.5 >75 % decrease <75 % decrease	mOS (months) 8 20 11 26 23 8	Pretreatment, post treatment levels of CA 19-9 are prognostic for survival Degree of decrease in CA 19-9 with treatment is predictive for survival
Lee et al. (2013)	Retrospective review, $N = 187$	Upper limit of normal: 37 Median 376	mOS (months) 12.4 vs. 13.5 months (in elevated CA 19-9 vs. lower) p value of 0.969	CA 19-9 levels did not correlate with stage or survival

(*continued*)

Table 4 (continued)

Paper/year	Description	CA 19-9 range U/mL[a]	Results	Conclusions in papers
Martin et al. (2012)	Retrospective review, $N = 123$	Preoperative: <37, ≥37 <37,≥37 <37, ≥37 <37, ≥37 Postoperative: <37, ≥3 Adv disease: 0–50 % decline >50 % decline	mOS (months) 36, 20 DFS 16.5, 7.6 LN + 13 %, 64 % T ≥ 3 cm 38 %, 93 % mOS 36, 20 mOS 8.5 11.916	Higher CA 19-9 levels perioperatively is prognostic for worse survival. Higher decline with therapy in advanced disease is prognostic and predictive
Nishida et al. (1999)	Retrospective review, $N = 75$	CA 19-9 doubling time: Range from <1 day to 313 days	Shorter doubling time associated with worse survival	CA 19-9 doubling time is prognostic
Bauer et al. (2013)	Pooled analysis of 6 prospective trials, $N = 212$	Median CA 19-9 level at baseline: ng/mL 1,077 (range 15–492.241) Below median Above median After 2 cycles of gemcitabine: <5 % increase ≥5 % increase	mOS (months), 5.8 3.7 mOS and TTP 10.3, 7.5 5.1, 3.5	Baseline CA 19-9 is a prognostic marker Increase in CA 19-9 after treatment is a negative predictive marker Decrease in CA 19-9 during treatment – no prognostic implication for survival
Haas et al. (2013)	Pooled analysis of 2 multicenter RCT phase II plus prospective data from a high volume cancer center, $N = 291$	Median pretreatment: 1,137 (range 6–100,000) ≤1,000 vs. >1,000 Decline (after 2 cycles) <50 % ≥50 %	Months: mOS: 9 6.1 vs. 4.0 mOS, mTTP 8.8, 5.4 11.9, 5.8	Pretreatment CA 19-9 is prognostic for survival and change in CA 19-9 levels during treatment is predictive
Katz et al. (2010)	Analysis of 2 phase II trials of patients with normal bilirubin receiving neoadjuvant CRT	Pretreatment: <37 Restaging: <61	Completing PD PPV 86 % NPV 28 % PPV 93 % NPV 28 %	Decision making for resectability should not be based on CA 19-9 levels due to low NPV even with high PPV

(*continued*)

Table 4 (continued)

Paper/year	Description	CA 19-9 range U/mL[a]	Results	Conclusions in papers
Haas et al. (2010)	Retrospective review of patients receiving second line chemotherapy, $N = 70$	CA 19-9 change within 1st 2 cycles: >20 %	Worse survival with HR of 2.00	CA 19-9 change is predictive
Reni et al. (2009)	Analysis of patients with pancreatic cancer on 5 trials, $N = 247$	Baseline: ≤37 38–1,167 >1,167	mOS (months): 15.5 11.9 8	Baseline CA 19-9 is an independent prognostic factor
Koom et al. (2009)	Retrospective review of patients with elevated CA 1-9 and pancreas cancer, $N = 69$	Pretreatment: >1,200 Posttreatment: >100 Decline ≤40 %	All associated with worse survival	Pretreatment, posttreatment, as well as decline in CA 19-9 are prognostic
Yoo et al. (2011)	Retrospective review of patients who underwent CRT, $N = 84$	Pretreatment: ≤400 >400	Tumor response %, early distant mets, MOS (months): 45.1, 19.6, 15.1 15.2, 42.4, 9.1	CA 19-9 is a prognostic marker

[a]Unless otherwise specified

CA 19-9 in Biliary Tract Cancers

Current NCCN guidelines suggest obtaining CA 19-9 levels as a part of workup for suspected intrahepatic cholangiocarcinoma as well as extrahepatic cholangiocarcinoma along with liver function studies, imaging studies, and interventional staging. CA 19-9 level serves as a useful prognostic biomarker in biliary tract cancers (Chung et al. 2011; Kawamata et al. 2013; Liu et al. 2010). In both intrahepatic and extrahepatic cholangiocarcinoma, the overall survival seems better in patients with lower initial CA 19-9 levels (Liu et al. 2012b). It is used in combination with other tumor markers such as CEA and CA 125 in the initial diagnosis, prognostication (Wang et al. 2013), and monitoring response to treatment (Woo et al. 2012). It could also predict tumor stage as well as resectability in conjunction with other staging studies (Juntermanns et al. 2010). CA 19-9 may be elevated in primary sclerosing cholangitis, which predisposes to cholangiocarcinoma and can predict adverse prognosis in this setting (Barr Fritcher et al. 2013; Sinakos et al. 2011; Venkatesh et al. 2013).

Gallbladder cancer is often diagnosed at an advanced stage, given its aggressive behavior and delayed diagnosis as its symptoms are similar to more benign etiologies such as chronic cholecystitis and cholelithiasis. CA 19-9 levels should be obtained as part of the initial diagnostic evaluation keeping in mind that baseline levels are more accurate following biliary decompression if the patient presented with signs and symptoms of obstruction. Similar to other malignancies, low or undetectable CA 19-9 levels following resection seem to be associated with a better prognosis and predict for lower TNM stage, R0 resection, and perineural invasion (D'Hondt et al. 2013; Pais-Costa et al. 2012).

It can be concluded that in biliary tract cancers, elevated preoperative CA 19-9 levels are independent predictors of decreased overall survival after successful resection or attempted resection and hence is prognostic across all stages of disease (Hatzaras et al. 2010).

CA 19-9 in Colorectal Cancer

Screening colonoscopy has proved to be an effective screening tool for early detection of colorectal cancer with a primary impact on prolonging survival of patients with early diagnosis. CEA is the most commonly used tumor marker in surveillance and monitoring of disease. CA 19-9 may also be increased in patients with colorectal cancer with higher levels linked to higher TNM stage and worse prognosis (Yu et al. 2013). There is insufficient data to recommend using CA 19-9 in the routine management of colorectal cancer (Bast et al. 2001).

CA 19-9 in Ovarian Cancer

CA 19-9 may be elevated in ovarian cancer, more commonly in mucinous tumors compared to nonmucinous ones (Ayhan et al. 2007; Dong et al. 2008). Only in mucinous ovarian tumors, CA 19-9 levels were more commonly associated with higher stage. This finding may be explained by the fact that CA 19-9 is a sialylated oligosaccharide that is most commonly found in circulating mucins in patients with malignancy. The presence of CA 19-9 detected by immunohistochemical staining in mucinous ovarian tumor and borderline mucinous tumors was found to be around 84 % (Motoyama et al. 1990). In borderline ovarian tumors, CA 19-9 was found to be elevated in the range of 40.9–57 % for mucinous tumors and 7.9–51.5 % for serous tumors (Ayhan et al. 2007; Engelen et al. 2000; Tamakoshi et al. 1996). In mature cystic teratomas, CA 19-9 could be elevated in up to 39 % of patients and is associated with higher likelihood of bilaterality (Dede et al. 2006).

In ovarian cancer, CA 19-9 levels along with CA 125 levels predict advanced clinical stage (both by TNM staging and FIGO), increased rates of lymph node involvement, and presence of occult neoplastic cells. Hence higher levels predict worse prognosis (Muramatsu et al. 2005). CA 19-9 measurement is especially useful in ovarian carcinoma with mucinous histology since serous type of cancer may fail to express the marker, with a positive rate up to 83.3 % in mucinous type versus 28.2 % in nonmucinous type (Gadducci et al. 1992). CA 19-9 alone cannot be recommended in the routine monitoring of patients with ovarian cancer. However, if initially elevated, it can be used concomitantly with other tumor markers, especially in combination with CA 125 or alone in patients who are negative for CA 125.

Utility in Other Malignancies

CA 19-9 can serve as an independent prognostic factor in other malignancies such as pseudomyxoma peritonei with higher levels following cytoreductive surgery and perioperative intraperitoneal chemotherapy which are typically associated with worse prognosis and overall survival (Koh et al. 2013).

CA 19-9 can also be found to be elevated in non-small lung cancers along with other tumor markers such as CEA and CA 125. However, given its lack of specificity and overall sensitivity when used alone, it should not be recommended for use in routine practice (Li et al. 2012).

CA 19-9 in Occult Primary

Current NCCN guidelines recommend considering obtaining CA 19-9 along with other tumor markers as part of the initial evaluation in biopsy-proven adenocarcinoma in the liver or patients with peritoneal disease when pancreatic or biliary tract primary is suspected.

Potential Applications to Prognosis, Other Diseases, or Conditions

CA 19-9 is a biomarker that has been extensively studied, primarily in pancreatic malignancy and biliary tract malignancies, and has been shown to be a prognostic factor in different stages of presentation. It has been used as a tumor marker to follow after resection of the primary malignancy to detect recurrence as well as to monitor response to therapy in the metastatic setting. Its utility has been studied extensively as a diagnostic tool, especially in pancreatic cancer, and has been demonstrated as having poor positive predictive value.

With ongoing research to understand the biology of several diseases, search for newer and more effective therapies, the development of a prognostic model with incorporation of several factors including CA 19-9 is the first step toward improving the outlook in several cancers, especially pancreatic cancer.

Summary Points

- CA 19-9 is a sialylated Lewis A group antigen and is positive only in patients with the Le $(a - B+)$ or Le $(a + B-)$ blood groups. About 5–10 % of the population will not test positive for CA 19-9.

- CA 19-9 is a useful biomarker and is the only FDA-approved biomarker in pancreatic cancer.
- It is relatively nonspecific and has a low predictive value as a screening tool in pancreatic cancer.
- It can be elevated in pancreatic cancer as well as other malignancies such as biliary tract cancers, gastric cancers, and ovarian cancers among others. The biomarker can also be elevated in nonmalignant conditions such as biliary obstruction secondary to other benign etiologies, pancreatitis, benign neoplasms of the pancreas, inflammatory hepatobiliary diseases, and thyroid disease among others.
- CA 19-9 has been shown to have a prognostic value, with higher levels being associated with worse prognosis, mainly in pancreatic cancer and other malignancies such as biliary tract cancers, ovarian tumors, especially in mucinous tumors.
- CA 19-9 is one of the biomarkers that can be considered during workup for occult primary when suspecting pancreaticobiliary origin.

References

Abdel-Misih SR, Hatzaras I, Schmidt C, Saab TB, Klemanski D, Muscarella P, Melvin WS, Ellison EC, Bloomston M. Failure of normalization of CA19-9 following resection for pancreatic cancer is tantamount to metastatic disease. Annals of Surgical Oncology, 2011;1:1116–21.

Alexander BM, Fernandez-Del Castillo C, Ryan DP, Kachnic LA, Hezel AF, Niemierko A, Willett CG, Kozak KR, Blaszkowsky LS, Clark JW, Warshaw AL, Hong TS. Intraductal papillary mucinous adenocarcinoma of the pancreas: clinical outcomes, prognostic factors, and the role of adjuvant therapy. Gastrointestinal Cancer Research, 2011;32:116–21.

Ayhan A, Guven S, Guven ES, Kucukali T. Is there a correlation between tumor marker panel and tumor size and histopathology in well staged patients with borderline ovarian tumors? Acta Obstetricia et Gynecologica, 2007;55:484–90.

Barr Fritcher EG, Voss JS, Jenkins SM, Lingineni RK, Clayton AC, Roberts LR, Halling KC, Talwalkar JA, Gores GJ, Kipp BR. Primary sclerosing cholangitis with equivocal cytology: Fluorescence in situ hybridization and serum CA 19–9 predict risk of malignancy. Cancer Cytopathology, 2013;48:708–17.

Barton JG, Bois JP, Sarr MG, Wood CM, Qin R, Thomsen KM, Kendrick ML, Farnell MB. Predictive and prognostic value of CA 19–9 in resected pancreatic adenocarcinoma. Journal of Gastrointestinal surgery, 2009;117:2050–8.

Bast Jr RC, Ravdin P, Hayes DF, Bates S, Fritsche Jr H, Jessup JM, Kemeny N, Locker GY, Mennel RG, Somerfield MR. 2000 update of recommendations for the use of tumor markers in breast and colorectal cancer: clinical practice guidelines of the American Society of Clinical Oncology. Journal of Clinical Oncology, 2001;53:1865–78.

Bauer TM, El-Rayes BF, Li X, Hammad N, Philip PA, Shields AF, Zalupski MM, Bekaii-Saab T. Carbohydrate antigen 19–9 is a prognostic and predictive biomarker in patients with advanced pancreatic cancer who receive gemcitabine-containing chemotherapy: a pooled analysis of 6 prospective trials. Cancer, 2013;152:285–92.

Berger AC, Garcia Jr M, Hoffman JP, Regine WF, Abrams RA, Safran H, Konski A, Benson 3rd AB, MacDonald J, Willett CG. Postresection CA 19–9 predicts overall survival in patients with pancreatic cancer treated with adjuvant chemoradiation: a prospective validation by RTOG 9704. Journal of clinical oncology, 2008;100:5918–22.

Berger AC, Winter K, Hoffman JP, Regine WF, Abrams RA, Safran H, Freedman GM, Benson 3rd AB, Macdonald J, Willett CG. Five year results of US intergroup/RTOG 9704 with postoperative CA 19–9 </=90 U/mL and comparison to the CONKO-001 trial. International Journal of Radiation Oncology biology, physics, 2012;133:291–7.

Chua TC, Liauw W, Morris DL. Early recurrence of pseudomyxoma peritonei following treatment failure of cytoreductive surgery and perioperative intraperitoneal chemotherapy is indicative of a poor survival outcome. International journal of colorectal diseases, 2012;68:381–9.

Chung MJ, Lee KJ, Bang S, Park SW, Kim KS, Lee WJ, Song SY, Chung JB, Park JY. Preoperative serum CA 19–9 level as a predictive factor for recurrence after curative resection in biliary tract cancer. Annals of Surgical Oncology, 2011;39:1651–6.

Dede M, Gungor S, Yenen MC, Alanbay I, Duru NK, Hasimi A. CA19-9 may have clinical significance in mature cystic teratomas of the ovary. International Journal of Gynecological Cancer, 2006;59:189–93.

Del Villano BC, Brennan S, Brock P, Bucher C, Liu V, McClure M, Rake B, Space S, Westrick B, Schoemaker H, Zurawski Jr VR. Radioimmunometric assay for a monoclonal antibody-defined tumor marker, CA 19–9. Clinical Chemistry, 1983;5:549–52.

D'Hondt M, Lapointe R, Benamira Z, Pottel H, Plasse M, Letourneau R, Roy A, Dagenais M, Vandenbroucke-Menu F. Carcinoma of the gallbladder: patterns of presentation, prognostic factors and survival rate. An 11-year single centre experience. EJSO- The journal of Cancer surgery, 2013;49:548–53.

Dong L, Cui H, Li XP, Sun LF, Chang XH, Liang XD, Zhu HL. Clinical value of serum CA19-9, CA125 and CP2 in mucinous ovarian tumor: a retrospective study of 273 patients. Zhonghua Fu Chan Ke Za Zhi, 2008;54:5–8.

Duraker N, Hot S, Polat Y, Hobek A, Gencler N, Urhan N. CEA, CA 19–9, and CA 125 in the differential diagnosis of benign and malignant pancreatic diseases with or without jaundice. Journal of Surgical Oncology, 2007;4:142–7.

Engelen MJ, de Bruijn HW, Hollema H, ten Hoor KA, Willemse PH, Aalders JG, van der Zee AG. Serum CA 125, carcinoembryonic antigen, and CA 19–9 as tumor markers in borderline ovarian tumors. Gynecologic Oncology, 2000;58:16–20.

Ferrone CR, Finkelstein DM, Thayer SP, Muzikansky A, Fernandez-delCastillo C, Warshaw AL. Perioperative CA19-9 levels can predict stage and survival in patients with resectable pancreatic adenocarcinoma. Journal of Clinical Oncology, 2006;87:2897–902.

Gadducci A, Ferdeghini M, Prontera C, Moretti L, Mariani G, Bianchi R, Fioretti P. The concomitant determination of different tumor markers in patients with epithelial ovarian cancer and benign ovarian masses: relevance for differential diagnosis. Gynecologic Oncology, 1992;61:147–54.

Haas M, Laubender RP, Stieber P, Holdenrieder S, Bruns CJ, Wilkowski R, Mansmann U, Heinemann V, Boeck S. Prognostic relevance of CA 19–9, CEA, CRP, and LDH kinetics in patients treated with palliative second-line therapy for advanced pancreatic cancer. Tumor Biology, 2010;168:351–7.

Haas M, Heinemann V, Kullmann F, Laubender RP, Klose C, Bruns CJ, Holdenrieder S, Modest DP, Schulz C, Boeck S. Prognostic value of CA 19–9, CEA, CRP, LDH and bilirubin levels in locally advanced and metastatic pancreatic cancer: results from a multicenter, pooled analysis of patients receiving palliative chemotherapy. Journal of cancer research Clinical Oncology, 2013;158:681–9.

Halm U, Schumann T, Schiefke I, Witzigmann H, Mossner J, Keim V. Decrease of CA 19–9 during chemotherapy with gemcitabine predicts survival time in patients with advanced pancreatic cancer. British Journal of Cancer, 2000;28:1013–6.

Hammad N, Heilbrun LK, Philip PA, Shields AF, Zalupski MM, Venkatramanamoorthy R, El-Rayes BF. CA19-9 as a predictor of tumor response and survival in patients with advanced pancreatic cancer treated with gemcitabine based chemotherapy. Asia-Pacific Journal of Clinical Oncology, 2010;137:98–105.

Hartwig W, Strobel O, Hinz U, Fritz S, Hackert T, Roth C, Buchler MW, Werner J. CA19-9 in Potentially Resectable Pancreatic Cancer: Perspective to Adjust Surgical and Perioperative Therapy. Annals of Surgical Oncology, 2013;10:2188–96.

Hatzaras I, Schmidt C, Muscarella P, Melvin WS, Ellison EC, Bloomston M. Elevated CA 19–9 portends poor prognosis in patients undergoing resection of biliary malignancies. HPB, 2010;51:5.

Herlyn M, Sears HF, Steplewski Z, Koprowski H. Monoclonal antibody detection of a circulating tumor-associated antigen. I. Presence of antigen in sera of patients with colorectal, gastric, and pancreatic carcinoma. Journal of Clinical Immunology, 1982;2:135–40.

Hernandez JM, Cowgill SM, Al-Saadi S, Collins A, Ross SB, Cooper J, Villadolid D, Zervos E, Rosemurgy A. CA 19–9 velocity predicts disease-free survival and overall survival after pancreatectomy of curative intent. Journal of Gastrointestinal surgery, 2009;90:349–53.

Hess V, Glimelius B, Grawe P, Dietrich D, Bodoky G, Ruhstaller T, Bajetta E, Saletti P, Figer A, Scheithauer W, Herrmann R. CA 19–9 tumour-marker response to chemotherapy in patients with advanced pancreatic cancer enrolled in a randomised controlled trial. The Lancet Oncology, 2008;140:132–8.

Hou JX, Yang XQ, Chen C, Jiang Q, Yang GL, Li Y. Screening the gastric cancer related tumor markers from multi-tumor markers protein chip with kappa coefficient and cost-effectiveness analysis. Hepatogastroenterology, 2011;36:632–6.

Humphris JL, Chang DK, Johns AL, Scarlett CJ, Pajic M, Jones MD, Colvin EK, Nagrial A, Chin VT, Chantrill LA, Samra JS, Gill AJ, Kench JG, Merrett ND, Das A, Musgrove EA, Sutherland RL, Biankin AV. The prognostic and predictive value of serum CA19.9 in pancreatic cancer. Annals of Oncology, 2012;99:1713–22.

Ishii H, Okada S, Sato T, Wakasugi H, Saisho H, Furuse J, Ishikawa O, Matsuno S, Yokoyama S. CA 19–9 in evaluating the response to chemotherapy in advanced pancreatic cancer. Hepatogastroenterology, 1997;27:279–83.

Juntermanns B, Radunz S, Heuer M, Hertel S, Reis H, Neuhaus JP, Vernadakis S, Trarbach T, Paul A, Kaiser GM. Tumor markers as a diagnostic key for hilar cholangiocarcinoma. European Journal of Medical Research, 2010;45:357–61.

Kamangar F, Dores GM, Anderson WF. Patterns of cancer incidence, mortality, and prevalence across five continents: defining priorities to reduce cancer disparities in different geographic regions of the world. Journal of Clinical Oncology, 2006;33:2137–50.

Katz A, Hanlon A, Lanciano R, Hoffman J, Coia L. Prognostic value of CA 19–9 levels in patients with carcinoma of the pancreas treated with radiotherapy. International Journal of Radiation Oncology, biology, physics, 1998;141:393–6.

Katz MH, Varadhachary GR, Fleming JB, Wolff RA, Lee JE, Pisters PW, Vauthey JN, Abdalla EK, Sun CC, Wang H, Crane CH, Lee JH, Tamm EP, Abbruzzese JL, Evans DB. Serum CA 19–9 as a marker of resectability and survival in patients with potentially resectable pancreatic cancer treated with neoadjuvant chemoradiation. Annals of Surgical Oncology, 2010;165:1794–801.

Kau SY, Shyr YM, Su CH, Wu CW, Lui WY. Diagnostic and prognostic values of CA 19–9 and CEA in periampullary cancers. Journal of American College of Surgeons, 1999;14:415–20.

Kawamata H, Yamashita K, Nakamura K, Katagiri H, Ishii K, Takahashi Y, Furuta K, Kumamoto Y, Watanabe M. Perineural invasion and preoperative serum CA19-9 as predictors of survival in biliary tract cancer. Anticancer research, 2013;40:583–94.

Kim JE, Lee KT, Lee JK, Paik SW, Rhee JC, Choi KW. Clinical usefulness of carbohydrate antigen 19–9 as a screening test for pancreatic cancer in an asymptomatic population. Journal of Gastroenterology and Hepatology, 2004;8:182–6.

Kim YC, Kim HJ, Park JH, Park DI, Cho YK, Sohn CI, Jeon WK, Kim BI, Shin JH. Can preoperative CA19-9 and CEA levels predict the resectability of patients with pancreatic adenocarcinoma? Gastroenterology, 2009;138:1869–75.

Kinsella TJ, Seo Y, Willis J, Stellato TA, Siegel CT, Harpp D, Willson JK, Gibbons J, Sanabria JR, Hardacre JM, Schulak JP. The impact of resection margin status and postoperative CA19-9 levels on survival and patterns of recurrence after postoperative high-dose radiotherapy with 5-FU-based concurrent chemotherapy for resectable pancreatic cancer. American Journal of Clinical Oncology, 2008;106:446–53.

Kochi M, Fujii M, Kanamori N, Kaiga T, Kawakami T, Aizaki K, Kasahara M, Mochizuki F, Kasakura Y, Yamagata M. Evaluation of serum CEA and CA19-9 levels as prognostic factors in patients with gastric cancer. Gastric Cancer, 2000;34:177–186.

Koh JL, Liauw W, Chua T, Morris DL. Carbohydrate antigen 19–9 (CA 19–9) is an independent prognostic indicator in pseudomyxoma peritonei post cytoreductive surgery and perioperative intraperitoneal chemotherapy. Journal of Gastrointestinal Oncology, 2013;62:173–81.

Kondo N, Murakami Y, Uemura K, Hayashidani Y, Sudo T, Hashimoto Y, Nakashima A, Sakabe R, Shigemoto N, Kato Y, Ohge H, Sueda T. Prognostic impact of perioperative serum CA 19–9 levels in patients with resectable pancreatic cancer. Annals of Surgical Oncology, 2010;112:2321–9.

Koom WS, Seong J, Kim YB, Pyun HO, Song SY. CA 19–9 as a predictor for response and survival in advanced pancreatic cancer patients treated with chemoradiotherapy. International Journal of Radiation Oncology, biology, physics, 2009;175:1148–54.

Koprowski H, Steplewski Z, Mitchell K, Herlyn M, Herlyn D, Fuhrer P. Colorectal carcinoma antigens detected by hybridoma antibodies. Somatic Cell Genetics, 1979;3:957–71.

Lee KJ, Yi SW, Chung MJ, Park SW, Song SY, Chung JB, Park JY. Serum CA 19–9 and CEA levels as a prognostic factor in pancreatic adenocarcinoma. Yonsei Medical Journal, 2013;146:643–9.

Li X, Asmitananda T, Gao L, Gai D, Song Z, Zhang Y, Ren H, Yang T, Chen T, Chen M. Biomarkers in the lung cancer diagnosis: a clinical perspective. Neoplasma, 2012;63:500–7.

Liu SL, Song ZF, Hu QG, Shan D, Hu SB, Li J, Zheng QC. Serum carbohydrate antigen (CA) 19–9 as a prognostic factor in cholangiocarcinoma: a meta-analysis. Frontiers of medicine in China, 2010;41:457–62.

Liu X, Cai H, Wang Y. Prognostic significance of tumor markers in T4a gastric cancer. World Journal of Surgical Oncology, 2012a;37:10:68.

Liu ZH, Chen Z, Ma LL, Li XH, Wang LX. Factors influencing the prognosis of patients with intrahepatic cholangiocarcinoma. Acta Gastro-enterologica Belgica, 2012b;42:215–8.

Locker GY, Hamilton S, Harris J, Jessup JM, Kemeny N, Macdonald JS, Somerfield MR, Hayes DF, Bast Jr RC. ASCO 2006 update of recommendations for the use of tumor markers in gastrointestinal cancer. Journal of Clinical Oncology, 2006;9:5313–27.

Lukaszewicz-Zajac M, Mroczko B, Gryko M, Kedra B, Szmitkowski M. Comparison between clinical significance of serum proinflammatory proteins (IL-6 and CRP) and classic tumor markers (CEA and CA 19–9) in gastric cancer. Clinical and experimental medicine, 2011;35:89–96.

Lundin J, Roberts PJ, Kuusela P, Haglund C. The prognostic value of preoperative serum levels of CA 19–9 and CEA in patients with pancreatic cancer. British Journal of Cancer, 1994;13:515–9.

Maisey NR, Norman AR, Hill A, Massey A, Oates J, Cunningham D. CA19-9 as a prognostic factor in inoperable pancreatic cancer: the implication for clinical trials. British Journal of Cancer, 2005;26:740–3.

Martin LK, Wei L, Trolli E, Bekaii-Saab T. Elevated baseline CA19-9 levels correlate with adverse prognosis in patients with early- or advanced-stage pancreas cancer. Medical Oncology (Northwood, London, England), 2012;148:3101–7.

Montgomery RC, Hoffman JP, Riley LB, Rogatko A, Ridge JA, Eisenberg BL. Prediction of recurrence and survival by post-resection CA 19–9 values in patients with adenocarcinoma of the pancreas. Annals of Surgical Oncology, 1997;18:551–6.

Motoyama T, Watanabe H, Takeuchi S, Watanabe T, Gotoh S, Okazaki E. Cancer antigen 125, carcinoembryonic antigen, and carbohydrate determinant 19–9 in ovarian tumors. Cancer, 1990;56:2628–35.

Muramatsu T, Mukai M, Sato S, Tajima T, Nagase E, Ikeda M, Goya K, Shida M, Hirasawa T, Murakami M, Shinozuka T. Clinical usefulness of serum and immunohistochemical markers in patients with stage Ia and Ic ovarian cancer. Oncology reports, 2005;60:861–5.

Nishida K, Kaneko T, Yoneda M, Nakagawa S, Ishikawa T, Yamane E, Nishioka B, Miyamoto Y, Takano H, Yoshikawa T, Kondo M. Doubling time of serum CA 19–9 in the clinical course of patients with pancreatic cancer and its significant association with prognosis. Journal of Surgical Oncology, 1999;151:140–6.

Paganuzzi M, Onetto M, Marroni P, Barone D, Conio M, Aste H, Pugliese V. CA 19–9 and CA 50 in benign and malignant pancreatic and biliary diseases. Cancer, 1988;66:2100–8.

Pais-Costa SR, Farah JF, Artigiani-Neto R, Franco MI, Martins SJ, Goldenberg A. Gallbladder adenocarcinoma: evaluation of the prognostic factors in 100 resectable cases in Brazil. ABCD = Brazilian archives of digestive surgery, 2012;50:13–19.

Park J, Lee KT, Jang TH, Seo YW, Lee KH, Lee JK, Jang KT, Heo JS, Choi SH, Choi DW, Rhee JC. Risk factors associated with the postoperative recurrence of intraductal papillary mucinous neoplasms of the pancreas. Pancreas, 2011;31:46–51.

Poruk KE, Gay DZ, Brown K, Mulvihill JD, Boucher KM, Scaife CL, Firpo MA, Mulvihill SJ. The clinical utility of CA 19–9 in pancreatic adenocarcinoma: diagnostic and prognostic updates. Current molecular medicine, 2013;1:340–51.

Reni M, Cereda S, Balzano G, Passoni P, Rognone A, Fugazza C, Mazza E, Zerbi A, Di Carlo V, Villa E. Carbohydrate antigen 19–9 change during chemotherapy for advanced pancreatic adenocarcinoma. Cancer, 2009;173:2630–9.

Saad ED, Machado MC, Wajsbrot D, Abramoff R, Hoff PM, Tabacof J, Katz A, Simon SD, Gansl RC. Pretreatment CA 19–9 level as a prognostic factor in patients with advanced pancreatic cancer treated with gemcitabine. International Journal of Gastrointestinal Cancer, 2002;25:35–41.

Safi F, Roscher R, Bittner R, Schenkluhn B, Dopfer HP, Beger HG. High sensitivity and specificity of CA 19–9 for pancreatic carcinoma in comparison to chronic pancreatitis. Serological and immunohistochemical findings. Pancreas, 1987;65:398–403.

Satake K, Takeuchi T, Homma T, Ozaki H. CA19-9 as a screening and diagnostic tool in symptomatic patients: the Japanese experience. Pancreas, 1994;7:703–6.

Siegel R, Naishadham D, Jemal A. Cancer statistics, 2013. A cancer Journal for clinicians, 2013;6:11–30.

Sinakos E, Saenger AK, Keach J, Kim WR, Lindor KD. Many patients with primary sclerosing cholangitis and increased serum levels of carbohydrate antigen 19–9 do not have cholangiocarcinoma. Clinical Gastroenterology and Hepatology, 2011;47:434–9.

Sugiura T, Uesaka K, Kanemoto H, Mizuno T, Sasaki K, Furukawa H, Matsunaga K, Maeda A. Serum CA19-9 is a significant predictor among preoperative parameters for early recurrence after resection of pancreatic adenocarcinoma. Journal of Gastrointestinal Surgery, 2012;135:977–85.

Tamakoshi K, Kikkawa F, Shibata K, Tomoda K, Obata NH, Wakahara F, Tokuhashi Y, Ishikawa H, Kawai M, Tomoda Y. Clinical value of CA125, CA19-9, CEA, CA72-4, and TPA in borderline ovarian tumor. Gynecologic Oncology, 1996;57:67–72.

Tempero MA, Uchida E, Takasaki H, Burnett DA, Steplewski Z, Pour PM. Relationship of carbohydrate antigen 19–9 and Lewis antigens in pancreatic cancer. Cancer research, 1987;256:5501–3.

Tsavaris N, Kosmas C, Papadoniou N, Kopterides P, Tsigritis K, Dokou A, Sarantonis J, Skopelitis H, Tzivras M, Gennatas K, Polyzos A, Papastratis G, Karatzas G, Papalambros A. CEA and CA-19.9 serum tumor markers as prognostic factors in patients with locally advanced (unresectable) or metastatic pancreatic adenocarcinoma: a retrospective analysis. Journal of Chemotherapy, 2009;139:673–80.

Ucar E, Semerci E, Ustun H, Yetim T, Huzmeli C, Gullu M. Prognostic value of preoperative CEA, CA 19–9, CA 72–4, and AFP levels in gastric cancer. Advances in therapy, 2008;38:1075–84.

Venkatesh PG, Navaneethan U, Shen B, McCullough AJ. Increased serum levels of carbohydrate antigen 19–9 and outcomes in primary sclerosing cholangitis patients without cholangiocarcinoma. Digestive diseases and sciences, 2013;46:850–7.

Wang Y, Li J, Xia Y, Gong R, Wang K, Yan Z, Wan X, Liu G, Wu D, Shi L, Lau W, Wu M, Shen F. Prognostic nomogram for intrahepatic cholangiocarcinoma after partial hepatectomy. Journal of Clinical Oncology, 2013;43:1188–95.

Waraya M, Yamashita K, Katagiri H, Ishii K, Takahashi Y, Furuta K, Watanabe M. Preoperative serum CA19-9 and dissected peripancreatic tissue margin as determiners of long-term survival in pancreatic cancer. Annals of Surgical Oncology, 2009;119:1231–40.

Willett CG, Daly WJ, Warshaw AL. CA 19–9 is an index of response to neoadjunctive chemoradiation therapy in pancreatic cancer. American Journal of Surgery, 1996;23:350–2.

Woo SM, Lee WJ, Han SS, Park SJ, Kim TH, Koh YH, Kim HB, Hong EK, Park JW, Kim CM. Capecitabine plus cisplatin as first-line chemotherapy for advanced biliary tract cancer: a retrospective single-center study. Chemotherapy, 2012;44:232–8.

Yoo T, Lee WJ, Woo SM, Kim TH, Han SS, Park SJ, Moon SH, Shin KH, Kim SS, Hong EK, Kim DY, Park JW. Pretreatment carbohydrate antigen 19–9 level indicates tumor response, early distant metastasis, overall survival, and therapeutic selection in localized and unresectable pancreatic cancer. International Journal of Radiation Oncology , biology, physics, 2011;181:623–30.

Yu H, Son GM, Joh YG. The clinical significance of preoperative serum levels of carbohydrate antigen 19–9 in colorectal cancer. Journal of Korean Surgical Society, 2013;52:231–7.

Zhang S, Wang YM, Sun CD, Lu Y, Wu LQ. Clinical value of serum CA19-9 levels in evaluating resectability of pancreatic carcinoma. World journal of Gastroenterology, 2008;64:3750–3.

Zhang D, Yu M, Xu T, Xiong B. Predictive Value of Serum CEA, CA19-9 and CA125 in Diagnosis of Colorectal Liver Metastasis in Chinese population. Hepato-gastroenterology, 2013;67:1297–301.

Ziske C, Schlie C, Gorschluter M, Glasmacher A, Mey U, Strehl J, Sauerbruch T, Schmidt-Wolf IG. Prognostic value of CA 19–9 levels in patients with inoperable adenocarcinoma of the pancreas treated with gemcitabine. British Journal of Cancer, 2003;29:1413–7.

PTTG (Securin) as Cancer Biomarker

9

Dimitrios N. Kanakis and Elmar Kirches

Contents

D.N. Kanakis (✉)
Department of Pathology, Medical Faculty, Democritus University of Thrace, Alexandroupolis, Greece
e-mail: aristoteles_stageira@yahoo.com; dkanakis@med.duth.gr

E. Kirches
Department of Neuropathology, Medical Faculty, Otto-von-Guericke University, Magdeburg, Germany
e-mail: elmar.kirches@med.ovgu.de

V.R. Preedy, V.B. Patel (eds.), *Biomarkers in Cancer, Biomarkers in Disease: Methods, Discoveries and Applications*,
DOI 10.1007/978-94-007-7681-4_19

Abstract

Pituitary tumor transforming gene (PTTG) has originally been discovered as a gene differentially expressed between rat pituitary tumor cells and normal rat pituitary tissue. It was rapidly recognized that PTTG mRNA and protein are much more abundant in various human tumor types as compared to the corresponding non-tumor tissue. The mammalian PTTG protein was found to be a securin, required for correct sister-chromatid separation and equal distribution of mitotic chromosomes to the daughter cells. Increased levels of the protein in tumor cells result in aneuploidy and DNA instability. The potential of PTTG to initiate and support tumor development was demonstrated in xenograft models. Transgenic mice finally proved a weak oncogenic potential of the gene. PTTG exhibits a vast impact on the transcriptome of tumor cells due to its ability to bind to general transcription factors, such as SP1, and to p53, which is of major importance for cell cycle regulation and apoptosis. Among the PTTG-regulated genes are some which are associated with tumor cell migration and invasion, corresponding to the metastasis-enhancing function of PTTG observed in xenograft models. In several human tumor types, high mRNA and protein levels of PTTG have been associated with increased proliferation index, with increased risk of metastases, and – most important – with lower overall survival. Due to the similarity of results among several clinical studies, including various types of solid tumors, it can be stated that PTTG is a valuable prognostic marker in aggressive human tumor diseases.

List of Abbreviations

ACTH	AdrenoCorticoTropic Hormone
ADH	AntiDiuretic Hormone
AFP	Alpha(α)-FetoProtein
bFGF	basic Fibroblast Growth Factor
ca.	"circa" (Latin) = approximately (English)
CAB	Combined Androgen Blockade
ccRCC	clear cell Renal Cell Carcinoma
cDNA	complimentary DNA
DNA	DeoxyriboNucleic Acid
e.g.	"exempli gratia" (Latin) = for example (English)
ECM	ExtraCellular Matrix
EGFP	Enhanced Green Fluorescent Protein
EGFR	Epidermal Growth Factor Receptor
EMT	Epithelial to Mesenchymal Transition
ESCC	Esophageal Squamous Cell Carcinoma
FAK	Focal Adhesion Kinase
FSH	Follicle-Stimulating Hormone
g	Gram
GAPDH	GlycerAldehyde-3-Phosphate DeHydrogenase
GBM	GlioBlastoma (Multiforme)

GH	Growth Hormone
HNSCC	Head and Neck Squamous Cell Carcinoma
HPF	High-Power Field
hPTTG	human PTTG
HR	High Risk
I	Iodine
i.e.	"id est" (Latin) = that is (English)
IDH1	Isocitrate DeHydrogenase 1
IHC	ImmunoHistoChemistry
LH	Luteinizing Hormone
M	Metastasis
MGMT	MethylGuanine-DNA MethylTransferase
MI	Mitotic Index
MMP	Matrix MetalloProteinase
mRNA	messenger RNA
MSH	Melanocyte-Stimulating Hormone
N	*(Lymph)*Node
NIS	Sodium-Iodide Symporter
NSCLC	Non-Small Cell Lung Carcinoma
p*(T,N,M)*	pathological*(T,N,M)*
PCNA	Proliferating Cell Nuclear Antigen
PCR	Polymerase Chain Reaction
PRL	Prolactin
pTNM	pathological Tumor-Node-Metastasis
PTTG	Pituitary Tumor Transforming Gene
p-*value*	probability-*value*
Rb	Retinoblastoma
RNA	RiboNucleic Acid
RT-PCR	Reverse Transcription-PCR
r-*value*	correlation coefficient
SCLC	Small Cell Lung Carcinoma
shRNA	short hairpin RNA
siRNA	short interfering RNA
SOP	Standard Operating Protocols
STAT	Signal Transducer and Activation of Transcription
STH	SomatoTropic Hormone
T	Tumor
TGF	Tumor Growth Factor
TIMP	Tissue Inhibitor of MetalloProtease
TSH	Thyroid-Stimulating Hormone
V	Vein
VEGF	Vascular Endothelial Growth Factor
WHO	World Health Organization
β-Gal	β-Galactosidase

Key Facts of Pituitary Gland

- Pituitary gland (hypophysis) is a bean-shaped organ, weighing ca. 0.6–0.8 g, which is situated within a bone-cavity – resembling a Turkish saddle (sella turcica) – located on the basis of the cranium.
- Pituitary gland is divided both from an anatomical and functional point of view mainly in two different parts, the anterior lobe (known as adenohypophysis) and the posterior lobe (known as neurohypophysis), whereas a rudimentary (in humans) intermediate lobe is located between them.
- Adenohypophysis produces and secretes a variety of hormones (i.e., Adreno-CorticoTropic Hormone [ACTH], Thyroid-Stimulating Hormone [TSH], Luteinizing Hormone [LH], Follicle-Stimulating Hormone [FSH], Growth Hormone [GH] or SomatoTropic Hormone [STH], and Prolactin [PRL]), regulating in this way the function of specific "target" organs.
- Neurohypophysis stores a couple of so-called neurohypophyseal hormones (namely, Oxytocin and AntiDiuretic Hormone [ADH] or Vasopressin), which are then released by the gland in the blood according to the needs of the organism.
- The intermediate lobe secretes Melanocyte-Stimulating Hormone (MSH) which – as the name implies – acts on the melanocytes of the skin.
- Pituitary gland stays in direct communication with the hypothalamus (an important structure lying above the gland and belonging to diencephalon ["interbrain"]). The latter both controls – through releasing and inhibiting hormones – the secretion of the hormones of adenohypophysis and also produces the neurohypophyseal hormones that reach the neurohypophysis via axonal transport.
- Due to the role of hypophysis as a regulator of the other hormone-producing organs, it is obvious that diseases (mainly benign tumors, so-called adenomas) affecting the gland can result either in excess or scarcity of certain hormones, leading subsequently to diverse endocrinologic conditions (e.g., Cushing's disease, acromegaly or gigantism, hypothyroidism, galactorrhea, amenorrhea, infertility and hypogonadism).

Definitions of Words and Terms

Aneuploidy Abnormality characterized by irregular number of chromosomes. Some chromosomes are represented by a higher or lower number of copies as compared to the normal somatic tissues of the species.

Apoptosis Known also as "programmed cell death", describes a process in which the cell uses its own cellular apparatus to commit suicide and thus a stable number of cells are retained or such cells are eliminated which threatens the survival of the organism.

Biomarker A molecule that is either present or absent or varies in abundance in a particular cell type/tissue and due to this fact may contribute either to the diagnosis of a disease or even to the estimation of therapeutic outcome.

Gene Knockdown Reduction of the expression level of a gene achieved either through manipulation of the genomic DNA or through the use of small RNA molecules, which interfere with gene expression, because they are complementary to critical sequence motifs of the messenger RNA.

Gene Promoter A region in the DNA sequence of a gene, in which RNA polymerase binds and initiates transcription.

Gene Silencing A mechanism used by the cell in order to inactivate a particular gene either at the transcriptional or translational level.

Oncogene A gene that is normally found in the cell (as a proto-oncogene) and which is responsible for the accomplishment of a particular cellular function. Various causes, such as increase in copy number or enhanced transcription, can lead this gene to acquire tumorigenic potential and thus transform normal cells into cancerous ones.

Predictive Factor A clinical or biological indicator that gives valuable information related to the likely benefit for the patient from a particular treatment.

Prognostic Factor A clinical or biological indicator that is used in order to estimate the progress and outcome of a disease in yet untreated individuals.

Pseudogene A region of genomic DNA that possesses sequence similarity to a functional gene, but cannot be translated into a functional protein, e.g., due to mutations.

RNA Interference (RNAi) Synonymous with Post-Transcriptional Gene Silencing (PTGS), describes a complex intracellular process carried out by highly specific double-stranded RNAs (dsRNAs) of about 20 nucleotides, which bind to messenger RNAs (mRNAs) with matching sequences, causing subsequently mRNA degradation.

Senescence Originates from the Latin word "senex" meaning "old age" or "old man" and is referred also as "biological aging". This yet not decoded process is recognized via certain features regarding individual cells ("cellular senescence") or the entire organism ("organismal senescence").

Transgenic Animal An animal that carries a foreign gene (incorporated through specific laboratory methods) in its own genome.

Tumor Suppressor Gene A gene that normally prevents the unrestrained cellular proliferation and thereby the development of cancer. However, when this gene is lost, mutated, or silenced, it loses its physiological function, which contributes together with other genetic changes to the formation of tumors.

Xenograft Model An experimental in vivo procedure by which tissue or cells of a species are transplanted to an immunocompromised animal (mostly mouse), in order to investigate the potential of the transplants to create tumors.

Introduction

In recent years, the pituitary tumor transforming gene (PTTG) has progressively gained interest as a potential prognostic marker in cancer. In the present chapter we aim to shortly introduce the discovery of the gene and the molecular functions of the encoded protein securin and to depict its role in biological processes relevant to cancer progression. In the second half of the chapter, we critically review the potential value of PTTG/securin as a determinant of clinical behavior and final outcome of tumor diseases.

Discovery of the Pituitary Tumor Transforming Gene

All basic discoveries regarding structure and expression of vertebrate PTTG and its oncogenic potential have already been published in the late 1990s. Much of this early work has been performed by Shlomo Melmed and colleagues at the Cedars-Sinai Research Institute (Los Angeles, USA).

The gene was initially discovered during a screening for small RNA fragments, which were differentially expressed between rat pituitary adenoma cells and normal pituitary tissue (Pei and Melmed 1997). A fragment selectively expressed in the tumor cells was used to isolate a complete cDNA from a rat pituitary adenoma cDNA library. The corresponding mRNA was confirmed to be highly expressed in the tumor tissue. In the same report the authors already demonstrated the oncogenic potential of the gene, because transfected mouse NIH3T3 fibroblasts were able to induce tumors when xenografted to immunodeficient mice. Having thus identified a new oncogene in rat pituitary tumors, the authors coined the term "pituitary tumor transforming gene". Only 2 years later, Melmed and colleagues reported the identification and chromosomal localization of a homologue human gene (Zhang et al. 1999a), later termed hPTTG-1, which was expressed more abundantly in pituitary adenoma tissues and carcinoma cells than normal human tissues (Zhang et al. 1999a, b; Saez et al. 1999), and was able to transform mouse fibroblasts into tumor initiating cells, just as it had been observed for its rat counterpart (Zhang et al. 1999a). Although PTTG-1 overexpression in various human cancers is meanwhile well established, the reason for this is not well understood until now. While a binding site for the general transcription factor SP1 in the PTTG-1 promoter had been recognized early (Pei 1998), it was only recently that the group of Shlomo Melmed demonstrated a role of PTTG as a functional downstream element of the transcription factor STAT 3 (Zhou et al. 2013), which itself possesses transforming properties. In parallel to the identification of hPTTG-1, a second member of the gene family (hPTTG-2) was described (Prezant et al. 1999), although it did not contribute much to the increased pool of PTTG mRNA in tumors. The gene hPTTG-2 is expressed at a low level in tumor cell lines and tissues (Prezant et al. 1999; Chen et al. 2000). Transcripts of a third homologue gene (hPTTG-3) were undetectable in human tissues at the level of Northern blots, suggesting that this locus may even represent a functionally inactive "pseudogene"

(Marques et al. 2005). In the following, we will thus use the designation PTTG instead of hPTTG-1, as it is done in most of the existing literature.

A first clue regarding the normal function of the PTTG-encoded protein in vertebrates came by the demonstration that the human gene product is identical with human securin, i.e., an inhibitor of sister-chromatid separation, which is required for the proper control of this process and insures genomic stability (Zou et al. 1999). While this finding suggested a relation of the oncogenic function of PTTG to chromosomal gains and losses, which are often observed in high-grade tumors, it was later shown that the protein clearly participates in transcriptional regulation of some tumor-relevant downstream genes. The earliest example was the induction of the well-known oncogene c-myc by binding of PTTG to its promoter (Pei 2001), suggesting that upregulation of c-myc participates in the oncogenic potential of increased securin levels. Later, the securin-mediated regulation of p21, the direct executor of the tumor suppressive functions of p53, was established as another possible route (Bernal et al. 2002; see section "Role as a Broad Regulator of the Transcriptome").

PTTG in Cancer

PTTG Is an Oncogene

Following the above mentioned early proof of the tumorigenic transformation of mouse fibroblasts by PTTG, the oncogenic potential of the gene in human cells was further confirmed by successful tumor induction in nude mice using xenografts of PTTG-transfected human embryonic kidney cells (Hamid et al. 2005). However, like most xenograft models, all these mouse models suffered from the disadvantage of non-orthotopic tumor growth under the skin of mice, following artificial inoculation with an initially high number of transfected cells. It was therefore meaningful that the group of Shlomo Melmed and other authors undertook huge efforts to construct serious genetic models to elucidate the role of PTTG in tumor development both inside and outside the pituitary gland.

It could be demonstrated that a targeted expression of the gene, i.e., under the control of a pituitary-specific promoter, led to focal pituitary hyperplasia, although no tumors were induced. However, if targeted overexpression of PTTG was achieved in mice with a heterozygous knockout of the well-known tumor suppressor Rb (retinoblastoma gene), a much higher frequency of tumors occurred in the anterior lobe of the pituitary, as compared to mice exhibiting solely the heterozygous loss of Rb (Donangelo et al. 2006). At this point there may have remained doubt regarding the true potential of PTTG in initiating tumors in mice, since a "partner gene" was required to lead from hyperplasia to tumor disease. While the contribution of both partners remained unclear, a dominating role of Rb may have been suggested, due to its apparently important role in cell cycle regulation and tumor development (Poznic 2009; Di Fiore et al. 2013). Recently, it could be clearly demonstrated that a more widespread

PTTG overexpression in several mouse tissues including lung, liver, kidney, spleen, and the female genitals indeed led to precancerous lesions and cancer, although the lesions were restricted to the female genital tract, indicating a limited ability of PTTG to induce cancer without the help of a "partner gene" (Fong et al. 2012). Histologically confirmed cancer occurred in a relatively small percentage of animals, i.e., 13–20 % depending on their age (Fong et al. 2012). At least since that publication there can be no doubt that PTTG acts as a true, though weak oncogene in mice. The observed overexpression of the gene in several human cancers is thus more likely to participate at some stage in tumor development than just to be a secondary event.

Basic Molecular PTTG Functions in Cancer not Restricted to Pituitary Adenomas

Role in Genetic Instability

Due to its early detected function as a securin, a role of PTTG overexpression in disturbed chromosomal segregation and aneuploidy in cancer cells could be suggested. In an approach to measure the cellular PTTG distribution, the time course of its degradation, and the cellular consequences in detail, the group of Shlomo Melmed used enforced overexpression of PTTG fused to enhanced green fluorescent protein (EGFP) in cancer cells lacking endogenous expression of the protein (Yu et al. 2003). A direct link could be demonstrated between the degree of expression of the transgene and the cytologic consequences visible by fluorescent microsopy. The transfected PTTG protein did not only co-localize with the mitotic spindle apparatus but was also visible and evenly distributed along the whole chromosomes. PTTG-EGFP, but not EGFP alone, was able to slow down and eventually block progression to the anaphase. If PTTG was expressed at sufficient levels, it could no longer be completely degraded prior to the onset of anaphase, thus disturbing or eventually blocking completely chromosomal segregation leading to severe aneuploidy. A clear quantitative correlation could be seen, since intermediate PTTG levels preferentially led to incomplete chromosomal segregation producing several micronuclei, while high levels resulted in a distribution of all chromosomes to only one daughter cell (macronucleus) while committing the second to cell death. Applying an undegradable mutant PTTG, the authors confirmed that indeed PTTG has to be tightly regulated in cells in order to allow a correct chromosomal segregation. Overexpression, as seen in many cancer cell types, will thus inhibit the ability of the cells to sufficiently control the amount of this securin, which in turn favors gross genomic instability (Fig. 1). These imbalances may include enhanced copy numbers of oncogenes or loss of tumor suppressor genes, thus playing a role in the generation of more malignant subsets of tumor cells.

However, PTTG induces genetic instability not only at the level of chromosomes but also at the level of short DNA stretches, as verified by a PCR-based approach (Kim et al. 2005). This pointed to a second mechanism, such as

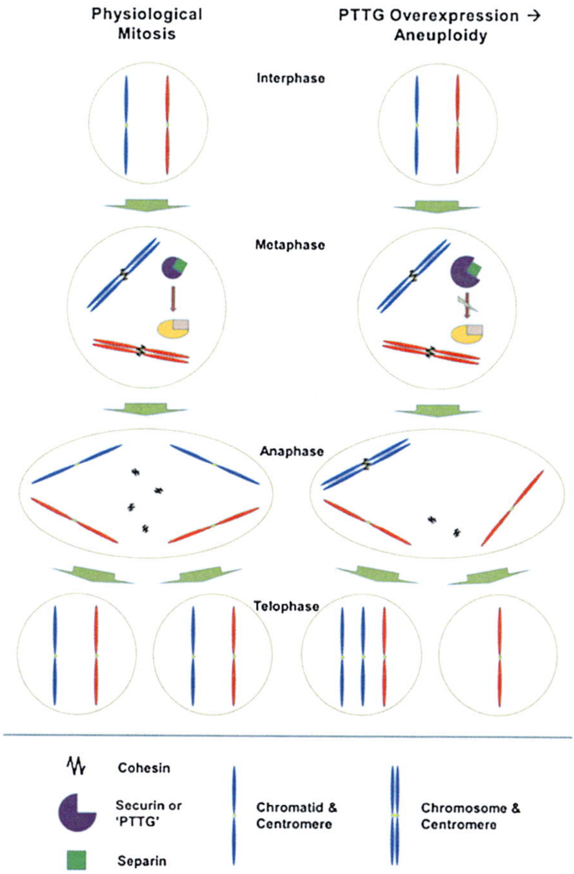

Fig. 1 Physiological and pathological function of PTTG. The *left side* of the scheme (Modified according to Yu et al. 2003) shows the physiological mitotic process, during which securin (PTTG) builds a complex with separin and as a result prevents the degradation of cohesins (hold sister chromatids bound) by the latter. At the end of metaphase, securin is degraded and in this way allows separin to act on cohesins causing their degradation and the subsequent release of chromatids which thus remain unbound and move in equal numbers to the newly formed daughter cells. The *right side* of scheme presents the impact of securin (PTTG) overexpression in the development of aneuploidy. Overexpressed PTTG retains separin tightly bound to itself, inhibiting in this manner the chromatids from being equally distributed in the daughter cells

disturbed DNA repair. In a first attempt to quantify this short distance genetic instability in human thyroid cancer tissues, the authors detected a high correlation between a PCR-defined instability index and mRNA levels of PTTG ($r = 0.8$, $p \leq 0.01$). These merely correlative results could be underpinned by transfection of thyroid cells with PTTG, showing a dramatic increase of the instability index. Later, a similar influence of the PTTG expression level on DNA instability was observed in colorectal cancer and PTTG transfection of colorectal cancer cells and human fibroblasts indeed resulted in an increase of the instability index (Kim et al. 2007). It could be shown that PTTG transfection reduced the activity of the etoposide-induced repair machinery for double-stranded DNA damage, which provided a possible explanation for the observed instability. High PTTG expression in tumors thus contributes to genetic instability on the level of DNA damage, which is invisible in cytologic/histologic stains. It may cause functional damage to many cellular proteins and gene promoters, thus having a broad impact in tumor biology.

Role as a Broad Regulator of the Transcriptome

While the above-cited changes may be mainly stochastic and do not lead to the understanding of molecular details participating in tumor development, more specific insights came from the growing evidence that PTTG acts as a transcriptional regulator of a broad panel of target genes, some of which are well-known to regulate basic cellular features, such as cell cycle and apoptosis, and to be important oncogenes or tumor suppressor genes.

The first proof that PTTG acts as a transcriptional regulator has come from the abovementioned role for c-myc induction, where PTTG is part of a promoter-binding protein complex (Pei 2001). Shortly thereafter, PTTG was shown to interact physically with the important tumor suppressor protein p53 (Bernal et al. 2002), which is well-known to be a key regulator of cell cycle progression and apoptosis and to have transactivating properties, exerting many of its functions via transcriptional regulation of the protein p21. The finding of functional complexes between p53 and PTTG was originally observed during phage-display screening and verified by co-immunoprecipitation. It pointed already strongly to a role of PTTG as a transcriptional regulator, which may be important in many tumor entities, not just in pituitary adenomas. Gel shift assays, which detect the ability of p53 to bind to a radioactive p53 motif of human DNA, revealed that this DNA-binding property is inhibited by PTTG in breast cancer. Accordingly, the promoter activity of all three tested p53-dependent target genes, involved in cell cycle progression and apoptosis, was decreased by PTTG (Bernal et al. 2002). Among those genes was p21, the most important executer of p53-dependent cell cycle regulation. Following transcriptional activation by p53, it suppresses cell cycle progression by inducing G_1 arrest. Inhibition of this process by PTTG thus stimulates tumor cell proliferation. The second target gene tested was BAX, which codes for a positive modulator of the mitochondrial apoptotic pathway, suggesting that high PTTG levels favor apoptotic resistance of tumor cells. The third gene, SFN, encoded an inhibitor of G_2–M transition, thus also supporting a pro-proliferative function of high PTTG levels.

A more generalized insight into the role of PTTG for the cancer cell transcriptome has come from a study, which did not use a screening for potential PTTG-binding proteins (phage display) as a starting point, but rather performed a search for PTTG-regulated gene promoters (Tong et al. 2007). This type of investigation suggested that PTTG binds (directly or indirectly) to more than 700 hundred promoters. As compared to the control group, PTTG interacting promoters were strongly enriched for sequences containing a binding motif for the general transcription factor SP1, suggesting a broad influence of PTTG in the transcriptome by forming complexes with SP1. A formation of such complexes in tumor cells could indeed be verified by co-immunoprecipitation of both proteins (Tong et al. 2007). Gel shift assays verified that PTTG can build a complex with SP1 bound to the corresponding SP1 consensus sequence in the DNA. Since the cell cycle regulator cyclin D3 had been found to be overrepresented in the original screening for PTTG-interacting promoters, the authors verified binding of PTTG-SP1 complexes to the cyclin D3 promoter. This goal was achieved by PCR amplification of the promoter sequence from immunoprecipitates of the protein complex (chip analysis). Upregulation of this cyclin is thus among the thinkable mechanisms, which may participate, independent from a loss of p53/p21-mediated inhibitory pathways, in a stimulation of cancer cell proliferation via PTTG.

Motility, Invasion, and Metastasis

In recent years, it has been shown that PTTG not only influences proliferation and survival of tumor cells and neovascularization but also regulates the migratory properties of tumor cells and its ability to remodel the extracellular matrix (ECM), thereby facilitating the spread of metastases. It seems that a switch of the epithelial character of the cells towards a mesenchymal character, the so-called epithelial to mesenchymal transition, (EMT) plays a significant role in this change (see section "Epidermal to Mesenchymal Transition").

In esophageal squamous cell carcinomas (ESCC), lymph node metastasis and poorer survival have been found to be significantly associated with PTTG overexpression (Fig. 2), leading the authors to investigate the influence of this oncogene on migration and metastasis in vitro and in a mouse model (Ito et al. 2008). PTTG knockdown by siRNA suppressed the migration of ESCC cell lines through pore membranes and the invasion into matrigel-covered membranes in transwell assays. Moreover, injection of siRNA-transfected cells into the foot-pads of nude mice and weekly repeated siRNA injections into the growing tumors to maintain PTTG suppression over 3 weeks resulted in a decrease of lymph node metastases, as revealed by histology. Gene expression arrays and data confirmation

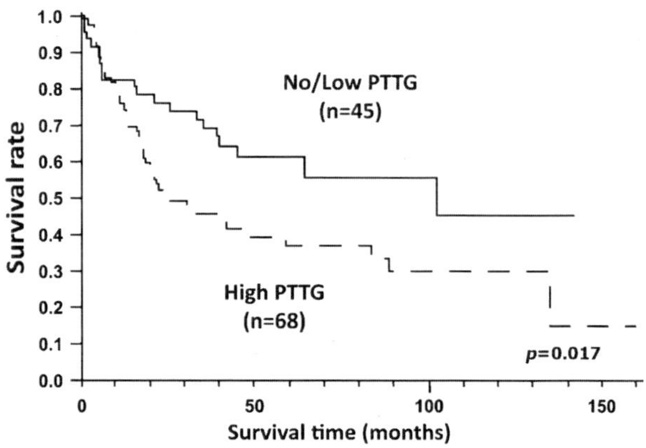

Fig. 2 **PTTG levels in contrariwise association with patients' survival in ESCC.** Kaplan-Meier curves demonstrating a significant difference ($p = 0.017$) in the survival rate of patients suffering from esophageal squamous cell carcinoma (ESCC) when comparing cases ($n = 45$) with no or low (+) PTTG expression in immunohistochemistry to those ($n = 68$) with a high one (++ or +++) (Modified according to Ito et al. 2008). The impact of PTTG on patient's survival was recently confirmed by an independent study (Zhang et al. 2013)

by quantitative real-time PCR revealed that several migration-associated genes were regulated by the siRNA (Ito et al. 2008). Correspondingly, transfection of an ESCC cell line with PTTG led to enhanced migration in transwell assays and to an increase of lymph node metastases, when tumor cells were injected into the tail vein of nude mice (Yan et al. 2009). PTTG transfection was shown to induce several genes associated with cell motility and ECM remodeling and invasion, such as S100A4 and galectin-1, while it suppressed the secretion of TIMP-1 and TIMP-2, two tissue inhibitors of matrix metalloproteinases (MMP) involved in ECM remodeling. The secretion of MMP-2 was enhanced by PTTG. Taken together, these results strongly supported a significant role of PTTG to enhance the migratory and invasive properties of carcinoma cells, although the precise molecular mechanisms are certainly still debatable.

Epidermal to Mesenchymal Transition

EMT has been implicated as a starting point in the progression of cancer to a metastatic state, because it generates a cell type of higher migratory and invasive ability within the tumor. EMT is characterized by the loss of epithelial markers, E-cadherin being lost early, and gain of mesenchymal markers, such as N-cadherin and vimentin. Moreover, the upregulation of some transcriptional repressors of E-cadherin, such as Snail, Slug, and Twist, is implicated in EMT (Zheng and Kang 2013; De Craene and Berx 2013). In the last few years, some evidence has accumulated on the one hand that PTTG induces EMT and on the other hand that this process plays a role for migratory activation of tumor cells.

Stable transfection of an ovarian epithelial tumor cell line with PTTG cDNA led to downregulation of E-cadherin and upregulation of Snail, Slug, and Twist and of TGF-β, a growth factor stimulating EMT (Shah and Kakar 2011), while transfection with an appropriate PTTG siRNA resulted in the opposite effect. A similar dependency of both marker sets on manipulated PTTG levels was observed in a cell line, derived from normal breast epithelium, and in two breast cancer cell lines (Yoon et al. 2012), which indicated that the oncogene may induce EMT in several types of normal or neoplastic epithelial cells. The PTTG-induced change of the marker sets in breast epithelial cells was paralleled by the expected enhancement of migratory properties (in vitro), although this did not clearly prove a consecutive chain of events leading from PTTG overexpression via EMT to a migratory stimulus.

While still hypothetical in large parts, Shah and colleagues recently provided an idea of how PTTG may induce EMT and cell migration, which was based on detailed molecular data obtained in lung cancer cell lines (Shah et al. 2012). In the focus of their model are integrins and the integrin-dependent focal adhesion kinase (FAK), which is needed to constitute the focal adhesion complex, required for remodeling of the actin cytoskeleton as a prerequisite of actively migrating cells. PTTG was shown to upregulate α_V and β_3 integrins on the mRNA level and the increase of the corresponding heterodimer in the plasma membrane was confirmed by fluorescence-activated cell sorting and immunostaining of the lung cancer cells. The expression and phosphorylation of FAK and the expression of other components of the focal adhesion complex were upregulated by PTTG. Treatment with α_V siRNA inhibited the migratory ability of lung cancer cells in a wound healing assay in vitro. At the same time PTTG led to a reorganization of the actin cytoskeleton compatible with EMT. The most important output from that study was the impact of PTTG on integrins and the focal adhesion complex, which are well known to play a major role in cell migration. On the other hand, it seems less clear at what point EMT is involved in PTTG-mediated migratory stimulation.

Taken together, PTTG is statistically associated with metastases in some tumor diseases and is likely to play an important role in tumor cell migration and invasion, while the impact of EMT in this setting requires further elucidation. Despite the lack of a precise knowledge, which ones of many thinkable molecular mechanisms are most important to link PTTG with tumor growth and metastases in vivo, clinical studies clearly revealed the oncogene as a prognostic marker in several cancers. This will be shown in the following sections.

Clinical Impact of PTTG

In the last years, special attention has been given in identifying new biomarkers, which could be used for either prognosis or prediction of various diseases. This target of research is more obvious and intensive in oncology than in any other field of medicine. As a consequence, a plethora of cancer biomarkers have been proposed recently, but their significance needs to be further elucidated. In this context the present effort aims to demonstrate, in the next two main subheadings both the prognostic and the predictive value of the above-described oncogene PTTG (mammalian securin), and to denote shortly its potential therapeutic applications, which began to become visible recently.

PTTG as a Prognostic Marker

The abundance of PTTG in various tumors raised the question whether this gene could be used in foreseeing the progression and the clinical outcome of a certain neoplastic condition. For this reason, several studies have been performed until now, and their results will be discussed in detail in the next paragraphs.

As it is fact with several other genes under investigation, concerning their role as cancer biomarkers, PTTG has also been primarily examined in tumors with a more aggressive biological behavior. This makes sense, since the aggressiveness of a tumor is widely accepted to present a reliable factor that correlates mostly with the prognosis of the disease. Aggressiveness is consecutively estimated in the first line by the use of various pathological and also – even though to a lesser extent – by some clinical parameters, according to well-established classifications and protocols.

Consequently, the cyto- and histopathological features which have been proved to be of particular importance in the evaluation of cancer's aggressiveness in the majority of organs are comprehensively described in the WHO (World Health Organization) classification of tumors and the pTNM (Tumor-Node-Metastasis) taxonomy. However, pTNM staging can neither be applied in tumors of the nervous system nor in hematological malignancies because of their unique morphology, though some of the basic criteria related to tumor's aggressiveness are included in the WHO grading of these neoplasms. According mainly to the WHO and pTNM criteria, the pathologist estimates in daily praxis a concrete number of cyto- and histopathological features as markers of tumor's aggressiveness and applies them as important prognosticators for disease's outcome and predictors of patient's survival. A synopsis of these factors could be as follows: (a) cellular and (b) vascular proliferation, (c) cellular dedifferentiation, (d) mitotic count (mitotic index – MI), (e) tumor necrosis/hemorrhage, and (f) cell's invasion/migration ability. As far as the last one is concerned, this comprises the potential of tumor cells to migrate and infiltrate the surrounding nonneoplastic tissue, their efficacy to enter the blood and lymphatic vessels, and also their capacity to produce metastases both in the regional and distant lymph nodes as well as in other organs.

The abovementioned factors have been investigated either alone or in combination in a variety of tumor diseases and were correlated with the expression levels (mRNA and/or protein) of PTTG and together with the latter with patient's survival. Due to the fact that some of these cyto- and histopathological characteristics represented preferable and constant prognostic factors in the majority of studies performed (in contrast to the clinical parameters that were partly dependent on the organ under investigation), the analysis and interpretation of the role of PTTG can be structured according to the issues cellular proliferation, vascular proliferation, and migration.

Cellular Proliferation

Under cellular proliferation is implied the ability of the cell to multiply and thus increase the number of its descendants in a particular tissue. Since a tumor represents an uncontrolled cell proliferation, which in turn is strictly associated with tumor development and growth, it is self-evident that a cancer biomarker should be capable of estimating the proliferative potential of a particular tumor. So far, only two markers, namely, Ki-67 and PCNA, have been proved to accomplish this criterion and have been established as confident in predicting the rate of a tumor growth.

In order to identify whether PTTG could also be used as a marker of cell proliferation or of advanced tumor stages, known to be characterized by enhanced cellularity and mitotic index, a couple of studies have been performed. In such a study carried out by Genkai et al. (2006), the expression level of PTTG protein was examined in three different grades of astrocytomas, namely, diffuse astrocytoma (WHO grade II), anaplastic astrocytoma (WHO grade III), and glioblastoma (WHO grade IV) by immunohistochemistry. Immunostaining for PTTG differed among these glioma subtypes, with increased staining in tumors of higher grade, i.e., higher mitotic index. In addition, a significant dependency of patient's overall survival from a PTTG immunostaining score was observed for glioblastomas, if patients were classified into two groups according to high or low PTTG score. Log-rank tests revealed a clearly longer survival of glioblastoma patients with low PTTG expression ($p \leq 0.05$). The protein may thus provide a basis for a further prognostic refinement within this group of highly malignant gliomas, which possesses a well-known potential for an extremely rapid proliferation of residual cells after resection. The result of log-rank tests remained significant, if the two most malignant stages of astrocytic tumor disease, i.e., anaplastic astrocytoma and glioblastoma, were pooled ($p \leq 0.01$) or if all gliomas were pooled ($p \leq 0.01$), while PTTG played no role for survival times in the slowly growing diffuse astrocytomas with a generally better prognosis. The immunohistochemical score used for this study had been calculated from a relative score of staining intensity, delivered by case-blinded observers, and the percentage of stained areas of the histologic slices. Similar results were obtained by Wondergem et al. (2012), who evaluated PTTG mRNA and protein levels in clear cell renal cell carcinomas (ccRCC). The examination showed a substantially increased amount of PTTG (mRNA and protein) in high-grade ccRCC (Fuhrman grades III/IV) as compared to low-grade tumors (Fuhrman grades I/II). Elevated PTTG mRNA expression was again inversely associated with patient's postoperative survival ($p \leq 0.01$) (Fig. 3). In ccRCC the enhanced expression of PTTG may be partly explained by the frequent amplification of chromosome arm 5q, which harbors this gene. In 29 patients of a large cohort with treated prolactin-secreting pituitary adenoma, Raverot and colleagues (2010) performed an analysis of several genes aiming to recognize possible candidates associated with pathological grade and disease progression. Although mRNA quantification by real-time PCR suggested that PTTG was upregulated remarkably in the most aggressive tumors (referred as aggressive-invasive), the result did not reach statistical significance on the basis of the small number of aggressive-invasive tumors in the cohort available for

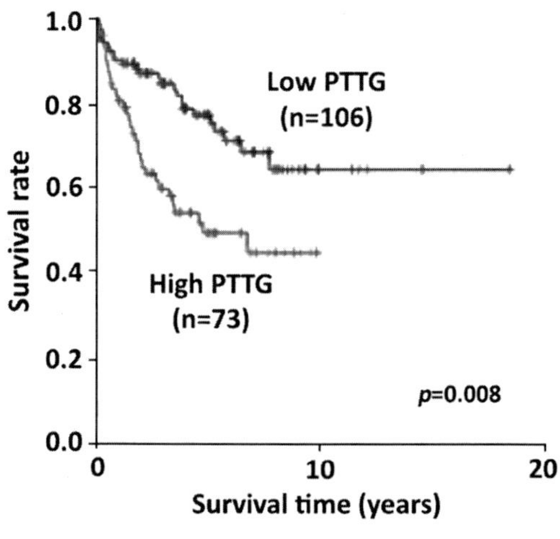

Fig. 3 PTTG expression inversely correlated with patients' survival in ccRCC. Kaplan-Meier curves showing PTTG mRNA expression being substantially, though inversely, associated ($p = 0.008$) with patient's survival in clear cell renal cell carcinoma (ccRCC) (Modified according to Wondergem et al. 2012)

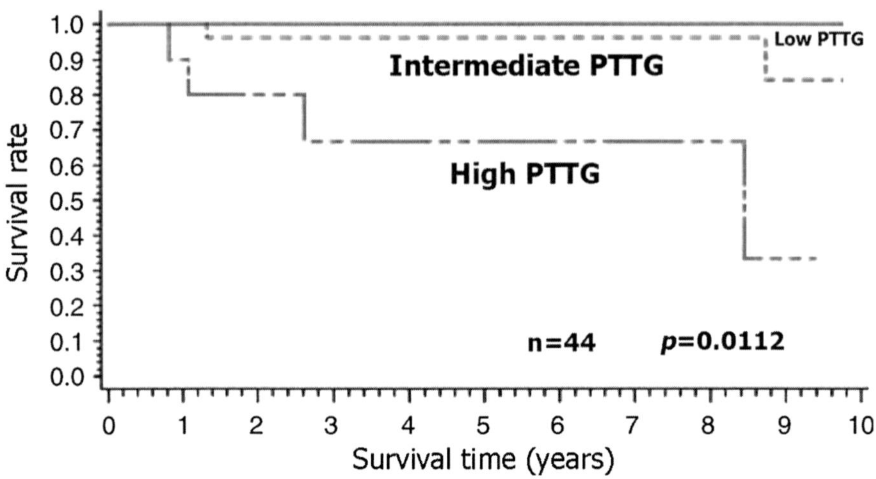

Fig. 4 The amount of PTTG as indicator (prognosticator) of survival in patients with breast cancer. Kaplan-Meier curves indicating a noteworthy association ($p = 0.0112$) concerning the amount of PTTG protein and the survival rate of patients suffering from breast cancer. When these cases were examined by immunohistochemistry for PTTG, three groups were built according to cutoff points of 10 % and 20 % immunopositive cells, namely, cases with low PTTG (<10 % positive cells), intermediate PTTG (>10 % and <20 % positive cells), and high PTTG (>20 % positive cells). The higher the PTTG immunoreactivity, the lower the survival rate of the patient, and vice versa (Modified according to Talvinen et al. 2008)

molecular analysis. However, PTTG was found to be significantly associated with the tumor recurrence ($p \leq 0.05$).

It is noteworthy to mention that, when PTTG was examined in breast cancer in parallel to the proliferative marker Ki-67 and to the number of mitoses, the former exhibited sometimes a better prognostic value in Cox regression analysis than the latter (Talvinen et al. 2008). By comparing PTTG and Ki-67, Talvinen and colleagues (2008) found the highest outcome advantage to be related to low PTTG immune expression, if tumors were grouped according to a content of more than 20 % or less than 10 % PTTG-positive cells (HR 7.1, $p \leq 0.05$). Only PTTG reached a prognostic value in Kaplan-Meier survival curves ($p \leq 0.05$) (Fig. 4). As a conclusion of the above mentioned, it could be suggested that PTTG possesses even a better potency than Ki-67 in predicting disease's outcome and patient's survival. In contrast to this suggested superiority of PTTG over Ki-67, another report performed in pituitary adenomas presented Ki-67 as the most reliable marker in estimating the recurrence potential of these tumors. Nevertheless, even in this study a good positive correlation existed between PTTG and Ki-67 ($r = 0.85, p \leq 0.001$) and higher PTTG expression was significantly associated with postsurgical recurrence of adenomas ($p \leq 0.01$), justifying once again its role as a disease prognosticator (Filippella et al. 2006). Recently, Jia et al. (2013) quantified both PTTG and PCNA mRNA in pituitary adenomas and confirmed a highly significant positive correlation between these two factors, but also their higher abundance in the invasive versus noninvasive tumors.

Vascular Proliferation

The formation of new blood vessels (angiogenesis) is closely related to the tumor's anaplastic behavior. Without a doubt, the needs of a neoplasm both in nutrients and oxygen supply, as it progresses to a larger tumor volume and a more rapidly growing, aggressive phenotype, become exponentially larger. Therefore, an extensive vascular network is required, which is actually achieved by the formation of new vessels. This process is guided by known angiogenic factors, vascular endothelial growth factor (VEGF), and basic fibroblast growth factor (bFGF) being two of the well-known proteins guiding angiogenesis. The importance of PTTG's possible connection with these markers is obvious in a number of studies that have been carried out till now, trying to identify such a link.

Soon after the isolation and characterization of PTTG, a report was published describing PTTG's ability to induce both expression and secretion of bFGF in NIH3T3 cells (Zhang et al. 1999a). Furthermore, the same group proposed a mechanism explaining this interaction, by demonstrating abolishment of bFGF stimulation after directed mutation of proline-rich residues in the PTTG protein. Several other investigations performed later also confirmed the existence of this close relationship between PTTG and bFGF. By using a semiquantitative RT-PCR, Heaney et al. (1999) revealed a concordant expression of these two factors ($r = 0.84$, $p \leq 0.01$) in a total of 41 human pituitary tumors. Subsequently, this observation was verified by our group ($r = 0.93$, $p \leq 0.01$) in a larger series of 103 pituitary adenomas using quantitative real-time PCR (Chamaon et al. 2009) (Fig. 5). The positive correlation between both mRNAs was also underpinned by the observation that the amounts of both mRNAs were dramatically increased in invasive pituitary adenomas as compared to noninvasive (Jia et al. 2013). Apart from this tumor entity, a study carried out in 62 hepatocellular carcinomas proved also a remarkable positive correlation, not only between mRNA expression of PTTG versus bFGF ($r = 0.78$, $p < 0.0001$) but also between PTTG versus VEGF ($r = 0.47$, $p = 0.0001$) as well as PTTG versus intratumoral microvessel density ($r = 0.80$, $p < 0.0001$) (Fujii et al. 2006). Moreover, in univariate and multivariate

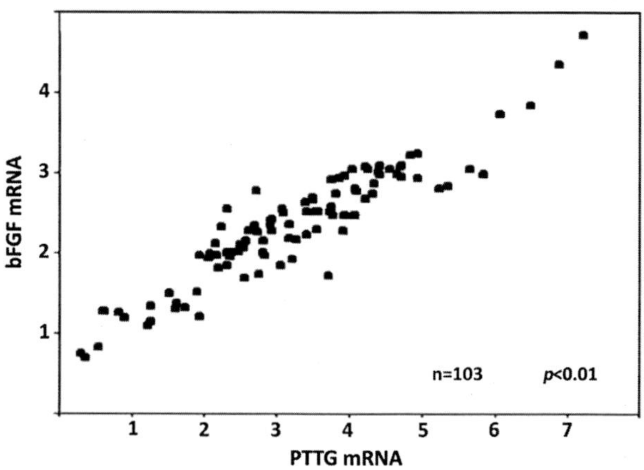

Fig. 5 Strong relation between PTTG and bFGF mRNAs in pituitary adenomas. Scattergram presenting a linear distribution and a significant correlation ($p < 0.01$), when the mRNA levels of PTTG and bFGF were plotted against each other, for a total of 103 pituitary adenomas, examined by quantitative real-time PCR (Modified according to Chamaon et al. 2009)

analyses, PTTG was found to possess superiority over the other variables examined (AFP [α-fetoprotein], tumor multiplicity, tumor size, vascular invasion, liver cirrhosis, and pathological stage) both in predicting disease-free and overall survival. In agreement with the results obtained by Fujii and colleagues (2006) with respect to PTTG and VEGF, another team also had evidenced a couple of years earlier the relationship between these two factors, by examining them both in in vitro and in ex vivo experiments (McCabe et al. 2002). This group noticed an induction of VEGF's expression by transfection of PTTG into human teratoma, breast carcinoma, and choriocarcinoma cell lines. Even more, by a stepwise increase of PTTG's amount during transfection of JEG-3 choriocarcinoma cells, a concordant and significantly correlated increase of VEGF mRNA was noted ($r^2 = 0.91$, $p \leq 0.001$). Finally, it was shown in the same study that PTTG induced upregulation of VEGF independently from bFGF; in other words this process is apparently the result of PTTG's direct influence on VEGF rather than an indirect consequence of bFGF's transactivation caused by PTTG (McCabe et al. 2002).

Migratory Ability of Tumor Cells

The invasive potential of a solid tumor represents a hallmark of its aggressiveness. It is reflected in the tumor's capacity to infiltrate the adjacent non-tumorous tissue and vasculature, but also in the ability to seed metastases into lymph nodes and other organs. It is obvious from the abovementioned, that the impact of a cancer biomarker is enhanced by its ability to distinguish neoplasms with a high potency of invasiveness, since the latter is related to the rate of disease progression and prognosis. Actually, the majority of the studies, aiming to establish PTTG as a cancer biomarker, dealt with the question whether this protein would be able to predict invasiveness.

Although esophageal carcinoma is not included among the five most common neoplasms, it is noteworthy that three independent reports were published concerning this particular tumor. Chronologically, Shibata and colleagues (2002) were the first who documented an outstanding positive association between PTTG and tumors of higher pathological stage (IV vs. 0–III, $p \leq 0.05$) as well as tumors with a higher lymph node status (pN; N4 vs. N0-3, $p \leq 0.01$). In addition, the results of univariate analysis recognized PTTG to be among other factors (pathological stage, tumor factor [T], nodal factor [N], and vein invasion [V]) a valuable predictor of patient's survival ($p \leq 0.05$). Some years later, a study performed in 113 esophageal squamous cell carcinomas (Ito et al. 2008) confirmed the power of high PTTG expression to distinguish tumors with regional lymph node metastasis (pN; $p \leq 0.05$), distant lymph node metastasis (pM; $p \leq 0.01$), and high total TNM score (pTNM; $p \leq 0.05$) from non-metastatic tumors or tumors of lower TNM score. Likewise, the potency of PTTG in predicting patient's survival was once more obvious ($p \leq 0.05$ in log rank test). However, this group and Yan and colleagues in a nearly simultaneous report (Yan et al. 2009) went a step further and revealed in vitro and in mouse experiments the ability of PTTG to promote cell migration/invasion and lymph node metastasis, as already depicted in section "Motility, Invasion and Metastasis." Besides esophageal cancer, also other organs of the gastrointestinal tract attracted the interest of the researchers. One of the earliest investigations (Heaney et al. 2000) examined PTTG expression in colorectal tumors and found it to be positively related to high tumor grades (Dukes' grades C/D vs. A/B; $p \leq 0.05$). Furthermore, by comparing carcinomas with regional lymph node invasion to others without, significantly higher PTTG values were noticed in the former group. Tumor's stage was also one of the parameters, together with alpha-fetoprotein and portal vein thrombosis, that was significantly associated with PTTG protein expression in a total of 65 hepatocellular carcinomas (Liang et al. 2011).

Two further studies carried out by Solbach et al., the first one (2004) in 72 breast cancers and the second (2006) in 89 squamous cell carcinomas of the head and neck (HNSCC), showed PTTG to be significantly associated with both lymph node status and tumor recurrence. Medullary thyroid carcinoma was in the focus of another investigation, which revealed positive correlations between PTTG (mRNA and protein) levels and tumor diameter as well as between PTTG mRNA expression and TNM status (Zatelli et al. 2010). Last but not least, in a large series of 136 small cell lung carcinomas (SCLC) and 91 non-small cell lung carcinomas (NSCLC), differing results were obtained (Rehfeld et al. 2006). In NSCLC, Pearson's correlation analysis showed a parallelism between PTTG expression, i.e., staining intensity of tumor cells, and extended lymph node involvement and distant metastases, a result which was in accordance with previous studies in other tumor diseases. Deviating results regarding a potential prognostic role of PTTG were detected for SCLC. Even though Cox regression model considered PTTG staining intensity as an independent prognostic factor in both tumor types ($p \leq 0.05$), its association with respect to patient's survival was completely opposite. Thus, PTTG expression was at the same time related to better (SCLC) and poorer (NSCLC) prognosis in patients with different histological types of lung cancer. Such contradictory results are probably due to different mechanisms underlying the genesis and progression of these lung cancer subtypes, which are underpinned by the well-known dissimilarities concerning their clinical behavior.

Perspectives for a Prognostic Application of PTTG in Clinical Practice

A critical review of the above-cited literature was performed, which excluded all studies merely demonstrating a correlation between PTTG and tumor grading, proliferation index, or other clinicopathologic or histologic findings without survival statistics. The remaining studies still clearly reveal that enhanced PTTG expression could be used as a potential prognostic marker, according to Kaplan-Meier statistics for tumor diseases occurring in various organs (Fig. 6). In malignant carcinomas and gliomas, i.e., in esophageal cancer (Shibata et al. 2002; Ito et al. 2008), clear cell renal cell carcinoma (Wondergem et al. 2012), breast cancer (Talvinen et al. 2008), anaplastic astrocytoma and glioblastoma (Genkai et al. 2006), and hepatocellular carcinoma (Fujii et al. 2006), enhanced PTTG expression characterized patients with shorter survival. In the less aggressive

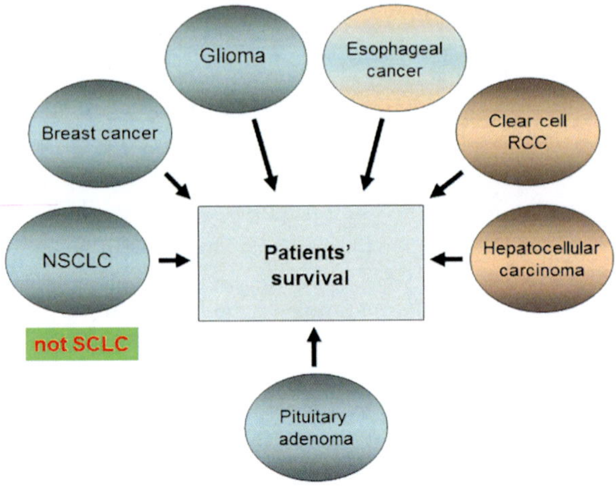

Fig. 6 PTTG's expression inversely associated with patients' survival in various tumors. The expression of PTTG above a threshold, which had been defined by immunohistochemistry (*blue color*), RNA-based protocols (*red color*), or both methods (*red and blue color*), was significantly associated with shorter recurrence-free survival (pituitary adenomas) or shorter overall survival (several malignant tumor diseases) according to Kaplan-Meier statistics. The large spectrum of cell types, from which these diseases originate, suggests a basic role of the oncogene PTTG in tumor disease. Small cell lung cancer (SCLC) exhibited an unexpected positive association between PTTG and survival. *NSCLC* non-small cell lung cancer. *RCC* renal cell carcinoma. The term "glioma" refers to anaplastic astrocytomas and glioblastomas

tumor disease, which had originally been associated with this oncogene, i.e., pituitary adenoma, enhanced PTTG expression identified patients with a shorter interval of recurrence-free survival (Filippella et al. 2006). Only in lung cancer, an opposite result was surprisingly observed for the group of small cell lung cancers (SCLC), i.e., shorter survival was evident for cases with lower PTTG expression (Rehfeld et al. 2006), which actually does not fit with the molecular role of PTTG as an oncogene. However, the group of non-small cell lung cancer (NSCLC) showed the expected inverse association between PTTG and survival time (Rehfeld et al. 2006). Taken together, these studies imply that PTTG is very likely to be a useful prognostic marker in a number of human tumor diseases, which may still grow over time. Nevertheless, a critical statement seems to be necessary regarding potential methodic problems associated with the introduction of PTTG as a marker in routine procedures, which are executable at pathological institutions.

Four of the above-cited studies (Fig. 6) used immunohistochemical staining (IHC) of routine paraffin sections, a method which clearly has the advantage of meeting the demands of routine processing of tissue samples, from surgical sample acquisition to routine processing in the histologic laboratory, i.e., embedding in paraffin blocks and preparation of histologic slices. No further efforts have to be taken and the relative stability of the protein does not warrant specific precautions during sampling. However, a major drawback of IHC seems to be the lack of standardization, which would clearly be required in order to validate IHC as a relevant procedure for measuring PTTG in clinical routine in the future. It is striking that all cited studies used different PTTG antibodies and some focused on nuclear staining (Filippella et al. 2006), while others used cytoplasmic staining (Ito et al. 2008). Although usually more than one case-blinded pathologists evaluated the stained sections, the precise criteria for IHC scoring differed among studies, e.g., by building classes for the percentage of PTTG-positive cells with somewhat differing borders (e.g., <10 %, 10–20 % and >20 % or <10 %, 10–30 % and >30 % of cells). Some scores were built by calculating the mean of scores suggested by three case-blinded observers, while in other cases pathologists discussed to find a final consensus, or the precise way of scoring was not sufficiently communicated in the publication. In one study (Filippella et al. 2006), the most representative high-power field per slice was subjected to counting of positive nuclei, although random sampling by using many high-power fields (HPFs) might have been an alternative choice. It is obvious that a meaningful standardization of quantitative IHC is difficult to achieve and its lack does not decrease the merits of the cited authors, who did their best to plan the study and analyze the sections carefully. However, a decision for quantitative IHC as the method of choice in a given tumor type would still require a better validated standard protocol for staining and scoring.

Alternatively, two of the cited studies used real-time PCR to quantify the mRNA of PTTG. This method required an aliquot of tumor tissue, which had been snap-frozen in liquid nitrogen immediately after surgical resection of the tumor to avoid RNA degradation. In general, this procedure necessitates fast isolation of RNA and synthesis of cDNA, which are less compatible with standard sampling and routine procedures of a histologic laboratory. While PTTG immunostains can be performed in serial sections, allowing a direct assignment of PTTG expression to histologically proven tumor areas, this is not possible with snap-frozen tumor material. Although probably a minor problem in large solid tumors, this missing spatial relationship is a major problem in small samples with doubtful tumor content (e.g., stereotactic biopsies of brain tumors). However, the major advantage of this method is an easier and better standardization, if standard operating protocols (SOP) for PCR and interpretation of results are established. Real-time PCR allows the determination of a quantitative threshold of PTTG expression, which optimally defines the groups of low expression (favorable prognosis) and high expression (unfavorable prognosis) for a given tumor type. A carefully validated protocol does not depend on the subjective interpretation of experienced observers. Nevertheless, such standard protocols would be required prior to clinical implementation of PTTG mRNA levels as a prognostic marker. For instance, the usage of a gene-specific fluorescent probe (Shibata et al. 2002) should be superior to SYBR Green-based PCR (Fujii et al. 2006), because the former possesses enhanced specificity compared to the latter. On the other hand, the idea of Fujii and colleagues (Fujii et al. 2006) is convincing, not to define the prognostic classes of high and low mRNA levels of PTTG solely by measuring the tumor samples, but by determining the fold increase of expression as compared to adjacent normal tissue (if available).

Yet, the usage of two or three reference genes would still enhance the reliability of results as compared to the usage of only a single "housekeeping" gene, such as GAPDH (Shibata et al. 2002) or β-actin (Fujii et al. 2006). Taken together, real-time PCR represents a highly sensitive and much more objective approach, but requires an appropriate apparatus, as well as appropriate sampling and sample processing, which are less compatible with established histopathologic routines. Data of PTTG expression extracted from the large datasets delivered by human genome expression arrays (Affymetrix) supported the usefulness of PTTG mRNA as a prognostic tool (Wondergem et al. 2012). However, the usage of such arrays will not be discussed here in detail, because it requires sophisticated technology and should not be superior to real-time PCR for the intended purpose, i.e., quantification of a single mRNA of interest.

Last but not least, future studies intended to validate standard operating protocols (SOP) for real-time PCR or IHC should at the same time evaluate the surplus – if any – which PTTG may have as a prognostic marker compared to other established or upcoming molecular markers in the same tumor type. As described above, some comparisons between PTTG and general proliferation markers had already been performed, although not with sufficiently standardized methods, in studies calculating Kaplan-Meier statistics. Comparisons with more tumor-type specific prognostic molecular markers would be important. They would help to better define the clinical benefit from introducing a new marker. This includes the detection of a special impact, which the new marker may have in groups of patients defined by molecular criteria with previously recognized significance in the given tumor disease. This aspect is especially important, if established molecular markers already guide the therapeutic regimens (e.g., lung cancer) or are suggested to do so in the near future (e.g., in older patients with glioblastoma).

This matter may first be illustrated in the field of anaplastic astrocytomas and glioblastomas (GBM), where PTTG was reported to possess a negative prognostic value (Genkai et al. 2006). There is a consensus that methylation of the promoter of the gene *MGMT* (methylguanine-DNA methyltransferase) (Chen et al. 2013) as well as inactivating missense mutations in codon 132 of the gene *IDH1* (isocitrate dehydrogenase 1) are favorable prognostic markers in glioblastomas (Hartmann et al. 2010, 2013; Cohen et al. 2013), although methodic details regarding the best way to determine promoter methylation of *MGMT* and choosing the most relevant promoter region to be analyzed are still debated. But, it became clear that lowered expression of MGMT mRNA (evaluated by real-time PCR) and the more easily accessible surrogate marker on the DNA level (promoter methylation) clearly identify a group of GBM with a more favorable outcome, i.e., longer progression-free and overall survival under treatment with radiotherapy and alkylating drugs. Due to the fact that the protein MGMT mediates resistance to alkylating drugs by removal of alkyl adducts from the DNA, methylation of the promoter improved the response to the current gold standard of GBM chemotherapy, namely, temozolomide (Hegi et al. 2005), and can thus be considered as a predictive marker, which is already on its way to guide future therapeutic decision-making in subgroups of GBM patients (Weller et al. 2012). Although, in the case of *IDH1*, the biochemical basis for a benefit from enzyme inactivation did not become clear and *IDH1* status does not guide therapeutic decisions, the presence of mutation in this gene currently seems to be the strongest prognostic molecular marker in GBM. This may be explained by the fact that the mutation is preferentially associated with a slower molecular pathway of GBM genesis, which leads to so-called secondary GBM via various pre-stages. Secondary GBM had been recognized since a long time to have a significantly longer median survival. Both variables, i.e., *MGMT* promoter methylation and *IDH1* mutation can reliably be assessed from routine paraffin sections, because these two features can be determined from chromosomal DNA. The most common *IDH1* mutation (in codon 132 of the gene), which comprises more than 95 % of cases, can be demonstrated in addition by IHC using a well-validated antibody. To estimate the prognostic benefit of a standardized PTTG measurement in GBM and other astrocytic tumors, a comparison with these two markers would be valuable. To name non-small cell lung cancer as another example, it may be meaningful to look separately for the prognostic value of PTTG on the one hand in patients with a wild-type EGFR (epidermal growth factor receptor) and on the other hand in patients with an EGFR mutation, the latter predicting them to respond well to EGFR antagonists, since both groups nowadays receive a different first-line chemotherapy. When asking for the clinical benefit of a new survival-associated marker, the different treatment of patients with and without EGFR mutation would have to be taken into account.

Currently, PTTG can thus be viewed as a promising marker in a spectrum of human tumors. However, protocols for its easy determination still need to be refined and standardized. A direct comparison with a few well-established predictive or prognostic markers will be required to better define a potential benefit of PTTG determination in a given tumor disease, but within different genetic groups of patients or within genetically stratified groups of patients, which already nowadays receive different treatments.

Therapeutic Aspects

Since the importance of PTTG for estimating disease outcome and patient's survival has been comprehensively discussed in the previous sections, it remains to be seen whether this protein could represent a therapeutic target, due to its suggested active involvement in tumor growth and metastatic spread. Numerous studies have tried to answer this particular question and they indeed recognized first hints for a potential role for PTTG as a target of treatment in various neoplasms.

The recognition of "RNA interference" as a reliable method in achieving "gene silencing" by the use of short interfering RNAs (siRNAs) has revealed new perspectives in the treatment of malignancy. Hence, nowadays there is an extensive experimentation in the targeting of oncogenes in tumor cells through the use of siRNAs. Using viral vectors, short hairpin RNAs (shRNAs) against virtually all thinkable targets can be expressed for some time in experimental solid tumors in animals to test the efficacy of gene silencing for any particular gene of interest.

Viral vectors could finally be used to introduce gene silencing shRNAs into residual human tumors or into the resection margins following surgery. Although still a "local" therapeutic approach, silencing of a relevant oncogene may be developed to a meaningful additional tool for cancer treatment in some tumor types. In view of that, almost all studies investigating the therapeutic implication of PTTG in different tumors were focused on silencing of this gene via RNA interference. The results of these preclinical studies in cell cultures and mouse models, although preliminary, warrant further observation and shall thus be described here in brief as an outlook beyond the role of PTTG as a prognostic marker.

One of the first efforts which confronted with this challenge was undertaken by Solbach and colleagues (2005), who investigated the effect of an antisense oligonucleotide, directed against PTTG mRNA, on the growth of HeLa-S3 human cervical cancer cells. They in fact observed an inhibition of proliferation in siRNA-transfected tumor cells as compared to controls. The proliferation of HepG2 and SMMC-7721 cells (hepatocyte carcinoma cell lines), transfected with siRNA (directed against PTTG mRNA), was also remarkably decreased compared to untransfected cells and those transfected with a negative control siRNA ($p \leq 0.01$) (Liang et al. 2011). In addition, other studies using RNA interference for PTTG silencing determined further the importance of this gene not only in proliferation but also in invasion and migration of tumor cells. In this context, Genkai and colleagues (2006) managed to suppress PTTG expression in three different glioma cell lines (U251, ON12 and T98G) and to achieve a striking inhibition of both, proliferation and invasion of glioma cells measured in vitro. Correspondingly, two esophageal carcinoma cell lines (EC9706 and KYSE) transfected with PTTG siRNA showed a significant decrease ($p \leq 0.05$) in their migratory and invasive capacity in vitro (Yan et al. 2009).

Two different reports published by the team of Kakar (2006 and 2007) proved that PTTG silencing was able to suppress tumor growth in nude mice. In the first case, transfection of H1299 lung tumor cells with PTTG siRNA resulted in a decrease of PTTG expression both on mRNA and protein level and inhibited colony formation in soft agar in the same cell line. Although the subsequent injection of H1299 cells (carrying PTTG siRNA) in nude mice also resulted in tumor development, there was a substantial difference in tumor mass of these animals (67.85 ± 45.87 mg) compared to mice with untransfected cells (232.12 ± 102.78) or cells transfected with a control siRNA (231.57 ± 83.76) (Kakar and Malik 2006). In their next study and opposite to their previous one, the same group generated stable constructs of PTTG siRNA and control siRNA introduced in a plasmid vector, instead of using a couple of siRNA oligos targeting PTTG mRNA. By using an ovarian cell line (A2780) as a recipient of their constructs, they observed a reduction of PTTG expression up to 50 % and colony formation up to 70 % in PTTG siRNA-treated cells compared to untransfected control and control-siRNA-transfected cells. Successive experimentation with two different PTTG siRNA clones (A2780 cells) in athymic nude mice revealed that partial silencing of PTTG could also result in the development of tumors in these animals and only the complete abolishment of PTTG expression was consistent with almost tumor-free animals; one out of five mice produced tumors at the site of inoculation, yet these latter were smaller in size than in the corresponding controls. A confirmation of their results was obtained further by the use of HCT116 wild-type and HCT116/PTTG (−/−) cells, after their subcutaneous injection in nude mice (El-Naggar et al. 2007).

Through the incorporation of PTTG siRNA in an adenoviral vector and the following transfection of an invasive hepatoma cell line (SH-J1) with this construct, Cho-Rok and colleagues (2006) achieved abolishment of endogenous PTTG, which concurrently promoted the apoptotic death of these cells. In a next step, they sought to evaluate the role of PTTG both in genesis and progression of tumors in vivo. For that reason, they transfected Huh-7 hepatoma cells with their construct and inoculated them in nude mice. Indeed, they noticed a pronounced suppression of tumor development from hepatoma cells carrying their PTTG siRNA. In a subsequent experiment, the authors injected their adenoviral vectors into preexisting tumors (3–5 mm in diameter), which had been initiated by subcutaneous inoculation of SH-J1 cells in nude mice. They observed that inhibition of PTTG expression was sufficient even to decelerate the growth rate of these preformed neoplasms (Cho-Rok et al. 2006), while a lower efficacy of tumor outgrowth in the previous experiment might have been influenced by an altered ability of PTTG-depleted Huh-7 cells to adhere and survive under the mouse skin, before tumor outgrowth can start. Above and beyond, Ito and colleagues (2008) experimented in a popliteal lymph node metastatic model in nude mice and proved that PTTG knockdown substantially reduced the metastatic potential of tumors in vivo, as described above in more detail (section "Motility, Invasion, and Metastasis.")

At least a few hints suggest that PTTG expression in tumors may not only be knocked down by RNA interference but also be attacked successfully by systemic drug application. Using luciferase reporter assays, Chintharlapalli et al. (2011) showed that two recently developed compounds, namely, CDODA-Me and CF_3DODA-Me, decreased the PTTG promoter activity in thyroid, colon, and pancreatic cancer cells. The drugs also managed to suppress PTTG expression both on mRNA and protein level, in four different thyroid cancer cell lines. Such findings may be starting points for the development of a PTTG-based pharmaceutical intervention.

PTTG may also influence the efficacy of known therapeutic agents, thus appraising its potential function as a predictive factor. In this context, a study published in Oncogene revealed a direct influence of PTTG in the expression of NIS (sodium-iodide symporter) and iodide uptake in vitro. In particular, the overexpression of PTTG caused a significant decrease in mRNA levels of NIS ($p \leq 0.001$), and this effect went hand in hand with a reduction in ^{125}I uptake in primary human thyrocytes ($p \leq 0.001$) (Boelaert et al. 2007). By suppressing cellular iodide accumulation, PTTG may diminish the efficacy of a radioiodide therapy.

Using a human colon carcinoma cell line (HCT116), Tong and colleagues (2011) demonstrated that the inhibition of DNA synthesis by the topoisomerase inhibitor doxorubicin and by the histone deacetylase inhibitor Trichostatin A were much more pronounced in HCT1116 cells with homozygous knockout of the PTTG gene as compared to wild-type cells. Further, by using β-galactosidase (β-Gal) staining as a marker of cellular senescence, they observed a positive β-Gal staining in the majority of treated HCT116 PTTG$^{-/-}$ cells as compared to 5 % staining in the controls.

The effect of PTTG-mediated senescence in conjunction with anticancer agents was confirmed also in vivo. Tumors, which developed after subcutaneous inoculation of HCT116 PTTG$^{-/-}$ cells in athymic mice, exhibited consistently a dramatically slower growth as their PTTG-expressing counterparts, as concluded from tumor volume estimation over 19 days and from the tumor weights, which were finally reached. Moreover, growth curves of doxorubicin-treated groups revealed a much better response of tumors with PTTG knockout. Staining for β-Gal activity demonstrated correspondingly an increased cellular senescence in the doxorubicin-treated tumors with PTTG knockout (Tong et al. 2011).

Last of all, a retrospective study of 64 patients, who underwent prostate needle biopsy and received combined androgen blockade (CAB) therapy, showed that the level of PTTG immunohistochemical expression could predict disease progression and patient's prognosis. Thus, the results of both univariate and multivariate analysis showed PTTG overexpression to be significantly correlated with decreased patient's disease-free survival after CAB treatment (Cao et al. 2012).

Concluding Remarks

It was shown above that PTTG was able to predict patient's survival not only in parallel to other widely accepted biomarkers but also independently. A number of in vitro and in vivo experiments suggested that PTTG may be a useful target for antineoplastic treatment either alone or in conjunction with other therapeutic regimens. In particular, the genetic silencing of this oncogene may be established in the future to a valuable method for decelerating the development of malignancies. The studies performed until now are promising and warrant further extension.

Summary Points

- Three homologous PTTG genes were found in humans at chromosomal loci 5q33 (hPTTG-1), 4p12 (hPTTG-2), and 8q22 (hPTTG-3).
- Only the homologue hPTTG-1 is significantly overexpressed in human tumors and is thus often referred simply as PTTG in the literature.
- PTTG functions as a securin, which assures equal distribution of chromosomes during mitosis. Enforced expression of abnormally high amounts of PTTG leads to aneuploidy and enhances DNA instability.
- PTTG builds complexes with transcription factors, thereby regulating many downstream genes, some of which are involved in cell cycle, apoptosis, angiogenesis, migration, and invasion.

- PTTG transforms normal cells into cells which develop tumors when xenografted to immunocompromised mice.
- PTTG silencing results in deceleration of tumor expansion both in vitro and in vivo.
- Experimental overexpression of PTTG in the mouse pituitary gland led to hyperplasia, but not to adenomas.
- PTTG is a "weak" oncogene in the mouse genital tract, inducing carcinoma development at a low rate.
- PTTG expression is associated with both tumor cell and vascular proliferation but also with neoplasm's invasion/migration capacity, thus effecting patient's survival in various tumor entities.
- PTTG exhibits notable interactions with some known antineoplastic regimens.

References

Bernal JA, Luna R, Espina A, et al. Human securin interacts with p53 and modulates p53-mediated transcriptional activity and apoptosis. Nat Genet. 2002;32:306–11.

Boelaert K, Smith VE, Stratford AL, et al. PTTG and PBF repress the human sodium iodide symporter. Oncogene. 2007;26:4344–56.

Cao XL, Gao JP, Xu Y, et al. Expression of pituitary tumor transforming gene 1 is an independent factor of poor prognosis in localized or locally advanced prostate cancer cases receiving hormone therapy. Asian Pac J Cancer Prev. 2012;13:3083–8.

Chamaon K, Kanakis D, Mawrin C, et al. Transcripts of PTTG and growth factors bFGF and IGF-1 are correlated in pituitary adenomas. Exp Clin Endocrinol Diabetes. 2009;118:121–6.

Chen L, Puri R, Lefkowitz EJ, et al. Identification of the human pituitary tumor transforming gene (hPTTG) family: molecular structure, expression, and chromosomal localization. Gene. 2000;248:41–50.

Chen Y, Hu F, Zhou Y, et al. MGMT promoter methylation and glioblastoma prognosis: a systemic review and meta-analysis. Arch Med Res. 2013;44:281–90.

Chintharlapalli S, Papineni S, Lee SO, et al. Inhibition of pituitary tumor-transforming gene-1 in thyroid cancer cell by drugs that decrease specificity proteins. Mol Carcinog. 2011;50:655–67.

Cho-Rok J, Yoo J, Jang YJ, et al. Adenovirus-mediated transfer of siRNA against PTTG1 inhibits liver cancer cell growth in vitro and in vivo. Hepatology. 2006;43:1042–52.

Cohen AL, Holmen SL, Colman H. IDH1 and IDH2 mutations in gliomas. Curr Neurol Neurosci Rep. 2013;13:345. doi:10.1007/s11910-013-0345-4.

De Craene B, Berx G. Regulatory networks defining EMT during cancer initiation and progression. Nat Rev Cancer. 2013;13:97–110.

Di Fiore R, D'Anneo A, Tesoriere G, et al. RB1 in cancer: different mechanisms of RB1 inactivation and alterations of pRb pathway in tumorigenesis. J Cell Physiol. 2013;228:1676–87.

Donangelo I, Gutman S, Horwath E, et al. Pituitary tumor transforming gene overexpression facilitates pituitary tumor development. Endocrinology. 2006;147:4781–91.

El-Naggar SM, Malik MT, Kakar S. Small interfering RNA against PTTG: a novel therapy for ovarian cancer. Int J Oncol. 2007;31:137–43.

Filippella M, Galland F, Kujas M, et al. Pituitary tumour transforming gene (PTTG) expression correlates with the proliferative activity and recurrence status of pituitary adenomas: a clinical and immunohistochemical study. Clin Endocrinol (Oxf). 2006;65:536–43.

Fong MY, Farghaly H, Kakar SS. Tumorigenic potential of pituitary tumor transforming gene (PTTG) in vivo investigated using a transgenic mouse model, and effects of cross breeding with p53 (+/−) transgenic mice. BMC Cancer. 2012;12:532. doi:10.1186/1471-2407-12-532.

Fujii T, Nomoto S, Koshikawa K, et al. Overexpression of pituitary tumor transforming gene 1 in HCC is associated with angiogenesis and poor prognosis. Hepatology. 2006;43:1267–75.

Genkai N, Homma J, Sano M, et al. Increased expression of pituitary tumor-transforming gene (PTTG)-1 is correlated with poor prognosis in glioma patients. Oncol Rep. 2006;15:1569–74.

Hamid T, Malik MT, Kakar SS. Ectopic expression of PTTG1/securin promotes tumorigenesis in human embryonic kidney cells. Mol Cancer. 2005;4:3.

Hartmann C, Hentschel B, Wick W, et al. Patients with IDH1 wild type anaplastic astrocytomas exhibit worse prognosis than IDH1-mutated glioblastomas, and IDH1 mutation status accounts for the unfavorable prognostic effect of higher age: implications for classification of gliomas. Acta Neuropathol. 2010;120:707–18.

Hartmann C, Hentschel B, Simon M, et al. Long-term survival in primary glioblastoma with versus without isocitrate dehydrogenase mutations. Clin Cancer Res. 2013;19:5146–57.

Heaney AP, Horwitz GA, Wang Z, et al. Early involvement of estrogen-induced pituitary tumor transforming gene and fibroblast growth factor expression in prolactinoma pathogenesis. Nat Med. 1999;5:1317–21.

Heaney AP, Singson R, McCabe CJ, et al. Expression of pituitary-tumor transforming gene in colorectal tumors. Lancet. 2000;355:716–9.

Hegi ME, Diserens AC, Gorlia T, et al. MGMT gene silencing and benefit from temozolomide in glioblastoma. N Engl J Med. 2005;352:997–1003.

Ito T, Shimada Y, Kan T, et al. Pituitary tumor-transforming 1 increases cell motility and promotes lymph node metastasis in esophageal squamous cell carcinoma. Cancer Res. 2008;68:3214–24.

Jia W, Lu R, Jia G, et al. Expression of pituitary tumor transforming gene (PTTG) in human pituitary macroadenomas. Tumour Biol. 2013;34:1559–67.

Kakar SS, Malik MT. Suppression of lung cancer with siRNA targeting PTTG. Int J Oncol. 2006;29:387–95.

Kim D, Pemberton H, Stratford AL, et al. Pituitary tumor transforming gene (PTTG) induces genetic instability in thyroid cells. Oncogene. 2005;24:4861–6.

Kim DS, Franklyn JA, Smith VE, et al. Securin induces genetic instability in colorectal cancer by inhibiting double-stranded DNA repair activity. Carcinogenesis. 2007;28:749–59.

Liang M, Chen X, Liu W, et al. Role of the pituitary tumor transforming gene 1 in the progression of hepatocellular carcinoma. Cancer Biol Ther. 2011;11:337–45.

Marques AC, Dupanloup I, Winckebosch N, et al. Emergence of young human genes after a burst of retroposition in primates. PLoS Biol. 2005;3:e357.

McCabe CJ, Boelaert K, Tannahill LA, et al. Vascular endothelial growth factor, its receptor KDR/Flk-1, and pituitary tumor transforming gene in pituitary tumors. J Clin Endocrinol Metab. 2002;87:4238–44.

Pei L. Genomic organization and identification of an enhancer element containing binding sites for multiple proteins in rat pituitary tumor-transforming gene. J Biol Chem. 1998;273:5219–25.

Pei L. Identification of c-myc as a down-stream target for pituitary tumor-transforming gene. J Biol Chem. 2001;276:8484–91.

Pei L, Melmed S. Isolation and characterization of a pituitary tumor-transforming gene (PTTG). Mol Endocrinol. 1997;11:433–41.

Poznic M. Retinoblastoma protein: a central processing unit. J Biosci. 2009;34:305–12.

Prezant TR, Kadioglu P, Melmed S. An intronless homolog of human proto-oncogene hPTTG is expressed in pituitary tumors: evidence for hPTTG family. J Clin Endocrinol Metab. 1999;84:1149–52.

Raverot G, Wierinckx A, Dantony E, et al. Prognostic factors in prolactin pituitary tumors: clinical, histological, and molecular data from a series of 94 patients with a long postoperative follow up. J Clin Endocrinol Metab. 2010;95:1708–16.

Rehfeld N, Geddert H, Atamna A, et al. The influence of the pituitary tumor transforming gene-1 (PTTG-1) on survival of patients with small cell lung cancer and non-small cell lung cancer. J Carcinog. 2006;5:4.

Saez C, Japon MA, Ramos-Morales F, et al. Hpttg is over-expressed in pituitary adenomas and other primary epithelial neoplasias. Oncogene. 1999;18:5473–6.
Shah PP, Kakar SS. Pituitary tumor transforming gene induces epithelial to mesenchymal transition by regulation of twist, snail, slug, and E-cadherin. Cancer Lett. 2011;311:66–76.
Shah PP, Fong MY, Kakar SS. PTTG induces EMT through integrin αVβ3-focal adhesion signaling in lung cancer cells. Oncogene. 2012;31:3124–35.
Shibata Y, Haruki N, Kuwabara Y, et al. Expression of PTTG (pituitary tumor transforming gene) in esophageal cancer. Jpn J Clin Oncol. 2002;32:233–7.
Solbach C, Roller M, Fellbaum C, et al. PTTG mRNA expression in primary breast cancer: a prognostic marker for lymph node invasion and tumor recurrence. Breast. 2004;13:80–1.
Solbach C, Roller M, Peters S, et al. Pituitary tumor-transforming gene (PTTG): a novel target for anti-tumor therapy. Anticancer Res. 2005;25:121–5.
Solbach C, Roller M, Eckerdt F, et al. Pituitary tumor-transforming gene expression is a prognostic marker for tumor recurrence in squamous cell carcinoma of the head and neck. BMC Cancer. 2006;6:242.
Talvinen K, Tuikkala J, Nevalainen O, et al. Proliferation marker securin identifies favourable outcome in invasive ductal breast cancer. Br J Cancer. 2008;99:335–40.
Tong Y, Tan Y, Zhou C, et al. Pituitary tumor transforming gene interacts with Sp1 to modulate G1/S cell phase transition. Oncogene. 2007;26:5596–605.
Tong Y, Zhao W, Zhou C, et al. PTTG1 attenuates drug-induced cellular senescence. PLoS One. 2011;6:e23754. doi:10.1371/journal.pone.0023754.
Weller M, Stupp R, Hegi ME. Personalized care in neuro-oncology coming of age: why we need MGMT and 1p/19q testing for malignant glioma patients in clinical practice. Neuro Oncol. 2012;14 Suppl 4:iv100–8. doi:10.1093/neuonc/nos206.
Wondergem B, Zhang Z, Huang D, et al. Expression of the PTTG-1 oncogene is associated with aggressive clear cell renal cell carcinoma. Cancer Res. 2012;72:4361–71.
Yan S, Zhou C, Lou X, et al. PTTG overexpression promotes lymph node metastasis in human esophageal squamous cell carcinoma. Cancer Res. 2009;69:3283–90.
Yoon CH, Kim MJ, Lee H, et al. PTTG1 oncogene promotes tumor malignancy via epithelial to mesenchymal transition and expansion of cancer stem cell population. J Biol Chem. 2012;287:19516–27.
Yu R, Lu W, Chen J, et al. Overexpressed pituitary tumor-transforming gene causes aneuploidy in live human cells. Endocrinology. 2003;144:4991–8.
Zatelli MC, Tagliati F, Amodio V, et al. Role of pituitary tumor transforming gene 1 in medullary thyroid carcinoma. Anal Cell Pathol (Amst). 2010;33:207–16.
Zhang X, Horwitz GA, Prezant TR, et al. Structure, expression, and function of human pituitary tumor-transforming gene (PTTG). Mol Endocrinol. 1999a;13:156–66.
Zhang X, Horwitz GA, Heaney AP, et al. Pituitary tumor transforming gene (PTTG) expression in pituitary adenomas. J Clin Endocrinol Metab. 1999b;84:761–7.
Zhang J, Yiang Y, Chen L, et al. Overexpression of pituitary tumor transforming gene (PTTG) is associated with tumor progression and poor prognosis in patients with esophageal squamous cell carcinoma. Acta Histochem. 2013. doi:10.1016/j.acthis.2013.09.01.
Zheng H, Kang Y. Multilayer control of the EMT master regulators. Oncogene. 2013. doi:10.1038/onc.2013.128.
Zhou C, Tong Y, Wawrowsky K, et al. PTTG acts as a STAT3 target gene for colorectal cancer cell growth and motility. Oncogene. 2013. doi:10.1038/onc.2013.16.
Zou H, McGarry TJ, Bernal T, et al. Identification of a vertebrate sister-chromatid separation inhibitor involved in transformation and tumorigenesis. Science. 1999;285:418–22.

U2 Small Nuclear RNA as a Biomarker in Cancer

10

Stephan A. Hahn, Hannah Zoellner, Abdelouahid Maghnouj, and Deepak B. Vangala

Contents

Abstract

Cancer is the second most common cause of death in western countries today. Despite of modern therapeutic approaches leading to longer survival rates, the only cure for the most solid tumors is resection of the entire tumor. However, cure is generally only possible in patients with limited disease without distant metastases. Therefore, detection of precancerous conditions or early cancer stages is crucial to reduce the mortality of cancer.

S.A. Hahn (✉) • H. Zoellner • A. Maghnouj
Department of Molecular Gastrointestinal Oncology, Ruhr-University Bochum, Molecular GI-Oncology (MGO), Bochum, Germany
e-mail: stephan.hahn@rub.de; hannah.zoellner@rub.de; abdelouahid.maghnouj@rub.de

D.B. Vangala
Department of Medicine and Department of Molecular Gastrointestinal Oncology, Ruhr-University Bochum, Knappschaftskrankenhaus, Bochum, Germany
e-mail: deepak.vangala@rub.de

V.R. Preedy, V.B. Patel (eds.), *Biomarkers in Cancer, Biomarkers in Disease: Methods, Discoveries and Applications*,
DOI 10.1007/978-94-007-7681-4_6

To date, blood-based biomarkers which can be assayed within the patient's clinical chemistry workup are the most frequently used markers for detecting cancer. Unfortunately, most of these markers are neither able to detect precancerous conditions nor early cancer stages at the required high sensitivity and specificity levels to be of use in any screening procedure.

Recently, RNA fragments derived from the noncoding RNA U2 snRNA were detected at elevated levels among others in the blood of patients suffering from pancreatic, colorectal, and non-small-cell lung cancer as compared to noncancerous controls. Sensitivity and specificity levels reached with the proposed U2 snRNA fragment detection assays were well above the levels reported for current noninvasive blood-based tumor markers used in clinical routine. U2 snRNA fragments proved to be highly stable in the serum and plasma from cancer patients and could be detected by a simple routine PCR-based assay, crucial requirements for an analyte to be successfully implemented into a clinical routine diagnostic procedure. Importantly, the fragments were also found to be significantly elevated in a fraction of early colon and lung cancer patients. Therefore, detection of U2 snRNA fragments in the blood cannot only be regarded as a novel strategy to detect cancer but may also hold promise for detecting some cancer types at a curable stage.

List of Abbreviations

Ago	Argonaute Protein
AUC	Area Under the Curve
BSiR	Branch Site-Interacting Region
CA19-9	Carbohydrate Antigen 19-9
CEA	Carcinoembryonic Antigen
CI	Confidence Interval
COPD	Chronic Obstructive Pulmonary Disease
CRC	Colorectal Carcinoma
Ct	Cycle Threshold
Cyfra 21-1	Cytokeratin 19 Fragments
EDTA	Ethylenediaminetetraacetic Acid
miRNA	MicroRNA
ncRNA	Noncoding RNA
NGS	Next-Generation Sequencing
NSCLC	Non-small-Cell Lung Cancer
PDAC	Pancreatic Ductal Adenocarcinoma
piRNA	PIWI-Associated RNAs
pre-mRNA	Precursor Messenger RNA
PSA	Prostate-Specific Antigen
qRT-PCR	Quantitative Real-Time Polymerase Chain Reaction
RNP	Ribonucleoprotein Particle
ROC	Receiver Operating Characteristic
rRNA	Ribosomal RNA

siRNA	Small Interfering RNA
snoRNA	Small Nucleolar RNAs
snRNA	Small Nuclear RNAs
snRNP	Small Nuclear Ribonucleoprotein Particle
tRNA	Transfer RNA
UICC	Union Internationale Contre Le Cancer

Key Facts of Noncoding RNAs as Biomarkers

- Noncoding RNAs (ncRNAs) can be used as biomarkers in pathological condition.
- A fragment of U2 snRNA (RNU2-1f) shows high potential as a diagnostic biomarker in various malignant conditions such as pancreatic cancer, colorectal cancer, or non-small-cell lung cancer.
- Functionally U2 snRNA plays a major role in splicing of pre-mRNA.
- Structurally miR-1246 which itself was described as biomarker in different cancers is identical to RNU2-1f.
- Current literature identified miR-1246 as a pseudo-miRNA and attributed miR-1246 data to RNU2-1f.

Definition of Words and Terms

Colorectal Cancer Colorectal cancer is the fourth most common cancer and ranks third in mortality statistics worldwide. It arises from the epithelial tissue of the large intestine with the vast majority of cases being adenocarcinomas. The molecular progression model of CRCs was first described by Fearon and Vogelstein at the end of the 1980s with the adenoma-carcinoma sequence being the general model for carcinogenesis for many years (Fearon and Vogelstein 1990). As adenomas are precancerous lesions which can be detected by colonoscopy, prevention and early detection of CRCs are possible. Unfortunately acceptance of preventive colonoscopy is not high in the general population, and many patients are diagnosed in advanced stages of the disease; hence the mortality rate is still high. That illustrates why even for a highly preventable disease, new and easy accessible noninvasive screening biomarkers could be valuable.

Pancreatic Cancer The majority of pancreatic carcinoma is thought to arise from the epithelial tissue of the pancreatic ducts. Pancreatic cancer is the 10th most common cancer but number 4 in cancer deaths with a devastating 5-year survival of about 5 % in advanced stages and less than 20 % in earlier stages. Early diagnosis through systematic screening is to date next to impossible, and most patients present in advanced stages of the disease due to the lack of early signs and symptoms and rapid progression of the disease.

Lung Cancer Lung cancer is the most common cause for cancer-associated death worldwide in male patients and the second most common cause in female patients. In 2008 13 % of all cancer patients suffered from lung cancer, and 18 % of all cancer-associated deaths were due to lung cancer. The major risk factor for the development of lung cancer is cigarette smoking, with some studies showing a decrease in incidence with reduction of smoking in the USA. Lung cancers are histologically classified in small-cell lung cancers (SCLC) and non-small-cell lung cancers (NSCLC). The latter comprise different tumor entities such as squamous cell carcinomas or adenocarcinomas. Lung cancer arises from the epithelium of the lung. Usually it is detected in advanced stages of disease leaving no option for curative treatment. Though early detection by computed tomography has been suggested by some authors, this has not found its way into daily clinical routine. Hence, new screening markers could aid enormously in early detection of lung cancer.

miRNA MicroRNAs are small (19–21 nt), noncoding, and highly conserved RNA molecules encoded in the genome. Associated with multiple proteins in a RNA-induced silencing complex (RISC), they regulate the expression of target genes by base-pairing with complementary sequences in the 3′-untranslated regions (3′-UTR) of their target mRNAs. Discovered in 1993, much effort has gone into understanding the function of miRNAs. To date, they have been described to act as key regulators of processes as diverse as early development, cell proliferation, apoptosis, and cell differentiation. A large body of evidence implicates aberrant miRNA expression patterns in most if not all human malignancies so that they provide potential as diagnostic, prognostic, and therapeutic tools.

ncRNA A noncoding RNA is a functional RNA that does not encode a protein. Noncoding RNAs include transfer RNAs (tRNAs), ribosomal RNAs (rRNAs), miRNAs, and snRNAs. The number of ncRNAs within the human genome is unknown, and many of the newly identified ncRNAs have not been validated for their function.

qRT-PCR The quantitative real-time PCR is a technique that enables reliable detection and quantification of products generated during each cycle of a PCR process. Compared to standard PCR, the process is monitored in real time as the amount of amplified cDNA is detected after each PCR cycle by the use of fluorescent markers. This ability to monitor the reaction during its exponential phase enables users to determine the initial amount of target with great precision. Fluorescent markers are used to measure the amount of cDNA. As the fluorescent markers are incorporated into the PCR product (amplicon), the fluorescent signal is directly proportional to the number of amplicon molecules generated in the exponential phase of the reaction. The most common fluorescent reporters are double-stranded DNA-binding dyes (e.g., SYBR Green) or dye molecules attached to PCR primers or probes that are incorporated into the product during amplification.

snRNP Small nuclear ribonucleic particles are components of the spliceosome. As the name suggests, they consist of RNA molecules (U snRNA) and proteins. The five most common kinds of snRNPs involved in splicing are U1, U2, U4, U5, and U6. They are named after their snRNA.

Spike-In Control Sample contaminants including co-extracted inhibitors such as ethylenediaminetetraacetic acid (EDTA) phenol, heparin, and ethanol can affect reaction steps in qRT-PCR. A spike-in control is used to identify the presence of those inhibitors and to measure sensitivity, accuracy, and biases of the qRT-PCR assay. As a spike-in, synthetic RNA molecules are added to the sample, purified, and reverse transcribed with the RNA sample, and the resulting cDNA is analyzed. Common spike-in controls are miRNA mimics of *C. elegans* that are distinguishable from endogenous human transcripts. To ensure accurate and reliable measurements via qRT-PCR, the use of a spike-in control is recommended.

Spliceosome The spliceosome (also called splicing body) is a large ribonucleoprotein complex that catalyzes the removal of introns (noncoding intervening sequences) from nuclear pre-mRNAs. This process is generally known as splicing. Each spliceosome is composed of the five U snRNA U1, U2, U4, U5, and U6 and a variety of associated proteins. These form complexes called snRNPs. The spliceosome must assemble anew on each intron.

U snRNA A class of eukaryotic small RNA molecules (100–215 nt) found in the nucleus as snRNPs and apparently involved in processing heterogeneous nuclear RNA. They became known as U snRNA because these RNAs appeared to be ubiquitous and were uridine rich. The most common U snRNAs are U1, U2, U4, U5, and U6.

Xenograft Model of generating human tumors through injection of human cancer cell lines or through implantation of tumor pieces in immunocompromised animals such as athymic nude mice. The tumors are usually generated subcutaneously and can then be either subject for further analysis, for example, testing of new substances with antitumor activity.

Introduction

Cancer is one of the major challenges in modern medicine. In 2008, approximately 12.8 million people suffered of a cancerous disease, and about 7.6 million people died due to cancer (Jemal et al. 2011). More than one third of people in the western world will suffer from cancer during lifetime.

The development of cancer is a complex process that involves the accumulation of genetic and epigenetic alterations, such as gene amplifications, chromosomal translocations, point mutations, and promoter methylation, respectively. Lifestyle and environmental or occupational factors can influence the transformation from a normal cell to a malignant cell. The hallmarks of these cells – as stated by Hanahan and Weinberg in 2011 – are a limitless replicative potential, self-sufficiency in growth signals and insensitivity to antigrowth signals, a sustained angiogenesis, evading apoptosis, and finally tissue invasion and metastasis (Hanahan and Weinberg 2011).

Modern therapeutic approaches have had a major impact on a wide variety of cancers leading to longer overall and disease- or progression-free survival rates. Nevertheless, resection of the entire tumor remains the only cure for the vast majority of solid tumors. Surgery as a curative measure is usually only possible in limited disease without distant metastases. Unfortunately, most patients present in advanced stages of the disease where a curative treatment is no longer possible. Therefore, screening for early cancer stages or precancerous conditions is a recognized preventive approach in many countries and currently the most effective way to reduce cancer mortality. Such screening approaches include ultrasound and mammography for breast cancer or colonoscopy for colorectal cancer. Unfortunately, for many other cancers, early detection methods are lacking. In addition, acceptance of patients to take part in invasive screening procedures such as colonoscopy is generally very low (Brenner et al. 2009; Taylor et al. 2011). Hence, the development of new biomarkers for noninvasive screening procedures is crucial to aid early diagnosis of cancers and to help in reducing mortality and morbidity especially in diseases such as lung or pancreatic cancer in which early detection and screening are to date next to impossible.

In recent years, miRNAs belonging to the family of noncoding RNAs (ncRNAs) have gained much attention as potential new biomarkers for noninvasive diagnostic procedures, not least because it was shown that miRNAs circulate in a cell-free form in body fluids. In addition, they proved to be very stable in blood, urine, stool, and other body fluids, what can be regarded as hostile environment for standard RNA molecules. Furthermore, even low amounts of miRNAs can be detected by quantitative real-time polymerase chain reaction (qRT-PCR) with high sensitivity and reproducibility at relatively low costs, making miRNAs good candidates for biomarkers arguably superior to protein markers (Madhavan et al. 2013; Valadi et al. 2007).

From the remaining noncoding RNA (ncRNAs) family members, which are PIWI-associated RNAs (piRNAs), small Cajal body-specific RNAs (scaRNAs), small nucleolar RNAs (snoRNAs), and small nuclear RNAs (snRNAs), only the latter two very recently surfaced as novel biomarkers. More specifically, fragments of U2 snRNA have been reported to function as a biomarker among others in pancreatic, colorectal, and lung cancer (Baraniskin et al. 2013; Mazières et al. 2013). Furthermore, three members of the snoRNAs (SNORD33, SNORD66, and SNORD76) were detected at elevated levels in lung patient plasma indicating their potential usefulness as a diagnostic cancer biomarker for non-small-cell lung cancer (Liao et al. 2010).

This chapter focuses on the potential use of U2 snRNA fragments as biomarker. First, the cell biological context where U2 snRNA is active is described. Second, the U2 snRNA genomic localization and the two current modes suggested for U2 snRNA fragment biogenesis are presented. Third, the sequence characteristics linked to an important aspect of the U2 snRNA fragment assay, which is the cross-reactivity with miR-1246 and miR-1290 molecules, will be discussed. Finally, the potential clinical use of the U2 snRNA fragment assay will be highlighted, laying focus on three common and often fatal cancers, which are pancreatic, colorectal, and lung carcinoma.

U2 snRNA and the Splicing Process of Pre-mRNAs

As mentioned above, fragments of U2 snRNA were recently discovered at increased levels in patient serum and plasma suffering from a variety of cancer types. U2 snRNA is highly abundant in cells and is essential for the splicing of pre-mRNA. For initiating splicing a spliceosome is formed. Today, two spliceosomes – the minor U12-dependent and the major U2-dependent complex (Will and Lührmann 2005), the latter being composed of >200 proteins – and five snRNAs which form four RNA-protein complexes, the so-called small nuclear ribonucleoprotein particles (snRNP), are known. These are named after their RNA component: U1, U2, U4/U6, and U5 snRNP. The protein components can be divided into common proteins that are present in all U snRNPs on the one hand and in specific proteins that are associated with individual snRNPs on the other hand. The common proteins are also known as Sm proteins. This family contains Sm motives which are necessary for Sm protein-protein interactions to form Sm protein complexes. Consequently, these complexes assemble around the conserved, uridyl-rich Sm site (Fig. 1)

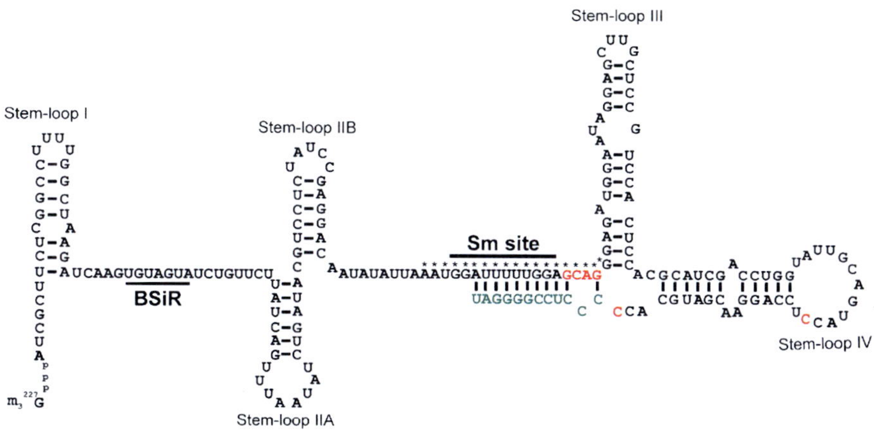

Fig. 1 Primary and secondary structure of the human U2 snRNA. Nucleotides indicated by *asterisks* correspond to the mature miR-1246 sequence. The *red* letters localize the sequence differences between U2-1 and U2-2 snRNAs. Stem loops are numbered with Roman numerals. The branch site-interacting region (*BSiR*) is underlined, and the Sm site is highlighted by a bar above the corresponding nucleotides. Letters marked in *green* correspond to the 3′-extended sequence newly discovered by Mazières et al.

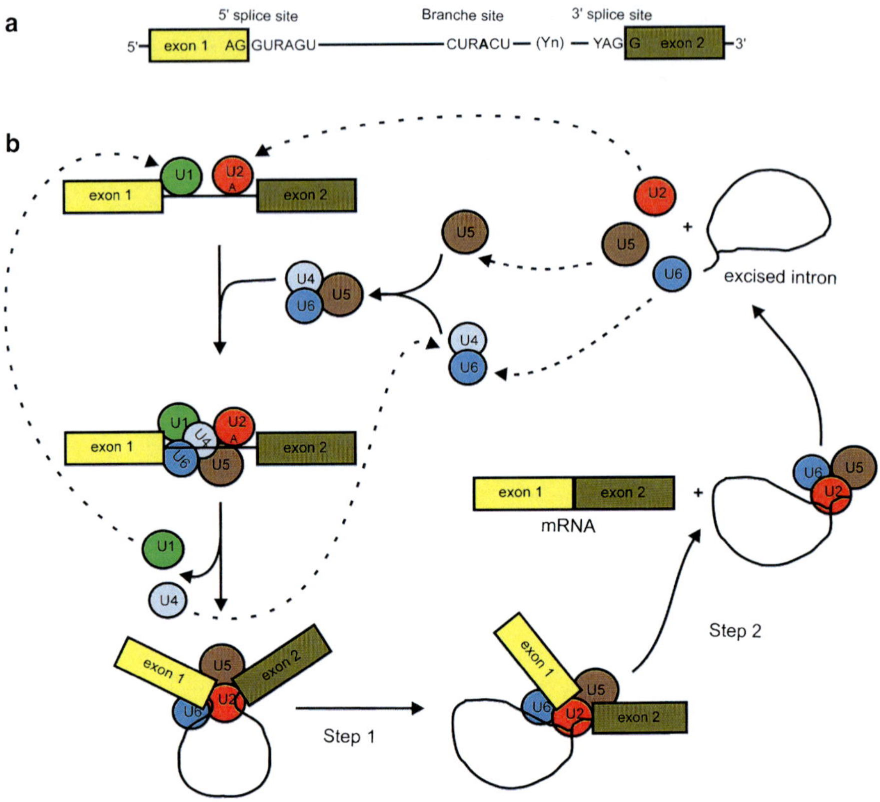

Fig. 2 **U2-type spliceosome and its conserved two-step splicing mechanism.** (**a**) Conserved sequences found at the 5′ and 3′ splice sites and branch site of U2-type pre-mRNA introns. The conserved sequences of human U2-dependant introns are shown, where Y = pyrimidine and R = purine. Exons (*boxes*), introns (*lettering* or *solid line*), the branch adenosine (*bold lettering*), and the polypyrimidine tract are indicated by (*Yn*). (**b**) Assembly and disassembly of the canonical two-step mechanism of pre-mRNA splicing pathway of the U2-dependent spliceosome. For simplicity, the ordered interactions of the snRNPs (indicated by *circles*), but not those of non-snRNP proteins, are shown. Exon and intron sequences are indicated by *boxes* and *solid lines*, respectively

present in the U snRNAs except U6 snRNA. As it will be discussed in more detail in a following paragraph, the interaction between Sm complex and the U2 snRNA Sm site may play together with the high abundance of the U2 snRNA, a role in the U2 snRNA fragment generation. The formation of the snRNPs occurs in the cytoplasm where the specific proteins also interact with the snRNPs immediately after translation. The snRNPs are then transferred into the nucleus. In addition to the snRNPs, at least another 100 splicing factors, the non-snRNPs, are required for the splicing process (Kambach et al. 1999). The splicing cycle follows an ordered pathway (Fig. 2).

Genomic Organization and Sequence Characteristics of U2 snRNA

There are two variants of U2 snRNA existing in the human genome: RNU2-1 and RNU2-2, located at 17q21.31 and 11q12.3, respectively. These genes of 187 nt are paralogous with differences being limited to four bases near the Sm protein-binding sequence and two point mutations at the 3′ end (Fig. 1). The RNU2-1 gene is arranged as a genomic cluster containing up to 30 clusters of tandem repeated copies, each repeat containing a single RNU2-1 gene, whereas the RNU2-2 gene is present at a single copy. In line with the higher copy number of RNU2-1, both the levels of U2-1 snRNA and its fragments detected to date in cells and blood are much higher compared to the levels of U2-2 snRNA and its fragments (Mazières et al. 2013). Therefore, the data reported are mainly focusing on RNU2-1 fragments (also termed RNU2-1f) as biomarker. Another important sequence characteristic of the RNU2-1 gene is that it contains at its 3′ region the proposed mature sequence of miR-1246 and – with only one mismatch – the sequence of miR-1290 (Fig. 3). Indeed, this fact led to the identification of U2 snRNA fragments as a biomarker for pancreatic and colorectal cancer. Baraniskin et al. (2013) analyzed sera from mice bearing human pancreatic cancer xenograft tumors to identify circulating miRNAs in a hybridization-based global miRNA array experiment. miR-1246 and miR-1290 were found to be able to discriminate between cancer-bearing and tumor-free control mice, a finding which was validated in serum samples from pancreatic and colon cancer patients. Similar results were subsequently also reported for lung cancer (Mazières et al. 2013). Unexpectedly, sequencing proved that the molecules found to be overrepresented in cancer serum are fragments of RNU2-1 and not miR-1246. The false detection of miR-1246/miR-1290 via the array experiment data can be explained by the cross-reactivity of the probes on the arrays due to the

```
snRNA-U2-1   ATCGCTTCTCGGCCTTTTGGCTAAGATCAAGTGTAGTATCTGTTCTTATCAGTTTAATAT
miR-1246     ------------------------------------------------------------
miR-1290     ------------------------------------------------------------

                                              *******************
snRNA-U2-1   CTGATACGTCCTCTATCCGAGGACAATATATTAAATGGATTTTTGGAGCAGGGAGATGGA
miR-1246     ---------------------------------AATGGATTTTTGGAGCAGG--------
miR-1290     -----------------------------------TGGATTTTTGGATCAGGA-------
                                                ************ ******

snRNA-U2-1   ATAGGAGCTTGCTCCGTCCACTCCACGCATCGACCTGGTATTGCAGTACCTCCAGGAACG
miR-1246     ------------------------------------------------------------
miR-1290     ------------------------------------------------------------

snRNA-U2-1   GTGCACCC
miR-1246     --------
miR-1290     --------
```

Fig. 3 Sequence relationship between U2-1 snRNA, miR-1246, and miR-1290. Common sequence regions are shown between human mature miR-1246 and RNU2-1 (*asterisk*) and miR-1290 and RNU2-1 (*dot*) high similarity between miR-1246 (100 % identical) and miR-1290 (one mismatch) and the RNU2-1 sequence (Fig. 3). Importantly, most commercially available miR-1290 and miR-1246 qRT-PCR assays are also cross-reactive with RNU2-1f (Baraniskin et al. 2013). Furthermore, deep sequencing revealed that miR-1246 and miR-1290 are a result of false mapping indicating that currently published data in the literature linked to either miR-1246 or miR-1290 should be assigned to RNU2-1 (Baraniskin et al. 2013; Mazières et al. 2013). Taking this into consideration, it is worth to mention that a recent manuscript proposed that circulating miR-1290 can be used for early diagnosis of pancreatic cancer, a finding likely also attributable to RNU2-1 (Li et al. 2013).

RNU2-1 Fragment Biogenesis and Stability

The mechanism behind the generation of the observed RNU2-1f is still poorly understood. Baraniskin et al. observed a rise in extracellular RNU2-1f concentration following induction of apoptosis both in a pancreatic and colon cancer cell line in vitro model but were unable to detect intracellular RNU2-1f. This led to the hypothesis that RNU2-1f is only generated as the consequence of a random RNA degradation process initiated within the apoptotic program (Fig. 4a). During this process, the Sm proteins which form a heteroheptameric ring structure surrounding the RNU2-1-Sm-binding site may help to prevent further degradation of RNU2-1 giving rise to the observed RNU2-1f. In addition, the facts that RNU2-1f were found to be resistant toward nuclease treatment and exhibited a partial stability toward protein as treatment suggested that RNU2-1f is not protected by its binding to proteins such as Argonaute2, as shown for many miRNAs (Arroyo et al. 2011). In consequence, it appears more likely that RNU2-1f are protected by their inclusion into a vesicle-like structure, such as apoptotic bodies (Fig. 4a). These structures are known to contain snRNPs (including U2-snRNA) and can be released into the peripheral blood via the compromised capillary network which is characteristic of tumor tissues (Biggiogera et al. 1997; Halicka et al. 2000). In line with the proposed link between apoptosis and RNU2-1f abundance, a recent study showed that photodynamic therapy which involves the light-induced activation of a photosensitizing compound to destroy tumor cells via dose-dependent induction of apoptosis was able to increase RNU2-1f abundance in an in vitro model (Bach et al. 2013). Furthermore, Palma et al. found RNU2-1f to be included in nucleosomes derived from breast cancer cell lines. In their model DNA-damage-induced apoptosis increased, similar to pancreatic and colon cancer lines, both the abundance of nucleosomes and RNU2-1f (Palma et al. 2012).

In contrast to the summarized data from above, Mazières et al. were able to identify cellular RNU2-1f. They also noted that the detected RNU2-1f exhibit a rather conserved sequence length, reminiscent of the so-called isomiRs, representing length variants observed for many miRNAs. In addition, a newly 3′ end sequence of RNU2-1 not present in the current RNA sequence databases was discovered by the deep sequencing effort of Mazières et al. This 3′ end is essential for U2 snRNA to be able to form a hairpin-like structure (Fig. 1) but awaits

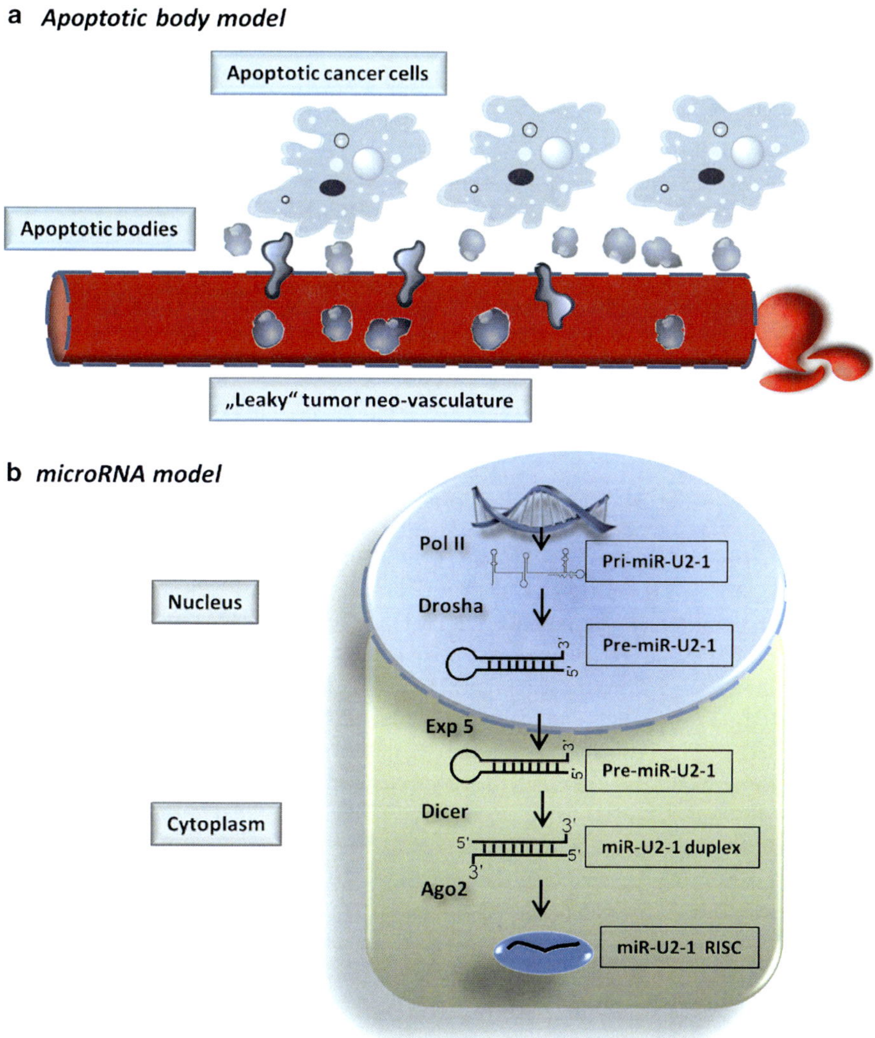

Fig. 4 Schematic illustration of the two currently suggested modes for RNU2-1f biogenesis

confirmation by independent sequencing efforts. Therefore, they concluded that it is more likely that RNU2-1 fragment generation is the end product of microRNA-like specific maturation steps than being formed in the course of the above introduced random degradation process during apoptosis (Fig. 4b). The hypothesis of specific processing was further supported by data from Burroughs et al. (2011)who identified Ago-bound fragments from U2 snRNA. In consequence, Mazières et al. named this sequence product miR-U2-1, a term which will for simplicity reasons not be used throughout this manuscript. Clearly, more work needs to be done to experimentally prove either of these hypotheses.

RNU2-1f in Serum of Pancreatic and Colorectal Cancer Patients

As mentioned above, RNU2-1f were first discovered in a patient-derived pancreatic carcinoma mouse xenograft model. Since the sequence of RNU2-1f is not contained in the mouse transcriptome, it was evident that the observed fragments released into the mouse bloodstream originated from the human tumor, suggesting them to be promising tumor biomarker candidates (Patent application SNRNA RNU2 – 1 ALS TUMORMARKER, 22 July 2011, European patent office, PCT/EP 2012/064321). In a comprehensive RNU2-1f qRT-PCR study using a cohort of 320 serum and plasma samples (80 pancreatic cancer, 111 colon cancer, and 129 controls), it was shown that correct discrimination between cancer and noncancerous samples is possible with a specificity and sensitivity of 97.7 % [95 % CI = (87.7, 99.9)] and 90.6 % [95 % CI = (80.7, 96.5)], respectively, with an area under the ROC curve (AUC) of 0.972. The data also showed a somewhat higher detection rate for pancreatic carcinoma (78/80 samples, 97.5 %) as compared to colon cancer (92/111 samples, 82.8 %; UICC stages II–IV). A similar high detection rate (AUC 0.96) was recently also reported for pancreatic cancer in comparison to normal controls with the use of a miR-1290 qRT-PCR assay (also cross-reactive with RNU2-1f, see above; Li et al. 2013). In this study, discrimination between chronic pancreatitis and pancreatic carcinoma was lower (AUC 0.81), suggesting that RNU2-1f measurements may not be optimal to discriminate between pancreatic carcinoma and chronic pancreatitis. Furthermore, abundance of RNU2-1f seemed to drop below the diagnostic threshold for most stage I pancreatic carcinomas. This is in line with the data reported for colorectal carcinoma (CRC) where RNU2-1f abundance did not reach the required abundance to enable the detection of UICC stage I cancers. Nevertheless, levels of RNU2-1f tended to be higher in more advanced CRC stages, indicating that there is a correlation between tumor mass and RNU2-1f serum levels, enabling the detection of CRC as early as UICC stage II with a high sensitivity of 81 %. An additional finding was that RNU2-1f levels dropped below the diagnostic threshold 5 to 14 days after resection of the tumor (Baraniskin et al. 2013), opening the possibility to use this biomarker for therapy response and relapse monitoring.

RNU2-1f in Lung Cancer

As already introduced above, Mazières et al. (2013) detected similar fragments of U2 snRNA in serum of lung cancer patients using next-generation sequencing (NGS). In order to search for the origin of RNU2-1f in serum of non-small-cell lung cancer (NSCLC) patients, they profiled 19 primary tumors as well as eight adjacent paired normal lung tissues by microRNA microarray analyses. This revealed a > threefold overexpression of RNU2-1f in most cancers compared to normal tissues, suggesting that lung cancer may indeed be at least in part the source of the augmented RNU2-1f concentration observed in patient sera. Subsequently, a larger cohort of controls and lung cancer patient ($N = 158$; controls without symptoms, COPD, not lung cancer; other lung disease, not lung cancer; COPD and lung cancer; lung cancer, not COPD) was tested. The authors verified that a significant overexpression of RNU2-1f was only detectable in lung cancer patients but not in patients with other lung diseases. The best sensitivity and specificity levels reached in their study were 72.6 % and 91.7 %, respectively, with an area under the curve (AUC) of 0.878. Mazières et al. also analyzed in a very small pilot study the ability of RNU2-1f to detect lung cancer in its very early stage of development. They included six stage I and seven stage II patients in their study. They observed increased RNU2-1f levels at stage I similar to stages III and IV but a somewhat unexpected significant decrease of the amount of RNU2-1f at stage II. They hypothesized that the transition from stage I to stage II induces or depends on very specific molecular mechanisms and gene-regulation mechanisms that involve RNU2-1f. These data hint toward the ability of detecting NSCLL as early as in UICC stage I by measuring RNU2-1f but have to be treated with caution until further verification in much larger and representative cohorts is provided.

RNU2-1f as Biomarker in Other Cancer Types

Currently, a limited number of additional solid tumor types, namely, cervical cancer and esophageal squamous cell carcinoma (Chen et al. 2013; Jones et al. 2012; Takeshita et al. 2013), were found to be associated with elevated RNU2-1f levels in patient serum. Not unexpectedly, RNU2-1f were detected in these studies via standard miRNA array technology leading to the misclassification of RNU2-1f as miR-1246. In line with the lung cancer data described above, RNU2-1f were also detected to be elevated in primary ovarian cancer but not in esophageal squamous cell carcinoma (ESCC) tissue.

For ESCC, 101 patients and 46 controls were analyzed via a RNU2-1f assay, and detection of ESCC was achieved with a sensitivity and specificity of 71.3 % and 73.9 %, respectively, and with an AUC of 0.754. RNU2-1f levels correlated in ESCC patients with the T- and M-stage, likely due to the increased tumor mass associated with more advanced T-stages as well as with metastatic disease, a finding which is in line with previous reports from colon and lung carcinoma (Baraniskin et al. 2013; Mazières et al. 2013). In addition, Takeshita et al. reported that RNU2-1f may serve as a prognostic marker for esophageal carcinoma. The 2-year overall survival rate for patients with lower serum levels of RNU2-1f was 77.3 % compared to 21.7 % for patients with higher levels. Lastly, they also noted an increased RNU2-1f level in the proximal lymph node, suggestive for draining of RNU2-1f via the lymphatic system.

For cervical carcinoma, RNU2-1f together with five additional miRNAs (miR-20a, miR-2392, miR-3147, miR-3162-5p, and miR-4484) were established as a marker panel predicting lymph node metastasis with sensitivity and specificity of 86 % and 85 %, respectively.

Although not yet tested in the patient setting, it is worth to mention that serum from mice carrying human breast cancer tissue was also positive for RNU2-1f, suggesting that breast cancer is a likely additional tumor type amenable via RNU2-1f blood testing (Pigati et al. 2010).

Besides the aforementioned epithelial cancer types, one malignant hematological disease, multiple myeloma, was also found to be linked to higher RNU2-1f serum levels compared to controls. The discriminatory value of miR-1246 was rather limited (AUC < 0.67) for multiple myeloma and controls (Jones et al. 2012).

Potential Applications of RNU2-1f Tests to Prognosis, Other Diseases, or Conditions

To date, RNU2-1f detection was firmly established in serum of six solid cancer types (lung, colon, pancreas, ovarian, esophageal, and possibly also breast cancer) and one hematological malignancy (multiple myeloma; Table 1). In the absence of prostate cancer, RNU2-1f seem to be positive in a significant fraction of tumors belonging to the major tumor types such as lung, colon, and breast cancer; the latter only provided the animal data that can be confirmed in the human setting. This rather "pan"-tumor-like mode of RNU2-1f release into patient serum clearly indicates that RNU2-1f are not a tumor type-specific diagnostic biomarker, rather a more general tumor screening marker. For RNU2-1f to be successfully used in the setting of a population-type cancer screening, a very low false-positive rate for RNU2-1f tests will be essential to prevent additional costs to the healthcare system generated by the imaging tests required during follow-up of false-positive patients. The reported false-positive rates for RNU2-1f in colon and pancreatic were very low indeed (~3 %). Combined with a >80 % sensitivity to detect UICC stage II colon cancer, serum RNU2-1f measurements can be considered a valid candidate to replace the currently used noninvasive fecal occult blood screening tool known for its overall lower performance characteristics. In contrast to this exceptionally high assay specificity reported by Baraniskin et al., false-positive detection rates for RNU2-1f measurements were in the range of 8–33 % in other studies (Jones et al. 2012; Mazières et al. 2013; Takeshita et al. 2013). Off note, all RNU2-1f reports published to date differ in the RNU2-1f detection technology and normalization procedure applied to their data (Table 1). Therefore, test system harmonization followed by larger studies will be necessary to firmly establish the false-positive rate for the RNU2-1f assay, critical to its potential usefulness as a population-based screening tool. An immediate and more cautious recommendation would be to use this assay for the screening of patients from familial cancer syndromes associated with a high risk for colon and pancreatic cancer or patients with other conditions known to significantly increase cancer risk, such as smoking for lung cancer or chronic inflammatory bowel disease for colon cancer. In this context, it is important to mention that neither acute nor chronic inflammation had a strong influence on RNU2-1f serum levels. In addition, the abundance of RNU2-1f in serum was not age dependent (Baraniskin et al. 2013).

Table 1 Synopsis of published RNU2-1f assay applications in various cancer types

Cancer type	Application	Analyte	Sensitivity	Specificity	AUC	2-year survival rate RNU2-1f high	2-year survival rate RNU2-1f low	Assay	Normalizer	References
CRC (UICC II–IV)	Carcinoma diagnosis	Serum	87.2 %	97.7 %	nr	na	na	Qiagen miR-1246 qRT-PCR assay	Cel-54 spike-in control	Baraniskin et al. (2013)
PDAC	Carcinoma diagnosis	Serum	96 %	97.7 %	nr	na	na	Qiagen miR-1246 qRT-PCR assay	Cel-54 spike-in control	Baraniskin et al. (2013)
NSCLC	Carcinoma diagnosis	Serum	79 %	80 %	0.84	na	na	Exiqon custom LNA qRT-PCR assay	Cel-39 spike-in control	Mazières et al. (2013)
ESCC	Carcinoma diagnosis	Serum	71.3 %	73.9 %	0.75	na	na	TaqMan miR-1246 qRT-PCR assay	miR-16	Takeshita et al. (2013)
ESCC	Prognosis	Serum	na	na	na	21.7 %	77.3 %	TaqMan miR-1246 qRT-PCR assay	miR-16	Takeshita et al. (2013)
CSCC[a]	Prediction[a] of lymph node metastasis	Serum	96.7 %[a]	95 %[a]	0.99[a]	na	na	Takara SYBR Premix Ex Taq™ II qRT-PCR assay[a]	miR-238 *C. elegans* spike-in and endogenous U6 control	Chen et al. (2013)
MM	MM diagnosis	Serum	56.4 %	80 %	0.66	na	na	TaqMan miR-1246 qRT-PCR assay	Absolute quantification	Jones et al. (2012)
BC	Carcinoma diagnosis	Ductal lavage	nr	nr	nr	na	na	Custom stem-loop qRT-PCR	Custom spike-in control	Pigati et al. (2010)

CRC colorectal carcinoma, *PDAC* pancreatic ductal adenocarcinoma, *NSCLC* non-small-cell lung cancer, *ESCC* esophageal squamous cell carcinoma, *CSCC* cervical squamous cell carcinoma, *MM* multiple myeloma, *BC* breast cancer, *AUC* area under the curve, *nr* not reported, *na* not applicable

[a]multi-miRNA assay (miR-1246, miR-20a, miR-2392, miR-3147, miR-3162-5p, and miR-4484)

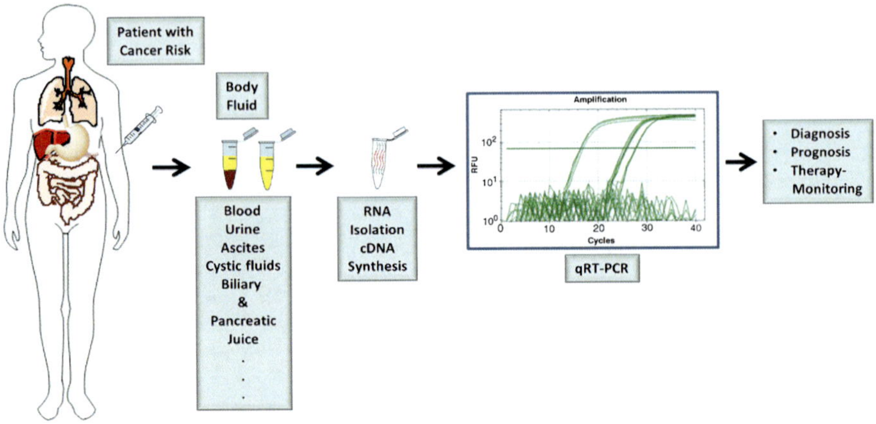

Fig. 5 Schematic workflow for RNU2-1f biomarker applications

Apart from serum and plasma, which have been successfully used for the detection of RNU2-1f, other body fluids are also potential sources to be used for RNU2-1f detection (Fig. 5). This would further increase the applicability of this new biomarker for cancer detection and help to localize the origin of RNU2-1f release to a certain organ or anatomic region. From the many body fluids (urine; stool; biliary and pancreatic juice; liquor cerebrospinalis; ascites; saliva; ductal fluids from the breast, pancreas, and biliary; cystic fluids) which are likely amenable to RNU2-1f detection, ductal lavages from the breast were already shown to contain RNU2-1f (Pigati et al. 2010). If confirmed in larger studies, it would open the possibility for women at high risk of breast cancer to use RNU2-1f measurements to supplement current early detection strategies.

Another potential clinical application is the use of RNU2-1f measurements to monitor the response to therapy in order to detect relapse or progression of the disease after the initial response. Results from three studies (Baraniskin et al. 2013; Mazières et al. 2013; Takeshita et al. 2013) showed a rapid decline of serum and plasma levels of RNU2-1f after surgical removal of tumors. Similarly one could assume declining levels of RNU2-1f in patients responding to chemotherapy or radiation and rising levels in patients with relapse of disease. In order to prove superiority of RNU2-1f detection to established serum markers already used in daily routine such as CEA in colorectal cancer, CA19-9 in pancreatic cancer, or Cyfra 21–1 in NSCLC, comparative studies are required.

Taken together, RNU2-1f are an emerging new pan-cancer biomarker which exhibit favorable characteristics for its successful implementation into the clinical routine, such as high stability in the serum and plasma and sensitive and specific detection via a standard PCR-based assay. Larger studies are now warranted in different cancerous and noncancerous conditions to fully explore and define its potential as a biomarker for diagnosis, prognosis, and therapy monitoring. Finally, a common standard RNU2-1f detection assay needs to be established to ensure comparability of study results.

Summary Points

- This chapter focuses on circulating fragments of the noncoding U2 snRNA (called RNU2-1f) as a novel biomarker for cancer.
- U2 snRNA plays a key role in the splicing of pre-mRNA and is therefore abundant in all eukaryotic cells.
- A large proportion of the identified U2 snRNA fragments share the same sequence with miR-1246, leading to the initial identification of RNU2-1f via miR-1246-specific assays.
- The current data in the literature support that miR-1246 is likely a pseudo-miRNA; thus miR-1246-related data should be attributed to U2 snRNA fragments.
- Elevated U2 snRNA fragment levels were to date reported in the blood of lung, pancreatic, colorectal, cervical, esophageal, and likely also breast cancer patients as well as in patients suffering from multiple myeloma.
- The present data suggest that a fragment of RNU2-1 is likely a new pan-tumor biomarker candidate which can be applied as a screening tool in cancer-risk populations and for therapy response and relapse monitoring and may also have some prognostic value.
- The high stability of RNU2-1 fragments warrants its evaluation in additional body fluids where tumors potentially drain RNU2-1f, such as urine; stool; biliary and pancreatic juice; liquor cerebrospinalis; ascites; saliva; ductal fluids from the breast, pancreas, and biliary; as well as cystic fluids.

References

Arroyo JD, Chevillet JR, Kroh EM, et al. Argonaute2 complexes carry a population of circulating microRNAs independent of vesicles in human plasma. Proc Natl Acad Sci U S A. 2011;108:5003–8. doi:10.1073/pnas.1019055108.

Bach D, Fuereder J, Karbiener M, et al. Comprehensive analysis of alterations in the miRNome in response to photodynamic treatment. J Photochem Photobiol B. 2013;120C:74–81. doi:10.1016/j.jphotobiol.2013.01.012.

Baraniskin A, Nöpel-Dünnebacke S, Ahrens M, et al. Circulating U2 small nuclear RNA fragments as a novel diagnostic biomarker for pancreatic and colorectal adenocarcinoma. Int J cancer. 2013;132:E48–57. doi:10.1002/ijc.27791.

Biggiogera M, Bottone MG, Martin TE, et al. Still immunodetectable nuclear RNPs are extruded from the cytoplasm of spontaneously apoptotic thymocytes. Exp Cell Res. 1997;234:512–20.

Brenner H, Hoffmeister M, Brenner G, et al. Expected reduction of colorectal cancer incidence within 8 years after introduction of the German screening colonoscopy programme: estimates based on 1,875,708 screening colonoscopies. Eur J Cancer (Oxford, England: 1990). 2009;45:2027–33. doi:10.1016/j.ejca.2009.02.017.

Burroughs AM, Ando Y, de Hoon ML, et al. Deep-sequencing of human Argonaute-associated small RNAs provides insight into miRNA sorting and reveals Argonaute association with RNA fragments of diverse origin. RNA Biol. 2011;8:158–77. doi:10.4161/rna.8.1.14300.

Chen J, Yao D, Li Y, et al. Serum microRNA expression levels can predict lymph node metastasis in patients with early-stage cervical squamous cell carcinoma. Int J Mol Med. 2013;32:557–67. doi:10.3892/ijmm.2013.1424.

Fearon EF, Vogelstein B. A genetic model for colorectal tumorigenesis. Cell. 1990;61:759–67.

Halicka HD, Bedner E, Darzynkiewicz Z. Segregation of RNA and separate packaging of DNA and RNA in apoptotic bodies during apoptosis. Exp Cell Res. 2000;260:248–56.

Hanahan D, Weinberg RA. Hallmarks of cancer: the next generation. Cell. 2011;144:646–74.

Jemal A, Bray F, Ferlay J. Global cancer statistics. 2011;61:69–90. doi:10.3322/caac.20107. Available

Jones CI, Zabolotskaya MV, King AJ, et al. Identification of circulating microRNAs as diagnostic biomarkers for use in multiple myeloma. Br J Cancer. 2012;107:1987–96. doi:10.1038/bjc.2012.525.

Kambach C, Walke S, Young R, et al. Crystal structures of two Sm protein complexes and their implications for the assembly of the spliceosomal snRNPs. Cell. 1999;96:375–87.

Li A, Yu J, Kim H, et al. MicroRNA array analysis finds elevated serum miR-1290 accurately distinguishes patients with low-stage pancreatic cancer from healthy and disease controls. Clin Cancer Res Off J Am Assoc Cancer Res. 2013. doi:10.1158/1078-0432.CCR-12-3092.

Liao J, Yu L, Mei Y, et al. Small nucleolar RNA signatures as biomarkers for non-small-cell lung cancer. Mol Cancer. 2010;9:198. doi:10.1186/1476-4598-9-198.

Madhavan D, Cuk K, Burwinkel B, Yang R. Cancer diagnosis and prognosis decoded by blood-based circulating microRNA signatures. Front Genet. 2013;4:116. doi:10.3389/fgene.2013.00116.

Mazières J, Catherinne C, Delfour O, et al. Alternative processing of the U2 small nuclear RNA produces a 19-22 nt fragment with relevance for the detection of non-small cell lung cancer in human serum. PLoS One. 2013;8:e60134. doi:10.1371/journal.pone.0060134.

Palma J, Yaddanapudi SC, Pigati L, et al. MicroRNAs are exported from malignant cells in customized particles. Nucleic Acids Res. 2012;40:9125–38. doi:10.1093/nar/gks656.

Patent application SNRNA RNU2 – 1 ALS TUMORMARKER, European patent office, PCT/EP 2012/064321, 22 July 2011

Pigati L, Yaddanapudi SCS, Iyengar R, et al. Selective release of microRNA species from normal and malignant mammary epithelial cells. PLoS One. 2010;5:e13515.

Takeshita N, Hoshino I, Mori M, et al. Serum microRNA expression profile: miR-1246 as a novel diagnostic and prognostic biomarker for oesophageal squamous cell carcinoma. Br J Cancer. 2013;108:644–52. doi:10.1038/bjc.2013.8.

Taylor DP, Cannon-Albright LA, Sweeney C, et al. Comparison of compliance for colorectal cancer screening and surveillance by colonoscopy based on risk. Genet Med Off J Am Coll Med Genet. 2011;13:737–43.

Valadi H, Ekström K, Bossios A, et al. Exosome-mediated transfer of mRNAs and microRNAs is a novel mechanism of genetic exchange between cells. Nat Cell Biol. 2007;9:654–9. doi:10.1038/ncb1596.

Will CL, Lührmann R. Splicing of a rare class of introns by the U12-dependent spliceosome. Biol Chem. 2005;386:713–24. doi:10.1515/BC.2005.084.

Part II

Bladder, Kidney, Liver and Lung

Centrosome Amplification as Biomarkers in Bladder Cancer Using Touch Biopsy and Bladder Washing Cytological Specimens

11

Hideyasu Matsuyama

Contents

Abstract

This chapter discusses the influence of chromosomal instability and its causative phenomenon, centrosome amplification (CA), and on patient prognosis; summarizes recent urine biomarker developments; and details their implications for prognosis and decision making in non-muscle-invasive bladder cancer (NMIBC). Several urine biomarkers have been reported as FDA-approved adjunctive tests for use in the initial diagnosis of bladder cancer and surveillance of patients with bladder cancer, and a few have been developed as markers for the prediction of patient outcome. CA is a compelling phenomenon that is closely associated with aneuploidy and tumorigenesis. Recent studies have revealed that overexpression of Aurora-A is a major cause of CA and that CA identified using bladder washing solution predicts disease progression in NMIBC. Other urine

H. Matsuyama (✉)
Department of Urology, Graduate School of Medicine, Yamaguchi University, Ube, Japan
e-mail: hidde@yamaguchi-u.ac.jp

V.R. Preedy, V.B. Patel (eds.), *Biomarkers in Cancer, Biomarkers in Disease: Methods, Discoveries and Applications*,
DOI 10.1007/978-94-007-7681-4_23

biomarkers, such as the combination of *FGFR3* mutation and Ki-67 (MIB-1) overexpression and UroVysion (multicolor fluorescence in situ hybridization kit for detecting copy number aberrations in chromosomes 3, 7, and 17, and the 9p21 locus), are promising for predicting disease progression and tumor recurrence in NMIBC. Further validation with a prospective multi-institutional study is needed for augmentation or replacement of conventional markers with new biomarkers for clinical management of patients with NMIBC.

List of Abbreviations

AURKA	Aurora Kinase A Gene
BRCA1	Breast Cancer Susceptibility Gene I
BWC	Bladder Washing Cytology
CA	Centrosome Amplification
CCND1	Cyclin D1 Gene
CGH	Comparative Genomic Hybridization
CIN	Chromosomal Instability
EAU	European Association of Urology
FDA	Food and Drug Administration
FISH	Fluorescence In Situ Hybridization
FGFR3	Fibroblast Growth Factor Receptor 3
MIBC	Muscle-Invasive Bladder Cancer
MSI	Microsatellite Instability
NMIBC	Non-muscle-Invasive Bladder Cancer
PBS	Phosphate-Buffered Saline
PLK-1	Polo-Like Kinase 1
Rb1	Retinoblastoma 1 Gene
ROS	Reactive Oxygen Species
TURBT	Transurethral Resection of the Bladder Tumor
XRCC2	X-ray Repair Complementing Defective Repair in Chinese Hamster Cells 2

Key Facts of Centrosome Amplification

- Centrosomes are organelles comprising the protein assembly of the major microtubule-organizing center that forms a bipolar spindle pole and plays a key role in the accurate segregation of chromosomes during mitosis.
- Alterations of cell cycle-related genes such as p53, AURA, and BubR1 cause CA defined as three or more centrosomes per cell.
- CA occurs frequently in a variety of malignancies, including bladder cancer, and causes chromosomal instability (CIN) with unfavorable prognosis.
- Specimens from presurgical touch preparations or BWC detect CA equally well and predict patient outcomes including recurrence and disease progression.

Definitions of Words and Terms

Aneuploidy Abnormal number of chromosomes.

Aurora-A A serine–threonine kinase with a variety of functions in centrosome maturation and separation, bipolar spindle assembly, chromosome alignment and the transition from prophase to metaphase, and cytokinesis. Overexpression of Aurora-A causes CA and tetraploidy, which eventually leads to CIN.

Cell Division Separation of a cell into two daughter cells.

Checkpoints Monitors of cell cycle progression that confirm that DNA replication (S phase) and segregation (mitosis) have occurred in an orderly fashion. Checkpoints delay the cell cycle until conditions are met or induce apoptosis under irreversible DNA damage or high levels of stress. Checkpoints are activated by DNA damage (G1, S, and G2/M checkpoint), stress responses (G1–G2 checkpoint), or mitotic disorders (mitotic checkpoint).

CIN Continuous gain or loss of chromosomes with structural chromosome aberrations in cell populations during abnormal cell division.

Cytokinesis Failure Inability to separate two daughter cells during cell division. Cytokinesis is a final stage of cell division via cleavage furrow formation, midbody maturation, and abscission of daughter cell. Failure to complete cytokinesis has been proposed to promote tumorigenesis via tetraploid formation.

Immunofluorescence Staining Fluorescence microscopy technique for visualizing cellular components with specific binding of fluorescent-labeled antibodies to antigens of interest.

Hybridization Association of two complementary DNA or RNA strands to form double-stranded molecules for detecting specific DNA or RNA sequences of interest.

Mitotic Spindle A football-shaped structure that appears temporarily during mitosis, which captures the chromosomes and pulls them to the opposite side of a dividing cell.

Polymerase Chain Reaction A technique to amplify a specific DNA segment through multiple cycles of DNA synthesis from a primer and a nucleic acid sequence of base pairs with a complementary template starting point.

Introduction

Bladder cancer is the second most common genitourinary cancer, and its management involves the greatest expenditure than that for other solid tumors, including surveillance costs after transurethral resection. Approximately 75 % of bladder cancer cases are low grade and non-muscle-invasive bladder cancer (NMIBC) for which transurethral resection of the bladder tumor is curative, whereas tumor recurrence and progression, defined as a muscle-invasive tumor when recurrent or the appearance of distant metastases, develop in 70 % and 15–30 % of these cases, respectively. Muscle-invasive bladder cancer, comprising the remaining 25 % of bladder cancer cases, has poor prognosis despite radical cystectomy (total removal of the bladder), with a 5-year survival of 50–60 %. This outcome highlights the urgent need for biomarkers predicting tumor progression in NMIBC (Netto and Cheng 2012).

Centrosomes are organelles comprising the protein assembly of the major microtubule-organizing center that forms the bipolar spindle pole and plays a central role in the accurate segregation of chromosome during mitosis. Thus, the number of centrosomes is strictly regulated by cell cycle-related proteins such as p53 (Fukasawa et al. 1996), STK15/BTAK/Aurora-A kinase (Zhou et al. 1998), Polo-like kinase (Li and Li 2006), or BubR1. Recent evidence has suggested that centrosome amplification (CA), which is defined as the presence of three or more centrosomes per cell, occurs frequently in a variety of malignancies, including urothelial cancer.

CA was first proposed in the early 1900s by Boveri, who stated that an excessive number of centrosomes lead to aneuploidy and cause cancer. Since then, CA has been associated with oncogenetic processes and accepted as a hypothesis of oncogenesis. Knudson (1971) introduced the two-hit theory in the 1970s; Rb1 was discovered as a tumor suppressor gene in the 1980s (Cavenee et al. 1983), and Vogelstein and colleagues proposed in the 1990s that multistep gene alterations transform tissue from adenoma into colorectal cancer. In 1997, Lengauer et al. proposed the concept of chromosomal instability (CIN), an early oncogenic event affecting proto-oncogene activation or the structural loss of tumor suppressor genes. The concept of CIN triggered the reevaluation of CA because aneuploidy changes cellular phenotypes more efficiently than gene mutation does (Duesberg 1999), and CA may lead to CIN by producing unequal segregation of chromosomes. Fujiwara et al. (2005) have shown direct association of CIN with oncogenesis in a study revealing that hyperploid cell (tetraploid)-associated CA induced by cytokinesis failure transforms p53−/− mammary epithelial cells into cancer cells in a mouse model. In this chapter, the clinical significance of CA in bladder cancer and new molecular biomarkers using urine (or cytological bladder washing) specimens for the prediction of tumor progression in NMIBC are discussed.

Mechanism of Centrosome Amplification

Centrosomes, organelles normally localized at the periphery of the nucleus, play a key role in cell division by forming bipolar spindle poles that anchor microtubules during mitosis (Fig. 1). To divide a cell into two daughter cells, a centrosome must duplicate once before the next mitosis. During S and G2, the procentrioles – central parts of centrosome – elongate, and two centrosomes mature and are generated by late G2 (Fig. 2). If centrosomes duplicate more than once within a cell cycle, CA occurs. CA is frequently seen in cells with cytokinesis failure owing to overexpression of Aurora-A kinase (Goepfert et al. 2002) or mutations of cell cycle regulator genes such as p53 (Kawamura et al. 2004). Cytokinesis is the final stage of cell division during which the two daughter cells separate completely. Failure of this process in mammals is associated with carcinogenesis. Cytokinesis failure causes tetraploid (binucleated) cell formation with simple centrosome duplication in G1. Although most tetraploid cells go into apoptosis due to G1 arrest, provided p53 is wild type and altered p53 produces CA in multinucleated cells owing to cell cycle progression (Fig. 3).

CA has several possible mechanisms: (1) Overduplication of centrioles during S phase; (2) cytokinesis failure – doubling of the genome as well as the number of centrosomes; (3) amplified centrosomes arising from de novo assembly and occurring independently of preexisting centrioles induced by overexpression of the pericentrin; (4) cell fusion, which occurs in both nonmalignant

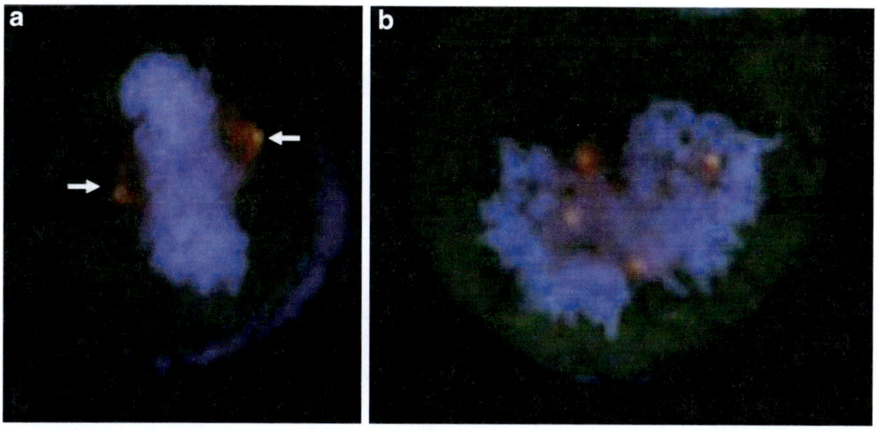

Fig. 1 Relationship between centrosome number and chromosomal segregation. Normal copy number of centrosomes (*arrow*) forms bipolar spindle pole. The microtubule is anchored between the spindle and chromosome on the equatorial plate, followed by the start of segregation (**a**). Centrosome amplification causes unequal segregation of chromosomes (**b**). Immunofluorescence staining was applied by using anti-pericentrin antibody for centrosomes (*orange*); chromosomes (*blue*) were counterstained with 4,6-diamidino-2-phenylindole (DAPI)

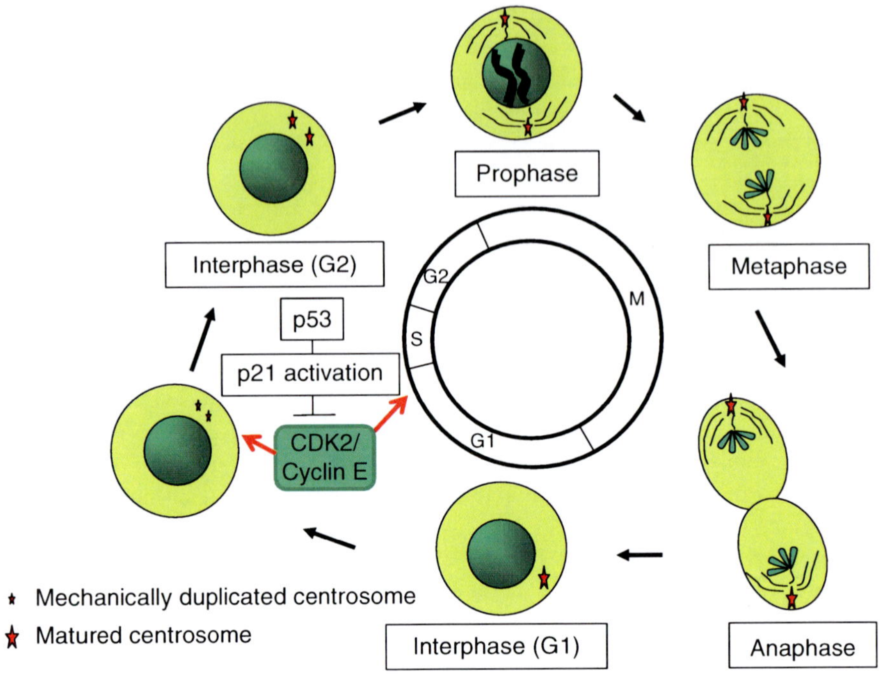

Fig. 2 Cell cycle and centrosomes. Centrosome duplication starts in late G1 by triggering CDK2/cyclin E expression, which is also a key event starting DNA synthesis and entrance into S phase. Centrosomes in late G2 are mechanically duplicated but not mature. Mature centrosomes are formed during S and G2 by proteins such as Aurora-A

(syncytial formation) and malignant tissues – e.g., human papillomavirus-induced cell fusion might trigger the development of cervical cancer; and (5) mitotic skipping (slippage) in which the cell cycle of malignant cells enters G1 phase owing to disturbances in the mitotic (or spindle) checkpoint or escape from mitotic catastrophe (Anderhub et al. 2012). Figure 3 depicts possible mechanisms of CA and the progression to aneuploid cells via a tetraploid cell. Recent studies have suggested that tetraploid cells may lead to malignant cells when combined with p53 mutation (Fukasawa et al. 1996; Kawamura et al. 2004; Fujiwara et al. 2005). Deregulation of mitotic checkpoints is also frequently reported to cause CA. BubR1, a checkpoint protein regulating the proper attachment of microtubules to the kinetochores of chromosomes, inhibits the onset of anaphase, which leads polyploid cells to mitotic catastrophe. Defects in BubR1 are known to contribute to CIN via chromosome destabilization through Polo-like kinase activation as well as CA. Interestingly, overexpression of BubR1 seems to confer a higher malignant potential to tumor cells because of its strong association with CIN, DNA aneuploidy, CA, and disease progression in bladder cancer. Alternatively, DNA damage by irradiation or cytotoxic reagents may cause CA if *BRCA1*, *XRCC2*, or DNA repair genes acquire genetic alterations. Such alterations provoke the G2/M

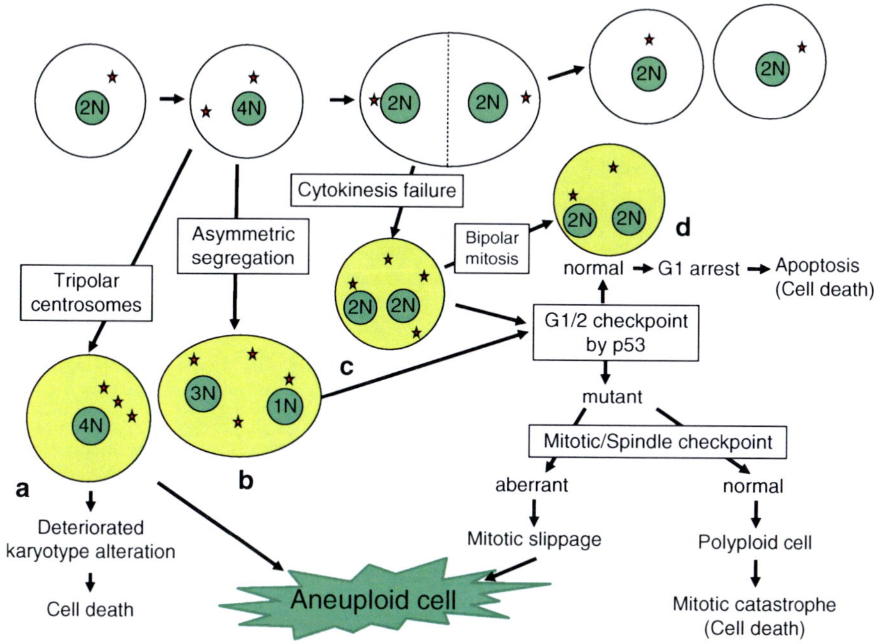

Fig. 3 Relationship between centrosome amplification and tetraploid cells. A sequence of white cells (*top line*) denotes cell division with normal DNA content and centrosomes. A substantial portion of tetraploid cells (*yellow*) arising from tripolar centrosomes owing to reduplication of one duplicated centrosome (*a*), asymmetric segregation owing to furrow regression (*b*), and cytokinesis failure owing to Aurora-A overexpression (*c*) will ultimately develop aneuploid cells if other checkpoints are disturbed. A small portion of tetraploid cells may reproduce permanent tetraploid cells owing to (pseudo-) bipolar mitosis (*d*). Star: centrosome, 2N: diploid cell, 4N: tetraploid cell

checkpoint, which results in cell arrest, allowing centrosomes to mature and gain duplication competency.

Whether CA arises as a consequence of oncogene-induced changes or initiates cancer formation in humans, it remains unclear. However, several studies have demonstrated that premalignant tissue harboring CA develops into tumors in an experimental mouse model (Bergmann et al. 2005). Taken together, the evidence suggests a causative role of CA in consequential aneuploidy and eventual tumor development (Anderhub et al. 2012).

Copy Number Aberrations and Centrosome Amplification

Accumulating evidence has suggested that nonrandom copy number aberrations of chromosomes 7, 9, and 17 and mutation of p53 (Sarkis et al. 1993) occur frequently in bladder cancer, and CA could cause copy number aberrations in chromosomes (aneuploidy) in bladder cancer (Kawamura et al. 2004;

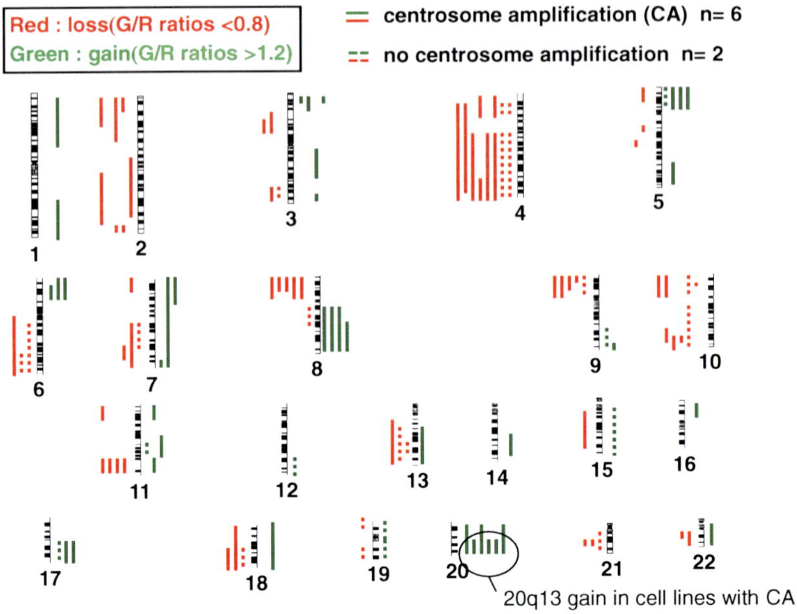

Fig. 4 Summary of array comparative genomic hybridization (array CGH) data in eight bladder cancer cell lines stratified by the status of centrosome amplification (*CA*). *Red* and *green lines* denote the loss and gain, respectively, of copy number of the corresponding region. Six cell lines with CA (*solid line*) demonstrated chromosomal gain of the 20q13 region, in which the Aurora-A gene (*AURA*) is located, whereas no copy number alteration on 20q13 was detected in two cell lines without CA (*dotted line*)

Yamamoto et al. 2004, 2006). The number of centrosomes seems to be directly proportional to the number of chromosomes in cells with CA, whereas large intercellular variation in chromosomal copy number is detected in cells with normal numbers of centrosomes. The data imply that each amplified centrosome plays a crucial role in chromosomal segregation, and cells without CA seem to depend on various pathways to induce aneuploidy in human bladder cell lines. Interestingly, cancer cells with four centrosomes more frequently display even numbers of chromosomes in cell lines showing both Aurora-A and p53 overexpression. As mentioned above, Aurora-A kinase overexpression may cause cytokinesis failure, which would produce an even number of centrosomes as well as tetraploid cells.

Figure 4 depicts data obtained with array comparative genomic hybridization (array CGH) stratified by the presence or absence of CA using eight established bladder cancer cell lines. A close association occurs between CA and gain of copy number of 20q13 on which *AURKA*, a gene encoding Aurora-A, is located. The data were confirmed in clinical bladder cancer specimens (Table 1), in which a significant correlation occurred among CA, 20q13 gain, and Aurora-A overexpression. Interestingly, all cases with 20q13 gain had CA. These data clearly demonstrate that overexpression of Aurora-A derived from the copy number gain of 20q13 is a

Table 1 Correlation among centrosome amplification, Aurora-A overexpression, and copy number gain of 20q13

		20q13 gain			Aurora-A overexpression		
		+	−	*P*-value	+	−	*P*-value
CA	+	30	19	<0.0001	43	6	<0.0001
	−	0	33		7	26	

causative mechanism of CA in clinical bladder cancer through cytokinesis failure (Yamamoto et al. 2004). Park et al. (2008) have reported that overexpression of *AURKA* (Aurora-A kinase) can cause both CA and aneuploidy in urothelial cells, and *AURKA* copy number is a promising biomarker for the detection of bladder cancer. This conclusion is supported by the results of another study that showed that 20q13 gain (Aurora-A overexpression), CA, or both have significant association with CIN, and patients with such alterations have significantly worse prognoses (Yamamoto et al. 2006).

Clinical Significance of Centrosome Amplification

Although CA has become a promising and pivotal phenomenon in both oncogenesis and cancer progression, few reports have described its clinical application as a prognostic biomarker. Yamamoto et al. (2004) have reported a striking association between CA caused by 20q13 gain (Aurora-A overexpression) and prognosis in bladder cancer. They detected CA under a fluorescent microscope by immunofluorescence staining with a mouse anti-γ-tubulin antibody and defined it as the presence of more than 5 % of a cell population in a specimen with three or more centrosomes per cell. A cutoff value of 5 % was set on the basis of a simple experiment using established bladder cancer cell lines. Two distinct groups with different biological characteristics have been identified. One group (six cell lines) was characterized by 20q13 gain on CGH and fluorescence in situ hybridization (FISH) and Aurora-A overexpression, with %CA (fraction of cell population with three or more centrosomes per cell) ranging from 6.1 % to 16 %. The other group (two cell lines) was characterized by no 20q13 gain and no Aurora-A overexpression, with %CA ranging from 0.7 % to 1.2 %.

Of clinical specimens from 50 patients with bladder cancer, 30 were positive for CA (CA+ patients). The mean %CA was 15.5 % in CA+ patients but only 1.7 % in CA− patients. CA was significantly associated with tumor grade, DNA ploidy (aneuploidy), CIN, recurrence, and disease progression. CIN was defined as more than 25 % of the average variant fractions, the sum of the fractions of non-modal chromosome number, in chromosomes 7, 9, and 17, with reference to the data of Lengauer et al. (1997). The mean variant fractions of chromosomes 7, 9, and 17 in patients with CA were 33.1 %, 34.6 %, and 34.0 %, whereas fractions of 9.4 %, 19.4 %, and 11.7 %, respectively, were found in those without CA ($p < 0.0001, p < 0.0005, p < 0.0001$, respectively). All of the 20 cases with aneuploidy were CA+. Tumor recurrence occurred in 23 of 43 patients with NMIBC. Multivariate analysis revealed CA+ as the strongest predictor for tumor recurrence.

Two types of genetic instabilities occur: (1) microsatellite instability (MSI) characterized by mutation of DNA repair genes with favorable prognosis and (2) CIN defined as tumors with a large intercellular variation in chromosomal copy number with poor prognosis. To elucidate the differences in biological characteristics between the two types of genetic instability in bladder cancer, Yamamoto et al. (2006) studied mismatched repair proteins (MLH1 and MSH2), Aurora-A, p53 protein, copy number of chromosomes 3, 9, 17, and 20q13, and CA in 100 bladder cancer specimens. Decreased expression level of either MLH1 or MSH2, surrogate markers for MSI, was detected in only 9 (9 %) cases with favorable prognosis and no association with CA, 20q13 gain, or overexpression of p53 or Aurora-A. Furthermore, MSI was a significant predictor of favorable progression-free survival. CIN cancer was detected in 49 (49 %) cases with unfavorable prognosis and significant association with CA, 20q13 gain, and overexpression of p53 and Aurora-A. CA proved to be the strongest predictor for disease progression on multivariate analysis.

The authors further grouped the 100 cases into group 1, with tumors displaying both 20q13 gain and CA (42 cases); group 2, with tumors displaying CA but no 20q13 gain (22); and group 3, with tumors lacking both 20q13 gain and CA (36). All MSI cases were included in group 3. Frequency of CIN was significantly different among the groups (group 1: 95.2 %, group 2: 31.8 %, and group 3: 5.6 %, $p < 0.0001$). Patients in group 3 had significantly better prognosis than those in groups 1 or 2. These results suggest that CA predicts patient prognosis, and the addition of an Aurora-A-related molecular marker may improve objective classification similar to that with molecular grading (van Rhijn et al. 2003). Figure 5 depicts cells with and without CIN, which were determined using FISH analysis. Likewise, positive correlation between CIN positivity, centrosome abnormalities, and *CCND1* (cyclin D1 gene) amplification has been reported in T1G3 bladder cancer (Del Rey et al. 2010). As mentioned previously, cyclin D1 overexpression is a key genetic event for not only CA but also cell cycle progression. Patients with *CCND1* amplification in primary bladder tumors had a significantly shorter overall survival.

Array-based CGH using 70 urothelial carcinomas demonstrated that the total DNA copy number aberrations and frequency of CIN were larger in tumors with CA than in those without CA, and these parameters were more closely associated with CA than with the subjectively assigned tumor grade. DNA copy number gains at 20p12.2, 5p15.2, 5p15.31, and 17q25.3 and losses at 17p12, 8p22, 2q37.3, 5q31.1, and 2q37.3 were more frequent in tumors with CA than in those without CA (Yamamoto et al. 2011). Figure 6 illustrates the hypothesis of the varying mechanism of CA in bladder cancer. Centrosome amplification may occur owing to Aurora-A overexpression through genotoxic stress such as reactive oxygen species, irradiation, or chemotherapy. This type of CA is temporary, however, and is abolished if p53 is intact. Although p53 is altered, polyploid (aneuploid) cells with CA enter mitotic catastrophe provided the mitotic checkpoint intact. A small

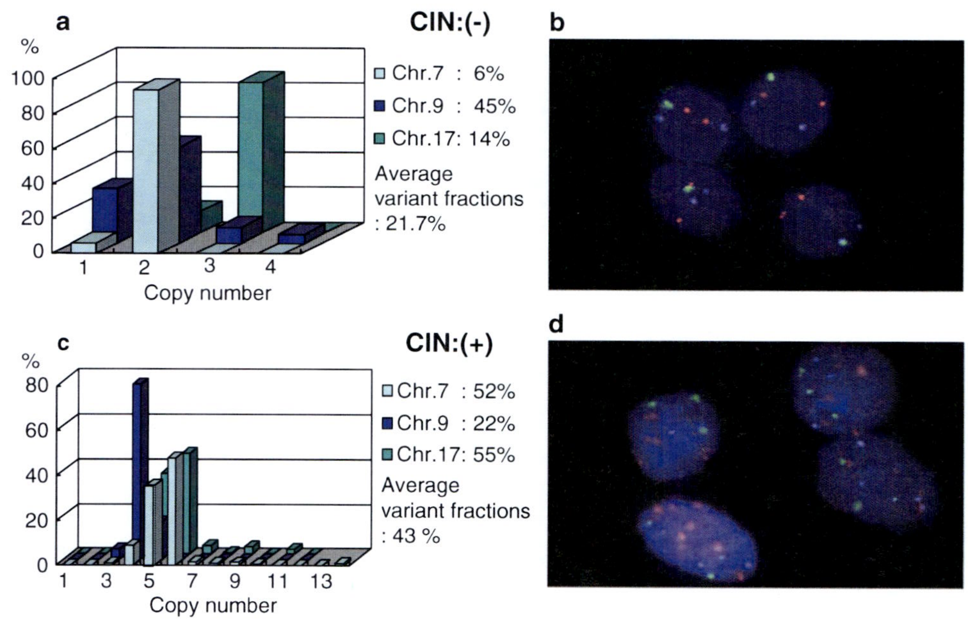

Fig. 5 Bladder cancer cell lines with and without chromosomal instability (*CIN*). CIN was defined as more than 25 % of the average variant fractions of chromosomes 7 (*red*), 9 (*green*), and 17 (*blue*) on fluorescence in situ hybridization (FISH). Histogram of the copy number of chromosomes 7, 9, and 17 in KK47 without CIN by an average variant fraction of 21.7 % (**a**) and in transitional cell carcinoma-sup with CIN by an average variant fraction of 43 % (**c**). Representative cells without (**b**) and with (**d**) CIN on FISH

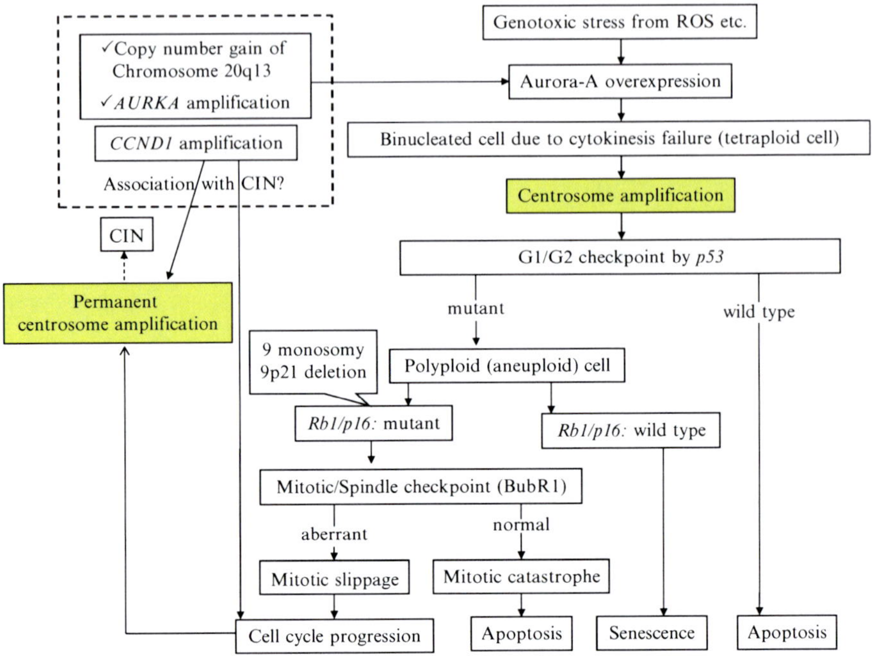

Fig. 6 Hypothesis of the mechanism of centrosome amplification in bladder cancer. *ROS* (reactive oxygen species), *Rb1* (retinoblastoma 1 gene), *CIN* (chromosomal instability), *CCND1* (cyclin D1 gene)

population of cells with CA advance to cell cycle progression (mitotic slippage), followed by acquisition of permanent CA, eventually resulting in CIN. Gain of copy number of chromosome 20q13 (or *AURKA* amplification) or *CCND1* amplification may follow a pathway to produce CA, likely in association with CIN (see Fig. 6).

Although the clinical significance of CA as a biomarker for patient prognosis has been reported, the specimens originated from touch biopsies that were prepared by gently pressing the resected tumor onto slide glass. Miyachika et al. (2013) first reported CA as a urine (bladder washing cytology [BWC]) biomarker for the prediction of disease progression in NMIBC. Figure 7 shows a representative case with CA determined using a touch biopsy specimen and a BWC specimen. In this study, the BWC specimen was prepared with a bladder washing solution of 90 mL of saline that was centrifuged at 1,500 rpm for 9 min, after which a drop of resuspended solution (phosphate-buffered saline) was placed onto a slide glass coated with poly-L-lysine. Immunofluorescence staining and CA determination were carried out according to a method as described elsewhere (Yamamoto et al. 2004). CA was identified (CA+) if >5 % of cells contained three centrosomes per cell (see Fig. 7) under an epifluorescence microscope (BX51; Olympus, Tokyo, Japan) equipped with triple band-pass filter.

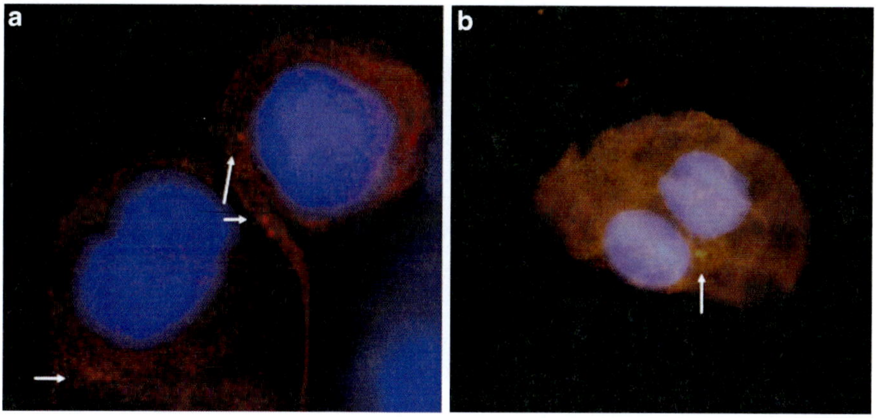

Fig. 7 Case presentation of centrosome amplification (CA) predicting disease progression. A 66-year-old man was diagnosed with non-muscle-invasive bladder cancer and underwent transurethral resection of the bladder tumor on February 13, 2007. The pathological diagnosis was transitional cell carcinoma (TCC), grade 3, pT1 (invaded into submucosal layer). Both a touch biopsy specimen from the tumor (**a**) and bladder washing specimen (**b**) showed three centrosomes (CA; *arrow*). The percentage of cells with CA in the touch (**a**) and bladder washing (**b**) specimens was 15 % and 17 %, respectively. Five months later, the patient displayed disease progression with the pathological diagnosis of TCC, grade 3, pT2 (muscle-layer invasion). Indirect immunofluorescence staining was performed using a rabbit pericentrin polyclonal antibody (Sigma, St. Louis, MO) followed by Alexa 594-conjugated goat anti-rabbit antibody (Molecular Probes, Eugene, OR) and counterstaining with 4′,6-diamidino-2-phenylindole (DAPI)

Disease progression was detected in 11.5 % (9 of 78) of NMIBC patients. Multivariate analysis revealed that CA in BWC specimens was the strongest predictor for disease progression (hazard ratio, 2.22; 95 % confidence interval [CI], 1.13–4.90; $p = 0.022$). Skepticism may arise about contamination with nonmalignant cells, including leukocytes or epithelial cells. Significant correlation in %CA was observed between BWC and touch biopsy preparation ($r = 0.56$, $p < 0.0001$), with a categorical concordance of CA status of 92.3 % between BWC and touch biopsy specimens (Miyachika et al. 2013). Aspiration specimens have yielded significantly higher %CA in cancer tissue compared with that in benign tissue in breast cancer (4.86 % vs. 2.77 %) (Guo et al. 2007). Taken together, CA in cancer cells seems more distinct than that in nonmalignant cells, even in specimens contaminated with nonmalignant cells.

Other Biomarkers Using Urine (Bladder Washing Cytology)

Urine biomarkers reported in the literature are listed in Table 2. NMP22 (Matritech Inc., Newton, MA), BTA stat (Polymedco Inc., Cortlandt Manor, NY), BTA TRAK® test (Polymedco Inc.), UroVysion® (Vysis–Abbott Laboratories,

Table 2 Urine biomarkers reported in the literature

Urinary marker	Clinical application	Target	Method	References
NMP22	Detection, surveillance	Nuclear matrix protein 22: nuclear mitotic apparatus protein	Qualitative point-of-care test	Grossman et al. (2005)
BTA stat	Detection, recurrence	Bladder tumor antigen: complement factor H-related protein	Immunochromatographic qualitative assay	Schroeder et al. (2004)
ImmunoCyt	Detection	Three fluorescent-labeled monoclonal antibodies	Immunofluorescence staining	Pfister et al. (2003)
Telomerase				
TRAP	Detection	Telomeric repeat amplification protocol	RT-PCR	Sanchini et al. (2005)
hTERT	Detection	Subunit of telomerase	RT-PCR	Melissourgos et al. (2003)
Lewis X	Detection	Blood group antigen	Immunocytochemical staining	Golijanin et al. (1995)
Survivin	Detection	Anti-apoptotic gene	qRT-PCR	Eissa et al. (2010)
Hyaluronic acid				
HA	Detection, recurrence	Extracellular glycosaminoglycan	Immunohistochemical staining, enzyme-linked immunosorbent assay-like assays	Lokeshwar et al. (2000)
HAase	Detection	Hyaluronidase: production of small fragment of HA	Enzyme-linked immunosorbent assay-like assay	Lokeshwar et al. (2000)
HYAL-1	Detection	Hyaluronoglucosaminidase-1: a specific HAase	qRT-PCR	Eissa et al. (2010)
HA/HAase	Detection		Two enzyme-linked immunosorbent assay-like assays	Lokeshwar (2002)
BLCA-4	Detection	Nuclear matrix protein specific to bladder cancer tissues	Sandwich immunoassay using two antibodies	Konety et al. (2000)
CertNDx	Detection, recurrence, molecular grading	FGFR 3, MMP-2, Twist-1, Nid-2, Vimentin, Ki-67	PCR-SSCP, Immunocytostaining	Knowles (2007), van Rhijn et al. (2003)
UroVysion	Detection, recurrence, progression	Chromosomes 3, 7, 17, 9p21	Fluorescence in situ hybridization	Sokolova et al. (2000), Matsuyama et al. (2013)

Des Plaines, IL), CertNDx™ (Predictive Biosciences, Lexington, MA), and ImmunoCyt™ test (DiagnoCure Inc., Quebec, Canada) have been approved by the FDA for urinary tumor marker testing. All urinary tests except ImmunoCyt™ are approved as adjuncts for the initial diagnosis of bladder cancer and surveillance of patients with bladder cancer in conjunction with standard procedures. NMP22 and BTA stat are point-of-care tests. Most urinary biomarkers have been established with the aim of increasing detection capability (sensitivity) compared with that of conventional urine cytology, particularly in low-grade/low-stage NMIBC. However, the cost, procedural complexity, or false positivity owing to inflammation of other tests may hamper their use as replacements for urine cytology as the gold standard in clinical practice.

Notably, CertNDx™ may become a promising urinary biomarker not only for detection but also for predicting patient outcome. Accumulating evidence has suggested that *FGFR3* mutation is strongly associated with low-grade/low-stage NMIBC (Knowles 2007) and is considered a potential biomarker for early recurrence (Hernandez et al. 2006). Molecular grading of urothelial cancer with Ki-67 (or MIB-1) and *FGFR3* is known to have superior predictive capability compared with that of pathological grade. Three molecular grades (mGs) are identified: mG1 (mutation; normal expression), favorable prognosis; mG2 (no mutation; normal expression), intermediate prognosis; and mG3 (no mutation; high expression), poor prognosis (van Rhijn et al. 2003). Urine can also be used to measure Ki-67 with quantitative reverse transcription polymerase chain reaction or immunocytological staining.

Multicolor FISH (Matsuyama et al. 1994) using urine or bladder washing cytological specimens was developed based on the numerical alterations of specific chromosomes such as 3, 7, 17, or 9p21 loci. UroVysion® can simultaneously detect such nonrandom numerical aberrations using several DNA probes labeled with various fluorescence colors and is now commercially available and commonly used in clinical management. Chromosome 9 alterations, which are frequent and well-known chromosomal aberrations in bladder cancer, are the earliest genetic alterations reported in the development of the malignancy (Knowles 2007), and monosomy of chromosome 9 may be linked with early recurrence of MNIBC (Tsukamoto et al. 2002). In particular, deletions in 9p21 (p16 locus) seem to be a promising prognostic marker for tumor progression (Kawauchi et al. 2009; Matsuyama et al. 2013). Urine cytology and FISH in post-Bacillus Calmette–Guerin using bladder washings solution seem to be predictive of failure of Bacillus Calmette–Guerin therapy in patients with NMIBC (Whitson et al. 2009). Matsuyama et al. (2013) have reported that higher variant fraction (the sum of the non-modal copy number fraction of each chromosome; see Fig. 5), defined as $\geq$16 %, and higher %deletion of 9p21 (fraction of null or one copy number of the 9p21 locus), defined as $\geq$12 %, may predict disease progression and recurrence, respectively, whereas the Maffezzini risk criteria failed to predict outcome. The authors examined BWC specimens collected just before bladder tumor resection in 118 patients, including tumor grade 1/2 and pTa in 70 (59.3 %) and 62 (52.5 %), respectively. Multivariate analysis showed that the % 9p21 loss ($>$12 %) was an independent prognostic factor for recurrence ($p < 0.001$; odds ratio, 3.24; 95 % CI,

1.85–5.62), and a mean variant fraction of >16 % was a prognostic factor for disease progression ($p = 0.048$; odds ratio, 6.07; 95 % CI, 1.02–57.45). As mentioned in the section on clinical significance of centrosome amplification, variant fraction is a parameter defining CIN (Lengauer et al. 1997). Evaluation of variant fraction may be a reasonable predictor of poor outcome in patients who develop CIN. UroVysion® may become a promising urine biomarker, not only for recurrence but also for disease progression in NMIBC.

MicroRNAs (miRNAs) are important regulatory molecules for developmental timing, stem cell division, and apoptosis, and they act as tumor suppressors or oncogenes. Dyrskjøt et al. (2009) identified several miRNAs, including miR-129, miR-133b, and miR-518c, with prognostic potential for predicting disease progression, and they found that miR-129 exerted significant growth inhibition and induced cell death with a direct link between miR-129 and the two putative targets GALNT1 and SOX4. MiRNA profile alterations as noninvasive diagnostic and prognostic tools will certainly be a new area of intense investigation in patients with bladder cancer.

Potential Applications to Prognosis

How can CA be applied to clinical practice? One example is the combination of conventional prognostic factors. In NMIBC, the European Association of Urology risk stratification model has been widely accepted into daily clinical practice. In this model, the risks of both recurrence and progression are estimated for individual patients by using a scoring system and risk tables. The model stratifies patients into low-, intermediate-, and high-risk groups according to the sum of the risk score of well-known conventional prognostic factors, including tumor size, number of tumors, prior recurrence, concurrent carcinoma in situ, tumor grade, and stage. Figure 8 depicts a Kaplan–Meier plot of progression-free survival in 87 Japanese NMIBC cases. Although the EAU risk model failed to predict disease progression, CA combined with tumor size (cutoff, 3 cm) may predict progression well. Because CA was significantly associated with tumor grade, stage, and carcinoma in situ but not with tumor size (data not shown), the combination of CA and tumor size may be complementary parameters for the prediction of disease progression.

Limitations of CA detection using urine include the presence of a relatively small population of cells with identifiable centrosomes, probably owing to protein degradation, and subjective observation in centrosome counting. This method must be validated in a second-stage, multicenter trial to verify its clinical significance.

Although molecular grading using a combination of *FGFR3* and Ki-67 (CertNDx) is also a promising biomarker, it is an order-made system in which clinicians must have urine specimens sent to a specific laboratory. The cost of the investigation may also hamper routine application of this technique. Detection of nonrandom chromosomal copy number aberrations by UroVysion may be the upcoming biomarker closest to reaching the clinical setting. Limitations of this technique include the need for large-cohort prospective validation and a trained technician for specimen preparation and signal counting, which may introduce inter-observer bias.

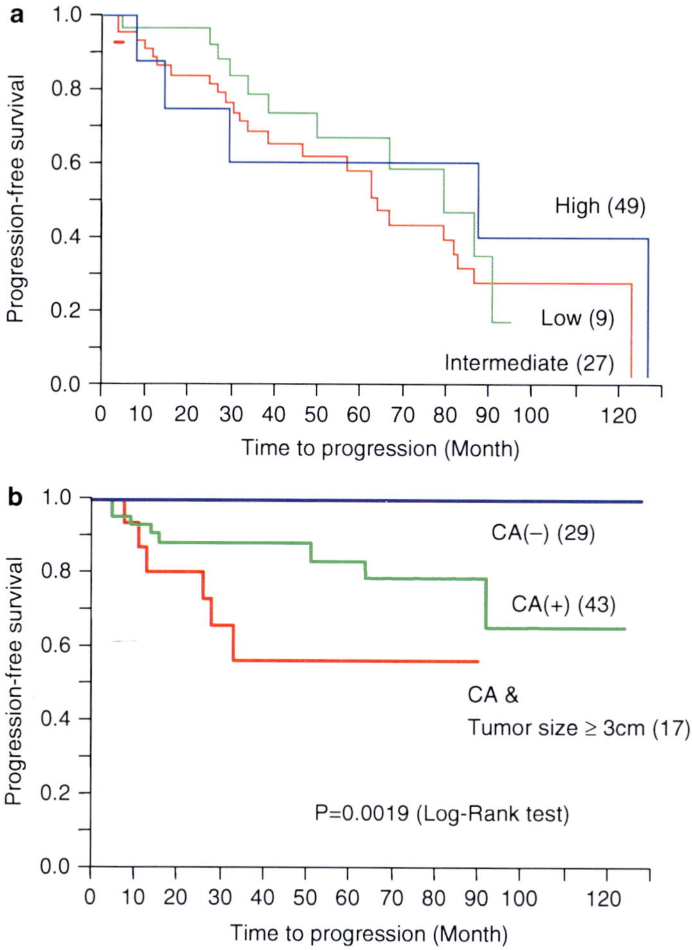

Fig. 8 Prediction of disease progression using the European Association of Urology (EAU) risk model (**a**) or the centrosome amplification (*CA*) model (**b**) in non-muscle-invasive bladder cancer. Significant difference of time to progression was observed among three risk groups stratified as low risk (CA– and tumor size < 3 cm), intermediate risk (CA+ and tumor size < 3 cm), and high risk (CA+ and tumor size ≥ 3 cm) (**b**), whereas no significant difference was observed between risk groups stratified using the EAU risk model (**a**). The number of patients is represented within parentheses

Conclusion

CA causes CIN, leading to tumor recurrence or disease progression in bladder cancer. Detection of CA provides crucial information about tumor recurrence and disease progression in bladder cancer. Further prospective multi-institutional trials are needed. Among several urine biomarkers, detection of copy number aberrations by UroVysion, molecular grading in combination with *FGFR3* mutation and Ki-67 overexpression, and miRNA may be promising new technologies in MNIBC.

Summary Points

1. Aneuploid cells with abnormal numbers of chromosomes occur frequently during cell division, and a small population of surviving cells that escape several cell cycle checkpoints can transform into malignant cells and confer tumors on further malignant phenotype and CIN.
2. CA seems to be a causative event of aneuploidy as well as CIN, and Aurora-A overexpression is among the strongest drivers of CA.
3. Detection of CA in bladder washing solution may be a promising biomarker for predicting patient prognosis.
4. Molecular grading using a combination of FGFR3, which is frequently seen as an early genetic event in NMIBC with relatively favorable prognosis, and Ki-67, the overexpression of which implicates poor prognosis, may be promising biomarkers.
5. Detection of chromosomal copy number aberrations by using multicolor FISH (UroVysion) may also serve as a next-generation biomarker not only for the detection and surveillance of tumors but also for the prediction of patient prognosis, including recurrence and disease progression in NMIBC.
6. MiRNA profile alterations will mark a new area of heavy investigation as noninvasive diagnostic and prognostic tools in NMIBC.

References

Anderhub SJ, Krämer A, Maier B. Centrosome amplification in tumorigenesis. Cancer Lett. 2012;322:8–17.

Bergmann S, Royer-Pokora B, Fietze E, et al. YB-1 provokes breast cancer through the induction of chromosomal instability that emerges from mitotic failure and centrosome amplification. Cancer Res. 2005;65:4078–87.

Cavenee WK, Dryja TP, Phillips RA, et al. Expression of recessive alleles by chromosomal mechanisms in retinoblastoma. Nature. 1983;305:779–84.

Del Rey J, Prat E, Ponsa I, et al. Centrosome clustering and cyclin D1 gene amplification in double minutes are common events in chromosomal unstable bladder tumors. BMC Cancer. 2010;10:280. doi:10.1186/1471-2407-10-280.

Duesberg P. Are centrosomes or aneuploidy the key to cancer? Science. 1999;284:2091–2.

Dyrskjøt L, Ostenfeld MS, Bramsen JB, et al. Genomic profiling of microRNAs in bladder cancer: miR-129 is associated with poor outcome and promotes cell death in vitro. Cancer Res. 2009;69:4851–60.

Eissa S, Swellam M, Shehata H, et al. Expression of HYAL1 and survivin RNA as diagnostic molecular markers for bladder cancer. J Urol. 2010;183:493–8.

Fujiwara T, Bandi M, Nitta M, et al. Cytokinesis failure generating tetraploids promotes tumorigenesis in p53-null cells. Nature. 2005;437:1043–7.

Fukasawa K, Choi T, Kuriyama R, et al. Abnormal centrosome amplification in the absence of p53. Science. 1996;271:1744–7.

Goepfert TM, Adigun YE, Zhong L, et al. Centrosome amplification and overexpression of aurora A are early events in rat mammary carcinogenesis. Cancer Res. 2002;62:4115–22.

Golijanin D, Sherman Y, Shapiro A, et al. Detection of bladder tumors by immunostaining of the Lewis X antigen in cells from voided urine. Urology. 1995;46:173–7.

Grossman H, Messing E, Soloway M, et al. Detection of bladder cancer using a point-of-care proteomic assay. JAMA. 2005;293:810–6.

Guo HQ, Gao M, Ma J, et al. Analysis of the cellular centrosome in fine-needle aspirations of the breast. Breast Cancer Res. 2007;9:R48.

Hernandez S, Lopez-Knowles E, Lloreta J, et al. Prospective study of FGFR3 mutations as a prognostic factor in nonmuscle invasive urothelial bladder carcinomas. J Clin Oncol. 2006;24:3664–71.

Kawamura K, Izumi H, Ma Z, et al. Induction of centrosome amplification and chromosome instability in human bladder cancer cells by p53 mutation and cyclin E overexpression. Cancer Res. 2004;64:4800–9.

Kawauchi S, Sakai H, Ikemoto K, et al. 9p21 index as estimated by dual-color fluorescence in situ hybridization is useful to predict urothelial carcinoma recurrence in bladder washing cytology. Hum Pathol. 2009;40:1783–9.

Knowles MA. Role of FGFR3 in urothelial cell carcinoma: biomarker and potential therapeutic target. World J Urol. 2007;25:581–93.

Knudson AG. Mutation and cancer: statistical study of retinoblastoma. Proc Natl Acad Sci U S A. 1971;68:820–3.

Konety BR, Nguyen TS, Brenes G, et al. Clinical usefulness of the novel marker BLCA-4 for the detection of bladder cancer. J Urol. 2000;164:634–9.

Lengauer C, Kinzler KW, Vogelstein B. Genetic instability in colorectal cancers. Nature. 1997;386:623–7.

Li JJ, Li SA. Mitotic kinases: the key to duplication, segregation, and cytokinesis errors, chromosomal instability, and oncogenesis. Pharmacol Ther. 2006;111:974–84.

Lokeshwar VB, Obek C, Pham HT, et al. Urinary hyaluronic acid and hyaluronidase: markers for bladder cancer detection and evaluation of grade. J Urol. 2000;163:348–56.

Lokeshwar VB, Schroeder GL, Selzer MG, et al. Bladder tumor markers for monitoring recurrence and screening comparison of hyaluronic acid-hyaluronidase and BTA-Stat tests. Cancer. 2002;95:61–72.

Matsuyama H, Pan Y, Mahdy EA, et al. p53 deletion as a genetic marker in urothelial tumor by fluorescence in situ hybridization. Cancer Res. 1994;54:6057–60.

Matsuyama H, Ikemoto K, Eguchi S, et al. Copy number aberrations using multicolour fluorescence in situ hybridization (FISH) for prognostication in non-muscle-invasive bladder cancer (NIMBC). BJU Int. 2013. doi:10.1111/bju.12232. [Epub ahead of print].

Melissourgos N, Kastrinakis NG, Davilas I, et al. Detection of human telomerase reverse transcriptase mRNA in urine of patients with bladder cancer: evaluation of an emerging tumor marker. Urology. 2003;62:362–7.

Miyachika Y, Yamamoto Y, Matsumoto H, et al. Centrosome amplification in bladder washing cytology specimens is a useful prognostic biomarker for non-muscle invasive bladder cancer. Cancer Genet. 2013;206:12–8.

Netto GJ, Cheng L. Emerging critical role of molecular testing in diagnostic genitourinary pathology. Arch Pathol Lab Med. 2012;136:372–90.

Park HS, Park WS, Bondaruk J, et al. Quantitation of Aurora kinase A gene copy number in urine sediments and bladder cancer detection. J Natl Cancer Inst. 2008;100:1401–11.

Pfister C, Chautard D, Devonec MJ, et al. Immunocyt test improves the diagnostic accuracy of urinary cytology: results of a French multicenter study. J Urol. 2003;169:921–4.

Sanchini MA, Gunelli R, Nanni O, et al. Relevance of urine telomerase in the diagnosis of bladder cancer. JAMA. 2005;294:2052–6.

Sarkis AS, Dalbagni G, Cordon-Cardo C, et al. Nuclear overexpression of p53 protein in transitional cell bladder carcinoma: a marker for disease progression. J Natl Cancer Inst. 1993;85:53–9.

Schroeder G, Lorenzo-Gomez MF, Hautmann SJ, et al. A side by side comparison of cytology and biomarkers for bladder cancer detection. J Urol. 2004;172:1123–6.

Sokolova IA, Halling KC, Jenkins RB, et al. The development of a multitarget, multicolor fluorescence in situ hybridization assay for the detection of urothelial carcinoma in urine. J Mol Diagn. 2000;2:116–23.

Tsukamoto M, Matsuyama H, Oba K, et al. Numerical aberrations of chromosome 9 in bladder cancer. A possible prognostic marker for early tumor recurrence. Cancer Genet Cytogenet. 2002;134:41–5.

van Rhijn BW, Vis AN, van der Kwast TH, et al. Molecular grading of urothelial cell carcinoma with fibroblast growth factor receptor 3 and MIB-1 is superior to pathologic grade for the prediction of clinical outcome. J Clin Oncol. 2003;21:1912–21.

Whitson J, Berry A, Carroll P, et al. A multicolour fluorescence in situ hybridization test predicts recurrence in patients with high-risk superficial bladder tumours undergoing intravesical therapy. BJU Int. 2009;104:336–9.

Yamamoto Y, Matsuyama H, Furuya T, et al. Centrosome hyperamplification predicts progression and tumor recurrence in bladder cancer. Clin Cancer Res. 2004;10:6449–55.

Yamamoto Y, Matsuyama H, Kawauchi S, et al. Biological characteristics in bladder cancer depend on the type of genetic instability. Clin Cancer Res. 2006;12:2752–8.

Yamamoto Y, Misumi T, Eguchi S, et al. Centrosome amplification as a putative prognostic biomarker for the classification of urothelial carcinomas. Hum Pathol. 2011;42:1923–30.

Zhou H, Kuang J, Zhong L, et al. Tumour amplified kinase STK15/BTAK induces centrosome amplification, aneuploidy and transformation. Nat Genet. 1998;20:189–93.

Microarrays and Renal Cell Cancer Biomarkers

12

Peter Schraml and Manfred Beleut

Contents

Both the authors contributed equally with all other contributors.

P. Schraml (✉)
Institute of Surgical Pathology, University Hospital Zurich, Zurich, Switzerland
e-mail: Peter.Schraml@usz.ch

M. Beleut (✉)
Qlaym Healthcare AG, Goettingen, Germany
e-mail: beleut@qlaym.com

V.R. Preedy, V.B. Patel (eds.), *Biomarkers in Cancer, Biomarkers in Disease: Methods, Discoveries and Applications*,
DOI 10.1007/978-94-007-7681-4_9

Abstract

The incidence of renal cell carcinoma (RCC) has steadily increased during the last decades. Although technological advances for early recognition of RCC exist, many tumors are accidentally detected, and clinical decision-making is still mainly based on morphological evaluation. Being a relatively chemotherapeutic-resistant and very heterogenic disease, the biological behavior of this tumor type is difficult to predict. Histologic subtyping, tumor staging, and grading are still the pathologic parameters with most valid prognostic and diagnostic significance. Novel high-throughput methodologies have been developed to depict the molecular constitution of individual tumors at the DNA, RNA, and protein levels in order to find relevant biomarkers for optimizing cancer patient care. In this chapter we recapitulate previous published efforts with different microarray platforms which were used to identify biomarkers in RCC. As a result, a large number of such markers, including pathways and gene signatures, have been described as promising biomarkers with significant prognostic and predictive value. However, at present and in contrast to other tumor types such as breast cancer, lung cancer, or melanoma, there is no RCC biomarker that can unrestrictedly be recommended for the use in routine diagnostics. In light of the increasing demand of targeted cancer therapies, vigorous biomedical studies will be needed to translate the molecular findings into clinical applications.

List of Abbreviations

ccRCC	Clear Cell Renal Cell Carcinoma
chRCC	Chromophobe Renal Cell Carcinoma
CGH	Comparative Genomic Hybridization
CNV	Copy Number Variant
CNA	Copy Number Aberration
FFPE	Formalin-Fixed Paraffin-Embedded
(F)ISH	(Fluorescence) In Situ Hybridization
IHC	Immunohistochemistry
miRNA	microRNA
pRCC	Papillary Renal Cell Carcinoma
RCC	Renal Cell Carcinoma
SNP	Single Nuclear Polymorphism
ADFP	Adipose Differentiation-Related Protein
AKT	Serine/Threonine Protein Kinase Akt (pAKT)
AMACR	Alpha-methylacyl-CoA Racemase
ANPEP	Alanyl (Membrane) Aminopeptidase
AP1M2	Adaptor-Related Protein Complex 1, mu 2 Subunit
ASCL2	Achaete-scute Complex Homolog 2
ATP5G2	ATP Synthase, H+ Transporting, Mitochondrial Fo Complex, Subunit C2 (Subunit 9)
B7H1	CD274 Molecule
BC029135	TMEM72 Transmembrane Protein 72

BCL2L2	BCL2-like 2
BIRC5	Baculoviral IAP Repeat-Containing 5
BNC1	Basonuclin 1
BRAF	v-Raf Murine Sarcoma Viral Oncogene Homolog B1
CA2	Carbonic Anhydrase II
CA9	Carbonic Anhydrase IX
CA12	Carbonic Anhydrase XII
CCDC8	Coiled-Coil Domain Containing 8
CD10	Membrane Metallo-Endopeptidase
CD95	Fas Cell Surface Death Receptor
CD151	CD151 Molecule (Raph Blood Group)
CDH1	Cadherin 1
CDKN1C	Cyclin-Dependent Kinase Inhibitor 1C (p57, Kip2)
CDKN2A	Cyclin-Dependent Kinase Inhibitor 2A
CK7	Keratin 7
CKS	CDC28 Protein Kinase
CLDN	Claudin 7
CMET	Met Proto-Oncogene (Hepatocyte Growth Factor Receptor)
COL14A1	Collagen, Type XIV, Alpha 1
COL15A1	Collagen, Type XV, Alpha 1
CORO6	Coronin 6
CSF1R	Colony-Stimulating Factor 1 Receptor
CST6	Cystatin E/M
DNMT DNA	(Cytosine-5-)-methyltransferase 1
DNMT3B DNA	(Cytosine-5-)-methyltransferase 3 Beta
DOC2	Dorsocross 2
EDNRB	Endothelin Receptor Type B
EGFR	Epidermal Growth Factor Receptor
ENST00000456816	Ensembl Gene Chr3:194014254–194030493
EPCAM	Epithelial Cell Adhesion Molecule
ERK	Mitogen-Activated Protein Kinase 1
EZH2	Enhancer of Zeste Homolog 2
FAM150A	Family with Sequence Similarity 150, Member A
FAM78A	Family with Sequence Similarity 78, Member A
FBN2	Fibrillin 2
FGF14	Fibroblast Growth Factor 14
FH	Fumarate Hydratase
FLCN	Folliculin
FLJ20171	Epithelial Splicing Regulatory Protein 1
FOXP1	Forkhead Box P1
FRA2	FOS-like Antigen 2
GNG4	Guanine Nucleotide Binding Protein (G Protein), Gamma 4

GPR56	G Protein-Coupled Receptor 56
GREM1	Gremlin 1
GRM6	Glutamate Receptor, Metabotropic 6
GSN	Gelsolin
GSTA	Glutathione S-Transferase Cluster
GSTA1	Glutathione S-Transferase Alpha 1
HER2	v-erb-b2 Erythroblastic Leukemia Viral Oncogene Homolog 2
HIF1	Hypoxia-Inducible Factor 1
HIF2	Endothelial PAS Domain Protein 1
HIG2	Hypoxia-Inducible Lipid Droplet-Associated
IKBA	Nuclear Factor Of Kappa Light Polypeptide Gene Enhancer in B-Cells Inhibitor, Alpha
KCNQ1	Potassium Voltage-Gated Channel, KQT-like Subfamily, Member 1
KHDRBS2	KH Domain Containing, RNA Binding, Signal Transduction-Associated 2
KI67	Antigen KI-67
KLHL35	Kelch-like Family Member 35
MAGEA9	Melanoma Antigen Family A, 9
MAL2	Mal, T-Cell Differentiation Protein 2 (Gene/Pseudogene)
MET	Met Proto-Oncogene (Hepatocyte Growth Factor Receptor)
MLC2	Myosin, Light Chain 2, Regulatory, Cardiac, Slow
MMP16	Matrix Metallopeptidase 16 (Membrane-Inserted)
MTOR	Mechanistic Target of Rapamycin (Serine/Threonine Kinase)
MYC	v-myc Myelocytomatosis Viral Oncogene Homolog (Avian)
NKX6-2	NK6 homeobox 2
NNMT	Nicotinamide *N*-methyltransferase
NR_024418	Uncharacterized LOC389332 *Homo sapiens*
NRG1	Neuregulin 1
P27	Proteasome (Prosome, Macropain) 26S Subunit, Non-ATPase, 9
P53	Tumor Protein p53
PACRG	PARK2 Co-regulated
PARK2	Parkinson protein 2, E3 Ubiquitin Protein Ligase (Parkin)
PAX2	Paired Box 2
PAX8	Paired Box 8
PBRM1	Polybromo 1
PCDH8	Protocadherin 8
PCDHAC1	Protocadherin Alpha Subfamily C, 1
PDGFR	Platelet-Derived Growth Factor Receptor

PDLIM4	PDZ and LIM Domain 4
PI3K	Phosphatidylinositol-4,5-bisphosphate 3-Kinase, Catalytic Subunit Alpha
POSTN	Periostin, Osteoblast Specific Factor
PRAC	Prostate Cancer Susceptibility Candidate
PROM2	Prominin 2
PRSS8	Protease, Serine, 8
PS6	Taste Receptor, Type 2, Member 63 Pseudogene
PTEN	Phosphatase and Tensin Homolog
PTPRJ	Protein Tyrosine Phosphatase, Receptor Type, J
PTTG1	Pituitary Tumor-Transforming 1
QPCT	Glutaminyl-Peptide Cyclotransferase
RGS5	Regulator of G-Protein Signaling 5
RIMS4	Regulating Synaptic Membrane Exocytosis 4
RPRM	Reprimo, TP53 Dependent G2 Arrest Mediator Candidate
SAV1	Salvador Homolog 1
SCUBE3	Signal Peptide, CUB Domain, EGF-like 3
SFRP1	Secreted Frizzled-Related Protein 1
SKP2	S-phase Kinase-Associated Protein 2, E3 Ubiquitin Protein Ligase
SLC13A5	Solute Carrier Family 13 (Sodium-Dependent Citrate Transporter), Member 5
SPARC	Secreted Protein, Acidic, Cysteine-Rich (Osteonectin)
STC2	Stanniocalcin 2
TFE3	Transcription Factor Binding to IGHM Enhancer 3
TGF	Transforming Growth Factor
TP2A	Topoisomerase (DNA) II Alpha 170 kDa
TRAIL(R)	Tumor Necrosis Factor (Ligand) Superfamily, Member 10 (Receptor)
TRH	Thyrotropin-Releasing Hormone
TRIM63	Tripartite Motif Containing 63, E3 Ubiquitin Protein Ligase
VCAM	Vascular Cell Adhesion Molecule
VCAM1	Vascular Cell Adhesion Molecule 1
VCAN	Versican
VEGFR	Kinase Insert Domain Receptor (a Type III Receptor Tyrosine Kinase)
VEZF1	Vascular Endothelial Zinc Finger 1
VHL	von Hippel-Lindau Tumor Suppressor, E3 Ubiquitin Protein Ligase
VIM	Vimentin
WNT3A	Wingless-Type MMTV Integration Site Family, Member 3A

X91348	*Homo sapiens* mRNA for KIAA1647 Protein
YAP1	Yes-Associated Protein 1
ZFHX1B	Zinc Finger E-Box Binding Homeobox 2
ZFP42 ZFP42	Zinc Finger Protein
ZNF154	Zinc Finger Protein 154
ZNF540	Zinc Finger Protein 540
ZNF671	Zinc finger protein 671
ZSCAN18	Zinc Finger and SCAN Domain Containing 18

Key Facts of Renal Cell Carcinoma

- Renal cell carcinoma (RCC) is a severe disease of the kidney.
- The growth pattern of the tumor and the tumor cells (histologic subtyping) and the size of the tumor (tumor stage) and the feature of the tumor cell nuclei (grading) are important parameters used by pathologists to characterize RCC.
- These parameters help to predict good and bad patient outcome.
- If the disease affects only the kidney, it can be cured with surgery (nephrectomy).
- If it has spread outside the organ, additional treatment is required.
- Traditional therapies (radio-, chemo-, immunotherapies) are rather ineffective.
- Abnormal alterations of genes or proteins in RCC may serve as biomarkers of this disease.
- Biomarkers are thought to optimize RCC patient care.

Definitions of Words and Terms

Biomarker Molecular and measureable indicator linked to a specific disease state, progress of a disease, or to the effects of a specific treatment.

Clustering Grouping a set of individuals (patients) according to molecular alterations (i.e., gene expression, methylation) and/or other parameters in order to distinguish patient subgroups with different molecular characteristics.

Epigenomics Study of modifications (i.e., DNA methylation) of the genome that influence gene activities without directly altering the DNA sequence.

Genomics Study of the structure and function of the entire genome of an individual.

Microarrays High-throughput tool for the simultaneous analysis of molecular parameters (i.e., human genes) of the same molecular type (DNA, RNA, protein).

Pathway Distinct cascade of biochemical reactions made by proteins.

Proteomics Study of the structure and function of proteins in a given setting.

Transcriptomics Study of RNA (i.e., gene expression) in a given cell population.

Introduction

About 2–3 % of all cancer diseases are renal cancers with an annual increase of about 2 % worldwide (Eble et al. 2004). In Europe around 60,000 cases are newly diagnosed and almost 20,000 patients succumb to this disease. More than 80 % of kidney cancers are renal cell carcinomas (RCC) which arise from renal tubular cells. Between 20 % and 30 % of the patients present with locally invasive or metastatic carcinoma at diagnosis. In addition, one-third of the patients who undergo surgical resection of organ-confined RCC will have a relapse. Most advanced RCC are insusceptible to cytokine, chemotherapies, or radiotherapies. The latter appear to be partly caused by a hypoxia-mediated resistance to radiotherapy and alkylating agents (Toffoli and Michiels 2008). As a consequence, the prognosis of advanced RCC is poor, which is reflected by a median survival rate of about 13 months for patients with metastatic disease (Cohen and McGovern 2005).

RCC is a very heterogeneous disease consisting of three main histological subtypes that are morphologically, prognostically, and genotypically different (Eble et al. 2004). With 80 % of all RCC, clear cell RCC (ccRCC) is the most frequent and aggressive subtype. The cytoplasm of tumor cells is enriched with neutral lipids, phospholipids, as well as with glycogen. Papillary RCC (pRCC) comprises approximately 10 % of RCC. The histology is characterized by epithelial cells forming papillae and tubules. pRCC is further subdivided into type 1 tumors with papillae covered by small cells with scanty cytoplasm and type 2 tumors with eosinophilic cytoplasm. About 5 % of RCC belongs to the chromophobe subtype (chRCC). This tumor is characterized by large polygonal cells with reticulated cytoplasm and prominent cell membranes. pRCC and chRCC have generally a better prognosis than ccRCC. Based on nephron-specific markers, it has been assumed that ccRCC and pRCC develop from proximal tubules, whereas chRCC originates from distal tubules. It is of note that sarcomatoid differentiation occurs in all three tumor subtypes, which is associated with poor patient outcome (Moch 2013).

Rare RCC subtypes are renal oncocytoma and multilocular cystic RCC which are considered benign neoplasms and collecting duct carcinoma, an extremely malignant tumor with frequent metastasis. In the last years new carcinoma types have been described such as TFE3 translocation carcinoma, mucinous tubular and spindle cell carcinoma, unclassified RCC, and additional tumor subtypes not yet considered in the WHO classification. All those cancers account for about 5 % of all RCC (Moch 2013).

Table 1 Most common chromosomal aberrations in RCC subtypes (Moch and Mihatsch 2002; Becker et al. 2013)

RCC subtype	Frequency (%)	Chromosomal gains	Chromosomal losses
Clear cell	80	5q, 7, 17	3p, 4q, 6q, 9p, 13q, 14q, Xq
Papillary	10	3, 7, 12q, 16q, 17, 20q	4, 9p, 13, 16, 17p, Y
Chromophobe	5		1, 2, 3, 6, 10, 13q, 17, 21
Oncocytoma	5		1, 6p, 14, 21, Y
Collecting duct	<1	13q	1p, 8p, 9p, 16p

Several diagnostic and prognostic (bio)markers exist which allow a better differentiation of RCC subtypes and possibly facilitate therapy decisions. For example, a diffuse, focal or absent expression pattern of cytokeratin 7 may help to better characterize RCC subtypes. Moreover, CD10, the RCC marker, but also PAX2 and PAX8 are recommended to assign metastasis of unclear origin to a primary RCC (Truong and Shen 2011). However, more detailed analyses are required to establish those markers as fully reliable for RCC diagnosis. In contrast to diagnostic biomarkers, the most important prognostic para-meters are represented by the RCC subtype, the tumor stage, and the nuclear differentiation grade (Eble 2004). The tumor stage category is the basis for all clinical decisions. Currently, the Fuhrman system is the commonly accepted system for grading RCC. It has been suggested, however, that this grading system is less suitable for chRCC and not applicable to mucinous, tubular, and spindle cell carcinoma and oncocytoma.

In order to better explain the molecular biology of RCC, restriction fragment length polymorphism, microsatellite analyses, and, finally, comparative genomic hybridization (CGH) were the methods of choice in the last decade of the twentieth century to identify chromosomal aberrations specific for the RCC subtypes. Loss of the short arm of chromosome 3p is the main characteristic feature of ccRCC. Subtype-specific but less prominent chromosomal alterations different to ccRCC were found in pRCC, chRCC, and other subtypes (Moch and Mihatsch 2002; Eble et al. 2004). Chromosomal losses are thought to contribute to the inactivation of tumor suppressor genes, whereas gains rather point to hyperactivated oncogenes. Chromosomal alterations described in RCC are summarized in Table 1.

Intense efforts contributed significantly to better understand the molecular biology of RCC. A crucial player in ccRCC tumor genesis is the von Hippel-Lindau (*VHL*) tumor suppressor gene which was cloned using tissue and cell lines from von Hippel-Lindau syndrome patients. Mutations and deletions of this gene were first described in patients with this disease which is characterized by a multitude of benign and malignant tumors, including ccRCC (Neumann et al. 1998). Surprisingly, in the vast majority of patients with sporadic ccRCC, chromosomal and gene alterations affecting *VHL* were also identified. The gene product of *VHL*, pVHL, exerts its function as multiadaptor protein in several pathways (Frew and Krek 2008) that are considered critical for cancer development and progression (Fig. 1).

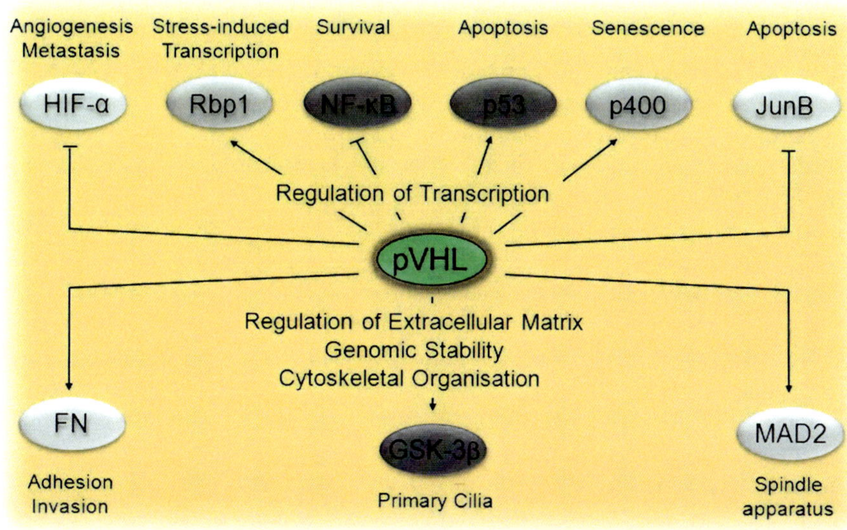

Fig. 1 The multiadaptor protein pVHL, its binding partners, and its functions in the biology of ccRCC

The best-described function of pVHL is its role as negative regulator of the hypoxia-inducible factor (HIF). Hydroxylation of the HIF subunits HIF-1α and HIF-2α by prolyl hydroxylases (PHD1-3) under normoxia facilitates the binding of pVHL and leads to ubiquitination and proteasomal degradation of HIFα. In ccRCC, both hypoxia and abrogation of pVHL function lead to HIF-α stabilization and consequently to HIF activation. HIF then promotes transcriptionally regulating programs toward angiogenesis and cell survival. HIF-responsive genes, such as *VEGFR* (vascular endothelial growth factor receptor), *PDGFR* (platelet-derived growth factor receptor), *CA9* (carbonic anhydrase 9), and many others, may represent therapeutic targets of locally advanced and metastatic ccRCC (Frew and Krek 2008). In contrast to hereditary and sporadic ccRCC in which pVHL's integrity is critical, the genes found to be involved in other hereditary forms of RCC (*CMET*, *FH* in pRCC; *FLCN* in chRCC) seem to play a minor role in the sporadic tumors (Eble et al. 2004). It is therefore much more challenging to identify molecular pathways with potential drug targets being responsible for the oncogenesis of these tumor subtypes.

The implementation of customized high-throughput microarray technologies at the beginning of this century has revolutionized the strategies that had been formerly used to identify cancer-causing genes and deregulated molecular pathways. Microarrays have been very useful in the essaying of molecules and the identification of biomarkers for different conditions. Their advantage is seen in the standardized procedure, the little material input, and the simultaneous comparison of a large amount of different molecules. Being built as compact chips, microarrays present well-defined immobilized probes binding to their target molecules. There are several platforms overall covering different fields of microarray analysis on the genomics, transcriptomics, and proteomics levels. The technologies have steadily improved with time and extend to different platforms such as single nuclear polymorphism (SNP) arrays, DNA methylation microarrays, tissue microarrays (TMA), and gene expression microarrays, the latter currently being the most commonly used microarray type.

The use of these technical high-throughput tools has dramatically increased data and knowledge about molecular mechanisms leading to RCC. They enabled the screening for markers in early stage and recurrent tumors after nephrectomy as well as for predictive markers for treatment response. In the following we describe microarray technology approaches that have been applied to uncover such potential RCC biomarkers.

Genomic Approaches

Array-Based CGH (aCGH) and SNP Arrays for Tracking Potential Chromosomal and Gene Marker Loci

In contrast to CGH in which normal metaphase chromosomes are used as hybridization targets, aCGH (Albertson et al. 2000) is performed with 100–200 kb DNA clones in array format. aCGH studies first applied to RCC have globally addressed the correct pathologic classification of benign and malignant neoplasia, focusing mainly on their use for diagnostic purposes (Wilhelm et al. 2002). By combining whole-genome amplification and genomic copy number analysis employing aCGH (Fiegler et al. 2007), it was possible to narrow down copy number changes to only a few Mb in microdissected 769P ccRCC cells. A summary illustration of published chromosomal and aCGH RCC data is shown in Fig. 2.

The data in Fig. 2 clearly demonstrate that in ccRCC distinct chromosomes are preferably affected and that losses and gains can occur on all chromosomes. Chromosomal losses may indicate the existence of one or more tumor suppressor

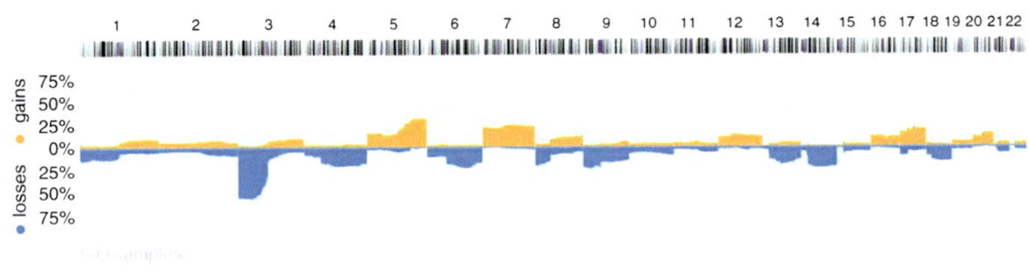

Fig. 2 CGH data of 599 ccRCC. Regional genomic CNAs are shown as percentage of analyzed cases. Note the higher frequency of distinct affected chromosomal regions. Genomic gains: *yellow*; Genomic losses: *blue* (With kind permission of Dr. Michael Baudis, Progenetix.org, Zurich University, Zurich, Switzerland)

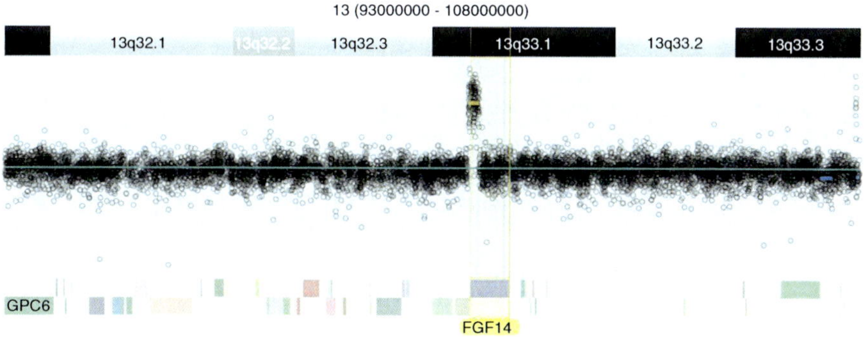

Fig. 3 DNA copy number analysis in one ccRCC in the chromosomal region 13q32.1-13q33.3 using a Genome-Wide Human SNP 6.0 array. SNPs are indicated by *circles*. Chromosomal gain of about 170 kb within the gene *FGF14* is shown

genes on the remaining parental chromosomes, whereas gains may point to abnormally active oncogenes. One such potential candidate is *SAV1* which was found frequently deleted on 14q22.1 in advanced high-grade ccRCC (Matsuura et al. 2011). SAV1 is a component of the Hippo pathway and negatively regulates YAP1 activity. It was thus hypothesized that this pathway may be relevant for RCC therapy.

aCGH was also used to find genetic markers associated with papillary renal cell tumor progression (Szponar et al. 2009). Three genetically defined developmental stages have been proposed with papillary renal cell adenoma characterized by combined trisomy of chromosomes 7 and 17, pRCC with additional changes without progression, and pRCC with deadly outcome characterized by 1q gain. This was independent of histological morphology and tumor size and suggested a classification system superior to morphological classification.

SNP arrays are ideal tools to assess copy number alterations in a much higher resolution compared to aCGH. An example of copy number variation is shown in Fig. 3. Using this technology (Monzon et al. 2008) identified both known characteristic chromosomal changes and additional copy number aberrations unique for each RCC analyzed. Even three RCCs with unclear subclassification could be assigned to oncocytoma and ccRCC by SNP array analysis. Data obtained from a similar study with unclassified RCC suggested that virtual karyotypes generated by SNP arrays help to increase diagnostic accuracy, particularly in morphologically challenging RCC in routine diagnostics (Kim et al. 2009).

However, genome-wide SNP array analysis not only confirmed large chromosomal aberrations already described by CGH and aCGH studies but also refined these affected regions and detected unknown microalterations (Chen et al. 2009). A comprehensive study with 80 ccRCC showed chromosomal losses spanning 3p21-36, 8p12-pter, 6q23.3-27, 14q24.1-qter, 9q32-qter, 10q22.3-qter, 9p13.3-pter, 4q28.3-qter, and 13q12.1-21.1. The smallest deletion had a size of 0.29 Mb on 8p12 containing *NRG1*. Concordance between SNP array data and gene expression was found for *FOXP1* on 3p and *PARK2* as well as for *PACRG* on 6q. The most frequent chromosome gains were at 5q32-ter with one tumor harboring a focal gain of 0.42 Mb in 5q35.3. Upregulation was observed for *CSF1R*. Additional gains were 1q25.1-qter, 7q21.13-qter, and 8q24.12-qter. These regions and genes may represent diagnostic, prognostic, and predictive biomarkers of ccRCC.

PTTG1, a recently discovered oncogene, was detected in amplified regions of 5q and was moreover associated with high tumor grade and poor patient prognosis. A depletion of this gene in functional in vitro studies demonstrated a decreased tumorigenic and invasive behavior, potentially pinpointing it as a novel therapeutic target (Wondergem et al. 2012).

By analyzing 112 ccRCC with SNP arrays, (Monzon et al. 2011) found a significant correlation between loss of chromosome 14q, gain of 8q, and worse patient outcome, particularly in patients with organ-confined ccRCC. 14q loss was associated with decreased *HIF-1α* mRNA and protein expression. It was concluded that 8q gain and MYC upregulation as well as 14q loss and HIF1A downregulation may serve as molecular markers of prognosis and personalized medicine for ccRCC patients.

DNA Methylation Arrays for Unmasking Silenced RCC Markers

DNA methylation is a chemical modification that primarily affects cytosine within CpG islands. Abnormal hypermethylated gene promoter regions in tumors can prevent transcription. These epigenetic events were first described for several tumor suppressor genes including *VHL* (Herman et al. 1994). In addition to deletions and mutations, hypermethylation of the VHL promoter can lead to gene silencing in up to 20 % ccRCC. The methylation status of a DNA sequence of interest is commonly determined either by using methylation-sensitive and methylation-nonsensitive restriction enzymes or by DNA bisulphite treatment which converts unmethylated cytosine to uracil but leaves methylated cytosine unaffected. Various DNA microarray approaches exist to investigate tumor-specific DNA methylation patterns.

The influence of histopathology and *VHL* mutation status to CpG methylation rates was explored in VHL-related and VHL-unrelated RCC by (McRonald et al. 2009). Forty-three genes were found methylated in over 20 % of RCC analyzed. CpG methylation was most prevalent in pRCC and least in ccRCC of VHL syndrome patients. Many of the genes preferentially methylated in pRCC were linked to TGF-beta or ERK/Akt signaling and may represent potential CpG methylation biomarkers for RCC.

In another epigenetic study high-density gene expression microarrays were used for analyzing the promoter methylation status of genes in 11 RCC cell lines (Morris et al. 2010). Of 28 selected genes *BNC1*, *PDLIM4*, *RPRM*, *CST6*, *SFRP1*, *GREM1*, *COL14A1*, and *COL15A1* showed frequent promoter hypermethylation in cell lines and tumor tissue, which was associated with transcriptional silencing. Functional studies demonstrated tumor suppressive properties of *BNC1*, *CST6*, *RPRM*, *SFRP1*, and *COL14A1*. *BNC1* or *COL14A1* methylation was associated with a poorer outcome which was independent of tumor size, stage, or grade. The authors concluded that these genes may be biomarkers for prognosis and RCC detection.

Using a bead-based methylation array platform (1,413 CpG loci in ~800 cancer-associated genes), (Avissar-Whiting et al. 2011) assessed DNA methylation profiles in RCC and associated these profiles with the expression of genes. The downregulation of *DNMT*, *DNMT3B*, *VEZF1*, and *EZH2* correlated with a high methylation status in RCC. A greater differential methylation between RCC and non-diseased kidney tissue was found with *EZH2*, a member of the polycomb repressive complex 2, and additional polycomb group targets. This work indicates how repressive marks on DNA and chromatin are deregulated in RCC which may contribute to the development of therapies or preventive strategies.

To identify frequently methylated and silenced marker genes, a more complex strategy was chosen by (Morris et al. 2011) who used methylated DNA immunoprecipitation and whole-genome array analysis in combination with high-density expression array analysis. Frequent promoter methylation was seen for *KLHL35*, *QPCT*, *SCUBE3*, *ZSCAN18*, *CCDC8*, *FBN2*, *ATP5G2*, *PCDH8*, and *CORO6*. Knockdown of *KLHL35*, *QPCT*, *SCUBE3*, *ZSCAN18*, *CCDC8*, and *FBN2* resulted in an anchorage-independent growth advantage. *SCUBE3* hypermethylation was correlated with increased risk of cancer death or relapse.

Arai et al. (2012) performed single-CpG-resolution analysis at 4830 CpG sites to uncover DNA methylation alterations during renal carcinogenesis using normal renal cortex tissue, noncancerous renal cortex tissue, and tumorous tissue samples. They identified RCC clusters with different methylation status, tumor aggressiveness, and survival rates. A CpG island methylator phenotype of RCC was identified with DNA hypermethylation of the CpG sites on 17 genes (*FAM150A*, *GRM6*, *ZNF540*, *ZFP42*, *ZNF154*, *RIMS4*, *PCDHAC1*, *KHDRBS2*, *ASCL2*, *KCNQ1*, *PRAC*, *WNT3A*, *TRH*, *FAM78A*, *ZNF671*, *SLC13A5*, and *NKX6-2*). They suggested that accumulation of DNA hypermethylation on specific CpG islands and genome-wide DNA hypomethylation may represent distinct pathways of renal carcinogenesis.

All chromosomal genetic and epigenetic changes occurring in RCC comprise mainly DNA losses and gains, specific gene mutations, as well as methylation of distinct DNA sequences. These abnormalities greatly influence the gene expression profile in a tumor and lead to the malignant, uncontrolled behavior of RCC. DNA microarray technology enables the study of such global gene expression patterns which give more insight into affected pathways and genes with known and unknown functions as well as their correlation with clinical data. The most important findings are described in the following chapter.

Transcriptomic Approaches

DNA Microarrays for Screening RCC-Specific Marker Expression Patterns

Gene expression microarrays have extensively been implemented in the stratification and restratification of RCC. As they simultaneously contain thousands of gene-specific probes, each experiment represents a global analysis of genes enabling an indirect illustration of upstream and downstream events, eventually leading to their manifestation on the gene expression level. Despite the uniqueness of individual RCC, sophisticated approaches with cDNA, cRNA, and customized DNA oligonucleotides microarrays have been used to identify common gene expression patterns and individual biomarkers associated with prognostic or predictive value.

Among the first published cDNA microarray studies on RCC, (Boer et al. 2001) investigated gene expression differences between 37 paired neoplastic and noncancerous renal epithelial specimens. Subsequent functional annotations pointed to 167 upregulated transcripts which participate in cell adhesion, signal transduction, and nucleotide metabolism processes. The identified 154 downregulated genes were primarily involved in mechanisms affecting small molecule transport, ion homeostasis, and oxygen metabolism. Genome-wide expression profiles in 10 ccRCC uncovered hypoxia-inducible protein-2 (HIG2) as novel putative diagnostic and therapeutic marker for ccRCC (Togashi et al. 2005). Functional analyses demonstrated HIG2's involvement in cell growth and Wnt signaling.

Further gene profiling of ccRCC identified signatures segregating this tumor subtype in subgroups with different prognostic characteristics. By analyzing 29 ccRCC, Takahashi et al. (Takahashi et al. 2001) identified a 40-gene signature which was able to separate tumors of nonaggressive and aggressive phenotype. In a prospective pilot study, the prediction even exceeded the accuracy of prediction by tumor staging. Other authors complemented this data by integrating ccRCC with similar numbers and the use of supervised and nonsupervised clustering methods. In particular, three groups (Vasselli et al. 2003; Jones et al. 2005; Kosari et al. 2005) reported the existence of distinct "metastatic signatures" already being present in the primary tumor. As candidate biomarkers *BIRC5*, *V-CAM* and genes coding for secreted proteins and membrane receptors were found correlated with cancer-specific survival, they were suggested potential therapeutic or diagnostic targets.

Among the 12 top-ranked genes which were the most tightly linked to positive outcome upon high-expression levels were *VCAM1*, *EDNRB*, and *RGS5* (Yao et al. 2008). It was concluded that a scoring system based on the expression levels of these genes may be useful in the prediction of survival for ccRCC patients. Recently, a panel of potential biomarkers for calculating the individual metastatic risk in ccRCC was proposed (Sanjmyatav et al. 2011). These genes resided in a cluster of 127 transcripts for increased metastasic probability involving prominent candidates, such as downregulated *CD151* and *IKBA* as well as upregulated *MMP16*, *B7H1*, *BCL2L2*, and *FRA2*.

In an attempt to gain biologic insight into VHL-dependent and VHL-independent ccRCC development, (Maina et al. 2005) compared the gene expression levels of VHL wild-type and VHL-null RCC cell lines. Eleven novel VHL/HIF targets, among them *CDKN1C*, *SPARC*, *GPR56*, *GNG4*, *MLC2*, and *DOC2*, were identified.

A meta-analysis of more than 480 ccRCC tumors pointed to a VHL-independent segregation into two subclasses termed ccA and ccB. ccA tumors had an overall better prognosis and were correlated to hypoxia and angiogenic processes, whereas ccB tumors had worse survival prognosis and displayed genes of epithelial-mesenchymal transition, wound healing, and cell cycle processes (Brannon et al. 2010). These data also indicate that the proposed subclassification system of ccRCC may provide prognostic information independent of standard clinical parameters.

Most of the microarray studies directly addressed the correlation of gene expression profiles to the histopathologic RCC subtypes. An example showing hierarchical clustering of genes in ccRCC and pRCC (Beleut et al. 2012) is shown in Fig. 4.

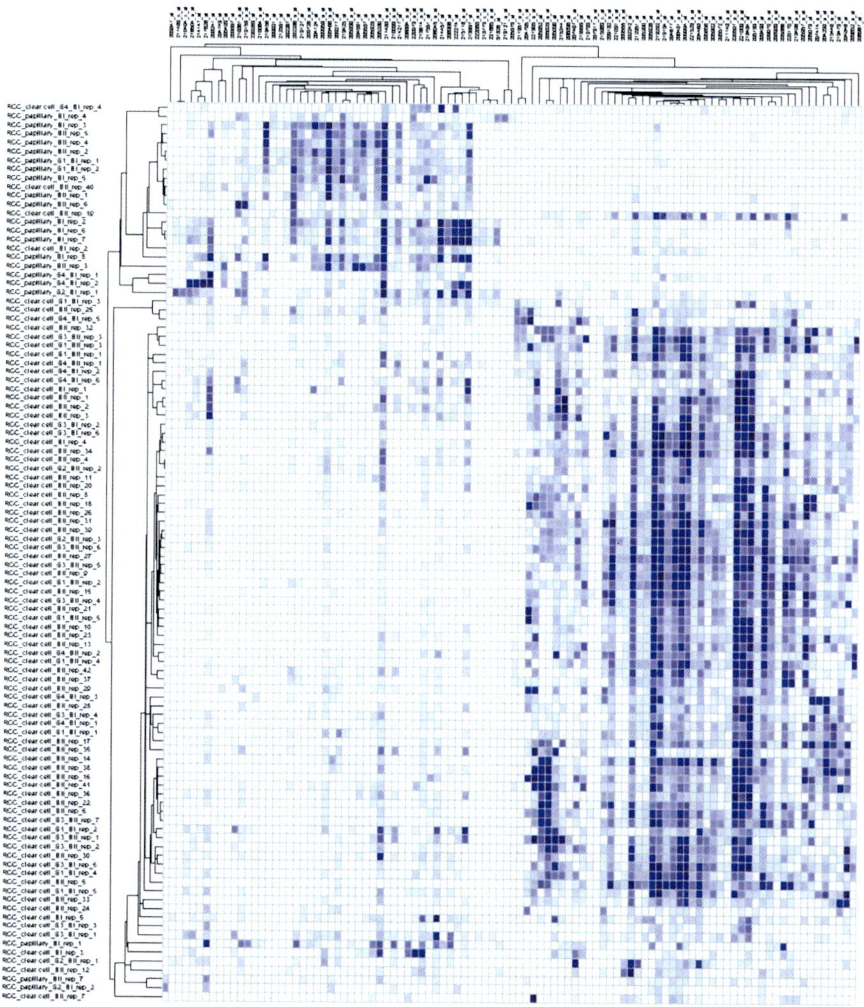

Fig. 4 Two-way supervised hierarchical clustering of a gene set distinguishing ccRCC and pRCC (own microarray data; see also (Beleut et al. 2012)). *blue*, relative increase; *white*, relative decrease of gene expression

Distinct gene expression patterns were found for all subtypes and up- or downregulated genes. *GSTA*, *NNMT*, and *ADFP* were highly expressed in ccRCC, *AMACR* in pRCC, and *CA2* in chRCC and proposed as diagnostic markers (Higgins et al. 2003; Takahashi et al. 2003; Yao et al. 2005). Critical biologic processes were suggested for ccRCC (angiogenic and immune response), oxidative phosphorylation for chRCC, and serine protease inhibitors as well as extracellular matrix products for pRCC (Schuetz et al. 2005). Other global gene expression patterns involving different candidates to further subclassify ccRCC did not only show subtype specificity, they were moreover able to separate tumor grades, thus confirming the histopathologic grading system on the molecular level (Skubitz et al. 2006; Maruschke et al. 2011).

Possible molecular variations of RCC in different countries were analyzed by Wozniak et al. (Wozniak et al. 2013). A cohort of 101 paired healthy and tumor samples from Eastern Europe were analyzed using gene expression microarrays. The data were set into relation with already existing RNA sequencing data derived from a publically available cohort of Western Europe/USA patients. 60 % downregulation and 74 % upregulation overlay were found between both cohorts. Subsequent biological characterization suggested common deregulations in metabolic and catabolic processes, excretion, oxidation reduction, ion transport and response to chemical stimulus, immune and inflammatory responses, response to hypoxia, stress, wounding, vasculature development, and cell activation.

Novel approaches to further complement the understanding of ccRCC carcinogenesis focused on the detection of aberrantly expressed clusters of long noncoding RNAs, supporting their involvement in tumorigenic processes. *ENST00000456816*, *X91348*, *BC029135*, and *NR_024418* are the most promising candidates (Yu et al. 2012).

Comprehensive gene expression profiling was also performed with RCC different to the clear cell subtype. By analyzing 34 pRCC using an Affymetrix GeneChip with 54,675 probe sets, two highly distinct molecular pRCC subclasses characterized by a seven-transcript predictor with morphologic correlation were identified (Yang et al. 2005). Class 1 pRCC tumors were defined by *CK-7* and class 2 tumors by *TP2A* expression. (Rohan et al. 2006) compared gene expression profiles of 9 chRCC and 9 benign oncocytoma. Five genes, *AP1M2*, *MAL2*, *PROM2*, *PRSS8*, and *FLJ20171*, were detected which discriminate chRCC from oncocytoma. Selective and differential expression of *MAL2* was observed in distal renal tubules as well as between chromophobe RCC and oncocytoma, respectively. Microarray analysis of two renal medullary carcinoma and 64 other RCC subtypes revealed a distinct molecular signature of this rare RCC (Yang et al. 2004). Eighteen genes were significantly overexpressed or underexpressed in renal medullary carcinoma compared with other types of renal tumors. The authors suggested that this tumor subtype should be treated as a special malignancy. Finally, whole-genome microarray expression profiling was performed on 4 *TFE3* translocation RCC and 48 other RCC subtypes (Camparo et al. 2008). More than 80 genes were significantly differentially expressed between renal translocation tumors and other RCC, with *TRIM63*, *GSTA1*, and *ANPEP* being the most prominent markers for this group of tumors.

Despite the tremendous amount of data of gene clusters and potential biomarkers identified to date, the agreement among these studies is mostly poor. The use of self-made microarrays and microarrays from different vendors and the lack of suited bioinformatics programs which select non-reliable samples, genes, and false positives as well as missing cross-platform validations may explain these strong discrepancies. A common valid conclusion about RCC biology and convincing biomarkers can therefore hardly be drawn.

miRNA Microarrays for Identifying RCC Key Players of Gene Regulation

miRNAs are considered as a novel type of biomarkers in human cancer. They represent short, single-stranded and noncoding RNAs consisting of approximately 22 nucleotides. miRNAs are considered as multipotent gene expression regulators being active mainly on the posttranscriptional level. Through binding to their target RNA, miRNAs may influence translation, induce RNA-degradation, but also positively stabilize their target for sustained gene expression products. The individual function of miRNAs is largely unknown. As shown in different cancer types, however, their expression patterns alter in healthy and diseased conditions. Therefore, miRNAs are considered as functional modulators facilitating the process of carcinogenesis on another molecular level. Ready-to-use and tailor-made miRNA arrays are available, enabling a large-scale analysis of multiple such targets to better understand global miRNA expression changes in a given tumor entity.

To date there are only few studies in which miRNA array technology has been applied to analyze RCC. Different research groups have independently demonstrated a preferred downregulation of miRNAs in primary RCC and metastatic tissue when compared to their healthy counterparts (Nakada et al. 2008; Yi et al. 2010; Wotschofsky et al. 2012; Duns et al. 2013). A total of 23 miRNAs were downregulated in metastatic tissue samples compared with normal tissue (Wotschofsky et al. 2012). Among them were miR-141 and miR-200c whose deregulation in ccRCC might be involved in suppression of *CDH1/E-cadherin* transcription via upregulation of transcriptional repressor ZFHX1B (Nakada et al. 2008). An up to 138-fold downregulation was observed for miR-200b, -363, -429, -200c, -514, and -141 (Jung et al. 2009), and (Duns et al. 2013) identified all members of the miR-200 family known to be involved in the epithelial to mesenchymal transition process significantly decreased in ccRCC. Surprisingly, the distinct alterations in miRNA expression were not found associated with clinicopathological factors, such as tumor stage, grade, or patient survival, suggesting a general implication of such modulators in the onset of RCC (Gottardo et al. 2007; Jung et al. 2009) rather than a sustained contribution in disease progression.

One consistently reappearing miRNA having a relative high-expression level upon hypoxia-induced signaling is miRNA-210. This candidate was identified as a VHL target to alter cell cycle progression, block apoptotic signaling cascades, and overall facilitate the process of carcinogenesis (Chen et al. 2010; Valera et al. 2011).

Its expression was significantly correlated with decreased prognosis in terms of overall patient survival in RCC (Neal et al. 2010). As relatively stable molecules, miRNA-1233, miRNA-378, and miRNA-451 were found in sera and proposed to constitute measurable biomarkers for the diagnosis of RCC (Wulfken et al. 2011; Redova et al. 2012).

One recent study investigated miRNA pattern alterations as a potential tool for improved histological stratification in 94 tumors including ccRCC, pRCC, chRCC, and oncocytoma (Youssef et al. 2011). The authors developed a robust classification system distinguishing different RCC subtypes according to unique miRNA signatures with an accuracy of up to 90 %.

Proteomic Approaches

Tissue Microarrays (TMA) for Evaluating Molecular Markers with Clinical Relevance in RCC

The invention of the TMA technology (Kononen et al. 1998) enabled researchers to validate promising gene candidates obtained from DNA microarray data by analyzing hundreds of tissue cores arrayed on a single glass slide. In the vast majority of the published studies, formalin-fixed tissue samples have been the material of choice to generate TMAs for investigating protein expression by immunohistochemistry and gene aberrations by FISH. A few groups showed that TMAs either consisting of FFPE or even frozen tissue specimen can be used for RNA ISH analysis, but the procedures and the interpretation of the results are rather time-consuming and sophisticated. The strategy of a typical TMA analysis is illustrated in Fig. 5. In light of the many published TMA studies and the restricted number of references provided by the editors of this book, we are focusing in the following on studies which describe highly significant outcomes in more than 200 analyzed ccRCC.

In one of the first RCC-TMA studies, 532 RCC were used to validate the clinical relevance of molecular changes detected by cDNA microarray analysis (Moch et al. 1999). In ccRCC vimentin expression was found significantly associated with poor patient prognosis. (Seligson et al. 2004) investigated EpCAM, an adhesion protein widely expressed in other human cancers and a candidate in therapy. Although strong expression was seen in only 10 % of 318 ccRCC, EpCAM positivity correlated with improved survival. These results were confirmed by (Eichelberg et al. 2013) who also observed no or only weak EpCAM expression in the majority of the 767 arrayed ccRCC. Positive EpCAM IHC was significantly linked to prolonged overall survival especially in patients with localized ccRCC.

To identify subtypes of ccRCC, (Shi et al. 2005) analyzed eight previously published tumor markers (CA9, CA12, Ki67, GSN, p53, EpCAM, PTEN, and VIM) in 307 ccRCC using random forest clustering for tumor profiling. They discovered two clusters corresponding to low- and high-grade tumors, a subgroup

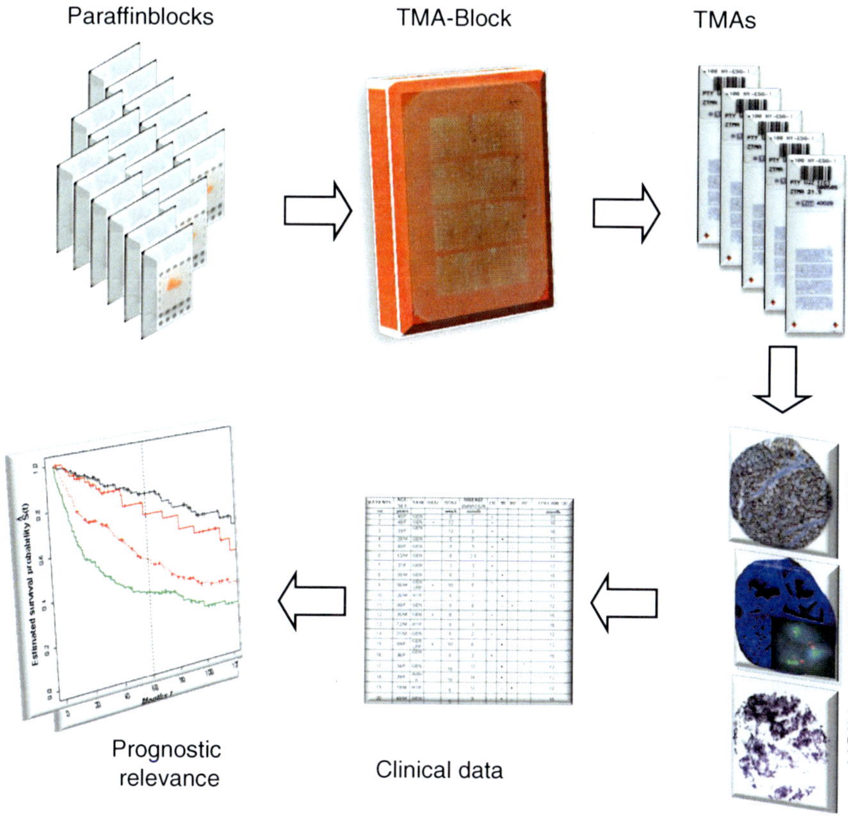

Fig. 5 TMA preparation and analysis for evaluating biomarkers with potential clinical relevance

of long-surviving patients, and two novel tumor subclasses in low-grade ccRCC. A strong correlation of high HIF-1a expression and worse survival was reported by (Klatte et al. 2007) who constructed a TMA with 308 ccRCC. By analyzing the mTOR pathway in 375 RCC, there was an association of nuclear pAKT expression with a favorable prognosis and cytoplasmic pAKT expression with a poor outcome (Pantuck et al. 2007). pAKT, PTEN, and pS6 were independent prognostic factors of tumor-specific survival. In a second and independent TMA study on 386 RCC, both cytoplasmic and nuclear pAKT levels were found as prognostic factors for shorter patient survival (Hager et al. 2009). Preferential increase of pAKT and decrease of PTEN expression in high-grade and high-stage RCC suggested therapeutic concepts based on PI3K/pAKT/mTOR pathway inhibitors. Finally, (Darwish et al. 2013) confirmed the importance of mTOR signaling in ccRCC by examining 9 mTOR pathway components in 419 nonmetastatic ccRCC. Their data showed that the cumulative number of aberrantly expressed mTOR pathway members correlated with tumor aggression and worse outcome which may support predictive exploration of the mTOR signaling cascade in ccRCC patients.

A TMA study with 318 RCC revealed Claudin-1, a tight junction protein, a prognosticator of shortened disease-specific survival in ccRCC patients (Fritzsche et al. 2008). The prognostic utility of the tumor suppressor p27 and its negative regulators Skp2 and Cks was studied in 482 RCC (Liu et al. 2008). Only low p27 expression served as independent prognostic factor for both cancer-specific survival and recurrence-free survival. IHC staining of the catalytic alpha subunit of the Na, K-adenosine triphosphatase in 317 ccRCC suggested this protein as clinical prognosticator for disease-specific death (Seligson et al. 2008). TRAIL and its receptors (TRAIL-R) were examined on a large TMA containing 838 RCC (Macher-Goeppinger et al. 2009). High TRAIL and TRAIL-R2 and low TRAIL-R4 expression were correlated with worse patient outcome. The authors conclude that TRAIL-R agonists may be of therapeutical relevance in patients with RCC.

Deep sequencing analysis of ccRCC revealed *PBRM1* as second most frequently mutated gene after VHL. An expression study of this histone/chromatin regulator in more than 300 RCC demonstrated that loss of PBRM1 was predominant in about 70 % of ccRCC and was associated to tumor stage, grade, and overall patient survival (Pawlowski et al. 2013). The authors suggested that molecular pathways deregulated by the inactivation of this protein may lead to new treatment strategies.

A comprehensive TMA analysis was performed by (Dahinden et al. 2010) who evaluated the expression patterns of 15 different proteins belonging to pathways controlled by pVHL and PTEN in over 800 ccRCC. They demonstrated that the use of advanced mathematical models for comprehensive TMA data analysis may clarify complex molecular contexts and may improve prediction of progression risk. For example, patients with intermediate grade ccRCC had a prolonged survival if the tumors were nuclear p27 and cytoplasmic PTEN positive but had inactive, non-phosphorylated ribosomal protein S6.

More recently even larger TMAs were applied to statistically better support the clinical relevance of single markers in RCC. Nuclear expression of the enhancer of EZH2 was defined as prognostic marker of poor cancer-specific survival in a TMA study with 520 RCC (Wagener et al. 2010). Similarly, a significant association between high CD95 expression, a member of the death receptor family, and patients with a poor clinical prognosis was observed (Macher-Goeppinger et al. 2011) by analyzing an RCC TMA with 617 tumors. (Morra et al. 2011) investigated the expression pattern of the extracellular matrix N-glycoprotein POSTN, a potential key player in tumor invasion in over 800 ccRCC patients. Increased presence of POSTN in tumor epithelia correlated with sarcomatoid differentiation and poor overall survival. High nuclear expression of melanoma-associated antigen MAGE-A9 was examined in 587 RCC and found independently associated with poor cancer-specific survival in patients with nonmetastatic RCC (Hatiboglu et al. 2012). The authors suggested MAGE-A9 assessment in decision-making regarding adjuvant therapy.

As the epidermal growth factor receptor (EGFR) represents an important therapeutic target, its role in RCC was determined by investigating 1,088 arrayed tumors (Minner et al. 2012). Both strong EGFR expression and high polysomy were observed in a small subset of ccRCC. The association with high tumor grade and stage suggested possible utility of anti-EGFR treatment.

cMET mutations were linked to pRCC with familial history (Eble et al. 2004). (Gibney et al. 2013) determined cMET expression by automated quantitative analysis on a TMA with 330 RCC. Strong c-Met expression may serve as independent predictor of survival in ccRCC patients suggesting cMET as a potential target of tyrosine kinase inhibition. Interestingly, PTPRJ, a negative regulator of tyrosine kinase receptors, including cMET, was found tightly linked to pVHL (Casagrande et al. 2013). As reliable antibodies against PTPRJ for immunostaining were not available, RNA-ISH was performed on an RCC-TMA. No or reduced PTPRJ mRNA expression had a less favorable outcome indicating that both PTPRJ downregulation and activation of cMET may be critical for ccRCC.

Combinations of Microarray Platforms Used to Validate Potential Biomarkers in RCC

In cancer research, the use of microarrays has generated huge data and enabled a simultaneous glance on multiple molecular parameters present in one single tumor at any given time point. However, one particular microarray platform can only provide information about molecules of the same sort (DNA or RNA or protein) and has therefore certain limitations about global biological insights on the whole molecular constitution of a tumor. To address this problem, very recent studies have begun to analyze cancers by generating data derived from different microarray platforms in parallel and integrate the results for further analyses. Some of those studies have also been focusing on RCC and give a more comprehensive picture on the complex molecular status of renal cancers.

To identify novel oncogenes and tumor suppressor genes relevant in RCC, Beroukhim et al. (Beroukhim et al. 2009) integrated data of chromosomal alterations and gene expression patterns from 90 tumors by using SNP and gene expression microarrays. Besides frequent 3p deletions mainly affecting VHL expression, CDKN2A and CDKN2B on the chromosome 9p deletion peak were also identified. Amplifications and accompanying increased gene expression levels of candidates on chromosome 7q22 as well as on the MYC locus on 8q24 were found in 30 % and 12 % of the tumors, respectively. The presence of at least eight additional oncogenes was predicted. A similar approach was used in another study which merely was focusing on 5q amplification peaks (Dondeti et al. 2012). The secreted glycoprotein STC2 and the proteoglycan VCAN were identified as potential oncogenes whose constant overexpression was shown to be sufficient to promote tumor genesis by limiting cell death.

The most detailed molecular depictions of RCC were achieved by (Sato et al. 2013) and The Cancer Genome Atlas Research Network (Creighton et al. 2013) who combined several microarray platforms. Novel and functional correlations between different molecular levels were unraveled by using array-based gene expression, copy number, and methylation analyses complemented by proteomics, sequencing, and clinicopathologic progression data. In line with current knowledge, VHL was reconfirmed as the main affected gene in ccRCC.

Interestingly, in both studies, the PI3K-AKT-mTOR signaling pathway was found recurrently affected, suggesting proteins of this pathway as potential therapeutic targets. A general change in metabolism mainly triggered by the deregulation of the pentose phosphate pathway, the glutamine transport, and acetyl-CoA carboxylase as well as altered miRNA activities through promoter methylation is currently regarded as the most relevant "pattern" for ccRCC biology.

In contrast to previous studies in which samples were mostly preselected according to clinicopathologic criteria, (Beleut et al. 2012) integrated SNP, gene expression, and tissue microarray data unbiased from regular tumor subgroup classification. Despite the molecular uniqueness of each RCC, the authors suggested the presence of common molecular "output" signatures which are independent of histological features in RCC and correlate with patient survival. A schematic illustration of the current and the proposed hypothesis is shown in Fig. 6. Based on these results it was concluded that any molecular alterations observed in each RCC are events which represent individual and functional modules, securing the achievement of distinct cancer-specific programs. This concept suggests a novel type of RCC classification with potential clinical relevance.

In summary, the use of different microarray technologies has revealed hundreds of genes as well as dozens of genetic profiles and pathways which are deregulated in RCC. Many of them are considered potential biomarkers of this cancer type which may further optimize and facilitate diagnosis, prognosis, and therapeutic decisions. For tailor-made therapies it will also be important not only to know the putative molecular key players but also to gain insight into the pathways and biological processes primarily affected in RCC. To get a clue, we used the Classification System PANTHER (http://www.pantherdb.org) for the organism of *Homo sapiens* to functionally group the entire list of RCC biomarkers described in this article as annotated by the databank under standard settings. In Fig. 7 the displayed output highlights the biological processes with the genes being involved. As expected, many processes seem to be crucial for development, progression, and metastasis of RCC. For individual RCC patient treatment (and probably for other cancer patients as well), it will therefore be essential to identify those biomarker alterations which allow to better predict the biologic tumor behavior.

Potential Applications to Prognosis, Other Diseases, or Conditions

Molecular biomarkers are thought to support the diagnosis, prognosis, and therapeutic strategies of RCC as well as to monitor tumor progression and recurrence. With the use of high-throughput microarrays, hundreds of biomarkers were identified and most of them were further evaluated for their potential use as prognostic and predictive factors in RCC. Some of them such as members of the VHL/HIF axis or the PI3K/AKT/mTOR pathway are promising but need vigorous validation to justify their clinical relevance. Predictive biomarkers such as HER2 amplification in breast cancer or activating gene mutations of EGFR and BRAF in lung cancer

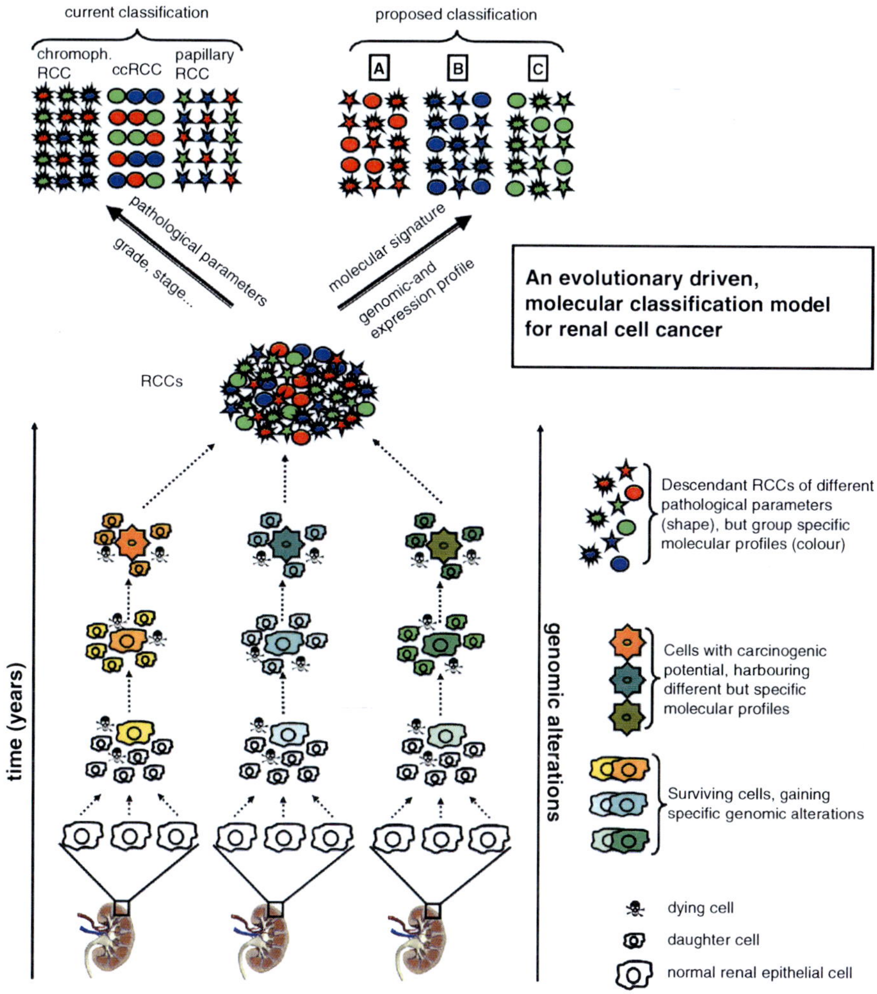

Fig. 6 Proposed model for a novel molecular classification of RCC independent of pathologic parameters

and melanoma, respectively, have not yet been identified in RCC. Moreover, all of the potential molecular RCC biomarkers described in the literature lack sufficient evidence to be unrestrictedly recommended for use in routine diagnostics. A huge amount of molecular information is available from RCC and many other human cancers, and a large number of genes have been reported as being cancer relevant. It is therefore not surprising that almost all of the human genes have already been identified as implicated ($n = 1{,}412$) or possibly implicated ($n = 26{,}292$) in cancer (http://atlasgeneticsoncology.org/). Furthermore, recent data obtained from next-generation sequencing technologies demonstrate that this number will still be rapidly increasing. Current cancer research and clinical trials often tend to focus

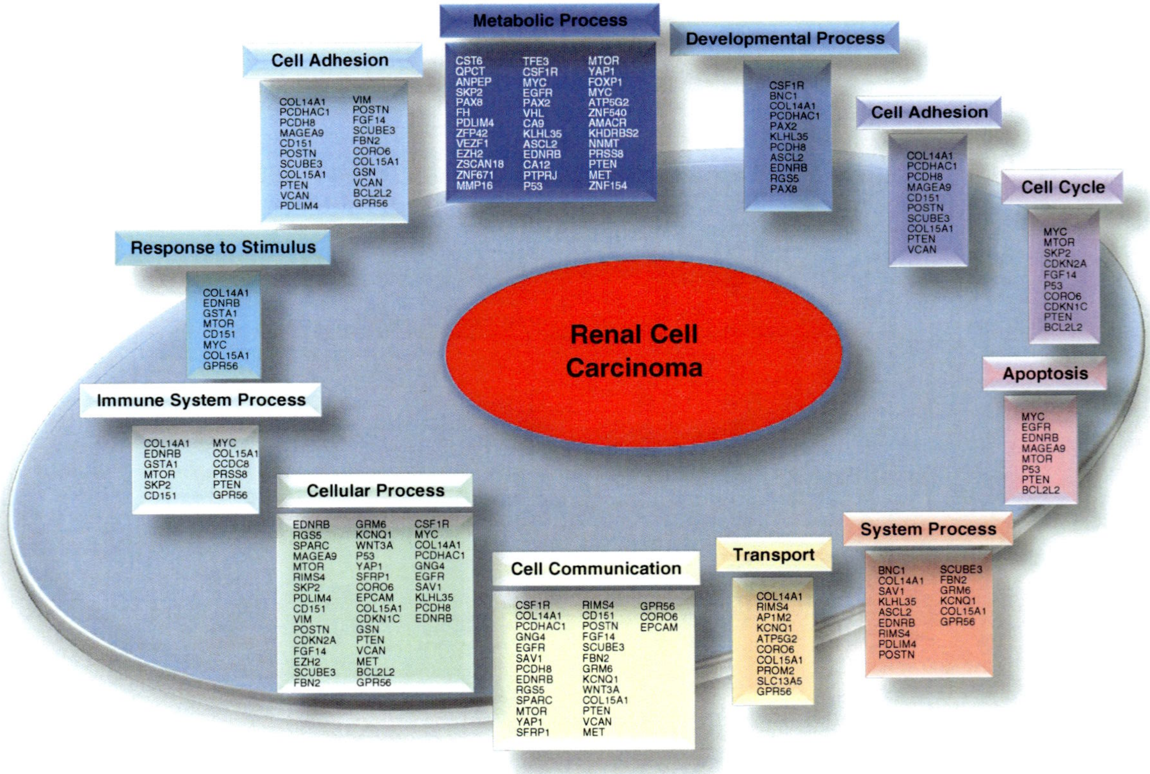

Fig. 7 Potential RCC biomarkers and their classification according to biological processes as suggested by the PANTHER Classification System database (http://www.pantherdb.org)

on single, relatively frequent molecular alterations ideally representing candidates with drug target potential. This rather isolated consideration of genes and pathways may fail to explain the more complex nature of carcinogenesis. As many genes and pathways proposed as being relevant in RCC are also found altered in other human cancers, it is tempting to speculate that the entity of molecular alterations (i.e., mutations, CNAs and methylation) existing in a single tumor would lead to common cancer-specific outputs (i.e., gene expression profiles) independent of histologic tumor classification. The application of this novel concept may imply additional potential impacts on cancer diagnostics and therapies.

Summary Points

- The biological behavior of RCC can still not be sufficiently predicted.
- Microarrays have been applied to identify molecular alterations at the DNA, RNA, and protein levels specific for RCC.
- Many potential biomarkers were identified and suggested to optimize diagnostics, prognosis, and treatment of RCC.
- None of these biomarkers is currently used in clinical routine.
- Pathways regulated by VHL/HIF and PI3K/AKT/mTOR seem to be crucial for RCC.
- Drugs targeting members of those pathways are currently used to treat RCC patients.
- Comprehensive biomedical studies and novel research concepts are needed to validate the prognostic and predictive value of molecular RCC biomarkers.

References

Albertson DG, Ylstra B, Segraves R, et al. Quantitative mapping of amplicon structure by array CGH identifies CYP24 as a candidate oncogene. Nat Genet. 2000;25:144–6.

Arai E, Chiku S, Mori T, et al. Single-CpG-resolution methylome analysis identifies clinicopathologically aggressive CpG island methylator phenotype clear cell renal cell carcinomas. Carcinogenesis. 2012;33:1487–93.

Avissar-Whiting M, Koestler DC, Houseman EA, et al. Polycomb group genes are targets of aberrant DNA methylation in renal cell carcinoma. Epigenetics. 2011;6:703–9.

Becker F, Junker K, Parr M, et al. Collecting duct carcinomas represent a unique tumor entity based on genetic alterations. PLoS One. 2013;8:e78137.

Beleut M, Zimmermann P, Baudis M, et al. Integrative genome-wide expression profiling identifies three distinct molecular subgroups of renal cell carcinoma with different patient outcome. BMC Cancer. 2012;12:310.

Beroukhim R, Brunet JP, Di Napoli A, et al. Patterns of gene expression and copy-number alterations in von-hippel lindau disease-associated and sporadic clear cell carcinoma of the kidney. Cancer Res. 2009;69:4674–81.

Boer JM, Huber WK, Sultmann H, et al. Identification and classification of differentially expressed genes in renal cell carcinoma by expression profiling on a global human 31,500-element cDNA array. Genome Res. 2001;11:1861–70.

Brannon AR, Reddy A, Seiler M, et al. Molecular stratification of clear cell renal cell carcinoma by consensus clustering reveals distinct subtypes and survival patterns. Genes Cancer. 2010;1:152–63.

Camparo P, Vasiliu V, Molinie V, et al. Renal translocation carcinomas: clinicopathologic, immunohistochemical, and gene expression profiling analysis of 31 cases with a review of the literature. Am J Surg Pathol. 2008;32:656–70.

Casagrande S, Ruf M, Rechsteiner M, et al. The protein tyrosine phosphatase receptor type J is regulated by the pVHL-HIF axis in clear cell renal cell carcinoma. J Pathol. 2013;229:525–34.

Chen M, Ye Y, Yang H, et al. Genome-wide profiling of chromosomal alterations in renal cell carcinoma using high-density single nucleotide polymorphism arrays. Int J Cancer. 2009;125:2342–8.

Chen Z, Li Y, Zhang H, et al. Hypoxia-regulated microRNA-210 modulates mitochondrial function and decreases ISCU and COX10 expression. Oncogene. 2010;29:4362–8.

Cohen HT, McGovern FJ. Renal-cell carcinoma. N Engl J Med. 2005;353:2477–90.

Creighton CJ, Morgan M, Gunaratne PH, et al. Comprehensive molecular characterization of clear cell renal cell carcinoma. Nature. 2013;499:43–9.

Dahinden C, Ingold B, Wild P, et al. Mining tissue microarray data to uncover combinations of biomarker expression patterns that improve intermediate staging and grading of clear cell renal cell cancer. Clin Cancer Res. 2010;16:88–98.

Darwish OM, Kapur P, Youssef RF, et al. Cumulative number of altered biomarkers in mammalian target of rapamycin pathway is an independent predictor of outcome in patients with clear cell renal cell carcinoma. Urology. 2013;81:581–6.

Dondeti VR, Wubbenhorst B, Lal P, et al. Integrative genomic analyses of sporadic clear cell renal cell carcinoma define disease subtypes and potential new therapeutic targets. Cancer Res. 2012;72:112–21.

Duns G, van den Berg A, van Dijk MC, et al. The entire miR-200 seed family is strongly deregulated in clear cell renal cell cancer compared to the proximal tubular epithelial cells of the kidney. Genes Chromosomes Cancer. 2013;52:165–73.

Eble JN, Sauter G, Epstein JI, et al. World Health Organization Classification of Tumours. Pathology and Genetics of Tumours of the Urinary System and Male Genital Organs. Lyon: IARC Press; 2004.

Eichelberg C, Chun FK, Bedke J, et al. Epithelial cell adhesion molecule is an independent prognostic marker in clear cell renal carcinoma. Int J Cancer. 2013;132:2948–55.

Fiegler H, Geigl JB, Langer S, et al. High resolution array-CGH analysis of single cells. Nucleic Acids Res. 2007;35:e15.

Frew IJ, Krek W. pVHL: a multipurpose adaptor protein. Sci Signal. 2008;1:pe30.

Fritzsche FR, Oelrich B, Johannsen M, et al. Claudin-1 protein expression is a prognostic marker of patient survival in renal cell carcinomas. Clin Cancer Res. 2008;14:7035–42.

Gibney GT, Aziz SA, Camp RL, et al. c-Met is a prognostic marker and potential therapeutic target in clear cell renal cell carcinoma. Ann Oncol. 2013;24:343–9.

Gottardo F, Liu CG, Ferracin M, et al. Micro-RNA profiling in kidney and bladder cancers. Urol Oncol. 2007;25:387–92.

Hager M, Haufe H, Kemmerling R, et al. Increased activated Akt expression in renal cell carcinomas and prognosis. J Cell Mol Med. 2009;13:2181–8.

Hatiboglu G, Pritsch M, Macher-Goeppinger S, et al. Prognostic value of melanoma-associated antigen A9 in renal cell carcinoma. Scand J Urol. 2012;47(4):311–22.

Herman JG, Latif F, Weng Y, et al. Silencing of the VHL tumor-suppressor gene by DNA methylation in renal carcinoma. Proc Natl Acad Sci U S A. 1994;91:9700–4.

Higgins JP, Shinghal R, Gill H, et al. Gene expression patterns in renal cell carcinoma assessed by complementary DNA microarray. Am J Pathol. 2003;162:925–32.

Jones J, Otu H, Spentzos D, et al. Gene signatures of progression and metastasis in renal cell cancer. Clin Cancer Res. 2005;11:5730–9.

Jung M, Mollenkopf HJ, Grimm C, et al. MicroRNA profiling of clear cell renal cell cancer identifies a robust signature to define renal malignancy. J Cell Mol Med. 2009;13:3918–28.

Kim HJ, Shen SS, Ayala AG, et al. Virtual-karyotyping with SNP microarrays in morphologically challenging renal cell neoplasms: a practical and useful diagnostic modality. Am J Surg Pathol. 2009;33:1276–86.

Klatte T, Seligson DB, Riggs SB, et al. Hypoxia-inducible factor 1 alpha in clear cell renal cell carcinoma. Clin Cancer Res. 2007;13:7388–93.

Kononen J, Bubendorf L, Kallioniemi A, et al. Tissue microarrays for high-throughput molecular profiling of tumor specimens. Nat Med. 1998;4:844–7.

Kosari F, Parker AS, Kube DM, et al. Clear cell renal cell carcinoma: gene expression analyses identify a potential signature for tumor aggressiveness. Clin Cancer Res. 2005;11:5128–39.

Liu Z, Fu Q, Lv J, et al. Prognostic implication of p27Kip1, Skp2 and Cks1 expression in renal cell carcinoma: a tissue microarray study. J Exp Clin Cancer Res. 2008;27:51.

Macher-Goeppinger S, Aulmann S, Tagscherer KE, et al. Prognostic value of tumor necrosis factor-related apoptosis-inducing ligand (TRAIL) and TRAIL receptors in renal cell cancer. Clin Cancer Res. 2009;15:650–9.

Macher-Goeppinger S, Bermejo JL, Wagener N, et al. Expression and prognostic relevance of the death receptor CD95 (Fas/APO1) in renal cell carcinomas. Cancer Lett. 2011;301:203–11.

Maina EN, Morris MR, Zatyka M, et al. Identification of novel VHL target genes and relationship to hypoxic response pathways. Oncogene. 2005;24:4549–58.

Maruschke M, Koczan D, Reuter D, et al. Putative biomarker genes for grading clear cell renal cell carcinoma. Urol Int. 2011;87:205–17.

Matsuura K, Nakada C, Mashio M, et al. Downregulation of SAV1 plays a role in pathogenesis of high-grade clear cell renal cell carcinoma. BMC Cancer. 2011;11:523.

McRonald FE, Morris MR, Gentle D, et al. CpG methylation profiling in VHL related and VHL unrelated renal cell carcinoma. Mol Cancer. 2009;8:31.

Minner S, Rump D, Tennstedt P, et al. Epidermal growth factor receptor protein expression and genomic alterations in renal cell carcinoma. Cancer. 2012;118:1268–75.

Moch H. An overview of renal cell cancer: pathology and genetics. Semin Cancer Biol. 2013;23:3–9.

Moch H, Mihatsch MJ. Genetic progression of renal cell carcinoma. Virchows Arch. 2002;441:320–7.

Moch H, Schraml P, Bubendorf L, et al. High-throughput tissue microarray analysis to evaluate genes uncovered by cDNA microarray screening in renal cell carcinoma. Am J Pathol. 1999;154:981–6.

Monzon FA, Hagenkord JM, Lyons-Weiler MA, et al. Whole genome SNP arrays as a potential diagnostic tool for the detection of characteristic chromosomal aberrations in renal epithelial tumors. Mod Pathol. 2008;21:599–608.

Monzon FA, Alvarez K, Peterson L, et al. Chromosome 14q loss defines a molecular subtype of clear-cell renal cell carcinoma associated with poor prognosis. Mod Pathol. 2011;24:1470–9.

Morra L, Rechsteiner M, Casagrande S, et al. Relevance of periostin splice variants in renal cell carcinoma. Am J Pathol. 2011;179:1513–21.

Morris MR, Ricketts C, Gentle D, et al. Identification of candidate tumour suppressor genes frequently methylated in renal cell carcinoma. Oncogene. 2010;29:2104–17.

Morris MR, Ricketts CJ, Gentle D, et al. Genome-wide methylation analysis identifies epigenetically inactivated candidate tumour suppressor genes in renal cell carcinoma. Oncogene. 2011;30:1390–401.

Nakada C, Matsuura K, Tsukamoto Y, et al. Genome-wide microRNA expression profiling in renal cell carcinoma: significant down-regulation of miR-141 and miR-200c. J Pathol. 2008;216:418–27.

Neal CS, Michael MZ, Rawlings LH, et al. The VHL-dependent regulation of microRNAs in renal cancer. BMC Med. 2010;8:64.

Neumann HP, Bender BU, Berger DP, et al. Prevalence, morphology and biology of renal cell carcinoma in von Hippel-Lindau disease compared to sporadic renal cell carcinoma. J Urol. 1998;160:1248–54.

Pantuck AJ, Seligson DB, Klatte T, et al. Prognostic relevance of the mTOR pathway in renal cell carcinoma: implications for molecular patient selection for targeted therapy. Cancer. 2007;109:2257–67.

Pawlowski R, Muhl SM, Sulser T, et al. Loss of PBRM1 expression is associated with renal cell carcinoma progression. Int J Cancer. 2013;132:E11–7.

Redova M, Poprach A, Nekvindova J, et al. Circulating miR-378 and miR-451 in serum are potential biomarkers for renal cell carcinoma. J Transl Med. 2012;10:55.

Rohan S, Tu JJ, Kao J, et al. Gene expression profiling separates chromophobe renal cell carcinoma from oncocytoma and identifies vesicular transport and cell junction proteins as differentially expressed genes. Clin Cancer Res. 2006;12:6937–45.

Sanjmyatav J, Steiner T, Wunderlich H, et al. A specific gene expression signature characterizes metastatic potential in clear cell renal cell carcinoma. J Urol. 2011;186:289–94.

Sato Y, Yoshizato T, Shiraishi Y, et al. Integrated molecular analysis of clear-cell renal cell carcinoma. Nat Genet. 2013;45:860–7.

Schuetz AN, Yin-Goen Q, Amin MB, et al. Molecular classification of renal tumors by gene expression profiling. J Mol Diagn. 2005;7:206–18.

Seligson DB, Pantuck AJ, Liu X, et al. Epithelial cell adhesion molecule (KSA) expression: pathobiology and its role as an independent predictor of survival in renal cell carcinoma. Clin Cancer Res. 2004;10:2659–69.

Seligson DB, Rajasekaran SA, Yu H, et al. Na, K-adenosine triphosphatase alpha1-subunit predicts survival of renal clear cell carcinoma. J Urol. 2008;179:338–45.

Shi T, Seligson D, Belldegrun AS, et al. Tumor classification by tissue microarray profiling: random forest clustering applied to renal cell carcinoma. Mod Pathol. 2005;18:547–57.

Skubitz KM, Zimmermann W, Kammerer R, et al. Differential gene expression identifies subgroups of renal cell carcinoma. J Lab Clin Med. 2006;147:250–67.

Szponar A, Zubakov D, Pawlak J, et al. Three genetic developmental stages of papillary renal cell tumors: duplication of chromosome 1q marks fatal progression. Int J Cancer. 2009;124:2071–6.

Takahashi M, Rhodes DR, Furge KA, et al. Gene expression profiling of clear cell renal cell carcinoma: gene identification and prognostic classification. Proc Natl Acad Sci U S A. 2001;98:9754–9.

Takahashi M, Sugimura J, Yang X, et al. Gene expression profiling of renal cell carcinoma and its implications in diagnosis, prognosis, and therapeutics. Adv Cancer Res. 2003;89:157–81.

Toffoli S, Michiels C. Intermittent hypoxia is a key regulator of cancer cell and endothelial cell interplay in tumours. FEBS J. 2008;275:2991–3002.

Togashi A, Katagiri T, Ashida S, et al. Hypoxia-inducible protein 2 (HIG2), a novel diagnostic marker for renal cell carcinoma and potential target for molecular therapy. Cancer Res. 2005;65:4817–26.

Truong LD, Shen SS. Immunohistochemical diagnosis of renal neoplasms. Arch Pathol Lab Med. 2011;135:92–109.

Valera VA, Walter BA, Linehan WM, et al. Regulatory effects of microRNA-92 (miR-92) on VHL gene expression and the hypoxic activation of miR-210 in clear cell renal cell carcinoma. J Cancer Educ. 2011;2:515–26.

Vasselli JR, Shih JH, Iyengar SR, et al. Predicting survival in patients with metastatic kidney cancer by gene-expression profiling in the primary tumor. Proc Natl Acad Sci U S A. 2003;100:6958–63.

Wagener N, Macher-Goeppinger S, Pritsch M, et al. Enhancer of zeste homolog 2 (EZH2) expression is an independent prognostic factor in renal cell carcinoma. BMC Cancer. 2010;10:524.

Wilhelm M, Veltman JA, Olshen AB, et al. Array-based comparative genomic hybridization for the differential diagnosis of renal cell cancer. Cancer Res. 2002;62:957–60.

Wondergem B, Zhang Z, Huang D, et al. Expression of the PTTG1 oncogene is associated with aggressive clear cell renal cell carcinoma. Cancer Res. 2012;72:4361–71.

Wotschofsky Z, Liep J, Meyer HA, et al. Identification of metastamirs as metastasis-associated microRNAs in clear cell renal cell carcinomas. Int J Biol Sci. 2012;8:1363–74.

Wozniak MB, Le Calvez-Kelm F, Abedi-Ardekani B, et al. Integrative genome-wide gene expression profiling of clear cell renal cell carcinoma in Czech Republic and in the United States. PLoS One. 2013;8:e57886.

Wulfken LM, Moritz R, Ohlmann C, et al. MicroRNAs in renal cell carcinoma: diagnostic implications of serum miR-1233 levels. PLoS One. 2011;6:e25787.

Yang XJ, Sugimura J, Tretiakova MS, et al. Gene expression profiling of renal medullary carcinoma: potential clinical relevance. Cancer. 2004;100:976–85.

Yang XJ, Tan MH, Kim HL, et al. A molecular classification of papillary renal cell carcinoma. Cancer Res. 2005;65:5628–37.

Yao M, Tabuchi H, Nagashima Y, et al. Gene expression analysis of renal carcinoma: adipose differentiation-related protein as a potential diagnostic and prognostic biomarker for clear-cell renal carcinoma. J Pathol. 2005;205:377–87.

Yao M, Huang Y, Shioi K, et al. A three-gene expression signature model to predict clinical outcome of clear cell renal carcinoma. Int J Cancer. 2008;123:1126–32.

Yi Z, Fu Y, Zhao S, et al. Differential expression of miRNA patterns in renal cell carcinoma and nontumorous tissues. J Cancer Res Clin Oncol. 2010;136:855–62.

Youssef YM, White NM, Grigull J, et al. Accurate molecular classification of kidney cancer subtypes using microRNA signature. Eur Urol. 2011;59:721–30.

Yu G, Yao W, Wang J, et al. LncRNAs expression signatures of renal clear cell carcinoma revealed by microarray. PLoS One. 2012;7:e42377.

Immunogenic Cell Death Markers in Liver Cancer

13

Nikolaus Kohles and Stefan Holdenrieder

Contents

Abstract

Primary and secondary liver cancers are still a major medical and social problem due to the often late diagnosis and poor prognosis. Therefore meaningful

N. Kohles
Department of Otorhinolaryngology, Helios-Klinikum Erfurt, Erfurt, Germany
e-mail: Nikolaus.Kohles@helios-kliniken.de

S. Holdenrieder (✉)
Institute of Clinical Chemistry and Clinical Pharmacology, University Hospital Bonn, Bonn, Germany
e-mail: Stefan.Holdenrieder@uni-bonn.de

V.R. Preedy, V.B. Patel (eds.), *Biomarkers in Cancer, Biomarkers in Disease: Methods, Discoveries and Applications*,
DOI 10.1007/978-94-007-7681-4_38

biomarkers for better diagnosis, therapy stratification, and monitoring are highly needed. Beyond conventional clinical and tumor markers, immunogenic cell death (ICD) markers are promising new candidates. They comprise an inhomogeneous group of molecules that are released from apoptotic or necrotic cells. In blood, these danger-associated molecular patterns (DAMPs) such as the high-mobility group box 1 protein (HMGB1) are able to exert activating and suppressive effects on the immunity system and promote tumor growth and invasiveness.

Here, we review the pathophysiology of primary and secondary liver cancer, the current therapeutic approaches, and the role of immunogenic cell death markers for the development and progression of cancer disease. Further, we report on their relevance as serum biomarkers for the diagnosis, estimation of prognosis, as well as the prediction and monitoring of response to cytotoxic therapy in cancer patients.

Key Facts

- Primary and secondary liver cancers are still a major medical and social problem because they often are diagnosed late and have a poor prognosis.
- Meaningful biomarkers for better diagnosis, therapy stratification, and monitoring are highly needed. Beyond conventional clinical and tumor markers, immunogenic cell death (ICD) markers are promising new candidates.
- ICD markers comprise an inhomogeneous group of molecules that are released from apoptotic or necrotic cells. In blood, these danger-associated molecular patterns (DAMPs) such as the high-mobility group box 1 protein (HMGB1), calreticulin, AFP, as well as nucleosomes are able to exert activating and suppressive effects on the immunity system and promote tumor growth and invasiveness.
- In the case of HMGB1, these immunologic effects are mediated by diverse toll-like receptors and the receptor of advanced glycation end products (RAGE).
- While circulating, HMGB1 and nucleosomes exert pro-immunogenic effects that may be enhanced when they are present in blood in form of HMGB1-nucleosome complexes; soluble RAGE and serum DNAse act as anti-immunogenic – by binding to HMGB1 as decoy receptor and by degrading nucleosomal DNA, respectively.
- In cancer patients, serum levels of HMGB1 and nucleosomes are found to be elevated and further increased already 24 h after cytotoxic therapies are applied. The extent of HMGB1 and nucleosome increase correlates with poor patient prognosis and poor response to locoregional therapies in patients with liver malignancies and in patients with diverse cancers during systemic therapies.
- In contrast, serum levels of sRAGE are decreased in cancer patients and further decline 24 h after therapeutic intervention. Low sRAGE levels correlate with poor prognosis and therapy response in diverse settings.
- Inclusion of ICD markers into large, prospective anticancer therapy trials is needed to validate these promising findings and to define biomarker-based procedures for a better individual management of cancer patients.

- Studies on the functional effects of immunogenic factors on tumor cells, immune cells, and cells of the tumor microenvironment will be conducted to identify new therapeutic approaches that improve the efficiency of cytotoxic therapies.

Introduction

Liver malignancies are a serious health problem worldwide. The liver can be affected by primary liver cancer, which arises in the liver, or by secondary liver cancer that originates from other sites and then spreads to the liver.

Primary liver cancer includes hepatocellular carcinoma (HCC), which is the most frequent form with 80–90 %, followed by cholangiocellular carcinoma with 10–15 %. Rare entities are hepatoblastoma (1–5 %) and sarcomas (<1 %) (Hamilton 2000). HCC is the fifth most common cancer in men and the eighth most common cancer in women worldwide with over 600,000 new cases each year. Concerning mortality, HCC accounts for the third most cause of cancer-related death with approximately 600,000 deaths each year (Parkin et al. 2005; MacSween et al. 2007).

In western countries, secondary liver malignancies are 40 times more frequent than primary liver malignancies, whereas primary liver malignancies prevail secondary liver malignancies in high-risk regions for HCC. The development of liver metastases is based on hematogenous dissemination via portal vein or via hepatic artery accordingly to the drainage of the primary neoplasia. The most liver metastases arise from colorectal cancers (CRC) due to the portal venous drainage. Further, liver metastases originate from primary neoplasia from upper gastrointestinal tract, like esophagus, stomach, gall bladder, and pancreas, and from breast, lung, and urogenital tract (Hamilton 2000). In this review, we will focus on the most frequent pathologies, HCC, and liver metastases from CRC and on biomarkers that are useful for diagnosis, prognosis, therapy prediction, and monitoring.

Hepatocellular Carcinoma (HCC)

As mentioned above, HCC is one of the most common cancers worldwide. The geographical extension of HCC is imbalanced in view of the different risk factors, like hepatitis B and C virus infections as well as alcohol abuse. The highest incidence rates are observed in Africa and Asia (20–40/100,000), whereas the incidence rates in Europe and the United States (6/100,000) are considerably lower. Nevertheless, the incidence of HCC is increasing in western countries in recent years, which depends on the increasing dissemination of hepatitis C virus (HCV) and on the rising alcohol abuse (Hamilton 2000). In Europe and the United States, median age at diagnosis is between 50 and 60 years, whereas HCC is diagnosed in the fourth and fifth decades of life in high-risk regions in Asia and Africa, respectively (Parkin et al. 2005). Most patients have at least two concomitant diseases such as chronic liver disease and HCC, and complex interactions between them have major implications for diagnosis, prognosis, and the management of HCC.

The diagnosis of HCC is usually made by combination of clinical, laboratory, imaging, and pathology examinations. Ultrasound, computed tomography (CT), and magnetic resonance imaging (MRI) are the most widely used diagnostic imaging modalities. In most cases, ultrasound is the first used modality, because it's widely available, noninvasive, and cheap. Detecting a suspicious lesion on ultrasound is followed by additional imaging studies to confirm the stage of the tumor (Gomaa et al. 2009).

The treatment of HCC includes surgical (liver resection, liver transplantation), locally ablative (percutaneous ethanol injection, radiofrequency ablation), intra-arterial (transarterial chemoembolization, selective internal radiation) as well as systemically cytotoxic (sorafenib) modalities. The first-line option for patients with a small resectable lesion in the non-cirrhotic liver is surgical resection.

In western countries, only about 5–15 % of patients are suitable for liver resection. Hepatic resection offers 5-year survivals of 60 % achievable in carefully selected patients (El-Serag et al. 2008). In cirrhotic patients, the best results are achieved by liver transplantation, if patients fulfill Milan criteria (single tumor $\leq$5 cm; two or three tumors, none >3 cm; no vascular invasion). 4-year survival rates up to 75 % were published (Mazzafero 1996). In patients, who are not suitable for surgery due to portal hypertension or comorbidity, ablative therapies are another therapy option. Percutaneous ethanol ablation (PEI) has an excellent outcome in patients with tumors <2 cm, where complete necrosis is achieved in most HCC lesions (Vilana et al. 1992). However, radiofrequency ablation (RFA) is currently more frequently used as ablative therapy option, as more favorable results are achieved in tumors >2 cm than by PEI.

Since many patients are asymptomatic in early stages, HCC is diagnosed in advanced stages of disease in 60–70 % of all patients. Here, curative therapy options are often not applicable and intra-arterial therapies are the best options available in palliative situations. The most widely used modality is transarterial chemoembolization (TACE), achieving partial response in 15–55 % of patients and improvement of median survival (Llovet 2003). A newer intra-arterial therapy for treatment of unresectable, multifocal HCC is selective internal radiation therapy (SIRT) that yielded similar results as observed by TACE treatment (Sangro et al. 2006). The multikinase inhibitor sorafenib is a new molecular targeted therapy option in patients, who are not suitable for interventional therapies anymore. Sorafenib showed better overall survival in comparison to best supportive care with good tolerance of drug (Villanueva et al. 2010).

Liver Metastases from Colorectal Cancer (CRC)

Most liver metastases arise from colorectal cancers due to the portal venous drainage. Colorectal cancer (CRC) is the most common gastrointestinal tumor and represents the third most common malignancy in the world with an estimated one million new cases and a half million deaths each year. The prognosis of CRC is better than in other carcinomas with a 5-year survival in Western Europe of 54 % (Parkin et al. 2005). While more immoderate consumption of meat, alcohol abuse, and smoking are well-known risk factors for CRC, vegetable nutrition is protective. Furthermore, chronic inflammatory bowel disease and genetic mutations arise the risk of developing CRC (Hamilton 2000).

Sixty percent of cases in patients suffering from CRC will develop liver metastases, and in 20 % of these, the liver represents the only site of the disease at death (Weiss et al. 1986). Synchronous liver metastases are detectable in 20–30 % of patients with CRC at diagnosis, while risk of developing metachronous liver metastases accounts to 10–30 % after 5 years dependent on primary tumor stage (Mentha et al. 2007; Nordlinger 2009). Surgical resection of liver metastases is the only curative possibility to obtain long-term survival. It is generally assumed that 10–15 % of patients with synchronous colorectal liver metastases will benefit from hepatic resection (Schlag et al. 2002).

In all kind of malignancies, staging of other organs is necessary for treatment decision. Thereby, the staging of the liver is an important aspect due to the high rates of secondary liver malignancies. The most widely used imaging modality for liver staging is ultrasound with a sensitivity of 71 % (Albrecht 1999). More expensive are CT and MRI that reach even higher sensitivities up to 90 %. While MRI plays an increasing role, CT is still the most commonly used method for hepatic imaging (Winterer et al. 2006).

Although metastases are often causes of death in malignancies, liver metastases of colorectal cancer or neuroendocrine tumors seem to be curable in certain cases. The precondition for curability is R0 resection of the lesion and the lack of extrahepatic metastases. However, only 15–20 % of CRC patients with hepatic metastases are primary resectable. In these cases, the 5-year survival amounts 20–45 % (Malafosse et al. 2001). For patients with unresectable disease, treatment with best supportive care alone is associated with a median survival of <10 months (Delaunoit et al. 2005). New local therapy options such as radiofrequency ablation (RFA) and cryotherapy are often performed when surgical resection is not feasible anymore. But also in these therapies, local recurrence rates are directly related to the diameter of the lesions treated and considerably increase in lesions over 4 cm (Seifert and Morris 1998). In disseminated liver metastases, surgical resection as well as RFA and cryotherapy cannot be applied anymore. In these cases SIRT or TACE are valuable alternatives to systemic chemotherapy (Jakobs et al. 2007; Vogl et al. 2007).

Locoregional Therapies

Interventional radiology plays an important role as palliative therapy or as bridging treatment before definite surgery or liver transplantation. Two options of locoregional therapies are transarterial chemoembolization (TACE) and selective internal radiation therapy (SIRT) for both HCC and colorectal liver metastases

(Llovet 2003; Jakobs et al. 2007; Vogl et al. 2007). Transarterial therapies comprise of a catheter-based group of procedures by which cytotoxic and/or embolic agents are intra-arterially directed to target tumor lesions. The efficiency of this approach is based on the unique dual blood supply of the liver. Whereas 90 % of the vascularization of tumor tissue is dependent on the hepatic artery, normal liver tissue is mainly delivered by the portal vein. This enables the application of high cytotoxic doses to the tumor while normal liver tissue is spared (Vogl et al. 2009).

In TACE, a solution of chemotherapy suspended in lipiodol, an oily contrast medium selectively retained within the tumor, is directly injected into the arteries supplying the tumor. This is followed by the obstruction of the feeding arteries with an embolizing agent. The combination of chemotherapeutic agent with embolic material extends the contact of the cytotoxic drug with the tumor and additionally causes ischemia in the tumor region. Such mixtures are able to dramatically increase the local concentration of the chemotherapeutic agent (Bruix et al. 2004). A number of chemotherapeutic cocktails have been used for TACE so far including doxorubicin, epirubicin, cisplatin, and mitomycin C. As there is little evidence for the superiority of any substance, the debate on the most appropriate drug is still controversial (Vogl et al. 2009). Nowadays, chemoembolization is the preferred treatment for palliation of unresectable HCC. Therefore, a pretherapeutic selection of the patients best responsive to TACE is required. An important aspect is the presence of sufficient liver function at treatment start. In patients with advanced liver disease, treatment-induced liver failure may offset the antitumoral effect or survival benefit of the intervention. Predictors of outcome are related to tumor burden (tumor size, vascular invasion, and AFP levels), liver functional impairment (Child-Pugh score, bilirubin), performance status (Karnofsky index, Eastern Cooperative Oncology Group (ECOG) performance status scale), and response to treatment. Interestingly, in a comparison of 12 liver staging systems, the Child-Pugh nominal liver staging system (including serum bilirubin level, serum albumin level, international normalized ratio (INR), ascites, and hepatic encephalopathy) was the most accurate in predicting survival of patients with unresectable HCC treated with TACE (Georgiades et al. 2006). Overall, the best candidates are patients with preserved liver function and asymptomatic lesions without vascular invasion or extrahepatic spread. In selected patients with well-preserved liver functions, TACE showed a statistically survival advantage in comparison to best supportive care (Llovet et al. 2002).

The main complication of TACE limiting its applicability is the postembolization syndrome (PES), which is characterized by nausea, vomiting, abdominal pain, and fever, occurring in 2–7 % of patients after the procedure. PES is probably caused by a combination of tissue and inflammation response to chemoembolization. The most serious complication is hepatic decompensation (Vogl et al. 2009).

Historically, radiation therapy had an extremely limiting role in the treatment of hepatic malignancies due to the very low tolerance of the liver to radiation. The application of conventional external beam radiotherapy for liver malignancies could be performed safely only up to 30–35 Gy, but such doses are not sufficient for eradication of tumor (Lawrence et al. 1995). However, initial experience with traditional external radiotherapy demonstrated palliation of symptoms in >50 % of patients and 20 % statistically significant tumor shrinkage indicating that liver malignancies seemed to be sensitive to radiation therapy (Dancey et al. 2000). Transarterial injection of radioembolic materials to the tumor-feeding artery combines the effect of radiotherapy and embolization, resulting in extremely high local tumor doses with an average of 200–300 Gy. Similar to TACE, normal liver tissue is spared due to the different blood supply of liver tissue, from the hepatic artery and the portal vein (Kennedy et al. 2004).

Unfortunately, some side effects may occur after SIRT application that are related to the liver or to other organs. The most frequent intrahepatic complication is postembolization syndrome (PES), including fatigue, nausea, abdominal pain, and sometimes fever. Furthermore, SIRT could cause radiation-induced liver disease with anicteric ascites, increased abdominal girth, and rapid weight gain with hypoalbuminemia. Extrahepatic complications are observed, when microspheres are shunted to other organs that eventually leads to radiation-induced pneumonitis or pancreatitis, ulceration, and even perforation of the stomach and duodenum (Ahmadzadehfar et al. 2010).

Effects of Locoregional Therapy on the Cellular Level

Both, TACE and SIRT, aim at destroying tumor cells by efficient induction of cell death. There are only few studies on the exact mechanism of cell death caused by TACE and SIRT. However, it is known from chemo- and radiotherapeutic studies that biochemical processes show time-, dose-, and cell type-dependent differences after cytotoxic stimuli. After high exposure to high chemo- or radiotherapeutic doses in the center of the lesion, cells will rapidly die by necrotic cell death. Other cells that are only slightly damaged will go into cell cycle arrest to enable repair processes (Plati et al. 2011). If they are not successful, those cells will die with some delay and present other morphological and biochemical features such as apoptosis or a mixture between both cell death types.

As mentioned above, TACE consists of the injection of a lipiodol-anticancer drug emulsion into the tumor's feeding arteries, followed by particle embolization. Bland embolization aims tumor ischemia, depriving it of nutrients, resulting in tumor cell necrosis and apoptosis. Besides controlling tumor growth, it preserves healthy liver tissue due to the livers dual blood supply (Llovet 2003; Brown et al. 2008). For TACE treatment, ischemia is an important part of therapy. It is known that cell death-related biomarkers such as nucleosomes are released during such ischemic events – as also found in cerebral stroke – already few hours after the onset into the blood circulation and showed maximum levels after 2–4 days (Geiger et al. 2006).

As chemotherapeutic agents of TACE, drugs like doxorubicin, epirubicin, or cisplatin were used in clinical trials, but to date, there is no evidence of the superiority of any single chemotherapeutic agent or any combination of them (Vogl et al. 2009). Both doxorubicin and its derivate epirubicin are anthracyclines, which cause DNA damage and kill cancer cells mainly by apoptosis (Lee et al. 2002). Both have the ability to bind to DNA and inhibit nucleic acid synthesis. This is achieved by DNA intercalation and results in protein-concealed DNA single- and double-strand breaks as a result of DNA topoisomerase II poisoning. Another way of cell death due to anthracycline therapy includes the production of reactive oxygen species (ROS) that react with intracellular components, like nucleic acids or proteins, and disrupt them (Ozkan 2004).

Similar to TACE treatment, SIRT causes tumor ischemia due to embolization as well. In consequence, nutrition of tumor is stopped resulting in apoptosis and necrosis. On the other hand, the β-emitter 90Y contributes to cell death, too. In vitro trials on leukemia cells showed that β-irradiation activates apoptosis pathways, including triggering of ligand/receptor pathways, mitochondrial activation, and caspase activation in leukemia cells (Friesen et al. 2003). De Nardo et al. supposed that low-dose β-irradiation leads to p53-dependent apoptotic cell death (De Nardo et al. 1995).

The effects of radiotherapy – single- and doubles-strand DNA breaks – are mediated directly, by activation of the CD95/Apo1/Fas receptor system and a proteolytic cascade of caspases, or by stimulation of the mitochondria, or by directed damage of the DNA (Friesen et al. 2003). After radiation therapy on bronchoepithelial and lung cancer cells, the release of nucleosomes reflects the extent of cell death (Holdenrieder et al. 2004): In irradiated lung cancer cells, a dosage of 30 Gy resulted in an early (after 24–48 h) and high maximum of apoptosis seen by elevated nucleosomes, while a dosage of 10 Gy leads to later (72 h) and less pronounced peak of apoptotic cell death. In the case of higher dosage, most cells are probably killed immediately after exposure to radiotherapy and are not able to activate any cell cycle repair mechanism. In lower dosage of irradiation, cells might still have the possibility to arrest their cell cycle and enable the repair of DNA damages. Only if they cannot be compensated appropriately, these cells will be determined to undergo cell death later on (Holdenrieder et al. 2004). Thereby, tumor cells showed a much more pronounced release of nucleosomes than normal bronchoepithelial cells pointing on a higher susceptibility to cytotoxic stimuli. In comparison to TACE treatment, we expected higher cell damage in SIR therapy due to higher lesions of tissue.

Cell Death Modalities

As mentioned, cytotoxic stimuli could lead to passive necrotic cell death including cellular swelling after gross cell damages and of active apoptotic cell death with activation of specific endonucleases that degrade the chromatin and including packaging of cellular substituents into apoptotic bodies before cellular demise. Of course, mixtures of both extreme types of cell death concerning morphological and biochemical features are observed as well. Further, cell death pathways that may play a role in the response to locoregional therapies are autophagy, mitotic catastrophe, paraptosis, and immunogenic cell death (Zitvogel et al. 2010).

Autophagy is an alternative and contrary mechanism to apoptosis by which cells respond to stressors such as hypoxia and starvation. Autophagy (self-eating) was found to be crucial for tumor cell survival particularly in established cancers to maintain viability in hypoxic, nutrient-limited microenvironments while it is inhibited during early carcinogenesis thus promoting tumor progression (Weiner and Lotze 2012). However, autophagy is not only used by tumor cells for self-protection; administration of chemotherapies to autophagy-competent tumor cells was also shown to induce tumor infiltration by antigen-presenting dendritic cells and cytotoxic T cells, which is mediated by the release of the DAMP adenosine triphosphate (ATP) from dying tumor cells (Weiner and Lotze 2012). ATP was demonstrated to bind to P2RX7 receptor on dendritic cells resulting in the assembly and activation of the NLRP3 inflammasome and subsequent secretion of IL-1 (Kepp et al. 2011). While chemotherapy-induced autophagic ATP release was critical for host-protective antitumor immune response, pericellular ATP levels were increased in autophagy-deficient tumors by administration of exogenous ATP or inhibition of ATP-degrading enzymes leading to improved chemotherapeutic responses in immunocompetent hosts (Michaud et al. 2011).

Immunogenic cell death, finally, is characterized by the stimulation of the immune system by products of degraded cells. After cancer cells underwent immunogenic cell death, e.g., as a consequence of exposure to chemotherapeutic agents such as anthracyclines, dendritic or other antigen-presenting cells engulf their corpses, process them, and present the resulting tumor antigens at the cellular surface to cytotoxic CD8+ T-cells or CD4+ T-helper cells. Those T-cells may directly attack residual tumor cells or stimulate the humoral immune system for efficient antitumor response (Zitvogel et al. 2010).

Biomarkers of Immunogenic Cell Death

Among the released proteins – so-called DAMPS – are, for example, calreticulin and adenosine triphosphate (ATP)), which are actively emitted by cells undergoing immunogenic cell death whereas others are emitted passively (e.g., high-mobility group box 1 (HMGB1)) (Krysko et al. 2013).

Calreticulin is a soluble protein in the lumen of the endoplasmatic reticulum, which is involved in several functions inside and outside the endoplasmatic reticulum, such as regulation of chaperone activity and Ca2+ homeostasis. The exposure of calreticulin on the outer plasma membrane of dying tumor cells is an important eat-me signal for phagocytes and dendritic cells to engulf tumor cells and their corpses. It has been shown that the exposure of calreticulin on the cell surface of cancer cells in response to anthracyclines is dependent on the endoplasmatic reticulum stress response associated with ROS production (Kepp et al. 2011).

A further important protein in immunogenic cell death is high-mobility group box 1 (HMGB1), a nuclear protein that is closely associated to the chromatin and plays an essential role in the regulation of transcription processes (Lotze and Tracey 2005; Bianchi 2009). In the blood circulation, HMGB1 is known to act as a danger-associated molecular pattern (DAMP) protein that binds to specific immune cells and promotes phagocytation and presentation of pathogenic cell death products and stimulation of immune responses (Lotze and Tracey 2005; Tesniere et al. 2008). Those effects are mediated by HMGB1 binding to specific receptors on dendritic or antigen-presenting cells such as the receptor of advanced glycation end products (RAGE) or the toll-like receptors 4 (TLR4) (Bianchi 2009; Park et al. 2006). In cancer diseases, tumor-related particles are phagocytized, processed intracellularly, and cross-presented at the cellular surface which leads to promotion of tumor-specific cytotoxic T-cell response (Sims et al. 2010; Tesniere et al. 2008; Kepp et al. 2009). During recent years, there is growing evidence that DAMP release during this form of "immunogenic cell death," which may be based on biochemical features of necrosis and apoptosis, is crucial for the sustained effects of chemotherapy (Kepp et al. 2009; Apetoh et al. 2008). Recently it was described that the oxidation status of HMGB1 is highly relevant for its immunostimulatory functions (Yang et al. 2012). This explains why HMGB1 can be protective to cancer development by inducing antineoplastic T-cell responses and, on the other hand, can promote tumor growth, neoangiogenesis, and metastatic spread (Campana et al. 2008).

The first identified receptor for HMGB1 was the multiligand receptor RAGE, which is regarded as a decoy marker if present in the circulation as soluble marker. Via RAGE and TLR-4 receptors, HMGB1 can induce maturation and homing of dendritic cells and inhibit the intracellular fusion of phagosomes and endolysosomes in dendritic cells thus facilitating the effective antigen cross-presentation at the cellular surface and the promotion of tumor-specific cytotoxic T-cell response. Signaling through RAGE leads to activation of the nuclear factor-kB (NF-kB) pathway and mitogen-activated protein (MAPK), which are important for cancer cell growth, invasion, and metastasis (Sims et al. 2010).

Another protein involved in cell death processes is DNase, which is not only involved in the hydrolysis of nuclear nucleosomal DNA after activation by caspases during apoptosis but as it also is present in blood and potentially important for the degradation of circulating nucleosomes (Zhang and Xu 2002).

Cell Death Markers in Blood Circulation

The measurement of markers of cell death and proliferation can provide information about the process of carcinogenesis and the response to antitumor treatment. Whenever apoptosis occurs under normal physiological conditions, most of the products of cell death are effectively removed by macrophages and neighboring cells. However, in pathological conditions of malignancy, this recycling system is impaired or overloaded. Consequently, cell death products can accumulate in appreciable quantity in the circulation where they can be potentially useful in the diagnosis, prognosis, and monitoring of disease (Beachy and Repasky 2008; Holdenrieder and Stieber 2009). Typical products of cell death are nucleosomes, complexes that are formed from a core particle of several histone components and DNA on the outside. During cell death, endonucleases preferentially bind to these easily accessible linking sites between the nucleosomes and cut the chromatin into multiple mono- and oligonucleosomes. In the cases of enhanced cell death, as during chemotherapy, they are also released into the circulation and can be detected specifically by ELISA techniques (Holdenrieder and Stieber 2009). The DNase is involved in the hydrolysis of nuclear nucleosomal DNA after activation by caspases during apoptosis. Furthermore, it is also present in blood and potentially important for the degradation of circulating nucleosomes (Zhang and Xu 2002).

Estimation of Response to Locoregional Therapy

Assessment of response to treatment is a key aspect in cancer therapy. Clinical symptoms, laboratory markers, or imaging modalities are possible parameters for determination of treatment success and decision of future therapy. The most widely used evaluation modality is imaging by ultrasound, CT, MRI, or positron emission tomography (PET). Evaluating the therapy response by imaging modalities, standard guidelines are helpful to improve comparability across different studies.

To date, the response evaluation criteria in solid tumors (RECIST) (Therasse et al. 2000) and the World Health Organization criteria (WHO criteria) (Miller et al. 1981) are often used for evaluation of response to treatment. Measurement of the largest diameter in one dimension (RECIST) and in two dimensions (WHO criteria) illustrates the basis of both methods. Both systems have shortcomings due to not considering neither tumor necrosis nor metabolic changes, which are the targets of all efficient locoregional therapies. Furthermore, vague form or diffuse dissemination of the tumors and changing contrast medium uptake in CT or MRI are not caught precisely with these measures (Jakobs et al. 2008). Therefore, the European Association for Study of the Liver (EASL) has proposed amendments to RECIST in patients with HCC: Only viable tumor (tumoral enhancement in the arterial phase) should be measured to assess response of target lesions. Determination of therapy response after locoregional therapy in patients with HCC by the use of lesion enhancement on contrast-enhanced CT is recommended as the standard modality by the EASL (Bruix et al. 2001). Regarding metabolic changes in tumor lesions, the use of fluorodeoxyglucose positron emission tomography (FDG-PET) seems to be superior to CT or MRI for evaluation of therapy response in patients with liver metastases from CRC or in patients with HCC undergoing TACE (Dierckx et al. 2009). Additionally, a considerable investigator-related error has to be mentioned. Therefore further investigations are needed to find out the best imaging modality for evaluation of therapy response. However, beyond treatment efficacy, improvement of survival and life quality is most relevant for the individual patient.

The Clinical Need of Prognostic and Predictive Markers

Because it is hard to identify patients who will benefit from locoregional treatment alone by clinical features, further indicators are needed that help to pretherapeutically estimate the prognosis of a single patient for progression-free and overall survival. And as the evaluation of therapy response by imaging techniques is only possible after several weeks or months, biomarkers that are able to prethera-peutically predict the efficiency of the treatment and to indicate the response to therapy already during the first days after application of TACE or SIRT are highly required.

Is has to be pointed out that prognostic markers are related to the survival outcome while predictive markers indicate therapy response. Biomarkers may be identical or different for both indications: An example for a predictive and prognostic marker is the estrogen receptor (ER) that plays a dual role in breast tumors; on the one hand, ER is a non-favorable prognostic marker as ER-negative tumors are associated with worse survival; on the other hand, ER is a predictive marker indicating potential response to antiestrogen drugs while virtually no response is noted in patients with ER-negative tumors. These predictive and prognostic markers before and during treatment are important for the therapeutic strategy meaning i) for the stratification of patients for efficient therapies and ii) for the early modification of treatment if it is not working sufficiently.

In order to reliably identify prognostic and predictive biomarkers for TACE and SIRT, prospective studies including a relevant number of cancer patients with a homogenous stage distribution, similar treatment, and well comparable staging of treatment success will be most useful. Furthermore, convenient time points of blood drawing before and during therapy, controlled preanalytical handling of blood samples, as well as the additional consideration of relevant clinical factors and biochemical markers are important criteria that affect the quality of those studies.

Immunogenic Cell Death Biomarkers in the Diagnosis of Liver Cancer

In tissue of liver cancer, HMGB1 was found to be highly expressed as compared with normal tissue and was associated with pathological grade and distant metastases. Knockdown of HMGB1 downregulated the expression of p-AKT, KI-67, and MMP-2 and inhibited liver cancer growth and metastasis (Dong et al. 2013). Indeed, higher levels of HMGB1 mRNA and protein were detected in liver cancer as compared with para-tumoral and normal tissue. High HMGB1 levels correlated with incomplete encapsulation, advanced tumor stage, and poor prognosis (Liu et al. 2012). A similar association of HMGB1 with clinicopathological features was reported by Jiang et al. who described a particular accumulation of HMGB1 in the nuclei of liver cancer cells (Jiang et al. 2012). Further, it was shown that HMGB1 is strongly released from necrotic cells that were treated by doxorubicin and enhances regrowth and metastasis of those cancer cells that had survived the chemotherapy via activation of RAGE (Luo et al. 2013). In addition, RAGE was found to be highly expressed on oval cells and to be a key regulator of oval cell activation and inflammation-associated liver carcinogenesis in mice (Pusterla et al. 2013). Parallel high expressions of HMGB1 and RAGE have already been found earlier in diverse malignant diseases among others in liver cancer (Kostova et al. 2010). While hypoxia is a common feature in solid tumors and contributes to tumor progression,

HMGB1 was found to play a key role in inducing an inflammatory response by activation of TLR-4 and RAGE pathways that led to stimulation of caspase-1 and proinflammatory cytokines IL-1β and IL-18 and finally promoted invasion and metastasis in liver cancer. Stable knockdown of HMGB1 attenuated these effects (Yan et al. 2012).

Whereas numerous studies have addressed the functional aspects of HMGB1, RAGE, and other ICD markers in cellular and animal models, only few studies have been published on the diagnostic relevance of immunogenic cell death serum biomarkers in liver malignancies so far. A study of Cheng et al. showed higher levels of HMGB1 in sera of 166 patients with hepatocellular carcinoma as compared with 62 patients with liver cirrhosis, 51 patients with chronic hepatitis, and 56 healthy persons. HMGB1 correlated with tumor size, stage, differentiation grade, and alpha-fetoprotein values (Cheng et al. 2008). Furthermore, it was shown that liver metastases derived from gastric cancer are associated with increased HMGB1 serum levels: In detail, pretherapeutic levels of HMGB1 in 227 patients undergoing gastroscopy were found to significantly discriminate different patient subgroups that will develop or have gastric cancer: while patients with nonmalignant gastric diseases (e.g., ulcers) had low HMGB1 levels, patients at high risk for gastric cancer (e.g., adenomas), those with early stage carcinoma, with locally advanced and those with metastastic gastric cancer exhibited increasing levels of HMGB1 in serum. Further, an association of HMGB1 levels with tumor size, lymph node status, and poor prognosis was shown. Thereby HMGB1 was superior than the established tumor marker carcinoembryonic antigen (Chung et al. 2009). In addition, HMGB1 serum levels were reported to be elevated in other cancers such as lung cancer (Shang et al. 2009; Naumnik et al. 2009) as well as in cervical cancer (Sheng et al. 2009; Table 1).

Immunogenic Cell Death Biomarkers During Cytotoxic Therapy in Liver Cancer

Although the implications of immunogenic cell death markers in the response to hypoxia and cytotoxic drugs and the association of high tissue ICD marker levels with poor prognosis are well known (Luo et al. 2013; Yan et al. 2012), only few studies have addressed the relevance of immunogenic cell death biomarkers circulating in the serum or plasma of patients with liver malignancies (i) for the monitoring of cytotoxic therapies, (ii) for the prediction of therapy response, and (iii) for the estimation of prognosis in a clinical setting.

Recently, we investigated several serum biomarkers involved in immunogenic cell death such as nucleosomes, DNAse activity, HMGB1, and RAGE in 49 advanced colorectal cancer patients with hepatic metastases who were treated by local elective internal radiation therapy (SIRT) and compared them with established cancer markers CEA and CA19-9, with cell death markers CYFRA 21-1 and LDH, with organ-related liver and pancreatic parameters as well as with the inflammatory marker CRP. These parameters were measured serially before and

Table 1 Clinical studies on immunogenic cell death markers in cancer disease

Malignancies	N	Marker	Time	Correlation with clinical features / progression/therapy response	Correlation with prognosis	Literature
HCC	166	HMGB1	Active disease	HMGB1-elevated versus nonmalignant liver diseases; positive correlation with cancer stage, size, and differentiation	Positive correlation with prognostic CLIP score	Cheng et al. (2008)
Gastric cancer	227	HMGB1	Active disease	HMGB1 in tumor patients is elavated; positive correlation with stage	High HMGB1 values correlate with poor prognosis	Chung et al. (2009)
NSCLC	145	HMGB1	Pre-/postoperative	Preoperative elevated, 1 month postoperative decreased; correlation with size and stage		Shang et al. (2009)
NSCLC	40	HMGB1	Pretherapeutic	HMGB1 is elevated in tumor patients		Naumnik et al. (2009)
Cervical cancer	284	HMGB1	Active disease	HMGB1 is higher in cancer recurrence than in healthy persons	High HMGB1 values correlate with short overall survival	Sheng et al. (2009)
Colorectal cancer with liver metastasis	49	HMGB1, sRAGE	Course (0 h, 24 h, 48 h) during SIRT therapy	HMGB1 is elavated after 24 h; sRAGE is decreased after 24 h; high HMGB1 values (0 h, 24 h) correlate with progression under therapy	High HMGB1 values (0 h, 24 h) correlate with short overall survival	Fahmueller et al. (2012)
HCC	50	HMGB1, sRAGE	Course (0 h, 24 h) during local TACE therapy	HMGB1 is elevated after 24 h; sRAGE is decreased after 24 h; low sRAGE values (0 h, 24 h) correlate with progression under therapy		Kohles et al. (2012)
Breast cancer	51	HMGB1, sRAGE	Course (0, 21, 84 days) during systemic neoadjuvant chemotherapy	sRAGE (0 h) is decreased in locally confined cancers; low sRAGE (0 h), high HMGB1 (0 h), and kinetics correlate with therapy response		Stoetzer et al. (2013)
Pancreatic cancer	78	HMGB1, sRAGE, nucleosomes	Course (0, 7, 14, 21, 28, 56 days) during systemic palliative chemotherapy	sRAGE (0 h) is decreased in pancreatic cancer; low sRAGE values (d56) correlate with progression under therapy	Low sRAGE, high HMGB1, and nucleosome values (different time points) correlate with poor prognosis	Wittwer et al. (2013)

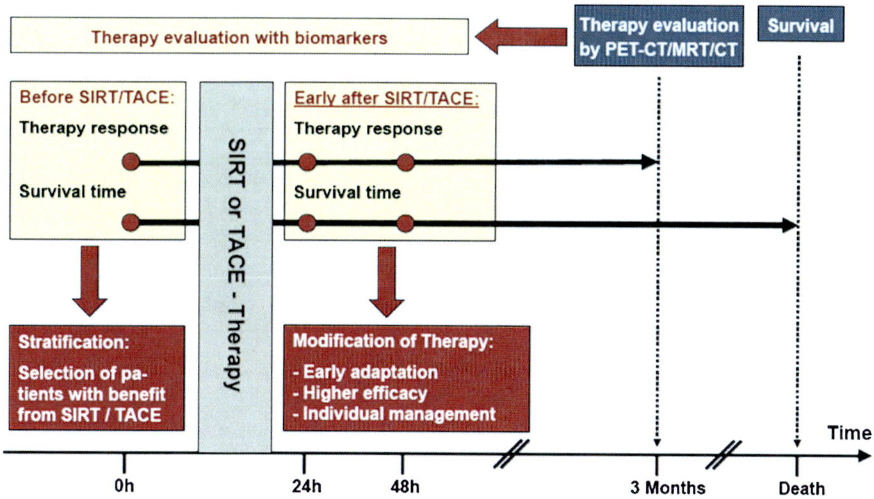

Fig. 1 Study setting for therapy monitoring, prediction of therapy response, and estimation of prognosis in liver malignancies

during the first days after SIRT to determine their relevance for the prediction of the radiologically evaluated therapy response after 3 months and with the patient survival. In addition, courses of some markers were closely followed already at the treatment day because the local damaging effects in the liver and the subsequent immune response after application of high doses of radioactively loaded microspheres into branches of the hepatic artery were expected to be strong and to occur timely after the therapeutic intervention (Fahmueller et al. 2012). Before the start of SIR therapy, levels of nucleosomes and HMGB1 were elevated in patients with liver cancer and particularly in patients with liver metastases from colorectal cancer while levels of sRAGE were slightly lower than that in healthy controls. Already 24 h after SIRT application, nucleosome and HMGB1 levels further increased significantly and showed a high correlation with each other. By contrast, sRAGE levels were decreased 24 h after SIRT (Fahmueller et al. 2013). Similar results with increases of nucleosomes 24 and 48 h after SIRT have also been found in patients with liver metastases from other tumor entities such as breast, pancreatic, cholangiocellular cancer, and carcinoids (Fehr et al. 2011, pp. 91–95). These consistent observations confirm the early release of the pro-immunogenic markers nucleosomes and HMGB1 and the reduced presence of anti-immunogenic markers sRAGE in circulation (Fig. 1).

In a similar study on 50 patients with hepatocellular cancer who were treated with transarterial chemoembolization (TACE) therapy, comparable courses with increases of nucleosomes (Kohles et al. 2011) and HMGB1 and decreases of RAGE and DNAse activity were found. Concerning tumor stage, significantly lower pretherapeutic RAGE levels were found in T3 than in T1 and T2 tumors while for the other markers and 24 h values, no correlation with tumor size was found (Kohles et al. 2012a).

Immunogenic Cell Death Biomarkers Predict Response to Therapy in Liver Cancer

Concerning the prediction of radiological response to SIRT in colorectal cancer patients with hepatic metastases, nucleosome levels (24 h after SIRT) were significantly elevated in progressive patients as compared with nonprogressive patients. In addition, other markers such as CYFRA 21-1, CEA, CA 19-9, AST, and LDH differentiated between response groups as well. With respect to patient survival, a multitude of markers showed prognostic relevance in univariate analyses. In multivariate analysis, the best prognostic model was obtained by the combination of nucleosomes (24 h), CRP, and AST (Fahmueller et al. 2012). In a second approach including also HMGB1, RAGE, and DNAse, HMGB1 levels 0 and 24 h after SIRT were found to be considerably higher in progressive patients as well. Interestingly, about 40 % of progressive patients had initial levels >10 ng/ml while all nonprogressive patients had lower HMGB1 values, which enables the specific and very early identification of a part of progressive patients (Fahmueller et al. 2013).

For evaluation of response to TACE therapy in patients with HCC, 71 therapies of 44 patients were included. Radiological staging investigations after a median of 70 days after TACE indicated 32 patients having stable disease or remission while 39 patients had progressive disease (Kohles et al. 2011). Although pretherapeutic values of circulating nucleosomes were not different in both responder groups, higher values of circulating nucleosomes were measured 24 h after treatment in patients with progressive disease compared to nonprogressive patients. In consequence, the percental changes of circulating nucleosomes between pretherapeutic values and 24 h values were significantly greater in the progressive group ($p < 0.001$) (Kohles et al. 2011). Besides nucleosomes, pretherapeutic and 24 h values of sRAGE indicated later response to therapy. Lower sRAGE levels were associated with progressive disease during therapy while DNase activity and HMGB1 levels did not indicate later response to therapy (Kohles et al. 2012b). Concerning clinical factors, tumor size and number of TACE cycles correlated with poor response. In a multivariate model, the combination of nucleosomes (24 h), alkaline phosphatase (24 h), and number of TACE cycles was the best model of predictive markers.

Immunogenic Cell Death Biomarkers Indicate Prognosis of Liver Cancer

Beyond response to a specific treatment, the estimation of prognosis is highly meaningful for the individual patient.

In the earlier mentioned SIRT study, HMGB1 levels before and 24 h after application had high prognostic value with high values being associated with shorter overall survival. In multivariate analysis, the combination of HMGB1 (24 h) and CRP (24 h) showed similar prognostic strength as compared with established prognostic liver markers in the earlier evaluation (Fahmueller et al. 2013).

In the TACE study, several markers have shown to be of prognostic value in univariate analysis such as CYFRA 21-1, AFP, LDH, AST, CHE, and bilirubin. Among immunogenic cell death markers, DNase activity revealed high prognostic impact: Low DNase activity levels measured before and 24 h after TACE were associated with more favorable outcome. HMGB1 and RAGE levels were not associated with prognosis. In multivariate analysis, the combination of DNase (24 h), CHE (24 h), and CYFRA 21-1 (24 h) yielded the best prognostic model (Kohles et al. 2013).

Application of Immunogenic Cell Death Biomarkers in Other Cancer Diseases

Immunogenic cell death biomarkers have been investigated in other clinical settings as well. In particular, it showed the high relevance of kinetic nucleosome measurements for the early prediction of therapy response and estimation in prognosis in patients with lung cancer, gastrointestinal, and gynecological cancers (Holdenrieder and Stieber 2009).

In addition, HMGB1 and RAGE were monitored in 51 patients with localized breast cancer receiving neoadjuvant chemotherapy (Stoetzer et al. 2013) as well as in 78 patients with advanced pancreatic cancer during palliative chemotherapy (Wittwer et al. 2013a). Similar to earlier findings, pretherapeutic high HMGB1 and low RAGE levels correlated with insufficient response to therapy in breast cancer patients and also HMGB1 kinetics revealed predictive potential while conventional tumor markers CEA and CA 15-3 did not have any predictive value (Stoetzer et al. 2013).

In pancreatic cancer patients, sRAGE and DNAse activity levels were lower than in the control group. Concerning therapy response, 42 patients with progressive disease had lower sRAGE levels during chemotherapy than those with stable disease status (Wittwer et al. 2013b). In addition, patients with low sRAGE and high HMGB1 levels had shorter time to progression and overall survival. High nucleosome levels at almost all time points investigated were prognostically unfavorable, too. Although established tumor markers CA 19-9, CEA, und CYFRA 21-1 showed high prognostic value as well, the new immunogenic cell death markers seem to be highly relevant tools for better therapy monitoring and estimation of patient prognosis.

Perspectives

Immunogenic cell death markers such as HMGB1 and sRAGE are involved in many acute and chronic pathophysiologic processes. In tumor disease, they play a key role in pathogenesis and in immune modulating functions that affect the maintenance of the inflammatory tumor microenvironment, the promotion of tumor growth, invasivity, angiogenesis, and metastazation. Due to their missing organ and tumor-specificity, circulating ICD blood biomarkers are hardly suitable for early and differential diagnosis of tumor diseases. However, elevated levels of soluble HMGB1 and nucleosomes and decreased sRAGE-levels may indicate later therapy response and prognosis of cancer patients. Further, early changes of serum levels after application of cytotoxic therapy may be meaningful for the early estimation of therapy response. Future clinical studies on large patient cohorts with diverse other cancers including immunogenic cell death biomarkers will show their usefulness in comparison with nowadays established biomarkers. In addition, it will have to be elucidated whether more specific assays, e.g., for diverse oxidized HMGB1 isoforms and nucleosomes with tumor-typical histone variants and modifications will further improve the clinical validity.

References

Ahmadzadehfar H, Biersack HJ, Ezziddin S. Radioembolization of liver tumors with yttrium-90 microspheres. Semin Nucl Med. 2010;40(2):105–21.

Albrecht T. Liver diagnostics. Conservative alternatives to CT? Interview by Petra Eiden. MMW Fortschr Med. 1999;141(41):14.

Apetoh L, Tesniere A, Ghiringhelli F, Kroemer G, Zitvogel L. Molecular interactions between dying tumor cells and the innate immune system determine the efficacy of conventional anticancer therapies. Cancer Res. 2008;68:4026–30.

Beachy SH, Repasky EA. Using extracellular biomarkers for monitoring efficacy of therapeutics in cancer patients: an update. Cancer Immunol Immunother. 2008;57(6):759–75.

Bianchi ME. HMGB1 loves company. J Leukoc Biol. 2009;86:573–6.

Brown DB, Cook RD, Kerr JR, Gould JE, Pilgram TK, Darcy MD. Chemoembolization of hepatocellular carcinoma: patient status at presentation and outcome over 15 years at a single center. AJR Am J Roentgenol. 2008;190(3):608–15.

Bruix J, Sherman M, Llovet JM, Beaugrand M, Lencioni R, Burroughs AK, Christensen E, Pagliaro L, Colombo M, Rodes J, et al. Clinical management of hepatocellular carcinoma. Conclusions of the Barcelona-2000 EASL conference. J Hepatol. 2001;35(3):421–30.

Bruix J, Sherman M, Llovet JM. Chemoembolization for hepatocellular carcinoma. Gastroenterology. 2004;127:179–88.

Campana L, Bosurgi L, Rovere-Querini P. HMGB1: a two-headed signal regulating tumor progression and immunity. Curr Opin Immunol. 2008;20:518–23.

Cheng BQ, Jia CQ, Liu CT, Lu XF, Zhong N, Zhang ZL, Fan W, Li YQ. Serum high mobility group box chromosomal protein 1 is associated with clinicopathologic features in patients with hepatocellular carcinoma. Dig Liver Dis. 2008;40(6):446–52.

Chung HW, Lee SG, Kim H, Hong DJ, Chung JB, Stroncek D, Lim JB. Serum high mobility group box-1 (HMGB1) is closely associated with the clinical and pathologic features of gastric cancer. J Transl Med. 2009;7:38.

Dancey JE, Shepherd FA, Paul K, Sniderman KW, Houle S, Gabrys J, Hendler AL, Goin JE. Treatment of nonresectable hepatocellular carcinoma with intrahepatic 90Y-microspheres. J Nucl Med. 2000;41(10):1673–81.

De Nardo GL, Kroger LA, Mirick GR, Lamborn KR, De Nardo SJ. Analysis of antiglobulin (HAMA) response in a group of patients with B-lymphocytic malignancies treated with 131I-Lym-1. Int J Biol Markers. 1995;10(2):67–74.

Delaunoit T, Alberts SR, Sargent DJ, Green E, Goldberg RM, Krook J, Fuchs C, Ramanathan RK, Williamson SK, Morton RF, Findlay BP. Chemotherapy permits resection of metastatic colorectal cancer: experience from Intergroup N9741. Ann Oncol. 2005;16:425–9.

Dierckx R, Maes A, Peeters M, Van de Wiele C. FDG PET for monitoring response to local and locoregional therapy in HCC and liver metastases. Q J Nucl Med Mol Imaging. 2009;53(3): 336–42.

Dong YD, Cui L, Peng CH, Cheng DF, Han BS, Huang F. Expression and clinical significance of HMGB1 in human liver cancer: knockdown inhibits tumor growth and metastasis in vitro and in vivo. Oncol Rep. 2013;29(1):87–94.

El-Serag HB, Marrero JA, Rudolph L, Reddy KR. Diagnosis and treatment of hepatocellular carcinoma. Gastroenterology. 2008;134(6):1752–63.

Fahmueller YN, Nagel D, Hoffmann RT, Tatsch K, Jakobs T, Stieber P, Holdenrieder S. Predictive and prognostic value of circulating nucleosomes and serum biomarkers in patients with metastasized colorectal cancer undergoing Selective Internal Radiation Therapy. BMC Cancer. 2012;12:5.

Fahmueller YN, Nagel D, Hoffmann RT, Tatsch K, Jakobs T, Stieber P, Holdenrieder S. Immunogenic cell death biomarkers HMGB1, RAGE, and DNAse indicate response to radioembolization therapy and prognosis in colorectal cancer patients. Int J Cancer. 2013;132 (10):2349–58.

Fehr Y, Holdenrieder S, Hoffmann RT, et al. Circulating nucleosomes in cancer patients with liver metastases undergoing selective internal radiation therapy using Yttrium-90 labelled microspheres. In: Gahan P, editor. Circulating nucleic acids in plasma and serum. New York/ Heidelberg: Springer; 2011. p. 91–5.

Friesen C, Lubatschofski A, Kotzerke J, Buchmann I, Reske SN, Debatin KM. Beta-irradiation used for systemic radioimmunotherapy induces apoptosis and activates apoptosis pathways in leukaemia cells. Eur J Nucl Med Mol Imaging. 2003;30(9):1251–61.

Geiger S, Holdenrieder S, Stieber P, Hamann GF, Bruening R, Ma J, Nagel D, Seidel D. Nucleosomes in serum of patients with early cerebral stroke. Cerebrovasc Dis. 2006;21 (1–2):32–7.

Georgiades CS, Liapi E, Frangakis C, Park JU, Kim HW, Hong K, Geschwind JF. Prognostic accuracy of 12 liver staging systems in patients with unresectable hepatocellular carcinoma treated with transarterial chemoembolization. J Vasc Interv Radiol. 2006;17(10):1619–24.

Gomaa AI, Khan SA, Leen ELS, Waked I, Taylor-Robinson SD. Diagnosis of hepatocellular carcinoma. World J Gastroenterol. 2009;15(11):1301–14.

Hamilton SR, Aaltonen L. World Health Organization classification of tumours: pathology and genetics of tumours of the digestive system. Lyon: IARC Press; 2000.

Holdenrieder S, Stieber P. Clinical use of circulating nucleosomes. Crit Rev Clin Lab Sci. 2009;46 (1):1–24.

Holdenrieder S, Stief J, Bergner A, Gamarra F, Mitlewski A, Nagel D, Huber RM, Stieber P. Nucleosomes indicate the in vitro radiosensitivity of irradiated bronchoepithelial and lung cancer cells. Tumor Biol. 2004;25(5–6):321–6.

Jakobs TF, Hoffmann RT, Poepperl G, Schmitz A, Lutz J, Koch W, Tatsch K, Lubiensky A, Reiser MF, Helmberger T. Mid-term results in otherwise treatment refractory primary or secondary liver confined tumours treated with selective internal radiation therapy (SIRT) using (90) Yttrium resin-microspheres. Eur Radiol. 2007;17(5):1320–30.

Jakobs TF, Hoffmann RT, Tatsch K, Trumm C, Reiser MF. Therapy response of liver tumors after selective internal radiation therapy. Radiologe. 2008;48(9):839–49.

Jiang W, Wang Z, Li X, Fan X, Duan Y. High-mobility group box 1 is associated with clinicopathologic features in patients with hepatocellular carcinoma. Pathol Oncol Res. 2012;18(2): 293–8.

Kennedy AS, Nutting C, Coldwell D, Gaiser J, Drachenberg C. Pathologic response and microdosimetry of Y-90 microspheres in man: review of four explanted whole livers. Int J Radiat Oncol Biol Phys. 2004;60(5):1552–63.

Kepp O, Tesniere A, Schlemmer F, Michaud M, Senovilla L, Zitvogel L, Kroemer G. Immunogenic cell death modalities and their impact on cancer treatment. Apoptosis. 2009;14:364–75.

Kepp O, Galluzzi L, Martins I, Schlemmer F, Adjemian S, Michaud M, Sukkurwala AQ, Menger L, Zitvogel L, Kroemer G. Molecular determinants of immunogenic cell death elicited by anticancer chemotherapy. Cancer Metastasis Rev. 2011;30(1):61–9.

Kohles N, Nagel D, Jüngst D, Durner J, Stieber P, Holdenrieder S. Relevance of circulating nucleosomes and oncological biomarkers for predicting response to transarterial chemoembolization therapy in liver cancer patients. BMC Cancer. 2011;11:202.

Kohles N, Nagel D, Jüngst D, Durner J, Stieber P, Holdenrieder S. Prognostic relevance of oncological serum biomarkers in liver cancer patients undergoing transarterial chemoembolization therapy. Tumour Biol. 2012a;33(1):33–40.

Kohles N, Nagel D, Jüngst D, Stieber P, Holdenrieder S. Predictive value of immunogenic cell death biomarkers HMGB1, sRAGE, and DNase in liver cancer patients receiving transarterial chemoembolization therapy. Tumour Biol. 2012b;33(6):2401–9.

Kohles N, Nagel D, Jüngst D, Stieber P, Holdenrieder S. DNase is a prognostic marker in liver cancer patients receiving transarterial chemoembolization therapy. Int J Clin Pharmacol Ther. 2013;51(1):80–3.

Kostova N, Zlateva S, Ugrinova I, Pasheva E. The expression of HMGB1 protein and its receptor RAGE in human malignant tumors. Mol Cell Biochem. 2010;337(1–2):251–8.

Krysko O, Løve Aaes T, Bachert C, Vandenabeele P, Krysko DV. Many faces of DAMPs in cancer therapy. Cell Death Dis. 2013;4:e631.

Lawrence TS, Robertson JM, Anscher MS, Jirtle RL, Ensminger WD, Fajardo LF. Hepatic toxicity resulting from cancer treatment. Int J Radiat Oncol Biol Phys. 1995;31(5):1237–48.

Lee TK, Lau TC, Ng IO. Doxorubicin-induced apoptosis and chemosensitivity in hepatoma cell lines. Cancer Chemother Pharmacol. 2002;49(1):78–86.

Liu F, Zhang Y, Peng Z, Gao H, Xu L, Chen M. High expression of high mobility group box 1 (hmgb1) predicts poor prognosis for hepatocellular carcinoma after curative hepatectomy. J Transl Med. 2012;10:135.

Llovet JM, Real MI, Montana X, Planas R, Coll S, Aponte J, Ayuso C, Sala M, Muchart J, Sola R, et al. Arterial embolisation or chemoembolisation versus symptomatic treatment in patients with unresectable hepatocellular carcinoma: a randomised controlled trial. Lancet. 2002;359 (9319):1734–9.

Llovet JM, Bruix J, Barcelona-Clinic Liver Cancer Group. Systematic review of randomized trials for unresectable hepatocellular carcinoma: chemoembolization improves survival. Hepatology. 2003;37(2):429–42.

Lotze MT, Tracey KJ. High-mobility group box 1 protein (HMGB1): nuclear weapon in the immune arsenal. Nat Rev Immunol. 2005;5:331–42.

Luo Y, Chihara Y, Fujimoto K, Sasahira T, Kuwada M, Fujiwara R, Fujii K, Ohmori H, Kuniyasu H. High mobility group box 1 released from necrotic cells enhances regrowth and metastasis of cancer cells that have survived chemotherapy. Eur J Cancer. 2013;49(3):741–51.

MacSween RNM, Burt AD, Portmann B. Pathology of the liver. 5th ed. London/ Edinburgh/New York: Churchill Livingstone; 2007.

Malafosse R, Penna C, Cunha AS, Nordlinger B. Surgical management of hepatic metastases from colorectal malignancies. Ann Oncol. 2001;12(7):887–94.

Mazzaferro V, Regalia E, Doci R, Andreola S, Pulvirenti A, Bozzetti F, Montalto F, Ammatuna M, Morabito A, Gennari L. Liver transplantation for the treatment of small hepatocellular carcinoma in patients with cirrhosis. N Engl J Med. 1996 Mar 14;334(11):693–9.

Mentha G, Majno P, Terraz S, et al. Treatment strategies for the management of advanced colorectal liver metastases detected synchronously with the primary tumor. Eur J Surg Oncol. 2007;33:76–83.

Michaud M, Martins I, Sukkurwala AQ, Adjemian S, Ma Y, Pellegatti P, Shen S, Kepp O, Scoazec M, Mignot G, Rello-Varona S, Tailler M, Menger L, Vacchelli E, Galluzzi L, Ghiringhelli F, di Virgilio F, Zitvogel L, Kroemer G. Autophagy-dependent anticancer immune responses induced by chemotherapeutic agents in mice. Science. 2011;334(6062): 1573–7.

Miller AB, Hoogstraten B, Staquet M, Winkler A. Reporting results of cancer-treatment. Cancer. 1981;47(1):207–14.

Naumnik W, Nilklinska W, Ossolinska M, et al. Serum levels of HMGB1, survivin, and VEGF in patients with advanced non-small cell lung cancer during chemotherapy. Folia Histochem Cytobiol. 2009;47:703–9.

Nordlinger B, Van Cutsem E, Gruenberger T, European Colorectal Metastases Treatment Group, Sixth International Colorectal Liver Metastases Workshop. Combination of surgery and chemotherapy and the role of targeted agents in the treatment of patients with colorectal liver metastases: recommendations from an expert panel. Ann Oncol. 2009;20(6):985–92.

Ozkan A, Fişkin K. Epirubicin HCl toxicity in human liver-derived hepatoma G2 cells. Pol J Pharmacol. 2004;56(4):435–44.

Park JS, Gamboni-Robertson F, He Q, Svetkauskaite D, Kim JY, Strassheim D, Sohn JW, Yamada S, Maruyama I, Banerjee A, et al. High mobility group box 1 protein interacts with multiple toll-like receptors. Am J Physiol Cell Physiol. 2006;290:917–24.

Parkin DM, Bray F, Ferlay J, Pisani P. Global cancer statistics, 2002. Cancer J Clin. 2005;55(2): 74–108.

Plati J, Bucur O, Khosravi-Far R. Apoptotic cell signaling in cancer progression and therapy. Integr Biol (Camb). 2011;3(4):279–96.

Pusterla T, Nèmeth J, Stein I, Wiechert L, Knigin D, Marhenke S, Longerich T, Kumar V, Arnold B, Vogel A, Bierhaus A, Pikarsky E, Hess J, Angel P. Receptor for advanced glycation endproducts (RAGE) is a key regulator of oval cell activation and inflammation-associated liver carcinogenesis in mice. Hepatology. 2013;58(1):363–73.

Sangro B, Bilbao JI, Boan J, Martinez-Cuesta A, Benito A, Rodriguez J, Panizo A, Gil B, Inarrairaegui M, Herrero I, et al. Radioembolization using 90Y-resin microspheres for patients with advanced hepatocellular carcinoma. Int J Radiat Oncol Biol Phys. 2006;66(3):792–800.

Schlag PM, Benhidjeb T, Stroszczynski C. Resection and local therapy for liver metastases. Best Pract Res Clin Gastroenterol. 2002;16(2):299–317.

Seifert JK, Morris DL. Prognostic factors after cryotherapy for hepatic metastases from colorectal cancer. Ann Surg. 1998;228(2):201–8.

Shang GH, Jia CQ, Tian H, et al. Serum high mobility group box protein 1 as a clinical marker for non-small cell lung cancer. Respir Med. 2009;103:1949–53.

Sheng X, Du X, Zhang X, et al. Clinical value of serum HMGB1 levels in early detection of recurrent squamous cell carcinoma of uterine cervix: comparison with serum SCCA, CAFRA 21-1, and CEA levels. Croat Med J. 2009;50:455–64.

Sims GP, Rowe DC, Rietdijk ST, Herbst R, Coyle AJ. HMGB1 and RAGE in inflammation and cancer. Annu Rev Immunol. 2010;28:367–88.

Stoetzer OJ, Fersching DM, Salat C, Steinkohl O, Gabka CJ, Hamann U, Braun M, Feller AM, Heinemann V, Siegele B, Nagel D, Holdenrieder S. Circulating immunogenic cell death biomarkers HMGB1 and RAGE in breast cancer patients during neoadjuvant chemotherapy. Tumour Biol. 2013;34(1):81–90.

Tesniere A, Panaretakis T, Kepp O, Apetoh L, Ghiringhelli F, Zitvogel L, Kroemer G. Molecular characteristics of immunogenic cancer cell death. Cell Death Differ. 2008;15:3–12.

Therasse P, Arbuck SG, Eisenhauer EA, Wanders J, Kaplan RS, Rubinstein L, Verweij J, Van Glabbeke M, van Oosterom AT, Christian MC, et al. New guidelines to evaluate the response to treatment in solid Tumors. J Natl Cancer Inst. 2000;92(3):205–16.

Vilana R, Bruix J, Bru C, Ayuso C, Solé M, Rodés J. Tumor size determines the efficacy of percutaneous ethanol injection for the treatment of small hepatocellular carcinoma. Hepatology. 1992;16(2):353–7.

Villanueva A, Minguez B, Forner A, Reig M, Llovet JM. Hepatocellular carcinoma: novel molecular approaches for diagnosis, prognosis, and therapy. Annu Rev Med. 2010;61:317–28.

Vogl TJ, Zangos S, Eichler K, Yakoub D, Nabil M. Colorectal liver metastases: regional chemotherapy via transarterial chemoembolization (TACE) and hepatic chemoperfusion: an update. Eur Radiol. 2007;17(4):1025–34.

Vogl TJ, Naguib NN, Nour-Eldin NE, Rao P, Emami AH, Zangos S, Nabil M, Abdelkader A. Review on transarterial chemoembolization in hepatocellular carcinoma: palliative, combined, neoadjuvant, bridging, and symptomatic indications. Eur J Radiol. 2009;72(3):505–16.

Weiner LM, Lotze MT. Tumor-cell death, autophagy, and immunity. N Engl J Med. 2012;366(12):1156–8.

Weiss L, Grundmann E, Torhorst J, Hartveit F, Moberg I, Eder M, Fenogliopreiser CM, Napier J, Horne CHW, Lopez MJ, et al. Hematogenous metastatic patterns in colonic-carcinoma – an analysis of 1541 necropsies. J Pathol. 1986;150(3):195–203.

Winterer JT, Kotter E, Ghanem N, Langer M. Detection and characterization of benign focal liver lesions with multislice CT. Eur Radiol. 2006;16(11):2427–43.

Wittwer C, Boeck S, Heinemann V, Haas M, Stieber P, Nagel D, Holdenrieder S. Circulating nucleosomes and immunogenic cell death markers HMGB1, sRAGE and DNAse in patients with advanced pancreatic cancer undergoing chemotherapy. Int J Cancer. 2013a;133(11): 2619–30.

Wittwer C, Boeck S, Heinemann V, Haas M, Stieber P, Nagel D, Holdenrieder S. Soluble receptor of advanced glycation end products (sRAGE) indicates response to chemotherapy in pancreatic cancer patients. Int J Clin Pharmacol Ther. 2013b;51(1):67–9.

Yan W, Chang Y, Liang X, Cardinal JS, Huang H, Thorne SH, Monga SP, Geller DA, Lotze MT, Tsung A. High-mobility group box 1 activates caspase-1 and promotes hepatocellular carcinoma invasiveness and metastases. Hepatology. 2012;55(6):1863–75.

Yang H, Lundbäck P, Ottosson L, Erlandsson-Harris H, Venereau E, Bianchi ME, Al-Abed Y, Andersson U, Tracey KJ, Antoine DJ. Redox modification of cysteine residues regulates the cytokine activity of high mobility group box-1 (HMGB1). Mol Med. 2012;18:250–9.

Zhang JH, Xu M. Apoptotic DNA fragmentation and tissue homeostasis. Trends Cell Biol. 2002;12:84–9.

Zitvogel L, Kepp O, Senovilla L, Menger L, Chaput N, Kroemer G. Immunogenic tumor cell death for optimal anticancer therapy: the calreticulin exposure pathway. Clin Cancer Res. 2010;16(12):3100–4.

Epigenetics and Biomarkers in Lung Cancer: Emerging Blood-Based Molecular Biomarkers for Detection and Monitoring

14

Athina Markou, Ioanna Sourvinou, Ioanna Balkouranidou, and Evi S. Lianidou

Contents

Abstract

Early detection and precise diagnosis of lung cancer are critical to select proper therapeutic treatments as early as possible. Toward this direction, the discovery and exploitation of novel innovative, non-invasive, and reliable tumor biomarkers are of vital importance. In this review, we present emerging blood-based molecular biomarkers that have been evaluated for the detection and

A. Markou • I. Sourvinou • I. Balkouranidou •
E.S. Lianidou (✉)
Analysis of Circulating Tumor Cells Lab, Laboratory of Analytical Chemistry, Department of Chemistry, University of Athens, Athens, Greece
e-mail: athina_markoy@yahoo.gr; jsourvin@gmail.com; ioannabalg@gmail.com; evilianidou@gmail.com

V.R. Preedy, V.B. Patel (eds.), *Biomarkers in Cancer, Biomarkers in Disease: Methods, Discoveries and Applications*,
DOI 10.1007/978-94-007-7681-4_35

monitoring of lung cancer. We specially focus on biomarkers based on a non-invasive liquid biopsy approach, such as circulating tumor cells (CTCs), circulating miRNAs, gene promoter methylation, and DNA mutations in cell-free circulating DNA.

List of Abbreviations

5-Aza-dC	5-Aza-2′-deoxycytidine
AD	Adenocarcinoma
ALK	Anaplastic Lymphoma Kinase
cfDNA	Cell-Free DNA
CTCs	Circulating Tumor Cells
DFI	Disease-Free Interval
EGFR	Epidermal Growth Factor Receptor
EGFR-TKIs	EGFR Tyrosine Kinase Inhibitors
LCM	Laser Cell Microdissection
miRNA	MicroRNA
MSP	Methylation-Specific PCR
NSCLC	Non-small Cell Lung Cancer
OS	Overall Survival
RT-qPCR	Reverse Transcription Quantitative PCR
SCC	Squamous Cell Carcinoma
SCLC	Small-Cell Lung Cancer

Key Facts

- A CTC can be used as "liquid biopsy" for the follow-up examinations of lung cancer patients. CTC molecular characterization has the potential to provide important information for the biology of metastasizing cancer cells which could further be utilized to guide individualized targeted treatments.
- Circulating cell-free tumor DNA (cfDNA) released from cancer cells into plasma represents an alternative important non-invasive liquid biopsy approach.
- miRNAs circulating in the blood have been evaluated as diagnostic and prognostic biomarkers, and it has been shown that they are associated with a clinical outcome in lung cancer patients.
- Tumor-associated mutations detectable in cfDNA circulating in the blood can now be used as lung cancer companion diagnostic biomarkers, including epidermal growth factor receptor (EGFR), KRAS, BRAF mutations, and EML4-anaplastic lymphoma kinase (ALK) rearrangements.

Definitions of Words and Terms

Liquid Biopsy This term refers to the non-invasive procedure where the peripheral blood can be used as a source of CTC or cell-free DNA to derive information useful for describing the status of a primary or metastatic tumor. It is extremely powerful, especially when the primary tumor is surgically removed.

Circulating Tumor Cells CTCs are cells that have escaped from a primary tumor or a metastatic site and circulate in the bloodstream.

Tumor Biomarker A **tumor biomarker** generally refers to a measured characteristic which may be used as an indicator of the presence of a tumor.

DNA Methylation Biomarker This term is describing the condition where a gene promoter (usually from a tumor suppressor or metastasis suppressor gene) is highly methylated in tumors, thus indicating the inactivation of the expression of this gene in cancer.

MicroRNA **miRNA** is a small noncoding RNA molecule (ca. 22 nucleotides) which functions in the transcriptional and post-transcriptional regulation of gene expression.

Introduction

Our understanding of cancer at the cellular and molecular level has increased exponentially during the last decade, not only by identifying many new targets for diagnosis and therapy but also by documenting the extraordinary heterogeneity within and between different cancers. Powerful genomic, proteomic, and epigenomic technologies provide now important and complementary information to get the full picture of this difficult puzzle. Mutational analysis of clinical material is now possible for hundreds of genes, and within the next few years, advances in next-generation sequencing promise to provide affordable whole genome data for each patient's cancer (Diamandis et al. 2013).

Lung cancer is clinically divided into two subtypes, small-cell lung cancer (SCLC, 10–15 % of lung cancer cases) and non-small cell lung cancer (NSCLC, 85–90 % of cases). Early detection of NSCLC, which is the more common and less aggressive of the two subtypes, has the highest potential for saving lives. As yet, no routine screening method that enables early detection exists, and this is a key factor in the high mortality rate of this disease (Anglim et al. 2008). Patients' survival depends significantly on early detection. For patients with operable stage IA, the 5-year survival can be as high as 55–80 % (Wang et al. 2010). Therefore, early detection and precise diagnosis are critical for the patients to receive proper therapeutic treatment as early as possible. In NSCLC, only small improvements in clinical outcome have been achieved, and this is very critical for stage I patients for whom there are no available biomarkers that will indicate high-risk patients which should receive adjuvant chemotherapy. However, focusing only on a median 5-year survival may ignore the substantial improvement in survival for subsets of patients treated with erlotinib or crizotinib for lung cancers that bear the appropriate genotypic changes in the epidermal growth factor receptor or anaplastic lymphoma kinase (Diamandis et al. 2013). Despite late advancements in lung cancer therapies, the prognosis for patients with advanced NSCLC remains poor, so innovative, non-invasive, sensitive, and reliable biomarkers still need to be discovered and exploited.

Tumor biomarkers can play an important role in cancer screening, diagnosis, prognosis, and therapeutic monitoring. Discovery and validation of novel biomarkers for early characterization of carcinomas is one of the main aims of contemporary cancer research. However, the journey of a cancer biomarker from the bench to the clinic is long, difficult, and challenging (Diamandis 2010). The major barriers that candidate tumor biomarkers need to overcome to reach the clinic have been recently clearly addressed (Pavlou et al. 2013). A number of important principles for both discovery and validation studies have been described with the goals of minimizing bias and optimizing the likelihood that an effective biomarker will be able to undergo definitive clinical evaluation. The European Group on Tumor Markers has recently presented guidelines (MONITOR) for designing studies on the validity of tumor markers for the serial monitoring of cancer patients, with the aim of showing whether monitoring improves outcomes, compared with other routinely used methods (Stenman 2013).

We now know that tumor growth is accompanied by changes at the DNA, RNA, miRNA, and protein levels. These changes can be used for the discovery and clinical evaluation of prognostic and predictive biomarkers for lung cancer. Epigenetic changes such as gene promoter methylation or point mutations that can be detected at the DNA level or differences in gene expression levels that can be assessed at the RNA level are now intensely being evaluated as cancer biomarkers. Based on the advances in our understanding of cancer at the molecular level over the last decade and on the new and breakthrough technologies that are now available, we could say that now is an appropriate time to translate and take advantage of this new knowledge to improve outcomes for cancer patients by identifying cancer subtypes for which prevention, early detection, and targeted therapy will affect patient outcomes substantially.

In this review, we describe the current knowledge concerning lung cancer biomarkers highlighting the exciting recent findings on the non-invasive liquid biopsy approach such as circulating tumor cells (CTCs), circulating miRNAs, and gene promoter methylation and DNA mutations in cell-free circulating DNA (Fig. 1).

The Liquid Biopsy Approach in Lung Cancer

The genetic profile of solid tumors is currently obtained from surgical or biopsy specimens; however, the latter procedure cannot always be performed routinely owing to its invasive nature. Information acquired from a single biopsy provides a spatially and temporally limited snapshot of a tumor and might fail to reflect its heterogeneity. Cancers are continuously evolving and acquire resistance to systemic treatment as a result of clonal evolution and selection. Serial biopsies to study

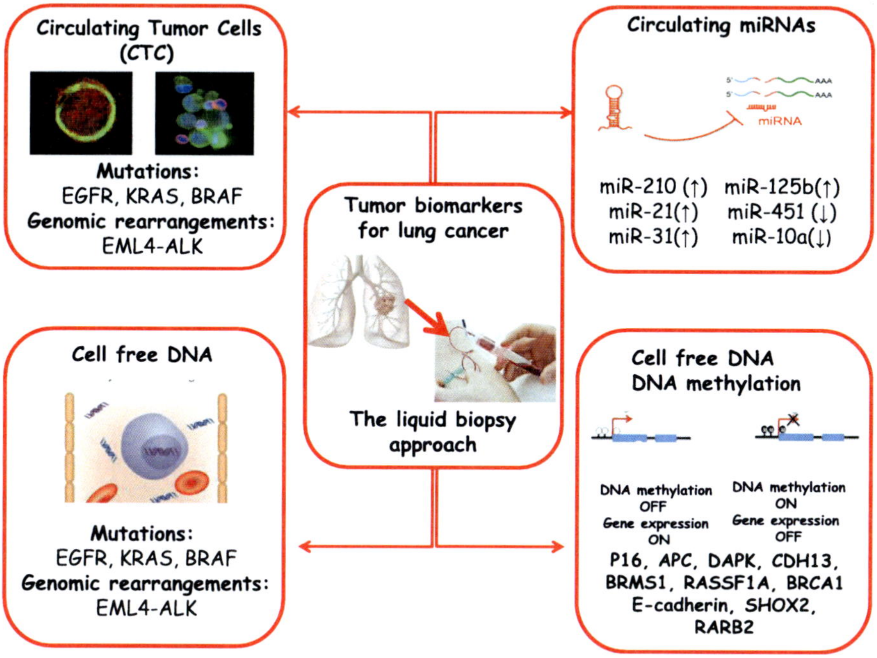

Fig. 1 Emerging blood-based molecular biomarkers for the detection and monitoring of lung cancer

genomic evolution as a result of therapy are difficult to obtain, since they are very invasive. Moreover, intra-tumor heterogeneity is additionally posing tremendous limitations.

A "liquid biopsy" or blood sample can provide the genetic landscape of all cancerous lesions (primary and metastases) as well as offering the opportunity to systematically track genomic evolution (Alix-Panabières and Pantel 2013; Crowley et al. 2013). There is now an urgent need for blood-based, non-invasive molecular tests to assist in the detection and diagnosis of cancers in a cost-effective manner at an early stage, when curative interventions are still possible. Additionally, blood-based diagnostics can classify tumors into distinct molecular subtypes and monitor disease relapse and response to treatment (Hanash et al. 2011).

There is increasing evidence that miRNAs play important and complex roles in human cancers, including lung cancer (Liu et al. 2004; Volinia et al. 2006; Hui et al. 2011). miRNAs are endogenous short noncoding RNAs that regulate gene expression by targeting mRNAs (Bagga et al. 2005), and their involvement in cancer and their potential as diagnostic, prognostic, and therapeutic tools have been recently reviewed (Maia et al. 2013; Iorio and Croce 2012; Markou et al. 2011). In lung cancer, miRNAs circulating in the blood have been evaluated as diagnostic and prognostic biomarkers (Markou et al. 2013; Keller et al. 2011; Boeri et al. 2011; Lin et al. 2012), and it is now clearly shown that they are associated with a clinical outcome (Markou et al. 2013; Zhu et al. 2011; Hu et al. 2010; Silva et al. 2011). With the aim at identifying new biomarkers of lung cancer, many investigators have carried out miRNA expression profiling studies firstly in cell lines and tissue samples and more recently in plasma and serum.

It was known since many years ago that tumor cells release circulating cell-free DNA (cfDNA) into the blood, but since the majority of circulating DNA is often not of cancerous origin, detection of cancer-associated alleles in the blood has long been impossible to achieve. Recent technological advances have overcome these restrictions, making it thus possible to identify both genetic and epigenetic aberrations in cfDNA. Cell-free nucleic acids circulating in the blood can now give important information as blood-based tumor biomarkers. In the past decade, a wealth of information indicating the potential use of circulating nucleic acids for cancer screening, prognosis, and the monitoring of the efficacy of anticancer therapies has emerged (Schwarzenbach et al. 2011). Recent studies have shown that genomic alterations in solid cancers can be characterized by massively parallel sequencing of circulating cell-free tumor DNA released from cancer cells into plasma, representing a non-invasive liquid biopsy. Especially, in NSCLC, where the acquisition of sufficient biopsy material is difficult and hinders the evolution of novel targeted therapies, a liquid biopsy approach is very promising. Murtaza et al. have recently shown that sequencing of cancer exomes in serial plasma samples can track the genomic evolution of metastatic cancers in response to therapy. By quantification of allele fractions in plasma, they identified increased representation of mutant alleles in association with the emergence of therapy resistance. Their results establish proof of principle that the exome-wide analysis of circulating tumor DNA could complement current invasive biopsy approaches to identify mutations associated with acquired drug resistance in advanced cancers (Murtaza et al. 2013).

Circulating Tumor Cells and Lung Cancer

Circulating tumor cells (CTCs) were the first to be proposed as "liquid biopsy" for follow-up examinations. The presence of CTCs in the peripheral blood has been linked with worse prognosis and early relapse in lung cancer. This topic is covered in detail in another chapter of this book (Chap. 2, "► Circulating Tumor Cells as Biomarkers in Cancer" by Ziman et al).

Circulating miRNAs as Blood-Based Biomarkers in Lung Cancer

Recently, the discovery of miRNAs in body fluids, such as serum and plasma, opens up the possibility of using them as non-invasive biomarkers of disease and therapy response. The use of circulating miRNAs as biomarkers of disease and therapy response and as diagnostic and prognostic markers in lung cancer is an extremely promising field since it can provide novel non-invasive tools for diagnosis, prognosis, and therapy response monitoring in lung cancer. Many research groups are working toward this direction in order to achieve diagnosis at early (asymptomatic if possible) stages for improving the survival rate of lung cancer patients which remains poor and to monitor the responsiveness of patients in chemotherapy leading to individualized therapies.

The first study which characterized miRNAs in serum of NSCLC patients employed Solexa sequencing and identified a specific expression pattern of 63 circulating miRNAs that were not detectable in healthy controls (Bianchi et al. 2011). Many other studies have indicated different serum or plasma miRNAs that are deregulated and can distinguish lung cancer patients from healthy donors (Chen et al. 2008, 2012; Tang et al. 2013; Hennessey et al. 2012).

The clinical significance of circulating miRNAs as prognostic biomarkers for the disease progress and lung cancer patients' outcome is demonstrated by a great number of research reports and by different technologies over the last years (Table 1). Zhu et al. showed that the expression levels of miR-96, miR-182, and miR-183 are positively correlated between specimens as well as that increased expression compared to healthy controls is associated with poor overall survival (Zhu et al. 2011). Another study focusing on genome-wide serum miRNA expression profiling by Solexa indicated that four miRNAs (miR-486, miR-30d, miR-1, and miR-499) were associated with the overall survival and thus were an independent prognostic factor for a clinical outcome (Hu et al. 2010). Using TaqMan low-density arrays for screening and RT-qPCR for validation, Silva et al. showed that decreased levels of miR-30e-5p and let-7f in plasma were associated with short DFI and OS, respectively (Silva et al. 2011). Finally, a very recent study has shown that high miR-21, decreased miR-10a, and increased miR-30e-5p expression levels in plasma of NSCLC patients are associated with shorter DFI and OS, respectively (Markou et al. 2013).

To demonstrate the potential role of miRNAs in early stage NSCLC, several groups have analyzed miRNA profiles in serum prior to and after lung cancer diagnosis (Keller et al. 2011). It has been recently reported that an miRNA signature could detect lung cancer at a very early stage, prior to the symptom occurrence. Boeri et al. analyzed the miRNA expression profile in plasma samples collected 1–2 years before the onset of the disease and at the time of computed tomography (CT) diagnosis and compared them with the ones of healthy smokers (Boeri et al. 2011). This miRNA signature could predict the development of lung cancer prior to diagnosis and has a strong diagnostic potential as samples were collected at the time-point of diagnosis. miRNA profiles were also compared between early (stage I/II) and advanced (stage IV) disease (Lin et al. 2012). Le et al. examined the expression of four miRNAs, miR-21, miR-24, miR-30d, and miR-205, in sera of pre- and postoperative lung cancer patients and normal volunteers and indicated that, except from the diagnostic value for the discrimination between patients and healthy individuals, increased expression levels of miR-21 and miR-24 have also the prognostic value for disease recurrence after surgery, while elevated miR-21 and miR-30d expression is also correlated with shorter overall survival in patients (Le et al. 2012). In another study, miRNA expression

Table 1 The clinical significance of circulating miRNAs as prognostic biomarkers for the disease progress and lung cancer patients' outcome

miRNA	Clinical significance	Sample	References
miR-125b(↑)	Association with poor prognosis	Serum	Cui et al. 2013; Yuxia et al. 2012
miR-30d (↑)	Association with short OS, prediction of disease recurrence	Serum	Hu et al. 2010; Le et al. 2012
miR-30e-5p(↓)	Association with short DFI	Plasma	Markou et al. 2013; Silva et al. 2011
miR-30e-5p(↑)	Association with short OS	Plasma	
miR-21(↑)	Association with poor outcome	Plasma	Markou et al. 2013; Boeri et al. 2011; Liu et al. 2004; Le et al. 2012
miR-21(↑)	Association with short OS, prediction of disease recurrence	Serum	
miR-182(↑)	Cancer patients vs. normal samples and further increase in patients with metastasis	Plasma	Zheng et al. 2011; Zhu et al. 2011
miR-182(↑)	Association with poor OS	Serum	
let-7f(↓)	Association with short OS	Plasma	Silva et al. 2011
miR-10a(↓)	Association with short DFI	Plasma	Markou et al. 2013
miR-486 (↑)	Association with poor OS	Serum	Hu et al. 2010
miR-1(↓)			
miR-499(↓)			
miR-96(↑)	Association with poor OS	Serum	Zhu et al. 2011
miR-183(↑)			
miR-155(↑)	Cancer patients vs. normal samples and further increase in patients with metastasis	Plasma	Zheng et al. 2011
miR-197(↑)			

levels were quantified in paired lung tumor tissues and plasma samples from stage I NSCLC patients by RT-qPCR, and the results showed a significant concordance in the expression of five miRNAs in both specimens. Four of these, miR-21, miR-126, miR-210, and miR-486-5p, could distinguish stage I NSCLC from healthy individuals and could also discriminate lung adenocarcinoma (AD) from squamous cell carcinoma (SCC) (Shen et al. 2011).

Many groups have shown that the expression levels of circulating miRNAs could alter during treatment with chemotherapy drugs. Increased levels of miR-21 in plasma of NSCLC patients are related to platinum-based chemotherapy resistance and to shorter DFI (Gao et al. 2012). The same tendency exhibits miR-125b as its high expression levels are indicative of non-responsiveness to cisplatin-based chemotherapy and are associated with poor survival (Cui et al. 2013; Yuxia et al. 2012). Expression levels of miR-155, miR-197, and miR-182 that are increased in lung cancer patients, including stage I patients, have a predictive value for responsiveness to chemotherapy, with the first two being further increased in patients with metastasis and decreased in patients responding to chemotherapy (Zheng et al. 2011).

After firstly identifying 12 miRNAs whose aberrant expressions in primary lung tumors were associated with early stage NSCLC, Shen et al. investigated whether these miRNAs could be used as potential plasma biomarkers for NSCLC. They found five miRNAs that displayed significant concordance in their expression levels in plasma and the corresponding tumor tissues. By using four miRNAs (miRNA-21, miRNA-126, miRNA-210, and miRNA-486-5p), they reported 86 % sensitivity and 96 % specificity in distinguishing NSCLC patients from healthy controls (Shen et al. 2011).

Promoter Hypermethylation of Tumor Suppressor Genes as a Lung Cancer Biomarker

DNA methylation has emerged as a highly promising biomarker and is being actively studied in multiple cancers. It is now widely known that aberrant DNA methylation within the promoter region initiates carcinogenesis and promotes cancer progression by activating oncogenes, suppressing tumor suppressor genes, and inducing chromosome instability (Esteller 2008). Since DNA is more stable than RNA or proteins, DNA methylation has a great potential to be established as a nucleic acid–based biomarker for many applications. The number of potential tumor biomarkers based on DNA methylation is rapidly increasing owing to the development of recent genome-wide approaches for their identification and functional analysis (Carmona and Esteller 2011; Heyn and Esteller 2012). Detection of these DNA methylation markers in cell-free DNA circulating in plasma or serum has led to many studies, evaluating the potential of getting precious information in a minimally invasive way, such as blood draw (Gormally et al. 2007). The sensitive and specific detection of tumor-specific DNA methylation patterns at distal sites makes DNA methylation a biomarker of choice for the clinical management of cancer patients (Table 2).

DNA Methylation Lung Cancer Biomarkers in Circulating Cell-Free DNA (cfDNA)

In the past decade, there are a multitude of promising studies which are demonstrating the hyper/hypomethylation of genes that are potentially useful in lung cancer diagnosis. The analysis of DNA methylation-based biomarkers in lung cancer is rapidly advancing, and a large number of potential lung cancer biomarkers have been identified (Anglim et al. 2008). To date, there are many studies on the potential of DNA methylation biomarkers in lung cancer management. Lung cancer is characterized by regional hypermethylation of promoters of well-known cancer-related genes, including RASSF1 (Fischer et al. 2007), CDKN2A (Damman et al. 2005), RARbeta (Virmani et al. 2000), MGMT (Zöchbauer-Müller 2012), APC, CDH13 (Kim et al. 2007), and BRMS1 (Yang et al. 2011). Many studies

Table 2 DNA methylation lung cancer biomarkers

Gene	Sample	Finding	References
RASSF1A	Bronchial washing	Hypermethylation of promoters provides 29 % detection of malignancy in false-negative cytology outcomes	Van der Drift et al. 2012
RASSF1A	Tumor tissues	Hypermethylation of promoters correlates with early recurrence and short survival	Fischer et al. 2007; Brock et al. 2008; Zhang et al. 2011
RASSF1A	cfDNA (plasma)	Highly methylated	Zhang et al. 2011; Ponomaryova et al. 2013; Begum et al. 2011
p16	Tumor tissues	Promoter hypermethylation was detected in 63 % of NSCLC	Brock et al. 2008; Bearzatto et al. 2002
p16	Bronchoalveolar lavage	Promoter hypermethylation was detected in NSCLCs	Ahrendt et al. 1999
p16	cfDNA (plasma)	Detected in 55 % of plasmas	Bearzatto et al. 2002
APC	Tumor tissues	Methylation of the promoter region in primary tumor and mediastinal lymph node biopsy samples strongly correlates with early recurrence and short survival	Damman et al. 2005; Brock et al. 2008; Zhang et al. 2011
APC	cfDNA (serum)	Aberrant methylation in serum DNA was accompanied by methylation in the matched tumor samples	Begum et al. 2011
CDH13	Tumor tissues	Methylation of the promoter predicts markedly worse prognosis in patients with stage I lung cancer ($P < 0.001$), similar to patients with stage III disease	Damman et al. 2005; Brock et al. 2008; Zhang et al. 2011
DAPK	Tumor tissues	Hypermethylated in drug-resistant derivatives from cell lines	Palmisiano et al. 2000
	Sputum	Promoter hypermethylation was detected in lung cancer	Palmisiano et al. 2000
BRCA1	Tumor tissues	BRCA1 promoter hypermethylation could provide information that is clinically relevant after adjuvant chemotherapy	Zhang et al. 2011
E-cadherin	Tumor tissues	Methylation of the promoter region strongly correlates with early recurrence and short survival	Brock et al. 2008
SHOX2	Bronchial aspirates	Methylation of the promoter could distinguish between malignant lung disease and controls at a sensitivity of 60 %	Dietrich et al. 2012; Kneip et al. 2011

(*continued*)

Table 2 (continued)

Gene	Sample	Finding	References
RARB2	Tumor tissues	Measurable differences between methylation levels in tumor and adjacent normal tissues and associations with clinical data	Virmani et al. 2000; Zhang et al. 2011
RARB2	cfDNA (plasma)	Highly methylated cfDNA isolated from plasma elevated two- to threefold in lung cancer patients compared with healthy donors	Ponomaryova et al. 2013
MGMT	Tumor tissues, sputum, serum	Hypermethylation of promoter aberrant methylation in serum DNA was accompanied by methylation in the matched tumor samples	Begum et al. 2011; Belinsky et al. 2005, 2006, 2007
BRMS1	Tumor tissues	Hypermethylation of promoter	Yang et al. 2011

illustrate measurable differences between methylation levels in tumor and adjacent normal tissues as well as associations with clinical data. DNA methylation can be used as a molecular prognostic biomarker of potentially curable stage I NSCLC (Brock et al. 2008). Methylation of the promoter region of four genes, p16, E-cadherin, Rassf1A, and APC, in primary tumor and lymph node biopsy samples strongly correlates with early recurrence and short survival (Brock et al. 2008). The validation of this and numerous other findings may allow restaging of NSCLC at a molecular level. On the other hand, lung cancer is also affected by global hypomethylation contributing to genomic instability (Daskalos et al. 2009) associating with poor outcome (Saito et al. 2010).

Cancer cell-specific methylated DNA has been found in the blood of cancer patients, indicating that cell-free DNA (cfDNA) circulating in the blood is a tumor-associated DNA marker that can be used as a minimally invasive diagnostic test. Nowadays, plasma or serum cell-free DNA may be the golden standard for the detection of DNA methylation biomarkers. Information on the methylation status of tumor suppressor genes in cfDNA is a very promising approach, since it can offer a useful tool for lung cancer diagnostics, the evaluation of cancer treatment efficiency, and the post-treatment monitoring.

Esteller et al. were one of the first that have shown already in 1999 that aberrant promoter hypermethylation of tumor suppressor genes could be detected in the serum DNA from NSCLC patients (Esteller et al. 1999). Bearzatto et al. have shown in 2002 that the p16 (INK4A) tumor suppressor gene that is inactivated in many solid tumors, including NSCLCs through promoter hypermethylation, could be detected in plasma with a highly sensitive methylation-specific PCR (MSP) assay. They reported that p16 (INK4A) promoter hypermethylation was detectable by this assay in 55 % of plasmas from patients with methylated tumors (Bearzatto et al. 2002).

Zhang et al. showed that the methylation analysis of a panel of five genes (APC, RASSF1A, CDH13, KLK10, and DLEC1) in plasma DNA reached a sensitivity of 83 % and a specificity of 74 % (Zhang et al. 2011). Ponomaryova et al. investigated the methylation status in blood samples of 32 healthy donors and 60 lung cancer patients before and after treatment with neoadjuvant chemotherapy followed by total tumor resection. Using quantitative methylation-specific PCR, they found that RASSF1A and RARB2 genes were highly methylated in cfDNA isolated from plasma and that cell surface-bound cfDNA was elevated two- to threefold in lung cancer patients compared with healthy donors, showing an 87 % sensitivity and 75 % specificity (Ponomaryova et al. 2013).

Recently, a phase I/II trial of combined epigenetic therapy with azacitidine and entinostat, inhibitors of DNA methylation and histone deacetylation, respectively, in extensively pretreated patients with recurrent metastatic NSCLC demonstrated that combined epigenetic therapy with low-dose azacitidine and entinostat results in objective, durable responses in patients with solid tumors. Demethylation of a set of 4 epigenetically silenced genes (CDKN2a, CDH13, APC, and RASSF1a) already known to be associated with lung cancer (Brock et al. 2008) was detectable with improved progression-free ($P = 0.034$) and overall survival ($P = 0.035$) (Juergens et al. 2011). Analysis of cfDNA in the plasma of these patients supports that detection of early demethylation in serial blood samples could be a potential predictor of clinical benefit from this therapy (Juergens et al. 2011). Evaluation of methylation changes in tumor DNA during cycle 1 of therapy as a predictor of clinical benefit should be included in future trials of epigenetically directed therapy (Juergens et al. 2011).

Begum et al. investigated the feasibility of detecting aberrant DNA methylation of some novel and known genes in the serum of lung cancer patients, by examining the tumor and the matched serum DNA for aberrant methylation of 15 gene promoters from 10 patients with primary lung tumors by using quantitative methylation-specific PCR. After testing this 15-gene set and identifying the more useful DNA methylation changes in serum, they tested the six most promising genes (APC, CDH1, MGMT, DCC, RASSF1A, and AIM1) for further elucidation of the diagnostic application of this panel of markers. They report that promoter hypermethylation of at least one of the genes studied was detected in all 10 lung primary tumors. In the majority of cases, aberrant methylation in serum DNA was accompanied by methylation in the matched tumor samples. This approach needs to be evaluated in a larger set of clinical samples to determine the role of this gene set in the early detection and surveillance of lung cancer (Begum et al. 2011).

DNA Methylation Lung Cancer Biomarkers in Bronchial Aspirates and Sputum

Abnormal hypermethylation has also been shown in sputum and bronchial washing samples that are both easily acquirable. p16 methylation in bronchoalveolar lavage was firstly shown already in 1999 (Ahrendt et al. 1999). More recently, RASSF1A methylation combined with KRAS mutations in bronchial washing is reported to provide 29 % detection of malignancy in false-negative cytology outcomes (Van der Drift et al. 2012). DNA methylation of SHOX2, as evaluated in 523 patients, could distinguish between malignant and benign lung disease, at high specificity (Schmidt et al. 2010). Two years later, the usefulness and analytical performance of an in vitro diagnostic kit which quantifies SHOX2 methylation in bronchial aspirates were described (Dietrich et al. 2012). SHOX2 methylation has also been detected in plasma cell-free DNA and could distinguish between malignant lung disease and controls at a sensitivity of 60 % (Kneip et al. 2011). A panel of potentially methylated genes has been examined, including DAPK, GATA5, MGMT, and PAX5beta (Palmisiano et al. 2000; Belinsky et al. 2005, 2006). However sputum or bronchial aspirates have certain limitations, as the variability of lung cell content, so the diagnostic efficiency of DNA markers in such samples is challenged by reports that can detect aberrant methylation in samples from cancer free controls (Hsu et al. 2007).

DNA Mutations in cfDNA as Companion Diagnostic Lung Cancer Biomarkers

Analysis of tumor-linked genetic alterations and especially gene mutations in various types of cancer are now being used for diagnostic, prognostic, and treatment purposes. More specifically, companion diagnostic tests are now being used in combination with specific therapies and can prospectively help predict responses to specific drugs or severe toxicity. Some successful examples include the detection of BRAF V600E mutations for vemurafenib in melanoma, EML4-ALK rearrangements for crizotinib and EGFR for erlotinib and gefitinib in NSCLC, KRAS against the use of cetuximab and panitumumab in colorectal cancer, ERBB2 (HER2/neu) for trastuzumab in breast cancer, and BCR-ABL for tyrosine kinase inhibitors in chronic myeloid leukemia. We believe that the co-development of new drugs with companion diagnostics will govern the progress in oncology in the immediate future. The role of companion biomarkers in guiding treatment in patients with cancer has been recently very nicely reviewed (Duffy and Crown 2013; Ong et al. 2012; Vincent et al. 2012) (Table 3).

Tumor-associated mutations detectable in the peripheral blood can now be used in the clinic after diagnosis, including the assessment of prognosis and early detection of disease recurrence, and as surrogates for traditional biopsies with the purpose of predicting response to treatments and the development of acquired resistance (Crowley et al. 2013). Recently, a number of remarkable studies have shown that cfDNA circulating in the blood can be isolated from plasma and allows for tumor-specific analyses, including epidermal growth factor receptor (EGFR), KRAS, BRAF mutations, and EML4-anaplastic lymphoma kinase (ALK) rearrangements. These biomarkers are currently used or evaluated as companion diagnostic biomarkers to select lung cancer patients that are eligible for molecular-targeted therapies.

Table 3 DNA mutations related to therapy response, detected in cell-free DNA isolated from lung cancer patients

Gene	Sample	Findings	References
EGFR mutations	Cell-free DNA (plasma)	Mutations could potentially be used to monitor EGFR-TKI therapy in association with the emergence of therapy resistance to gefitinib	Murtaza et al. 2013; Sakai et al. 2013
EGFR mutations	CTC	CTCs that carried EGFR mutations known to cause drug resistance had faster disease progression than CTCs who lacked the mutation	Maheswaran et al. 2008
KRAS mutations	Cell-free DNA (plasma)	Mutation carriers had significantly shorter OS and PFS compared to the wild-type patients	Nygaard et al. 2013
BRAF mutations	Cell-free DNA (plasma/serum)	Mutations occur in 4 % of NSCLCs; 50 % are non-V600E	Cardarella et al. 2013
EML4-ALK rearrangements	Tumor tissues	Functional ALK rearrangements were mutually exclusive with EGFR and KRAS mutations in a large Western patient population. This lack of overlap was also observed in ALK-positive cancers with acquired resistance to crizotinib	Gainor et al. 2013; Lee et al. 2013; Peters et al. 2013
EML4-ALK rearrangements	CTC	CTCs harboring a unique ALK rearrangement and mesenchymal phenotype may arise from the clonal selection of tumor cells that have acquired the potential to drive metastatic progression of ALK-positive NSCLC	Pailler et al. 2013

EGFR: It is now known that a secondary EGFR mutation, the substitution of threonine 790 with methionine (T790M), leads to acquired resistance to reversible EGFR-tyrosine kinase inhibitors (EGFR-TKIs). EGFR mutations may also have indirect value as predictors of sensitivity to chemotherapy and to radiotherapy and molecularly targeted agents (Vincent et al. 2012). Murtaza et al. have recently identified in plasma an increased representation of a resistance-conferring mutation in EGFR following treatment with gefitinib in association with the emergence of therapy resistance. Their results establish a proof of principle that exome-wide analysis of circulating tumor DNA could complement current invasive biopsy approaches to identify mutations associated with acquired drug resistance in advanced cancers (Murtaza et al. 2013). A non-invasive method for detecting T790M mutation would be desirable to direct patient treatment strategy. Sakai et al. detected the T790M mutation status in plasma samples obtained after treatment with an EGFR-TKI in 21 of the 75 plasma samples (28 %). When patients under 65 years of age who had a partial response were grouped according to their plasma T790M mutation status, the Progression Free Survival (PFS) of the T790M-positive patients ($n = 11$) was significantly shorter than that of the T790M-negative patients ($n = 29, P = 0.03$), indicating that the plasma T790M mutation status could potentially be used to monitor EGFR-TKI therapy (Sakai et al. 2013). Plasma is a better source of tumor-derived cfDNA than serum for the detection of EGFR alterations in lung tumor patients (Vallée et al. 2013).

KRAS: Very recently, in a prospective biomarker trial, Nygaard et al. investigated the prognostic value of plasma-mutated KRAS in patients with NSCLC and found that patients with a detectable plasma-KRAS mutation had a significantly shorter OS and DFI compared to the wild-type (WT) patients. The presence of KRAS mutations in plasma may be a marker of poor prognosis and may also hold predictive value. However, further validation of these results in an independent cohort is necessary (Nygaard et al. 2013).

EML4-ALK rearrangements: ALK gene rearrangements define a distinct molecular subset of NSCLC. Recently, several case reports and small series have reported that ALK rearrangements can overlap with other oncogenic drivers in NSCLC and in crizotinib-naïve and crizotinib-resistant cancers. Gainor et al. have very recently reviewed clinical genotyping data from 1,683 patients with NSCLC and investigated the prevalence of concomitant EGFR or KRAS mutations among patients with ALK-positive NSCLC. They report that functional ALK rearrangements were mutually exclusive with EGFR and KRAS mutations in a large Western patient population. This lack of overlap was also observed in ALK-positive cancers with acquired resistance to crizotinib (Gainor et al. 2013). The recent approval of crizotinib for the treatment of ALK-rearranged advanced NSCLC in the USA and other countries has provoked intense interest in ALK rearrangements as oncogenic drivers and promises to revolutionize the way in which NSCLC is diagnosed and treated. The therapy was approved by the US FDA in August 2011 and received conditional marketing approval by the European Commission in October 2012 for advanced NSCLC. A break-apart Fluorescence In Situ Hybridization (FISH)-based assay was jointly approved with crizotinib by the FDA. This assay and an immunohistochemistry assay that uses a D5F3 rabbit monoclonal primary antibody were also approved for marketing in Europe in October 2012. While ALK rearrangement has relatively low prevalence, a clinical benefit is exhibited in more than 85 % of patients with median progression-free survival of 8–10 months. In a recent paper, Lee et al. described the therapy and alternative test strategies for identifying NSCLC patients who are likely to respond to therapy with crizotinib, including key issues for effective and efficient testing. The key economic considerations regarding the joint companion diagnostic and therapy are also presented. Given the observed clinical benefit and relatively high cost of crizotinib therapy, companion diagnostics should be evaluated relative to response to therapy versus correlation alone whenever possible, and both high inter-rater reliability and external quality assessment programs are warranted (Lee et al. 2013; Peters et al. 2013).

BRAF: BRAF mutations are found in a subset of NSCLC. Cardarella et al. examined the clinical characteristics and treatment outcomes of patients with NSCLC harboring BRAF mutations. Using DNA sequencing and after screening 883 patients with NSCLC, they found that BRAF mutations occur in 4 % of NSCLC and half are non-V600E. Prospective trials are ongoing to validate BRAF as a therapeutic target in NSCLC (Cardarella et al. 2013).

Conclusions: Future Challenges

The discovery and exploitation of novel innovative, non-invasive, and reliable tumor biomarkers for lung cancer, based on a non-invasive liquid biopsy approach, such as CTCs, circulating miRNAs, gene promoter methylation, and DNA mutations in cell-free circulating DNA, are very promising for the clinical management of this disease in the near future. However, great expectations that cancer biomarkers could revolutionize cancer diagnosis and treatment have not been fulfilled up to now (Buchen 2011). A point of consideration is that despite the growing number of relevant studies in the area of developing novel lung cancer biomarkers, the potential of these novel biomarkers cannot be precisely estimated. Few of these studies can singly provide adequate validation, while a meta-analysis is almost impossible due to the large diversity of sample processing protocols, detection methods, DNA extraction methods, inclusion criteria, etc. There is still a great need to further validate these promising biomarkers in large numbers of patients, cross validate these findings in different labs, and further calculate their diagnostic sensitivity and specificity, as well as the positive and negative predictive values before their final approval for patient management.

Summary Points

- The discovery and exploitation of novel, innovative, non-invasive, and reliable tumor biomarkers are of vital importance toward the early detection and precise diagnosis of lung cancer. This is very critical to select proper therapeutic treatments as early as possible.
- Emerging blood-based molecular biomarkers for lung cancer, based on the non-invasive liquid biopsy approach, such as CTCs, circulating miRNAs, gene promoter methylation, and DNA mutations in cell-free circulating DNA, are now very promising.
- However, there is still a great need to further validate these promising biomarkers in a large number of patients, cross validate these findings in different labs, and further calculate their diagnostic sensitivity and specificity, as well as the positive and negative predictive values before their final approval for patient management.

References

Ahrendt SA, Chow JT, Xu LH, et al. Molecular detection of tumor cells in bronchoalveolar lavage fluid from patients with early stage lung cancer. J Natl Cancer Inst. 1999;91:332–9.

Alix-Panabières C, Pantel K. Circulating tumor cells: liquid biopsy of cancer. Clin Chem. 2013;59:110–8.

Anglim PP, Alonzo TA, Laird-Offringa IA. DNA methylation-based biomarkers for early detection of non-small cell lung cancer: an update. Mol Cancer. 2008;7:81.

Bagga S, Bracht J, Hunter S, et al. Regulation by let-7 and lin-4 miRNAs results in target mRNA degradation. Cell. 2005;122:553–63.

Bearzatto A, Conte D, Frattini M, et al. p16(INK4A) hypermethylation detected by fluorescent methylation-specific PCR in plasmas from non-small cell lung cancer. Clin Cancer Res. 2002;8:3782–7.

Begum S, Brait M, Dasgupta S, et al. An epigenetic marker panel for detection of lung cancer using cell-free serum DNA. Clin Cancer Res. 2011;17:4494–503.

Belinsky SA, Klinge DM, Dekker JD, et al. Gene promoter methylation in plasma and sputum increases with lung cancer risk. Clin Cancer Res. 2005;11:6505–11.

Belinsky SA, Liechty KC, Gentry FD, et al. Promoter hypermethylation of multiple genes in sputum precedes lung cancer incidence in a high risk cohort. Cancer Res. 2006;66:3338–44.

Belinsky SA, Grimes MJ, Casas E, et al. Predicting gene promoter methylation in non small cell lung cancer by evaluating sputum and serum. Br J Cancer. 2007;96:1278–83.

Bianchi F, Nicassio F, Marzi M, et al. A serum circulating miRNA diagnostic test to identify asymptomatic high-risk individuals with early stage lung cancer. EMBO Mol Med. 2011;3:495–503.

Boeri M, Verri C, Conte D, et al. MicroRNA signatures in tissues and plasma predict development and prognosis of computed tomography detected lung cancer. Proc Natl Acad Sci U S A. 2011;108:3713–8.

Brock MV, Hooker CM, Ota-Machida E, et al. DNA methylation markers and early recurrence in stage I lung cancer. N Engl J Med. 2008;358:1118–28.

Buchen L. Missing the mark. Nature. 2011;471:428–32.

Cardarella S, Ogino A, Nishino M, Butaney M, Shen J, Lydon C, et al. Clinical, pathologic, and biologic features associated with BRAF mutations in non-small cell lung cancer. Clin Cancer Res. 2013;19:4532–40.

Carmona FJ, Esteller M. DNA methylation in early neoplasia. Cancer Biomark. 2011;9:101–11.

Chen X, Ba Y, Ma L, et al. Characterization of microRNAs in serum: a novel class of biomarkers for diagnosis of cancer and other diseases. Cell Res. 2008;18:997–1006.

Chen X, Hu Z, Wang W, et al. Identification of ten serum microRNAs from a genome-wide serum microRNA expression profile as novel noninvasive biomarkers for nonsmall cell lung cancer diagnosis. Int J Cancer. 2012;130:1620–8.

Crowley E, Di Nicolantonio F, Loupakis F, et al. Liquid biopsy: monitoring cancer-genetics in the blood. Nat Rev Clin Oncol. 2013;10:472–84.

Cui EH, Li HJ, Hua F, et al. Serum microRNA 125b as a diagnostic or prognostic biomarker for advanced NSCLC patients receiving cisplatin-based chemotherapy. Acta Pharmacol Sin. 2013;34:309–13.

Damman R, Strunnikova M, Schagdarsurengin U, et al. CpG island methylation and expression of tumor-associated genes in lung carcinoma. Eur J Cancer. 2005;41:1223–36.

Daskalos A, Nikolaidis G, Xinarianos G, et al. Hypomethylation of retrotransposable elements correlates with genomic instability in non-small cell lung cancer. Int J Cancer. 2009;124:81–7.

Diamandis EP. Cancer biomarkers: can we turn recent failures into success? J Natl Cancer Inst. 2010;102:1462–7.

Diamandis EP, Bast RC, Lopez-Otín C. Conquering cancer in our lifetime: new diagnostic and therapeutic trends. Clin Chem. 2013;59:1–3.

Dietrich D, Kneip C, Raji O, et al. Performance evaluation of the DNA methylation biomarker SHOX2 for the aid in diagnosis of lung cancer based on the analysis of bronchial aspirates. Int J Oncol. 2012;40:825–32.

Duffy MJ, Crown J. Companion biomarkers: paving the pathway to personalized treatment for cancer. Clin Chem. 2013;59:1447–56.

Esteller M. Epigenetics in cancer. N Engl J Med. 2008;358:1148–59.

Esteller M, Sanchez-Cespedes M, Rosell R, et al. Detection of aberrant promoter hypermethylation of tumor suppressor genes in serum DNA from non-small cell lung cancer patients. Cancer Res. 1999;59:67–70.

Fischer JR, Ohnmacht N, Rieger N, et al. Prognostic significance of RASSF1A promoter methylation on survival of non-small cell lung cancer patients treated with gemcitabine. Lung Cancer. 2007;56:115–23.

Gainor JF, Varghese AM, Ou SH, Kabraji S, Awad MM, Katayama R, et al. ALK rearrangements are mutually exclusive with mutations in EGFR or KRAS: an analysis of 1,683 patients with non-small cell lung cancer. Clin Cancer Res. 2013;19:4273–81.

Gao W, Lu X, Liu L, et al. MiRNA-21: a biomarker predictive for platinum-based adjuvant chemotherapy response in patients with non-small cell lung cancer. Cancer Biol Ther. 2012;13:330–40.

Gormally E, Caboux E, Vineis P, et al. Circulating free DNA in plasma or serum as biomarker of carcinogenesis: practical aspects and biological significance. Mutat Res. 2007;635:105–17.

Hanash SM, Baik CS, Kallioniemi O. Emerging molecular biomarkers–blood-based strategies to detect and monitor cancer. Nat Rev Clin Oncol. 2011;8:142–50.

Hennessey PT, Sanford T, Choudhary A, et al. Serum microRNA biomarkers for detection of non-small cell lung cancer. PLoS One. 2012;7:e32307.

Herman JG, Baylin SB, Brock MV, Rudin CM. Combination epigenetic therapy has efficacy in patients with refractory advanced non-small cell lung cancer. Cancer Discov. 2011;1(7): 598–607.

Heyn H, Esteller M. DNA methylation profiling in the clinic: applications and challenges. Nat Rev Genet. 2012;13:679–92.

Hsu HS, Chen TP, Wen CK, et al. Multiple genetic and epigenetic biomarkers for lung cancer detection in cytologically negative sputum and a nested case–control study for risk assessment. J Pathol. 2007;213:412–9.

Hu Z, Chen X, Zhao Y, et al. Serum microRNA signatures identified in a genome-wide serum microRNA expression profiling predict survival of non-small-cell lung cancer. J Clin Oncol. 2010;28:1721–6.

Hui A, How C, Ito E, et al. Micro-RNAs as diagnostic or prognostic markers in human epithelial malignancies. BMC Cancer. 2011;11:500.

Iorio MV, Croce CM. MicroRNA dysregulation in cancer: diagnostics, monitoring and therapeutics. A comprehensive review. EMBO Mol Med. 2012;4:143–59.

Juergens RA, Wrangle J, Vendetti FP, et al, Combination epigenetic therapy has efficacy in patients with refractory advanced non-small cell lung cancer. Cancer Discov. 2011;1(7):598–607.

Keller A, Leidinger P, Gislefoss R, et al. Stable serum miRNA profiles as potential tool for non-invasive lung cancer diagnosis. RNA Biol. 2011;8:506–16.

Kim DS, Cha SI, Lee JH, et al. Aberrant DNA methylation profiles of non-small cell lung cancers in a Korean population. Lung Cancer. 2007;58:1–6.

Kneip C, Scmhidt B, Seegenbarth A, et al. SHOX2 DNA methylation is a biomarker for the diagnosis of lung cancer in plasma. J Thorac Surg. 2011;6:1632.

Le HB, Zhu WY, Chen DD, et al. Evaluation of dynamic change of serum miR-21 and miR-24 in pre- and post-operative lung carcinoma patients. Med Oncol. 2012;29:3190–7.

Lee JA, Bubendorf L, Stahel R, Peters S. Testing for anaplastic lymphoma kinase rearrangement to target crizotinib therapy: oncology, pathology and health economic perspectives. Expert Rev Anticancer Ther. 2013;13:625–36.

Lin Q, Mao W, Shu Y, et al. A cluster of specified microRNAs in peripheral blood as biomarkers for metastatic non-small-cell lung cancer by stem-loop RT-PCR. J Cancer Res Clin Oncol. 2012;138:85–93.

Liu CG, Calin GA, Meloon B, et al. An oligonucleotide microchip for genome-wide microRNA profiling in human and mouse tissues. Proc Natl Acad Sci U S A. 2004;101:9740–4.

Maheswaran S, Sequist LV, Nagrath S, et al. Detection of mutations in EGFR in circulating lung-cancer cells. N Engl J Med. 2008;359(4):366–77.

Maia BM, Rocha RM, Calin GA. Clinical significance of the interaction between non-coding RNAs and the epigenetics machinery: challenges and opportunities in oncology. Epigenetics. 2013;9:75–80.

Markou A, Liang Y, Lianidou E. Prognostic, therapeutic and diagnostic potential of microRNAs in non-small cell lung cancer. Clin Chem Lab Med. 2011;49:1591–603.

Markou A, Sourvinou I, Vorkas PA, et al. Clinical evaluation of microRNA expression profiling in non small cell lung cancer. Lung Cancer. 2013;81:388–96.

Murtaza M, Dawson SJ, Tsui DW, et al. Non-invasive analysis of acquired resistance to cancer therapy by sequencing of plasma DNA. Nature. 2013;497:108–12.

Nygaard AD, Garm Spindler KL, Pallisgaard N, et.al. The prognostic value of KRAS mutated plasma DNA in advanced non-small cell lung cancer. Lung Cancer. 2013;79:312–7.

Ong FS, Das K, Wang J, et al. Personalized medicine and pharmacogenetic biomarkers: progress in molecular oncology testing. Expert Rev Mol Diagn. 2012;12:593–602.

Pailler E, Adam J, Barthélémy A, et al. Detection of circulating tumor cells harboring a unique ALK rearrangement in ALK-positive non-small-cell lung cancer. J Clin Oncol. 2013;31(18):2273–81.

Palmisiano WA, Divine KK, Saccomano G, et al. Predicting lung cancer by detecting aberrant promoter methylation in sputum. Cancer Res. 2000;60:5954–8.

Pavlou MP, Diamandis EP, Blasutig IM. The long journey of cancer biomarkers from the bench to the clinic. Clin Chem. 2013;59:147–57.

Peters S, Taron M, Bubendorf L, Blackhall F, Stahel R. Treatment and detection of ALK-rearranged NSCLC. Lung Cancer. 2013;81:145–54.

Ponomaryova AA, Rykova EY, Cherdyntseva NV, et al. Potentialities of aberrantly methylated circulating DNA for diagnostics and post-treatment follow-up of lung cancer patients. Lung Cancer. 2013;81:397–403.

Saito K, Kawakami K, Matsumoto I, et al. Long interspersed nuclear element 1 hypomethylation is a marker of poor prognosis in stage IA non-small cell lung cancer. Clin Cancer Res. 2010;16:2418–26.

Sakai K, Horiike A, Irwin DL, et al. Detection of epidermal growth factor receptor T790M mutation in plasma DNA from patients refractory to epidermal growth factor receptor tyrosine kinase inhibitor. Cancer Sci. 2013;104:1198–204.

Schmidt B, Liebenberg V, Diethrich D, et al. SHOX2 DNA methylation is a biomarker for the diagnosis of lung cancer based on bronchial aspirates. BMC Cancer. 2010;3:600.

Schwarzenbach H, Hoon DS, Pantel K. Cell-free nucleic acids as biomarkers in cancer patients. Nat Rev Cancer. 2011;11:426–37.

Shen J, Todd NW, Zhang H, et al. Plasma microRNAs as potential biomarkers for non-small-cell lung cancer. Lab Invest. 2011;91:579–87.

Silva J, García V, Zaballos Á, et al. Vesicle-related microRNAs in plasma of nonsmall cell lung cancer patients and correlation with survival. Eur Respir J. 2011;37:617–23.

Stenman UH. Validating serum markers for monitoring of cancer. Clin Chem. 2013;59:4–5.

Tang D, Shen Y, Wang M, et al. Identification of plasma microRNAs as novel noninvasive biomarkers for early detection of lung cancer. Eur J Cancer Prev. 2013;22:540–8.

Vallée A, Marcq M, Bizieux A, et al. Plasma is a better source of tumor-derived circulating cell-free DNA than serum for the detection of EGFR alterations in lung tumor patients. Lung Cancer. 2013;82:373–4.

Van der Drift M, Prinsen C, Knuiman J, et al. Diagnosing peripheral lung cancer: the additional value of RASSF1A methylation and KRAS mutation analyses in washings in non diagnostic bronchoscopy. Chest. 2012;141:169–75.

Vincent MD, Kuruvilla MS, Leighl NB, et al. Biomarkers that currently affect clinical practice: EGFR, ALK, MET, KRAS. Curr Oncol. 2012;19:S33–44.

Virmani AK, Rathi A, Zochbauer-Muller S, et al. Promoter methylation and silencing of the retinoic acid receptor-beta gene in lung carcinomas. J Natl Cancer Inst. 2000;92:1303–7.

Volinia S, Calin GA, Liu CG, et al. A microRNA expression signature of human solid tumors defines cancer gene targets. Proc Natl Acad Sci U S A. 2006;103:2257–61.

Wang T, Nelson RA, Bogardus A, et al. Five-year lung cancer survival: which advanced stage non small cell lung cancer patients attain long term survival? Cancer. 2010;116:1518–25.

Yang J, Shen Y, Liu B, et al. Promoter methylation of BRMS1 correlates with smoking history and poor survival in non small cell lung cancer patients. Lung Cancer. 2011;74:305–9.

Yuxia M, Zhennan T, Wei Z. Circulating miR-125b is a novel biomarker for screening non-small-cell lung cancer and predicts poor prognosis. J Cancer Res Clin Oncol. 2012;138:2045–50.

Zhang Y, Wang R, Song H, Huang G, Yi J, et al. Methylation of multiple genes as a candidate biomarker in non-small cell lung cancer. Cancer Lett. 2011;303:21–8.

Zheng D, Haddadin S, Wang Y, et al. Plasma microRNAs as novel biomarkers for early detection of lung cancer. Int J Clin Exp Pathol. 2011;4:575–86.

Zhu W, Liu X, He J, et al. Overexpression of members of the microRNA-183 family is a risk factor for lung cancer: a case control study. BMC Cancer. 2011;11:393.

Zöchbauer-Müller S. Genome-wide miRNA expression profiling identifies miR-9-3 and miR-193a as targets for DNA methylation in non-small cell lung cancers. Clin Cancer Res. 2012;18:1619–29.

Maspin Staining and Its Use as Biomarker in Lung Cancer

15

Rossana Berardi, Francesca Morgese, Agnese Savini, Azzurra Onofri, and Stefano Cascinu

Contents

Abstract

Maspin is a member of the serine protease inhibitor/non-inhibitor superfamily (serpin), and it is implicated in inhibition of tumor invasion, cell migration, angiogenesis and then metastasis, promotion of apoptosis, and cell adhesion. The role of maspin is different in distinct types of tumor for site and histology. There is a limited number of studies which have investigated the biological activity of maspin in primary lung cancer.

The majority of studies found that maspin expression is enhanced in squamous cell carcinoma of the lung where it is correlated with good prognosis and its lack is associated with higher metastasis risk and poor outcome. Complete and standardized methods to study maspin are necessary in order to evaluate its

R. Berardi (✉) • F. Morgese • A. Savini • A. Onofri • S. Cascinu
Medical Oncology Unit, Università Politecnica delle Marche, Azienda Ospedaliero-Universitaria, Ospedali Riuniti Umberto I – GM Lancisi – G Salesi, Ancona, Italy
e-mail: r.berardi@univpm.it; francesca-morgese@libero.it; agnese.sav@libero.it; azzurraonofri@libero.it; s.cascinu@univpm.it

V.R. Preedy, V.B. Patel (eds.), *Biomarkers in Cancer, Biomarkers in Disease: Methods, Discoveries and Applications*,
DOI 10.1007/978-94-007-7681-4_36

therapeutic implications and to understand how different subcellular distributions and epigenetic alterations could be helpful for a shared interpretation of results.

List of Abbreviations

AC	Adenocarcinoma
ATF2	Activating Transcription Factor 2
ECM	Extracellular Matrix
MVD	Microvessel Density
N	Nuclear
N + C	Nuclear + Cytoplasmic
NSCLC	Non-small Cell Lung Cancer
OS	Overall Survival
SCC	Squamous Cell Carcinoma
SCLC	Small Cell Lung Cancer
VEGF	Vascular Endothelial Growth Factor
VM	Vasculogenic Mimicry
vs.	Versus

Key Facts

Key Facts of Lung Cancer

- Lung cancer is the leading cause of death due to cancer worldwide, despite the recent progresses in the diagnosis and treatment.
- There are different histological type of lung cancer: non-small cell lung cancer (predominantly adenocarcinoma and squamous carcinoma) and small cell lung cancer.
- Complete surgical resection of the primary tumor and local nodal metastasis is the only potentially curative treatment, but the prognosis of patients who undergo radical surgery remains poor.
- In advanced or metastatic lung cancer, chemotherapy is the main treatment strategy next to the recent use of biologic drugs.
- The recent progresses in molecular biology lead up to find biological and molecular markers that may impact on the choice of therapy.

Key Facts of Maspin

- Maspin is a protein with different biological activity in various types of cancer.
- Maspin is a member of the serine protease superfamily.
- Protease and protease inhibitors play important roles in the progression of malignant tumors as protease may promote tumor invasion and/or metastasis through degradation of extracellular matrix and protease inhibitors antagonize the process.

- Tumor invasion means the ability of cancer cells to penetrate through the membranes that separate them from healthy tissues and blood vessels.
- Metastasis means the spread of cancer cells to other parts of the body from an original site, usually by way of the blood vessels or lymphatics.
- Maspin can have different tissue distributions: intracellular localization (nuclear or cytoplasmatic or both) or extracellular localization (secreted form).
- Role of maspin was studied in different cancer.
- Maspin expression correlates to favorable prognosis in lung cancer especially in squamous carcinoma.

Definitions of Word and Terms

Vascular Endothelial Growth Factor A signal protein that is implicated in angiogenesis and growth of tumor invasion and metastasis. Solid tumors cannot grow beyond a limited size without an adequate blood source.

p53 Tumor suppressor protein that regulates the cell cycle, described as "the guardian of the genome." It is involved in preventing cancer. Apoptosis, genomic stability, and inhibition of angiogenesis are the principal functions of p53 gene, which has several mechanisms: DNA repair in the presence of damage/mutation, cell cycle arrest at the G1/S regulation point, and promotion of programmed cell death, if DNA damage seems to be irreparable. If the p53 gene is damaged, tumor suppression is severely reduced.

Microvessel Density A quantitative evaluation to assess the tumor vessel number in a particular tumor tissue using endothelial antibodies. High MVD has been found to be associated with poor outcome.

Prognosis A measure of the probable natural course and outcome of a disease.

Introduction

Tumor progression seems to be promoted by protease and protease inhibitors. In fact, protease plays a role in tumor invasion and/or process of metastasis through degradation of extracellular matrix (ECM) with implication of integrin, and protease inhibitors antagonize this phenomenon.

Maspin is a member of the serine protease inhibitor/non-inhibitor superfamily (serpin), like plasminogen activator inhibitors 1 and 2 and α1-antitrypsin, which was first isolated and described as a 42 kDa protein with tumor-suppressing activity in human mammary epithelial cells (Zou et al. 1994). Its gene is located on chromosome 18q21.3–q23.

Serpin structure presents a reactive center loop (RCL), a peptide stretch that is located 9–15 residues amino-terminal to the reactive site peptide bond. RCL allows the reactive site to obtain an optimal configuration for binding and subsequent inhibiting target protease.

The conformational change takes the name of "stressed-to-relaxed" transition. Maspin, however, contains a relatively short, divergent, not highly conserved, hydrophobic RCL, not able to perform this modification. Finally maspin takes place into the non-inhibitory category of the large serpin superfamily and leads us to focus on its genetic alterations, on its expression in different cancer types, and how the different subcellular localizations may alter the prognostic significance (Law et al. 2005; Beecken et al. 2000; Pemberton et al. 1995).

Another important feature of maspin is the G α-helix (G-helix), an internal salt bridge or the P1 position of the reactive center loop. The maspin G-helix is able to an "open and closed" conformational change shaping a new distribution of charged residues into the molecule. The effect of maspin on cell migration required an intact G-helix, and the function of maspin protein can be mimicked by a short protein which is equivalent of this structural element. Maspin and the 15-mer G-helix peptide are linked to α1 integrins and β1 integrin subunit for their effects on cell migration (D'Andrea et al. 2006). In particular the maspin action in cell migration needed of the inactivation of β1 integrins (Cella et al. 2006; Ravenhill et al. 2010).

Integrins α5 and α3 could reduce the invasive phenotype of cancer cells, inhibition of cell surface-associated urokinase-type plasminogen activator and fibrinogen-bound tissue-type plasminogen activator, and interaction with type I and III collagen. Their changes could contribute to induce cell adhesion (Latha et al. 2005; Biliran and Sheng 2001; Blacque and Worrall 2002).

Maspin seems to inhibit angiogenesis and endothelial cell motility in vitro and in vivo and it seems to increase tumor cell apoptosis through promotion of the mitochondrial permeability. All these properties may be correlated to tumor suppressor activity of maspin (Zhang et al. 2000).

Therefore, the presence of maspin may contribute to the inhibition of tumor metastasis with the detachment and invasion of tumor cells through the basement membrane and stroma (Affara and Coussens 2007; Sheng 2005; Jang et al. 2008; Fig. 1).

Several works indicate, however, that maspin tumor suppressor activity is conditioned by its nuclear localization in cancer cells. In fact, the maspin bind to chromatin is necessary to prevent cells from metastasizing (Goulet et al. 2011; 2012).

About subcellular distribution, maspin is predominantly cytoplasmic but it also localizes to other cellular compartments and it's secreted. Secreted maspin could bind to extracellular matrix components. Alternatively, it is possible that maspin exerts its role only in the nucleus with regulation of genes or chromatin and thus indirectly it affects the cell-matrix interaction and is released only as a consequence of cell damage or necrosis (Zhang et al. 1999; Pemberton et al. 1997; Khalkhali-Ellis 2006; Khalkhali-Ellis and Hendrix 2007; Goulet et al. 2011; Teoh et al. 2010; Sood et al. 2002; Fig. 2).

Histone deacetylation, cytosine methylation and loss of gene function through chromatin accessibility seem to be the tissue-specific way of epigenetical changes of maspin expression. These alterations could explain different prognostic significance of maspin expression. Maspin expression, furthermore, has been detected

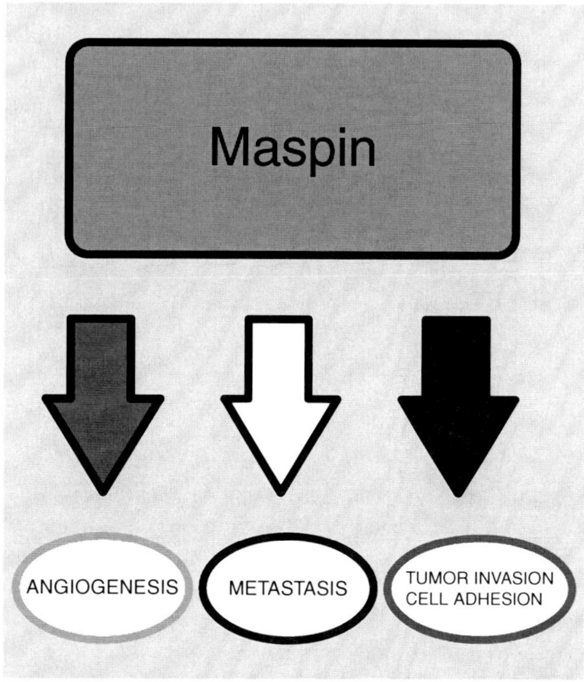

Fig. 1 Role of maspin in tumor

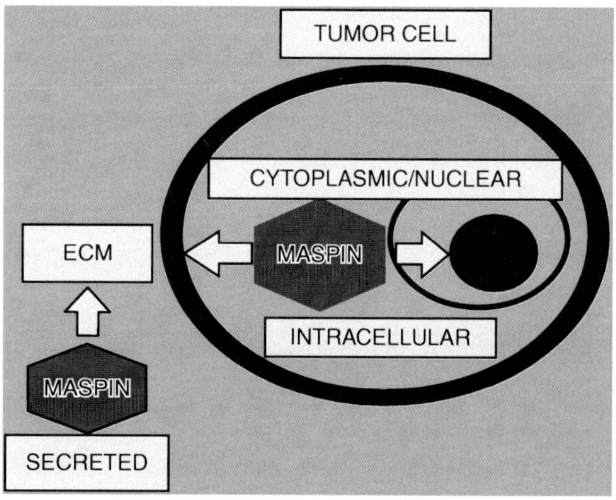

Fig. 2 Subcellular and extracellular distribution of maspin

not only in several types of tumor cells but it is expressed predominantly by epithelial cells in distinct manner (Beltran and Blancafort 2011; Wu et al. 2010; Bodenstine et al. 2012).

Downregulation on maspin expression is often present in breast, prostate, gastric, and melanoma epithelial cancer cells, while pancreatic, gallbladder, colorectal, and thyroid cancers usually overexpress maspin, thus confirming that it may have

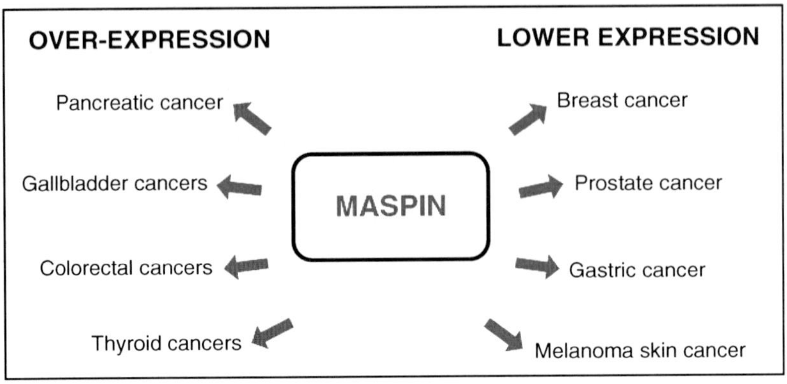

Fig. 3 Maspin expression in different types of tumor

different activity in various cell types (Fig. 3). Maspin has distinct subcellular localization in cancer cells (cytoplasmic, nuclear or both cytoplasmic-nuclear expression), with different interactions with extracellular matrix. Studies focused to interpret discordant expression and also significance of maspin protein are warranted (Seftor et al. 1998; Klasa-Mazurkiewicz et al. 2009; Lockett et al. 2006; Chen et al. 2005).

There is a limited number of studies which have investigated the role of maspin in primary lung cancer where the mechanism of action of maspin remains yet to be elucidated (Frey et al. 2009; Takanami et al. 2008; Nakagawa et al. 2006).

Non-small cell lung cancer (NSCLC) is the leading cause of death due to cancer worldwide, despite the recent progresses in the diagnosis and treatment (Jemal et al. 2011). Radical surgical resection of the primary tumor and local nodal metastasis is the only potentially curative treatment; nevertheless, the prognosis of patients who undergo radical surgery still remains poor with a 5-year survival rate ranging from 25 % to 40 % (Capewell and Sudlow 1990; Naruke et al. 1998; Van Raemdonck et al. 1992).

The recent studies in molecular biology lead up to find many biological and molecular markers that may be correlated with patient outcome and that may guide on the choice of treatment.

Potential Applications to Prognosis, Other Diseases, or Condition

In this section, the evidence that supports the clinical utility of maspin as a marker for stratifying the prognosis of different subtypes of lung cancer and, possibly, predicting the effectiveness of lung cancer therapy is elucidated.

Several studies showed that maspin influence the response to cell death in lung cancer cells and then inhibits the survival pathway (Nam and Park 2010).

Maspin has been found significantly expressed in primary lung cancer samples, and in particular, it is higher in squamous cell carcinoma (SCC).

Bircan et al. investigated maspin, p53, and VEGF expression in 63 patients with different histological lung carcinoma: SCC, adenocarcinoma (AC), and small cell lung carcinoma (SCLC).

The rate was significantly higher in NSCLC and in particular in SCC and AC than SCLC ($p = 0.0001$, $p = 0.0001$, $p = 0.038$, respectively). In ACs, maspin-positive cases had a significantly higher T status compared to negative cases ($p = 0.036$). In SCC, the stage of disease was positively correlated with p53 ($p = 0.007$) and negatively correlated with VEGF expression ($p = 0.013$). At multivariate analysis, stage of disease emerges as a significant independent prognostic parameter in NSCLC ($p = 0.031$) (Bircan et al. 2010).

Furthermore, in lung cancer maspin biological functions have been connected to its subcellular localization. In particular, a nuclear, opposed to a combined nuclear and cytoplasmic localization, has been associated with increased survival in NSCLC.

Lonardo et al. studied maspin expression in a model of transformation of bronchial epithelial cells and in 123 resected NSCLC. SCC showed almost exclusively a combined nuclear-cytosolic stain. In contrast, nuclear maspin, but not combined nuclear-cytoplasmic maspin, significantly correlated with low histological grade, lower proliferative rate, absence of invasion and negative p53 stain in AC (Lonardo et al. 2006).

Frey et al. investigated the role of maspin in 80 adenocarcinomas. Nuclear versus combined nuclear-cytoplasmic expression of masp was related to favorable histological and molecular features of lung adenocarcinoma and also, in early stage, improved prognosis.

Immunohistochemistry for maspin demonstrated immunoreactivity in 75/80 cases. Forty-seven of them revealed nuclear, while 28 combined nuclear + cytoplasmic staining. Five cases were negative.

No statistical correlation between maspin expression pattern and age or gender was detected. Mean survival, for stage I cases only, was higher for the nuclear compared with nuclear + cytoplasmic group. A statistically significant survival advantage for cases with only nuclear expression was shown in stage I, but not in advanced stages.

Finally maspin subcellular expression was related with histological grade and selected molecular markers. A statistically significant association of nuclear maspin was observed in low histological grade, negative p53 expression, and lower proliferative rate. The mean proliferative rate of cases with nuclear maspin was 36.6 %, while that of nuclear + cytoplasmic cases was 56.9 %. A highly significant association between nuclear maspin expression and low VEGF-A expression levels was also present (Frey et al. 2009).

Woenckhaus et al. investigated maspin subcellular localization and p53 expression in 487 lung cancer samples. Remarkably, nuclear ($p = 0.04$) and cytoplasmic ($p = 0.001$) maspin staining in at least 10 % of tumor cells was observed more frequently in primary SCCs than in other tumor types. However, no correlation was shown between maspin expression and tumor stage and nodal status. Only nuclear maspin immunoreactivity in at least 10 % of tumor cells was significantly associated with positive p53 staining ($p = 0.006$) (Woenckhaus et al. 2007).

Hirai et al. examined 112 lung cancer specimens. Cytoplasmic staining pattern was present in AC and SCC. The cytoplasmic positive rate was 77.8 % (42 out of 54 specimens) for the stage III group and 36.2 % (21 of 58 specimens) for the stage I group ($p < 0.0001$). Three-year survival rates after surgery were 30.8 % for the maspin-positive group and 71.1 % for the maspin-negative group ($p = 0.007$). Multivariate analysis showed that maspin expression was an independent prognostic factor for overall survival in patients with NSCLC. No correlation between maspin and p53 expression in cancer cells could be observed. The results of this study suggest that overexpression of maspin in cytoplasm may be a useful marker of tumor progression and unfavorable prognosis for overall survival in patients with NSCLC. Furthermore, maspin expression in cytoplasm appears to be unaffected by p53 (Hirai et al. 2005).

Recently, another study showed that maspin expression, with nuclear or cytoplasmic localization, together with smoking history, could represent prognostic factors in NSCLC.

In 424 samples, univariate analysis showed a positive correlation between maspin expression and SCC ($p < 0.0001$).

No correlation with stage of disease or lymph nodes involvement was noted, while an association with smoking history was documented. A higher cytoplasmic maspin expression was observed in smokers than in nonsmokers or former smokers ($p = 0.0041$), while no differences were evident in nuclear expression. Nuclear expression of maspin was also found to be an independent prognostic factor.

Interestingly, a statistically significant longer overall survival was present in patients with higher as compared with lower expression of nuclear maspin ($p = 0.0098$) and a significant poorer overall survival was observed in patients with a higher intensity of cytoplasmic staining ($p = 0.024$). Similarly, significant results were obtained in the different histotypes. In particular, a longer overall survival was showed in patients with higher versus lower nuclear maspin expression both in AC ($p = 0.012$) and in SCC ($p = 0.0095$) (Berardi et al. 2012).

In another recent study, Wu et al. examined maspin expression in NSCLC and its relationship to vasculogenic mimicry (VM). A total of 160 NSCLC specimens were analyzed. The loss of maspin expression correlated to the invasion and metastasis of NSCLC, and a positive relationship to VM in NSCLC was demonstrated ($p < 0.05$) (Wu et al. 2012; Table 1).

Again, Nakagawa et al., Katakura et al., and Takanami et al. showed that enhanced maspin expression was a significant and an independent factor in predicting a favorable prognosis in lung SCC. In particular Nakagawa et al. studied maspin expression along with intratumoral microvessel density, proliferative activity and p53 status in 210 consecutive patients with stage I–IIIA NSCLC. The incidence of strong maspin expression was significantly higher in SCC ($p < 0.001$) than in other histological types. The incidence of aberrant expression of p53 was significantly higher in maspin-strong than in maspin-weak tumors ($p = 0.005$). Univariate analysis showed that enhanced maspin expression was a significant factor in predicting a favorable prognosis in SCC patients, (5-year survival rates, 70.1 % for maspin-strong tumors and 41.5 % for maspin-weak tumors; $p = 0.014$), which was confirmed in a multivariate analysis ($p = 0.032$) (Nakagawa et al. 2006).

Table 1 Maspin expression in normal lung tissue. This table lists maspin expression in normal lung tissue and its correlation with microvessel density in the tumor, survival, stage, grading, and presence of lymph node metastasis

Authors	N. patients	Maspin expression	Prognostic implications
Wu et al. (2012)	20 normal tissue	51.9 % negative maspin	Negative maspin = higher vasculogenic mimicry and microvessel density, lower OS, high stage, high grade, lymph node metastasis
		100 % positive maspin	

Moreover, Katakura et al. examined 55 resected NSCLC patients. Maspin expression in SCC was significantly higher than that in AC ($p = 0.011$). Univariate and multivariate analysis confirmed that a high maspin expression was an independent and significant factor to predict a favorable overall survival ($p = 0.042$ and $p = 0.031$, respectively) (Katakura et al. 2006).

Takanami et al. investigated maspin expression in 181 patients with curatively resected NSCLC to determine maspin correlation with the microvessel density (MVD) level and prognosis. In SCC, there was no significant difference between maspin expression status and MVD, but strong maspin expression was an independent factor in predicting a favorable prognosis in SCC patients ($p = 0.01$) (Takanami et al. 2008; Tables 2 and 3).

Finally, some studies showed that maspin inhibits survival by inactivating Akt phosphorylation, and this could influence the response to cell death in lung cancer cells. The activating transcription factor 2, also known as ATF2, linked to transactivator domains was able to demethylate the maspin promoter. Consistently, co-treatment of ATF-transduced cells with methyltransferase inhibitors enhanced maspin expression as well as induction of tumor cell apoptosis.

Therefore, lung cancer cells lacking maspin would be resistant to chemotherapeutic drugs such as doxorubicin or etoposide, implying that treatment strategies based on the level of maspin might improve the efficacy of these chemotherapeutic drugs (Beltran and Blancafort 2011).

Methods

The specimens are usually formalin fixed. Histological sections are deparaffinized and analyzed by immunohistochemistry, using standard streptavidin-biotin-peroxidase techniques, with diaminobenzidine as the chromogen. Immunohistochemistry is performed using different types of IHC Detection Systems and NCL-maspin primary antibody.

All the neoplastic area presents in the slides is considered and both cytoplasmic and nuclear stainings are evaluated. In some studies, for example, for the nuclear-cytoplasmic staining, the cases are classified, according to the positive neoplastic cells, as follows: negative (<5 %), low positive (5–50 %), and high positive (>50 %). Moreover, in the positive cases, the intensity of the staining was also considered and subjectively scored by the two pathologists as 1+ (low), 2+ (medium), and 3+ (high).

Table 2 Maspin expression in different lung cancer histotypes. This table lists maspin expression in different lung cancer histotypes and its prognostic implications, according to several studies. In particular in squamous cell carcinoma (SCC), in adenocarcinoma (AC), in non-small cell lung cancer (NSCLC), and small cell lung cancer (SCLC)

Authors	N. patients	Maspin expression	Prognostic implications
Lonardo et al. (2006)	46 SCC	100 % positive maspin	Positive maspin = almost exclusively nuclear position
	77 AC	93.5 % positive maspin	Positive nuclear maspin in SCC = low grade, low proliferative rate, absence of invasion, negative p53 vs. nuclear-cytoplasmic position
Nakagawa et al. (2006)	210 NSCLC	73.7 % positive maspin in SCC	Positive maspin = 70.1 % 5-year OS
		26.3 % negative maspin in SCC	Negative maspin = 41.5 % 5-year OS
Woenckhaus et al. (2007)	487 tissue microarrays	72.3 % positive maspin	Positive nuclear maspin = 63.9 % SCC, 16.9 % AC
		65.3 % positive nucleus	Positive cytoplasmic maspin = 78.2 % SCC, 6.8 % AC
		37.8 % positive cytoplasm	
Takanami et al. (2008)	181 NSCLC	40.8 % positive maspin	Positive maspin in SCC = 52.2 % 5-year OS
		65.7 % positive maspin in SCC	Negative maspin in SCC = 24 % OS 5-year OS
		34.3 % negative maspin in SCC	
		22.8 % positive maspin in AC	
		59.2 % negative maspin	
Frey et al. (2009)	80 AC	93.7 % positive maspin	Positive nuclear maspin = 36.6 % proliferative rate, stage I OS: 87.7 ± 6.9 months, 42.5 % moderate and poor differentiation, 25.5 % p53 +, 4.2 % high VEGF
		62.6 % positive nucleus	
		37.3 % positive cytoplasm – nucleus	Positive cytoplasmic maspin = 56.9 % proliferative rate, stage I OS: 58.7 ± 6.5 months, 71.4 % moderate and poor differentiation, 53.5 % p53 +, 39.2 % high VEGF
Bircan et al. (2010)	28 SCC	89.3 % positive maspin	
	18 AC	77.8 % positive maspin	
	17 SCLC	52.9 % positive maspin	

Table 3 Maspin expression in lung cancer. This table shows maspin expression in non-small cell lung cancer (NSCLC) in unselected patient populations and its prognostic implications in terms of survival, tumor stage, grading, and presence of lymph node metastasis

Authors	N. patients	Maspin expression	Prognostic implications
Hirai et al. (2005)	112 NSCLC	55.3 % positive maspin	Positive maspin = 77.8 % positive cytoplasm stage III and 36.2 % positive cytoplasm stage I
		44.7 % negative maspin	
Katakura et al. (2006)	55 NSCLC	Not found	Positive maspin = 67.7 % 5-year OS
			Negative maspin = 41.4 % 5-year OS
Berardi et al. (2012)	439 NSCLC	85.6 % positive maspin	Positive maspin = longer OS
		22.8 % positive nucleus	Positive nuclear maspin = independent prognostic factor
		44 % positive cytoplasm	Positive cytoplasmic maspin = especially smokers, lower OS than nuclear position
		14.4 % negative maspin	Negative maspin = lower OS
Wu et al. (2012)	160 NSCLC	48.1 % positive maspin	Positive maspin = lower vasculogenic mimicry and microvessel density, longer OS, low stage, low grade, low lymph node metastasis

Instead, in other works, maspin immunoreactivity was defined as positive if at least 10 % of tumor cells showed at least moderate staining intensity. The cutoff value of 10 % was chosen for categorization of cytoplasmic and nuclear maspin expression.

It is important to notice that the nuclear expression is an important objective parameter, while the cytoplasmic maspin expression depends more on the pathologist's reading.

Another way to study maspin expression, in particular its mRNA levels, is represented by quantitative real-time PCR (qRT-PCR) or reverse transcription PCR. Protein expression and cellular localization were analyzed by immunofluorescence.

Conclusion

Although maspin expression correlates to favorable prognosis in lung cancer, especially in SCC, further studies are warranted for defining its role and its therapeutic implications. To this objective could be used, in future studies, both techniques PCR and IHC. The IHC could be used as a standardized method to assess the degree of expression, and intracellular localization of maspin and pCR might serve to identify if the presence of epigenetic alterations may explain conflicting results. In addition, the predominance of maspin expression in NSCLC with squamous histology can stimulate a discussion in the field of molecular biology on the phenotypic and genotypic characteristics of this particular disease.

Summary Points

1. Maspin is a member of the serine protease inhibitor/non-inhibitor superfamily (serpin).
2. Maspin promotes tumor invasion and/or metastasis through degradation of ECM.
3. Maspin is a marker for stratifying the prognosis of different subtypes of lung cancer and, possibly, predicting the effectiveness of lung cancer therapy.
4. Maspin has been found significantly expressed in primary lung cancer samples and in particular it is higher in squamous cell lung cancer.
5. Enhanced maspin expression was a significant and independent factor in predicting a favorable prognosis in lung squamous cell carcinoma.

References

Affara NI, Coussens LM. IKKα at the crossroads of inflammation and metastasis. Cell. 2007;129(1):25–6.

Beecken WD, Kramer W, Jonas D. New molecular mediators in tumor angiogenesis. J Cell Mol Med. 2000;4(4):262–9.

Beltran AS, Blancafort P. Reactivation of MASPIN in non-small cell lung carcinoma (NSCLC) cells by artificial transcription factors (ATFs). Epigenetics. 2011;6(2):224–35. Epub 1 Feb 2011.

Berardi R, Santinelli A, Onofri A, Brunelli A, Pierantoni C, Pisa E, et al. Maspin expression is a favorable prognostic factor in nonsmall cell lung cancer. Anal Quant Cytol Histol. 2012;34(2):72–8.

Biliran Jr H, Sheng S. Pleiotrophic inhibition of pericellular urokinase-type plasminogen activator system by endogenous tumour suppressive maspin. Cancer Res. 2001;61(24):8676–82.

Bircan A, Bircan S, Kapucuoglu N, Songur N, Ozturk O, Akkaya A. Maspin: VEGF and p53 expression in small biopsies of primary advanced lung cancer and relationship with clinicopathologic parameters. Pathol Oncol Res. 2010;16(4):553–61. doi:10.1007/s12253-010-9259-5. Epub 28 Mar 2010.

Blacque OE, Worrall DM. Evidence for a direct interaction between the tumor suppressor serpin, maspin, and types I and III collagen. J Biol Chem. 2002;277:10783–8. Epub 11 Jan 2002.

Bodenstine TM, Seftor REB, Khalkhali-Ellis Z, Seftor EA, Pemberton PA, Hendrix MJ. Maspin: molecular mechanisms and therapeutic implications. Cancer Metastasis Rev. 2012;31(3–4):529–51. doi:10.1007/s10555-012-9361-0.

Capewell S, Sudlow M. Performance and prognosis in patients with lung cancer. Thorax. 1990;45:951–6.

Cella N, Contreras A, Latha K, Rosen JM, Zhang M. Maspin is physically associated with [beta]1 integrin regulating cell adhesion in mammary epithelial cells. FASEB J. 2006;20(9):1510–2. Epub 23 May 2006.

Chen EI, Florens L, Axelrod FT, Monosov E, Barbas 3rd CF, Yates 3rd JR, et al. Maspin alters the carcinoma proteome. FASEB J. 2005;19(9):1123–4. Epub 27 Apr 2005.

D'Andrea LD, Del Gatto A, Pedone C, Benedetti E. Peptide-based molecules in angiogenesis. Chem Biol Drug Des. 2006;67(2):115–26.

Frey A, Soubani AO, Adam AK, Sheng S, Pass HI, Lonardo F. Nuclear, compared with combined nuclear and cytoplasmic expression of maspin, is linked in lung adenocarcinoma to reduced VEGF-A levels and in Stage I, improved survival. Histopathology. 2009;54(5):590–7. doi:10.1111/j.1365-2559.2009.03260.x. Epub 20 Mar 2009.

Goulet B, Kennette W, Ablack A, Postenka CO, Hague MN, Mymryk JS, et al. Nuclear localization of maspin is essential for its inhibition of tumor growth and metastasis. Lab Invest. 2011;91(8):1181–7. doi:10.1038/labinvest.2011.66. Epub 18 Apr 2011.

Goulet B, Chan G, Chambers AF, Lewis JD. An emerging role for the nuclear localization of maspin in the suppression of tumor progression and metastasis. Biochem Cell Biol. 2012;90(1):22–38. doi:10.1139/o11-053. Epub 2 Nov 2011.

Hirai K, Koizumi K, Haraguchi S, Hirata T, Mikami I, Fukushima M, et al. Prognostic significance of the tumor suppressor gene maspin in non-small cell lung cancer. Ann Thorac Surg. 2005;79(1):248–53.

Jang HL, Nam E, Lee KH, Yeom S, Son HJ, Park C. Maspin polymorphism associated with apoptosis susceptibility and in vivo tumorigenesis. Int J Mol Med. 2008;22(3):333–8.

Jemal A, Bray F, Center MM, Ferlay J, Ward E, Forman D. Global cancer statistics. CA Cancer J Clin. 2011;61:69–90. doi:10.3322/caac.20107. Epub 4 Feb 2011.

Katakura H, Takenaka K, Nakagawa M, et al. Maspin gene expression is a significant prognostic factor in resected non-small cell lung cancer (NSCLC). Maspin in NSCLC. Lung Cancer. 2006;51(3):323–8. Epub 6 Jan 2006.

Khalkhali-Ellis Z. Maspin: the new frontier. Clin Cancer Res. 2006;12:7279–83.

Khalkhali-Ellis Z, Hendrix MJ. Elucidating the function of secreted maspin: inhibiting cathepsin D-mediated matrix degradation. Cancer Res. 2007;67(8):3535–9.

Klasa-Mazurkiewicz D, Narkiewicz J, Milczek T, Lipińska B, Emerich J. Maspin overexpression correlates with positive response to primary chemotherapy in ovarian cancer patients. Gynecol Oncol. 2009;113(1):91–8. doi:10.1016/j.ygyno.2008.12.038. Epub 3 Feb 2009.

Latha K, Zhang W, Cella N, Shi HI, Zhang M. Maspin mediates increased tumor cell apoptosis upon induction of the mitochondrial permeability transition. Mol Cell Biol. 2005;25:1737–48. doi:10.1128/MCB. 25.5.1737-1748.2005.

Law RH, Irving JA, Buckle AM, Ruzyla K, Buzza M, Bashtannyk-Puhalovich TA, et al. The high resolution crystal structure of the human tumor suppressor maspin reveals a novel conformational switch in the G-helix. J Biol Chem. 2005;280(23):22356–64.

Lockett J, Yin S, Li X, Meng Y, Sheng S. Tumor suppressive maspin and epithelial homeostasis. J Cell Biochem. 2006;97(4):651–60.

Lonardo F, Li X, Siddiq F, Singh R, Al-Abbadi M, Pass HI, et al. Maspin nuclear localization is linked to favorable morphological features in pulmonary adenocarcinoma. Lung Cancer. 2006;51(1):31–9. Epub 12 Sep 2005.

Nakagawa M, Katakura H, Adachi M, Takenaka K, Yanagihara K, Otake Y, et al. Maspin expression and its clinical significance in non-small cell lung cancer. Ann Surg Oncol. 2006;13(11):1517–23.

Nam E, Park C. Maspin suppresses survival of lung cancer cells through modulation of Akt pathway. Cancer Res Treat. 2010;42(1):42–7. doi:10.4143/crt.2010.42.1.42. Epub 31 Mar 2010. Epub 3 Mar 2010.

Naruke T, Goya T, Tsuchiya R, Suemasu K. Prognosis and survival in resected lung carcinoma based on the new international staging system. J Thorac Cardiovasc Surg. 1998;96:440–7.

Pemberton PA, Wong DT, Gibson HL, Kiefer MC, Fitzpatrick PA, Sager R, et al. The tumor suppressor maspin does not undergo the stressed to relaxed transition or inhibit trypsin-like serine proteases evidence that maspin is not a protease inhibitory serpin. ASBMB. 1995;270(26):15832–7.

Pemberton PA, Tipton AR, Pavloff N, Smith J, Erickson JR, Mouchabeck ZM, Kiefer MC, et al. Maspin is an intracellular serpin that partitions into secretory vesicles and is present at the cell surface. J Histochem Cytochem. 1997;45:1697–70613.

Ravenhill L, Wagstaff L, Edwards DR, Ellis V, Bass R. G-helix of maspin mediates effects on cell migration and adhesion. J Biol Chem. 2010;285(47):36285–92. doi:10.1074/jbc.M110.177253. Epub 13 Sep 2010.

Seftor RE, Seftor EA, Sheng S, Pemberton PA, Sager R, Hendrix MJC. Maspin suppresses the invasive phenotype of human breast carcinoma. Cancer Res. 1998;58(24):5681–5.

Sheng S. Maspin: a novel serine protease inhibitor. Cancer Growth Progression. 2005;15:407–18.

Sood AK, Fletcher MS, Gruman LM, Coffin JE, Jabbari S, Khalkhali-Ellis Z, et al. The paradoxical expression of maspin in ovarian carcinoma. Clin Cancer Res. 2002;8(9):2924–32.

Takanami I, Abiko T, Koizumi S. Expression of maspin in non-small-cell lung cancer: correlation with clinical features. Clin Lung Cancer. 2008;9(6):361–6. doi:10.3816/CLC.2008.n.052.

Teoh SS, Whisstock JC, Bird PI. Maspin (SERPINB5) is an obligate intracellular serpin. J Biol Chem. 2010;285(14):10862–9. doi:10.1074/jbc.M109.073171. Epub 1 Feb 2010.

Van Raemdonck DE, Schneider A, Ginsberg RJ. Surgical treatment for higher stage non-small cell lung carcinoma. Ann Thorac Surg. 1992;54:999–1013.

Woenckhaus M, Bubendorf L, Dalquen P, Foerster J, Blaszyk H, Mirlacher M, et al. Nuclear and cytoplasmic Maspin expression in primary non-small cell lung cancer. J Clin Pathol. 2007;60(5):483–6. Epub 12 May 2006.

Wu Y, Alvarez M, Slamon DJ, Koeffler P, Vadgama JV. Caspase 8 and maspin are downregulated in breast cancer cells due to CpG site promoter methylation. BMC Cancer. 2010;10:32. doi:10.1186/1471-2407-10-32.

Wu S, Yu L, Cheng Z, Zhou L, Tao Y. Expression of maspin in nonsmall cell lung cancer and its relationship to vasculogenic mimicry. J Huazhong Univ Sci Technolog Med Sci. 2012;32(3):346–52. doi:10.1007/s11596-012-0060-4. Epub 9 Jun 2012.

Zhang M, Magit D, Botteri F, Shi HY, He K, Li M, et al. Maspin plays an important role in mammary gland development. Dev Biol. 1999;215:278–87. doi:10.1006/dbio.1999.9442.

Zhang M, Volpert O, Shi YH, Bouck N. Maspin is an angiogenesis inhibitor. Nat Med. 2000;6:196–9.

Zou Z, Anisowicz A, Hendrix MJ, Thor A, Neveu S, Sheng S, et al. Maspin, a serpin with tumour-suppressing activity in human mammary epithelial cells. Science. 1994;263(5146):526–9. doi:10.1126/science.8290962.

Part III

Brain

LGR5 as Marker in Brain Cancer

16

Susumu Nakata, Emma Phillips, and Violaine Goidts

Contents

Abstract

WHO classification of tumors of the central nervous system (CNS) is the standard basis for brain cancer diagnosis. It is primarily based on histopathological findings and some parameters such as frequency of mitotic malignant cells and existence of necrosis, providing a guideline for treatments of patients.

S. Nakata
Division of Oncological Pathology, Aichi Cancer Center Research Institute, Nagoya, Japan
e-mail: notsusumo@gmail.com

E. Phillips • V. Goidts (✉)
Division of Molecular Genetics (B060), German Cancer Research Center (DKFZ), Heidelberg, Germany
e-mail: e.phillips@dkfz.de; v.goidts@dkfz.de; v.goidts@dkfz-heidelberg.de

V.R. Preedy, V.B. Patel (eds.), *Biomarkers in Cancer, Biomarkers in Disease: Methods, Discoveries and Applications*,
DOI 10.1007/978-94-007-7681-4_11

Gliomas, the most frequently occurring brain tumor group, are particularly heterogeneous, showing a variety of cellular morphologies, molecular aberrations, and biological behavior. This fact has driven intensive investigations on searching for biomarkers for better stratification of gliomas and has resulted in the discovery of specific expression of the leucine-rich repeat-containing G-protein-coupled receptor 5 (LGR5) in multiple adult tissue stem cells. This is particularly relevant, as tumors with a low level of differentiation are associated with especially poor prognosis. Although inadequate choices of therapeutics for glioma patients currently make biomarkers' utility for glioma patients limited, recent advances are shedding light not only on the heterogeneity of glioma tumors within and across the subtypes, but also on the heterogeneity between malignant cells within the individual tumors.

List of Abbreviations

AP1	Activator Protein 1
ChIP	Chromatin Immunoprecipitation
CIC	Capicua Transcriptional Repressor
CNS	Central Nervous System
EMSA	Electrophoretic Mobility Shift Assay
EPHA2	Ephrin Type-A Receptor 2
G-CIMP	Glioma-CpG Island Methylator Phenotype
GSC	Glioblastoma Stem Cell
IDH	Isocitrate Dehydrogenase
L1CAM	L1 Cell Adhesion Molecule
LGR5	Leucine-Rich Repeat-Containing G-Protein-Coupled Receptor 5
LHX2	LIM Homeobox 2
LOH	Loss of Heterozygosity
MAPK	Mitogen-Activated Protein Kinase
MGMT	O^6-Methylguanine-DNA Methyltransferase
PFKFB4	Fructose-2,6-biphosphatase 4
PFS	Progression-Free Survival
RB	Retinoblastoma
RNAi	RNA Interference
WHO	World Health Organization

Key Facts of Brain Cancer

- There are over 130 types of brain tumor listed by WHO.
- The most common type of primary brain tumor is glioma.
- Symptoms of brain cancer include headaches, nausea, seizures, personality changes, visual problems, memory loss, and speech disturbances.
- Brain cancer is the number 2 cancer killer of children and young adults (after leukemia).

- The 5-year survival rate for adult patients with (malignant) brain cancer is around 10 %.
- Brain cancer is usually treated by surgical resection, radiation therapy, chemotherapy, or a combination of these.

Definitions of Words and Terms

Tumor Heterogeneity Cellular differences within a single tumor due to variations in cell lineage.

Epigenetics The study of changes in gene expression caused by mechanisms other than changes in the underlying DNA sequence. Examples include promoter methylation and histone modification.

Next-Generation Sequencing Modern method of high-throughput DNA sequencing which has allowed the sequencing of cancer genomes and helped identify many important mutations.

Chemotherapy Classical cancer therapy involving delivery of chemical agents that target highly proliferating cells by inducing DNA damage.

Progression-Free Survival The length of time during and after treatment during which the disease does not get worse. Usually spans from the date of diagnosis until recurrence, second malignancy, or death.

CpG Island Areas of DNA with high content of adjacent cytosine and guanine bases. Can be modified by methylation in glioma to give the glioma-CpG island methylator phenotype.

Cancer Stem Cells Tumor cells reminiscent of normal stem cells in terms of the cardinal stem cell properties of self-renewal capacity and ability to generate differentiated daughter cells. Seem to play a major role in driving tumor growth and recurrence in glioma.

Tissue Microarray Array assembly of hundreds of tissue cores in paraffin blocks which allows multiplex histological analysis.

Loss of Heterozygosity Occurs when one allele is lost by a deletion mutation, or a chromosome is lost from a chromosome pair, resulting in abnormal hemizygosity.

Transplantation Assay In vivo assay carried out by transplanting increasingly diluted single-cell preparations to measure stem cell (tumor-initiating cell) frequency.

Tumor Sphere Culture System Tumor stem cells from organs including the breast, colon, and brain can be grown in suspension culture in a serum-free medium, supplemented with growth factors. Under these conditions, tumor spheres are formed, small cell clusters containing tumor stem cells and some of their progeny.

Tumor Microenvironment This is the cellular environment surrounding a tumor, including immune cells, blood vessels, stromal cells, extracellular matrix, and signaling molecules. The composition of this microenvironment can affect the fate of the tumor, and in turn, the tumor can influence its microenvironment by exerting certain signals.

Wnt Pathway Signal transduction pathway which regulates key aspects of cell fate determination, cell polarity, organogenesis, neural patterning, and cell migration during embryonic development. Also plays a role in carcinogenesis.

Chromatin Immunoprecipitation Analysis A technique to determine the DNA binding site of a particular protein based on crosslinking the protein of interest to chromatin and sequencing the bound DNA fragment.

Electrophoretic Mobility Shift Assay A gel retardation assay used to determine whether a protein can bind a given DNA/RNA sequence. If the protein binds, the nucleic acid migrates much more slowly in an agarose gel, resulting in a "band shift."

Introduction

The World Health Organization (WHO) classification of tumors of the central nervous system (CNS) currently provides the most important basis for differential diagnosis of CNS tumors and subsequent clinical decisions about treatment (Louis et al. 2007). It is primarily based on histopathological findings and various parameters such as frequency of mitosis and existence of necrosis, providing a guideline for treatment. This process involves estimating the tumor cell of origin based on the cell morphology and tissue structure that the tumor actually resembles. Glial tumors are very heterogeneous in terms of cell morphology and molecular basis. Despite the established WHO classification system, some CNS tumor cases have had very different outcomes than what was expected according to the classification. Therefore, intensive effort has gone into identifying certain molecular makers, which could improve tumor diagnosis and classification and allow optimization of treatment for each patient (Weller et al. 2013). Our understanding of biomarkers in tumors in the CNS is dramatically changing. This is mainly due to the major progress made in the following three areas.

Firstly, progress made in CNS tumor genetics has provided a wealth of information on gene mutations, copy number aberrations, and epigenetics found in patients' tumors. For instance, intensive investigations on 1p/19q codeletion, MGMT promoter methylation, and IDH1/2 mutation have had a major impact on the stratification of glioma cases (Watanabe et al. 2009; Weller et al. 2012; Yip et al. 2012). Furthermore, the development of global high-throughput analysis, including next-generation sequencing, has helped to identify molecular aberrations accumulated in tumor cells. Global expression profiling allows the stratification of cases according to global expression pattern rather than one or a few molecular markers (Verhaak et al. 2010; Sturm et al. 2012).

Secondly, genetically modified glioma mouse models have provided information on concrete gene sets that can induce gliomagenesis in vivo and formed the basis for the tumor subtyping according to aberrant genetics that contribute to the carcinogenesis (Holland et al. 2000; Alcantara Llaguno et al. 2009).

Finally, developments in developmental biology technology have deepened our understanding on the process of development and homeostasis generated from tissue stem cells. This has led to identification of stem cell-related and regulating genes as biomarkers for the stratification of the gliomas. Today, the established databases of glioma cohorts with clinical information in the public platform facilitate rapid feedback from the identification of these biomarkers, indicating their impacts on the patients' outcomes. However, the actual clinical use of biomarkers is still limited. One recently discovered biomarker is LGR5, which is specifically expressed in multiple adult tissue stem cells and correlates with prognosis in glioma.

Molecular Biology of Glioma

Classification of Glioma

A comprehensive review by David Louis provides an excellent overview of the most recent edition of the CNS tumor WHO classification system (Louis et al. 2007). Here we describe the classification of the main types of glioma (Fig. 1). As stated above, the WHO classification of gliomas is predominantly based on the cytogenetic origin of the tumor cells, coupled with the grade of malignancy. The predominant cell type and the pathological features in glioma are mainly determined by light microscopy and immunohistochemistry. Astrocytes are supportive glial cells with essential functions in synaptic transmission and information processing by neuronal circuit functions (Sofroniew and Vinters 2010). Tumors of astrocytic origin include diffuse pilocytic astrocytoma, astrocytoma, anaplastic astrocytoma, and glioblastoma. Tumors arising from oligodendrocytes, the myelinating cells of the CNS, include oligodendroglioma and anaplastic oligodendroglioma. Such tumors sometimes have areas which resemble the astrocytic tumors and are hence known as oligoastrocytomas. Ependymal cells, which form the lining of the ventricles in the brain, can give rise to the ependymomas. These include subependymoma, myxopapillary ependymoma, ependymoma, and anaplastic ependymoma.

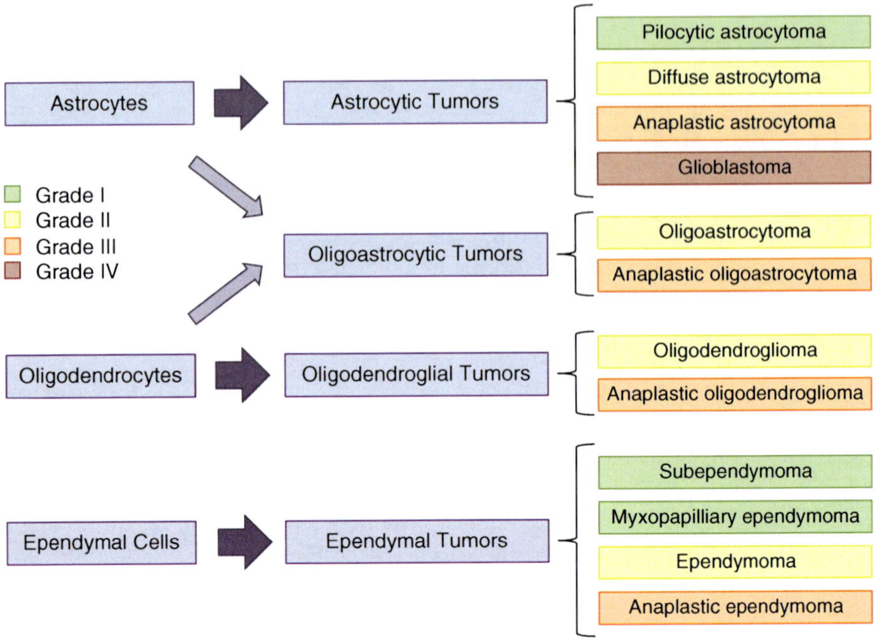

Fig. 1 WHO classification of glioma. The WHO classification of glioma divides the tumors into astrocytoma, oligodendroglioma, oligoastrocytoma, and ependymoma, depending on their cytogenetic origin. Within each subgroup, tumors are split into four different grades: I (*green*), II (*yellow*), III (*orange*), and IV (*red*)

Established Biomarkers in Glioma

1p19q Deletion

In oligodendroglial tumors, patients with codeletion of chromosome 1p and 19q have a relatively favorable outcome, making this chromosomal aberration one of the most important molecular markers for optimizing therapy. A recent study showed that 1p/19q codeletion results in the loss of heterozygosity (LOH) of the gene CIC, a potential inhibitory regulator of Ras/MAPK pathway. This mutation has a high incidence (53–83 %) in 1p/19q codeleted oligodendroglioma cases and suggests that CIC could be a tumor suppressor gene targeted by the codeletion (Bettegowda et al. 2011; Sahm et al. 2012; Yip et al. 2012).

MGMT Methylation

DNA alkylating agents such as nitrosourea or temozolomide are standard chemotherapeutic drugs that are commonly used for glioma patients. These agents exert antitumor activities by inducing guanine alkylation of genomic DNA. For more than a decade, the O^6-methylguanine-DNA methyltransferase gene (MGMT), which removes alkylation from guanine, has been recognized as a strong prognostic biomarker for glioma patients. Expression levels of MGMT are predominantly regulated via the methylation status of the promoter region. Patients with MGMT promoter methylation show better outcome represented by progression-free survival (PFS) from chemotherapy with temozolomide, while patients without methylation benefit more from radiation therapy. In some glioma cases, broad CpG islands throughout the genome are modified with methylation, which is known as the glioma-CpG island methylator phenotype (G-CIMP). Glioma cases with G-CIMP usually display MGMT promoter methylation, meaning MGMT promoter-methylated glioma might be part of the G-CIMP-positive group of glioma.

IDH1/2 Mutation

IDH mutations are present in both astrocytic and oligodendrocytic tumors. It seems that this gene aberration is an early event in tumorigenesis, with subsequent loss of 1p19q leading to oligodendrocytic differentiation and subsequent mutations in p53 leading to astrocytic differentiation (Watanabe et al. 2009). IDH-mutated gliomas often show G-CIMP, unlike gliomas with wild-type IDH. This is because the molecular function of IDH is directly related to CpG methylation, mediated by increased levels of 2-hydroxyglutarate (Turcan et al. 2012). Most importantly, IDH mutation status has been shown to be a better indicator of prognosis than histopathological classification, with IDH-mutated glioblastoma WHO grade IV patients doing better than IDH-wild-type anaplastic astrocytoma grade III patients. Hence, IDH-mutated gliomas are now thought to represent a distinct group of gliomagenesis, regardless of histomorphological features, i.e., direction of differentiation. This finding indicates that molecular profiling probably reflects the process of carcinogenesis and can potentially reveal biomarkers for patients' benefit.

Glioblastoma

Glioblastoma is the highest-grade glioma and is associated with extremely poor prognosis. The mean survival after diagnosis is in the range of 1 year, despite aggressive multimodal treatment (Stupp et al. 2007). Most glioblastoma arise de novo (primary glioblastoma), without detection of an antecedent tumor, although some glioblastoma progress from lower-grade gliomas (secondary glioblastoma). These two types of glioma have marked molecular differences, most notably in IDH1 mutation status, which occurs almost exclusively in secondary glioblastoma (Parsons et al. 2008). Intensive studies are underway to improve glioblastoma therapy, and the theme of personalized therapy is emerging as a crucial factor for achieving this goal. Major advances in high-throughput technology in the last decade have facilitated large-scale projects for integrated analysis of genomic or all exon sequencing, global gene expression profiling, and genomic copy number analysis on large cohorts of glioma tumors. Such techniques have the potential to identify all molecular aberrations accumulated in glioma tumors, which include candidates for therapeutic molecular targets. Of note, the tyrosine kinase receptor signaling pathway involving the Ras/PI3K/Akt axis, p53 pathway, and RB pathway have been found to be the major pathways that comprise the central targets for glioblastoma pathogenesis (TCGA Research Network 2008). Furthermore, Verhaak and colleagues were able to stratify glioblastoma into four groups: proneural, classical, mesenchymal, and neural, based on PDGFRA/IDH1, EGFR, and NF1 genomic abnormalities. It was shown that patient response to aggressive therapy differs by subtype (Verhaak et al. 2010). In addition, Sturm and colleagues stratified glioblastoma based on epigenetic modifications, which revealed six subgroups. Two of these are specific to pediatric glioblastoma, involving histone modifications. The other four subgroups were designated IDH, RTKI, mesenchymal, and RTKII and largely correlate with the grouping described by Verhaak and colleagues (Sturm et al. 2012). Studies such as these highlight the importance of markers for achieving the most effective tumor therapy. As described in this chapter, LGR5 has recently emerged as a promising marker for glioblastoma, which could greatly impact the efficacy of therapy for particular patients.

The Cancer Stem Cell Model

Theoretically there are three models used to describe cellular heterogeneity in a tumor. A traditional view is demonstrated by the stochastic model, which states that every cell in the population has the same potential to form tumors (Fig. 2a). More recently, a more complex model has been proposed, which suggests the existence of one or several subpopulations of cells within a tumor, which are capable of self-renewal and therefore have high tumor-initiating potential. Such populations could have variable genetic and epigenetic makeup: genetic mutations may enable the formation of completely new cell populations, whereas epigenetic changes could allow the formation of progeny with limited fate (Fig. 2b). Much evidence has been gathered in the last decade to support the existence of a small subpopulation of cancer cells that are capable of self-renewal and tumor initiation, as described in the aforementioned complex model. These are known as cancer stem cells. The first evidence for their existence was provided in hematological cancer (Lapidot et al. 1994; Bonnet and Dick 1997) and later extended to other solid tumors. Glioblastoma stem cells (GSCs) were identified and isolated around 10 years ago (Singh et al. 2003). Cancer stem cells are defined by their capabilities for self-renewal and differentiation. Technically, these characteristics have been demonstrated by transplantation assay using immunocompromised mice, combined with enrichment of the stem cell population via cell-surface marker expression. An example of a brain cancer stem cell marker is LGR5, which is described in detail in the next section.

Histopathological diagnosis in most cancer entities, including brain cancer, has shown that less-differentiated tumors are more aggressive, often with a rapid growth phenotype, and consequently result in poor prognosis. Clinical experience has also shown that tumors which have fewer cells with morphological features of normal terminally differentiated cells are more difficult to treat. In line with this,

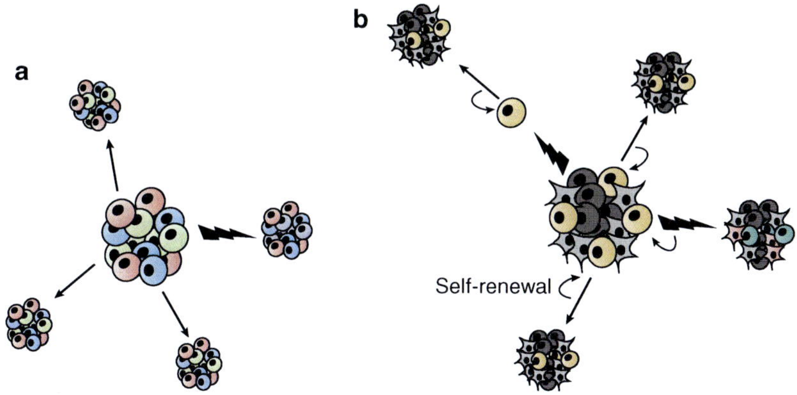

Fig. 2 Models of tumor heterogeneity. (**a**) The clonal evolution model, also known as stochastic model, postulates that all tumor cells are equally tumorigenic. Tumor heterogeneity is achieved through genetic and/or epigenetic alterations (indicated by a *flash*). (**b**) In the cancer stem cell model of tumor growth, only a subset of tumor cells, the so-called cancer stem cells (in *orange*), has the ability to self-renew and to give rise to progenitors with limited proliferative potential, which are able to differentiate. In addition, epigenetic changes potentially due to microenvironmental factors can influence the tumor cell phenotype and function (indicated by *flashes*)

GSCs have been shown to be particularly resistant to both chemo- and radiotherapy (Bao et al. 2006a, b); in this way they could be considered to be responsible for patient relapse. Targeting GSCs should cause the tumor to lose its ability to generate new cells, leading to complete tumor degeneration.

LGR5: A Potential Tumor Prognosis Marker

Structure and Function

One of the milestones in the field of the adult tissue stem cell research in recent years has been the discovery of specific expression of the leucine-rich repeat-containing G-protein-coupled receptor 5 (LGR5) in multiple adult tissue stem cells.

LGR5, also known as GPR49, is a member of the largest family of cell-surface molecules involved in signaling, the G-protein-coupled receptors (GPCRs).

LGR5 is ~144 kb long and is located on chromosome 12 at position 12q22-q23. It encodes a protein that harbors seven transmembrane domains (Fig. 3), and experimental evidence shows that the mature receptor protein contains up to 17 leucine-rich repeats, each composed of 24 amino acids. For several years, the exact molecular function and the ligand of LGR5 were unknown. Indeed, LGR4, LGR5, and LGR6 were considered to be "orphan" receptors. Recently, however, several groups have identified the R-spondins, soluble protein modulators of the canonical Wnt/β-catenin signaling pathway, as ligands for LGR5 (Carmon et al. 2011; de Lau et al. 2011; Glinka et al. 2011). After binding R-spondin, LGR5 forms a protein

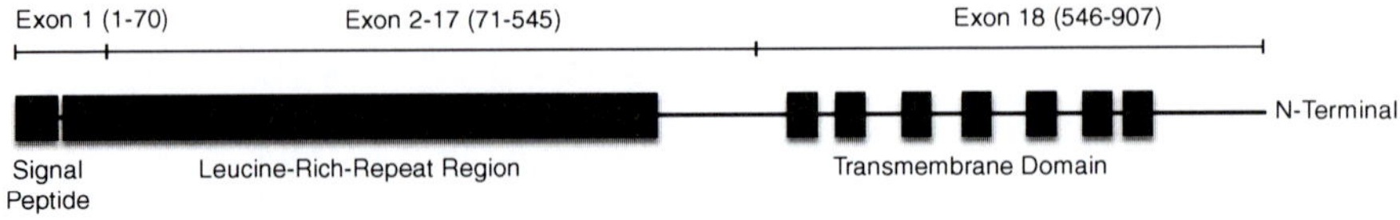

Fig. 3 Scheme depicting the structure of the LGR5 protein. *Numbers* indicate amino acid length of the different exons within the protein

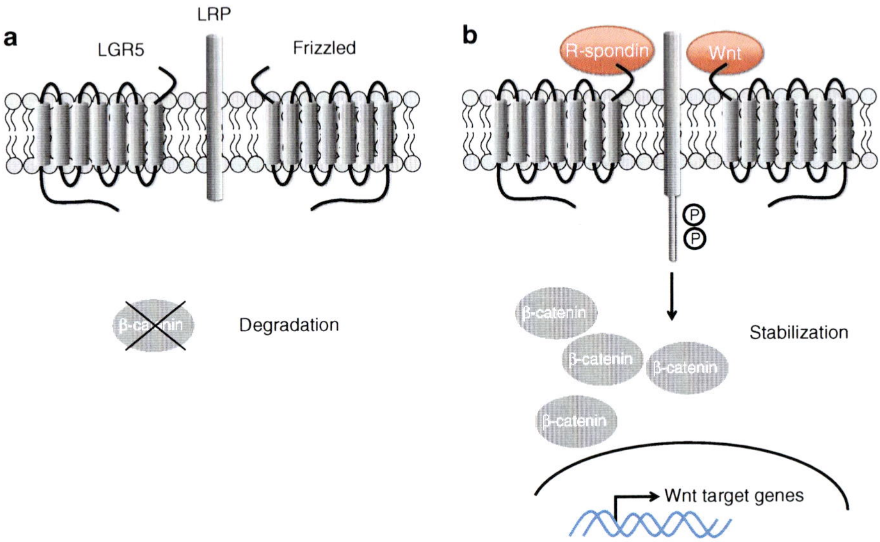

Fig. 4 (**a**) On the absence of a ligand, β-catenin is marked for degradation by phosphorylation. (**b**) Upon R-spondin binding, LGR5 recruits the LRP–Frizzled receptor complex, which binds to Wnt ligands, leading to the phosphorylation of LRP (Lipoprotein receptor-related proteins). β-catenin is then stabilized and can accumulate and, ultimately, translocates into the nucleus (Based on Birchmeier (2011), by permission of Wiley Publishers)

complex with Frizzled–LRP5/6, which positively regulates Wnt signaling (Fig. 4). Moreover, LGR5 was identified as a downstream target gene of the Wnt pathway that is regulated in a Tcf4-dependent manner (Barker et al. 2007).

A lineage-tracing technique using Lgr5 promoter activity in transgenic mouse models proved the existence of Lgr5^{+ve} stem cells in several adult tissues, such as the intestine, colon, stomach, hair follicle, cochlea, and tongue epithelium. In these tissues, it was shown that Lgr5^{+ve} stem cells are maintained over a long period of time and substantially generate all of the lineage cells in the tissue.

It is now broadly accepted that the R-spondin–Lgr5 complex functions as a Wnt pathway modulator, probably forming a positive feedback loop for the Wnt pathway in the stem cell compartment.

To date, several regulatory mechanisms for LGR5 expression have been identified, depending on the cellular context. In the intestine, Ascl2, a basic helix–loop–helix transcription factor that binds to the Lgr5 promoter and which is indispensible for maintenance of intestinal stem cells, exhibits a restricted expression pattern in the stem cell compartment (van der Flier et al. 2009). Inhibition of proto-oncogene c-Jun, a member of the AP1 signaling pathway, decreases Lgr5 expression in intestinal stem cells, together with Wnt pathway target genes (Sancho et al. 2009). Indeed, c-Jun binds to an intronic region of the Lgr5 gene locus and transactivates Lgr5 expression when phosphorylation-mediated activation of AP1 signaling occurs (Aguilera et al. 2011). This indicates that Lgr5 expression is regulated by cross talk of Wnt and AP1 signaling pathways in intestinal stem cells. In hair follicle progenitor cells, the Lim-homeodomain transcription factor Lhx2 binds to the Lgr5 promoter, as shown by ChIP analysis, and negatively regulates its expression (Mardaryev et al. 2011). GATA6 is one of the transcription factors that binds to Lgr5 promoter, as demonstrated by cell-based EMSA. In parallel, modulation of GATA6 expression results in the regulation of Lgr5 expression. This phenomenon was supported by the demonstration that GATA6 and Lgr5 are co-localized in chondrogenesis in mouse embryos (Alexandrovich et al. 2008).

LGR5 in Cancer

The new model of tumorigenesis suggesting the existence of a small subpopulation of cells uniquely capable of generating tumors led to the reconsideration of known stem cell markers in the context of tumor biology.

In that respect, many recent studies have shown the importance of the molecular function of LGR5 in several solid tumors and its use as a biomarker.

In adenoma cells, a Wnt pathway enhancer, prostaglandin E2, increases LGR5 protein but not mRNA levels independently of β-catenin, indicating the existence of posttranslational regulation of LGR5 protein expression and conditional regulation of *LGR5* rather than a function in a stem cell context (Al-Kharusi et al. 2013). Interestingly, it has been shown that *LGR5* expression can be epigenetically regulated and that methylation of its promoter causes repression of *LGR5* expression in some colon cancer cells (de Sousa et al. 2011). In other cellular contexts, inhibition and activation of the Sonic-hedgehog signaling pathway are capable of modulating *LGR5* expression in basal cell carcinoma cells, a SHH-related skin cancer entity (Tanese et al. 2008).

However, in colon cancer cells, LGR5 could function as negative regulator of the Wnt pathway, which is contradictory to findings in intestinal stem cells (Walker et al. 2011).

LGR5 in Glioma

LGR5 is expressed in the cancer stem cell fractions of glioblastoma and breast cancer. Interestingly, various lines of spheroid culture derived from breast

(Oskarsson et al. 2011), colorectal (Vermeulen et al. 2008), and glioblastoma (Nakata et al. 2013) tumors exhibit high expression of the *LGR5* gene. This suggests that tumorsphere cultures might be particularly suitable for the study of tumor cell behaviors that are driven by developmental signaling pathways such as the Wnt pathway. It was recently reported that in independent lines of neurosphere culture derived from glioblastoma, inhibition of *LGR5* gene expression caused significant programmed cell death, resulting in the exhaustion of the neurospheres (Mao et al. 2013; Nakata et al. 2013). In parallel to the induction of apoptosis, several stemness-related genes, developmental signaling pathway-related genes (including the Wnt and Sonic-hedgehog pathways), and cell cycle regulatory genes (such as L1CAM, FZD3, PATCH1, and CDKN1B) were significantly modulated (Nakata et al. 2013). Interestingly, inhibition of LGR5 causes a decrease in *PFKFB4* expression, which was recently identified as an indispensable gene for the glioblastoma stem-like cell fraction (Goidts et al. 2012). PFKFB4 mediates the process of glycolysis in cells that are adapted to hypoxic conditions. This might suggest that deficiency of LGR5 leads to improper adaptation to the hypoxic microenvironment.

Potential Applications in Prognosis and Other Diseases or Conditions

On the basis of its specific expression in stem cell fractions, LGR5 was used to enrich the cancer stem cell fraction in colorectal cancer (Kemper et al. 2012) and also proved to be a good prognosis marker for glioma patients (Nakata et al. 2013).

However, the immunolabeling-based detection of proteins is subject to many technical issues. Indeed, reproducibility of the results might be impaired due to variable methods for fixation, subjective interpretation of results, and limitation of sampling area. It is therefore essential to standardize the methods used and to increase the number of samples. In that respect, tissue microarrays containing multiple samples from each tumor have proven to be a useful and powerful tool to detect protein expression in hundreds of tissue samples under identical fixation and staining conditions. Establishment and preparation of large-scale tissue microarrays coupled with clinical information, including patients' outcome, require a lot of effort from many scientists and a great deal of resources. The tissue-based evaluation of molecules has the important advantage of availability of information on intercellular heterogeneity within tumor tissues. Indeed, information from genome-wide gene expression profiling of tumors is based on the assumption that an abundant gene product should play a more important biological role and reflects an average of the region sampled, losing information on intercellular heterogeneity. Therefore it is possible that lowly expressed but important players are missed in the process of the high-throughput exploration, particularly in the context of the cancer stem cell model. To facilitate more efficient feedback from accumulating evidence on potential biomarkers for clinical applications generated in basic cancer research, multiinstitutional collaborations to reserve controlled tumor specimens that can be partially used for tissue microarray preparation would be very important.

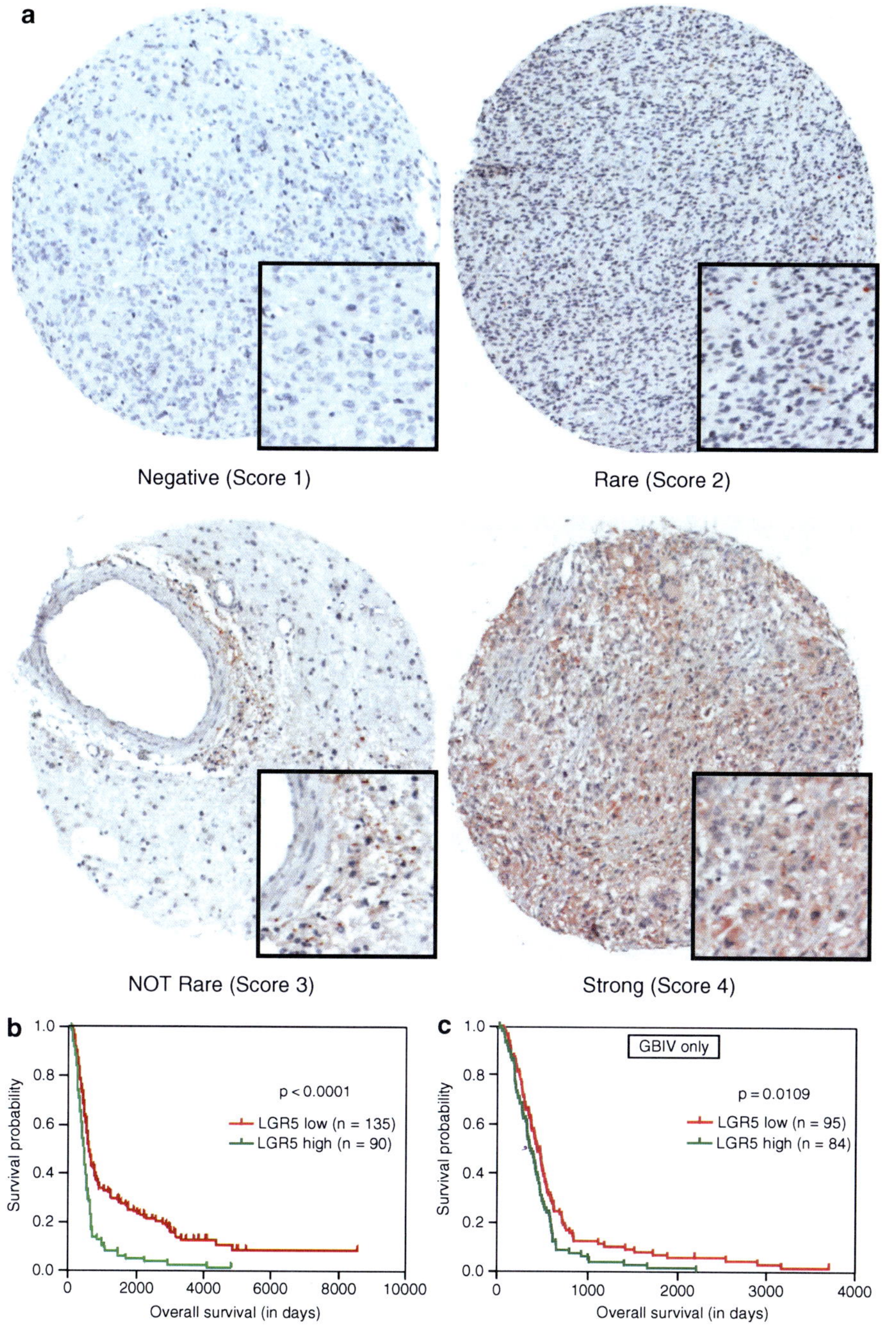

Fig. 5 (**a**) Representative immunohistochemistry staining of LGR5 on tissue microarrays from glioblastoma patients. (**b**) Kaplan–Meier analysis showing the significant association of LGR5 expression with overall survival rate in all glioma tumors. Low- and high-expression groups were

In addition, automatic image scanning systems for a large area of array slides for evaluation of tissue microarray results are also necessary to ensure identical conditions upon signal capture.

A further caveat in the study of biomarkers on tissue microarrays is the availability of suitable antibodies for immunohistochemistry. Hence, it is of utmost importance to have reliable positive and negative controls.

For the establishment of LGR5 staining in glioma, the antibodies against LGR5 were controlled with human normal small intestine tissues as a positive control, and shRNA-mediated knockdown cells as a negative control. In addition, identical staining patterns with two independent antibodies targeting different epitopes of the LGR5 protein were confirmed (Ernst et al. 2011; Nakata et al. 2013).

LGR5 expression analysis shows that a higher proportion of LGR5^{+ve} cells in glioma tissues correlates with poor outcome for glioma patients. The tissue microarray-based immunostaining of a large cohort of nearly 300 glioma cases demonstrated that LGR5 expression in glioma tissue shows typically four types of pattern (Fig. 5 and Table 1). Firstly, there are cases in which LGR5 signal is not detected at all. These cases suggest that some gliomas are independent of LGR5 and driven by LGR5^{-ve} cancer stem cells. Secondly, in some cases, only a few LGR5^{+ve} cells are scattered between the abundant LGR5^{-ve} cells. In these cases, each LGR5^{+ve} cell often resides solely as a single cell. These two types of pattern are considered as LGR5-low cases. The third pattern of LGR5 expression markedly exhibits clusters of LGR5^{+ve} cells, often gathered around blood vessels and damaged necrotic tissue. Over 10 % of the tumor cells are LGR5^{+ve} but accompanied with considerable number of negative cells. The fourth pattern is that the vast majority of tumor cells (over 70 %) are strongly LGR5^{+ve}. Only approximately 3 % of glioma cases displayed the fourth pattern of LGR5 expression. These nine cases were all grade IV glioblastoma, which is in line with the idea that expression of LGR5 is increased in higher-grade glioma cases. No distinct clinical parameters characterizing these rare cases specifically could be identified, probably due to an inadequate number of cases.

It has recently been reported that LGR5 immunoreactivity on glioma tissues correlates with WHO tumor grades, and LGR5 knockdown in established glioma cell lines blocks formation of tumor spheres and in vivo xenograft formation (Wang et al. 2014). The adverse effect of the LGR5 gene expression in glioma tumor cases is also supported by other cancer entities including colon, gastric, and skin cancers. In colon cancer cells, expression of LGR5 correlates with poor prognosis (Wu et al. 2012).

Fig. 5 (continued) separated according to the strength of the staining. Score *1* and *2* were grouped and considered as low expression. Score *3* and *4* represented the sections with a high LGR5 protein expression. (**c**) Kaplan–Meier analysis showing the association of LGR5 expression with overall survival in patients with glioblastoma grade IV (Reproduced from Nakata et al. (2013) by permission of Wiley Publishers)

Table 1 Expression of LGR5 in human gliomas as determined by Tissue Microarray (TMA) staining (Reproduced from Nakata et al. (2013) by permission of Wiley Publishers)

	LGR5 expression[a]	
Clinical grading	Low (%)	High (%)
WHO grade II	87	13
WHO grade III	86	14
WHO grade IV	53	47

[a]LGR5 expression level of the tumor sections is defined as low when less than 10 % of the cells are positive for LGR5 and as high when more than 10 % of the tumor section is positively stained

Conclusion

Glioma is a very heterogeneous tumor entity. The borders of each subtype in the WHO classification are very unclear. Although histopathology-based classification is very useful for the categorization of clinical cases, there are accumulating findings indicating that molecular basis should be considered for the stratification of cases.

An emerging large body of evidence indicates that stem cell-related genes, such as LGR5, are promising biomarkers for the stratification of glioma cases. In order to establish their use in the clinic, it is necessary to reproducibly and stably show a stem cell-related gene product at the protein level. It would be more meaningful if expression analysis of stem cell marker genes on tissue-based detection could be integrated with next-generation sequencing, global expression profiling, and copy number aberration analysis data, together with 1p/19q codeletion, MGMT promoter methylation, and IDH1/2 mutation in the same large cohort. Currently, inadequate therapeutic choice renders biomarkers in glioma of limited use for actually benefiting glioma patients. Therefore, it is important that large-scale analyses should also be carried out intensively in low-grade gliomas, aiming at extracting patients who should undergo intensive therapy. In addition to secondary glioblastoma, since it is relatively difficult to collect a large number of cases with defined clinical history for low-grade glioma, multiinstitutional studies in international collaborations are strongly desired.

Summary Points

- Gliomas are tumors of the CNS which are traditionally classified based on the cytogenetic origin into astrocytic, oligodendrocytic, and ependymal tumors.
- Certain genetic mutations and chromosomal aberrations have also proved useful for glioma classification and prognosis, such as codeletion of 1p19q, MGMT methylation, and IDH1/2 mutation.
- Advances in high-throughput technology have allowed further stratification based on genetic and epigenetic aberrations, which often have prognostic effect and facilitate the choice of therapy.

- Gliomas are highly heterogeneous, and low differentiation has been shown to correlate with poor prognosis.
- After their identification in the late 1990s, cancer stem cells are now believed to have a major role in tumor recurrence due to their resistance to chemo- and radiotherapy.
- Therefore it is of utmost importance to identify and target this population of tumor cells, stressing the importance of cancer stem cell biomarker identification.
- LGR5 is one such biomarker, being highly upregulated in cancer stem cells.
- LGR5 has huge potential as a glioma prognosis marker, although technical issues surrounding immunolabeling-based detection of proteins must be addressed.

References

Aguilera C, Nakagawa K, Sancho R, Chakraborty A, Hendrich B, Behrens A. c-Jun N-terminal phosphorylation antagonises recruitment of the Mbd3/NuRD repressor complex. Nature. 2011;469:231–5.

Alcantara Llaguno S, Chen J, Kwon CH, et al. Malignant astrocytomas originate from neural stem/progenitor cells in a somatic tumor suppressor mouse model. Cancer Cell. 2009;15:45–56.

Alexandrovich A, Qureishi A, Coudert AE, et al. A role for GATA-6 in vertebrate chondrogenesis. Dev Biol. 2008;314:457–70.

Al-Kharusi MR, Smartt HJ, Greenhough A, et al. LGR5 promotes survival in human colorectal adenoma cells and is upregulated by PGE2: implications for targeting adenoma stem cells with NSAIDs. Carcinogenesis. 2013;34:1150–7.

Bao S, Wu Q, McLendon RE, et al. Glioma stem cells promote radioresistance by preferential activation of the DNA damage response. Nature. 2006a;444:756–60.

Bao S, Wu Q, Sathornsumetee S, et al. Stem cell-like glioma cells promote tumor angiogenesis through vascular endothelial growth factor. Cancer Res. 2006b;66:7843–8.

Barker N, van Es JH, Kuipers J, et al. Identification of stem cells in small intestine and colon by marker gene Lgr5. Nature. 2007;449:1003–7.

Bettegowda C, Agrawal N, Jiao Y, et al. Mutations in CIC and FUBP1 contribute to human oligodendroglioma. Science. 2011;333:1453–5.

Birchmeier W. Stem cells: orphan receptors find a home. Nature. 2011;476:287–8.

Bonnet D, Dick JE. Human acute myeloid leukemia is organized as a hierarchy that originates from a primitive hematopoietic cell. Nat Med. 1997;3:730–7.

Carmon KS, Gong X, Lin Q, Thomas A, Liu Q. R-spondins function as ligands of the orphan receptors LGR4 and LGR5 to regulate Wnt/beta-catenin signaling. Proc Natl Acad Sci U S A. 2011;108:11452–7.

de Lau W, Barker N, Low TY, et al. Lgr5 homologues associate with Wnt receptors and mediate R-spondin signalling. Nature. 2011;476:293–7.

de Sousa EMF, Colak S, Buikhuisen J, et al. Methylation of cancer-stem-cell-associated Wnt target genes predicts poor prognosis in colorectal cancer patients. Cell Stem Cell. 2011;9:476–85.

Ernst A, Aigner M, Nakata S, et al. A gene signature distinguishing CD133hi from CD133-colorectal cancer cells: essential role for EGR1 and downstream factors. Pathology. 2011;43:220–7.

Glinka A, Dolde C, Kirsch N, et al. LGR4 and LGR5 are R-spondin receptors mediating Wnt/beta-catenin and Wnt/PCP signalling. EMBO Rep. 2011;12:1055–61.

Goidts V, Bageritz J, Puccio L, et al. RNAi screening in glioma stem-like cells identifies PFKFB4 as a key molecule important for cancer cell survival. Oncogene. 2012;31:3235–43.
Holland EC, Celestino J, Dai C, Schaefer L, Sawaya RE, Fuller GN. Combined activation of Ras and Akt in neural progenitors induces glioblastoma formation in mice. Nat Genet. 2000;25:55–7.
Kemper K, Prasetyanti PR, De Lau W, Rodermond H, Clevers H, Medema JP. Monoclonal antibodies against Lgr5 identify human colorectal cancer stem cells. Stem Cells. 2012;30:2378–86.
Lapidot T, Sirard C, Vormoor J, et al. A cell initiating human acute myeloid leukaemia after transplantation into SCID mice. Nature. 1994;367:645–8.
Louis DN, Ohgaki H, Wiestler OD, et al. The 2007 WHO classification of tumours of the central nervous system. Acta Neuropathol. 2007;114:547 (vol 114, pg 97, 2007).
Mao XG, Song SJ, Xue XY, et al. LGR5 is a proneural factor and is regulated by OLIG2 in glioma stem-like cells. Cell Mol Neurobiol. 2013;33:851–65.
Mardaryev AN, Meier N, Poterlowicz K, et al. Lhx2 differentially regulates Sox9, Tcf4 and Lgr5 in hair follicle stem cells to promote epidermal regeneration after injury. Development. 2011;138:4843–52.
Nakata S, Campos B, Bageritz J, et al. LGR5 is a marker of poor prognosis in glioblastoma and is required for survival of brain cancer stem-like cells. Brain Pathol. 2013;23:60–72.
Oskarsson T, Acharyya S, Zhang XH, et al. Breast cancer cells produce tenascin C as a metastatic niche component to colonize the lungs. Nat Med. 2011;17:867–74.
Parsons DW, Jones S, Zhang X, et al. An integrated genomic analysis of human glioblastoma multiforme. Science. 2008;321:1807–12.
Sahm F, Koelsche C, Meyer J, et al. CIC and FUBP1 mutations in oligodendrogliomas, oligoastrocytomas and astrocytomas. Acta Neuropathol. 2012;123:853–60.
Sancho R, Nateri AS, de Vinuesa AG, et al. JNK signalling modulates intestinal homeostasis and tumorigenesis in mice. EMBO J. 2009;28:1843–54.
Singh SK, Clarke ID, Terasaki M, et al. Identification of a cancer stem cell in human brain tumors. Cancer Res. 2003;63:5821–8.
Sofroniew MV, Vinters HV. Astrocytes: biology and pathology. Acta Neuropathol. 2010;119:7–35.
Stupp R, Hegi ME, Gilbert MR, Chakravarti A. Chemoradiotherapy in malignant glioma: standard of care and future directions. J Clin Oncol. 2007;25:4127–36.
Sturm D, Witt H, Hovestadt V, et al. Hotspot mutations in H3F3A and IDH1 define distinct epigenetic and biological subgroups of glioblastoma. Cancer Cell. 2012;22:425–37.
Tanese K, Fukuma M, Yamada T, et al. G-protein-coupled receptor GPR49 is up-regulated in basal cell carcinoma and promotes cell proliferation and tumor formation. Am J Pathol. 2008;173:835–43.
TCGA Research Network. Comprehensive genomic characterization defines human glioblastoma genes and core pathways. Nature. 2008;455:1061–8.
Turcan S, Rohle D, Goenka A, et al. IDH1 mutation is sufficient to establish the glioma hypermethylator phenotype. Nature. 2012;483:479–83.
van der Flier LG, van Gijn ME, Hatzis P, et al. Transcription factor achaete scute-like 2 controls intestinal stem cell fate. Cell. 2009;136:903–12.
Verhaak RG, Hoadley KA, Purdom E, et al. Integrated genomic analysis identifies clinically relevant subtypes of glioblastoma characterized by abnormalities in PDGFRA, IDH1, EGFR, and NF1. Cancer Cell. 2010;17:98–110.
Vermeulen L, Todaro M, de Sousa Mello F, et al. Single-cell cloning of colon cancer stem cells reveals a multi-lineage differentiation capacity. Proc Natl Acad Sci U S A. 2008;105:13427–32.
Walker F, Zhang HH, Odorizzi A, Burgess AW. LGR5 is a negative regulator of tumourigenicity, antagonizes Wnt signalling and regulates cell adhesion in colorectal cancer cell lines. PLoS One. 2011;6:e22733.

Wang D, Zhou J, Fan C, et al. Knockdown of LGR5 suppresses the proliferation of glioma cells in vitro and in vivo. Oncol Rep. 2014;31:41–9.

Watanabe T, Nobusawa S, Kleihues P, Ohgaki H. IDH1 mutations are early events in the development of astrocytomas and oligodendrogliomas. Am J Pathol. 2009;174:1149–53.

Weller M, Stupp R, Hegi ME, et al. Personalized care in neuro-oncology coming of age: why we need MGMT and 1p/19q testing for malignant glioma patients in clinical practice. Neuro Oncol. 2012;14 Suppl 4:iv100–8.

Weller M, Pfister SM, Wick W, Hegi ME, Reifenberger G, Stupp R. Molecular neuro-oncology in clinical practice: a new horizon. Lancet Oncol. 2013;14:e370–9.

Wu XS, Xi HQ, Chen L. Lgr5 is a potential marker of colorectal carcinoma stem cells that correlates with patient survival. World J Surg Oncol. 2012;10:244.

Yip S, Butterfield YS, Morozova O, et al. Concurrent CIC mutations, IDH mutations, and 1p/19q loss distinguish oligodendrogliomas from other cancers. J Pathol. 2012;226:7–16.

Using 2D-DIGE-MS to Identify Biomarkers for Brain Cancer

17

Hirendra Nath Banerjee and Mukesh Verma

Contents

Abstract

This review discusses about identification and characterization of biomarkers in brain cancer utilizing proteomic analysis which is a powerful tool for the discovery of cancer molecular markers. Proteomic analysis allows the characterization of proteins at pictogram level with mass spectrometry (MS) and changes in the levels inherent to the pathophysiology of any cell type, tissue, or whole organism. Protein markers identified by this approach could discriminate cancerous from

H.N. Banerjee (✉)
Department of Biological Sciences and Pharmaceutical Sciences,
Elizabeth City State University/University of North Carolina, Elizabeth City, NC, USA
e-mail: docbanerjee@hotmail.com; bhirendranath@mail.ecsu.edu

M. Verma
Methods and Technologies Branch, Epidemiology and Genetics Research Program, Division of Cancer Control and Population Sciences, National Cancer Institute (NCI), National Institutes of Health (NIH), Rockville, MD, USA
e-mail: vermam@mail.nih.gov

V.R. Preedy, V.B. Patel (eds.), *Biomarkers in Cancer, Biomarkers in Disease: Methods, Discoveries and Applications*,
DOI 10.1007/978-94-007-7681-4_22

normal cells. As demonstrated here, proteomic analysis may be efficiently used to identify new indicators for the diagnosis and prognosis of cancer progression. The 2D-DIGE method has been one of the mainstream technologies used for proteomic investigations. In this method, proteins are separated in the first dimension according to charge by isoelectric focusing, followed by separation in the second dimension according to molecular weight, using polyacrylamide gel electrophoresis. Using this approach, up to 1,000 protein spots could be separated and visualized in a single experiment. Gels of different samples are compared and analyzed using computer software, and differentially expressed protein spots are then excised and identified using MS. In this manuscript, we reviewed the relevance of biomarkers in brain cancers and cancer proteomics and the possibility of application of 2D-DIGE-MS method in discovery of potential biomarkers in brain cancers especially glioblastoma multiforme (GBM) which has high rate of recurrence and resistance to chemotherapy.

Key Facts

For the early detection of brain cancer diagnosis, 2D-DIGE technology offers promise. This technology is simple to use and shows high specificity and sensitivity, and proteomic biomarkers isolated using this technology may be useful in diagnosis, treatment, and prognosis of brain tumors.

Definitions of Words and Terms

Biomarker A biomarker is a measurable substance in an organism whose levels correlate with the initiation and/or progression of a disease or abnormal condition due to exposure to abnormal conditions, infection, or other external stimuli.

Brain tumor A brain tumor is an intracranial solid neoplasm within the brain or the central spinal canal.

Epigenetics Epigenetics is the study of inherited changes in gene expression caused by mechanisms other than changes in DNA sequence.

2D-DIGE (Two-dimensional difference gel electrophoresis) Two-dimensional difference gel electrophoresis is a technique to separate proteins first based on their molecular weight (in one dimension) and then based on their isoelectric focusing point (in the second dimension).

Methylation DNA methylation involves addition of a methyl group to the fifth position of the pyrimidine cytosine, and this modification is inheritable.

Prognosis Prognosis is a prediction of the probable course and outcome of a disease.

Proteomics Proteomics is a branch of biotechnology which involves application of molecular biology technologies for analyzing the structure, function, and interaction of proteins produced by a cell or a group of cells of an organism.

RNAi RNA interference or RNAi is a system within living cells that involves miRNA and siRNA activity, which helps to control which genes are active and how active they are.

Tumor grade All gliomas, except GBM, range from well-differentiated tumors (low grade) to anaplastic, which are, completely chaotic, undifferentiated (high grade). High-grade tumors are more aggressive and are associated with lower survival rates. In terms of surviving the disease, the grade of the tumor is the most important feature.

Introduction

Brain tumors are a heterogeneous group of central nervous system neoplasms that arise within or adjacent to the brain. Some are curable by surgical resection, but many cannot be eradicated by current treatments, and, when they are, disabling neurological injury often ensues. Moreover, the location of the tumor within the brain has a profound effect on the patient's symptoms, surgical therapeutic options, and likelihood of obtaining a definitive diagnosis. The location of the tumor in the brain also markedly alters the risk of neurological toxicities that alter the patient's quality of life.

At present, brain tumors are detected by imaging only after the onset of neurological symptoms. No early detection strategies are in use, even in individuals known to be at risk for specific types of brain tumors by virtue of their genetic makeup. Current histopathological classification systems, which are based on the tumor's presumed cell of origin, have been in place for nearly a century and were updated by the World Health Organization in 1999. Although satisfactory in many respects, they do not allow accurate prediction of tumor behavior in the individual patient nor do they guide therapeutic decision-making as precisely as patients and physicians would hope and need. Current imaging techniques provide meticulous anatomical delineation and are the principal tools for establishing that neurological symptoms are the consequence of a brain tumor. Little research has been done on whether early detection improves an individual's prognosis, lessens long-term side effects, and reduces costs associated with treatment. There is some indication that this might be the case. The earlier a brain tumor is detected, the smaller the tumor and the less likely that the tumor has significantly infiltrated normal brain tissue. This increases the chance that the tumor can be totally or almost totally resected during surgery which could be an important factor in an individual's prognosis. A smaller tumor also means that a smaller area of the brain will need to be subjected to radiotherapy, minimizing the adverse effects of radiation.

Even if early diagnosis is found to be advantageous, at this point there is not an accessible, efficient, cost-effective early screening tool. A simple detection test that looks for a biomarker of a brain tumor would be incredibly valuable as testing could be done repeatedly, on a wide scale, and relatively inexpensively. In the following sections, we have discussed about different types of brain cancer and different markers which are generally used for early detection of cancer and make a case of the advantages of using proteomics-based markers in diagnosis of brain cancers, especially glioblastoma multiforme (GBM).

Different Kinds of Brain Cancers

The World Health Organization (WHO) has nine categories of primary brain tumors, which are based on the types of cells in which the tumors originate. Gliomas are primary brain tumors that are made up of glial cells – cells that provide important structural support for the nerve cells in the brain. Infiltrative astrocytoma and GBM account for nearly 85 % of all brain tumors, with the remainder spread among the other seven types (Yurtsever et al. 2013). Different tumor types and cell origins are presented in Table 1.

Different Biomarkers Used in Brain Cancer Detection

Tumor markers are substances that are produced by cancer cells or by other cells of the body in response to cancer or certain benign (noncancerous) conditions. Most tumor markers are made by normal cells as well as by cancer cells; however, they are produced at much higher levels in cancerous conditions (Verma 2012). These substances can be found in the blood, urine, stool, tumor tissue, or other tissues or bodily fluids of some patients with cancer. Biomarkers for cancer diagnosis may belong to different categories described below.

Most tumor markers are proteins. However, more recently, patterns of gene expression and changes to DNA have also begun to be used as tumor markers. Markers of the latter type are assessed in tumor tissue specifically. Thus far, more than 20 different tumor markers have been characterized and are in clinical use. Some are associated with only one type of cancer, whereas others are associated with two or more cancer types. There is no "universal" tumor marker that can detect any type of cancer. There are some limitations to the use of tumor markers (described later on in this chapter). Sometimes, noncancerous conditions can cause the levels of certain tumor markers to increase. In addition, not everyone with a particular type of cancer will have a higher level of a tumor marker associated with that cancer. Moreover, tumor markers have not been identified for every type of cancer. Along with proteomic biomarkers, which we'll discuss in details, some other biomarkers have potential in brain cancer diagnosis and prognosis, and we have discussed about these biomarkers below.

Genetic biomarkers. These biomarkers contain alterations in genome which could arise as a result of polymorphism, mutation, deletion, translocation, or change

Table 1 Different types of brain cancers and their origin

Tumor type	Cell of origin
Infiltrative astrocytoma	Astrocytes
Pilocytic astrocytoma	Astrocytes
Oligodendroglioma	Oligodendrocytes
Mixed oligoastrocytoma	Oligodendrocytes and astrocytes
Glioblastoma multiforme (GBM)	Astrocytes and other brain cell types (astroblasts, spongioblasts)
Ependymoma	Ependymocytes
Medulloblastoma	Primitive neural cell
Meningioma	Meninges

in copy number of chromosomes. Chromosome 10q and chromosome 17 statuses were utilized for risk associated with adult medulloblastoma (Kool et al. 2012).

Epigenetic biomarkers. Epigenetic biomarkers are those markers which do not involve alteration in gene sequence and structure, but these biomarkers reflect alteration in gene expression in cancer of different types, including brain cancer (Verma 2012). Four major components of epigenetics are DNA methylation, histone modifications, miRNA expression, and chromosomal compaction and relaxation. *PTEN* and *MGMT* hypermethylation in the promoter region was reported in glioblastoma (Yurtsever et al. 2013). In pediatric brain tumors, *TERT* hypermethylation was reported a diagnostic biomarker (Diede 2013).

Proteomic biomarkers. A number of proteomic biomarkers associated with brain cancer have been identified (Lemee et al. 2013). Those which showed promise are being validated in large sample size so that they can be used in clinic. Recently, glial fibrillary acidic protein (GFAP) antibody present in the serum was proposed as a biomarker for glioma (Wei et al. 2013). Other brain cancer biomarkers are discussed throughout the text.

Glyco-biomarkers. Oligosaccharides (mono- and polysaccharides) constitute different genes involved in regulation of brain tumors (Moskal et al. 2009). Some of the glycobiological biomarkers have potential to be used in brain cancer diagnosis. Depending on the posttranslation modifications, different kinds of sugars bind to the protein, and generally their complexity and number are associated with the progression of the cancer development (Wade et al. 2013).

Imaging biomarkers. Magnetic resonance-based diagnosis of brain tumors, especially at metastasis stage, was reported recently (Yang et al. 2013). A sensitivity of 81 % and specificity of 98.2 % were obtained by this technology.

Lipid biomarkers. Glycolipids were used as biomarkers of cisplatin treatment response in brain cancer cells (Pan et al. 2011). Two prominent markers in this study were uridine diphospho-*N*-acetylglucosamine (UDP-GluNAc) and uridine diphospho-*N*-acetylgalactosamine (UDP-GalNAc). These markers were identified using the nuclear magnetic resonance spectroscopy.

Metabolomic biomarkers. Metabolites are considered true representative of physiology (Verma et al. 2013). The role of choline metabolism was demonstrated in astrocytoma (McNight et al. 2011). Phosphocholine (PC) and glycerophosphocholine (GPC) were evaluated in astrocytoma tumor samples. Results indicated that levels of PC and GPC reflect grade of the tumor.

Different Tests Based on Biomarkers for Detection of Brain Cancers

The following are the clinically accepted tests using biomarkers for diagnosis and prognosis of brain cancers.

MGMT methylation test. The MGMT methylation test can be useful in predicting how effective chemotherapy treatment is likely to be for the patient and can be used to help plan a suitable, individualized treatment plan. *MGMT* is a gene that is responsible for the coding of a protein involved in DNA repair. The *MGMT* test is used to determine the levels of activity of the MGMT protein. Since it is involved in DNA repair, the MGMT protein can disturb the action of some chemotherapy drugs (such as Temozolomide). It does this by taking away the point at which the chemotherapy attacks most effectively. Higher levels of the MGMT protein can therefore lower the effectiveness of some chemotherapy drugs.

1p/19q test. The 1p/19q test may predict long-term survival in people who have some types of brain tumor. The test can also be useful in diagnosing some types of brain tumors and in making decisions about the most appropriate treatment type. The 1p/19q test looks at genetic changes to chromosome numbers 1 and 19 in tumor cells and whether these genes are complete or have a section missing (which is known as "loss of heterozygosity").

IDH-1 test. The *IDH-1* test may predict long-term survival in people who have many types of brain tumor. It may also be useful in predicting how effective a particular treatment is likely to be. A mutation in the *IDH-1* gene has been found in a large number of astrocytomas, oligodendrogliomas, and secondary glioblastomas. For people with high-grade glioma, mutations to the *IDH-1* gene are often linked with longer-term survival rates. It is not yet clear, however, how mutations to the *IDH-1* gene link to outcomes for people with low-grade brain tumors. In addition to long-term survival rates, scientists have looked at whether the *IDH-1* gene mutation predicts treatment outcomes. Further research needs to be carried out before clear conclusions can be drawn, but it looks possible that chemoradiotherapy (a combination of chemotherapy and radiotherapy) may be more effective for people who have the *IDH-1* mutation than those who do not.

BRAF test. The BRAF test (along with other investigations) can sometimes help to determine whether a tumor is a pilocytic astrocytoma (a type of grade 1 tumor) rather than another type of (non-pilocytic) astrocytoma if there is uncertainty. The B-raf protein is important because it sends signals to help direct the growth of cells within our body. Signals sent from the BRAF gene to the cells is known as the "BRAF pathway." Research has found that some brain tumors (some types of grade 1 and 2 astrocytoma, including grade 1 pilocytic astrocytoma) sometimes have a fault with their *BRAF* gene. The fault leads to the BRAF gene permanently sending signals that make cells divide and create copies of themselves. This uncontrolled growth of cells forms a tumor. BRAF testing is only clinically useful in a few selected tumor types and is most commonly used to determine whether a tumor is a pilocytic astrocytoma.

Use of 2D-DIGE-MS in Detecting Brain Cancers

Basic principle of 2D-DIGE and methodology. The 2D-DIGE method is a technique where two different protein samples (e.g., control and disease) and, optionally, one reference sample (e.g., control and disease pooled together) are labeled with one of three spectrally different fluorophores: cyanine (Cy)2, 3, or 5 (Kang et al. 2009). These fluorophores have the same charge, similar molecular weight and distinct fluorescent properties, allowing their discrimination during scanning using appropriate optical filters (Epstein et al. 2013). Two types of cyanine dyes are available: CyDye DIGE Fluor (GE Healthcare, Uppsala, Sweden) minimal dye and CyDye DIGE Fluor saturation dye. The minimal dye labels a small percentage of available lysine residues and causes minimal change in the electrophoretic mobility pattern of the protein, whereas the saturation dye labels all available cysteine residues and is, therefore, more sensitive but causes electrophoretic mobility shift of labeled proteins (Epstein et al. 2013). Various types of samples could be used for 2D-DIGE, such as serum, plasma, cell lysates, and proteins extracted from patient tissue samples. Labeled sample pairs (with or without the pooled reference sample) are then mixed together and run on a single gel. A significant improvement in this technique compared to previous techniques is that the same pooled reference sample is used for all gels within an experiment and serves as a common internal reference for normalization and spot matching. The gel is scanned by a fluorescent scanner at three different wavelengths for Cy2 (488 nm), Cy3 (532 nm), and Cy5 (633 nm), and a gel image for each of the different samples is obtained.

Advantages of using 2D-DIGE in identification of brain cancer biomarkers. Since samples from control and disease are run in the same gel, variation between gels is minimized and difficulties associated with the correct matching of protein spots across different gels are reduced. Moreover, normalization and relative quantification of protein spots are greatly simplified and have increased accuracy because the same internal reference sample is used for all gels. Other advantages of the DIGE technology include its excellent sensitivity comparable to those of post-run fluorescent stains, a linear dynamic range of over four orders of magnitude and its being fully compatible with mass spectrometry (MS). Few examples of protein biomarkers identified and characterized by 2D-DIGE are shown in Table 2.

Challenges inherent in 2D-DIGE technique and potential solutions. 2D-DIGE still has limitations because proteins with extreme isoelectric focusing points, large molecular weights, low solubility (hydrophobic proteins), and low copy numbers are poorly represented owing to it being 2D-DIGE based in nature. This technique is also mainly used for the discovery of novel biomarkers, and careful validations of such markers are required using alternative techniques, such as

Table 2 Differentially expressed peptides/proteins in GBM samples identified by MALDI mass spectrometry after 2D-DIGE analysis

Spot label	Name of the protein	Accession number	Molecular weight of protein (kDa)	PI of protein	Fold changed
1	Lactotransferrin precursor	IPI00298860	80	8.50	**6.55**
2	Fibrinogen beta chain precursor	IPI00298497	57	8.54	**9.43**
3	Glucose-regulated protein 78	P11021	78	5.10	2.6

immunohistochemistry (IHC) or Western blot. Moreover, equipments such as fluorescent scanners, are required for image acquisition, which incurs additional costs. Whether potential biomarkers identified using 2D-DIGE could be successfully validated is greatly related to the careful planning of experiments, correct matching and selection of protein spots across gels, and application of appropriate statistical analysis methods.

Analysis of data and associated features. Results from 2D-DIGE gels are commonly analyzed using commercially available softwares. In a study that compared three commonly used DIGE analysis software packages, Kang et al. (2009) concluded that although the three softwares performed satisfactorily with minimal user intervention, significant improvements in the accuracy of analysis could be achieved by optimizing software settings and performing manual corrections during spot detection and gel matching. Moreover, it was suggested that results concerning the magnitude of differential expression between protein spots after statistical analysis by such softwares must be examined with care. The choice of appropriate statistical methods for the analysis of DIGE data should be conducted in several studies. It was reported that the use of normalization methods utilizing local background correction resulted in dye-specific bias during quantification of low-intensity spots and was resolved by implementation of an "offset/scale" normalization method (Melchior et al. 2009). Furthermore, in order to identify statistically significant changes in protein expression, the application of univariate statistical methods, such as the Student's *t*-test, would be inappropriate as these tests do not account for multiple testings and lead to large numbers of false-positive results. This problem could be addressed by the use of statistical methods that apply a false discovery rate (FDR) for the determination of significance. In this method, q-values are calculated for all protein spots. The q-value of each spot corresponds to the expected proportion of false-positives that would be incurred if the change in expression level of that particular protein spot was determined to be significant. Advantages of this approach include ease of use, maintenance of power while being tolerant of between-feature dependency, and option to the researcher to select an appropriate FDR according to study requirements. However, this approach was found to be only applicable to DIGE experiments using a two-dye labeling scheme as a three-dye labeling approach violated the assumption of data independence required for statistical analysis. Other statistical tests that have been applied for the analysis of DIGE results include significance analysis of microarrays, principal components analysis, and partial least squares discriminant analysis.

Proteomic biomarkers isolated from glioblastoma cell line and underlying mechanistic regulation. In our laboratory, we have published on identification of several novel peptides/proteins when we performed a 2D-DIGE experiment with glioblastoma cell line in comparison to healthy astrocytes (Banerjee et al. 2012). Collett et al. reported findings from five glioblastoma patients and identified several novel proteins using this technique. They found 51 protein spots significantly upregulated in GBM samples, and MS identified 22 proteins. The differential expression of a selected protein set was first validated by Western blotting and then tested on large cohorts of GBM specimens and non-tumor tissues, using immunohistochemistry and real-time reverse transcriptase polymerase chain reaction (RT-PCR). Blood proteins emerged as a significant group highlighting the high angiogenesis capacity of GBM. This is emphasized here that GBM tumors are highly vascular tumors, and this study analyzed the proteome of the whole GBM sample extract, without removing the blood vessels (Collet et al. 2011).

In eukaryotic cells, mitochondria and endoplasmic reticulum form two endomembrane networks which interact closely with each other to control metabolic flow, protein transport, intracellular signaling, and cell death. In normal glial cells, besides their essential role of adenosine triphosphate (ATP) generation to produce energy, mitochondria are also involved in the regulation of cellular proliferation and apoptosis. The important consequences of mitochondrial dysfunction in glioma in these three areas were highlighted in a recent study. It is not surprising to find some mitochondrial or endoplasmic reticulum proteins differentially expressed in GBM and in nontumorous samples. Collett et al. reported that 2D-DIGE analysis and immunohistochemistry study revealed two mitochondrial enzymes, aldehyde dehydrogenase (ALDH) and Mn-SOD, which are highly expressed in GBM: on average in a series of 50 GBM samples, 69 % of tumor cells were ALDH positive and 81 % were Mn-SOD (superoxide dismutase) positive. Mn-SOD expression has recently been suggested as a potential GBM prognostic marker because the lack of overexpression is found in 3-year survival group patients compared to short-term survival patients (Dokic et al. 2012). These results confirmed earlier work which correlated shortest median survival with high Mn-SOD enzyme expression level in GBM patients. ALDH is a potential biomarker for neural stem cells and tumor initiator cells (TICs). ALDH could therefore be a good candidate for best TIC enrichment in GBM and an early diagnostic biomarker. Thakkar et al. (2011) used this 2D-DIGE technique as a comprehensive proteomic study to assess the effect of inhibiting two different regulatory mechanisms of telomerase in glioma. RNAi was used to target hTERT and hsp90α genes. Inhibition of telomerase activity resulted in downregulation of various cytoskeletal proteins with correlative evidence of the involvement of telomerase in regulating the expression of vimentin. Inhibition of telomerase via sihTERT resulted in the downregulation of vimentin expression in glioma cell lines in a grade-specific manner. This study identified a novel downstream role of telomerase in regulating the expression of vimentin, thereby affecting tumor progression and metastasis.

Potential Applications to Prognosis, Other Diseases or Conditions

Among other brain cancers, Zanini et al. (2011) reported application of this 2D-DIGE technique to detect different protein profiles in medulloblastoma (MDB) that may be clinically relevant and to check the correspondence of histological classification of MDB with the resulting proteomic profiles. Eighty-six unique proteins were identified and compared to histology by them with the determination of proteins expressed by single histotypes and of a smaller number of proteins shared by two or three histotypes. The sharp difference of protein expression was found to be in agreement with the WHO histological classification, with the identification of type-specific proteins with limited overlapping between histotypes.

Concluding Remarks

High-grade gliomas are the most common brain tumors in adults, and due to difficulties associated with their management, they make the fourth biggest cause of cancer death. Major efforts in neuro-oncology research are needed for this tumor type and more progress in treatment efficacy should be achieved as has been achieved for other cancers in recent years. In addition to the urgent need to identify novel effective drug targets against malignant gliomas, the search for glioma biomarkers and grade-specific protein signatures will provide a much needed contribution to diagnosis, prognosis, treatment decision, and assessment of treatment response. Over the past years glioma proteomics has been attempted at different levels, including proteome analysis of patient biopsies and bodily fluids, glioma cell lines, and animal models. Initial proteomic studies aiming at the identification of biomarkers and molecular targets for glioma were mostly small scale classically stained gel-based approaches. In recent years, more large-scale approaches adopting MS/MS-based proteomics are reported. The aim of the present proteomic review was to highlight potential new glioblastoma tumor antigen identification by the 2D-DIGE technique. This is a very powerful technique which allows controls and experimental samples run together on the same gel with an internal reference, each sample being labeled with a different cyanine. Using the DeCyder software, gel images can be analyzed to identify statistically significant differences in protein expression between different samples on a limited number of gels. This technique is very useful for applications requiring accurate quantization and direct differential proteomic analysis of normal and abnormal tissues. However, no proteomic technique is currently able to reveal the complete human proteome; therefore, the choice of the technique should be guided by the specific research question, and ideally a combination of complementary techniques should be applied. Novel technologies are now starting to be applied to glioma proteomics and will undoubtedly improve the sensitivity, specificity, and reproducibility of the results. It should be kept in mind though that an analysis will only be as good and as relevant as the starting material from which it was derived; therefore, attention should be paid to collect biospecimens. Despite some experimental shortcomings, the 2D-DIGE technique could be an effective tool in proteomic studies to search for novel diagnostic and prognostic biomarkers in the dangerous brain cancer GBM with a very high mortality rate and also other brain tumors described in the review.

Summary Points

- Biomarkers which can detect brain tumors early in their development are needed.
- Progress has been made in identification of potential biomarkers of different brain tumor types although only few have been validated.
- Proteomic biomarkers are superior to other kinds of biomarkers because they represent functional aspects of a gene and most of the drugs are directed toward proteins.
- Epigenetic biomarkers are also promising, and research should be conducted to evaluate specificity and sensitivity of these markers when used in combination with other biomarkers in the same patient.
- 2D-DIGE technique has several advantages (such as ease to use, high sensitivity, detection limit in pictogram range) to identify brain tumor markers.

References

Banerjee HN, Mahaffey K, Riddick E, Banerjee A, Bhowmik N, Patra M. Search for a diagnostic/prognostic biomarker for the brain cancer glioblastoma multiforme by 2D-DIGE-MS technique. Mol Cell Biochem. 2012;367:59–63.

Collet B, Guitton N, Saïkali S, Avril T, Pineau C, Hamlat A, Mosser J, Quillien V. Differential analysis of glioblastoma multiforme proteome by a 2D-DIGE approach. Proteome Sci. 2011;9:5956–9.

Diede SJ. TERT hypermethylation: biomarker in paediatric brain tumors. Lancet Oncol. 2013;14:447–8.

Dokic I, Hartmann C, Herold-Mende C, Régnier-Vigouroux A. Glutathione peroxidase 1 activity dictates the sensitivity of glioblastoma cells to oxidative stress. Glia. 2012;60:1785–800.

Epstein MG, Reeves BD, Matty WS, et al. Enhanced sensitivity employing zwitterionic and pI balancing dyes (Z-CyDyes) optimized for 2-D gel electrophoresis based on side chain modifications of CyDye fluorophores. New tools for use in proteomics and diagnostics. Bioconjug Chem. 2013;24:1552–61.

Kang Y, Techanukul T, Mantalaris A, et al. Comparison of three commercially available DIGE analysis software packages: minimal user intervention in gel-based proteomics. J Proteome Res. 2009;8:1077–84.

Kool M, Korshunoy A, Pfister SM. Update on molecular and genetic alterations in adult medulloblastoma. Memo. 2012;5:228–32.

Lemee JM, Com E, Clavreul A, et al. Proteomic analysis of glioblastomas: what is the best brain control sample? J Proteomics. 2013;85:165–73.

McNight TR, Smith KJ, Chu PW, et al. Choline metabolism, proliferation, and angiogenesis in nonenhancing grades 2 and 3 astrocytoma. J Magn Reson Imaging. 2011;33:808–16.

Melchior K, Tholey A, Heisel S, Keller A, Lenhof HP, Meese E, et al. Proteomic study of human glioblastoma multiforme tissue employing complementary two-dimensional liquid chromatography- and mass spectrometry-based approaches. J Proteome Res. 2009;8:4604–14.

Moskal JR, Kroes RA, Dawson G. The glycobiology of brain tumors: disease relevance and therapeutic potential. Expert Rev Neurother. 2009;9:1529–45.

Pan X, Willim M, Mirbahai L, et al. In vitro metabonomic study detects increases in UDP- GlcNAc and UDP- GalNAc, as early phase markers of cisplatin treatment response in brain tumor cells. J Proteome Res. 2011;10:3493–500.

Thakkar D, Shervington L, Shervington A. Proteomic studies coupled with RNAi methodologies can shed further light on the downstream effects of telomerase in glioma. Cancer Invest. 2011;29:113–22.

Verma M. Epigenetic biomarkers in cancer epidemiology. Methods Mol Biol. 2012;863:467–80.

Verma M, Khoury MJ, Ioannidis JP. Opportunities and challenges for selected emerging technologies in cancer epidemiology: mitochondrial, epigenomic, metabolomic and telomerase profiling. Cancer Epidemiol Biomarkers Prev. 2013;22:189–200.

Wade A, Robinson AE, Engler JR, et al. Proteoglycans and their role in brain cancer. FEBS J. 2013;280:2399–417.

Wei P, Zhang W, Yang LS, et al. Serum GFAP autoantibody as an ELISA-detectable glioma marker. Tumour Biol. 2013;34:2283–92.

Yang S, Nam Y, Kim MO, et al. Computer-aided detection of metastatic brain tumors using magnetic resonance black-blood imaging. Invest Radiol. 2013;48:113–9.

Yurtsever A, Haydaroglu A, Biray-Avci C, et al. Assessment of genetic markers and glioblastoma stem-like cells in activation of dendritic cells. Hum Cell. 2013;26:105–13.

Zanini C, Mandilli G, Pulera F, et al. Analysis of different medulloblastoma histotypes by two-dimensional gel and MALDI-TOF. Childs Nerv Syst. 2011;27:2077–83.

Imaging Biomarkers in Preclinical Studies on Brain Tumors

18

Caroline Chung

Contents

Abstract

There is a growing role for neuroimaging in the multidisciplinary management of brain tumors. Beyond anatomical imaging, additional functional and physiological imaging capabilities introduce the potential to interrogate characteristics of the tumor that can aid in diagnosis, guide treatment decisions, and better evaluate response to treatment in a timely manner. This chapter highlights

C. Chung (✉)
Department of Radiation Oncology, University of Toronto/University Health Network-Princess Margaret Cancer Centre, Toronto, ON, Canada
e-mail: caroline.chung@rmp.uhn.on.ca; caroline.chung.md@gmail.com

V.R. Preedy, V.B. Patel (eds.), *Biomarkers in Cancer, Biomarkers in Disease: Methods, Discoveries and Applications*,
DOI 10.1007/978-94-007-7681-4_46

preclinical investigation that facilitates translation of these promising functional and physiological imaging measures including perfusion and diffusion magnetic resonance imaging (MRI) and molecular and metabolic imaging with positron emission tomography (PET) and spectroscopy.

List of Abbreviations

ADC	Apparent Diffusion Coefficient
AIF	Arterial Input Function
BOLD	Blood Oxygen Level Dependent
CT	Computed Tomography
DCE	Dynamic Contrast Enhanced
DSC	Dynamic Susceptibility Weighted
DTI	Diffusion Tensor Imaging
DWI	Diffusion-Weighted Imaging
GBM	Glioblastoma
GFP	Green Fluorescence Protein
MRI	Magnetic Resonance Imaging
MVD	Microvessel Density
PET	Positron Emitted Tomography
RANO	Response Assessment in Neuro-oncology
rCBV	Relative Cerebral Blood Volume
SPECT	Single-Photon Emission Computed Tomography
SUV	Standard Uptake Value
VEGF	Vascular Endothelial Growth Factor

Key Facts of Glioblastoma (GBM)

- GBM is a malignant primary brain tumor that arises from glial cells in the brain.
- Despite aggressive therapy with surgery, radiation, and temozolomide chemotherapy, GBM remains incurable, and survival with GBM is in the range of 12–18 months for patients who are well enough to tolerate this aggressive combined treatment.
- For patients who are not fit enough for this treatment, single modality treatment with radiation or chemotherapy may be offered. In some patients, supportive care alone may be offered to minimize treatment toxicity and maximize quality of life.
- Further characterization of the tumor based on molecular and genetic profiling presents the potential to personalize treatment.
- Imaging biomarkers have the potential to further guide personalized treatment based on individual responses to novel therapy.
- Particularly with the introduction of newer targeted treatments (e.g., Avastin – a monoclonal antibody to vascular endothelial growth factor (VEGF)), additional imaging studies may help determine whether there is true tumor response or if there is pseudoresponse (i.e., radiological improvement in conventional imaging studies that do not reflect underlying pathological response)

- Animal models allow for efficient investigation of novel treatments and imaging biomarkers so that only the most promising treatments and biomarkers are investigated in clinical trials.

Definitions of Words and Terms

Angiogenesis Formation of new blood vessels form from preexisting vessels.

Apparent Diffusion Coefficient (ADC) Magnitude of diffusion (of water molecules) within tissue.

Arterial Input Function (AIF) Representative flow of contrast agent within the representative vessel perfusing the tumor used to calculate perfusion parameters in dynamic perfusion imaging.

Fractional Anisotropy (FA) Scalar value between zero and one that describes the degree of anisotropy (directional dependence) of a diffusion process.

K^{trans} The rate constant of the movement of the contrast agent from the intravascular space to the extravascular space.

Multiparametric Use of multiple parameters (measurements); often used in terms of imaging studies with multiple quantitative measurements.

Orthotopic Graft of tissue in its natural environment (e.g., glioma tumor implanted intracranially).

Relative Cerebral Blood Volume (rCBV) Cerebral blood volume in a region of interest relative to normal brain (typically contralateral white matter).

Standard Uptake Value (SUV) Ratio of tissue radioactivity concentration and the injected activity over the body weight.

Vascular Endothelial Growth Factor (VEGF) A signaling protein that stimulates vasculogenesis and angiogenesis.

Xenograft A tissue graft from a donor of a different species from the recipient.

Introduction

There is growing multidisciplinary involvement in the management of all brain tumors, an increasing role of neuroimaging to guide the management of brain tumors by providing information that aids diagnosis, treatment, and evaluation of treatment response. Advances in multimodal neuroimaging capabilities have introduced the potential to develop novel tools to interrogate changes in the structure and physiology of both the tumor and its microenvironment in response to treatments that may serve as biomarkers to guide optimal coordination of multidisciplinary care.

Surgery is a core component in the diagnosis and treatment of brain tumors. Advances in intraoperative imaging, functional imaging, and neuronavigation have improved the ability to achieve more complete resections and to minimize surgical morbidity. These imaging tools not only help to characterize the tumor tissue but also provide information regarding the surrounding brain tissue. For example, diffusion tensor imaging can help delineate fiber tracks from the motor cortex such that surgeons can avoid disrupting these pathways thereby minimizing morbidity after resection.

Radiotherapy is a mainstay treatment of brain tumors, either in conjunction with surgery or as the primary treatment. With technological advances in treatment planning software and radiation delivery platforms, radiation can be delivered with incredible precision. In order to maximally benefit from high-precision radiotherapy, accurate delineation of the treatment target is critical. This relies on high-quality imaging and image interpretation with an understanding of what the imaging features represent, particularly when multiparametric imaging is utilized for radiotherapy planning.

To date, the evaluation of brain tumors has largely been based on anatomical imaging, and radiological response to treatments has been based on reduction in tumor size. For example, standard response criteria including the McDonald criteria and Response Assessment in Neuro-oncology (RANO) criteria have utilized two-dimensional tumor measurements, either on CT or MRI. The introduction of additional neuroimaging techniques including multiparametric MRI and molecular imaging with various PET tracers has added a new layer of complexity that comes with greater capability to interrogate the tumor in order to noninvasively characterize functional and metabolic features, cell density ,and vasculature and appreciate heterogeneity within the tumor (Yamasaki et al. 2010; Lemasson et al. 2011). These novel techniques not only help provide additional detail in the radiological characterization of brain tumors, there are also growing studies investigating the association of these radiological features with underlying pathophysiological changes in the tumor. This relationship allows these imaging features to serve as useful imaging biomarkers that may be prognostic and/or predictive for multimodal treatments such that they can help guide personalized therapy for brain tumors (Dhermain et al. 2010a, b).

Just as in vitro studies are often used to screen tumor cell line sensitivity to particular systemic agents, preclinical investigation of imaging biomarkers helps identify the most promising imaging measures and guides the application of these measures in the clinical setting. In particular, preclinical studies help overcome the limitations of clinical trials including the ability to acquire serial tissue samples to correlate imaging changes to tumor pathophysiology. This is particularly helpful in the brain tumor research, where repeated biopsies are less feasible in the clinical

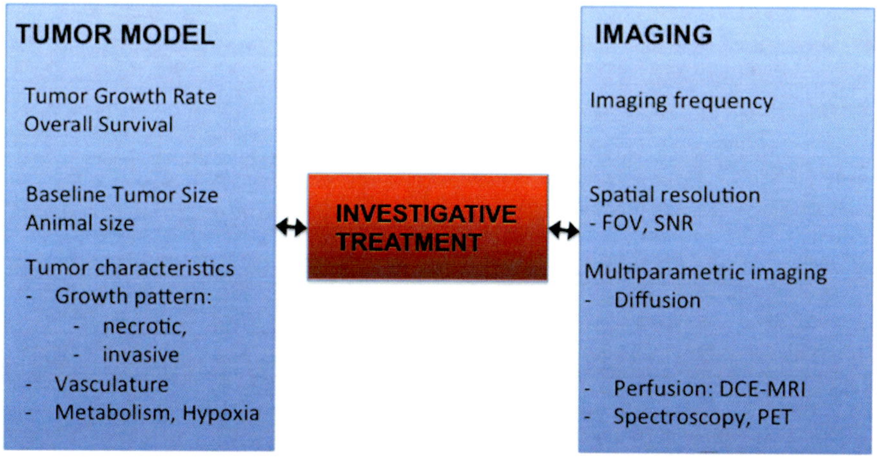

Fig. 1 Schematic diagram summarizing factors to be considered in preclinical imaging biomarker studies. *FOV* field of view, *SNR* signal-to-noise ratio, *DCE-MRI* dynamic contrast-enhanced magnetic resonance imaging, *PET* positron emission tomography

setting compared to other cancer sites. This chapter highlights how animal tumor models provide the platform to investigate imaging biomarkers of response to therapy, including changes in the tumor vasculature, metabolism, and microenvironment (Fig. 1).

Brain Tumor Models for Imaging Biomarker Discovery

The translational value of preclinical research relies on the overall preclinical study design, including the choice of the tumor model. Significant work has been focused on developing effective animal models for high-grade glioma, the most common primary malignant brain tumors in adults. Table 1 summarizes a list of recommended criteria provided by a recent expert review on valid brain tumor models for the investigation of new anticancer agents.

The two main types of mouse brain tumor models are endogenous (or spontaneous) and exogenous (or xenograft). Spontaneous tumor models tend to better recapitulate the biological behavior of human brain tumors with representative interaction between the tumor and the brain microenvironment. But spontaneous tumors tend to develop in variable locations in the brain and can even develop at multiple foci in single animals, which raises challenges for investigation of localized therapies such as radiation or surgery.

Xenograft tumor models tend to develop single tumors that can be grown subcutaneously or orthotopically in the original host organ. Evidence supports that orthotopic solid tumor models have greater similarity in histopathological features and gene expression profiles to human tumors and reflect clinical tumor behavior better than their subcutaneous counterparts, even when the same cell lines

Table 1 Recommended criteria for a valid brain tumor model for the investigation of new anticancer agents (Aldape et al. 2006)

Tumor development
Derived from glial cells and grow as a stable cell line
Able to propagate in vivo by serial transplantation
Tumor growth
Does not extend beyond the brain
Have a predictable and reproducible tumor growth rate that allows for adequate assessment of treatment effect
Tumor behavior
Have a predictable and reproducible tumor take and growth rate that allows for adequate assessment of treatment effect
Have a response to conventional treatment that is predictive of the behavior of the human counterpart

are used (Camphausen et al. 2005a). This greater resemblance in orthotopic models is thought to be due to factors in the microenvironment that influence gene expression as the tumor develops and even in response to treatment such as radiation (Camphausen et al. 2005a, b).

More recently, transplantable models derived from genetically engineered mouse models have been developed to have high penetrance and predictable tumor growth while maintaining the histological, molecular, and genetic features of human brain tumors. These transplantable models have introduced promising tools for preclinical investigation of new therapies and corresponding biomarkers (Smilowitz et al. 2007).

Without the aid of improved imaging tools, a major limitation of intracranial tumor models compared to subcutaneous models is the inability to easily and noninvasively measure tumor size. Advances in various imaging modalities have been introduced to assist and improve murine brain tumor model investigation including optical imaging with bioluminescence, fluorescence and near-infrared optical imaging, CT, multiparametric MRI, SPECT, and PET (Lyons 2005).

Despite the central role of surgical resection in the management of brain tumors, most animal models fail to incorporate tumor resection (Fomchenko and Holland 2006; Jacobs et al. 2011). Clinically, additional tools have improved intraoperative image guidance to achieve better tumor resections while minimizing functional loss, which has improved outcomes in brain tumor patients (Krammer and Plaetzer 2008; Stummer et al. 2006). To better simulate the current clinical scenario and provide greater translational value from preclinical studies, preclinical model platforms that incorporate surgical resection into the treatment paradigm for the investigation of novel GBM therapies in murine brain tumor models have been developed (Akbar et al. 2009; Kauer et al. 2012; Bello et al. 2002). These surgical models have incorporated optical and MRI image guidance, as in clinical cases, for tumor resection followed by postoperative noninvasive imaging to monitor for tumor recurrence (Kauer et al. 2012). These surgical models have also used intraoperative GFP fluorescence to allow for better visualization of the borders of the tumor and this approach as demonstrated better surgical removal, achieving greater than 90 % resection of GBM tumors, similar to the advantages reported from using ALA in the clinical setting (Kauer et al. 2012).

The introduction of these models not only help investigate the impact of greater surgical debulking on survival with brain tumors, it facilitates investigation of multimodal therapy. For example, preclinical investigation of the optimal sequence or combinations of multimodal therapy approaches would allow us to invest and translate only the most promising regimens for clinical trial investigation (Hess 1999; Metcalfe and Grant 2001). Several preclinical studies using these models have reported investigation of novel approaches for postoperative therapy in gliomas including the use of a biodegradable gel matrix for local temozolomide delivery in the tumor bed and implantation of encapsulated therapeutic stem cells in the tumor resection cavity (Akbar et al. 2009; Kauer et al. 2012).

Ongoing challenges of translating the findings of preclinical research using brain tumor models to the clinical setting include the variability in the particular animal models used, treatment dose and timing variations, and differences in the route of drug administration and potential biases with non-blinded outcomes assessment, which can overestimate the efficacy of new treatments (Amarasingh et al. 2009). Imaging biomarkers may facilitate a bridge between findings from various tumor models and patient studies in order to improve the translational value of brain tumor model research.

Role of Imaging Biomarkers in Preclinical Studies

Neuroimaging is an ideal translational bridge from preclinical to clinical research because a number of imaging modalities have been investigated both clinically and preclinically, including CT, multiparametric MRI (DCE, DSC, DWI, DTI, spectroscopy), PET, and SPECT. In the preclinical setting, optical imaging in conjunction with bioluminescence, fluorescence, and near-infrared optical imaging has also been investigated as measures of noninvasively monitoring tumor growth longitudinally.

MRI

Clinically, MRI is the most commonly used imaging modality utilized to evaluate brain tumors as it provides the best-detailed soft-tissue neuroanatomic imaging. It also offers the capability of acquiring multiparametric imaging including DWI, DCE, DSC, BOLD, and MR spectroscopy to evaluate tumor cell density, tumor metabolism, vascularity and vascular physiology, and tissue oxygenation.

There have been promising studies demonstrating the role of MRI to serially monitor tumor growth and evaluate changes in tumor characteristics over time (Bock et al. 2003, 2005; Dazai et al. 2004; Chung et al. 2013; Jalali et al. 2014). A challenge of longitudinal MRI studies in murine models can be the length of time required for each MRI study, which can limit the number of mice than can be followed concurrently. Groups have demonstrated the feasibility of multiple-mouse imaging techniques in order to facilitate larger preclinical imaging studies (Bock et al. 2003, 2005). In particular, multiple-mouse imaging techniques allow for efficient screening for tumor development in intracranial xenograft models. But single-mouse acquisitions with high-field MRI have generally produced higher-quality images (Cha et al. 2003; Nelson et al. 2003). More recently, Bock et al. demonstrated a multiple-mouse technique in a high-field multiple-mouse MRI system that produced similar high-quality images while achieving a much higher throughput for screening intracranial tumor models using weekly high-resolution 3D whole brain T2- and T1-weighting MR image acquisition. With the assistance of new software packages that assist in co-registration, image segmentation, and automated image analysis for multiple-mouse MRI, large preclinical studies that utilize high-resolution anatomical imaging are now feasible (Hingtgen et al. 2013). Multiparametric MRI studies that evaluate additional tumor characteristics including vascular perfusion and permeability, tissue density, and metabolism generally remain limited to single-mouse MRI.

Anatomical MRI

A major strength of preclinical MR imaging studies is the ease of acquiring postmortem high-resolution MR images. In the postmortem setting, long scan times are less of a concern, and any motion associated with respiration and cardiac pulse is eliminated. Preclinical studies have used postmortem images to correlate with pathology and gather in situ phenotypic information, also referred to as "MR histology" (Nieman et al. 2005). The Visible Mouse Project demonstrated the ability to acquire FSE T2-weighted images with a 100-μm isotropic resolution with a scan time of fewer than 3 h, which could be compared to the matched histological slides as shown in Fig. 2 (Johnson et al. 2002).

Correlations of MR imaging features with immunohistopathological features are valuable for providing a basis of interpreting subsequent serial imaging studies. Radaelli et al. characterized the MR imaging features of two commonly used xenograft tumors, U87MG and U251 (Radaelli et al. 2009). In this study, Radaelli described U251 tumors to have ill-defined infiltrative margins, necrosis, and peritumoral edema, resembling the human counterpart. In contrast, U87MG tumors were generally round, well-demarcated tumors that morphologically resembled brain metastases rather than primary high-grade glioma. In addition, it was noted that the U87MG tumors had strong gadolinium enhancement that correlated to intense neoangiogenesis, thereby identifying this tumor model as a potentially useful tool for evaluating response to anti-angiogenic agents.

For intracranial tumor models, anatomical MRI is often used to screen for tumor development, particularly if an efficient process such as multimouse MRI screening is available. As there can be variability in baseline tumor size, some studies have started treatment only once tumors reached a specific size. The alternative approach

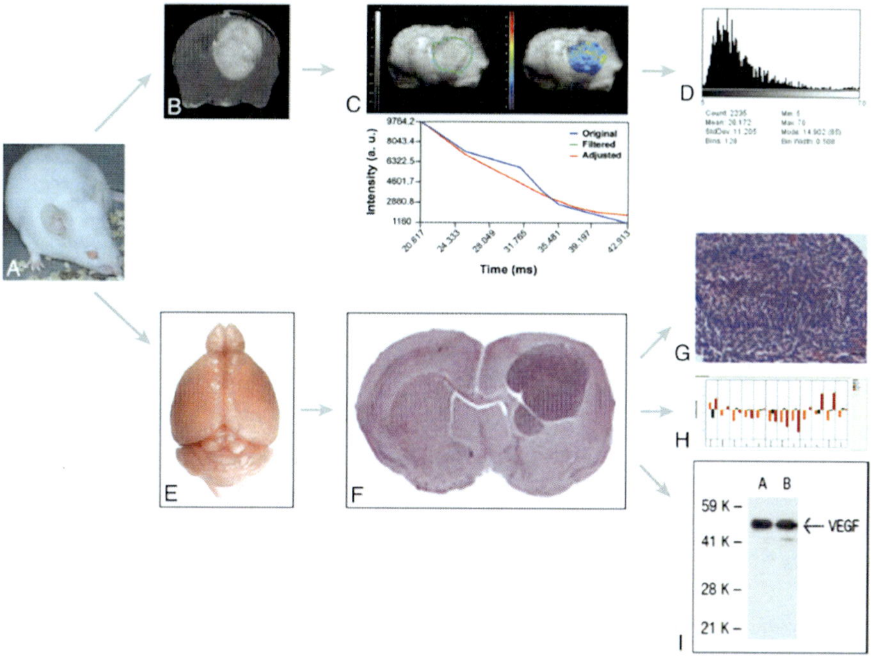

Fig. 2 Representative images of mouse magnetic resonance imaging, histology and genomic information (With permission from A. Borges and AJNR) (Borges et al. 2012)

could be to stratify mice to treatment arms based on tumor size in order to avoid biases in the results due to imbalance in baseline tumor size.

Perfusion MRI

Specific MRI acquisition parameters can be used to further characterize tumor vascular physiology and angiogenesis. As increased angiogenesis is a feature of more aggressive tumors in the brain, perfusion MRI has the potential to serve as a prognostic factor. In terms of treatment, with the introduction of anti-angiogenic therapy in the treatment of cancer including brain tumors, perfusion imaging has been investigated as promising biomarkers that predict treatment response.

Dynamic Contrast-Enhanced MRI

Dynamic contrast-enhanced MRI helps characterize the leakage of contrast across tumor vasculature, which reflects the functional and architectural changes that can occur with tumor-associated angiogenesis and vasculogenesis. It generally involves injection of a small molecular weight contrast agent that extravasates into the extracellular and extravascular spaces when the blood-brain barrier is disrupted around tumor and image acquisition at a high temporal resolution (Li et al. 2010).

Analysis of the DCE-MRI data requires the use of a model, typically an established equilibrium exchange model that can estimate vascular permeability into and out of the extravascular space as well as tumor blood volume (Li et al. 2010). These estimated measures rely on several factors including the choice of the exchange model that is used and the additional variables that are included in these models such as arterial input function (AIF). For example, the use of a population value for AIF versus individual measurement for AIF can potentially impact the kinetic parameters derived from the exchanges model both in the preclinical and clinical setting (Li et al. 2011). Additionally, the nature of the contrast agent can be associated with different kinetics in terms of tumor uptake and clearance (Adzamli et al. 2003). Therefore, interpretation of these findings can be challenging across preclinical studies, across clinical studies, and for translation from preclinical to clinical studies.

Preclinical studies have demonstrated correlation between maximum vascular permeability measured using DCE-MRI and Evans blue extravasation in murine xenograft models of glioblastoma, suggesting it to be a useful noninvasive measure of vascular permeability (Cha et al. 2003). Particularly in the preclinical setting when very small tumors are under investigation, it is important to note that tumors typically reach their limits of oxygen and nutrient diffusion by 1–2 mm^3 in volume beyond which angiogenesis is initiated to allow for further tumor growth (Jain et al. 2007). Veeravagu et al. has described a temporal correlation between DCE-MRI changes and histological changes with increasing microvessel density (MVD) and genetic expression of VEGF and angiotensin 1 and 2, consistent with angiogenesis in a murine GL261 C57Bl/6 orthotopic xenograft glioblastoma model (Veeravagu et al. 2008). These findings suggest a temporal relationship between tumor growth and angiogenesis and that perhaps imaging biomarkers could help guide the optimal timing of introducing anti-angiogenic agents, which in the preclinical setting could be further investigated with correlative histology.

Many investigators have focused on measuring relative differences in DCE-MRI parameters, such as K^{trans} and iAUC, while using a standardized approach for image acquisition and analysis in order to account for variability in the imaging conditions and to better compare measurements across treatment groups or over time from pretreatment baseline to posttreatment (Chung et al. 2013). Using this approach, a number of studies in murine brain tumor models have demonstrated changes in iAUC, K^{trans}, and rCBV following treatment with anti-angiogenic, anti-VEGF, and anti-vascular therapies, both as monotherapy and in combination with radiation and other cytotoxic chemotherapeutic agents (Chung et al. 2013; Sun et al. 2004).

In general, anti-angiogenic agents that target vascular endothelial growth factor (VEGF) cause a reduction in K^{trans} and iAUC, which is consistent with the expected decrease in vascular permeability with these agents (Bradley et al. 2009; Hillman et al. 2009; O'Connor et al. 2008; Sorensen et al. 2009). In contrast, K_{ep}, which reflects the efflux of the contrast agent from the tumor tissue back into the vasculature, has been variable even when other measures of vascular response to anti-angiogenic agents were observed (Zwick et al. 2009). This may be due to the dependence of K_{ep} on both K^{trans} and v_e (the volume of extravascular extracellular space per unit volume of tissue) (Tofts et al. 1999).

Table 2 Studies of perfusion imaging biomarker dynamics in response to anti-angiogenic agents in intracranial animal models of brain tumors

Study	Model	Agent	Finding
Hoff et al. (2012)	9L glioma cell line, intracranial, rats	VEGF-Trap	Decrease in K^{trans}, K_{ep}, and V_p
Muldoon et al. (2011)	UW28 glioma, LX-1 small cell lung carcinoma, MDA-MB231BR-HER2 breast carcinoma cell lines, intracranial, athymic nude rats	Intetumumab (monoclonal antibody targeting α_v-integrins)	Intetumumab increased permeability
		Bevacizumab (monoclonal antibody targeting VEGF)	Bevacizumab decreased permeability
			Control tumors had no significant change in permeability
Bradley et al. (2009)	C6 glioma, intracranial, rats	Cediranib (tyrosine kinase inhibitor targeting	Decrease in K^{trans} and iAUC
Chung et al. (2013)	U87 glioma, intracranial, NOD/SCID mice	Sunitinib Radiation	Temporary decrease in K^{trans} with sunitinib alone, sustained decrease in K^{trans} with sunitinib + radiation
Jalali et al. (2014)	U87 glioma, intracranial, NOD/SCID mice	Sunitinib VEGF-Trap B20 (murine monoclonal antibody to VEGF, murine equivalent to bevacizumab)	Complete loss of enhancement with VEGF-Trap and B20 resulting in inability to measure DCE parameters, reduction in K^{trans} with sunitinib

VEGF vascular endothelial growth factor, iAUC initial area under the curve

Following radiation therapy to brain tumors, short-term rises in K^{trans} have been reported as early as within the first 3 days, which may reflect acute breakdown of the blood-brain barrier with ionizing radiation exposure (Chung et al. 2013). These studies have also demonstrated long-term decreases in K^{trans} after the short-term rise in K^{trans} following radiation. The temporary acute rise in K^{trans}, reflecting a temporary increase in vascular permeability, may be due to an inflammatory reaction, acute endothelial cell apoptosis, and increased expression of pro-angiogenic cytokines in response to radiation. The resolution of this acute rise and subsequent fall in K^{trans} may reflect reduction in microvasculature from loss of endothelial cells, which has been described in previous reports that have reported reductions in microvessel density and microvascular perfusion following radiotherapy (de Lussanet et al. 2005).

Table 2 highlights a number of preclinical studies investigating a range of various anti-angiogenic compounds administered as monotherapy and in combination with radiation for which DCE-MRI measures were followed serially. It is apparent that there can be variability in permeability and perfusion changes in response to different anti-angiogenic agents, even with similar presumed mechanisms and molecular targets. A number of additional factors can contribute to variability in DCE-MRI results including the particular tumor model used for experimentation, the specific contrast agent used, the volume and injection speed for contrast administration, the MRI acquisition parameters (temporal and spatial resolution), the model used for data analysis and assumptions made in the model as well as the timing of treatment relative to tumor volume, and the overall physiology of the animal.

Dynamic Susceptibility-Weighted MRI

Dynamic susceptibility-weighted contrast-enhanced MRI (DSC-MRI or perfusion-weighted imaging) is typically used to assess tumor relative cerebral blood volume (rCBV). High rCBV is thought to indicate neovascularization and therefore suggest the presence of viable tumor (Russell et al. 2009; Law et al. 2008). This measurement has shown potential as an imaging biomarker of response to therapy in human glioblastoma and has also been shown to help differentiate tumor progression from pseudoprogression in glioblastoma (Hu et al. 2009; Gahramanov et al. 2011). In order to improve the accuracy of DSC-MRI, a blood-pool contrast agent such as ferumoxytol iron oxide nanoparticles has been used to minimize leakage artifacts (Gahramanov et al. 2011; Varallyay et al. 2009).

Using DSC-MRI, preclinical studies have demonstrated a correlation between rCBV and specific histopathological features including the MVD and CD31 staining in glioma xenograft models (Cha et al. 2003). In general, rCBV is elevated relative to normal brain tissue at all stages of tumor progression, and heterogeneity in rCBV is observed within the tumor. As tumors develop and grow, the rCBV in the tumor periphery is generally higher than in the center, and this has been attributed to increased vessel co-option and dilation at the tumor margins early in tumor development and angiogenesis at the tumor margins with central necrosis later in tumor development (Cha et al. 2003).

Various anti-angiogenic agents have been evaluated using DSC. Bevacizumab, a monoclonal antibody to vascular endothelial growth factor (VEGF), has been shown to dramatically reduce blood volume and vascular permeability within a short time frame of drug administration in multiple preclinical and clinical studies (Jalali et al. 2014; Varallyay et al. 2009). This has been associated with rapid improvement in symptoms in patients but has not translated to improvement in survival in glioblastoma patients (Chinot et al. 2014; Gilbert et al. 2014).

Diffusion MRI

Diffusion-Weighted MRI

Diffusion-weighted imaging (DWI) measures the Brownian motion of molecules, predominantly water in human tissue, which reflects the underlying tissue structure (Ross et al. 2003). In a tumor, water diffusion can be heterogeneous due to the presence of tumor necrosis and apoptosis resulting in areas of variable cellular density. The primary measure of DWI is the apparent diffusion coefficient (ADC), which is sensitive to changes in cellular size, extracellular volume, membrane permeability, and stromal changes (Ross et al. 2003; Hamstra et al. 2008; Woodfield et al. 2010). A recent clinical study compared histology from precise stereotactic biopsies of human gliomas with ADC and found that cell density in gliomas were strongly inversely correlated with ADC, $R^2 = 0.7933$ ($p < 0.0001$). This has led to the concept of "cellularity maps" using ADC to noninvasively estimate cellular proliferation in human gliomas (Ellingson et al. 2010).

Therefore, changes in ADC following treatment have been attributed to changes in cellular density and appear to be a promising biomarker of treatment response. In preclinical studies, rises in ADC have been associated with positive tumor response to a range of anticancer therapies (Ross et al. 2003; Hamstra et al. 2008; Chenevert et al. 1997, 2000; Roth et al. 2004), and even dose-dependent changes in ADC have been observed for specific systemic agents (Chenevert et al. 2000; Jennings et al. 2002; Zhao et al. 1996). Following cytotoxic treatment, the increase in water diffusion, which has been consistently observed in tumors, likely reflects processes such as increased cellular apoptosis and death. Other measures reflecting changes in extracellular water content, including changes in tumor T1 and T2, have been observed following cytotoxic treatment, but ADC appears to be the most sensitive measure of cytotoxic therapy response (Chenevert et al. 2000).

Very early changes in mean ADC were observed in preclinical studies of murine brain tumor models treated with both radiation and sunitinib (Chung et al. 2013). Larocque et al. investigated rising doses of radiation and found a strong correlation between an early rise in ADC and subsequent tumor growth rate (Larocque et al. 2009). A subsequent study of radiation with or without sunitinib in a murine glioblastoma model confirmed the same correlation between rise in ADC and subsequent tumor growth rate in various treatment groups but also in individual mice (Chung et al. 2013) (Fig. 3). With higher-resolution DWI and particularly for larger tumors, the use of ADC maps and histograms provide additional information about the spatial heterogeneity of ADC and measure the regional differences in treatment response (Moffat et al. 2004). Shifts in the ADC histogram to higher values have also indicated positive responses to treatment, whereas shifts to lower ADC values have been associated with negative responses.

Diffusion Tensor Imaging

Diffusion tensor imaging (DTI) is an MR acquisition that provides information about the microstructures of ordered biological tissues in terms of total magnitude of diffusion tensor (L) as well as the isotropic (p) and anisotropic (q) components. It has shown significant benefit clinically by providing information about the relationship between brain tumors and the surrounding white matter tracts to guide neurosurgical resections in order to maximize the functional status of patients postoperatively (Vassal et al. 2014). Both in clinical and preclinical studies, it has

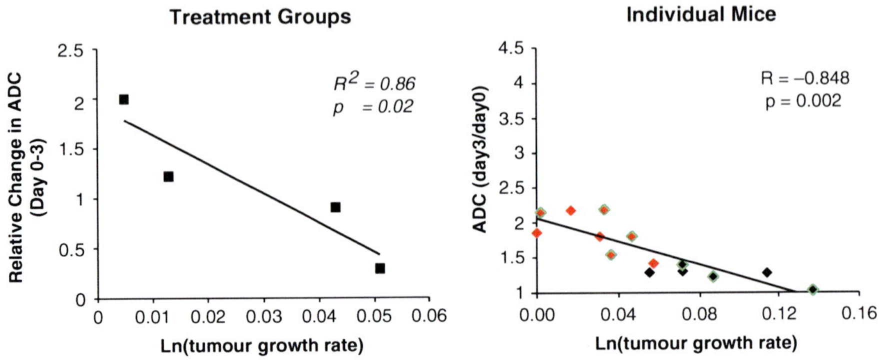

Fig. 3 Correlation between early rise in ADC at day 3 of treatment and tumor growth rate. A moderately strong correlation was observed both for treatment groups (*left*) and individual mice (*right*) treated with radiation, sunitinib, radiation + sunitinib, and placebo (control) (Chung et al. 2013)

also been demonstrated that DTI can detect invasion of cells into the adjacent brain tissue beyond the margins demonstrated on conventional imaging thereby raising the potential to guide more extensive tumor resections (Wang et al. 2013).

In addition to distinguishing tumor margins from surrounding normal brain, early clinical and preclinical studies have shown the there are significant differences in anisotropy within subregions of the tumor that reflect areas of greater cellular density and necrosis as well as in areas of tumor that are higher in grade (Wang et al. 2013; Smitha et al. 2013). In a preclinical study evaluating three murine glioblastoma tumor models, the solid portions of tumor were found to have higher degrees of anisotropy compared to the necrotic regions, and this was histologically confirmed with demonstration of well-organized tumor cells at the tumor rims, which formed circular patterns in the 9L and F98 tumors and a radial pattern in GBM22 tumors. This raises the potential for using DTI as an imaging biomarker within the pretreatment setting to noninvasively determine the tumor grade to guide overall management and identify subregions of tumor to guide potential local therapies. Following radiation therapy, a growing challenge is distinguishing acute radiation-related radiological changes on conventional MRI, and DTI has shown the potential differentiate early toxicity from radiation treatment from tumor progression in the murine glioma models (Wang et al. 2013; Haris et al. 2008).

Molecular Imaging

The development of novel targeted anticancer agents demands parallel advances in methods to rapidly assess their therapeutic efficacy. Small-animal PET has been used to evaluate the use of ^{18}F-fluoro-deoxy-D-glucose (FDG) radiotracer to predict the therapeutic efficacy of a number of anticancer agents in rat glioma models. Assadian et al. detected differences in early FDG-PET response as early as 3 days following treatment using relative changes in standardized uptake value (SUV) over the course of treatment. In this study, SUV values significantly decreased in tumors treated with a hypoxia-inducible factor-1a inhibitor, YC-1, compared with control tumors, whereas no significant SUV change was noted following a proapoptotic agent NS1619, the combination of YC-1 and NS1619, or temozolomide. This difference in early FDG-PET response was consistent with greater tumor volume decreases in this arm compared to the control arm and significantly lower levels of glucose transporter-1 (GLUT-1) expression in the YC-1–treated tumors on immunohistochemistry. This study suggested that FDG-PET could help determine the therapeutic efficacy of novel agents at an early time point following treatment administration in a preclinical glioma model (Assadian et al. 2008). Subsequently, a study of BCNU and BCNU + dexamethasone in 9L gliosarcoma tumors in rats reported that treatment-associated inflammation in response to tumor therapy may result in an increase in tumor FDG uptake associated with histological presence of glucose-consuming activated macrophages and that this inflammatory response should be considered when interpreting FDG-PET biomarker results (Galban et al. 2010).

Beyond FDG, a number of additional promising radiotracers are under investigation for PET in neuro-oncology (Table 3). These include ^{18}F-fluoro-L-thymidinem (FLT) and ^{11}C-methylmethionine as markers of increased transport and proliferation in brain tumors, fluorine-labeled misonidazole to investigate hypoxia, and annexin V to image apoptosis, respectively (Dhermain et al. 2010a; Jacobs et al. 2002a, b, 2005; Wester 2007). Novel tracers under early investigation include ^{11}C-radiolabeled antisense oligonucleotide to visualize glial fibrillary acidic protein messenger ribonucleic acid expression, ^{123}I-VEGF to visualize VEGF receptor, and O-(2-[^{18}F]fluoroethyl)-L-tyrosine and/or methyl-[^{11}C]-L-methionine to visualize amino acid metabolism (Jacobs et al. 2002a; Derlon et al. 2000; Hutterer et al. 2011).

Table 3 Positron emission tomography (PET) radiotracers under preclinical investigation in brain tumors (Dhermain et al. 2010a; Jacobs et al. 2002a, b, 2005; Wester 2007; Derlon et al. 2000; Hutterer et al. 2011)

Radiotracer	Functional investigation
18F-fluorodeoxyglucose	Glucose metabolism
18F-fluoro-L-thymidine (FLT)	Transport and proliferation in brain tumors Amino acid metabolism
11C-methlymethionine (C-MET)	Transport and proliferation in brain tumors Amino acid metabolism
18F-misonidazole (F-MISO)	Hypoxia
18F-FAZA	Hypoxia
18F-labeled annexin V	Apoptosis
11C-radiolabeled antisense oligonucleotide	Glial fibrillary acidic protein messenger ribonucleic acid (mRNA) expression

Several preclinical studies have shown that ^{18}F-FLT-PET may be a useful early biomarker of treatment response. In particular, in both subcutaneous and intracranial murine glioma models of temozolomide-sensitive glioblastoma tumors, [^{18}F] FLT-PET was able to detect a significant difference in tumor/brain ratio for tumors treated with temozolomide or DMSO (control) as early as day 2 of treatment (subcutaneous model $p = 0.01$; intracranial model $p = 0.01$) (Viel et al. 2013). When FLT was compared with FDG in intracranial glioma models using U87 and U251 tumors treated with temozolomide and/or bevacizumab, FDG was less predictive for treatment efficacy than was FLT in both tumor models ($p < 0.001$) (Corroyer-Dulmont et al. 2013).

Tumor hypoxia has been associated with more aggressive tumor behavior including increased invasion, proliferation, migration, angiogenesis, and resistance to treatment. Both MRI and molecular imaging have been investigated to noninvasively measure tumor oxygenation prior to treatment and serially over the course of treatment. To date, the most promising single imaging measure for hypoxia in the brain appears to be PET imaging by using the ^{18}F-labeled misonidazole radiotracer (Pacheco-Torres et al. 2011). However, multimodal and multiparametric imaging investigating the vascular physiology and metabolic features of the tumor associated with the presence of hypoxia may serve as a stronger biomarker in terms of predictability for therapeutic efficacy but also to guide ongoing treatment, as this multimodal approach will provide a better understanding of the tumor microenvironment.

Beyond the use of specific radiotracers, particularly when a vascular-targeted agent is under investigation, dynamic uptake of the tracer can be evaluated to obtain measures of vascular permeability (Corroyer-Dulmont et al. 2013). Additionally, a number of studies have incorporated multimodal, multiparametric imaging to acquire multiple imaging biomarker measures within the same tumors in order to improve efficiency of biomarker investigation, to compare the capabilities of each modality, and to investigate the added benefit of using a composite measure that incorporates measures from the various imaging studies. For example, in the preclinical study comparing FDG and FLT radiotracers, additional imaging measures including anatomical, diffusion, and perfusion MRI parameters were collected as response biomarkers to temozolomide and/or bevacizumab, and although FLT was a sensitive predictor of treatment efficacy, the predictability was enhanced through a combination of these imaging biomarkers (Corroyer-Dulmont et al. 2013).

Metabolic Imaging

Tumor metabolomics introduces a novel, promising area of imaging biomarkers. Tumor metabolism can be measured in vivo using MR spectroscopy or ex vivo in tissue samples using mass spectrometry. The benefit of spectroscopy is that it can be done in vivo, and for this reason, it provides additional spatial information with the potential to generate a metabolic map of the entire tumor, which can be repeated to evaluate serial changes over time. Using both MR spectroscopy and mass spectrometry, Griffin et al. have profiled metabolites in animal models of brain tumors and have found good correlation between specific metabolic imaging phenotypes and specific tumor type, proliferation index, metabolic activity, and cell death (Griffin and Kauppinen 2007).

Currently, the use of 1H, 31P, and 13C MR spectroscopy allows imaging of a wide range of metabolites that belong to different classes of compounds, reflecting various cellular processes including tumor metabolism and cell death. For example, 13C spectra estimates glycolytic and oxidative metabolism. Metabolic profiling of lipids by 1H-MRspectroscopy can discriminate cell death mechanisms with the presence of saturated lipids indicating cell death by necrosis and presence of polyunsaturated fatty acids indicating apoptosis.

Potential Applications to Prognosis, Other Diseases, or Conditions

Novel imaging biomarkers can help better characterize brain tumors to guide initial therapy and allow early evaluation of therapeutic response, rather than waiting for traditional therapeutic endpoints. This can enable adaptive therapeutic approaches with timely secondary interventions to improve tumor control outcomes and minimize treatment-related morbidities from pursuing inefficient therapies. Preclinical investigation of imaging biomarkers facilitates an efficient approach to identify promising predictive or prognostic parameters and to identify optimal combinations of multimodal imaging biomarker measures prior to clinical translation. In addition, preclinical investigation allows for histopathological correlation that can be particularly challenging in brain tumors, where the tumor is not readily accessible for serial biopsies.

Ongoing Challenges

There are a number of ongoing challenges in the discovery of imaging biomarkers in the preclinical setting and subsequent translation of these imaging biomarkers to the clinical setting. A number of factors can impact the findings of imaging biomarker studies. These include the acquisition parameters, such as spatial resolution, temporal resolution for dynamic studies, and field of view as well as the data analysis approach utilized. In the preclinical setting, additional factors including the particular choice of animal and tumor model can further impact the findings. Finally, the overall study design including the specicfic treatment parameters such as treatment doses and schedules and the relative timing of imaging biomarker measurement can all impact the results and interpretation of the findings (Nieman et al. 2005).

Summary Points

- In order to maximize the translational value of preclinical research, the overall preclinical study design, including choice of the tumor model, should be considered carefully.
- High-field multiple-mouse MRI systems have introduced a method for high-throughput screening and anatomical monitoring of intracranial tumor models
- Preclinical studies have correlated tumor vascular features such as microvessel density with perfusion imaging parameters including K^{trans} and relative cerebral blood volume (rCBV), which appear to be promising biomarkers of response to anti-angiogenic therapy.
- Preclinical and clinical data support the correlation of diffusion imaging measures (apparent diffusion coefficient (ADC), anisotropy) with cellular density, and changes in these measures may reflect early response to therapy.
- Molecular and metabolic imaging approaches to interrogate tumor metabolism, hypoxia, and cell death have shown promising histological correlation in preclinical studies.
- The use of multimodal imaging information appears to be most predictive for therapeutic efficacy, and a composite measure may serve as a stronger imaging biomarker.

References

Adzamli K, Yablonskiy DA, Chicoine MR, Won EK, Galen KP, Zahner MC, et al. Albumin-binding MR blood pool agents as MRI contrast agents in an intracranial mouse glioma model. Magnet Reson Med Off J Soc Magnet Reson Med/Soc Magnet Reson Med. 2003;49(3):586–90. PubMed PMID: 12594765, Epub 2003/02/21. eng.

Akbar U, Jones T, Winestone J, Michael M, Shukla A, Sun Y, et al. Delivery of temozolomide to the tumor bed via biodegradable gel matrices in a novel model of intracranial glioma with resection. J Neurooncol. 2009;94(2):203–12. PubMed PMID: 19337695, Epub 2009/04/02. eng.

Aldape KD, Colman H, James CD. Models of malignant glioma. Drug Discov Today. 2006;3(2):6.

Amarasingh S, Macleod MR, Whittle IR. What is the translational efficacy of chemotherapeutic drug research in neuro-oncology? A systematic review and meta-analysis of the efficacy of BCNU and CCNU in animal models of glioma. J Neurooncol. 2009;91(2):117–25. PubMed PMID: 18813876, Epub 2008/09/25. eng.

Assadian S, Aliaga A, Del Maestro RF, Evans AC, Bedell BJ. FDG-PET imaging for the evaluation of antiglioma agents in a rat model. Neuro Oncol. 2008;10(3):292–9. PubMed PMID: 18430796, Pubmed Central PMCID: 2563051.

Bello L, Giussani C, Carrabba G, Pluderi M, Lucini V, Pannacci M, et al. Suppression of malignant glioma recurrence in a newly developed animal model by endogenous inhibitors. Clin Cancer Res. 2002;8(11):3539–48. PubMed PMID: 12429645, Epub 2002/11/14. eng.

Bock NA, Konyer NB, Henkelman RM. Multiple-mouse MRI. Magnet Reson Med Off J Soc Magnet Reson Med/Soc Magnet Reson Med. 2003;49(1):158–67. PubMed PMID: 12509832, Epub 2003/01/02. eng.

Bock NA, Nieman BJ, Bishop JB, Mark HR. In vivo multiple-mouse MRI at 7 Tesla. Magnet Reson Med Off J Soc Magnet Reson Med/Soc Magnet Reson Med. 2005;54(5):1311–6. PubMed PMID: 16215960, Epub 2005/10/11. eng.

Borges AR, Lopez-Larrubia P, Marques JB, Cerdan SG. MR imaging features of high-grade gliomas in murine models: how they compare with human disease, reflect tumor biology, and play a role in preclinical trials. AJNR Am J Neuroradiol. 2012;33(1):24–36. PubMed PMID: 22194368.

Bradley DP, Tessier JJ, Lacey T, Scott M, Jurgensmeier JM, Odedra R, et al. Examining the acute effects of cediranib (RECENTIN, AZD2171) treatment in tumor models: a dynamic contrast-enhanced MRI study using gadopentate. Magn Reson Imaging. 2009;27(3):377–84. PubMed PMID: 18814988.

Camphausen K, Purow B, Sproull M, Scott T, Ozawa T, Deen DF, et al. Influence of in vivo growth on human glioma cell line gene expression: convergent profiles under orthotopic conditions. Proc Natl Acad Sci U S A. 2005a;102(23):8287–92. PubMed PMID: 15928080, Pubmed Central PMCID: 1142119, Epub 2005/06/02. eng.

Camphausen K, Purow B, Sproull M, Scott T, Ozawa T, Deen DF, et al. Orthotopic growth of human glioma cells quantitatively and qualitatively influences radiation-induced changes in gene expression. Cancer Res. 2005b;65(22):10389–1093. PubMed PMID: 16288029, Epub 2005/11/17. eng.

Cha S, Johnson G, Wadghiri YZ, Jin O, Babb J, Zagzag D, et al. Dynamic, contrast-enhanced perfusion MRI in mouse gliomas: correlation with histopathology. Magnet Reson Med Off J Soc Magnet Reson Med/Soc Magnet Reson Med. 2003;49(5):848–55. PubMed PMID: 12704767, Epub 2003/04/22. eng.

Chenevert TL, McKeever PE, Ross BD. Monitoring early response of experimental brain tumors to therapy using diffusion magnetic resonance imaging. Clin Cancer Res. 1997;3(9):1457–66. PubMed PMID: 9815831.

Chenevert TL, Stegman LD, Taylor JM, Robertson PL, Greenberg HS, Rehemtulla A, et al. Diffusion magnetic resonance imaging: an early surrogate marker of therapeutic efficacy in brain tumors. J Natl Cancer Inst. 2000;92(24):2029–36. PubMed PMID: 11121466.

Chinot OL, Wick W, Mason W, Henriksson R, Saran F, Nishikawa R, et al. Bevacizumab plus radiotherapy-temozolomide for newly diagnosed glioblastoma. N Engl J Med. 2014;370(8):709–22. PubMed PMID: 24552318.

Chung C, Jalali S, Foltz W, Burrell K, Wildgoose P, Lindsay P, et al. Imaging biomarker dynamics in an intracranial murine glioma study of radiation and antiangiogenic therapy. Int J Radiat Oncol Biol Phys. 2013;85(3):805–12. PubMed PMID: 22929856, Epub 2012/08/30. eng.

Corroyer-Dulmont A, Peres EA, Petit E, Guillamo JS, Varoqueaux N, Roussel S, et al. Detection of glioblastoma response to temozolomide combined with bevacizumab based on muMRI and muPET imaging reveals [18F]-fluoro-L-thymidine as an early and robust predictive marker for treatment efficacy. Neuro Oncol. 2013;15(1):41–56. PubMed PMID: 23115160, Pubmed Central PMCID: 3534417.

Dazai J, Bock NA, Nieman BJ, Davidson LM, Henkelman RM, Chen XJ. Multiple mouse biological loading and monitoring system for MRI. Magnet Reson Med Off J Soc Magnet Reson Med/Soc Magnet Reson Med. 2004;52(4):709–15. PubMed PMID: 15389955, Epub 2004/09/25. eng.

de Lussanet QG, Backes WH, Griffioen AW, Padhani AR, Baeten CI, van Baardwijk A, et al. Dynamic contrast-enhanced magnetic resonance imaging of radiation therapy-induced microcirculation changes in rectal cancer. Int J Radiat Oncol Biol Phys. 2005;63(5):1309–15. PubMed PMID: 16125874, Epub 2005/08/30. eng.

Derlon JM, Chapon F, Noel MH, Khouri S, Benali K, Petit-Taboue MC, et al. Non-invasive grading of oligodendrogliomas: correlation between in vivo metabolic pattern and histopathology. Eur J Nucl Med. 2000;27(7):778–87. PubMed PMID: 10952489.

Dhermain FG, Hau P, Lanfermann H, Jacobs AH, van den Bent MJ. Advanced MRI and PET imaging for assessment of treatment response in patients with gliomas. Lancet Neurol. 2010a;9(9):906–20. PubMed PMID: 20705518, Epub 2010/08/14. eng.

Dhermain F, Saliou G, Parker F, Page P, Hoang-Xuan K, Lacroix C, et al. Microvascular leakage and contrast enhancement as prognostic factors for recurrence in unfavorable low-grade gliomas. J Neurooncol. 2010b;97(1):81–8. PubMed PMID: 19727561, Epub 2009/09/04. eng.

Ellingson BM, Malkin MG, Rand SD, Connelly JM, Quinsey C, LaViolette PS, et al. Validation of functional diffusion maps (fDMs) as a biomarker for human glioma cellularity. J Magn Reson Imaging. 2010;31(3):538–48. PubMed PMID: 20187195, Pubmed Central PMCID: 2903058, Epub 2010/02/27. eng.

Fomchenko EI, Holland EC. Mouse models of brain tumors and their applications in preclinical trials. Clin Cancer Res. 2006;12(18):5288–97. PubMed PMID: 17000661, Epub 2006/09/27. eng.

Gahramanov S, Raslan AM, Muldoon LL, Hamilton BE, Rooney WD, Varallyay CG, et al. Potential for differentiation of pseudoprogression from true tumor progression with dynamic susceptibility-weighted contrast-enhanced magnetic resonance imaging using ferumoxytol vs gadoteridol: a pilot study. Int J Radiat Oncol Biol Phys. 2011;79(2):514–23. PubMed PMID: 20395065, Pubmed Central PMCID: 3111452, Epub 2010/04/17. eng.

Galban CJ, Bhojani MS, Lee KC, Meyer CR, Van Dort ME, Kuszpit KK, et al. Evaluation of treatment-associated inflammatory response on diffusion-weighted magnetic resonance imaging and 2-[18F]-fluoro-2-deoxy-D-glucose-positron emission tomography imaging biomarkers. Clin Cancer Res. 2010;16(5):1542–52. PubMed PMID: 20160061, Pubmed Central PMCID: 2843556, Epub 2010/02/18. eng.

Gilbert MR, Dignam JJ, Armstrong TS, Wefel JS, Blumenthal DT, Vogelbaum MA, et al. A randomized trial of bevacizumab for newly diagnosed glioblastoma. N Engl J Med. 2014;370(8):699–708. PubMed PMID: 24552317.

Griffin JL, Kauppinen RA. Tumour metabolomics in animal models of human cancer. J Proteome Res. 2007;6(2):498–505. PubMed PMID: 17269706.

Hamstra DA, Galban CJ, Meyer CR, Johnson TD, Sundgren PC, Tsien C, et al. Functional diffusion map as an early imaging biomarker for high-grade glioma: correlation with conventional radiologic response and overall survival. J Clin Oncol. 2008;26(20):3387–94. PubMed PMID: 18541899.

Haris M, Kumar S, Raj MK, Das KJ, Sapru S, Behari S, et al. Serial diffusion tensor imaging to characterize radiation-induced changes in normal-appearing white matter following radiotherapy in patients with adult low-grade gliomas. Radiat Med. 2008;26(3):140–50. PubMed PMID: 18683569.

Hess KR. Extent of resection as a prognostic variable in the treatment of gliomas. J Neurooncol. 1999;42(3):227–31. PubMed PMID: 10433106, Epub 1999/08/05. eng.

Hillman GG, Singh-Gupta V, Zhang H, Al-Bashir AK, Katkuri Y, Li M, et al. Dynamic contrast-enhanced magnetic resonance imaging of vascular changes induced by sunitinib in papillary renal cell carcinoma xenograft tumors. Neoplasia. 2009;11(9):910–20. PubMed PMID: 19724685.

Hingtgen S, Figueiredo JL, Farrar C, Duebgen M, Martinez-Quintanilla J, Bhere D, et al. Real-time multi-modality imaging of glioblastoma tumor resection and recurrence. J Neurooncol. 2013;111(2):153–61. PubMed PMID: 23242736, Pubmed Central PMCID: 3548430, Epub 2012/12/18. eng.

Hoff BA, Bhojani MS, Rudge J, Chenevert TL, Meyer CR, Galban S, et al. DCE and DW-MRI monitoring of vascular disruption following VEGF-Trap treatment of a rat glioma model. NMR Biomed. 2012;25(7):935–42. PubMed PMID: 22190279, Epub 2011/12/23. eng.

Hu LS, Baxter LC, Smith KA, Feuerstein BG, Karis JP, Eschbacher JM, et al. Relative cerebral blood volume values to differentiate high-grade glioma recurrence from posttreatment radiation effect: direct correlation between image-guided tissue histopathology and localized dynamic susceptibility-weighted contrast-enhanced perfusion MR imaging measurements. AJNR Am J Neuroradiol. 2009;30(3):552–8. PubMed PMID: 19056837, Epub 2008/12/06. eng.

Hutterer M, Nowosielski M, Putzer D, Waitz D, Tinkhauser G, Kostron H, et al. O-(2-18F-fluoroethyl)-L-tyrosine PET predicts failure of antiangiogenic treatment in patients with recurrent high-grade glioma. J Nuclear Med. 2011;52(6):856–64. PubMed PMID: 21622893.

Jacobs AH, Dittmar C, Winkeler A, Garlip G, Heiss WD. Molecular imaging of gliomas. Mol Imaging. 2002a;1(4):309–35. PubMed PMID: 12926228.

Jacobs AH, Winkler A, Dittmar C, Gossman A, Deckert M, Kracht L, et al. Molecular and functional imaging technology for the development of efficient treatment strategies for gliomas. Technol Cancer Res Treat. 2002b;1(3):187–204. PubMed PMID: 12622512.

Jacobs AH, Thomas A, Kracht LW, Li H, Dittmar C, Garlip G, et al. 18F-fluoro-L-thymidine and 11C-methylmethionine as markers of increased transport and proliferation in brain tumors. J Nuclear Med. 2005;46(12):1948–58. PubMed PMID: 16330557.

Jacobs VL, Valdes PA, Hickey WF, De Leo JA. Current review of in vivo GBM rodent models: emphasis on the CNS-1 tumour model. ASN Neuro. 2011;3(3):e00063. PubMed PMID: 21740400, Pubmed Central PMCID: 3153964, Epub 2011/07/12. eng.

Jain RK, di Tomaso E, Duda DG, Loeffler JS, Sorensen AG, Batchelor TT. Angiogenesis in brain tumours. Nat Rev Neurosci. 2007;8(8):610–22. PubMed PMID: 17643088.

Jalali S, Chung C, Foltz W, Burrell K, Singh S, Hill R, et al. MRI biomarkers identify the differential response of glioblastoma multiforme to anti-angiogenic therapy. Neuro Oncol. 2014;16(6):868–79. PubMed PMID: 24759636, Pubmed Central PMCID: 4022230, Epub 2014/04/25. eng.

Jennings D, Hatton BN, Guo J, Galons JP, Trouard TP, Raghunand N, et al. Early response of prostate carcinoma xenografts to docetaxel chemotherapy monitored with diffusion MRI. Neoplasia. 2002;4(3):255–62. PubMed PMID: 11988845, Pubmed Central PMCID: 1531699, Epub 2002/05/04. eng.

Johnson GA, Cofer GP, Gewalt SL, Hedlund LW. Morphologic phenotyping with MR microscopy: the visible mouse. Radiology. 2002;222(3):789–93. PubMed PMID: 11867802, Epub 2002/02/28. eng.

Kauer TM, Figueiredo JL, Hingtgen S, Shah K. Encapsulated therapeutic stem cells implanted in the tumor resection cavity induce cell death in gliomas. Nat Neurosci. 2012;15(2):197–204. PubMed PMID: 22197831, Pubmed Central PMCID: 3601490, Epub 2011/12/27. eng.

Krammer B, Plaetzer K. ALA and its clinical impact, from bench to bedside. Photochem Photobiol Sci. 2008;7(3):283–9. PubMed PMID: 18389144, Epub 2008/04/05. eng.

Larocque MP, Syme A, Yahya A, Wachowicz K, Allalunis-Turner J, Fallone BG. Temporal and dose dependence of T2 and ADC at 9.4 T in a mouse model following single fraction radiation therapy. Med Phys. 2009;36(7):2948–54. PubMed PMID: 19673193, Epub 2009/08/14. eng.

Law M, Young RJ, Babb JS, Peccerelli N, Chheang S, Gruber ML, et al. Gliomas: predicting time to progression or survival with cerebral blood volume measurements at dynamic susceptibility-weighted contrast-enhanced perfusion MR imaging. Radiology. 2008;247(2):490–8. PubMed PMID: 18349315, Pubmed Central PMCID: 3774106, Epub 2008/03/20. eng.

Lemasson B, Christen T, Tizon X, Farion R, Fondraz N, Provent P, et al. Assessment of multiparametric MRI in a human glioma model to monitor cytotoxic and anti-angiogenic drug effects. NMR Biomed. 2011;24(5):473–82. PubMed PMID: 21674650, Pubmed Central PMCID: 3351072, Epub 2011/06/16. eng.

Li X, Rooney WD, Varallyay CG, Gahramanov S, Muldoon LL, Goodman JA, et al. Dynamic-contrast-enhanced-MRI with extravasating contrast reagent: rat cerebral glioma blood volume determination. J Magn Reson. 2010;206(2):190–9. PubMed PMID: 20674422, Pubmed Central PMCID: 2946221, Epub 2010/08/03. eng.

Li X, Welch EB, Arlinghaus LR, Chakravarthy AB, Xu L, Farley J, et al. A novel AIF tracking method and comparison of DCE-MRI parameters using individual and population-based AIFs in human breast cancer. Phys Med Biol. 2011;56(17):5753–69. PubMed PMID: 21841212, Pubmed Central PMCID: 3176673.

Lyons SK. Advances in imaging mouse tumour models in vivo. J Pathol. 2005;205(2):194–205. PubMed PMID: 15641018, Epub 2005/01/11. eng.

Metcalfe SE, Grant R. Biopsy versus resection for malignant glioma. Cochrane Database Syst Rev. 2001;3, CD002034. PubMed PMID: 11687008, Epub 2001/11/01. eng.

Moffat BA, Hall DE, Stojanovska J, McConville PJ, Moody JB, Chenevert TL, et al. Diffusion imaging for evaluation of tumor therapies in preclinical animal models. MAGMA. 2004;17(3–6):249–59. PubMed PMID: 15580371.

Muldoon LL, Gahramanov S, Li X, Marshall DJ, Kraemer DF, Neuwelt EA. Dynamic magnetic resonance imaging assessment of vascular targeting agent effects in rat intracerebral tumor models. Neuro Oncol. 2011;13(1):51–60. PubMed PMID: 21123368, Pubmed Central PMCID: 3018910.

Nelson AL, Algon SA, Munasinghe J, Graves O, Goumnerova L, Burstein D, et al. Magnetic resonance imaging of patched heterozygous and xenografted mouse brain tumors. J Neurooncol. 2003;62(3):259–67. PubMed PMID: 12777077.

Nieman BJ, Bock NA, Bishop J, Chen XJ, Sled JG, Rossant J, et al. Magnetic resonance imaging for detection and analysis of mouse phenotypes. NMR Biomed. 2005;18(7):447–68. PubMed PMID: 16206127, Epub 2005/10/06. eng.

O'Connor JP, Jackson A, Asselin MC, Buckley DL, Parker GJ, Jayson GC. Quantitative imaging biomarkers in the clinical development of targeted therapeutics: current and future perspectives. Lancet Oncol. 2008;9(8):766–76. PubMed PMID: 18672212.

Pacheco-Torres J, Lopez-Larrubia P, Ballesteros P, Cerdan S. Imaging tumor hypoxia by magnetic resonance methods. NMR Biomed. 2011;24(1):1–16. PubMed PMID: 21259366.

Radaelli E, Ceruti R, Patton V, Russo M, Degrassi A, Croci V, et al. Immunohistopathological and neuroimaging characterization of murine orthotopic xenograft models of glioblastoma multiforme recapitulating the most salient features of human disease. Histol Histopathol. 2009;24(7):879–91. PubMed PMID: 19475534, Epub 2009/05/29. eng.

Ross BD, Moffat BA, Lawrence TS, Mukherji SK, Gebarski SS, Quint DJ, et al. Evaluation of cancer therapy using diffusion magnetic resonance imaging. Mol Cancer Ther. 2003;2(6):581–7. PubMed PMID: 12813138, Epub 2003/06/19. eng.

Roth Y, Tichler T, Kostenich G, Ruiz-Cabello J, Maier SE, Cohen JS, et al. High-b-value diffusion-weighted MR imaging for pretreatment prediction and early monitoring of tumor response to therapy in mice. Radiology. 2004;232(3):685–92. PubMed PMID: 15215551, Epub 2004/06/25. eng.

Russell SM, Elliott R, Forshaw D, Golfinos JG, Nelson PK, Kelly PJ. Glioma vascularity correlates with reduced patient survival and increased malignancy. Surg Neurol. 2009;72(3):242–6. PubMed PMID: 19329156, discussion 6–7. Epub 2009/03/31. eng.

Smilowitz HM, Weissenberger J, Weis J, Brown JD, O'Neill RJ, Laissue JA. Orthotopic transplantation of v-src-expressing glioma cell lines into immunocompetent mice: establishment of a new transplantable in vivo model for malignant glioma. J Neurosurg. 2007;106(4):652–9. PubMed PMID: 17432718, Epub 2007/04/17. eng.

Smitha KA, Gupta AK, Jayasree RS. Total magnitude of diffusion tensor imaging as an effective tool for the differentiation of glioma. Eur J Radiol. 2013;82(5):857–61. PubMed PMID: 23394764.

Sorensen AG, Batchelor TT, Zhang WT, Chen PJ, Yeo P, Wang M, et al. A "vascular normalization index" as potential mechanistic biomarker to predict survival after a single dose of cediranib in recurrent glioblastoma patients. Cancer Res. 2009;69(13):5296–300. PubMed PMID: 19549889, Pubmed Central PMCID: 2824172, Epub 2009/06/25. eng.

Stummer W, Pichlmeier U, Meinel T, Wiestler OD, Zanella F, Reulen HJ, et al. Fluorescence-guided surgery with 5-aminolevulinic acid for resection of malignant glioma: a randomised controlled multicentre phase III trial. Lancet Oncol. 2006;7(5):392–401. PubMed PMID: 16648043, Epub 2006/05/02. eng.

Sun Y, Schmidt NO, Schmidt K, Doshi S, Rubin JB, Mulkern RV, et al. Perfusion MRI of U87 brain tumors in a mouse model. Magnet Reson Med Off J Soc Magnet Reson Med/Soc Magnet Reson Med. 2004;51(5):893–9. PubMed PMID: 15122670, Epub 2004/05/04. eng.

Tofts PS, Brix G, Buckley DL, Evelhoch JL, Henderson E, Knopp MV, et al. Estimating kinetic parameters from dynamic contrast-enhanced T(1)-weighted MRI of a diffusable tracer:

standardized quantities and symbols. J Magn Reson Imaging. 1999;10(3):223–32. PubMed PMID: 10508281.

Varallyay CG, Muldoon LL, Gahramanov S, Wu YJ, Goodman JA, Li X, et al. Dynamic MRI using iron oxide nanoparticles to assess early vascular effects of antiangiogenic versus corticosteroid treatment in a glioma model. J Cereb Blood Flow Metab. 2009;29(4):853–60. PubMed PMID: 19142191, Pubmed Central PMCID: 2747492, Epub 2009/01/15. eng.

Vassal F, Boutet C, Lemaire JJ, Nuti C. New insights into the functional significance of the frontal aslant tract-An anatomo-functional study using intraoperative electrical stimulations combined with diffusion tensor imaging-based fiber tracking. Brit J Neurosurg. 2014;28(5):685–7. PubMed PMID: 24552256.

Veeravagu A, Hou LC, Hsu AR, Cai W, Greve JM, Chen X, et al. The temporal correlation of dynamic contrast-enhanced magnetic resonance imaging with tumor angiogenesis in a murine glioblastoma model. Neurol Res. 2008;30(9):952–9. PubMed PMID: 18662497, Epub 2008/07/30. eng.

Viel T, Schelhaas S, Wagner S, Wachsmuth L, Schwegmann K, Kuhlmann M, et al. Early assessment of the efficacy of temozolomide chemotherapy in experimental glioblastoma using [18F]FLT-PET imaging. PLoS One. 2013;8(7):e67911. PubMed PMID: 23861829, Pubmed Central PMCID: 3701682.

Wang S, Qiu D, So KF, Wu EX, Leung LH, Gu J, et al. Radiation induced brain injury: assessment of white matter tracts in a pre-clinical animal model using diffusion tensor MR imaging. J Neurooncol. 2013;112(1):9–15. PubMed PMID: 23334608.

Wester HJ. Nuclear imaging probes: from bench to bedside. Clinical Cancer Res. 2007;13(12):3470–81. PubMed PMID: 17575209.

Woodfield CA, Tung GA, Grand DJ, Pezzullo JA, Machan JT, Renzulli 2nd JF. Diffusion-weighted MRI of peripheral zone prostate cancer: comparison of tumor apparent diffusion coefficient with Gleason score and percentage of tumor on core biopsy. AJR Am J Roentgenol. 2010;194(4):W316–22. PubMed PMID: 20308476, Epub 2010/03/24. eng.

Yamasaki F, Sugiyama K, Ohtaki M, Takeshima Y, Abe N, Akiyama Y, et al. Glioblastoma treated with postoperative radio-chemotherapy: prognostic value of apparent diffusion coefficient at MR imaging. Eur J Radiol. 2010;73(3):532–7. PubMed PMID: 19250783. Epub 2009/03/03. eng.

Zhao M, Pipe JG, Bonnett J, Evelhoch JL. Early detection of treatment response by diffusion-weighted 1H-NMR spectroscopy in a murine tumour in vivo. Br J Cancer. 1996;73(1):61–4. PubMed PMID: 8554985, Pubmed Central PMCID: 2074297, Epub 1996/01/01. eng.

Zwick S, Strecker R, Kiselev V, Gall P, Huppert J, Palmowski M, et al. Assessment of vascular remodeling under antiangiogenic therapy using DCE-MRI and vessel size imaging. J Magn Reson Imaging. 2009;29(5):1125–33. PubMed PMID: 19388117.

Part IV

Breast and Prostate

Breast Cancer: Serum TPS as a Biomarker 19

Dong-Young Noh, Soo Kyung Ahn, Hyeong-Gon Moon,
Wonshik Han, and Jisun Kim

Contents

Abstract

Cytokeratin tumor markers are traditionally used as serological markers in various epithelial cell-associated carcinomas, such as breast, lung, colorectal, and bladder cancer. Cytokeratin reflects the proliferative activity of tumor cells (Barak et al. 2004).

D.-Y. Noh (✉) • S.K. Ahn • H.-G. Moon • W. Han • J. Kim
Division of Breast and Endocrine, Department of Surgery, College of Medicine, University of Ulsan, Asan Medical Center, Sonpa-gu, Seoul, South Korea
e-mail: dynoh@snu.ac.kr; dynoh56@gmail.com; sooahn79@naver.com; sooahn79@gmail.com; moonhgsurgi@gmail.com; hanw@snu.ac.kr; leticeclear@naver.com

V.R. Preedy, V.B. Patel (eds.), *Biomarkers in Cancer, Biomarkers in Disease: Methods, Discoveries and Applications*,
DOI 10.1007/978-94-007-7681-4_37

Tissue polypeptide-specific antigen (TPS) is a cytokeratin marker that quantitates a critical epitope structure of peptide in serum associated with human cytokeratin 18. TPS is detected using the monoclonal antibody, M3 (Bonfrer et al. 1994; Rydlander et al. 1996, D' Alessandro et al. 2001). The M3 epitope is related to the proliferative activity of the tumor (O'Hanlon et al. 1996). Since the well-known serum tumor markers in breast cancer, including CA 15-3 and CEA, do not reflect proliferative activity, TPS may be more beneficial as a prognostic indicator.

TPS has consistently been reported as an effective serum marker for providing prognostic information and establishing patient responses to therapy. A main limitation of TPS is that it is not "organ specific," which impedes diagnostic utility. Additionally, TPS levels are altered according to inflammation conditions, such as liver cirrhosis, ovulation, and menopausal status. Further clinical studies are required to fully establish the clinical utility of TPS, both alone and in combination with other established prognostic markers.

List of Abbreviations

CEA	Carcinoembryonic Antigen
ER	Estrogen Receptor
HER2	Human Epidermal Growth Factor Receptor 2
MCA	Mucinous Carcinoma-Associated Antigen
NSCLC	Non-small-Cell Lung Cancer
PR	Progesterone Receptor
TPA	Tissue Polypeptide Antigen
TPS	Tissue Polypeptide-Specific Antigen

Key Facts of TPS

- Bjorklund and Bjorklund (1957) initially developed a monoclonal antibody (M3) specific for tissue polypeptide antigen (TPA).
- TPA measures cytokeratins 8, 18, and 19 in serum samples, and TPS detects a defined epitope structure on human cytokeratin 18 using the M3 monoclonal antibody.
- The M3 epitope of tissue polypeptide antigen is related to proliferation activity of the tumor.
- Measurement of TPS was completed with a one-step solid phase radiometric sandwich assay based on an immunochemical technique using a commercially available test kit for TPS.
- TPS is a well-documented cytokeratin tumor marker in various epithelial cell-associated carcinomas, such as breast, ovarian, prostate, and gastrointestinal cancer.
- A potential problem is that TPS is a recognized nonspecific marker.

Definitions of Words and Terms

Cytokeratin Belongs to the intermediate filament (IF) protein family. Upon release from proliferating or apoptotic cells, cytokeratin provides a useful marker of epithelial malignancies, including breast, colorectal, lung, head-and-neck, and bladder cancer.

Serum Tumor Marker A substance found in the blood that can be elevated in malignancy. The potential uses of serum markers include aiding early diagnosis, determining prognosis, prospectively predicting response or resistance to specific therapies, surveillance after primary surgery, and monitoring therapy in patients with advanced disease.

Prognostic Marker Factors are involved in tumor metastasis and disease progression in the absence of intervening therapy, distinct from predictive markers, which are associated with response to particular therapy.

CEA Abbreviation for carcinoembryonic antigen, a glycosyl phosphatidyl inositol (GPI) cell surface-anchored glycoprotein involved in cell adhesion. CEA may be increased in colorectal, gastric, pancreatic, lung, and breast cancer, as well as some noncancerous conditions, such as ulcerative colitis, Crohn's disease, and liver cirrhosis.

CA 15-3 Abbreviation for cancer antigen 15-3 derived from MUC1. This is the most widely used marker for breast cancer and useful for monitoring therapy in advanced breast cancer that is not assessable with existing clinical or radiological procedures.

Introduction

Despite numerous studies worldwide, a limited number of single biomarkers have been identified for use in breast cancer management over several years, including estrogen receptor (ER), progesterone receptor (PR), and human epidermal growth factor receptor 2 (HER2). These established markers in breast cancer require tissue samples. The majority of research on cancer prognostic markers to date has focused on tissue, although serum is more readily available than tumor tissue. OncotypeDX® and MammaPrint® are among the most widely used tissue-based prognostic markers in breast cancer.

Serum tumor markers are easily accessible and require a less invasive procedure than biopsy or surgery. Thus, serum tumor markers that afford independent prognostic information are of significant value. The most widely used serum markers in breast cancer, CA 15-3 and carcinoembryonic antigen (CEA), do not reflect proliferative activity. In contrast, cytokeratin tumor markers measure proliferative activity, one of the most important phenotypic characteristics of tumor

Table 1 Serum tumor markers in breast cancer. A list of the most widely used serum tumor markers in breast cancer

Marker	Protein(s) detected
CEA	CEA
CA 15-3	MUC-1
TPA	Fragments of cytokeratins 8, 18, and 19
TPS	Fragments of cytokeratin 18
HER-2 (shed form)	Extracellular form of HER-2

TPA tissue polypeptide antigen, *TPS* tissue polypeptide-specific antigen

aggressiveness, and may thus be more beneficial as a prognostic indicator than the serum tumor markers reported earlier (Table 1).

The most widely applied cytokeratin tumor markers include tissue polypeptide antigen (TPA), CYFRA 21-1, and tissue polypeptide-specific antigen (TPS). TPA may be effectively applied to estimate cytokeratins 8, 18, and 19 in serum samples (Weber et al. 1984), which was initially described by Bjorklund and Bjorklund (1957). The group additionally developed a monoclonal antibody (M3) specific for TPA (Bjorklund 1992). TPS detects a defined epitope structure on human cytokeratin 18 using the M3 monoclonal antibody, while CYFRA 21-1 measures soluble keratin 19 fragments in the circulation (Bodenmuller et al. 1994). The clinical value of these markers lies in the early detection of recurrence and assessment of the efficacy of therapeutic response in epithelial carcinomas, such as breast, colorectal, lung, head-and-neck, and bladder cancer.

In the current study, we have described the clinical application of TPS as a biomarker in breast cancer.

Serum TPS as a Useful Biomarker in Breast Cancer

Tissue polypeptide-specific antigen (TPS) was originally identified in human carcinomas and tumor cell lines using antibodies directed toward insoluble tumor material shown to stain cytoskeletal intermediate filaments in HeLa cells. Intermediate filament types I and II constitute cytokeratins (acidic and basic proteins, respectively). To date, 20 distinct cytokeratins have been identified in the cytoskeleton of epithelial tissue and are further subdivided into types I and II, based on sequence homology. Cytokeratins 1–8 constitute the type II group (53–68 kDa, neutral to basic protein components), while cytokeratins 9–20 constitute the type I group (40–56 kDa, acidic proteins) (Kerif et al. 2003; Osborn et al. 1982; Fuchs et al. 1994). The cytokeratins are paired into heterodimers, each containing one type I and one type II, which are further organized into filamentous structures via side-by-side alignment to form tetramers and higher cytokeratin polymers with coiled-coil dimeric structures through further end-to-end associations (Parry et al. 1999; Hatzfeld et al. 1985; Coulombe et al. 2002).

Tissue polypeptide antigen is proposed to be immunologically related to a mixture of non-epidermal cytokeratins 8, 18, and 19 (Bjorklund and Bjorklund, 1957). Earlier monoclonal mapping of a fraction of tissue polypeptide antigen revealed the presence of 35 antigenic determinants. Two epitopes were shown to be related to tumor cell activity. Monoclonal antibodies against these epitope structures were raised in mice with human carcinoma preparations. The monoclonal antibody specific for TPS was raised against the M3 epitope of tissue polypeptide antigen that is related to tumor proliferative activity. TPS is a well-documented cytokeratin tumor marker found in various epithelial cell-associated carcinomas, such as breast, ovarian, prostate, and gastrointestinal cancer.

Conflicting results on the value of TPS as a serum tumor marker in breast cancer have been documented to date. Given et al. (2000) showed that TPS fails to act as an effective predictive factor in breast cancer, compared to CA 15-3. In patients receiving neoadjuvant chemotherapy, TPS was inversely associated with histologic grade, and only pretreatment CA 15-3 levels were correlated with higher recurrence rate (Bottini et al. 1957). On the other hand, other published reports suggest that TPS acts as a marker of recurrence and metastasis (Giai et al. 1995).

Serum TPS Aids in Early Diagnosis

Hwa and coworkers (2008) reported the utility of TPS in detection of primary breast cancer. Earlier, D'Alessandro et al. (2001) reported that in combination with CA 15-3, TPS increases the overall sensitivity of breast cancer diagnosis. The complementarity between CA 15-3 and TPS was further confirmed in a longitudinal study, where the increase in sensitivity was obtained by combining assessment of TPS with CA15-3 yielding a 12.7 % increase in overall sensitivity in the case of local recurrence. Furthermore, TPS provided additional information to both mammography and CA 15-3 data in the detection of breast cancer (Barak et al. 1995).

Determination of Prognosis

TPS appears to have utility as a marker of recurrence and metastases, according to published reports. O'Hanlon et al. (1996) demonstrated that TPS is elevated with disease stage in breast cancer, and levels are significantly higher in patients with locoregional recurrence and increased to an even greater extent in patients with metastases. Patients with elevated TPS during follow-up were more likely to experience disease progression on further follow-up. In a recent study, Ahn et al. 2013 suggested that elevated preoperative serum TPS is associated with poor breast cancer outcomes. The group assayed preoperative serum TPS levels in 1,477 breast cancer patients. Age (>45 years), tumor size (>2 cm), nodal metastasis, negative progesterone receptor, and human epidermal growth factor receptor 2 were associated with elevated TPS. Moreover, elevated TPS was related to poor disease-free survival ($p < 0.001$) and overall survival ($p < 0.001$). Preoperative TPS was identified as a significant prognostic marker for survival, especially in luminal A subtype patients. The researchers proposed that highly proliferative tumors expressing elevated preoperative TPS in the luminal A subtype are more aggressive and result in increased risk of recurrence or death.

Surveillance After Primary Treatment

Bjorklund et al. (1996) conducted a large review including 3,000 cases. Compared to CEA, MCA (mucinous carcinoma-associated antigen), and CA15-3, TPS was the only marker that exhibited an immediate decrease when therapy was effective and increase upon inadequate treatment response. Specifically, upon decrease in TPS to normal levels, applied therapy was effective and tumor activity growth was decreased. However, both CEA and CA15-3 remained elevated due to the continued presence of tumor mass.

Additionally, TPS appeared to indicate clinical outcomes (remission, progression) faster than either CA 15-3 or CEA in metastatic breast cancer patients with different types of routine treatments, and combined determination of CA 15-3 and TPS in monitoring therapy in metastatic breast cancer was recommended. In a European multicenter study, TPS, CA15-3, and CEA were serially measured in 129 metastatic breast cancer patients during a 6-month treatment period. After 6 months of follow-up, patients were divided into four groups according to the UICC criteria for treatment response. Forty-six patients with a more favorable prognosis (complete remission, partial remission, or stable disease) were followed up for an extended period. In 30 of the 46 patients, at least one marker had increased at the end of the 6-month period by at least 25 % (TPS in 54 %, CA 15-3 in 20 %, CEA in 20 %). These 30 patients subsequently developed disease progression. Prognostic sensitivity for TPS, CA 15-3, and CEA was 83 %, 30 %, and 30 %, respectively. The combination of TPS and CA 15-3 increased overall sensitivity to 96 % (Van Dalen et al. 1996,1998).

Monitoring Response to Therapy in Advanced Disease

In two retrospective studies, TPS was evaluated as a marker for clinical follow-up of patients subjected to chemotherapy and/or interferon-based immunotherapy. The results suggest that TPS is a sensitive marker with a longer lead time to recurrence than both CA15-3 and CEA. The prognostic information imparted by circulating TPS levels at the beginning of the study before treatment correlated significantly with longer survival times (Barak et al.1994, 1997).

In a prospective study, (Barak et al. 1998a and 1998b) evaluated the utility of TPS in predicting response to Taxol administered as second-line treatment in 87 advanced breast cancer patients. TPS, as well as CEA and CA15-3, was measured before, during, and after Taxol treatment. The three-marker combination provided higher sensitivity than each single marker. Significant correlations of TPS levels with response and prognosis were observed. Specifically, 29 %, 41 %, and

60 % of the patients showed a decrease of at least 50 % in CEA, CA15-3, and TPS, respectively. Survival was significantly correlated with low pretreatment TPS levels. Pre-Taxol levels for TPS and CEA were further analyzed with multivariate Cox regression analysis, where the difference in relative risk was statistically significant only for TPS (2.1 vs. 1). TPS provides important reliable information in advanced breast cancer regarding Taxol treatment efficacy and survival prognosis (Barak et al. 2004).

Limitations

A potential problem with TPS is that it is a recognized nonspecific marker. TPS is elevated in inflammatory conditions, particularly liver cirrhosis (Van Dalen, 1992). In addition, TPS may be markedly elevated at the time of ovulation (Inaba et al. 1993), and serum TPS levels are altered according to menopausal status.

Conclusions

In conclusion, TPS is a valuable serum marker for breast cancer that aids in early diagnosis, determining prognosis, surveillance after primary surgery, and monitoring therapy in patients with advanced disease, although the precise mechanisms are unclear at present. The serum TPS level may thus be combined with established prognostic factors for clinical use in predicting patient outcomes, improving ineffective treatments, and facilitating individualization of therapy for breast cancer patients.

Potential Applications in Prognosis, Other Diseases, and Conditions

TPS has been employed as a serum tumor marker in various other epithelial cell-associated carcinomas, such as ovarian, pancreatic, colorectal, and lung cancer. The majority of studies have reported the utility of TPS in combination with established prognostic markers for different cancer types. The lack of sensitivity and organ specificity of TPS signifies that it is not a suitable marker for early diagnosis. However, a number of studies have concluded that the prime utility of TPS is in monitoring treatment and providing early indications of recurrence and tumor progression.

Ovarian Cancer

A combination of CA 125, the best available marker for ovarian cancer, with TPS has been shown to increase the sensitivity for monitoring therapy and add prognostic value. In a prospective European multicenter trial, 212 ovarian cancer patients (FIGO stage I-IV) were analyzed. In the subgroup of patients with FIGO stages III + IV, cutoff levels of CA 125 (35 kU/l) and TPS (80 kU/l) after chemotherapy were excellent discriminators of survival ($p < 0.0001$). The combined value of CA 125 and TPS cutoff points showed better correlation with survival rates (63 % vs. 17 %, $p = 0.0004$). The researchers concluded that TPS and CA 125 levels after chemotherapy are excellent discriminators of overall survival in patients with advanced ovarian cancer (Van Dalen et al. 1999). The prognostic values of TPS and CA 125 after three cycles of chemotherapy were further analyzed by the group (Van Dalen et al. 2000). Their data suggest that only CA 125 and TPS values below the discriminatory level after three cycles of chemotherapy indicate favorable prognosis in FIGO III and IV ovarian cancer patients.

Several studies examining the utility of CA 125 and TPS in ascetic fluid from cancer patients have concluded that high levels of both markers indicate metastatic spread (Barak et al. 1993; Chechlinska et al. 2003; Sedlaczek et al. 2002).

Pancreatic Cancer

The study by Slesak et al. (2000) supports the ability of TPS and CA 19-9 to discriminate between pancreatic adenocarcinoma and chronic pancreatitis. The researchers concluded that TPS is potentially useful in differential diagnosis between pancreatic adenocarcinoma and chronic pancreatitis with significantly higher sensitivity and specificity, compared to CA 19-9. Additionally, TPS was shown to be helpful in monitoring the proliferative process in patients with chronic pancreatitis.

Colorectal Cancer

Berglund and coworkers (2002) evaluated the reliability and validity of the serum markers, TPS, CEA, VEGF (vascular endothelial growth factor), and bFGF (basic fibroblast growth factor), in monitoring palliative chemotherapy in advanced colorectal cancer patients ($n = 87$). They concluded that repeated measurements of TPS are of clinical relevance in monitoring chemotherapy in advanced colorectal cancer patients, but cannot precisely predict which patients will have positive outcomes.

Lung Cancer

Several studies have suggested that TPS is significant prognostic marker in patients with non-small-cell lung cancer (NSCLC). The groups of Barak and Nismen (Nisman et al. 1998a and 1998b) concluded that independent of the histological type, including adenocarcinoma, squamous cell carcinoma, and large-cell carcinoma, TPS is a better prognostic marker than CYFRA 21-1 and CEA in NSCLC.

Multivariate analysis of survival showed that only TPS is an independent prognostic factor in patients with squamous cell carcinoma. Furthermore, TPS was identified as a useful marker for detecting relapse (Devine et al. 1994; Pujol et al. 1996; Ebert and Muley 1998; Stieber et al. 1993).

Summary Points

- This chapter focuses on TPS as a valuable tumor marker in breast cancer.
- Tissue polypeptide-specific antigen (TPS) is one of the cytokeratin markers.
- TPS quantitates the critical epitope structure of a peptide in serum associated with human cytokeratin 18.
- TPS is detected using the monoclonal antibody, M3. The M3 epitope is related to the proliferative activity of the tumor.
- TPS plays a role as a marker of recurrence and metastasis according to some published reports.
- A limitation of TPS is that it is not "organ specific," which limits diagnostic utility.
- The serum TPS level may be combined with established prognostic factors for clinical use in predicting patient outcomes, improving ineffective treatments, and facilitating individualization of therapy for breast cancer patients.

References

Ahn SK, Moon HG, Ko E, et al. Preoperative serum tissue polypeptide-specific antigen is a valuable prognostic marker in breast cancer. Int J Cancer. 2013;132(4):857–81.

Barak V, Anteby SO, Edelman D, Halperin T, Roisman I, Perez T. CA 125 – the ovarian cancer tumor marker. Israeli Cancer J Bamah. 1993;17:10–4.

Barak V, Nisman B, Roisman I, Hubert A, Burde B, Peretz T. TPS in evaluation of response to Taxol and interferon therapy in breast cancer patients. J Tumor Marker Oncol. 1994;9:89.

Barak V, Gimmon Z, Libson Y, et al. Breast cancer detection by mammography, CA 15-3 and TPS. J Tumor Marker Oncol. 1995;10:51–2.

Barak V, Nisman B, Roisman I, et al. TPS in assessing response to therapy and prognosis of breast cancer patients treated with interferons. J Tumor Marker Oncol. 1997;12:17–26.

Barak V, Nisman B, Roisman I, Hubert A, Peretz T. Clinical utility of TPS in breast cancer. Tumor Biol. 1998a;19:59.

Barak V, Nisman B, Hubert A, Peretz T. TPS-prognosticator in breast cancer. Anticancer Res. 1998b;18:4982.

Barak V, Goike H, Panaretakis KW, et al. Clinical utility of cytokeratins as tumor markers. Clin Biochem. 2004;37:529–40.

Beresford MJ, Wilson GD, Makris A. Measuring proliferation in breast cancer: practicalities and applications. Breast Cancer Res. 2006;8:216.

Berglund A, Molin D, Larsson A, Einarsson R, Glimelius B. Tumor markers as early predictors of response to chemotherapy in advanced colorectal carcinoma. Ann Oncol. 2002;13:1430–7.

Bjorklund B, Bjorklund V. Antigenicity of pooled human malignant and normal tissues by cytoimmunological technique: presence of an insoluble heat-labile tumor antigen. Inst Arch Allergy. 1957;10:153–84.

Bjorklund B, Einarsson R. TPS (tissue polypeptide specific antigen) in oncologic practice: a review with reference to 3000 cases of breast cancer. Tumordiagn Ther. 1996;17:67–73.

Bjorklund B, Tumor-markers TPA. TPA-S and cytokeratins- a working hypothesis. Tumor diagnTher. 1992;13:78–80.

Bodenmuller H, Ofenloch-Hahnle B, Lane EB, et al. Lung cancer-associated keratin 19 fragments: development and biochemical characterisation of the new serum assay Enzymun-Test CYFRA 21–1. Int J Biol Markers. 1994;9:75–81.

Bonfrer JM, Groeneveld EM, Korse CM, et al. Monoclonal antibody M3 used in tissue polypeptide-specific antigen assay for the quantification of tissue polypeptide antigen recognizes keratin 18. Tumour Biol. 1994;15:210–22.

Bottini A, Berruti A, Tampellini M, et al. Influence of neoadjuvant chemotherapy on serum tumor markers CA 15–3, MCA, CEA, TPS and TPA in breast cancer patients with operable disease. Tumour Biol. 1997;18:301–10.

Chechlinska M, Kaminska J, Kowalska M, Radziszewski J, Steffen J. The origin of cytokines, soluble cytokine receptors and CA125 in ascitic fluids and sera of ovarian cancer patients. Tumor Biol. 2003;24:76.

Coulombe PA, Omary MB. "Hard" and "soft" principles defining the structure, function and regulation of keratin intermediate filaments. Curr Opin Cell Biol. 2002;14:110–22.

D'Alessandro R, Roselli M, Ferroni P, et al. Serum tissue polypeptide specific antigen (TPS): a complementary tumor marker to CA 15–3 in the management of breast cancer. Breast Cancer Res Treat. 2001;68:9–19.

Devine PL, Yarker J, Fong K, et al. Serum markers CASA, CEA, CYFRA 21-1, MSA, NSE, TPA and TPS in lung cancer. Int J Oncol. 1994;4:1129–35.

Ebert W, Muley T. Cyfra 21-1, TPS and NSE in the follow-up of non-small (NSCLC) and small cell lung cancer (SCLC). Anticancer Res. 1998;18:4983.

Fuchs E, Weber K. Intermediate filaments: structure, dynamics, function and disease. Ann Rev Biochem. 1994;63:345–82.

Giai M, Roagna R, Ponzone R, et al. TPS and CA15-3 serum values as a guide for treating and monitoring breast cancer patients. Anticancer Res. 1995;15:2711–6.

Given M, Scott M, Mc Grath JP, et al. The predictive of tumour markers CA 15–3, TPS and CEA in breast cancer recurrence. Breast. 2000;9:277–80.

Hatzfeld M, Franke WW. Pair formation and promiscuity of cytokeratins: formation in vitro of heterotypic complexes and intermediate-sized filaments by homologous and heterologous recombinations of purified polypeptides. J Cell Biol. 1985;101:1826–41.

Hwa HL, Kuo WH, Chang LY, et al. Prediction of breast cancer and lymph node metastatic status with tumour markers using logistic regression models. J Eval Clin Pract. 2008;14:275–80.

Inaba N, Fukasawa I, Okajima Y, et al. Immunoradiometrical measurement of tissue polypeptide specific antigen (TPS) in normal, healthy, nonpregnant and pregnant Japanese women. Asia Oceania J Obstet Gynaecol. 1993;19:459–66.

Kirfel J, Magin TM, Reichelt J. Keratins: a structural scaffold with emerging functions. Cell Mol Life Sci. 2003;60:56–71.

Nisman B, Lafair J, Heching N, Lyass O, Baras M, Barak V. Evaluation of tissue polypeptide specific antigen, CYFRA 21-1 and carcinoembryonic antigen in non small cell lung carcinoma: does the combined use of cytokeratin markers give an additional information? Cancer. 1998a;10:1850–9.

Nisman B, Lafair J, Heshing N, Lyass O, Peretz T, Barak V. Prognostic value of CEA, Cyfra 21-1 and TPS in different subtypes of lung cancer. Anticancer Res. 1998b;18:4982.

O'Hanlon DM, Kerin MJ, O'Boyle C, et al. Tissue polypeptide specific antigen (TPS) in breast cancer – an initial evaluation. Eur J Surg Oncol. 1996;22:38–41.

Osborn M, Weber K. Intermediate filaments: cell-type specific markers in the differentiation and pathology. Cell. 1982;31:303–6.

Parry D, Steinert PM. Intermediate filaments: molecular architecture, assembly, dynamics and polymorphism. Q Rev Biophys. 1999;32:99–187.

Pujol JL, Grenier J, Parrat E, et al. Cytokeratins as serum markers in lung cancer: a comparison of Cyfra 21-1 and TPS. Am J Respir Crit Care Med. 1996;154:725–33.

Rydlander L, Ziegler E, Bergman T, et al. Molecular characterization of a tissue-polypeptide-specific-antigen epitope and its relationship to human cytokeratin 18. Eur J Biochem. 1996;241:309–14.

Schuurman JJ, Bong SB, Einarsson R. Determination of serum tumor markers TPS and CA 15–3 during monitoring of treatment in metastatic breast cancer patients. Anticancer Res. 1996;16:2169–72.

Sedlaczek P, Frydecka I, Gabrys M, van Dalen A, Einarsson R, Harlozinska A. Comparative analysis CA125, tissue polypeptide specific antigen, and soluble Interleukin-2 receptor alpha levels in sera, cyst, and ascitic fluids from patients with ovarian carcinoma. Cancer. 2002;95:1886–93.

Slesak B, Harlozinska-Szmyrka A, Knast W, Sedlaczek P, van Dalen A, Einarsson R. Tissue polypeptide specific antigen (TPS), a marker for differentiation between pancreatic carcinoma and chronic pancreatitis. Cancer. 2000;89:83–8.

Stieber P, Dienemann H, Hasholzner U, et al. Comparison of cytokeratin fragment 19 (CYFRA 21-1), tissue polypeptide antigen (TPA) and tissue polypeptide specific antigen (TPS) as tumour markers in lung cancer. Eur J Clin Chem Clin Biochem. 1993;31:689–94.

Van Dalen A. TPS in breast cancer – a comparative study with carcinoembryonic antigen and CA 15–3. Tumour Biol. 1992;13:10–7.

Van Dalen A, Heering KJ, Barak V, et al. Treatment response in metastatic breast cancer: a multicenter study comparing UICC criteria and tumor marker changes. Breast. 1996;5:82–8.

Van Dalen A, Barak V, Cremaschi A, et al. The prognostic significance of increasing marker levels in metastatic breast cancer patients with clinically complete remission, partial remission or stable disease. A multicenter study. Int J Biol Markers. 1998;13:10–5.

Van Dalen A, Favier J, Baumgartner L, et al. Prognostic significance of CA 125 and TPS levels after chemotherapy in ovarian cancer patients. Anticancer Res. 1999;19:2523–6.

van Dalen A, Favier J, Burges A, et al. Prognostic significance of CA 125 and TPS levels after 3 chemotherapy courses in ovarian cancer patients. Gynecol Oncol. 2000;79:444–50.

Weber K, Osborn M, Moll R, Wiklund B, Luning B. Tissue polypeptide antigen (TPA) is related to the non-epidermal keratins 8, 18 and 19 typical of simple and non-squamous epithelia: re-evaluation of a human tumor marker. EMBO J. 1984;3:2707–14.

CD133 as Biomarker in Breast Cancer

20

Tasuku Matsuoka and Masakazu Yashiro

Contents

Abstract

Breast cancer is one of the most common malignant diseases worldwide. Prognosis of breast cancer is still poor despite the diagnostic and therapeutic progress in recent years. In order to decrease breast cancer-related deaths, many studies are aimed at identifying novel screening- and prognosis-related biomarkers. Cancer stem cells (CSCs) are characterized by the capacity for self-renewal, tumorigenesis, and differentiation. Due to the role of cancer stem cells in tumor initiation and treatment failure, studies of CSC markers have been of great interest. CD133, five transmembrane single-chain glycoproteins, has been successfully used as a stem cell marker to identify and isolate CSCs in malignant tumors. CD133 can also be used to predict tumor metastasis, patient survival and

T. Matsuoka • M. Yashiro (✉)
Department of Surgical Oncology, Osaka City University Graduate School of Medicine, Osaka, Japan
e-mail: m4808279@med.osaka-cu.ac.jp; m9312510@med.osaka-cu.ac.jp

V.R. Preedy, V.B. Patel (eds.), *Biomarkers in Cancer, Biomarkers in Disease: Methods, Discoveries and Applications*,
DOI 10.1007/978-94-007-7681-4_24

resistance to therapy. This chapter provides an overview of the evidence regarding the existence and function of CD133 in breast cancers in the context of the experimental and clinical data. It also discusses CD133 as a possible target for breast cancer therapy.

List of Abbreviations

ALDH	Aldehyde Dehydrogenase
CSCs	Cancer Stem Cells
DFS	Disease-Free Survival
HIF	Hypoxic Inducible Factor
NAC	Neoadjuvant Therapy
OS	Overall Survival
TGF-β	Transforming Growth Factor-beta
TNBC	Triple-Negative Breast Cancer
Wnt	Wingless Related

Introduction

Breast cancer is a heterogeneous disease comprising various receptor subtypes associated with different biological features, clinical outcome, and response to therapy (Di Cosimo and Baselga 2010). Tumor markers (e.g., carcinoembryonic antigen) are used as primary screening tools, in combination with mammography and sonography in patients testing positive. However, there are currently no tests or biomarkers available for use in early stage tumors that may impact long-term survival (Table 1).

Increasing evidence has recently suggested that a subpopulation of cells exist in tumors, termed cancer stem cells (CSCs). Recent studies have demonstrated that tumors are not recognized as homogeneous masses of proliferating cells, but as heterogeneous tissues containing a hierarchy of cells derived from a single CSC (Clarke et al. 2006). CSCs are also believed to be responsible for tumor initiation, metastasis, and resistance to treatments (Clarke et al. 2006). Numerous data indicate the presence of CSCs in various solid tumors (Visvader and Lindeman 2008). Cell surface markers, such as CD133, CD44, CD24, epithelial cell adhesion molecule (EpCAM), THY1, and ABCB5, are proven to be useful for the determination of CSCs (Bomken et al. 2010). One of the most widely used methods for the isolation of CSCs from tumors is based on cell surface markers such as CD133, CD24, CD29, CD44 (Al-Hajj et al. 2003), and enzyme aldehyde dehydrogenase 1 (ALDH1) (Vermeulen et al. 2008; Visvader and Lindeman 2008).

Success of isolating CSC markers in breast cancer has also become an important issue, particularly in the context of potential therapeutic targeting (Al-Hajj et al. 2003). However, although several studies have shown the presence of breast CSCs based on cell surface marker profiles, a consensus on their characterization is still in progress. CD133 is one of the most frequently used biomarkers in

Table 1 Key fact of breast cancer. This table lists the key facts of breast cancer including the heterogeneity of breast cancer, the classification, and the current problem in detecting the early stage of breast tumors

Breast cancer is a complex and heterogeneous disease consisting of various receptor subtypes
The current classification of breast cancer is based on the pattern of expression of the hormone receptors
Estrogen receptor and/or progesterone receptor and human epidermal receptor 2 (Her2) identify three major breast cancer subtypes
Luminal tumors are hormone receptors positive and Her2 negative
Another subtype is Her2-amplified tumors
Tumors with a lack of expression of the three receptors are termed triple-negative breast cancer. Although the mortality of breast cancer is improving, that of triple-negative breast cancer (TNBC) remains precisely high
There are currently no tests or biomarkers available in the early stage of breast tumors which cause long-term survival

Table 2 Key fact of cancer stem cells (CSCs). This table lists the key facts of CSCs including the concept of CSCs, the role, and the importance in targeting CSCs

CSCs are characterized by self-renewal, infinite proliferation, differentiation potential, and high oncogenicity
CSCs are responsible for tumor initiation, metastasis, and resistance to chemo- and radiotherapy
Cell surface markers, such as CD44, CD24, epithelial cell adhesion molecule (EpCAM), THY1, and ABCB5, are proven to be useful for the separation of CSCs
The success in isolating CSC marker in cancer is an important issue particularly in the context of potential therapeutic targeting

CSC-related research for the identification of stem cells from cancerous tissues (Irollo and Pirozzi 2013), and its prognostic value has also been found in many cancers (Collins et al. 2005; Hermann et al. 2007; Ricci-Vitiani et al. 2007; Singh et al. 2004; Suetsugu et al. 2006; Tirino et al. 2009; Table 2).

The search for new prognostic and predictive biomarkers in breast cancer is of interest because patients respond to treatment differently and show variation in prognosis according to subtype (Chavez-MacGregor and Gonzalez-Angulo 2012). In this review, we summarize the latest research findings on the relevance of CD133 in breast cancer initiation and progression, highlighting its potential diagnostic and prognostic applications.

Role of CD133

CD133 is a glycoprotein also known as prominin 1 (Corbeil et al. 2001) or AC133 (Yin et al. 1997). It defines a population of somatic stem and progenitor cells as a marker of the hematopoietic and nervous systems. CD133 is a member of the five transmembrane single-chain glycoprotein family and localizes in cellular plasma membrane protrusions such as microvilli and primary cilia (Fig. 1). It is encoded by

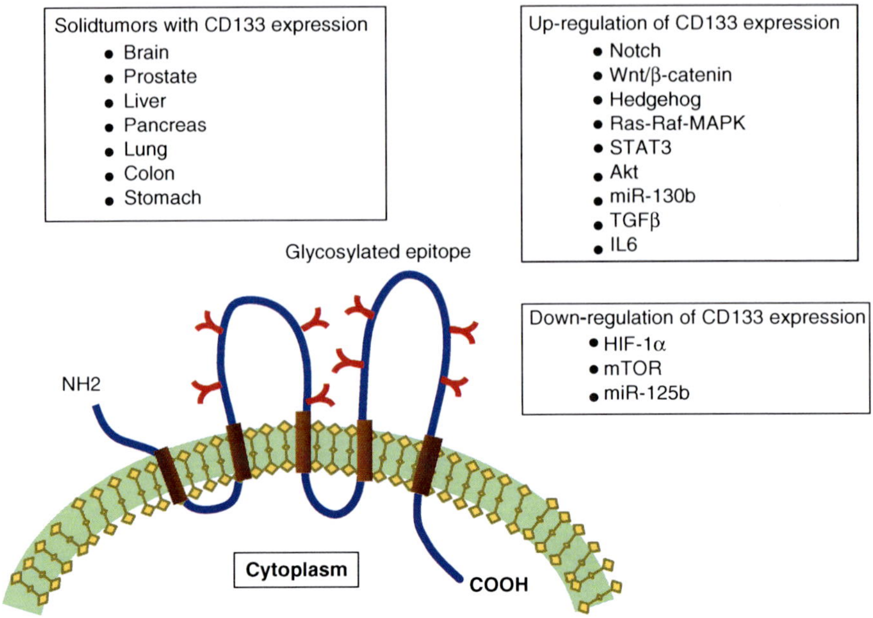

Fig. 1 **Structure and regulation of CD133**. The CD133 protein is a member of five transmembrane single-chain glycoproteins consisting of 865 amino acids, and its molecular weight is about 120 kDa. The molecular structure of CD133 includes one extracellular NH2 terminal, two big extracellular annuli, five membrane-spanning domains, two small intracellular annuli containing rich cysteines, and one intracellular COOH structure. CD133 expression is regulated by several signaling pathways. Some cytokines are also positively associated with the expression of CD133

up to 27 exons of the *PROM1* gene mapped on chromosome 4p15, which are subject to alternative splicing (Yin et al. 1997). Transcription of CD133 is driven by five tissue-specific alternative promoters, resulting in the formation of differentiated spliced mRNA isoforms and CD133 variants with distinct cytoplasmic C-terminal domains. CD133 is recognized as a marker for identification and isolation of specific cell subpopulations, being used as a putative CSC population from malignant tumors of the brain (Singh et al. 2004), prostate (Collins et al. 2005), liver (Suetsugu et al. 2006), pancreas (Hermann et al. 2007), lung (Tirino et al. 2009), and colon (Ricci-Vitiani et al. 2007). CD133-expressing tumor cells sustain the capability of CSC properties, to self-renew in culture, to differentiate into cells similar to the original tumor, and to form tumors in animal xenografts (Fig. 2). Accumulating evidence suggests the growing significance of CD133 as a marker for the major CSC phenotype.

To elucidate the molecular function of CD133, many investigators have analyzed CD133-positive and CD133-negative subpopulations of different cell lines and demonstrated that CD133+ cells have stemness properties such as self-renewal, differentiation ability, and tumorigenicity (Shmelkov et al. 2005; Tirino et al. 2008, 2009).

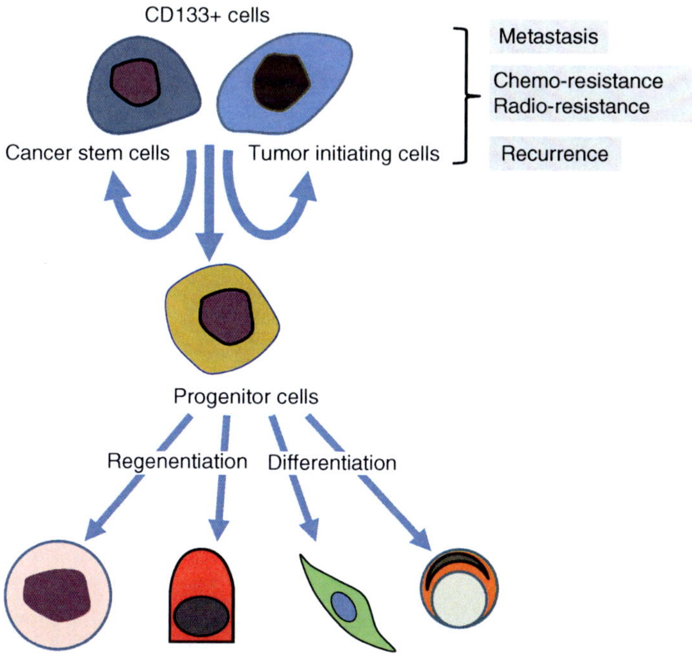

Fig. 2 The role of CD133 cells. CD133+ progenitor or stem cells are activated to self-renew, proliferate, and differentiate in order to repair the damage. CD133+ CSCs are responsible for tumor metastasis, chemo- or radio-resistance, and recurrence

Moreover, it has been demonstrated that CD133+ cells are more resistant to radiation and standard chemotherapy than CD133− cells. In contrast, other studies have shown that CD133− cells can also initiate the same characteristics as those positive for CD133+ (Meng et al. 2009). Hence, certain inconsistencies between published data on CD133 function can be attributed to the difference of opinion with regard to its main role as a specific marker of CSCs. Key facts of CD133 were summarized in Table 3.

The oxygen microenvironment influences stem cell development and maintenance (Mohyeldin et al. 2010), and the most appealing hypothesis in support of this finding is that stem cells may possibly benefit from hypoxic niches where oxidative DNA damage is reduced. Upregulation of a CD133+ CSC subpopulation was demonstrated in the brain tumor cultures under low oxygen concentrations (Platet et al. 2007). In contrast, in gastric and colorectal cancer cell lines, the *CD133* mRNA expression was downregulated at 0.1 % oxygen (Matsumoto et al. 2009), suggesting that observations cannot be generalized. In particular, the level of CD133 expression was positively correlated with the increasing level of hypoxic inducible factor (HIF). HIF-1α regulates the expression of several members of the Notch signaling pathway, CD133, and markers of basal lineage in mammary tumors (Schwab et al. 2012).

Table 3 Key fact of CD133. This table lists the key facts of CD133 including the structure, the expressed cancer cells, function, and the problem as CSC biomarker

CD133, originally known as AC133, is a glycoprotein also known in humans and rodents as prominin 1
CD133 is a member of five transmembrane single-chain glycoproteins and localizes to cellular plasma membrane protrusions
CD133 is used as a putative CSC population from malignant tumors of the brain, prostate, liver, pancreas, lung, stomach, and colon
CD133+ cells have stemness properties such as self-renewal, differentiation ability, and retained tumor-initiating capacity. CD133+ cells are resistant to radiation and chemotherapy
CD133 is upregulated in several malignant tumors, suggesting that CD133 might be a specific surface molecule of CSCs
Other studies demonstrated that CD133− cells can also initiate the same characteristics of those positive for CD133+. Other functional, still unknown markers and/or environmental factors might cause this discrepancy

Regulation of CD133

Several pathways, including the wingless-related (Wnt), transforming growth factor-beta (TGF-β), Notch, and Hedgehog signaling pathways (Roy and Majumdar 2012), have been shown to be correlated with the CD133 expression in malignant tumors. The Wnt pathway plays a pivotal role in the proliferation and maintenance of CSCs. Wnt signaling interfered with the CD133 expression in Wnt-conditioned culture media (Nikolova et al. 2007) and enhanced a CD133+ population in Wnt3-treated prostaspheres (Bisson and Prowse 2009). TGF-β1 was shown to be capable of upregulating the CD133 expression specifically within the Huh-7 hepatocellular carcinoma cell line in a time- and dose-dependent manner (You et al. 2010). MicroRNA (miRNA) profiling showed that miRNA, miR-130b (Ma et al. 2010), and miR-125b (Shi et al. 2012) are involved in the regulation of CD133 expression in a various cells. Forcing the expression of miR-130b in CD133− cells increased resistance to therapy, self-renewal, and tumorigenicity in vivo, whereas upregulation of miR-125b inhibited the invasive ability of CD133+ glioblastoma cells.

The CD133 expression is also regulated by epigenetic factors. Methylation of the CD133 promoter repressed CD133 gene transcription, whereas demethylation of the CD133 gene has been demonstrated in various human malignancies, including colorectal cancer (Hibi et al. 2009), gastric cancer (Hibi et al. 2010), glioblastoma (Tabu et al. 2008), and ovarian cancer (Baba et al. 2009). TGF-β1 inhibited the expression of DNA methyltransferases 1 and 3β and induced the demethylation of promoter-1 of CD133 (You et al. 2010).

In addition, CD133+ CSCs may be associated with the Ras–Raf (Kemper et al. 2012), STAT3 (Lin et al. 2011), Akt, and mitogen-activated protein kinase (Wang et al. 2010). In breast cancer, IL-6 also induced loss of methylation at CD133 promoter region 1 and the CD44 proximal promoter, enhancing CD133 and CD44 gene transcription in basal-like breast cancer (D'Anello et al. 2010).

CD133 as a Diagnostic Marker in Breast Cancer

CD133 was first reported to identify CSCs in brain tumors (Singh et al. 2004). Subsequently, in a study on colon cancer, tumorigenic CSCs were found to be included among a high-density CD133+ population (Ricci-Vitiani et al. 2007). Initial reports on breast CSCs described the use of CD44+/CD24^{low} / ALDH1+ cells to select CSCs (Al-Hajj et al. 2003; Ginestier et al. 2007). Although the investigation of CD133 as a surface marker in the breast CSCs is still in progress, CD133 remains a promising candidate among several proposed stem-like markers.

Studies examining the association between breast cancer and CS133 are summarized in Table 4. To the best of our knowledge, the first report of the potential use of CD133 as a diagnostic marker in breast cancer was in 2008 (Storci et al. 2008; Wright et al. 2008), when its expression was shown to correlate with clinicopathological factors. The positive expression of CD133 in invasive ductal carcinoma was shown by immunohistochemistry to be related to the tumor size and stage and lymph node metastasis (Liu et al. 2009). In addition, CD133+ immunoreactivity was found to be correlated with the tumor size and nodal involvement in 74 unselected tumors (Liu et al. 2009). Another study described how CD133+ tumor cells were associated with younger women, high tumor grade, and negative hormone receptors, regarded as features of more aggressive tumors (Currie et al. 2013). In addition, the hypoxia marker CAIX was also found to be associated with CD133+ tumors. On the other hand, CD133 was highly expressed in inflammatory breast cancer, a particularly lethal form of breast cancer characterized by exaggerated lymphovascular invasion. Single CD133+ cells demonstrated a capacity for both proliferation and the ability of recapitulating the unique temporal phenotype (Xiao et al. 2008). Furthermore, a CD326−/CD45− fraction of patients with elevated SNAIL1 and ZEB1 transcripts also had a higher percentage of ALDH+/CD133+ cells in their blood than those with normal SNAIL1 and ZEB1 expression (Giordano et al. 2012). Another study revealed that a third population of xenograft-initiating cells enriched in CD44+/CD49f^{high}/CD133^{high}/ER-negative breast cancer cells showed an elevated tumorigenicity and self-renewal in vivo (Meyer et al. 2010).

Although mortality rates in breast cancer are improving because of developments in diagnosis and therapy, those in triple-negative breast cancer (TNBC) remain high (Bauer et al. 2007). Thus, the characterization of TNBC may be important for evaluating patient outcomes and for developing a molecular-based therapeutic strategy. One recent study revealed that CD133+ immunoreactivity was correlated with the tumor size and nodal involvement in 67 cases of TNBC (Zhao et al. 2011). The CD133 expression was significantly associated with the expression of the cell cycle progression inhibitor, geminin, in particular for TNBC. This association between the expression of CD133 and geminin could be useful in molecular stratification (Di Bonito et al. 2012a). CD133 was significantly hypomethylated in TNBC versus non-TNBC in 91 American Joint Committee on Cancer stage I–III primary breast cancer tumors. Methylation status levels of

Table 4 Experimental studies performed to study CD133 in breast cancer. This table lists the experimental studies performed to study CD133 in breast cancer

Category	Authors	Material	Results
Diagnosis	Lehmann C et al.	Cell lines	The cell lines isolated from human breast cancer tumors did not expressed CD133
	Currie MJ et al.	Tumor specimens	CD133+ tumor cells were associated with younger women, high tumor grade, and negative hormone receptors. No significant relationships were observed between the markers studied and survival for 5 years
	Giordano A et al.	Tumor specimens	The CD326−/CD45− fraction of patients with elevated SNAIL1 and ZEB1 transcripts also had a higher percentage of ALDH+/CD133+ cells in their blood than patients with normal SNAIL1 and ZEB1 expression
	Di Bonito M et al.	Tumor specimens	CD133 expression was significantly associated to cell cycle progression inhibitor, geminin, in particular for TNBC. CD133 expression was associated with ductal breast cancer histotype and Ki67 expression
	Kagara N et al.	Tumor specimens	CD133 was significantly hypomethylated in TNBC versus non-TNBC in 91 primary breast cancer tumors
	Liu TJ et al.	Cell lines/tumor specimens	CD133+ phenotype was positively associated with vasculogenic mimicry in breast cancer specimen
	Schwab LP et al.	Cell lines	CD133 expression was reduced in HIF-1alpha-null cells and in tumorspheres. Tumorsphere formation was enhanced in CD133hi versus CD133neg cells sorted from PyMT tumors
	Zhao P et al.	Tumor specimens	CD133+ immunoreactivity has been correlated with tumor size and nodal involvement in 67 triple-negative tumors
	D'Anello L et al.	Cell lines	IL-6 elicits the loss of methylation at the CD133 promoter region 1, enhancing CD133 gene transcription in basal-like breast cancer
	Meyer MJ et al.	Tumor specimens	A population of xenograft-initiating cells enriched in CD44^{pos}CD49f^{hi}CD133/2^{hi}
			ER-negative breast cancer cells display heightened tumorigenicity and self-renewal in vivo
	Liu Q et al.	Tumor specimens	The expression of CD133 in breast cancer was shown to correlate with clinicopathological factors. CD133+ immunoreactivity has been correlated with the tumor size and nodal involvement
	Xiao Y et al.	Cell lines/tumor specimens	CD133 was highly expressed in inflammatory breast cancer. CD133+ cells demonstrated a capacity for both proliferation and the ability of recapitulating the temporal phenotype

(*continued*)

Table 4 (continued)

Category	Authors	Material	Results
	Wright MH et al.	Cell lines	Brca1 breast tumors contain distinct CD44 +/CD24- and CD133+ cells with cancer stem cell characteristics
	Storci G et al.	Cell lines/ tumor specimens	Tumor tissues of breast cancer expressing high levels of SLUG mRNA express high levels of CD133
Prognosis	Aomatsu N et al.	Tumor specimens	CD133 expression in breast cancer patients treated with epirubicin followed by paclitaxel was associated with survival. Recurrence was more frequent in patients with CD133-positive tumors compared with negative ones
	Giuffre G et al.	Tumor specimens	CD133 expression is associated with the appearance of distant metastases
	Ieni A et al.	Tumor specimens	CD133 showed a highly significant value regarding metastatic localizations in the bone
	Yan X et al.	Tumor specimens	CD133 gene signature distinguishes higher-grade breast cancers from their lower-grade counterparts
Chemoradiotherapy response	Liu H et al.	Cell lines	CD133 mRNA expression levels in tamoxifen-resistant breast cancer cells were significantly higher than those in wild-type cells
	Nadal R et al.	Tumor specimens	Enrichment of CK+/CD133+ CTCs in nonluminal breast cancer subtypes was observed after systemic therapy
	Di Bonito M et al.	Tumor specimens	CD133 expression was heterogeneous in different carcinomas but was strikingly hyperexpressed in a tubulolobular variant of breast cancer
	Achuthan S et al.	Cell lines	Therapy-resistant cells displayed higher CD133 and Oct-4 expression in breast cancer cell lines
	Mine T et al.	Cell lines	The numbers of $CD44^{hi}$ $CD24^{lo}$, $CD44^{hi}$ $CD133^{+}$, and $CD24^{lo}$ $CD133^{+}$ cells in gemcitabine-, paclitaxel-, and 5-fluorouracil-resistant breast cancer lines are higher compared with drug-sensitive lines
Therapeutic target	Koshio J et al.	Cell lines	An immunogenic protein, DEAD/H (Asp–Glu–Ala–Asp/His) box polypeptide 3, X-linked (DDX3X), is preferentially expressed in CD133(+) tumor cells, including breast cancer cells
	Swaminathan SK et al.	Cell lines	Tumor regrowth during free paclitaxel was significantly lower when paclitaxel was delivered through polymeric nanoparticles targeting CD133
	Sun B et al.	Cell lines	The sodium butyrate-resistant cells showed the expression of CD133
	Sun J et al.	Cell lines	Suppression of CD133 activity by LS-7 reduced the migration of breast cancer cell lines

CD133 could serve as surrogate biomarkers for identifying TNBC (Kagara et al. 2012). Liu et al. showed that lymph node metastasis and higher histological grade were correlated with the CD133 expression, with the CD133+ rate much higher in TNBC than in the luminal and HER2+ subtypes. This finding suggests that CD133+ is closely associated with TNBC. Moreover, the CD133+ phenotype was positively associated with vasculogenic mimicry in breast cancer specimens (Liu et al. 2013).

CD133 as a Prognostic Marker in Breast Cancer

Several studies have demonstrated the use of CD133 as a marker predictive of postoperative recurrence; CD133 is found not only in primary tumors but also in metastatic tumors such as liver metastases in the colon cancer cells. Aomatsu N. et al. examined the association between survival and the CD133 expression in patients with breast cancer treated with epirubicin followed by paclitaxel (Aomatsu et al. 2012). DFS and OS in patients with CD133-positive tumors were significantly shorter than in patients with CD133-negative tumors prior to neoadjuvant therapy (NAC). In contrast, the ALDH1 expression did not correlate with regard to DFS and OS. Univariate and multivariate regression analysis indicated that the CD133 expression prior to NAC was an independent prognostic factor for DFS. In agreement with this, the expression of CD133 corresponded to the tumor size, clinical stage, and lymphatic metastasis. The CD133 expression was found to be related to the overall survival and disease-free survival in patients with TNBC (Zhao et al. 2011). Values of CD133 were highly significant with regard to metastatic localizations in bone by multivariate analysis; CD133 emerged as the only independent prognostic variable (Ieni et al. 2011). However, no significant differences were observed in DFS or OS for patients with tumors expressing any of the three stem cell markers studied, including CD133 (Currie et al. 2013). Discrepancies among studies can result from differences in patient characteristics, study design, or the use of commercial antibodies, which may lead to high background interference. More uniform studies should be performed to elucidate these issues.

Several studies have shown a significant correlation between prognosis and the CD133 expression. Evidence from clinical studies showed that the expression of CD133 is associated with a poor prognosis in patients with advanced colon cancer (Li et al. 2009). Intercomparison among gene expression profiles showed that the CD133 gene signature identifies an aggressive subtype of glioblastoma seen in younger patients and characterized by shorter duration of survival (Yan et al. 2011), and it was reported that the CD133+/CD44+ subpopulation is responsible for this metastasis (Chen et al. 2011). Among several CSC markers, CD133 was immunohistochemically shown to be more highly expressed in patients with distant metastasis of node-negative invasive breast carcinoma, suggesting that it may be a useful biomarker candidate in tumor metastasis (Giuffre et al. 2011).

CD133 as a Biomarker in Chemoradiotherapeutic Response in Breast Cancer

Sensitivity to drug therapy and radiation is considered to be responsible for the poor response to current anticancer drugs (Tentes et al. 2010), and CSCs are believed to contribute to resistance to cytotoxic therapies (Clarke et al. 2006). An association between CSCs and chemoresistance in breast cancer cells has been shown in vitro (Achuthan et al. 2011; Di Bonito et al. 2012b; Liu et al. 2006; Nadal et al. 2013). In glioma, CD133 selected for a population of cells exhibited radiation resistance, and CD133+ cells exhibited increased clonogenic survival (Bao et al. 2006), with one clinical study providing supportive evidence for this hypothesis (Ong et al. 2010).

Our data revealed that the CD133 expression is significantly related to chemosensitivity. Recurrence was more frequent in patients with CD133+ tumors compared with CD133−, suggesting that CD133 may be a useful marker in predicting the effectiveness of NAC and recurrence of breast cancer (Aomatsu et al. 2012). The numbers of $CD44^{high}$, $CD24^{low}$, and CD133+ cells in gemcitabine-, paclitaxel-, and 5-fluorouracil-resistant breast cancer lines, respectively, were higher compared with corresponding drug-sensitive lines (Mine et al. 2009). A recent study showed that the CD133 expression is associated with ductal breast cancer histotype and Ki67 expression. The authors also mentioned the importance of the detection of stem cell niches by CD133 in all phenotypic variants of breast carcinoma (Di Bonito et al. 2012b). The CD133 mRNA expression levels in tamoxifen-resistant breast cancer cells were significantly higher than those in wild-type cells (Liu et al. 2006). Enrichment of cytokeratin+/CD133+ circulating tumor cells in nonluminal breast cancer subtypes was observed after systemic therapy, suggesting a potential role in resistance to therapy (Nadal et al. 2013). Therapy-resistant cells displayed higher CD133 and Oct-4 expression in breast cancer cell lines (Achuthan et al. 2011), suggesting that CD133 is a good predictor of resistance in chemoradiation therapy.

Therapeutic Insights into Targeting CD133

Several attempts have been made to use CD133 in cancer treatment, with successful targeting in hepatocellular and gastric cancer xenografts reported (Smith et al. 2008). These data suggest that CD133, in addition to its role as a CSC marker, is an important cancer therapeutic target. CD133 monoclonal antibody conjugated by cytolethal distending toxin preferentially inhibited the growth of CD133+ cancer cell lines derived from head and neck carcinomas (Damek-Poprawa et al. 2011), whereas siRNAs decreased the number of CD133 molecules in melanoma cells (Rappa et al. 2008). Cell growth, cell motility, and spheroid-forming capacity were inhibited as a result of downregulation of CD133. In addition, nanotubes conjugated with CD133 monoclonal antibodies blocked the self-renewal character of CD133+ glioblastoma cells (Wang et al. 2011).

DEAD/H (Asp–Glu–Ala–Asp/His) box polypeptide 3, X-linked (DDX3X) is a major immunogenic target protein of CD133+ melanoma cells. Vaccination with synthesized DDX3X protein exhibited therapeutic efficacy against established skin melanoma, effecting curing of the tumor. Because DDX3X is expressed in breast cancer cells, this finding indicates that anti-DDX3X immunotherapy may be a promising strategy (Koshio et al. 2013). Tumor growth was lower when paclitaxel was delivered through polymeric nanoparticles targeting CD133 (Swaminathan et al. 2013). Cells resistant to sodium butyrate, a potent histone deacetylase inhibitor and anticancer agent, showed the expression of CD133. The CD133+ group presents a higher level of c-MET, and a combination treatment regimen of MET siRNA and sodium butyrate efficiently inhibited breast cancer progression (Sun et al. 2012a). The possibility of targeting breast CSCs by CD133 inhibition provides a novel therapeutic approach in the treatment of breast tumors.

Future Perspectives

Limitations of CD133 as a Breast Cancer Biomarker

Although CD133 has been used as a marker to identify CSCs, contradictory results have been reported in several recent studies. In colon cancer, the CD133 expression was not restricted to tumor initiation (Shmelkov et al. 2008) because it did not distinguish the entire population of tumor-initiating cells. CD133− glioma cells proved tumorigenic in nude rats, and CD133+ cells were obtained from these tumors, suggesting that the CD133 expression may not be required for brain tumor initiation (Wang et al. 2008). These findings raise a major issue about the validity of CD133 as a marker for CSCs. In breast cancer, established CSC markers are not indicative of in vivo tumorigenicity, and the cell lines S2 and S2N isolated from human breast cancer tumors did not express CD133 (Lehmann et al. 2012). The authors of this paper suggest that other functional, hitherto unknown, markers and/or environmental factors may impact increased tumorigenicity in breast cancer, and further studies have been conducted in several kinds of tumor to investigate this discrepancy (Kawamoto et al. 2010; Liao et al. 2010).

Future Perspectives

Because CD133 cannot be used as a specific marker to characterize CSCs in breast cancer for a precise detection of the stemness of cancer cells, other markers should be used in combination with CD133. ALDH+/CD133+ cells generated tumor initiation more strongly than ALDH+/CD133− cells (Huang et al. 2009). The incidence of tumor cells positive for stem cell-like and more differentiated cell markers varies according to the tumor subtype and histological stage (Park et al. 2010). For example, cytokeratin+/CD133+ CTCs were significantly associated with non-amplified HER2 and primary tumors with slow proliferation index. This finding indicates genetic heterogeneity in promoting diversity for the expression of stem cell markers in cancer cells. $ALDH^{high}$/CD44+/CD133+ cells showed enhanced tumorigenicity and metastasis relative to ALDH(low)/D44(low/−) cells (Croker et al. 2009).

However, it remains to be elucidated which combination of these markers is optimal to identify CSC or shows biological characters consistent with CSCs. Moreover, little is known about the function of CD133 (e.g., what is the ligand and downstream signaling of CD133?). Whether CD133 participates in the biological behavior of CSC or merely acts as a marker of CSC phenotype is unclear. Although it remains a challenge to incorporate the regulatory and functional data of CD133, several recent studies have identified these questions. CD133 may play a role in cell polarity and integration via cell–cell and cell–matrix interactions (Giebel et al. 2004). shRNA-mediated downregulation had profound effects on human CD133-expressing malignant melanoma cells. CD133 knockdown slowed cell growth, reduced cell motility, and decreased the formation of spheroids under stem cell-like growth conditions. In vivo, the downregulation of CD133 reduced the capacity of cells to metastasize (Rappa et al. 2008). LS-7 (amino acid sequence, LQNAPRS) is a specific binding peptide targeting mouse CD133. The suppression of CD133 activity by LS-7 reduced migration in the breast cancer cell line MA782. In addition, the high specificity and affinity of LS-7 to mCD133 showed that the expression of only c-MET and STAT3 decreased in breast cancer cells exposed to LS-7 (Sun et al. 2012b). Similarly, agar-selected cells (designated GI-AGR) were homogeneous for CD44+ and CD133+ and were fivefold more invasive than the parental GI-101A cells (Guo et al. 2011). These findings may provide new insights into the clarification of the mechanism of CD133 and strategies in breast cancers through its use.

Summary Points

- CD133, a five transmembrane single-chain glycoprotein, is successfully used as a stem cell marker to identify and isolate cancer stem cells in malignant tumors.
- It can be also be used to predict tumor metastasis, patient survival, and resistance to therapy.
- Prognosis of breast cancer is still poor despite the diagnostic and therapeutic progress in recent years.
- This paper reviews the evidence regarding the existence and function of CD133 in breast cancers in the context of experimental and clinical data.
- We also discuss its potential use as a possible target in breast cancer therapy.

Acknowledgments This study is partially funded by KAKENHI (Grant-in-Aid for Scientific Research, Nos. 23390329).

References

Achuthan S, Santhoshkumar TR, Prabhakar J, et al. Drug-induced senescence generates chemoresistant stemlike cells with low reactive oxygen species. J Biol Chem. 2011;286: 37813–29.

Al-Hajj M, Wicha MS, Benito-Hernandez A, et al. Prospective identification of tumorigenic breast cancer cells. Proc Natl Acad Sci U S A. 2003;100:3983–8.

Aomatsu N, Yashiro M, Kashiwagi S, et al. CD133 is a useful surrogate marker for predicting chemosensitivity to neoadjuvant chemotherapy in breast cancer. PLoS One. 2012;7:e45865.

Baba T, Convery PA, Matsumura N, et al. Epigenetic regulation of CD133 and tumorigenicity of CD133+ ovarian cancer cells. Oncogene. 2009;28:209–18.

Bao S, Wu Q, McLendon RE, et al. Glioma stem cells promote radioresistance by preferential activation of the DNA damage response. Nature. 2006;444:756–60.

Bauer KR, Brown M, Cress RD, et al. Descriptive analysis of estrogen receptor (ER)-negative, progesterone receptor (PR)-negative, and HER2-negative invasive breast cancer, the so-called triple-negative phenotype: a population-based study from the California cancer Registry. Cancer. 2007;109:1721–8.

Bisson I, Prowse DM. WNT signaling regulates self-renewal and differentiation of prostate cancer cells with stem cell characteristics. Cell Res. 2009;19:683–97.

Bomken S, Fiser K, Heidenreich O, et al. Understanding the cancer stem cell. Br J Cancer. 2010;103:439–45.

Chavez-MacGregor M, Gonzalez-Angulo AM. Breast cancer in 2012: new drugs, new knowledge, new targets. Nat Rev Clin Oncol. 2012;10:75–6.

Chen KL, Pan F, Jiang H, et al. Highly enriched CD133(+)CD44(+) stem-like cells with CD133(+) CD44(high) metastatic subset in HCT116 colon cancer cells. Clin Exp Metastasis. 2011;28:751–63.

Clarke MF, Dick JE, Dirks PB, et al. Cancer stem cells–perspectives on current status and future directions: AACR workshop on cancer stem cells. Cancer Res. 2006;66:9339–44.

Collins AT, Berry PA, Hyde C, et al. Prospective identification of tumorigenic prostate cancer stem cells. Cancer Res. 2005;65:10946–51.

Corbeil D, Fargeas CA, Huttner WB. Rat prominin, like its mouse and human orthologues, is a pentaspan membrane glycoprotein. Biochem Biophys Res Commun. 2001;285:939–44.

Croker AK, Goodale D, Chu J, et al. High aldehyde dehydrogenase and expression of cancer stem cell markers selects for breast cancer cells with enhanced malignant and metastatic ability. J Cell Mol Med. 2009;13:2236–52.

Currie MJ, Beardsley BE, Harris GC, et al. Immunohistochemical analysis of cancer stem cell markers in invasive breast carcinoma and associated ductal carcinoma in situ: relationships with markers of tumor hypoxia and microvascularity. Hum Pathol. 2013;44:402–11.

D'Anello L, Sansone P, Storci G, et al. Epigenetic control of the basal-like gene expression profile via Interleukin-6 in breast cancer cells. Mol Cancer. 2010;9:300.

Damek-Poprawa M, Volgina A, Korostoff J, et al. Targeted inhibition of CD133+ cells in oral cancer cell lines. J Dent Res. 2011;90:638–45.

Di Bonito M, Cantile M, Collina F, et al. Overexpression of cell cycle progression inhibitor geminin is associated with tumor stem-like phenotype of triple-negative breast cancer. J Breast Cancer. 2012a;15:162–71.

Di Bonito M, Collina F, Cantile M, et al. Aberrant expression of cancer stem cells marker prominin-1 in low-grade tubulolobular breast carcinoma: a correlative study between qRT-PCR, flow-cytometric and immunohistochemistry analysis [corrected]. J Breast Cancer. 2012b;15:15–23.

Di Cosimo S, Baselga J. Management of breast cancer with targeted agents: importance of heterogeneity. [corrected]. Nat Rev Clin Oncol. 2010;7:139–47.

Giebel B, Corbeil D, Beckmann J, et al. Segregation of lipid raft markers including CD133 in polarized human hematopoietic stem and progenitor cells. Blood. 2004;104:2332–8.

Ginestier C, Hur MH, Charafe-Jauffret E, et al. ALDH1 is a marker of normal and malignant human mammary stem cells and a predictor of poor clinical outcome. Cell Stem Cell. 2007;1:555–67.

Giordano A, Gao H, Anfossi S, et al. Epithelial-mesenchymal transition and stem cell markers in patients with HER2-positive metastatic breast cancer. Mol Cancer Ther. 2012;11:2526–34.

Giuffre G, Adamo V, Ieni A, et al. Hematopoietic progenitor cells (HPCs) in node-negative invasive breast carcinomas: immunohistochemical analysis and clinico-pathological correlations. Pathol Res Pract. 2011;207:487–91.

Guo L, Fan D, Zhang F, et al. Selection of brain metastasis-initiating breast cancer cells determined by growth on hard agar. Am J Pathol. 2011;178:2357–66.

Hermann PC, Huber SL, Herrler T, et al. Distinct populations of cancer stem cells determine tumor growth and metastatic activity in human pancreatic cancer. Cell Stem Cell. 2007;1:313–23.

Hibi K, Sakata M, Kitamura YH, et al. Demethylation of the CD133 gene is frequently detected in advanced colorectal cancer. Anticancer Res. 2009;29:2235–7.

Hibi K, Sakata M, Kitamura YH, et al. Demethylation of the CD133 gene is frequently detected in early gastric carcinoma. Anticancer Res. 2010;30:1201–3.

Huang EH, Hynes MJ, Zhang T, et al. Aldehyde dehydrogenase 1 is a marker for normal and malignant human colonic stem cells (SC) and tracks SC overpopulation during colon tumorigenesis. Cancer Res. 2009;69:3382–9.

Ieni A, Giuffre G, Adamo V, et al. Prognostic impact of CD133 immunoexpression in node-negative invasive breast carcinomas. Anticancer Res. 2011;31:1315–20.

Irollo E, Pirozzi G. CD133: to be or not to be, is this the real question? Am J Transl Res. 2013;5:563–81.

Kagara N, Huynh KT, Kuo C, et al. Epigenetic regulation of cancer stem cell genes in triple-negative breast cancer. Am J Pathol. 2012;181:257–67.

Kawamoto H, Yuasa T, Kubota Y, et al. Characteristics of CD133(+) human colon cancer SW620 cells. Cell Transplant. 2010;19:857–64.

Kemper K, Versloot M, Cameron K, et al. Mutations in the Ras-Raf Axis underlie the prognostic value of CD133 in colorectal cancer. Clin Cancer Res. 2012;18:3132–41.

Koshio J, Kagamu H, Nozaki K, et al. DEAD/H (Asp–Glu–Ala–Asp/His) box polypeptide 3, X-linked is an immunogenic target of cancer stem cells. Cancer Immunol Immunother. 2013;62:1619–28.

Lehmann C, Jobs G, Thomas M, et al. Established breast cancer stem cell markers do not correlate with in vivo tumorigenicity of tumor-initiating cells. Int J Oncol. 2012;41:1932–42.

Li CY, Li BX, Liang Y, et al. Higher percentage of CD133+ cells is associated with poor prognosis in colon carcinoma patients with stage IIIB. J Transl Med. 2009;7:56.

Liao Y, Hu X, Huang X, et al. Quantitative analyses of CD133 expression facilitate researches on tumor stem cells. Biol Pharm Bull. 2010;33:738–42.

Lin L, Liu Y, Li H, et al. Targeting colon cancer stem cells using a new curcumin analogue, GO-Y030. Br J Cancer. 2011;105:212–20.

Liu G, Yuan X, Zeng Z, et al. Analysis of gene expression and chemoresistance of CD133+ cancer stem cells in glioblastoma. Mol Cancer. 2006;5:67.

Liu Q, Li JG, Zheng XY, et al. Expression of CD133, PAX2, ESA, and GPR30 in invasive ductal breast carcinomas. Chin Med J (Engl). 2009;122:2763–9.

Liu TJ, Sun BC, Zhao XL, et al. CD133+ cells with cancer stem cell characteristics associates with vasculogenic mimicry in triple-negative breast cancer. Oncogene. 2013;32:544–53.

Ma S, Tang KH, Chan YP, et al. miR-130b Promotes CD133(+) liver tumor-initiating cell growth and self-renewal via tumor protein 53-induced nuclear protein 1. Cell Stem Cell. 2010; 7:694–707.

Matsumoto K, Arao T, Tanaka K, et al. mTOR signal and hypoxia-inducible factor-1 alpha regulate CD133 expression in cancer cells. Cancer Res. 2009;69:7160–4.

Meng X, Li M, Wang X, et al. Both CD133+ and CD133− subpopulations of A549 and H446 cells contain cancer-initiating cells. Cancer Sci. 2009;100:1040–6.

Meyer MJ, Fleming JM, Lin AF, et al. CD44posCD49fhiCD133/2hi defines xenograft-initiating cells in estrogen receptor-negative breast cancer. Cancer Res. 2010;70:4624–33.

Mine T, Matsueda S, Li Y, et al. Breast cancer cells expressing stem cell markers CD44+ CD24 lo are eliminated by Numb-1 peptide-activated T cells. Cancer Immunol Immunother. 2009;58:1185–94.

Mohyeldin A, Garzon-Muvdi T, Quinones-Hinojosa A. Oxygen in stem cell biology: a critical component of the stem cell niche. Cell Stem Cell. 2010;7:150–61.

Nadal R, Ortega FG, Salido M, et al. CD133 expression in circulating tumor cells from breast cancer patients: Potential role in resistance to chemotherapy. Int J Cancer. 2013;133:2398–407.

Nikolova T, Wu M, Brumbarov K, et al. WNT-conditioned media differentially affect the proliferation and differentiation of cord blood-derived CD133+ cells in vitro. Differentiation. 2007;75:100–11.

Ong CW, Kim LG, Kong HH, et al. CD133 expression predicts for non-response to chemotherapy in colorectal cancer. Mod Pathol. 2010;23:450–7.

Park SY, Lee HE, Li H, et al. Heterogeneity for stem cell-related markers according to tumor subtype and histologic stage in breast cancer. Clin Cancer Res. 2010;16:876–87.

Platet N, Liu SY, Atifi ME, et al. Influence of oxygen tension on CD133 phenotype in human glioma cell cultures. Cancer Lett. 2007;258:286–90.

Rappa G, Fodstad O, Lorico A. The stem cell-associated antigen CD133 (Prominin-1) is a molecular therapeutic target for metastatic melanoma. Stem Cells. 2008;26:3008–17.

Ricci-Vitiani L, Lombardi DG, Pilozzi E, et al. Identification and expansion of human colon-cancer-initiating cells. Nature. 2007;445:111–5.

Roy S, Majumdar AP. Signaling in colon cancer stem cells. J Mol Signal. 2012;7:11.

Schwab LP, Peacock DL, Majumdar D, et al. Hypoxia-inducible factor 1alpha promotes primary tumor growth and tumor-initiating cell activity in breast cancer. Breast Cancer Res. 2012;14: R6.

Shi L, Wan Y, Sun G, et al. Functional differences of miR-125b on the invasion of primary glioblastoma CD133-negative cells and CD133-positive cells. Neuromolecular Med. 2012;14:303–16.

Shmelkov SV, Meeus S, Moussazadeh N, et al. Cytokine preconditioning promotes codifferentiation of human fetal liver CD133+ stem cells into angiomyogenic tissue. Circulation. 2005;111:1175–83.

Shmelkov SV, Butler JM, Hooper AT, et al. CD133 expression is not restricted to stem cells, and both CD133+ and CD133− metastatic colon cancer cells initiate tumors. J Clin Invest. 2008;118:2111–20.

Singh SK, Hawkins C, Clarke ID, et al. Identification of human brain tumour initiating cells. Nature. 2004;432:396–401.

Smith LM, Nesterova A, Ryan MC, et al. CD133/prominin-1 is a potential therapeutic target for antibody-drug conjugates in hepatocellular and gastric cancers. Br J Cancer. 2008;99:100–9.

Storci G, Sansone P, Trere D, et al. The basal-like breast carcinoma phenotype is regulated by SLUG gene expression. J Pathol. 2008;214:25–37.

Suetsugu A, Nagaki M, Aoki H, et al. Characterization of CD133+ hepatocellular carcinoma cells as cancer stem/progenitor cells. Biochem Biophys Res Commun. 2006;351:820–4.

Sun B, Liu R, Xiao ZD, et al. c-MET protects breast cancer cells from apoptosis induced by sodium butyrate. PLoS One. 2012a;7:e30143.

Sun J, Zhang C, Liu G, et al. A novel mouse CD133 binding-peptide screened by phage display inhibits cancer cell motility in vitro. Clin Exp Metastasis. 2012b;29:185–96.

Swaminathan SK, Roger E, Toti U, et al. CD133-targeted paclitaxel delivery inhibits local tumor recurrence in a mouse model of breast cancer. J Control Release. 2013;171:280–7.

Tabu K, Sasai K, Kimura T, et al. Promoter hypomethylation regulates CD133 expression in human gliomas. Cell Res. 2008;18:1037–46.

Tentes IK, Schmidt WM, Krupitza G, et al. Long-term persistence of acquired resistance to 5-fluorouracil in the colon cancer cell line SW620. Exp Cell Res. 2010;316:3172–81.

Tirino V, Desiderio V, d'Aquino R, et al. Detection and characterization of CD133+ cancer stem cells in human solid tumours. PLoS One. 2008;3:e3469.

Tirino V, Camerlingo R, Franco R, et al. The role of CD133 in the identification and characterisation of tumour-initiating cells in non-small-cell lung cancer. Eur J Cardiothorac Surg. 2009;36:446–53.

Vermeulen L, Todaro M, de Sousa MF, et al. Single-cell cloning of colon cancer stem cells reveals a multi-lineage differentiation capacity. Proc Natl Acad Sci U S A. 2008;105:13427–32.

Visvader JE, Lindeman GJ. Cancer stem cells in solid tumours: accumulating evidence and unresolved questions. Nat Rev Cancer. 2008;8:755–68.

Wang YK, Zhu YL, Qiu FM, et al. Activation of Akt and MAPK pathways enhances the tumorigenicity of CD133+ primary colon cancer cells. Carcinogenesis. 2010;31:1376–80.

Wang CH, Chiou SH, Chou CP, et al. Photothermolysis of glioblastoma stem-like cells targeted by carbon nanotubes conjugated with CD133 monoclonal antibody. Nanomedicine. 2011;7:69–79.

Wang J, Sakariassen PØ, Tsinkalovsky O, et al. CD133 negative glioma cells form tumors in nude rats and give rise to CD133 positive cells. Int J Cancer. 2008;122:761–8.

Wright MH, Calcagno AM, Salcido CD, et al. Brca1 breast tumors contain distinct CD44+/CD24- and CD133+ cells with cancer stem cell characteristics. Breast Cancer Res. 2008;10:R10.

Xiao Y, Ye Y, Yearsley K, et al. The lymphovascular embolus of inflammatory breast cancer expresses a stem cell-like phenotype. Am J Pathol. 2008;173:561–74.

Yan X, Ma L, Yi D, et al. A CD133-related gene expression signature identifies an aggressive glioblastoma subtype with excessive mutations. Proc Natl Acad Sci U S A. 2011;108:1591–6.

Yin AH, Miraglia S, Zanjani ED, et al. AC133, a novel marker for human hematopoietic stem and progenitor cells. Blood. 1997;90:5002–12.

You H, Ding W, Rountree CB. Epigenetic regulation of cancer stem cell marker CD133 by transforming growth factor-beta. Hepatology. 2010;51:1635–44.

Zhao P, Lu Y, Jiang X, et al. Clinicopathological significance and prognostic value of CD133 expression in triple-negative breast carcinoma. Cancer Sci. 2011;102:1107–11.

Prognostic and Predictive Biomarkers for Castration Resistant Prostate Cancer

21

Jing Li and Andrew J. Armstrong

Contents

J. Li
Duke University and Cancer Institute, Durham, NC, USA

A.J. Armstrong (✉)
Duke Cancer Institute, Duke Prostate Center, Divisions of Medical Oncology and Urology, Duke University School of Medicine, Durham, NC, USA
e-mail: andrew.armstrong@duke.edu

V.R. Preedy, V.B. Patel (eds.), *Biomarkers in Cancer, Biomarkers in Disease: Methods, Discoveries and Applications*,
DOI 10.1007/978-94-007-7681-4_13

Abstract

Despite significant advances in diagnosis and management, prostate cancer is still a leading cause of cancer-related death in men. Castration-resistant prostate cancer (CRPC) is defined by disease progression despite androgen deprivation and castrate levels of testosterone. There have been a rapidly increasing number of new systematic agents which have been approved by the USFDA for men with metastatic CRPC, based on the results of successful phase 3 trials of a diverse range of agents with immunomodulatory, hormonal, bone-targeting, and microtubule-targeting mechanisms of action. Therefore, it is becoming essential to understand the optimal and rational combination and sequences of these treatments in the clinic, as well as to identify patients most likely to benefit from a specific treatment. Minimizing harms and costs of ineffective therapies is an equally important goal. Predictive biomarkers linked to relevant clinical outcomes are thus needed in drug development in CRPC, and there is an increasing need for these biomarkers to guide a clinician's decision. We discuss in this chapter existing and emerging prognostic and predictive biomarkers in CRPC and future directions of biomarker development in men with CRPC.

Key Facts

Key Facts of CRPC

- Despite high response rates to androgen deprivation therapy in men with advanced and recurrent prostate cancer, almost all will develop lethal castration-resistant metastatic disease.
- Based on the concept that reactivated androgen- and AR-based pathways still continue to stimulate CRPC progression, abiraterone acetate and enzalutamide were developed and play a significant role in the management of men with metastatic CRPC. Predictive biomarkers based on this biology may aid in patient selection for these therapies.

- Chemotherapy choices for CRPC patients initially include docetaxel, with cabazitaxel or mitoxantrone as second line choices, with multiple available prognostic biomarkers; predictive biomarkers remain to be validated prospectively.

Key Facts of CTCs

- CTCs are cells that have shed into the vasculature from a primary or metastatic tumor, circulate in the blood, and are considered seeds for primary tumors to metastasize to distant place.
- CTCs had been observed for the first time in 1869, but were not objectively measured and quantified in the clinic until recent years, and have emerged as a novel biomarker of prognosis and platform for predictive biology across multiple solid tumor types, both before and during systemic therapies.
- CTCs are considered a "liquid biopsy" which can provide live real-time information about the patient's disease status and biology, and thus, there is great potential for CTCs to provide predictive information about tumor biology that may inform on therapeutic decision-making.

Definitions of Words and Terms

AR-V (Androgen Receptor Variants) AR-V results from premature stop codons due to nonsense mutations or from alternative splicing with the frequent retention of a cryptic exonic sequence.

Biomarker A biomarker is an objectively measured and evaluated tumor or host characteristic to be used as an indicator of normal biological or pathogenic processes or pharmacological responses to a therapeutic intervention.

BSI (Bone Scan Index) Quantitative measurement of the tumor-bone metastatic burden as percentage of total skeletal mass.

CTC (Circulating Tumor Cell) While there are multiple definitions used in research, the USFDA defines a CTC to be a nucleated cell > 4 um in diameter isolated from whole blood using EpCAM-based ferromagnetic antibody and also lacking the leukocyte marker CD45. This definition has been used in clinically validating the Cellsearch assay as a prognostic biomarker in men with mCRPC.

miRNA An miRNA is a small noncoding RNA molecule found in both plants and animals, which functions in transcriptional and posttranscriptional regulation of gene expression.

CRPC (Castration-resistant prostate cancer) Progressive disease despite castrate levels of serum testosterone, usually manifested as a rise in serum PSA despite therapy or progression either radiographically or based on symptoms.

Introduction

The introduction of biomarkers for disease diagnosis and management has been a revolution in the practice of oncology. Biomarkers of import in oncology are indicators of a biological state, objectively measurable and reproducible, and must relate to specific pathogenic processes or responses to therapeutic intervention. A biomarker is defined as a characteristic that is an objectively measured indicator of normal or pathogenic biological process or pharmacologic response to treatment. Biomarkers can be proteins, metabolites, RNA, DNA, epigenetic modifications of DNA, quantitative surveys of symptoms or pain scores, quantified radiographic images or changes in tumor characteristics, or patient-reported outcomes. Biomarkers can facilitate care at screening, diagnosis, prognosis determination, epidemiology studies, and new drug development. Biomarkers through prediction also help identify appropriate patients for specific treatment and assess disease response to treatment. Biomarkers can be prognostic, predictive, surrogate, or pharmacodynamic in nature (Table 1). A **prognostic biomarker** reflects disease outcome independent of therapy (natural history), while a **predictive biomarker** indentifies the likelihood of benefit from a specific therapy. There are a number of prognostic biomarkers in men with CRPC, but there are no validated predictive biomarkers to guide therapeutic decision-making at the time of this writing. In addition, **surrogate biomarkers** of OS are still uncertain in clinical trials of men with metastatic CRPC and are beyond the scope of the current chapter. Certain biomarkers are additionally used for determining drug mechanism or metabolism,

Table 1 Classification of biomarkers

Biomarker type	When biomarker is measured	Implication of biomarker
Prognostic	Prior to or after treatment	Provides information on the likelihood of a disease outcome independent of therapy (natural history)
Predictive	Prior to treatment if to be used to predict future response, but can be measured following treatment to determine predictive value on therapy	Identifies the likelihood of benefit from a specific treatment
Surrogate	During or after treatment completion	Provides an early indicator of treatment outcomes that is highly associated with the more relevant clinical end point and thus estimates the treatment effect on the final clinical end point Requires validation across trials

which are called **pharmacodynamic biomarkers**, which will not be further discussed in this chapter.

As an example to demonstrate the importance of mechanism and disease state in determining the relevance of a biomarker, an elevated serum PSA level has been used as marker of diagnosis and prognosis for prostate cancer in decades and carries prognostic weight across all known disease states (localized disease, recurrence, metastatic disease, CRPC). However, it does not always reflex the benefits of a specific treatment. For example, sipuleucel-T treatment prolongs overall survival in metastatic CRPC patients but has only modest effect on PSA level (Kantoff et al. 2010), while bevacizumab with docetaxel resulted in more deep PSA declines but did not significantly improve survival (Kelly et al. 2012). Another example of the disconnection between PSA changes and survival is radium-223 chloride, which demonstrated an overall survival (OS) benefit in men with bone-predominant symptomatic mCRPC, but with no clear impact on PSA levels (Parker et al. 2011). Therefore, new quantifiable biomarkers are needed to help determine the benefits of treatment. Novel biomarkers can also help provide an understanding into the complex biology of CPRC, identify men more likely to benefit to a given therapy, identify patients with early response or progression to optimize outcomes, and accelerate development of new therapeutics and improve clinical outcomes. The purpose of this chapter is to examine the current status of CRPC biomarkers.

Established Prognostic Biomarkers in CRPC

Prognostic biomarkers may be useful as an aid to informing upon treatment decisions given that more aggressive therapies such as chemotherapy or clinical trials may be pursued if survival is anticipated to be short, while less aggressive therapies such as secondary hormonal therapies and immunomodulatory therapies may be pursued if the burden of disease is lower. This section below introduces the established and validated pretreatment and posttreatment prognostic biomarkers in CRPC (Table 2).

PSA and PSA Kinetics

Serum PSA is secreted by prostate cancer cells under the regulation of androgen receptor (AR) transcriptional direction. Serum PSA levels are an established prognostic biomarker across multiple disease states in prostate cancer that reflects the burden of disease, and PSA level is a confirmed independent prognostic risk factor for CRPC mortality that is included in all current prognostic models (Armstrong et al. 2007a; Halabi et al. 2003; Vollmer et al. 1998). PSA changes reflect patients' response to chemotherapy or hormonal agents and provide prognostic information for individual patients over time. PSA nadir and declines in PSA in men with hormone-sensitive metastatic prostate cancer are independent predictors of survival (Hussain et al. 2006). However, caution must be considered in the interpretation of

Table 2 Established and validated prognostic biomarkers in men with metastatic CRPC. *CRP* C-reactive protein, *NLR* neutrophil to lymphocyte ratio, *LDH* lactate dehydrogenase, *CTC* circulating tumor cell, *PSA* prostate-specific antigen, *PFS* progression-free survival

Pretreatment prognostic factors	Posttreatment prognostic factors
PSA	PSA decline
PSA kinetics	Pain improvement
CTC enumeration	Quality of life changes
Anemia	Decrease of CTC to <5
LDH	Worsening anemia
Bone turnover biomarkers	Increased LDH
Inflammation biomarkers (CRP, NLR)	Type of progression, PFS
Performance status	
Visceral metastatic disease (liver > lung)	
Albumin	
Pain (requiring narcotic analgesia)	
Number of disease sites, bone scan index	
Age	
Gleason score in primary	
Chromogranin A	
Type of progression (PSA, bone scan, measurable disease)	
Testosterone level	

PSA level changes after therapy, as the PSA level change is variably dependent on the mechanism of action of different treatments. For example, sipuleucel-T improved OS in CRPC, but had only a modest effect on short-term PSA levels (Kantoff et al. 2010). In docetaxel-treated CRPC patients, the improvement in OS correlates moderately well with early PSA declines within the first 3 months of treatment (Armstrong et al. 2007b; Petrylak et al. 2006). The majority of novel hormonal therapies (enzalutamide, abiraterone acetate) result in early drops in PSA which are highly prognostic and directly related to the mechanism of action of these agents. Therefore, interpretation of PSA level changes must be based on the treatment mechanism and time of sampling.

Early changes in PSA (blips, transient rises) may be observed with cytotoxic therapies. For example, in 15 % of men with mCRPC treated with docetaxel, early rises in the first 3–4 cycles of chemotherapy were observed, followed by a subsequent fall in PSA with continued therapy (Berthold et al. 2008a). These early changes were not adversely prognostic, indicating that these transient changes should not be a reason for docetaxel discontinuation. Prospective evaluation of PSA level changes in clinical trials across a range of drug mechanisms is needed, given that in certain contexts where the correlation is strongest, PSA is strongly associated with survival benefit, such as with hormonal therapies. PCWG2 (Prostate Cancer Working Group) includes guidelines on the reporting of PSA changes and progression metrics, but de-emphasizes these changes as definitive outcomes or sole end points of trials to decide on changes in therapy or declaration of treatment

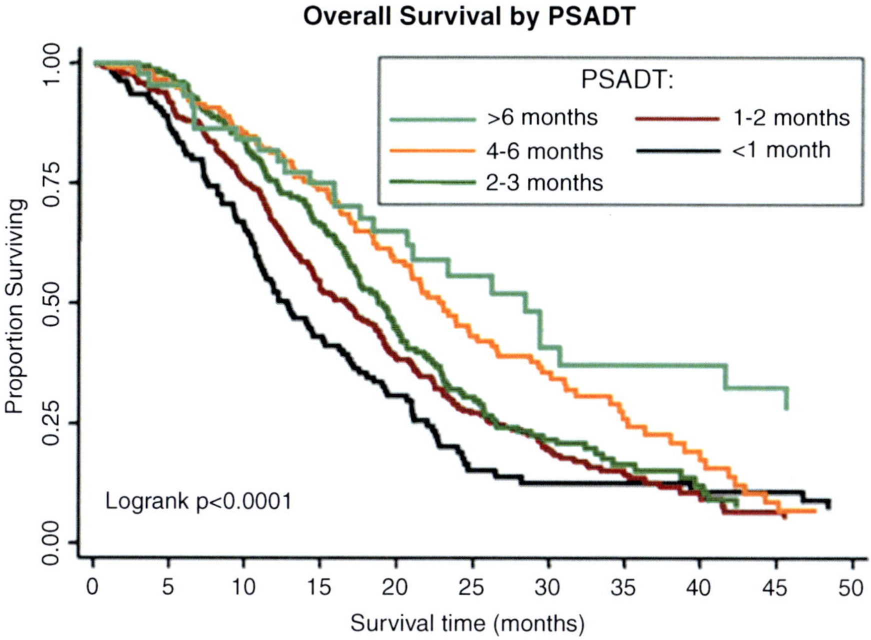

Fig. 1 The relationship between PSA doubling time (PSADT) and overall survival prognosis in men with mCRPC (Reproduced with permission from Armstrong et al. Clin Cancer Res. 2007;13:6396–403). Kaplan-Meier estimated the overall survival according to PSADT inTAX327 cohort ($n = 686$, 518 events). Median PSADT is 55 days in this study. PSADT is separated into five cohorts: >6 months ($n = 44$; median overall survival not reached; mean overall survival, 25 months), 3–6 months ($n = 118$; median overall survival not reached; mean overall survival, 22.5 months), 2–3 months ($n = 151$; median overall survival, 20.7 months), 1–2 months ($n = 264$; median overall survival, 18.6 months), and <1 month ($n = 109$; median overall survival, 13.3 months)

failure (Scher et al. 2008). Most of the transient PSA increases occur in the first 3 months of chemotherapy. Therefore, early PSA level changes following chemotherapy in men with mCRPC should be incorporated with the overall clinical assessment including pain and radiographic changes; and isolated early PSA change alone should not result in decisions to stop a systemic therapy.

PSADT (PSA doubling time) is the time necessary for the serum PSA level to double. PSADT or PSA velocity (slope) together with PSA level can help identify high-risk non-metastatic CRPC for early metastatic development, by representing the burden of disease and pace of the disease progression (Smith et al. 2005). For example, men with a PSADT $<$ 8 months or a PSA $>$ 10–20 with M0 CRPC have a high risk of metastasis development within 1–2 years. In metastatic CRPC, PSADT together with PSA is independent prognostic for OS (Armstrong et al. 2007a; Petrylak et al. 2006). Reduction in PSA velocity in docetaxel-treated CRPC also suggests a more favorable prognosis (Armstrong et al. 2007a). The relationship between PSADT and overall survival prognosis in mCRPC is shown in Fig. 1. In asymptomatic metastatic CRPC, rapid PSADT is a poor prognostic marker, indicating the need for therapeutic intervention (Armstrong et al. 2007a). PSADT needs to be cautiously interpreted since PSADT may change over time without intervention or with a placebo effect and as more data points accumulate (regression to the mean). In addition, PSA levels may slowly climb during therapy with novel hormonal agents such as abiraterone or enzalutamide following an initial response (PSA drift), and this may be quite prolonged in some men with CRPC in the absence of other clinical signs of progression. Thus, PSA levels and kinetics have a complex and often confusing relationship with tumor biology, prognosis, and response to therapies.

About 15–20 % of metastatic prostate cancer patients have a very low serum PSA level (Thompson et al. 2004), particularly those with neuroendocrine or small cell prostate histology. Histologic appearance of small cell or neuroendocrine prostate cancer has both prognostic and predictive value, as these tumors generally have a poor prognosis, make little PSA, exhibit viscerotropic spread, and have a much reduced sensitivity to hormonal therapies (Beltran et al. 2011). These tumors may exhibit Rb loss, aurora kinase A, and N-Myc amplification, accompanied by reduced AR signaling, indicating that these tumors are a distinct but often clonally derived clinical variant entity of CRPC. The optimal definition in terms of clinical phenotype and molecular genotype remains to be established. However, in these cases, PSA levels may not reflect the disease status well when neuroendocrine histology is present. Instead, other biomarkers (serum chromogranin A or carcinoembryonic antigen (CEA) or LDH levels, CTC enumerations, posttreatment radiologic changes, or pain and symptom relief) rather than PSA should be explored (Sasaki et al. 2005; Spiess et al. 2007).

In summary, PSA level changes should be interpreted in the context of overall clinical picture including the mechanism of the given treatment, pain, radiographic changes, and other biomarker changes.

Bone Turnover Biomarkers

Bone is the most common site of metastasis in prostate cancer, impacting over 90 % of men at autopsy. The effects of bone metastasis can be indirectly measured by bone turnover markers, including bone type 1 collagen breakdown product N-telopeptide (Ntx), tartrate-resistant acid phosphatase 5b, serum type 1C-telopeptide, osteopontin, bone alkaline phosphatase, and others (Jung et al. 2011). These biomarkers reflect both osteoblastic activity (e.g., bone alkaline phosphatase) and osteoclastic activity (e.g., Ntx, C-telopeptides such as aminoterminal propeptide of procollagen type I (P1NP) and beta-isomer of carboxiterminal telopeptide of collagen I (b-CTX)). Agents that impede this tumor-bone stromal interaction such as zoledronic acid and denosumab delay the development of skeletal-related events in CRPC. Persistent activation of Ntx was observed despite zoledronic acid therapy in bone metastatic CRPC. RANKL antagonism with denosumab was demonstrated to reduce these bone turnover markers, which is accompanied by superiority in the prevention of skeletal-related events when compared with zoledronic acid.

Even though the predictive role for these biomarkers is still unknown, the bone turnover marker levels are clearly prognostic for survival and correlate with meaningful clinical outcomes such as skeletal-related events, cancer progression, and survival (Saylor et al. 2013). The issue of measurement of these bone biomarkers in CRPC has been extensively reviewed elsewhere (Saylor et al. 2013). Here we give a brief review of the prognostic value of bone turnover markers.

Effective cytotoxic chemotherapy or radiopharmaceutical therapy results in reduction of bone turnover markers. Bone alkaline phosphatase (BAP) is an established prognostic marker in CRPC. In docetaxel-treated CRPC patients, reduction in total alkaline phosphatase is an independent prognostic biomarker and may also provide survival benefit in the absence of PSA level decline (Sonpavde et al. 2010). The elevated baseline level of BAP may be predictive for survival benefit with radium-223 treatments, and posttreatment BAP reductions are highly associated with improvements in survival with radium-223 chloride (Parker et al. 2013). Ntx has been evaluated recently as a potential prognostic biomarker in CRPC. Many groups have demonstrated that elevated urinary Ntx is a prognostic indicator for increased bone metastasis-related complications, disease progression, and death in prostate cancer patients (Brown et al. 2005; Coleman et al. 2005). Bone turnover markers have an established prognostic and potentially a predictive role with bone-targeted antiresorptive agents such as zoledronic acid and denosumab, in which lack of normalization of bone biomarkers with these agents has been associated with a higher risk of skeletal-related events and death (Piedra et al. 2013).

While prognostic, levels of bone turnover markers during therapy may also have therapeutic implications for the escalation or deescalation of osteoclast-targeted therapy (Saylor et al. 2013). While not prospectively validated, suboptimal bone turnover marker suppression could be taken as a cue to escalate therapeutic intensity, and marker suppression beyond the regular dosing interval of zoledronic acid or denosumab may provide a rationale for less frequent dosing. However, this approach using these bone biomarkers to guide therapy has not been prospectively tested in clinical trials and is not recommended at this time.

In conclusion, measurement of baseline and serial levels of bone turnover biomarkers during the CRPC treatment provides prognostic information, and serial measurements can update this prognostic relevance in the context of chemotherapy and bone-targeted agents. Active investigations are ongoing to clarify and validate the utility of measuring Ntx and other bone turnover markers as prognostic and predictive biomarkers in men with CRPC across a range of systemic agents such as bone-targeting agents such as denosumab, zoledronic acid, and radium-223.

Hemoglobin

Anemia in prostate cancer patients is due to multiple factors including bone metastasis, long-term androgen deprivation therapy, renal disease, chemotherapy toxicity, and blood loss (e.g., hematuria). Degree of anemia is a strong independent prognostic biomarker for docetaxel-related PSA declines, tumor response rates, and overall survival in CPRC (Halabi et al. 2003; Smaletz et al. 2002). Degree of anemia is included in almost every prognostic model (e.g., modern nomograms in docetaxel-treated CRPC) and in the CRPC risk-based classification score, together with progression by bone scan, visceral metastases, and significant pain (Armstrong et al. 2010a). Severity of anemia reflects both the disease burden and the response to treatment. Therefore, monitoring hemoglobin has prognostic implications in men with CRPC and provides an updated prognosis based on the development of anemia due to disease progression.

Lactate Dehydrogenase (LDH)

LDH is part of the cellular glycolysis and gluconeogenesis pathway, generating lactate from pyruvate or vice versa, depending on cellular energy needs. Cancer cell proliferation favors aerobic glycolysis pathways, which produce LDH. Rapid tumor growing induces elevated LDH through hypoxia, tissue necrosis, and oncogenic signaling; therefore, LDH is an independent prognostic biomarker in multiple tumors including CRPC. In men with mCRPC, elevated LDH is one of the strongest prognostic factors for survival, and increased LDH level likely reflects advanced tumor burden or an aggressive proliferative phenotype in CRPC (Halabi et al. 2003). Combinations of LDH measurements with other biomarkers including PSA or CTC may improve the clinical utility of LDH as risk stratification and prognostication (Scher et al. 2011a). In addition, increase in LDH level after treatment may be predictive for poor treatment response (Halabi et al. 2007). We have recently shown that elevated levels of LDH are predictive for the benefit of PI3K/mTOR pathway inhibition in patients with poor risk metastatic renal cell carcinoma treated with temsirolimus (Armstrong et al. 2012), which may be related to tumor burden, angiogenesis dependence, tumor metabolic profiles, or PI3K/mTOR regulation of LDH levels itself. Thus, LDH may have potential to be a relatively easy to measure predictive biomarker for oncogenic pathway targeting of tumor metabolism. Therefore, serial measurement of LDH during treatment and in the context of clinical trials is useful and strongly recommended. However, we do not recommend that changes in therapy be made based on isolated changes in LDH, given the lack of prospective study using LDH to inform clinical decision making.

CTC Enumeration

Hematogenous metastasis of solid tumors involves spread of invasive carcinoma cells followed by extravasated colony establishment. The USFDA defines the Cellsearch-based CTC to be a nucleated cell >4 um in diameter isolated from whole blood using EpCAM-based ferromagnetic antibody and also lacking the leukocyte marker CD45 (Allard et al. 2004), and the Cellsearch assay remains the only FDA approved CTC enumeration method in oncology. Multiple techniques are available to enrich CTCs. Representing the "seeds" of cancer metastasis and behaving as a real-time liquid biopsy, CTC enumerization and characterization are promising alternatives to tumor biopsies to detect, investigate, and monitor progression of solid tumors. Enumeration of CTCs has been shown to be prognostic for OS in many tumors including CRPC (de Bono et al. 2008).

Currently, CellSearch (Veridex LLC) is the only FDA-approved assay for patient use in prostate cancer CTC capture. In CellSearch, CTCs are captured by using EpCAM conjugated ferrofluid. The captured cells are then defined by immunofluorescent staining with a 4′,6-diamidino-2-phenylindole (DAPI) in nucleus surrounded by cytoplasm expressing cytokeratins CK8, CK18, or CK19, but no expression of CD-45 (Shaffer et al. 2007) (Fig. 2a). The CTC number in CRPC is established as an independent prognostic factor before treatment, four or fewer cells per 7.5 ml of blood related to favorable prognosis, whereas five or more cells per 7.5 ml of blood associated with an unfavorable prognosis (de Bono et al. 2008) (Fig. 2b). A decrease in the CTC counts to less than five after treatment is associated with improvement in OS (Fig. 2c). In addition, CTC measurement may complement other prognostic factors, such as visceral disease, PSA, and pain (Bitting et al. 2013). The USFDA indicates currently that it is used as "an aid in the monitoring of patients in conjunction with other clinical methods" (FDA 2008), which illustrates the prognostic importance of CTC enumeration over time, both before and during systemic therapy. CTC flare has not been observed to date, and CTC enumeration changes may occur earlier than PSA declines, with some studies suggesting improvements in survival association with early CTC changes as compared with PSA declines (de Bono et al. 2008). While CTC declines are prognostic, the exact level of CTC decline that has the strongest association with survival is not known. In addition, using CTC to define progression in CRPC is also not prospectively validated at this time, but CTC enumeration may be particularly useful when early clinical, PSA, and radiographic changes are discordant (Scher et al. 2011b). Recent studies also suggest that CTCs may reflect survival benefit to serve as a potential surrogate biomarker for OS (Scher et al. 2011b). There are multiple studies going on to determine whether CTC combined with other biomarkers (e.g., LDH, hemoglobin, PSA level) increases the prognostic significance and can be used as surrogate end point in future CPRC clinical trials.

The use of CTCs is not limited to CTC detection. In addition, CTC visualization will enable direct measurement of the tumor biology and assess biomarkers directly in tumor cells. For example, identification of ERG, AR, and PTEN gene status in circulating tumor cells from patients with CRPC suggests that personalization of therapy using biomarker guidance like therapy directed against AR or PI3 kinase pathway is possible. For example, CTCs captured through the Adnatest method and assayed for AR-variant 7 (AR-V7) were recently shown to be highly prognostic and predictive of novel hormonal therapy efficacy (see below for discussion). Thus, CTC collection may provide a liquid biopsy for precision medicine and the use of additional predictive biomarkers for drug sensitivity. The use of these CTC biomarkers will be context dependent and requires prospective validation.

One major limitation in the study of CTCs is the lack of detection of CTCs in many men with mCRPC (>50 %). Some CTCs express not only markers for

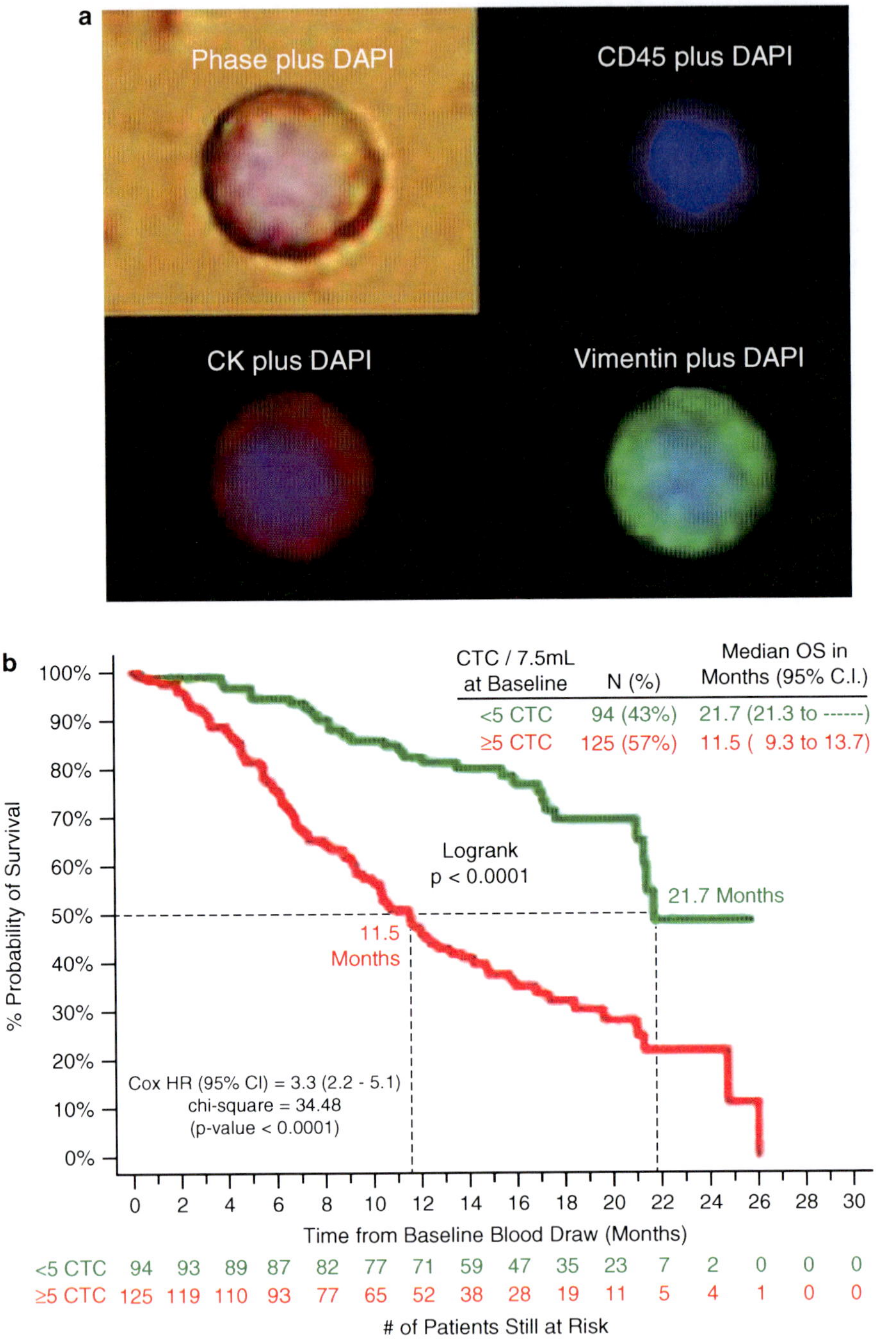

Fig. 2 (continued)

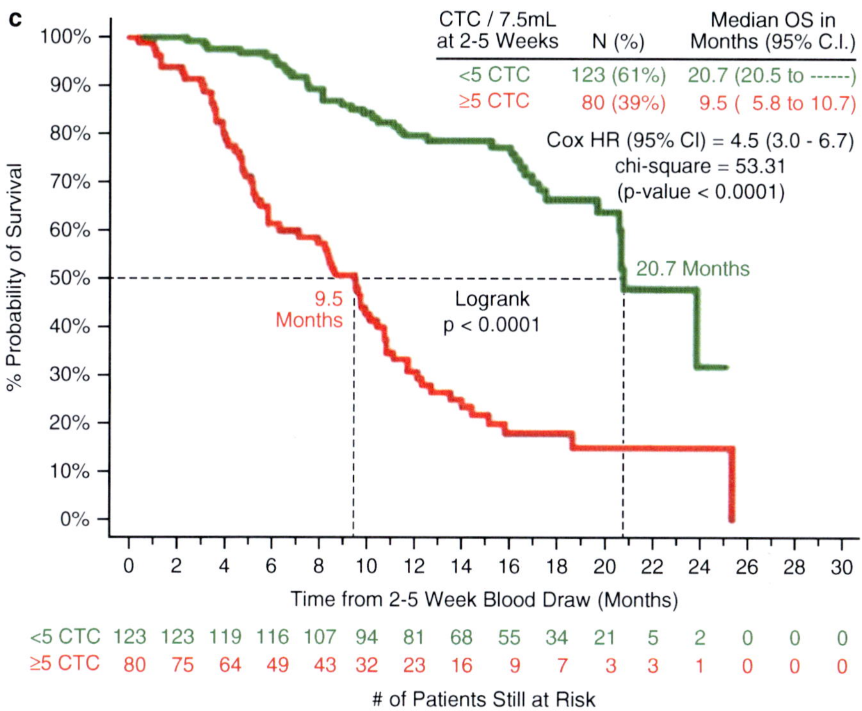

Fig. 2 CTC captured in CRPC patients by EpCAM using CellSearch and prognostic value of CTCs in CRPC. (**a**) CTC captured by EpCAM from men with CRPC (reproduced from Armstrong AJ et al. Mol Cancer Res. 2011; 9:997–1007). This is example of an EpCAM-captured CTC from a man with CRPC. The CTC is DAPI, CK and vimentin positive, and is differentiated from leukocytes by the lack of CD45 expression. (**b**) Kaplan-Meier estimated of probability of OS of CRPC patients with favorable (<5) and unfavorable (>5) CTCs before initiation of therapy (reproduced from de Bono J et al, Clin. Cancer Res.2008; 14, 6302–6309). (**c**) Kaplan-Meier estimates of probabilities of OS of CRPC patients with favorable (<5) and unfavorable (>5) CTC 2 to 5 weeks after initiation of therapy (reproduced from de Bono J et al, Clin. Cancer Res. 2008; 14, 6302–6309)

epithelial cells but also stemness and mesenchymal markers (Armstrong et al. 2011). This heterogeneity in CTCs may explain partly the escape of detection of CTCs in CRPC by using the standard epithelial antigen-based technology. Improvements in CTCs captured by novel capture antibodies (e.g., mesenchymal antigens), flow cytometry, or novel CTC chip designs or in the use of cell-free methods such as circulating tumor DNA or RNA will help further exploration in using this liquid biopsy approach and its prognostic and predictive role in CRPC.

Inflammatory Biomarkers

Chronic inflammation induces carcinogenesis through irreversible cellular and DNA damage by generation of free radicals and the promotion of cell growth by

DNA and cellular replication (Hussain et al. 2003). CRP is a sensitive marker of acute inflammation and tissue damage. Elevated CRP is reported to be associated with shorter OS and predicts a lower probability of PSA response to docetaxel-based therapy in CRPC (Prins et al. 2012). In addition, elevated CRP level was validated as adversely prognostic in a multivariate model in men with mCRPC treated with docetaxel chemotherapy and improved the ability of this model to discriminate survival outcomes (Pond et al. 2012). Thus, CRP may be a sensitive and easy to use biomarker in the clinic to provide prognostic information and should be measured in research studies in order to develop improved prognostic models. However, the incorporation of CRP into novel nomograms and prognostic models requires prospective validation before routine measurements of CRP can be recommended in men with mCRPC in the clinic. The neutrophil to lymphocyte ratio (NLR) is an easily measured and reproducible inflammation marker, which is prognostic in several cancers including CRPC. One retrospective study reported that patients with a pretreatment NLR $<=3$ had a higher response rate to treatment with the CYP17 inhibitor ketoconazole and longer PFS interval (Keizman et al. 2012).

Albumin

Pretreatment serum albumin levels provide useful prognostic significance in cancer and have been implicated as an independent prognostic factor in various cancers including CRPC (Smaletz et al. 2002). Low albumin levels may be a measure of nutritional status or a marker of chronic illness and inflammation, reflecting underlying disease burden and aggressiveness. Low pretreatment albumin level was reported to be prognostic for increased risk of death and short survival in men with CRPC (Smaletz et al. 2002). With its independent prognostic value, albumin is included in the modified Glasgow prognostic score in prostate cancer, together with Gleason score, PSA, and CRP (Shafique et al. 2013).

Pain

Pain has been identified as an important prognostic indicator of overall survival in men with metastatic CRPC (Armstrong et al. 2007a; Halabi et al. 2008). In Halabi's study, the median survival times were 17.6 months and 10.2 months in men with low and high pain scores, respectively. The same study also reported that pain was inversely associated with likelihood of prostate-specific antigen decline, objective response, and time to bone progression. Pain responses have also been strongly associated with improvements in survival with docetaxel chemotherapy and with abiraterone acetate therapy (Armstrong et al. 2007b). Pain measurement is subjective and patient reported; however, quantifiable measures of pain assessment are available and validated and under current evaluation as an intermediate endpoint for regulatory approval for novel systemic agents such as the c-met/VEGFR2 inhibitor cabozantinib. The limitations of pain response as an objective biomarker include issues of durability of response, the association of this outcome with survival, the variability of this biomarker from day to day and even within a single day in a given patient, and the fact that analgesic therapy can reduce pain independent of a treatment effect. However, despite these limitations, pain assessment and improvements in the context of analgesic use and accounting for this normal variability remain of direct importance to both patients and providers. The presence of pain has therapeutic implications, as men with asymptomatic mCRPC are candidates for immunotherapy with sipuleucel-T, while men with symptomatic bone metastatic CRPC are candidates for radium-223 therapy. Thus, pain represents one of the most important clinical biomarkers in CRPC, as it is clearly associated with death, morbidity, and therapeutic decision-making in the clinic.

Quality of Life

Men with CRPC may have a variety of symptoms that lead to reduced quality of life (QoL). A retrospective study used the TAX-327 database to address whether PSA, pain, and QoL response predict for overall survival (Berthold et al. 2008a). This study demonstrated that symptoms other than pain contribute to impaired QoL in men with CRPC, and those with minimal symptoms have better prognosis and prolonged survival. By using the same TAX-327 database, Berthold et al. also reported that patients with a Karnofsky performance status (KPS) $\geq$ 90 % lived approximately 8 months longer than those with a KPS $\leq$ 80 % (Berthold et al. 2008b). Halabi et al. developed and validated a pretreatment prognostic model to stratify patients with CRPC and found that performance status, together with Gleason sum, LDH, PSA, and alkaline phosphatase, was a significant prognostic factor of overall survival (Halabi et al. 2003), and functional status is captured in current nomograms as an independent prognostic measure associated with mortality (Logothetis et al. 2012). Objective QOL measures can also be captured as patient reported outcomes that go beyond the traditional functional status assessments by clinicians. QOL outcomes are being reported commonly in phase 3 trials of men with mCRPC and reflect a direct measure of patient benefit over time from these agents. Objective and validated scales that can be used include survey instruments and reported patient reported outcomes (PRO) using NCI's Common Toxicity-PRO scales. Therefore, QoL represents an important prognostic biomarker that can be objectively measured in CRPC and is associated with survival rate.

Pattern of Metastatic Spread

The most frequent metastatic sites in prostate cancer are the bone and pelvic and abdominal lymph nodes. Visceral metastases (e.g., liver, lungs) are less commonly seen (~25 % of men with mCRPC) but are commonly found at autopsy in over half of patients who die of mCRPC. Men with non-metastatic (M0) CRPC have a heterogeneous but more favorable prognosis measured in 3–6 years, while men with isolated nodal mCRPC have a survival estimate of 2–3 years (Armstrong et al. 2010b). Bone-only metastatic disease is relatively common and carries an intermediate prognosis of 1.5–2 years depending on disease setting (Armstrong et al. 2010b). The presence of visceral involvement is a known adverse prognostic factor for men with metastatic prostate cancer when compared with patients with only bone and/or lymph node disease. In the TAX 327 study, 22 % of patients with visceral disease died on average 6 months earlier than those without visceral metastases (Berthold et al. 2008). Liver metastases were reported to carry even greater influence than overall visceral metastases (Armstrong et al. 2010b) and had a worse prognosis than men with isolated pulmonary metastases. Neuroendocrine differentiation of the prostate cancer is an independent poor prognostic marker and is often associated with visceral metastases (Huang et al. 2006). The presence of visceral metastasis, together with absolute PSA nadir on ADT, time to PSA nadir, and duration of hormone sensitivity, was reported to be independently prognostic and predictive of adverse survival from CRPC to death (Humphreys et al. 2013). Because if its independent prognostic value, visceral metastases are included in many prognostic risk stratification nomograms for men with CRPC (Armstrong et al. 2007a; Halabi et al. 2003; Smaletz et al. 2002). Visceral disease is important clinically for treatment decision-making, as the presence of visceral metastases is currently exclusionary for the use of sipuleucel-T immunotherapy and radium-223 radiopharmaceutical therapy.

Tumor Histology

The morphologic variants of prostatic carcinoma are relatively uncommon, but the histology type of prostate cancer has independent prognostic value and is associated with different disease progression pattern and prognosis. Neuroendocrine differentiation is a common feature of prostatic adenocarcinomas and is usually determined by immunoreactivity for neuroendocrine markers (e.g., chromogranin A, neuron specific enolase) (Vashchenko and Abrahamsson 2005). Neuroendocrine differentiation is associated with castrate-resistant status and worse prognosis in CRPC (Berruti et al. 2010). In Komiya's study, neuroendocrine differentiation was evaluated in men with hormone-sensitive and castration-resistant prostate cancer, by using IHC staining in the biopsied prostate tissue. This study reported that neuroendocrine differentiation was observed more frequently in CRPC vs. hormone-sensitive prostate cancer and was associated with a worse prognosis (Komiya et al. 2013). Recent efforts to define this anaplastic variant of prostate cancer using neuroendocrine biomarkers and other biomarkers suggest that these men have a worse prognosis, despite the use of platinum or taxane doublet therapies, and new therapies are needed (Aparicio et al. 2013). By RNA sequencing, IHC, and fluorescence in situ hybridization (FISH), Beltran et al. discovered significant overexpression and gene amplification of AURKA and MYCN in 40 % of neuroendocrine prostate cancer which has enhanced sensitivity to aurora kinase inhibitor therapy both in vitro and in vivo (Beltran et al. 2011). These tumors may also have loss of RB function and PI3K pathway activation, suggesting genomic complexity that may require multiple targeting agents. Therefore, the histology type of CRPC has independent prognostic value and may be predictive to patient's response to particular treatment. However, a molecularly-defined subtype that captures this biology, rather than the variable histology seen with anaplastic or neuroendocrine PC, is needed.

Emerging Prognostic Biomarkers in CRPC

The identification and validation of other multipurpose biomarker assays is crucial to individualizing management of CRPC and improving models that better discriminate outcomes. Intense research efforts to identify novel pathobiology-based biomarkers are ongoing and should lead to improvement in cancer prognosis and management of the therapeutic response of CRPC patients. This section summarizes the emerging prognostic biomarkers in CRPC (Table 3).

Novel Imaging Biomarkers

The bone is the most common metastasis site of prostate cancer. Bone metastases are the primary cause of morbidity and mortality in the CRPC population, developing in 80–90 % of patients with prostate cancer (Bubendorf et al. 2000). Bone scans (TcM-99) can often be subjective, and clinical reports of these scans do not quantify the disease burden in a manner that is usable as a biomarker. In addition, early bone scan changes such as flare or healing reactions may lead to misclassification of response as progression, a phenomenon commonly observed in men with mCRPC treated with active agents (Scher et al. 2008). Thus, methods are needed to objectify bone burden of metastatic disease and changes over time.

Researchers in MSKCC developed the bone scan index (BSI) to quantitatively measure the tumor-bone metastatic burden as percentage of total skeletal mass. A study by Imbriaco et al. enrolled 191 patients with progressive CRPC and showed inferior survival as BSI increased (Imbriaco et al. 1998). The manual BSI measurement is very reproducible, though time consuming and tedious. Automated methods for interpreting bone scans and calculating BSI are under development. Ulmet et al. developed computer-assisted BSI measure and reported that BSI is a valuable metric for estimating metastatic burden in patients with advanced prostate cancer (Ulmert et al. 2012). The same team also reported that automated BSI calculation, like its manual counterpart, is a valuable clinical parameter in patients with progressive prostate cancer. In another study, pretreatment and posttreatment BSI was found to be highly associated with survival, and posttreatment changes in BSI were reported to correlate most with the outcome; a doubling of BSI conferred an almost twofold increase in the risk of death (Dennis et al. 2012). Recently, the first

Table 3 Emerging prognostic biomarkers in CRPC

Emerging prognostic biomarkers	Potential application in CRPC
Bone scan index	Prognostic for survival
PET with different tracers (F-18, choline, DHT)	Quantify primary and metastatic diseases
Androgen receptor splice variants	Prognostic for low response and short time to progression and survival with abiraterone acetate and enzalutamide
Molecular genotypes	Serve as predictors for specific therapies, may be prognostic for aggressive clinical course
Whole-blood RNA profiles	Stratify patients into distinct prognostic groups
Circulating miRNA	Differentiate localized PCa and mCRPC subtypes
Circulating cytokines/ chemokines	Useful biomarkers for early detection or spread of cancer
Disseminated tumor cells (DTCs)	Prognostic for recurrence after localized therapies

randomized study of men with mCRPC to include BSI measures over time was reported (Armstrong et al. 2013). In this trial, a novel immunomodulatory agent, tasquinimod, was compared with placebo, in men with mCRPC. Importantly, this trial validated BSI as prognostic for survival and found that BSI tracked with other prognostic biomarkers of disease burden such as alkaline phosphatase. BSI measures will need to account for transient worsening of BSI changes due to healing/ flare as well by automating the measures of new lesions over time with the intensity of existing lesions. Further study of the BSI thresholds for determining progression in mCRPC within phase III clinical trials is needed to confirm the value of BSI.

A variety of tracers are being explored in PET imaging that has shown promise as potential prognostic biomarkers in CRPC. PET imaging results can serve as a potential prognostic and predictive biomarkers, because of its ability to quantify primary and metastatic lesions in PET scan to estimate the disease burden and response to treatments. 18 F- FDG-PET is a marker of tumor glycolytic rate with established prognostic benefit in oncology (Morris et al. 2005); however, prostate cancers typically have low metabolic and proliferative rates even in the metastatic setting, and measuring glycolysis has been less reliable in this disease than other solid tumors and lymphomas. For this reason, other modalities are being pursued. 18 F-sodium fluoride (NaF) is a high affinity bone-seeking agent that could enhance traditional bone scanning if employed in replace of the single photon 99 m Tc agents. In Even-Sapir's study, planar bone scintigraphy, bone SPECT, NaF PET, and NaF PET/CT in patients with localized high-risk or metastatic prostate cancer were compared. The sensitivity and specificity for detection of bone metastasis was higher in NaF PET/CT than in the others (Even-Sapir et al. 2006). Additional metabolic agents such as 18 F-FACBC, 18 F-choline, and 11 C-methionine have been studied extensively as PET tracer in prostate cancer. In addition, 18 F-FDHT and novel tracers such as 89 Zr-J591 are under development for probing the AR signaling pathway. To validate PET imaging to be prognostic biomarker for CRPC, all steps in the imaging need to be validated including uniform tracer production and administration, acquisition of images, data collection, data processing, and data interpretation.

Novel CTC and Disseminated Tumor Cell (DTC) Enumeration Methods

Ozkumur et al. engineered an automated platform, called the "CTC-iChip," that captured both EpCAM+ and EpCAM− cancer cells, by using whole blood from patients with prostate, lung, breast, pancreatic, and colorectal cancers. The CTC-iChip is able to process large volumes of patient blood to obtain not just EpCAM + CTCs but also the EpCAM−CTCs (Ozkumur et al. 2013). This CTC-iChip could be a promising addition to the CRPC CTCs study. The high-throughput, efficient, and automatable CTC capture technology will enable the integration of CTC-based diagnostics into the clinical management of CRPC. Multiple other technologies are in development to enumerate and characterize cells based on negative exclusion, novel capture antibodies (e.g., mesenchymal), or size/cell property mechanisms. Each of these methods must go through a rigorous prospective validation.

Over 90 % of prostate cancer is considered localized at the time of diagnosis, and the rate of biochemical recurrence (PSA) after radical prostatectomy is 20–30 %. The mean time from PSA recurrence to clinical metastasis is 8 years (Pound et al. 1999). These facts suggest the presence and persistence of disseminated tumor cells (DTC) prior to metastatic progression. Since prostate cancer metastasizes predominantly in the bone, some researchers explored assays to enrich and identify DTC from the bone marrow of men with prostate cancer. Weckermann et al. analyzed the bone marrow aspirate for cytokeratin-positive cells and reported that cytokeratin-positive cells in the bone marrow aspirate are prognostically relevant when detected before radical prostatectomy and patients with cytokeratin-positive cells in bone marrow before surgery may therefore benefit from adjuvant therapies (Weckermann et al. 2009). By using immunostaining with fluorescein isothiocyanate (FITC)-labeled anti-BerEP4 antibodies and phycoerythrin conjugated anti-CD45 antibody, Morgan et al. refined a sensitive assay that enriches and identifies DTC (BerEP4 positive and CD-45 negative) from the bone marrow of men with prostate cancer and reported that persistence of DTC after radical prostatectomy in no evidence disease patients was a potential independent prognostic factor for later recurrence (Morgan et al. 2009). Further studies are needed to define which men with DTCs go on to recur and escape dormancy and whether the measurement of DTCs at diagnosis or upon recurrence has value over other clinical factors already measured.

Molecular Genotype of Prostate Cancer Cells

Somatic genomic alterations contribute to cancer development, progression, and prognosis by altering the function of genes or pathways that are important for tumorigenesis, metastasis, and resistance to therapies. Several genomic alterations have been identified in CRPC which may serve as predictors of prognosis and progression.

Constitutively, active androgen receptor variants (AR-V) lacking the ligand binding domain (LBD) may promote the development of CRPC. Recent study reported that expression of AR-V is prevalent in CRPC. Two most abundantly expressed variants are AR-V1 and AR-V7, whose mRNA showed an average 20-fold higher expression in CRPC when compared with castrate-sensitive prostate cancer. Hörnberg et al. reported that higher expression of AR-V7 predicted biochemical recurrence following surgical treatment and CRPC with bone metastases has the increased expression of AR splice variants AR-V1, AR-V7, and AR-V567es (Hörnberg et al. 2011). This study also reported that the expression of the AR-V567es and very high levels of the AR-V7 is found in individuals with particularly poor prognosis. The results from this study suggest a novel mechanism for the development of CRPC and the possible role of AR-V as novel prognostic biomarkers and therapeutic targets. While measurement of these AR variants is not part of routine practice at the time, ongoing studies to develop and qualify AR variant assessment tools are ongoing and may provide useful information prognostically.

PTEN (phosphatase and tensin homologue) is a negative regulator of the phosphatidylinositol 3-kinase (PI3K)/AKT survival pathway and a tumor suppressor, which is frequently deleted in prostate cancer. Alteration of the PTEN/PI3K pathway is observed in CRPC; however, its exact role is not clear (Mulholland et al. 2011). PTEN genomic deletion has been detected in human tissues representing all stages of prostate cancer with higher frequency in metastatic prostate cancer and CRPC (Yoshimoto et al. 2006). It was also reported that CRPC and early biochemical recurrence were associated with reduced immunoreactivity of PTEN and AR in the prostate cancer samples harvested before treatment initiation (El Sheikh et al. 2008). The addition of an inhibitor of PI3K/mTOR to the standard androgen ablation treatment of CRPC may therefore be beneficial to patients with PTEN-deleted tumor. Detection of the PTEN deletion status in tumor tissue obtained from men with CRPC could potentially provide important prognostic value for response to inhibitor of PI3K/mTOR. Additional studies will help to determine its efficacy as a prognostic biomarker and as a predictive marker to identify patients who could benefit from emerging PI3K pathway-targeted therapies or who may be resistant to hormonal therapies.

Retinoblastoma (RB) as a tumor suppressor plays functions in multiple tissues to protect against tumor development. Substantive clinical evidence showed that RB protects against prostate cancer progression, and preclinical modeling demonstrates that RB loss in human tumor xenografts promotes the transition of prostate cancer to castration-resistant disease state (Aparicio et al. 2011). These suggest that RB status is a solid candidate for development as a prognostic marker and predictive marker of response to therapy that might guide therapeutic decisions. Loss of Rb may lead to CRPC and predict for lack of response to cell cycle inhibitors, and thus the benefit of chemotherapy or cell cycle inhibitors may be optimized in men with intact Rb function (Comstock et al. 2013; Sharma et al. 2010).

Whole-Blood RNA Profiles

Measurements of broad gene transcription expression profiles of blood cells in whole-blood collections in men with mCRPC may provide useful prognostic information related to host microenvironmental and macroenvironmental changes during tumor progression. For example, prostate cancer bone marrow invasion affects hematopoiesis by competing with primitive hemopoietic cell niches; circulating through the neoplastic tissue could influence the whole-blood gene expression. Chromosomal aberrations and epigenetic changes have been identified in peripheral blood mononuclear cells from patients with solid tumors including prostate cancer. The prognostic value of whole-blood expression profiling of CRPC patients has been studied recently. Olmos D et al. compared whole-blood gene expression profiles among patients with early prostate cancer and patients with CPRC. An expression profile with nine-gene signature was derived to identify patients with CRPC and was associated with CRPC, high-burden disease, and poor outcome (Olmos et al. 2012). This result suggested that gene expression signatures identified by whole-blood gene profiling could help stratify patients with CRPC into distinct prognosis groups. Ross R et al. reported a different six-gene model to separate patients with CRPC into low-risk group with a median survival of more than 34.9 months and a high-risk group with a median survival of 7.8 months (Ross et al. 2012). The majority of these genes identified in these profiles were reflective of T cell, NK cell, immature red blood cell, and monocytic function, indicating the importance of immune response and bone marrow invasion in determining prognosis. However, the independent value of measuring either or both of these relatively expensive RNA profiles has not been prospectively established in large datasets, and the value of measuring these novel assays has not been shown to improve existing nomogram assessments in mCRPC. In addition, the predictive value of these signatures in the context of immunologic and hormonal chemotherapies is also unknown and requires prospective study. In conclusion, whole-blood RNA transcript-based model could be an effective prognostic biomarker in CRPC and is worthy of future research.

Circulating miRNA

MicroRNAs (miRNAs) are $\sim$22 nucleotide-long, single-stranded, noncoding RNAs. MicroRNAs are essential regulators of gene expression and play critical roles in physiological and pathological process. Recent studies showed that miRNA is deregulated in human cancers and may have potential value of being used as prognostic biomarkers in cancer. In one study, the author compared plasma levels of miRNAs in localized prostate cancer vs. mCRPC and identified selected combinations of miRNAs that appear to be able to differentiate localized prostate cancer from mCRPC (Watahiki et al. 2013). This study indicated that expression levels of plasma miRNAs may be useful as predictive and prognostic biomarkers, particularly those associated with AR signaling (e.g., miR-21, miR-31) and with cancer metastasis (miR-200 family). Larger patient cohorts are required to confirm the potential utility of circulating miRNA profiling as biomarkers in the context of other established clinical biomarkers.

Circulating Cytokines/Chemokines

Cytokines are signaling molecules that are key mediators of inflammation or an immune response. Constitutive exposure to high levels of pro-inflammatory cytokines is thought to be pro-tumorigenic. Chemokines are a subgroup of cytokines that recruit leukocytes to sites of inflammation by chemotaxis. Altered levels of circulating inflammatory cytokines have been found in most cancers, including CRPC (Seruga et al. 2008). Elevated levels of circulating IL6 have been associated with decreased overall survival or disease-free recurrence in metastatic prostate cancer (Ebrahimi et al. 2004). Subudhi et al. reported a risk group classification based on two serum cytokines (M-CSF and IL-10) and log CTC, which predicted survival in men with progressive CRPC. Therefore, these cytokines may serve as prognostic biomarker for clinical benefit (Subudhi et al. 2013). Another study reported significantly greater increases in 10 cytokines from baseline in nonresponder with CRPC after one cycle of chemotherapy compared with those who responded to treatment (Mahon et al. 2011). Among these 10 cytokines, increases in IL8 and gamma-IFN levels by more than 40 % from baseline were associated with poorer OS, and higher baseline MIC-1 levels also predicted shorter OS and potentially docetaxel resistance. Therefore, early changes in circulating levels of cytokines may behave as prognostic biomarker for chemoresistance in men with CRPC.

Potential Predictive Biomarkers in CRPC

Predictive biomarkers help identify the likelihood of patients to benefit from a specific therapy and offer the hope of individualized therapy. In CRPC, a number of prognostic biomarkers are available to guide risk stratification; however, there is no confirmed predictive biomarkers. With the number of newly approved and emerging therapeutic agents, it is important to develop new predictive biomarkers to guide oncologists in making therapeutic decisions and matching the right patient to the right therapy sequence at a given time. We discuss here the potential predictive biomarkers in CRPC and how these potential predictive markers can be developed in clinical trials (Table 4).

CTC Biomarkers

CTC enumeration is prognostic, but the value of CTC as predictive biomarkers is unknown. Recent prospective studies have shown that changes in CTC number after 4, 8, or 12 weeks of chemotherapy were more strongly predictive of survival

Table 4 Potential predictive biomarkers in CRPC

Potential predictive biomarkers	Potential predictive application in CRPC
AR-variants (i.e. AR-v7) or mutations	Predict lack of benefit with abiraterone acetate or enzalutamide
CTC count decrease with treatment	Predict future survival and response to treatment
TMPRSS2:ERG	Predict better response to ADT
High N-cadherin expression	Early biochemical failure and clinical recurrence
Baseline adrenal androgens	Predict benefit from androgen biosynthesis inhibitor
Tubulin mutations	Selection of microtubule-based therapies
High bone turnover markers	Benefit with denosumab or zoledronic acid
Lower baseline PSA	Benefit from Sipuleucel-T
PTEN loss	Enrich for benefit with PI3K pathway inhibitors
RB loss	Increased risk of transition to CRPC, sensitivity to cell cycle inhibition (resistance)
c-met activity	Enrich for benefit with c-met inhibitors
Ras/raf mutations	Potential benefit with ras pathway inhibitors (i.e., sorafenib, vemurafenib)
DNA repair defects (BRCA2)	Enrich for benefit with poly-ADP ribose polymerase (PARP) inhibitors
Myc amplification	Cell-cycle inhibitors (anti-proliferation agents)
Neuroendocrine phenotype	Aurora kinase inhibition sensitivity

than PSA changes in men with CRPC (Scher et al. 2009). The feasibility of CTCs as an easily obtained tissue for molecular analysis by techniques such as FISH and RT-PCR has been explored to investigate the ERG, AR, and PTEN expression in CTCs from men with CRPC. Danila et al. reported that the frequency of detection of the TMPRSS2-ERG fusion in CTCs by RT-PCR from patients with metastatic CRPC was 37 % and the androgen-driven TMPRSS2-ERG fusion in CTCs is a potential predictive biomarker of sensitivity to abiraterone (Danila et al. 2011). AR amplification is infrequent in primary and/or diagnostic tumor specimens in prostate cancer, but is detected in up to 50 % of castration-resistant lesions (Holzbeierlein et al. 2004). AR genomic amplification and copy number gain have been documented in CTCs from men with CRPC (Attard et al. 2009). AR amplification and copy number gain, occurring under the selective pressure of androgen deprivation therapy, have the potential predictive value for sensitivity to second-generation AR antagonist (Danila et al. 2011). Attard et al. also reported a significant heterogeneity of PTEN loss in CTCs from men with CRPC by using FISH (Attard et al. 2009). The status of PTEN loss in CTCs from men with CRPC may be predictive for patients' response to small molecule inhibitors of the phosphatidylinositol-3-kinase (PI3K)/PTEN. Although using the CTC molecular profile is promising as predictive biomarker for men with CRPC, full qualification will ultimately require analytical validation of the assays and new prospective trials to explore the relationship between molecular profile and clinical outcome.

Potential Predictive Biomarkers of Response to Hormonal Therapies

Androgen deprivation is the main treatment for CRPC. Enhanced androgen receptor signaling and androgen synthesis are essential steps in the CRPC progression and are the focus for intervention and drug development and recent approvals of abiraterone acetate and enzalutamide. Resistance to these therapies and androgen deprivation therapy (ADT) in general has been linked to the presence of AR variants that have truncated or spliced C-terminal regions, in which the ligand binding domain for androgens has been disrupted. AR splice variants have been linked to early CRPC progression, and assays for the common AR variants are under evaluation in CTCs and tissue specimens to help guide hormonal therapy selection and predict response or resistance to therapy (Chen et al. 2004). Assays for specific AR variants and AR mutations in CTCs or tissue or whole blood are in the process of being evaluated and objectively measured and qualified in the context of novel hormonal agents as predictive biomarkers.

Multiple AR gene rearrangements and AR variants have been reported in CRPC. These variants lack the ligand binding domain and constitutively signal in the absence of androgen and are not currently inhibited by AR antagonists. AR variants may be functional drivers of CRPC progression and treatment resistance development (Ware et al. 2014). Androgen receptor variant 7 (AR-V7) is one such key variant with a known protein product in which the C-terminal ligand binding domain is lost, the N-terminal transactivating and DNA binding domains are retained, a novel cryptic exon 3 is gained, and constitutive activity as a transcription factor in a ligand-independent manner is observed. Antonarakis ES et al reported that AR-V7 was reliably detected in CTCs as measured by a modified Adnatest from men with mCRPC. Detection of AR-V7 in CTC was strongly associated with enzalutamide and abiraterone resistance (Antonarakis et al. 2014) including lack of PSA declines and short progression free survival in approximately 60 patients. Among enzalutamide treated men, the rate of a 50 % or greater PSA decline was 0 % in AR-V7 positive patients compared with 53 % in AR-V7 negative patients ($P = 0.004$); PSA progression-free survival (PFS) was shorter in ARV-7 positive patients (1.4 months vs. 6.0 months; $P<0.001$). Similar results were seen in abiraterone treated men with mCRPC, in which AR-V7–positive patients had lower PSA response rates (0 % vs. 68 %, $P = 0.004$) and a shorter PSA PFS (1.3 months vs. not reached; $P<0.001$). These data require confirmation studies in larger prospective multicenter trials but suggest that AR-v7 is highly associated as a predictive biomarker of the lack of efficacy with novel hormonal agents such as enzalutamide or abiraterone acetate.

In addition, recent findings suggest that full length AR nuclear translocation and activity is microtubule dependent, while AR variants exhibit variable microtubule dependence. Thadani-Mulero et al reported that AR-V7 expressing LuCap 23.1 tumor xenografts in noncastrate SCID mice demonstrated docetaxel resistance given that this variant lacks the microtubule binding domain important for full length AR nuclear translocation (Thadani-Mulero et al. 2014). This result indicated that mCRPC predominantly expressing ARv7 may be resistant to taxane chemotherapy. Other AR-variants, such as AR-v567es, remain microtubule dependent and possess this domain, suggesting a degree of taxane sensitivity based on the specific AR-variant present. Taken together, AR-V7 is likely a potential predictive biomarker for resistance to enzalutamide, abiraterone acetate and possibly to taxane. The data on taxane sensitivity has not yet been validated clinically.

Clinical validation of these predictive biomarkers are ongoing through a PCF global treatment sciences challenge award entitled "Development of Circulating Molecular Predictors of Chemotherapy and Novel Hormonal Therapy Benefit in Men with Metastatic Castration Resistant Prostate Cancer (mCRPC)" (Clinicaltrial.gov NCT02269982), and prospective trials such as TAXYNEGY (NCT01718353) using CTC biomarkers to predict taxane sensitivity. These studies will help to further validate the potential predictive role of AR-V7.

PSA is an AR-regulated protein secreted by prostate cancer cells; therefore, the PSA level reflects not only the tumor burden in CRPC but also the level of AR transcriptional activity, although some AR variants may not regulate PSA production to the same degree. PSA is an independent prognostic biomarker for survival in CRPC, but PSA levels have not been shown prospectively to be predictive of the benefits of any specific therapy. There is some suggestion that lower PSA levels may be predictive of the benefit with immunotherapy (e.g., sipuleucel-T) for men with metastatic asymptomatic CRPC (Schellhammer et al. 2013), possibly reflecting the greater ability to harness immune responses in men with lower disease burden. In addition, novel hormonal agents such as abiraterone and enzalutamide have not been studied in the more anaplastic or neuroendocrine prostate cancer phenotype in which PSA levels are quite low and are typically AR independent, and thus, these men would be predicted to be resistant to these agents. Therefore, PSA itself may be a predictive biomarker of AR pathway activity and the benefit of AR pathway-directed therapies and may also be a measure of disease burden and the relative benefits of immunotherapy. These findings require prospective validation.

Transmembrane protease, serine 2 (TMPRSS2) encodes for an androgen-regulated, prostate-specific protease. In about two thirds of prostate cancer, TMPRSS2 fuses to ETS-related gene (ERG) or other oncogenes within the ETS family, which results in ERG overexpression (Tomlins et al. 2005). It was hypothesized that this overexpression predicts better response to androgen deprivation therapy. However, in a phase II postchemotherapy study, the presence of the fusion in CTCs did not predict for response to treatment with abiraterone (Danila et al. 2011). Further prospective studies are needed to evaluate the potential predictive value of ERG overexpression. Higher level of baseline adrenal androgens is thought to predict for benefit from treatment with androgen biosynthesis inhibitor. However, a survival benefit with abiraterone was seen even in men with low levels of baseline adrenal androgen levels (Ryan et al. 2012). This hypothesis is under evaluation in a phase III retrospective randomized trial of abiraterone + prednisone vs. placebo + prednisone (Ryan et al. 2012).

Potential Predictive Biomarkers of Response to Chemotherapy

Taxanes cause stabilization of cellular microtubules and mitosis phase arrest and finally lead to cell death by apoptosis. One study reported that elevated class III beta-tubulin expression is independently prognostic and is under investigation as a predictor of resistance to taxane chemotherapy (Ploussard et al. 2010). There is an ongoing prospective study on acetylated tubulin and microtubule dynamics in CTCs to predict response of men with prostate cancer to docetaxel chemotherapy (Nanus et al. 2012). Other biomarkers of docetaxel resistance such as MIC-1, clusterin, BCL-2 levels, cytochrome P450 genetic variants, loss of epithelial phenotype, and stemness pathways are also under evaluation. Domingo-Domenech's study provided evidence for that inhibition of Notch and Hedgehog signaling in hormone refractory prostate cancer depletes a subpopulation of cells responsible for acquired docetaxel resistance (Domingo-Domenech et al. 2012). By inducing docetaxel-resistant DU-145 PC cells in culture, Marín-Aguilera compared global gene expression between docetaxel-sensitive and docetaxel-resistant cell lines and found that exposing parental cells to TGF-b1 increased their survival in the presence of docetaxel. The result suggested a role of the TGF-b superfamily in conferring docetaxel resistance (Marín-Aguilera et al. 2012). It was also reported that men with prostate cancer carrying two copies of the CYP1B1*3 polymorphic variant had a poor prognosis after docetaxel-based therapies compared with others carrying at least one copy of the CYP1B1*1 allele (Sissung et al. 2008). This finding provided evidence that CYP1B1*3 may be a predictive marker for estimating docetaxel efficacy in men with prostate cancer. By comparing protein profiling between docetaxel-sensitive PC3 cells and docetaxel-resistant PC3 cells, Zhao et al. identified MIC-1 and AGR2 as, respectively, upregulated and downregulated in docetaxel-resistant cells, and the result suggested that both AGR2 and MIC-1 play a potential predictive role in docetaxel resistance in CRPC (Zhao et al. 2009).

Potential Predictive Biomarkers of Response to Bone-Targeted Agents

Bone turnover markers are confirmed to be prognostic for CRPC; however, their predictive value has not been validated yet. Bone turnover markers such as Ntx, tartrate-resistant acid phosphatase 5b, C-telopeptide, alkaline phosphatase, and osteopontin have been evaluated as potential predictive biomarkers in multiple studies of zoledronic acid or denosumab in patients with bone metastases (Coleman et al. 2005; Jung et al. 2011). Pretreatment elevations in BAP appear to associate with the relative survival improvements associated with radium-223, suggesting a potential predictive role for this biomarker (Parker et al. 2013). Posttreatment BAP reductions are also highly associated with improvements in survival in men with metastatic prostate cancer treated by radium-223 chloride (Parker et al. 2013), which indicates the predictive value of posttreatment

BAP in men with CRPC treated with radium-223 chloride. Urinary Ntx is reported to be associated with skeletal complications, disease progression, and death (Brown et al. 2005). Prospective validation of these predictive uses of bone turnover markers in the context of bone-targeted therapies is needed; however, currently, treatment selection for these agents is not recommended based on elevations or changes in these biomarkers given the lack of prospective validation.

Potential Predictive Biomarkers of Response to Immunotherapy

Sipuleucel-T is a therapeutic vaccine and is FDA approved for minimally symptomatic men with metastatic CRPC. However, there is no validated predictive marker to help select patient who may derive benefit from this treatment. Sipuleucel-T was reported to be more beneficial in patients with lower baseline PSA than those with higher PSA level (Schellhammer et al. 2013). This indicates sipuleucel-T therapy may work better in early state when disease burden is low and immunologic tolerance is less. McNeel DG et al. reported that posttreatment eosinophilia predicted prolonged survival with sipuleucel-T therapy (McNeel et al. 2012). Further evaluation of predictive immunologic biomarkers is needed given the rapid progression in emerging immunotherapy in prostate cancer, particularly immune checkpoint therapies (CTLA-4 and PD-1/PD-L1 inhibition) and targeted vaccines.

Potential Predictive Biomarkers of Targeted Therapy

Cabozantinib is an inhibitor of the receptor tyrosine kinase c-met and VEGFR-2. Antitumor activity of cabozantinib has been reported in multiple tumors including prostate cancer (Hussain et al. 2011). C-met overexpression or activity may be predictive for benefit from cabozantinib treatment given the lack of observed efficacy of this agent in improving survival in unselected groups of men with mCRPC. Additional studies are needed to confirm the predictive role of c-met in CRPC. PI3K pathway is activated by loss of PTEN or other phosphatases or gains in activating genes. The aberrancies in PI3K pathway are seen in almost 100 % men with CRPC (Taylor et al. 2010). However, loss of PTEN or other activation of PI3K pathway has not been found to be predictive to clinical outcomes. Validation of predictive value of PI3K pathway inhibitor in CRPC needs prospective evaluation in clinical trials. LDH elevation is a predictive biomarker for OS in patients treated with mTOR inhibitor (e.g., temsirolimus) in renal cell carcinoma (Armstrong et al. 2012). Whether or not LDH serves the similar predictive role in CRPC needs prospective clinical trials to confirm associations with benefit to PI3K pathway inhibition. KRAS and BRAF mutations are known to rarely occur in prostate adenocarcinomas (Chao et al. 2006). However, KRAS pathway activation is commonly observed in mCRPC (Karantanos et al. 2013).

Sorafenib was reported to improve bony metastatic lesions, though interpretation of the study result is complicated by discordant radiographic and PSA responses (Dahut et al. 2008). This result suggested that sorafenib may have a role in patients with metastatic bone lesions, due to its inhibition of the ERK/mitogen-activated protein kinase pathway. Vemurafenib is proved to improve rates of overall and progression-free survival in patients with previously untreated melanoma with the BRAF V600E mutation (Chapman et al. 2011). Whether or not vemurafenib has similar value in prostate cancer is under study. Status of mutations in KRAS and BRAF may be used as predictive marker to help identify men with CRPC who may benefit from sorafenib or vemurafenib. The RB is a critical mediator of cell cycle progression and is functionally inactivated in the majority of human cancers, including prostatic adenocarcinoma. Twenty five percent to 50 % of prostatic adenocarcinomas harbor aberrations in RB pathway (Sharma et al. 2007). In Sharma's study, RB-deficient cells failed to elicit a cytostatic response when challenged with androgen ablation, AR antagonist, or combined androgen blockade. In the contrary, RB-deficient prostate cancer cells showed enhanced susceptibility to cell death induced by a selected subset of cytotoxic agents including antimicrotubule agents and a topoisomerase inhibitor. Therefore, the RB deficiency status can be potentially predictive for response to androgen deprivation or cytotoxin agents in men with CRPC. The cyclin/cyclin-dependent kinase (CDK)/RB-axis is a critical modulator of cell cycle entry and is aberrant in many human cancers including prostate cancer. PD-0332991 is a selective CDK4/6 inhibitor and was reported to effectively limit proliferation of hormone-sensitive and CRPC cells in vitro (Comstock et al. 2013). This PD-mediated inhibition of prostate cancer proliferation is dependent on the presence of RB. RB disruption might be predictive for the development of resistance to therapeutic agents that inhibit CDK4/6 activity (Comstock et al. 2013). Based on the fact that RB is commonly disrupted in CRPC (Sharma et al. 2010), early-stage prostate cancer patients with functional RB have a greater benefit from CDK4/6 inhibition; in the contrary, men with CRPC would be predicted to be resistant to CDK inhibition.

Conclusions

Prostate cancer has a complex molecular etiology and a prolonged disease course. Although most men initially respond to androgen deprivation therapy, most will eventually become castration resistant and develop lethal metastases. CRPC is a group of heterogeneous diseases, both in clinical manifestations and outcomes, requiring an individualized approach to both patient care and trial design. Given the increasing number of molecularly targeted and expensive systemic therapies, improving patient selection is critical to maximize benefit and minimize harms and costs. A major challenge in CRPC is how to define a molecular taxonomy that incorporates the clinical presentation or phenotype prospectively and in real time using tissue- or blood-based assays to define a homogeneous population and to evaluate specific therapies in these specific contexts. With the increasing number of treatment choices in CRPC, risk stratification and predictive biomarkers will help in the selection of patients who will be more likely to benefit from a specific treatment. Composite studies of multiple biomarkers will provide evidence for improved risk stratification, prognostication, and therapeutic decisions. The clinical utility of biomarkers in CRPC is dependent on the clinical context (e.g., prognosis, prediction, and surrogacy), the mechanism of action of a therapy, and how the biomarker will affect on the therapy decision. There are no credentialed predictive or surrogate biomarkers in CRPC yet as of 2015, but many are under evaluation. More rigorous studies on CRPC biomarkers are needed to facilitate new drug development and help promote more intelligent use of systemic therapies with most benefit and least harm.

Potential Applications to Other Diseases and Conditions

Advances in human genetics and tumor biology together with the development of drugs for specific targets hold promise for a new era of personalized oncology treatment. The essence of personalized oncology treatment relies on the use of precision biomarkers that define the disease in question biologically. Development of new biomarkers is important for all cancers, particularly for those with lethal potential. For example, there is growing evidence that CTCs are prognostic for OS in multiple malignancies including prostate cancer, breast cancer, and colorectal cancer (Budd et al. 2006; Cristofanilli et al. 2004; Tol et al. 2010). In breast cancer, the number of CTCs before treatment is reported to be an independent predictor of PFS and OS in patients with metastatic breast cancer (Cristofanilli et al. 2004). The CTC count before and during treatment also independently predicts PFS and OS in colorectal patients treated with chemotherapy plus targeted agents (Tol et al. 2010). With the improvement of CTC capturing technique, CTC biomarker characterization through genomic or protein-based application should contribute to guiding specific targeted therapy and personalized medicine in multiple malignancies.

Summary Points

- This chapter focuses on the introduction of biomarkers in CRPC and future development in biomarker in CRPC.
- Composite uses of multiple prognostic biomarkers in men with mCRPC help to risk stratify, prognosticate, and inform on therapeutic decision-making.
- Prognostic biomarkers provide insights on the natural history of disease with many emerging prognostic biomarkers under study in men with CRPC.
- There are no validated predictive biomarkers to date in men with CRPC, although this is an area of active research, including measurements in tumor tissue, whole blood, and circulating tumor cells.

References

Allard WJ, Matera J, Miller MC, et al. Tumor cells circulate in the peripheral blood of all major carcinomas but not in healthy subjects or patients with nonmalignant diseases. Clin Cancer Res. 2004;10:6897–904.

Antonarakis ES, Lu C, Wang H, Luber B, et al. AR-V7 and resistance to enzalutamide and abiraterone in prostate cancer. N Engl J Med. 2014;371(11):1028-38.

Aparicio A, Den R, et al. Time to stratify? The retinoblastoma protein in castrate-resistant prostate cancer. Nat Rev Urol. 2011;8(10):562–8.

Aparicio A, Harzstark A, et al. Platinum-based chemotherapy for variant castrate-resistant prostate cancer. Clin Cancer Res. 2013;19:3621–30.

Armstrong AJ, Garrett-Mayer ES, et al. A contemporary prognostic nomogram for men with hormone-refractory metastatic prostate cancer: a TAX327 study analysis. Clin Cancer Res. 2007a;13:6396–403.

Armstrong AJ, Garrett-Mayer E, et al. Prostate-specific antigen and pain surrogacy analysis in metastatic hormone- refractory prostate cancer. J Clin Oncol. 2007b;25:3965–70.

Armstrong AJ, Tannock IF, et al. The development of risk groups in men with metastatic castration-resistant prostate cancer based on risk factors for PSA decline and survival. Eur J Cancer. 2010a;46:517–25.

Armstrong AJ, Garrett-Mayer E, et al. Prediction of survival following first-line chemotherapy in men with castration-resistant metastatic prostate cancer. Clin Cancer Res. 2010b;16:203–11.

Armstrong AJ, Marengo MS, Oltean S, et al. Circulating tumor cells from patients with advanced prostate and breast cancer display both epithelial and mesenchymal markers. Mol Cancer Res. 2011;9:997–1007.

Armstrong AJ, George DJ, Halabi S. Serum lactate dehydrogenase predicts for overall survival benefit in patients with metastatic renal cell carcinoma treated with inhibition of mammalian target of rapamycin. J Clin Oncol. 2012;30:3402–7.

Armstrong AJ, et al. Association of bone scan index (BSI) with prognostic biomarkers and survival in men with metastatic castration-resistant prostate cancer (mCRPC) enrolled in a prospective randomized controlled trial of tasquinimod. J Clin Oncol. 2013;31:(suppl; abstr 5081).

Attard G, Swennenhuis JF, et al. Characterization of ERG, AR and PTEN gene status in circulating tumor cells from patients with castration-resistant prostate cancer. Cancer Res. 2009;69:2912–8.

Beltran H, Rickman DS, et al. Molecular characterization of neuroendocrine prostate cancer and identification of new drug targets. Cancer Discov. 2011;1:487–95.

Berruti A, Vignani F, et al. Prognostic role of neuroendocrine differentiation in prostate cancer, putting together the pieces of the puzzle. Open Access J Urol. 2010;2:109–24.

Berthold DR, Pond GR, et al. Treatment of hormone-refractory prostate cancer with docetaxel or mitoxantrone: relationships between prostate-specific antigen, pain, and quality of life response and survival in the TAX-327 study. Clin Cancer Res. 2008a;14:2763–7.

Berthold DR, Pond GR, et al. Docetaxel plus prednisone or mitoxantrone plus prednisone for advanced prostate cancer: updated survival in the TAX 327 study. J Clin Oncol. 2008b;26:242–5.

Bitting RL, Healy P, et al. Evaluation of clinical phenotype, survival, and circulating tumor cell (CTC) enumeration in men with metastatic castration-resistant prostate cancer (mCRPC). J Clin Oncol. 2013;31 Suppl. Abstract 5031.

Brown JE, Cook RJ, Major P, et al. Bone turnover markers as predictors of skeletal complications in prostate cancer, lung cancer, and other solid tumors. J Natl Cancer Inst. 2005;97:59–69.

Bubendorf L, Schopfer A, et al. Metastatic patterns of prostate cancer: an autopsy study of 1589 patients. Hum Pathol. 2000;31:578–83.

Budd G, Cristofanilli M, Ellis M, et al. Circulating tumor cells versus imaging – predicting overall survival invmetastatic breast cancer. Clin Cancer Res. 2006;12:6403–9.

Chao NU, Choi M, et al. BRAF and KRAS mutations in prostatic adenocarcinoma. Int J Cancer. 2006;119(8):1858–62.

Chapman PB, Hauschild A, Robert C, et al. Improved survival with vemurafenib in melanoma with BRAF V600E mutation. N Engl J Med. 2011;364:2507–16.

Chen CD, Welsbie DS, Tran C, et al. Molecular determinants of resistance to antiandrogen therapy. Nat Med. 2004;10:33–9.

Coleman RE, Major P, Lipton A, et al. Predictive value of bone resorption and formation markers in cancer patients with bone metastases receiving the bisphosphonate zoledronic acid. J Clin Oncol. 2005;23:4925–35.

Comstock CES, Augello MA, et al. Targeting cell cycle and hormone receptor pathways in cancer. Oncogene. 2013;32(48):5481–5491.

Cristofanilli M, Budd GT, Ellis MJ, et al. Circulating tumor cells, disease progression and survival in metastatic breast cancer. N Engl J Med. 2004;351:781–91.

Dahut WL, Scripture C, et al. A phase II clinical trial of sorafenib in androgen-independent prostate cancer. Clin Cancer Res. 2008;14(1):209–14.

Danila DC, Anand A, Sung CC, et al. TMPRSS2-ERG status in circulating tumor cells as a predictive biomarker of sensitivity in castration-resistant prostate cancer patients treated with abiraterone acetate. Eur Urol. 2011;60:897–904.

de Bono JS, Scher HI, et al. Circulating tumor cells predict survival benefit from treatment in metastatic castration-resistant prostate cancer. Clin Cancer Res. 2008;14:6302–9.

de la Piedra C, Alcaraz A, et al. Usefulness of bone turnover markers as predictors of mortality risk, disease progression and skeletal-related events appearance in patients with prostate cancer with bone metastases following treatment with zoledronic acid: TUGAMO study. Br J Cancer. 2013;108:2565–72.

Dennis ER, Jia X, et al. Bone scan index: a quantitative treatment response biomarker for castration-resistant metastatic prostate cancer. J Clin Oncol. 2012;30:519–24.

Domingo-Domenech J, Vidal S, et al. Suppression of acquired docetaxel resistance in prostate cancer through depletion of notch and hedgehog-dependent tumor-initiating cells. Cancer Cell. 2012;22:373–88.

Ebrahimi B, Tucker SL, et al. Cytokines in pancreatic carcinoma: correlation with phenotypic characteristics and prognosis. Cancer. 2004;101:2727–36.

El Sheikh SS, Romanska HM, et al. Predictive value of PTEN and AR coexpression of sustained responsiveness to hormonal therapy in prostate cancer – a pilot study. Neoplasia. 2008;10:949–53.

Even-Sapir E, Metser U, et al. The detection of bone metastases in patients with high risk prostate cancer: 99mTc-MDP planar bone scintigraphy, single and multifield of view SPECT, 18 F- fluoride PET and 18 F-fluoride PET/CT. J Nucl Med. 2006;47:287–97.

FDA. CellSearch(TM) Circulating Tumor Cell Kit. Premarket notification – expanded indications for use – metastatic prostate cancer. http://www.accessdata.fda.gov/cdrh_docs/pdf7/K073338.pdf (2008).

Halabi S, Small EJ, et al. Prognostic model for predicting survival in men with hormone-refractory metastatic prostate cancer. J Clin Oncol. 2003;21:1232–7.

Halabi S, Ou S, Vogelzang NJ, et al. The prognostic value of change in hemoglobin (HGB), LDH and PSA levels at 3 months from baseline in men with castrate recurrent prostate cancer [abstract]. American Society of Clinical Oncology Prostate Cancer Symposium; 2007 Feb 22–24; Orlando.

Halabi S, Vogelzang NJ, Kornblith AB, et al. Pain predicts overall survival in men with metastatic castration-refractory prostate cancer. J Clin Oncol. 2008;26:2544–9.

Holzbeierlein J, Lal P, et al. Gene expression analysis of human prostate carcinoma during hormonal therapy identifies androgen-responsive genes and mechanisms of therapy resistance. Am J Pathol. 2004;164:217–27.

Hörnberg E, Ylitalo EB, et al. Expression of androgen receptor splice variants in prostate cancer bone metastases is associated with castration-resistance and short survival. PLoS One. 2011;6:e19059.

Huang J, Yao JL, di Sant'Agnese PA. Immunohistochemical characterization of neuroendocrine cells in prostate cancer. Prostate. 2006;66:1399–406.

Humphreys MR, Fernandes KA, Sridhar SS. Impact of age at diagnosis on outcomes in men with castrate-resistant prostate cancer (CRPC). J Cancer. 2013;4(4):304–14.

Hussain SP, Hofseth LJ, Harris CC. Radical causes of cancer. Nat Rev Cancer. 2003;3:276–85.

Hussain M, Tangen CM, et al. Absolute prostate-specific antigen value after androgen deprivation is a strong independent predictor of survival in new metastatic prostate cancer: data from Southwest Oncology Group Trial 9346 (INT-0162). J Clin Oncol. 2006;24:3984–90.

Hussain M, Smith MR, Sweeney C, et al. Cabozantinib (XL184) in metastatic castration-resistant prostate cancer (mCRPC): results from a phase II randomized discontinuation trial. ASCO 2011 annual meeting. J Clin Oncol. 2011;29S. Abstract 4516.

Imbriaco M, Larson SM, et al. A new parameter for measuring metastatic bone involvement by prostate cancer: the Bone Scan index. Clin Cancer Res. 1998;4:1765–72.

Jung K, Miller K, et al. Bone turnover markers as predictors of mortality risk in prostate cancer patients with bone metastases following treatment with zoledronic acid. Eur Urol. 2011;59:604–12.

Kantoff PW, Higano CS, et al. Sipuleucel-T immunotherapy for castration-resistant prostate cancer. N Engl J Med. 2010;363:411–22.

Karantanos T, et al. Prostate cancer progression after androgen deprivation therapy: mechanisms of castrate resistance and novel therapeutic approaches. Oncogene. 2013;32:5501–11.

Keizman D, Gottfried M, et al. Castration-resistant prostate cancer patients treated with ketoconazole: pretreatment neutrophil-to-lymphocyte ratio in metastatic association with outcome and predictive nomogram. Oncologist. 2012;17:1508–14.

Kelly WK, Halabi S, et al. Randomized, double-blind, placebo-controlled phase III trial comparing docetaxel and prednisone with or without bevacizumab in men with metastatic castration-resistant prostate cancer: CALGB 90401. J Clin Oncol. 2012;30:1534–40.

Komiya A, Yasuda K, et al. The prognostic significance of loss of the androgen receptor and neuroendocrine differentiation in prostate biopsy specimens among castration-resistant prostate cancer patients. Mol Clin Oncol. 2013;1:257–62.

Logothetis CJ, Basch E, Molina A, et al. Effect of abiraterone acetate and prednisone compared with placebo and prednisone on pain control and skeletal-related events in patients with metastatic castration-resistant prostate cancer: exploratory analysis of data from the COU-AA-301 randomised trial. Lancet Oncol. 2012;13(12):1210–7.

Mahon KL, Chatfield MD, et al. Cytokines' profiles to predict chemotherapy outcome in castration-resistant prostate cancer (CRPC). ASCO annual meeting proceedings (Post-Meeting Edition). J Clin Oncol. 2011;29 Suppl:4598.

Marín-Aguilera M, Codony-Servat J, et al. Identification of docetaxel resistance genes in castration-resistant prostate cancer. Mol Cancer Ther. 2012;11:329–39.

McNeel DG, Lin DW, Gardner T, et al. Correlation of increased eosinophil count following sipuleucel-T treatment with outcome in patients with metastatic castrate-resistant prostate cancer. J Clin Oncol. 2012;30(suppl; abstract 4650).

Morgan T, Lange P, et al. Disseminated tumor cells in prostate cancer patients after radical prostatectomy and without evidence of disease predicts biochemical recurrence. Clin Cancer Res. 2009;15:677–83.

Morris MJ, Akhurst T, et al. Fluorodeoxyglucose positron emission tomography as an outcome measure for castrate metastatic prostate cancer treated with antimicrotubule chemotherapy. Clin Cancer Res. 2005;11:3210–6.

Mulholland D, Tran L, et al. Cell autonomous role of PTEN in regulating castration-resistant prostate cancer growth. Cancer Cell. 2011;19:792–804.

Nanus DM, Loftus M, Akhtar NH, et al. Prospective analysis of prostate cancer (PC) circulating tumor cells (CTCs) to predict response to docetaxel (DOC) chemotherapy. J Clin Oncol. 2012;30(Suppl 5; abstract 100).

Olmos D, Brewer D, Clark J, et al. Prognostic value of blood mRNA expression signatures in castration-resistant prostate cancer: a prospective, two-stage study. Lancet Oncol. 2012; 11:1114–24.

Ozkumur E, Shah A, et al. Inertial focusing for tumor antigen–dependent and –independent sorting of rare circulating tumor cells. Sci Transl Med. 2013;5(179):179ra47.

Parker C, Heinrich D, et al. Overall survival benefit of radium-223 chloride (alpharadin) in the treatment of patients with symptomatic bone metastases in castration-resistant prostate cancer (CRPC): a phase III randomized trial (ALSYMPCA). Eur J Cancer. 2011;47 Suppl 2. Abstract 1LBA.

Parker C, Nilsson S, et al. Alpha emitter radium-223 and survival in metastatic prostate cancer. N Engl J Med. 2013;369:213–23.

Petrylak DP, Ankerst DP, Jiang CS, et al. Evaluation of prostate- specific antigen declines for surrogacy in patients treated on SWOG 99-16. J Natl Cancer Inst. 2006;98:516–21.

Ploussard G, Terry S, Maille P, et al. Class III beta-tubulin expression predicts prostate tumor aggressiveness and patient response to docetaxel-based chemotherapy. Cancer Res. 2010; 70:9253–64.

Pond GR, Armstrong AJ, Wood BA, et al. Ability of C-reactive protein to complement multiple prognostic classifiers in men with metastatic castration resistant prostate cancer receiving docetaxel-based chemotherapy. BJU Int. 2012;110(11 Pt B):E461–8.

Pound CR, Partin AW, et al. Natural history of progression after PSA elevation following radical prostatectomy. JAMA. 1999;281:1591–7.

Prins RC, Rademacher BL, et al. C-reactive protein as an adverse prognostic marker for men with castration-resistant prostate cancer (CRPC): confirmatory results. Urol Oncol. 2012;30:33–7.

Ross RW, Galsky MD, Scher HI, et al. A whole-blood RNA transcript based transcript based prognostic model in men with castration-resistant prostate cancer: a prospective study. Lancet Oncol. 2012;11:1105–13.

Ryan CJ, Li J, Kheoh T, et al. Baseline serum adrenal androgens are prognostic and predictive of overall survival (OS) in patients (pts) with metastatic castrate-resistant prostate cancer (mCRPC): results of the COU-AA-301 phase 3 randomized trial. Cancer Res. 2012;72:S1. Abstract LB-434.

Sasaki T, Komiya A, Suzuki H, et al. Changes in chromogranin A serum levels during endocrine therapy in metastatic prostate cancer patients. Eur Urol. 2005;48:224–30.

Saylor PJ, Armstrong AJ, et al. New and emerging therapies for bone metastases in genitourinary cancers. Eur Urol. 2013;63:309–20.

Schellhammer PF, Chodak G, et al. Lower baseline prostate-specific antigen is associated with a greater overall survival benefit from sipuleucel-T in the Immunotherapy for Prostate Adenocarcinoma Treatment (IMPACT) trial. Urology. 2013;81:1297–302.

Scher HI, Halabi S, Tannock I, et al. Design and end points of clinical trials for patients with progressive prostate cancer and castrate levels of testosterone: recommendations of the Prostate Cancer Clinical Trials Working Group. J Clin Oncol. 2008;26:1148–59.

Scher H, Jia X, et al. Circulating tumour cells as prognostic markers in progressive, castration-resistant prostate cancer: a reanalysis of IMMC38 trial data. Lancet Oncol. 2009;10:233–9.

Scher HI, Morris MJ, Basch E, Heller G. End points and outcomes in castration-resistant prostate cancer: from clinical trials to clinical practice. J Clin Oncol. 2011a;29:3695–704.

Scher HI, Heller G, Molina A, et al. Evaluation of circulating tumor cell (CTC) enumeration as an efficacy response biomarker of overall survival (OS) in metastatic castration-resistant prostate cancer (mCRPC): planned final analysis (FA) of COU-AA-301, a randomized double-blind, placebo-controlled phase III study of abiraterone acetate (AA) plus low-dose prednisone (P) post docetaxel (Meeting Abstracts). J Clin Oncol. 2011b;29:LBA4517.

Seruga B, Zhang H, et al. Cytokines and their relationship to the symptoms and outcome of cancer. Nat Rev Cancer. 2008;8:887–99.

Shaffer DR, Leversha MA, et al. Circulating tumor cell analysis in patients with progressive castration-resistant prostate cancer. Clin Cancer Res. 2007;13:2023–9.

Shafique K, Proctor M, et al. The modified Glasgow prognostic score in prostate cancer: results from a retrospective clinical series of 744 patients. BMC Cancer. 2013;13:292–300.

Sharma A, Comstock CES, et al. Retinoblastoma tumor suppressor status is a critical determinant of therapeutic response in prostate cancer cells. Cancer Res. 2007;67:6192–203.

Sharma A, Yeow WS, et al. The retinoblastoma tumor suppressor controls androgen signaling and human prostate cancer progression. J Clin Invest. 2010;120:4478–92.

Sissung T, Danes R, et al. Association of the CYP1B1*3 allele with survival in patients with prostate cancer receiving docetaxel. Mol Cancer Ther. 2008;7:19–26.

Smaletz O, Scher HI, Small EJ, et al. Nomogram for overall survival of patients with progressive metastatic prostate cancer after castration. J Clin Oncol. 2002;20:3972–82.

Smith MR, Kabbinavar F, Saad F, et al. Natural history of rising serum prostate-specific antigen in men with castrate nonmetastatic prostate cancer. J Clin Oncol. 2005;23:2918–25.

Sonpavde G, Pond GR, Berry WR, et al. Serum alkaline phosphatase changes predict survival independent of PSA changes in men with castration-resistant prostate cancer and bone metastasis receiving chemotherapy. Urol Oncol. 2010;5:607–13.

Spiess PE, Pettaway CA, Vakar-Lopez F, et al. Treatment outcomes of small cell carcinoma of the prostate: a single-center study. Cancer. 2007;110:1729–37.

Subudhi SK, Heller G, et al. Sera cytokine levels to predict survival in men with progressive castration-resistant prostate cancer. J Clin Oncol. 2013;13 Suppl. Abstract 5083.

Taylor BS, Schultz N, Hieronymus H, et al. Integrative genomic profiling of human prostate cancer. Cancer Cell. 2010;18:11–22.

Thadani-Mulero M, Portella L, Sun S, Sung M, et al. Androgen receptor splice variants determine taxane sensitivity in prostate cancer. Cancer Res. 2014;74(8):2270–82.

Thompson IM, Pauler DK, Goodman PJ, et al. Prevalence of prostate cancer among men with a prostate-specific antigen level $<$ or $=$ 4.0 ng per milliliter. N Engl J Med. 2004;350:2239–46.

Tol J, Koopman M, et al. Circulating tumour cells early predict progression-free and overall survival in advanced colorectal cancer patients treated with chemotherapy and targeted agents. Ann Oncol. 2010;21:1006–12.

Tomlins SA, Rhodes DR, Perner S, et al. Recurrent fusion of TMPRSS2 and ETS transcription factor genes in prostate cancer. Science. 2005;310:644–8.

Ulmert D, Kaboteh R, Fox JJ, et al. A novel automated platform for quantifying the extent of skeletal tumour involvement in prostate cancer patients using the bone scan index. Eur Urol. 2012;62:78–84.

Vashchenko N, Abrahamsson PA. Neuroendocrine differentiation in prostate cancer: implications for new treatment modalities. Eur Urol. 2005;47:147–55.

Vollmer RT, Dawson NA, Vogelzang NJ. The dynamics of prostate specific antigen in hormone refractory prostate carcinoma: an analysis of cancer and leukemia group B study 9181 of megestrol acetate. Cancer. 1998;83:1989–94.

Ware KE, Garcia-Blanco MA, Armstrong AJ, Dehm SM. Biologic and clinical significance of androgen receptor variants in castration resistant prostate cancer. Endocr Relat Cancer. 2014;21(4):T87–103.

Watahiki A, Macfarlane R, et al. Plasma miRNAs as biomarkers to identify patients with castration-resistant metastatic prostate cancer. Int J Mol Sci. 2013;14:7757–70.

Weckermann D, Polzer B, et al. Perioperative activation of disseminated tumor cells in bone marrow of patients with prostate cancer. J Clin Oncol. 2009;27:1549–56.

Yoshimoto M, Cutz JC, et al. Interphase FISH analysis of PTEN in histologic sections shows genomic deletions in 68 % of primary prostate cancer and 23 % of high-grade prostatic intraepithelial neoplasias. Cancer Genet Cytogenet. 2006;169:128–37.

Zhao L, Lee BY, et al. Identification of candidate biomarkers of therapeutic response to docetaxel by proteomic profiling. Cancer Res. 2009;69:7696–703.

Part V

Cervix and Uterus

Mitosis Targets as Biomarkers in Cervical Cancer

22

Jaime Berumen, Ana María Espinosa, Ingrid Medina, and Mariano Guardado

Contents

Abstract

The effectiveness of a preventive human papillomavirus (HPV) vaccination for reducing the cervical cancer (CC) burden will likely not be known for 30 years. Current screening methods for detecting high-grade cervical intraepithelial neoplasias (CIN2/3) and CC (CIN2+) have low sensitivity (Pap test) or low specificity (HPV tests). Improved procedures for CC screening and treatment are therefore required. Based on comparisons with healthy cervical epithelium,

J. Berumen (✉)
Departamento de Medicina Experimental, Facultad de Medicina, Universidad Nacional Autonoma de Mexico, Mexico city, Mexico

Unidad de Medicina Genomica, Hospital General de Mexico, Mexico city, Mexico
e-mail: jaimeberumen@hotmail.com; jaimeberumen@yahoo.com.mx

A.M. Espinosa • I. Medina • M. Guardado
Unidad de Medicina Genomica, Hospital General de Mexico, Mexico city, Mexico
e-mail: anaesga@hotmail.com; medmarin@unam.com; jos_mariano@hotmail.com

V.R. Preedy, V.B. Patel (eds.), *Biomarkers in Cancer, Biomarkers in Disease: Methods, Discoveries and Applications*,
DOI 10.1007/978-94-007-7681-4_25

the genes most upregulated and enriched in CC are those involved in mitosis. Some of these upregulated genes might be good candidates for CC screening or survival markers or as potential therapeutic targets. In this chapter, we analyze the benefits and limitations of current methods used for early CC detection, the evidence that demonstrates that the most enriched genes in CC are those involved in mitosis, the mechanism that regulates mitosis and its relationship with HPV, and our experimental evidence suggesting that some mitosis genes might be good markers for screening and survival in CC. In addition, we discuss the need to develop less expensive and more efficient methods that can be automated for large-scale application in poor and developing countries. We also discuss the potential use of the markers for other types of cancers and as potential therapeutic targets.

List of Abbreviations

APC/C	Anaphase-Promoting Complex
AUC	Area Under the Curve
CC	Cervical Cancer
Cdks	Cyclin-Dependent Kinases
CIN	Cervical Intraepithelial Neoplasia
DNA	Deoxyribonucleic Acid
DSB	Double-Strand Breaks
ELISA	Enzyme-Linked Immunosorbent Assay
FDA	US Food and Drug Administration
FIGO	International Federation of Gynecology and Obstetrics
H&E	Hematoxylin and Eosin Stain
HC2	Hybrid Capture 2 Technology
HPV	Human Papillomavirus
HR	Hazard Ratio
IH	Immunohistochemistry
mRNA	Messenger Ribonucleic Acid
NPV	Negative Predictive Value
Pap	Papanicolaou Test
PPV	Positive Predictive Value
qRT-PCR	Quantitative Reverse-Transcription PCR
RMA	Robust Multi-array Average
ROC	Receiver-Operating Characteristic

Key Facts of Microarray Technology

- A microarray consists of an orderly arrangement of small probes of genetic material that are chemically synthesized on a solid surface. The precise location where each probe is synthesized is called a cell, and a microarray contains thousands of cells. A microarray experiment can be used to explore thousands of genes simultaneously.

- There are different types of microarrays. DNA microarrays are used to explore single-nucleotide polymorphisms (SNPs). RNA microarrays are used to explore gene expression. There are also tissue microarrays for the detection of proteins by immunohistochemistry and immunofluorescence.
- Some applications of microarrays include the identification of differential gene expression, splicing variants, changes in the methylation patterns, germ line and somatic mutations, genotype, and changes in gene copy number.
- Microarray technology is based on hybridization of nucleic acids. In the case of expression microarrays, the experiment starts with the total RNA to be explored. It is then converted to cDNA, transcribed in vitro, fragmented, and labeled. Subsequently, the microarray is hybridized with the labeled material for 16 h at a constant temperature of 45 °C, followed by washing and staining. The intensity signal of each probe is then read with a special fluorescent reader.
- In order to eliminate experimental biases, microarray expression signals are normalized prior to conducting statistical analysis. One of the most commonly used algorithms to accomplish this, is the robust multi-array average (RMA), which is based on equalizing the median signal intensity of each microarray. The accuracy of the algorithm increases with the number of analyzed microarrays.
- One of the objectives of an expression microarray is the identification of genes that are differentially expressed between an experimental condition and a control group. Such genes may be used as biomarkers for screening, diagnosis, prognosis, and treatment decisions.
- Validation of microarray experiments is indispensable. The predominant technology used to validate expression microarrays is quantitative reverse-transcription PCR.

Definitions of Words and Terms

Anaphase Bridges Chromatin fibers that connect two separated chromosomes resulting from the presence of dicentric chromosomes that are formed by the fusion of two telomere-deficient fragments. This phenomenon occurs commonly in cancer because of the lack of ligation of DNA double-strand breaks.

Aneuploidy Structural alterations of the genome characterized by an abnormal number of chromosomes.

Area Under the Curve (AUC) The area under the curve of a receiver-operating characteristic (ROC) graph, which is designed to select the best signal cutoff value for detecting the greatest number of true positive samples (cases, sensitivity) and the lowest number of true negative samples (controls, specificity). The higher the value of the AUC, the higher the discriminative power of the algorithm.

Cervical Intraepithelial Neoplasia (CIN) Noninvasive cervical epithelial lesions characterized by abnormal growth and neoplastic changes in cell morphology.

CINs are classified by the fraction of affected epithelium as measured from the basal to the apical side of the epithelium, CIN1, CIN2, and CIN3 representing 1/3, 2/3, or the full cervical epithelium, respectively.

FIGO Stage A clinical classification system of tumors based on tumor characteristics such as size, degree of invasion, spread to lymph nodes, and metastasis. FIGO was established by the International Federation of Gynecology and Obstetrics.

Hematoxylin and Eosin Stain (H&E) A histological stain that combines a basic (hematoxylin) and an acid (eosin) dye that enables the identification of cellular structures with a light microscope. The stain is used commonly in histologic and pathologic analyses because the procedure is rapidly performed and inexpensive.

Hybrid Capture 2 Technology (HC2) A DNA hybridization technique performed in a liquid solution to detect human papillomavirus DNA obtained from cervical samples, such as exudates and tumor biopsies. It is useful as an initial screening methodology.

Negative Predictive Value (NPV) The probability of being free of the disease if the result of the diagnostic test is negative.

Positive Predictive Value (PPV) The probability of having the disease if the result of the diagnostic test is positive.

Potential Therapeutic Target A deregulated gene that has a high power of discrimination between cancer and control samples and that is extremely important for cancer development. Blocking such a gene might delay or prevent cancer cell proliferation or tumor growth.

Quantitative Reverse Transcription PCR (qRT-PCR) A quantitative DNA technology based on amplification of genomic material by the polymerase chain reaction (PCR) that is used to assess the level of gene expression by measuring the amplified product in each growth cycle with fluorescently labeled probes.

Introduction

The human papillomavirus (HPV) is the main causal factor in the development of invasive cervical cancer (CC), being found in nearly 100 % of these tumors (Schiffman et al. 2011). CC develops through the progression of preinvasive cervical intraepithelial neoplasia (CIN), which is histologically graded as mild (CIN1), moderate (CIN2), or severe (CIN3) dysplasia. CC develops predominately from CIN3 and CIN2 but rarely from CIN1, with estimated progression rates from these lesions to CC of 12 %, 5 %, and 1 %, respectively (Ostor 1993).

Currently, there are vaccines on the market that prevent infection by oncogenic HPV types 16 and 18, which are associated with 65–70 % of CCs worldwide (de Sanjose et al. 2010). These vaccines are highly efficient at preventing infection and high-grade CINs (CIN2/CIN3) (Lehtinen et al. 2012). However, vaccinated women must continue to participate in early detection programs for CC because the vaccines can only protect against certain virus types, and it is not known for how long the immune protection against the targeted virus remains (Romanowski 2011). In many countries, preventive vaccines for HPV16 and HPV18 have been incorporated into a national vaccination program for girls from 9 to 12 years of age (Cuzick 2010; Markowitz et al. 2007). However, because the peak incidence of CC occurs in women 45–50 years old, the effectiveness of these preventive vaccination programs on reducing the incidence of CC will not be known for 30 years. Therefore, it is necessary to improve the procedures for CC screening and treatment. Because each year 530,000 new CC cases and 275,000 CC deaths are reported worldwide, the mortality-to-incidence ratio is approximately 50 % (Hwang and Shroyer 2012; Ferlay et al. 2008).

For many years, the Papanicolaou (Pap) test has been the most important screening procedure for early detection of CC, and its massive application in developed countries has decreased the incidence of CC by more than 50 % in the last 40 years (McCrory et al. 2009). Women with abnormal Pap test results are referred for colposcopy to confirm, reject, or clarify the diagnosis with histopathological analysis. Unfortunately, the average sensitivity of cytology for detection of CIN lesions is only 50–60 %, although the specificity is very high at approximately 90 % (Wright 2007). Since HPV is essential for the development of CC, several procedures to detect the HPV genome have been incorporated into CC screening. Hybrid Capture 2 technology (HC2) is the methodology most frequently used for screening, particularly for measuring high-risk virus. This method, approved by the Food and Drug Administration (FDA) in the United States, demonstrates higher sensitivity but lower specificity than conventional cytology for detecting CIN2 lesions or higher (CIN2+). HC2 has an average sensitivity of 95 % (range, 62–98 %) for detecting high-grade lesions and invasive cancer. However, HC2 has low specificity for CIN2+, especially in young women, because the majority of detected infections are not associated with neoplastic lesions (Leinonen et al. 2009; Whitlock et al. 2011). In women over the age of 30 years, the specificity is higher, but it varies among studies because of its partial dependence on the prevalence of HPV in the study population (Giorgi-Rossi et al. 2012). In most studies, the positive predictive value (PPV) is less than 20 %, which is consistent with the percentage of infected women having high-grade lesions. The high sensitivity and high negative predictive value (NPV) of HPV DNA tests for the detection of CIN2+ lesions suggest that this test could be used to extend screening intervals. However, the low specificity of HPV DNA tests would increase the number of follow-up tests and colposcopy referrals, thereby increasing the cost of screening (Leinonen et al. 2009).

Therefore, there is an obvious need to develop new methods for early detection of CC with high sensitivity and specificity. Multiple tumor markers associated with

CIN2+ have been identified, in particular *CDKN2A*, *TOP2A*, and *MCM2*. However, these markers have been proposed not for screening but for diagnosis, prognosis, or clinical management (Natunen et al. 2011). Although several studies have used microarrays to identify genes associated with cervical cancer (Narayan et al. 2007; Gius et al. 2007; Zhai et al. 2007; Pyeon et al. 2007; Biewenga et al. 2008; Buitrago-Pérez et al. 2009), most have been insufficient for identifying screening markers because they employed an insufficient design, such as heterogeneous samples positive for different or undetermined HPV types and/or a small number of tumors and controls.

It is important to emphasize that the primary value of CC biomarkers and the goal of developing procedures for cervical screening are to improve the specificity rather than the sensitivity relative to HPV testing (Hwang and Shroyer 2012). Primary HPV DNA screening with cytology triage increases the specificity to an extent similar to that of conventional cytology (Markowitz et al. 2007; Leinonen et al. 2009). However, use of this procedure in developing countries creates logistical problems because a high percentage of women who test positive for HPV do not return for a cytological follow-up or because of the handling difficulties associated with a sample taken for cytology at the first visit. In addition, the procedure appears to be impractical because it cannot be automated. The simultaneous use of HC2 for high-risk viruses with a molecular method that can distinguish CIN2+ from CIN1− would increase the specificity and PPV and would provide the advantages of speed and automation potential compared to triaged cytology.

Use of p16 for Clinical Diagnosis but not for Screening Cervical Cancer

Of the markers associated with CC, the tumor suppressor protein p16 has been the most widely studied (Hwang and Shroyer 2012). This protein accumulates in the nucleus and cytoplasm of cells transformed by high-risk HPVs and is usually detected by immunohistochemistry (IH). The amount of p16 is related to the severity of cervical neoplasia and is considered to be a marker of CIN2+. p16 has been used successfully to classify HPV-related diseases. Lower interobserver variations have been reported for IH detection of p16 in punch and cone biopsies than for diagnosis with hematoxylin and eosin (H&E)-stained sections. Recently, p16 has emerged as a sensitive and specific diagnostic tool to detect CIN2+ lesions in cervical cytology specimens (Hwang and Shroyer 2012). p16 consistently exhibits high sensitivity (80–95 %) for detection of CIN2+, but its specificity is lower (ca. 50 %) than that of cytology (Tsoumpou et al. 2009). The low specificity is because p16 is expressed in approximately 38 % of low-grade CIN lesions, i.e., those infected with high-risk HPV types (Tsoumpou et al. 2009). The relatively low specificity and the need for a pathologist to interpret the IH results are the major reasons contributing to the fact that p16 has not been widely adopted for primary screening. Recently, Wentzensen et al. developed enzyme-linked immunosorbent assay (ELISA) method to detect p16 protein in cell lysates of cervix exudates, which provides a sensitivity and specificity for the identification of high-risk lesions of 84–87 %, respectively (Wentzensen et al. 2006).

Mitosis is the Main Phase of the Cell Cycle Altered in Cervical Cancer

The cell cycle is the primary process altered in CC; it is ranked highest in all published CC studies that have analyzed biological processes (Buitrago-Pérez et al. 2009). Similarly, in two studies of CC, in which we analyzed the expression of 8,638 genes with the HG-Focus microarray (Espinosa et al. 2013) or 21,034 genes with the HG 1.0 ST microarray from Affymetrix, the cell cycle process was the most enriched and appeared at the top of the lists of gene datasets that were analyzed with the Database for Annotation, Visualization and Integrated Discovery (DAVID) tool at medium stringency (Table 1). However, in both datasets, the M-phase processes were the most enriched (labeled in red in Table 1) when the analyses were conducted at high stringency, suggesting that the M phase is the main altered cell cycle phase in CC. According to the IH data, approximately 30 % of tumor cells in CC might be in the M phase (Espinosa et al. 2013). These findings are consistent with the in vitro alterations in the cell cycle and mitosis caused by HPV (Teissier et al. 2007; Moody and Laimins 2010), and they correlate with other CC studies (Teissier et al. 2007). The E6 and E7 oncoproteins of high-risk HPVs induce numerous mitotic defects, including multipolar mitoses, chromosomal missegregation, anaphase bridges, and aneuploidy. Although cells with abnormal mitosis are normally targeted for cell death, E6 and E7 act cooperatively to allow cells with abnormal centrosomes to accumulate by relaxing the G2/M checkpoint response and inhibiting apoptotic signaling (Moody and Laimins 2010). In agreement with these data, the canonical pathways G2/M DNA damage checkpoint regulation and role of CHK proteins in cell cycle checkpoint control were ranked at the second and fifth positions, respectively, of the altered canonical pathways in CC (Espinosa et al. 2013). Furthermore, E6 and E7 induce mechanisms that also avoid the mitosis checkpoint. The E6 and E7 genes have been shown to induce overexpression of CDC20 and UBCH10, which activates the APC/C ubiquitin ligase complex (Patel and McCance 2010). The finding of the enrichment of positive regulation of ubiquitin–protein ligase activity during the mitotic cell cycle in CC is consistent with the in vitro results (Espinosa et al. 2013).

A total of 128 genes of the mitosis phase were identified in two series of CCs studied in Mexico: 72 with HG-Focus microarray, 114 with HG 1.0 ST microarray, and 58 genes shared with both. The non-supervised hierarchical clustering performed with both sets of gene expression values clearly separated the cancer samples from those of the control group (Fig. 1). Interestingly, all but four genes involved in mitosis were upregulated (Fig. 2). Eleven of those genes (*CCNB2, CDK1, CDC20, CDKN3, CKS2, MKI67, NUSAP1, PRC1, SMC4, SYCP2,* and *ZWINT*), together with some genes used previously as markers for CC (*CDKN2A,*

Table 1 DAVID functional annotation cluster analysis at medium stringency of genes deregulated in cervical cancer. The table shows the 10 most enriched biological processes in the set of deregulated genes in cervical cancer obtained both with HG-Focus (panel A) and HG 1.0 ST (panel B) microarrays and analyzed with the DAVID tool

Cluster	Enrichment score[a]	Biological process	No. of genes	*p*-value	Fold change[b]
A. Deregulated genes in 43 CC identified with HG-Focus ($n = 997$)					
1	19.92	Cell cycle	140	2.1E-30	2.8
		M phase	72	2.0E-20	3.4
		Mitosis (1)	51	1.4E-15	3.6
2	11.59	DNA metabolic process	99	4.3E-24	3.1
		DNA repair	51	4.0E-11	2.8
3	9.53	Regulation of ubiquitin–protein ligase activity during mitotic cell cycle (2)	30	6.3E-17	6.6
		Anaphase-promoting complex-dependent proteasomal ubiquitin-dependent protein catabolic process	28	4.5E-16	6.8
4	7.97	Response to chemical stimulus	150	9.8E-14	1.8
5	7.26	Spindle organization	21	6.8E-13	7.3
		Cytoskeleton organization	57	3.7E-07	2.1
6	5.53	Developmental process	268	5.6E-08	1.3
		Cell differentiation	129	7.1E-03	1.2
7	5.5	Negative regulation of nucleobase, nucleoside, nucleotide, and nucleic acid metabolic process	51	1.6E-03	1.6
8	5.38	Interphase	24	1.7E-07	3.6
		G1/S transition of mitotic cell cycle	13	1.7E-04	3.6
9	5.23	Embryonic development	66	2.7E-06	1.8
10	4.89	Regulation of cell cycle	61	1.1E-13	2.9
		Regulation of mitosis	13	1.7E-04	3.6
B. Deregulated genes in 48 CC identified with HG 1.0 ST ($n = 1{,}812$)					
1	29.47	Cell cycle	200	4.3E-41	2.7
		M phase	114	8.5E-36	3.6
		Mitosis (1)	83	4.9E-29	3.9
2	9.19	DNA metabolic process	112	1.9E-17	2.3
		DNA repair	63	4.4E-10	2.3
3	8.06	Chromosome segregation	36	2.0E-15	4.6
		Mitotic sister chromatid segregation	19	7.3E-10	5.5
4	7.62	Microtubule cytoskeleton organization	39	9.2E-09	2.8
		Cytoskeleton organization	54	3.6E-08	2.2

(continued)

Table 1 (continued)

Cluster	Enrichment score[a]	Biological process	No. of genes	p-value	Fold change[b]
5	6.87	DNA packaging	45	2.3E-16	4.0
		Chromosome organization	92	2.4E-10	2.0
6	6.74	Meiosis	31	4.9E-09	3.3
		Meiotic cell cycle	31	8.3E-09	3.2
7	5.31	Developmental process	387	1.3E-08	1.3
		Cell differentiation	196	5.9E-04	1.2
8	4.73	Response to chemical stimulus	172	3.1E-06	1.4
9	4.17	Regulation of cell cycle	69	1.0E-09	2.2
		Regulation of mitosis	16	1.9E-04	3.0
10	3.94	Angiogenesis	31	6.1E-05	2.2

[a]Enrichment score is the -log10 of the average p-value of the terms in the cluster. [b]Fold change is the ratio of the proportion of genes in the tested list versus the Human Gene Reference database. The clusters in red were enriched in a functional annotation cluster analysis at highest stringency

MCM2, *TOP2A*, and *PCNA*), were validated with quantitative reverse-transcription polymerase chain reaction (qRT-PCR) mostly in HPV16-positive CC and healthy cervical epitheliums (Espinosa et al. 2013). The box plots (Fig. 3) clearly show the difference in gene expression between the cancer and control groups ($p < 1 \times 10^{-15}$ for all genes, Mann–Whitney U test).

The mitosis genes identified in both series of tumors participate in several of the subprocesses of mitosis, primarily formation and control of mitotic use, regulation of the metaphase-to-anaphase transition, chromosome segregation, cytokinesis, and mitotic entrance/exit (Fig. 4). While activation of cyclin-dependent kinases (Cdks) drives cells into mitosis, mitotic exit depends on inhibition of Cdk activity and dephosphorylation of proteins phosphorylated by Cdks. The activity of Cdks is inhibited primarily through degradation of mitotic cyclins by the anaphase-promoting complex (APC/C) and accumulation of Cdk inhibitor proteins. Five (CDK1, CCNB2, CDC20, CDKN3, and PRC1) of the eleven mitosis proteins validated in a previous paper (Espinosa et al. 2013) appear to be essential in these processes. Cyclin B2 (CCNB2) and cyclin B1 (CCNB1) bind to CDK1 (CDC2) to form the complex M-CDK, which is essential for control of the cell cycle at the G2/M transition. However, while cyclin B1-CDK1 causes chromosome condensation, reorganizes microtubules, and disassembles the nuclear lamina and the Golgi apparatus, cyclin B2-CDK1 is restricted to the cytoplasm and disassembles the Golgi apparatus during mitosis (Gong and Ferrell 2010). Consistent with these data, cyclin B2 was localized exclusively in the cytoplasm of the CCs examined in our study (Espinosa et al. 2013). Interestingly, the expression of cyclin B1 in these tumors did not differ from that in the control samples. Degradation of cyclin B1 by APC/C, a key regulator of the metaphase-to-anaphase transition, allows progression of mitosis from metaphase to anaphase (Gong and Ferrell 2010). While *CCNB2* has been scantily associated with CC (Buitrago-Pérez et al. 2009), it has also been

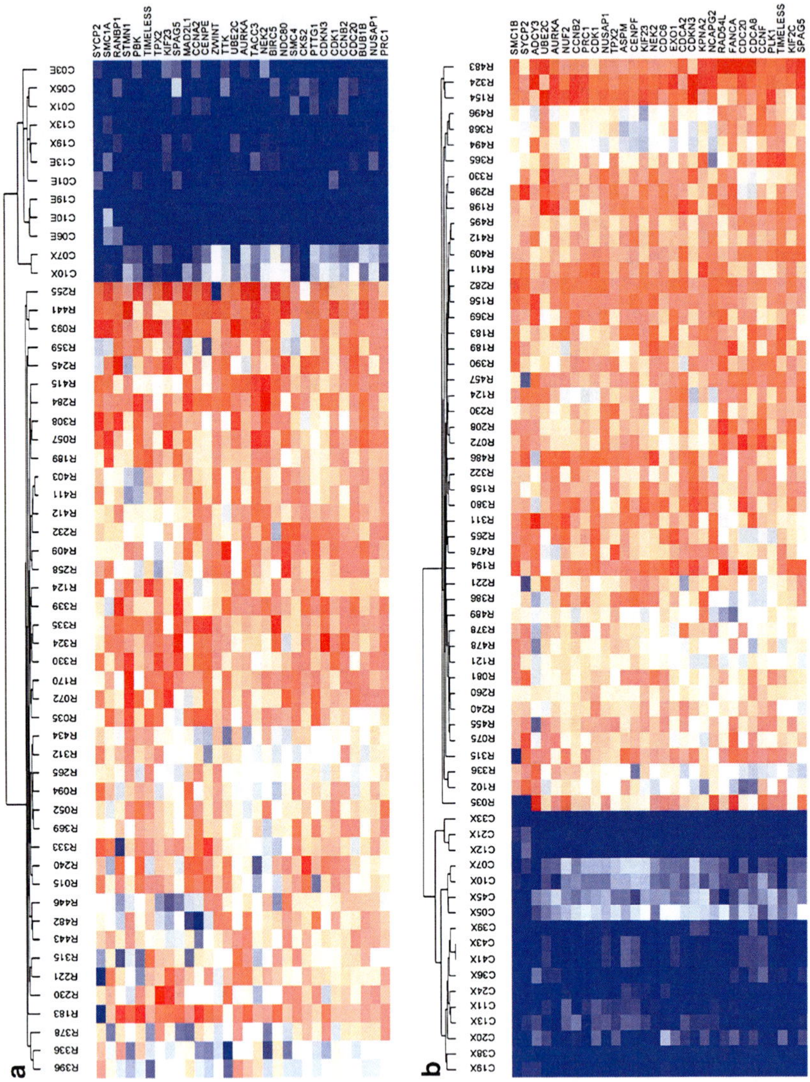

Fig. 1 (continued)

reported to be associated with other types of cancer. For example, it is upregulated in cancers of the colon (Park et al. 2007), lung, and digestive tract (Mo et al. 2010).

An increased amount of CDC20, a key regulatory protein of the APC/C complex during anaphase, could explain the absence of cyclin B1. UBE2C (also known as UBCH10) was also found to be increased in CC (Espinosa et al. 2013). Both CDC20 and UBE2C are required for full ubiquitin ligase activity of the APC/C complex and may confer substrate specificity upon the complex. CDC20 is negatively regulated by MAD2L1 and BUB1B (also known as BUBR1). In metaphase, the MAD2L1-CDC20-APC/C ternary complex is inactive, whereas in anaphase, the CDC20-APC/C binary complex is active in degrading substrates. Interestingly, the MAD2L1 and BUB1B transcripts were also increased in CC (Espinosa et al. 2013), suggesting that the corresponding proteins could be increased, thereby preventing activation of APC/C. However, part of the CDC20 protein could remain free to bind and activate APC/C, as has been shown in transfected cells expressing E6 and E7 proteins (Patel and McCance 2010). Upregulated CDC20 has been found in lung, pancreatic, and gastric cancers (Nakayama and Nakayama 2006), as well as in CC (Teissier et al. 2007).

CDKN3 is a dual-specificity protein phosphatase of the Cdc14 phosphatase group that interacts with CDK1 (CDC2) and inhibits its activity (Demetrick et al. 1995). CDKN3 and other Cdc14 phosphatases have not been well studied, but they appear to be essential for antagonizing Cdk activity in late mitosis, allowing cells to exit mitosis and enter telophase. Regulation of cytokinesis may be the one conserved function of the Cdc14 phosphatases. Although overexpression of CDKN3 has been associated with inhibition of cell proliferation in colon cancer cell lines (Galamb et al. 2010), it has been found to be overexpressed in breast, prostate, and lung cancers (MacDermed et al. 2010; Julien et al. 2011; Taylor et al. 2010). In the previous report of the association of *CDKN3* with cervical cancer, *CDKN3* was shown to behave as an oncogene (Espinosa et al. 2013). However, it has been proposed that CDKN3 is a tumor suppressor of mitosis control (Nalepa et al. 2013).

PRC1 is essential for control of the spatiotemporal formation of the midzone and successful cytokinesis (Subramanian et al. 2010). It is required for kinesin family member 14 (KIF14) (Gruneberg et al. 2006) and polo-like kinase 1 (PLK1) (Lens et al. 2010) localization to the central spindle and midbody. Suppression of PRC1 blocks cell division. Transcription of *PRC1* is repressed by p53 and is one of the routes by which p53 stops the cell cycle at the G2/M checkpoint (Li et al. 2004).

Fig. 1 Segregation of tumor and control samples according to the mitosis gene expression profile. Unsupervised hierarchical cluster analysis using the expression values of the top 30 genes deregulated from mitosis as identified with either the HG-Focus (**panel a**: 43 CCs and 12 healthy cervical epitheliums) or the HG 1.0 ST (**panel b**: 48 CCs and 17 healthy cervical epitheliums) microarray. Each row represents a gene, and each column represents a sample. The length and the subdivision of the branches represent relationships among the samples based on the intensity of gene expression. The cluster is color-coded using *red* for upregulation, *blue* for downregulation, and *white* for unchanged expression

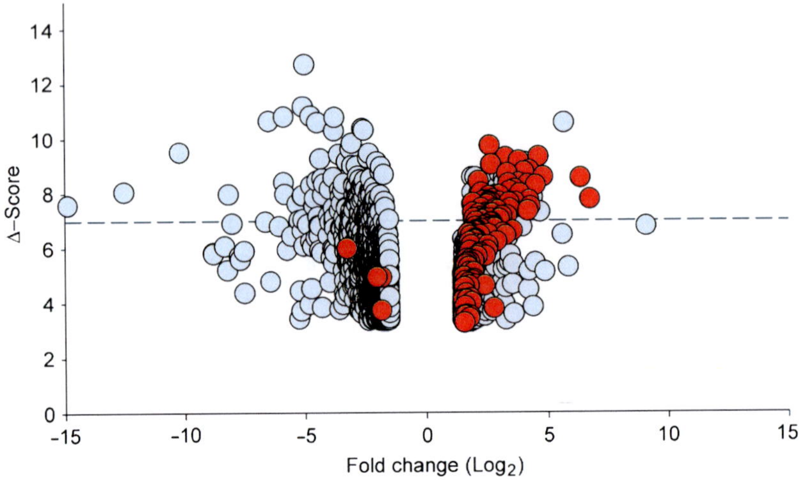

Fig. 2 Distribution of deregulated genes involved in mitosis according to fold change (FC) and Δ-score. The 1812 deregulated genes (circles) found in tumors of cervical cancer with the HG 1.0 ST microarray are shown in a volcano plot. The x-axis represents the FC of gene expression (tumor/control) expressed in $\log_2$ values, and the y-axis shows the absolute value of the Δ-score, which is equivalent to the t value in a student's t-test, calculated by the significance analysis of microarrays (SAM) method. A higher value of the Δ-score correlates with greater statistical significance. Log_2 FC values were positive in overexpressed genes and negative in underexpressed genes. The *black dashed lines* show the cutoff point for the most significant genes. The 128 genes of mitosis identified with HG-Focus and HG 1.0 ST microarrays are shown as *red circles*. The *gray circles* in the background represent deregulated genes not involved in mitosis

Because the E6 oncoprotein of HPV16 induces degradation of p53 in proteasomes, it is likely that in cervical carcinomas PRC1 is overexpressed via this mechanism. PRC1 has been reported to be associated with liver cancer (Wang et al. 2011) and CC (Zhai et al. 2007).

NUSAP1 is a nucleolar-spindle-associated protein that plays a role in spindle microtubule organization. The gene for NUSAP1 has not been associated with CC but has been found to be upregulated in breast cancer and melanoma (Kretschmer et al. 2011).

SYCP2 is a major component of the synaptonemal complex, which promotes the repair of double-strand breaks (DSBs) by the homologous recombination pathway in meiosis (Li et al. 2011). The high levels of *SYCP2* expression in the CCs examined in our previous work (Espinosa et al. 2013) suggest that DSBs are very common in some CC samples and that SYCP2 might be involved in DSB repair via the stimulation of the homologous recombination pathway. Interestingly, *SYCP2* has been found to be upregulated in CC (Buitrago-Pérez et al. 2009) and oropharyngeal squamous cell carcinomas positive for HPV16 but not in HPV-negative carcinomas (Martinez et al. 2006).

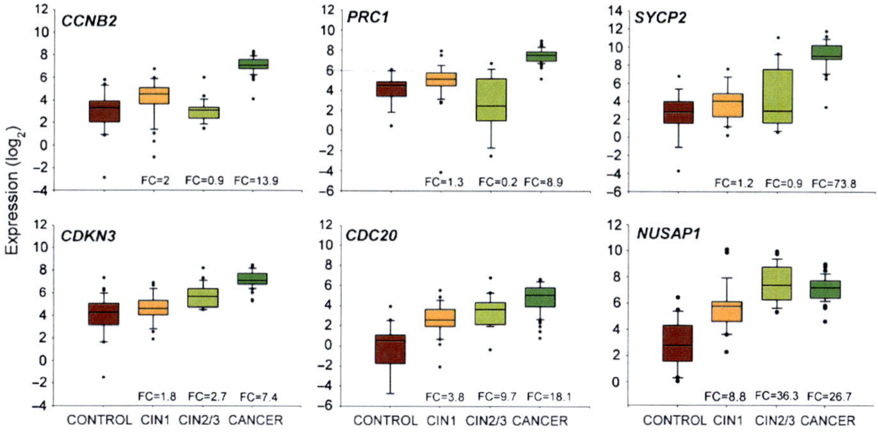

Fig. 3 **Validation of gene expression of six genetic markers by qRT-PCR**. The intensity of gene expression, expressed in $\log_2$ values, is shown in box plots. Expression of the six genes (*CCNB2*, *PRC1*, *SYCP2*, *CDKN3*, *CDC20*, and *NUSAP1*) is compared among four groups: healthy cervical epitheliums (normal, $n = 25$), low-grade CIN (CIN1, $n = 29$), high-grade CIN (CIN2/3, $n = 21$), and invasive CC (cancer, $n = 44$). The upper and lower boundaries of the boxes represent the 75th and 25th percentiles, respectively. The *black line* within the box represents the median value, and the whiskers represent the minimum and maximum values that lie within 1.5× the interquartile range from the end of box. Values outside this range are represented by *black circles*. The fold change (FC) in expression was calculated by dividing the median of each pathological group by the median of the control group

Mitosis as a Source of Targets for Screening and Survival in Cervical Cancer

The genes involved in mitosis were not only the most enriched in CC but also the most different in terms of expression fold change and Δ-score (statistical significance) when compared with control samples (red circles in Fig. 2). Therefore, these genes are good candidates to be tested as markers for screening and survival or as potential therapeutic targets. Furthermore, several of the 15 markers validated in our previous study either have not been identified previously (*CDKN3, NUSAP1*, and *SMC4*) or have been identified rarely in other studies (*CCNB2, CDC20, CKS2, PRC1*, and *SYCP2*). By contrast, genes not associated with mitosis have been identified in many studies (*CDKN2A, MCM2, TOP2A*, and *PCNA*) (Buitrago-Pérez et al. 2009).

Markers for Cervical Cancer Screening

In order to establish the potential value of these genes as markers in CC by defining a line of separation between cancer and control group signals, cutoff values were established by analyzing receiver-operating characteristic (ROC) curves.

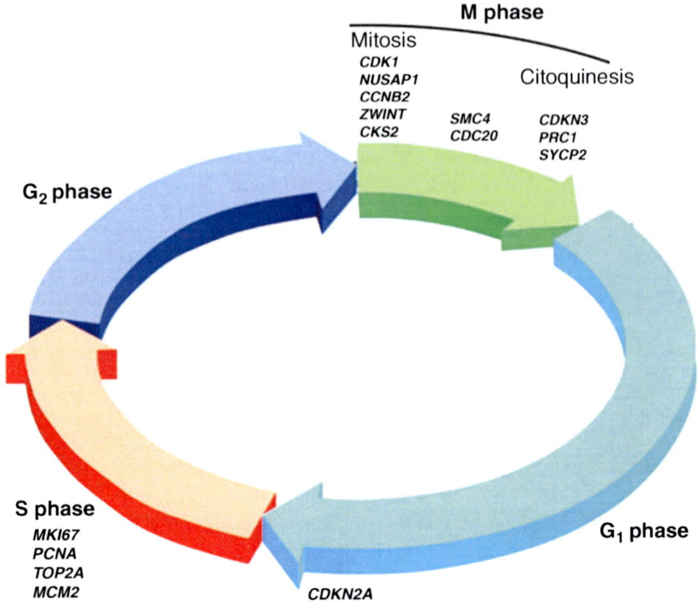

Fig. 4 Localization of the 15 genes described in this chapter in the cell cycle phases. The cell cycle phases and the genes altered in cervical cancer described in this chapter. All but four genes (*TOP2A*, *PCNA*, *MCM2*, and *CDKN2A*) participate in mitosis

In general, ROC curves with an area under the curve (AUC) $\leq$ 0.75 are not clinically useful, whereas an AUC of 0.97 has very high clinical value (Fan et al. 2006). The AUC for 10 genes (*CDKN2A*, *MKI67*, *PRC1*, *CDC2*, *CCNB2*, *SYCP2*, *PCNA*, *NUSAP1*, *CDC20*, and *CDKN3*) was $\geq$0.97 (Table 2). In fact, most of these genes had a sensitivity and specificity greater than 95 %, suggesting that they might be good screening markers that could distinguish healthy samples from invasive cancers. Interestingly, this subset included six genes involved in mitosis that had not been reported to be associated with CC (*NUSAP1* and *CDKN3*) or that had been only rarely reported to be associated with CC (*PRC1*, *SYCP2*, *CCNB2*, and *CDC20*).

For screening tests, it is important to detect not only CC but also high-grade lesions (CIN2/3) and to distinguish them from low-grade CIN lesions (CIN1) and healthy controls. To investigate whether these genes can differentiate CIN2+ from CIN1−, their expression was analyzed in two additional groups of samples: 29 low-grade CINs and 21 high-grade CINs (Espinosa et al. 2013). According to the median and distribution of the data shown in the box plots of Fig. 3, the six markers could be classified into two groups. The first group included markers linked exclusively (*CCNB2* and *PRC1*) or mostly (*SYCP2*) to invasion, which clearly differentiated invasive tumors from high-grade CIN, low-grade CIN, and normal cervices. The specificity for detecting only CC, and no other lesions, ranged from 0.85 (*SYCP2*) to 0.98 (*CCNB2*). The second group included the other three genes

Table 2 **ROC analysis and calculus of sensitivity, specificity, and predictive values.** The table shows calculations of predictive values, specificity, and sensitivity for 15 genes validated in cervical tumors and healthy controls. Eleven of the genes are involved in mitosis

			Controls ($n = 25$)		Cervical cancer ($n = 44$)							
Genes	AUC	Cutoff value[a]	FPF	TNF	TPF	FNF	*p*-value[b]	Sensitivity	Specificity	PPV	NPV	Youden index[c]
CDKN2A	0.996	18	0	25	42	2	$<1 \times 10^{-10}$	0.95	1	100	92.6	0.95
CCNB2	0.995	58	0	25	43	1	$<1 \times 10^{-10}$	0.98	1	100	96.2	0.98
MKI67	0.995	79	0	25	43	1	$<1 \times 10^{-10}$	0.98	1	100	96.2	0.98
PRC1	0.995	80	0	25	43	1	$<1 \times 10^{-10}$	0.98	1	100	96.2	0.98
CDK1	0.995	85	0	25	42	2	$<1 \times 10^{-10}$	0.95	1	100	92.6	0.95
SYCP2	0.992	115	0	25	42	2	$<1 \times 10^{-10}$	0.95	1	100	92.6	0.95
NUSAP1	0.99	48	1	24	43	1	$<1 \times 10^{-10}$	0.98	0.96	97.7	96	0.94
PCNA	0.99	100	0	25	42	2	$<1 \times 10^{-10}$	0.95	1	100	92.6	0.95
CDC20	0.971	3	3	22	42	2	$<1 \times 10^{-10}$	0.95	0.88	93.3	91.7	0.83
CDKN3	0.97	83	1	24	41	3	$<1 \times 10^{-10}$	0.93	0.96	97.6	88.9	0.89
SMC4	0.96	431	1	24	40	4	$<1 \times 10^{-10}$	0.91	0.96	97.6	85.7	0.87
TOP2A	0.866	128	5	20	43	1	$<1 \times 10^{-10}$	0.98	0.8	89.6	95.2	0.78
MCM2	0.846	121	4	21	40	4	2.5×10^{-9}	0.91	0.84	90.9	84	0.75
ZWINT	0.827	59	7	18	39	5	1.1×10^{-6}	0.89	0.72	84.8	78.3	0.61
CKS2	0.815	239	5	20	35	9	5×10^{-6}	0.8	0.8	87.5	69	0.6

AUC area under the curve, *FPF* false-positive fraction, *TNF* true-negative fraction, *TPF* true-positive fraction, *FNF* false-negative fraction, *PPV* positive predictive value, *NPV* negative predictive value

[a]Optimal cutoff values (ng/ml) were selected according to the ROC analysis

[b]Chi-square test

[c]J= sensitivity - specificity - 1

(*CDC20*, *NUSAP1*, and *CDKN3*), the expression of which tended to increase from the control to the CC group (*CDC20* and *CDKN3*) or the high-grade CIN group (*NUSAP1*). These three genes could distinguish CIN2+ lesions from CIN1− lesions ($p < 1 \times 10^{-15}$, Mann–Whitney *U* test [MW]). It is clear that genes in the first group would not be good markers for screening since they could not distinguish high-grade CIN and CC lesions from low-grade CIN lesions and control samples. Therefore, ROC analysis was performed to explore the potential of the genes in the second group (*CDC20*, *CDKN3*, and *NUSAP1*) together with *CDKN2A* as markers for screening. None of them had AUC values equal to or greater than 0.97; the highest AUC value was obtained with *CDKN2A* (0.92), followed by *NUSAP1* (0.917), *CDKN3* (0.91), and *CDC20* (0.86). However, the new markers (*NUSAP1* and *CDKN3*) showed slightly greater sensitivity than *CDKN2A* but lower specificity (Fig. 5). The sensitivity and specificity did not increase significantly when data for the individual markers were combined (Espinosa et al. 2013).

NUSAP1, CDKN3, or CDKN2A might be good candidates to use with HC2 as a first-line strategy in a screening program. The goal of our previous study (Espinosa et al. 2013) was to perform a feasibility evaluation of mRNA levels of novel genes in cervical samples as diagnostic markers to identify high-grade CIN or invasive lesions with high sensitivity and specificity. However, the sensitivities reported in that analysis were probably greater than those likely to be found in clinical practice because patients with CIN2+ have a higher proportion of cervical cancer (which is easy to identify) than would be expected in any screening setting. By contrast, the specificity appears to be underestimated, given that a large proportion of CIN1− had CIN1. Therefore, we did not expect to obtain conclusive data on the sensitivity, specificity, or predictive values of the assays. Additional studies of a screening population are needed to determine the levels of *CDKN3*, *NUSAP1*, or *CDC20* mRNA or protein in cervical samples, to obtain information about the predictive values, and to define the optimal trade-off between sensitivity and specificity for the detection of CIN2+.

Markers for Cervical Cancer Survival

One way to investigate whether or not these molecular targets are associated with CC progression is to conduct a survival study. Therefore, a survival analysis using qRT-PCR expression values of the 15 validated markers and International Federation of Gynecology and Obstetrics (FIGO) staging was conducted on 42 patients with HPV16-positive CC whose progress was followed for at least 3.5 years after diagnosis and initial treatment (Espinosa et al. 2013). This sample included individuals at FIGO stages IB1 ($n = 16$), IB2 ($n = 14$), IIA ($n = 1$), IIB ($n = 9$), and IIIB ($n = 2$). The overall survival rate for the whole sample was 79.6 % and for FIGO stages IB1, IB2, IIA, IIB, and IIIB was 100 %, 69.2 %, 0 %, 85.7 %, and 0 %, respectively. These differences were statistically significant ($p < 0.001$, log-rank test, Fig. 6). Of the 15 genes analyzed using Kaplan–Meier survival curves, only *CDKN3* was associated with poor survival ($p = 0.004$, log-rank test; Fig. 6).

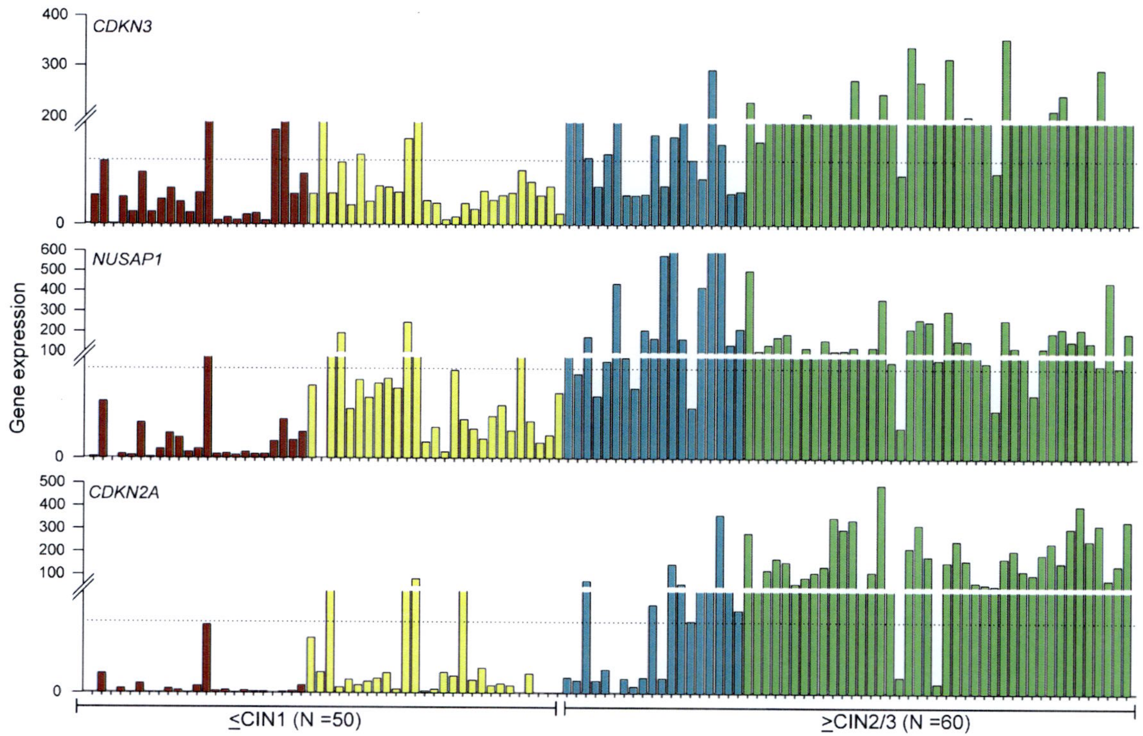

Fig. 5 **Cutoff values of gene expression intensity for *NUSAP1, CDKN3,* and *CDKN2A*.** Gene expression intensity of the individual samples and the cutoff values (*dashed lines*) calculated by using the ROC method. The first group (CIN1-, $n = 50$) included 23 healthy cervical epitheliums (*red bars*) and 27 low-grade lesions (*yellow bars*), and the second group (CIN2+, $n = 60$) included 19 high-grade lesions (*blue bars*) and 41 CCs positive for HPV16 (*green bars*). Markers *CDKN3* and *NUSAP1* showed slightly greater sensitivity than *CDKN2A*, but the opposite was true for specificity. Graphed values represent the median intensity of triplicate experiments normalized with an internal control (*GAPDH*)

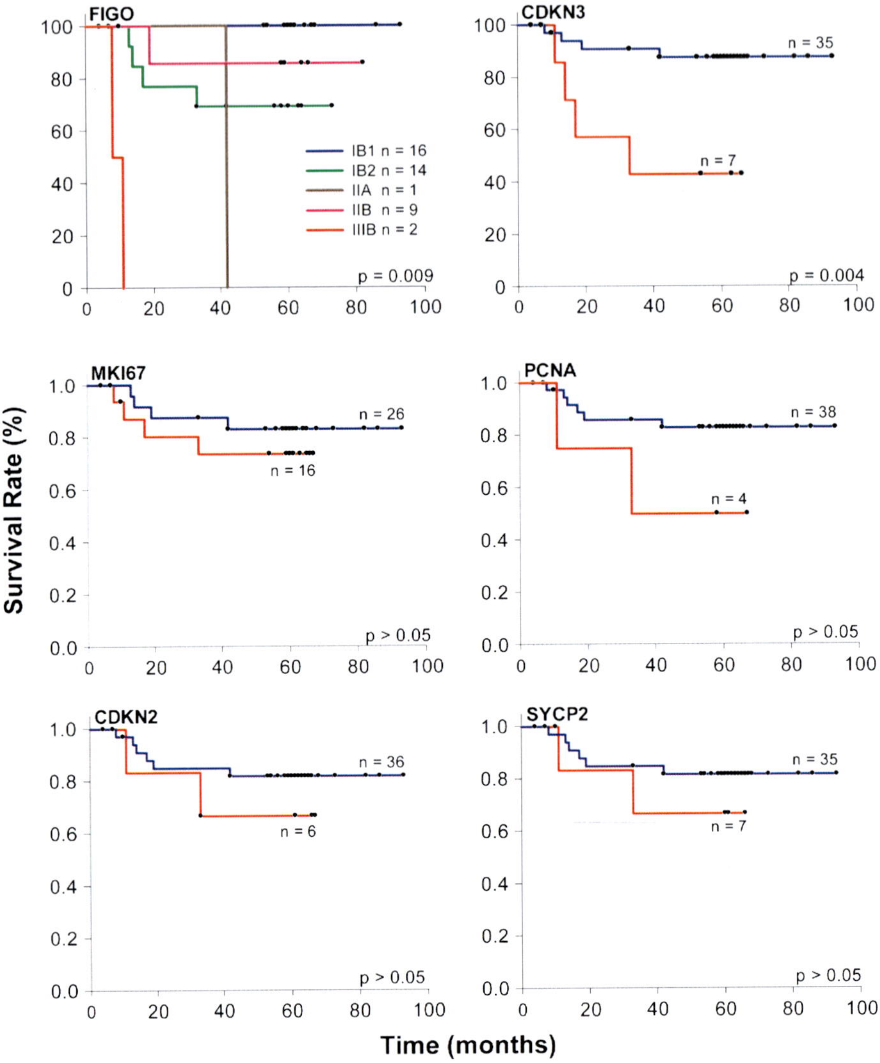

Fig. 6 The Kaplan–Meier survival curves for FIGO staging and *CDKN3, MKI67, PCNA, CDKN2*, and *SYCP2* genes. Patients were followed for at least 42 months. For gene expression, cancer patients with higher (*red line*) and lower (*blue line*) expression fold-change values were compared. The cutoff values were calculated with the ROC method. The *p*-values were calculated by comparing the curves with the log-rank test. Censored patients are labeled with *black dots*, but only four of them were censored before the minimal period of follow-up (42 months)

The overall survival rate of patients with higher levels of *CDKN3* (fold change > 15) was 42.9 %, and the median survival time was 22 months. By contrast, those with lower levels of *CDKN3* had an overall survival rate of 87.5 %. FIGO staging and *CDKN3* expression were analyzed together using Cox proportional hazard models, and *CDKN3* remained invariably significant with a hazard ratio (HR) of 5.9 (95 % confidence interval (CI), 1.4–23.8, $p = 0.01$). These results suggest that *CDKN3* could be a prognostic factor for survival that is independent of FIGO staging. However, a larger sample size is needed to confirm these results.

Potential Applications to Diagnosis, Prognosis, and Other Diseases or Conditions

A system for early detection of CC must be efficient and inexpensive. The markers proposed in our previous work (Espinosa et al. 2013) and this chapter (CDKN3, NUSAP1) have a sensitivity and specificity of approximately 90 %. However, the initial discoveries were made by analyzing mRNA of tumors and controls with traditional qRT-PCR, which is performed in four steps and costs approximately 50 USD. Because analysis of these markers with traditional qRT-PCR would be neither inexpensive nor easy, cheaper, easier, and high-performance screening methods that can be automated must be developed. Because our previous work using IH demonstrated that proteins encoded by the genes proposed as markers were overexpressed in tumors, ELISA methodology meets these requirements. However, it must be shown that the measurement of CDKN3 and NUSAP1 proteins by ELISA has a sensitivity and specificity similar to that of qRT-PCR analysis of mRNA. Another possibility would be to develop a cheaper qRT-PCR procedure that can be automated, for example, the use of a one-step qRT-PCR procedure that would allow simultaneous synthesis of cDNA and quantitative PCR in the same tube. Three markers labeled with different fluorochromes could be used simultaneously: one to detect high-grade lesions (NUSAP1 or CDKN3), another to detect exclusively invasive lesions (PRC1 or CCNB2), and an internal control. This methodology, besides to detect the CIN2+ lesions (NUSAP1 or CDKN3), could detect already invasive lesions (PRC1 or CCNB2), which deserve an immediate clinical attention. The cost of such a system, including RNA purification, produced in high volume would be approximately 5–10 USD. A low-cost system with high sensitivity and specificity could be easily adopted for the early detection of cervical cancer in poor and developing countries. However, validation of the system would require comparison with cytology and HPV testing in a large sample (ca. 5,000) of unselected women who regularly attend an early cancer detection program.

The association of CDKN3 with lower survival of CC patients clearly indicates that this gene is involved in the progression of CC. CDKN3 mRNA measurements might serve as a good predictive marker to assess patient survival and tumor aggressiveness. Depending on the clinical stage of the disease, invasive CC is treated currently with surgery, chemotherapy, radiotherapy, or a combination of these therapies. The success of conventional therapies and patient survival diminishes as the disease progresses to more advanced stages (Andrae, et al. 2012). In fact, the percentage of women who survive 5 years decreases from 93 % for stage IA to 15 % for stage IVB (www.cancer.org). The level of CDKN3 mRNA could be used to select women who need to be treated more aggressively with additional neoadjuvant chemotherapy. Appropriate clinical trials should investigate the clinical value of measuring CDKN3 mRNA as an indicator for additional specific cancer therapy.

In contrast to other types of cancer, for which several specific molecular drugs have been developed (Torti and Trusolino 2011), there are no specific molecular-targeted therapies for CC. The majority of specifically targeted cancer drugs are directed toward mutated proteins, especially protein kinases (Knight et al. 2012), but some drugs also target normal proteins that are overexpressed, such as HER2/neu in breast cancer (Saxena and Dwivedi 2012). The first step in developing a specific molecular drug is identifying universal molecular targets that are present in patients with CC and absent in healthy women. Inhibition of mitosis is a well-known strategy to combat cancers. Drugs that perturb the process of cell division have proven to be effective anticancer therapies. Well-known examples of these drugs, such as taxanes and vinca alkaloids, perturb the formation of the mitotic spindle. However, they have remarkably low therapeutic indices and narrow therapeutic windows. Their efficacy is restricted because they also perturb the microtubule network of nondividing cells, causing neurotoxic effects and affecting endothelial cell function. To resolve these issues, a new generation of antimitotic agents has been developed that target kinesins and kinases that play unique roles in mitosis, such as KIF11, PLK1, and aurora kinase A (AURKA) (Lens et al. 2010). Interestingly, the transcripts of these three genes were upregulated in the CCs evaluated; *AURKA* ranked in 19th place, *KIF11* ranked in 72nd place, and *PLK1* ranked in 263rd place (Espinosa et al. 2013). Therefore, the new generation of antimitotic drugs could be tested for treating cervical cancer. In addition to testing exiting drugs, several factors make CDKN3 a potential target for treating CC. First, CDKN3 is involved in mitosis; second, it is overexpressed in CC, averaging seven times higher than expression in the healthy cervix; and third, it is associated with low survival in CC patients, suggesting that it is associated with aggressive tumors. However, it remains to be demonstrated that CDKN3 is indispensable for tumor growth and that small drugs that inhibit CDKN3 function in tumor cells can be discovered.

Consistent with our data, *CDKN3*, along with other genes, has been found to be associated with lower survival of patients with lung adenocarcinomas (MacDermed et al. 2010; Tang et al. 2013). In addition, *CDKN3* has been shown to be essential for in vitro neoplastic growth of cells derived from hepatocellular carcinoma (Xing et al. 2012). Therefore, the clinical utility of *CDKN3* as a potential drug target and as a diagnostic tool to evaluate survival and select patients for more aggressive treatments could also be evaluated in lung cancer and hepatocellular carcinoma.

Summary Points

- The effect of preventive human papillomavirus (HPV) vaccination on the reduction of the cervical cancer (CC) burden will not be known for 30 years. Current methods for screening have low sensitivity (Pap test) or low specificity

(HPV tests) for the detection of high-grade cervical intraepithelial neoplasias (CIN2/3) and CC (CIN2+). Therefore, it remains necessary to improve the procedures for CC screening and treatment.

- The tumor suppressor protein p16 is one of the most widely studied markers associated with CC. The amount of p16 is related to the severity of cervical neoplasia and is considered a marker of CIN2+. However, the relatively low specificity of this marker and the need for a pathologist to interpret the test results are the major reasons that this marker has not been adopted for primary screening.
- The most upregulated and enriched genes in cervical cancer, compared with healthy cervical epithelium, are those involved in mitosis. Some mitotic genes might be good candidates as markers for screening or survival or as potential therapeutic targets.
- Six genes from mitosis were recently discovered to be associated with CC (*CCNB2*, *PRC1*, and *SYCP2*) and also with CIN2/3 (*CDC20*, *NUSAP1*, and *CDKN3*).
- The sensitivity and specificity of *CDKN3* and *NUSAP1* to detect CIN2+ was approximately 90 %. Therefore, they may be potential targets for the development of novel screening methods.
- *CDKN3* was also associated with poor CC patient survival, and it was independent of clinical stage. Therefore, *CDKN3* might serve as both a screening tool and a survival marker.

References

Andrae B, Andersson T, Lambert P, et al. Screening and cervical cancer cure: population based cohort study. BMJ Br Med J. 2012;344:e900.

Biewenga P, Buist M, Moerland P, et al. Gene expression in early stage cervical cancer. Gynecol Oncol. 2008;108:520–6.

Buitrago-Pérez A, Garaulet G, Vázquez A, et al. Molecular signature of HPV-induced carcinogenesis: pRb, p53 and gene expression profiling. Curr Genomics. 2009;10:26–34.

Cuzick J. Long-term cervical cancer prevention strategies across the globe. Gynecol Oncol. 2010;117:S11–4.

de Sanjose S, Quint W, Alemany L, et al. Human papillomavirus genotype attribution in invasive cervical cancer: a retrospective cross-sectional worldwide study. Lancet Oncol. 2010;11:1048–56.

Demetrick D, Matsumoto S, Hannon GJ, et al. Chromosomal mapping of the genes for the human cell cycle proteins cyclin C (CCNC), cyclin E (CCNE), p21 (CDKN1) and KAP (CDKN3). Cytogenet Cell Genet. 1995;69:190–2.

Espinosa A, Alfaro A, Roman E, et al. Mitosis is a source of potential markers for screening and survival and therapeutic targets in cervical cancer. PLoS One. 2013;8:e55975.

Fan J, Upadhye S, Worster A. Understanding receiver operating characteristic (ROC) curves. CJEM. 2006;8:19–20.

Ferlay J, Shin H, Bray F, et al. Cancer Incidence and Mortality Worldwide: IARC Cancer Base No. 10. International Agency for Research on Cancer. 2008; 2010. http://globocan.iarc.fr

Galamb O, Spisák S, Sipos F, et al. Reversal of gene expression changes in the colorectal normal-adenoma pathway by NS398 selective COX2 inhibitor. Br J Cancer. 2010;102:765–73.

Giorgi-Rossi P, Franceschi S, Ronco G. HPV prevalence and accuracy of HPV testing to detect high-grade cervical intraepithelial neoplasia. Int J Cancer. 2012;130:1387–94.

Gius D, Funk M, Chuang E, et al. Profiling microdissected epithelium and stroma to model genomic signatures for cervical carcinogenesis accommodating for covariates. Cancer Res. 2007;67:7113–23.

Gong D, Ferrell J. The roles of cyclin A2, B1, and B2 in early and late mitotic events. Mol Biol Cell. 2010;21:3149–61.

Gruneberg U, Neef R, Li X, et al. KIF14 and citron kinase act together to promote efficient cytokinesis. J Cell Biol. 2006;172:363–72.

Hwang S, Shroyer K. Biomarkers of cervical dysplasia and carcinoma. J Oncol. 2012;2011:507286.

Julien S, Dubé N, Hardy S, et al. Inside the human cancer tyrosine phosphatome. Nat Rev Cancer. 2011;11:35–49.

Knight Z, Lin H, Shokat K. Targeting the cancer kinome through polypharmacology. Nat Rev Cancer. 2012;12:130–7.

Kretschmer C, Sterner A, Siedentopf F, et al. Identification of early molecular markers for breast cancer. Mol Cancer. 2011;10:15.

Lehtinen M, Paavonen J, Wheeler C, et al. Overall efficacy of HPV-16/18 AS04-adjuvanted vaccine against grade 3 or greater cervical intraepithelial neoplasia: 4-year end-of-study analysis of the randomised, double-blind PATRICIA trial. Lancet Oncol. 2012;13:89–99.

Leinonen M, Nieminen P, Kotaniemi L, et al. Age-specific evaluation of primary human papillomavirus screening vs conventional cytology in a randomized setting. J Natl Cancer Inst. 2009;101:1612–23.

Lens S, Voest E, Medema R. Shared and separate functions of polo-like kinases and aurora kinases in cancer. Nat Rev Cancer. 2010;10:825–41.

Li C, Lin M, Liu J. Identification of PRC1 as the p53 target gene uncovers a novel function of p53 in the regulation of cytokinesis. Oncogene. 2004;23:9336–47.

Li X, Bolcun E, Schmenti J. Genetic evidence that synaptonemal complex axial elements govern recombination pathway choice in mice. Genetics. 2011;189:71–82.

MacDermed D, Khodarev N, Pitroda S, et al. MUC1-associated proliferation signature predicts outcomes in lung adenocarcinoma patients. BMC Med Genomics. 2010;3:16.

Markowitz L, Dunne E, Saraiya M, et al. Quadrivalent human papillomavirus vaccine: recommendations of the Advisory Committee on Immunization Practices (ACIP). MMWR Recomm Rep. 2007;56:1–24.

Martinez I, Wang J, Hobson K, et al. Identification of differentially expressed genes in HPV-positive and HPV-negative oropharyngeal squamous cell carcinomas. Eur J Cancer. 2006;43:415–32.

McCrory D, Matchar D, Bastian L, et al. Evaluation of cervical cytology. Evid Rep Technol Assess (Summ). 2009;1999:1–6.

Mo M, Chen Z, Li J, et al. Use of serum circulating CCNB2 in cancer surveillance. Int J Biol Markers. 2010;25:236–42.

Moody C, Laimins L. Human papillomavirus oncoproteins: pathways to transformation. Nat Rev Cancer. 2010;10:550–60.

Nakayama K, Nakayama K. Ubiquitin ligases: cell-cycle control and cancer. Nat Rev Cancer. 2006;6:369–81.

Nalepa G, Barnholtz-Sloan J, Enzor R, et al. The tumor suppressor CDKN3 controls mitosis. J Cell Biol. 2013;201:997–1021.

Narayan G, Bourdon V, Chaganti S, et al. Gene dosage alterations revealed by cDNA microarray analysis in cervical cancer: identification of candidate amplified and overexpressed genes. Genes Chromosomes Cancer. 2007;46:373–84.

Natunen K, Lehtinen J, Namujju P, et al. Aspects of prophylactic vaccination against cervical cancer and other human papillomavirus-related cancers in developing countries. Infect Dis Obstet Gynecol. 2011;2011:675858.

Ostor A. Natural history of cervical intraepithelial neoplasia: a critical review. Int J Gynecol Pathol. 1993;12:186–92.

Park S, Yu G, Kim W, et al. NF-Y-dependent cyclin B2 expression in colorectal adenocarcinoma. Clin Cancer Res. 2007;13:858–67.

Patel D, McCance D. Compromised spindle assembly checkpoint due to altered expression of Ubch10 and Cdc20 in human papillomavirus type 16 E6- and E7-expressing keratinocytes. J Virol. 2010;84:10956–64.

Pyeon D, Newton M, Lambert P, et al. Fundamental differences in cell cycle deregulation in human papillomavirus–positive and human papillomavirus–negative head/neck and cervical cancers. Cancer Res. 2007;67:10163–72.

Romanowski B. Long term protection against cervical infection with the human papillomavirus: review of currently available vaccines. Hum Vaccin. 2011;7:161–9.

Saxena R, Dwivedi A. ErbB family receptor inhibitors as therapeutic agents in breast cancer: current status and future clinical perspective. Med Res Rev. 2012;32:166–215.

Schiffman M, Wentzensen N, Wacholder S, et al. Human papillomavirus testing in the prevention of cervical cancer. J Natl Cancer Inst. 2011;103:368–83.

Subramanian R, Wilson E, Arthur C, et al. Insights into antiparallel microtubule crosslinking by PRC1, a conserved non motor microtubule binding protein. Cell. 2010;142:433–43.

Tang H, Xiao G, Behrens C, et al. A 12 gene set predicts survival benefits from adjuvant chemotherapy in non-small lung cancer patients. Clin Cancer Res. 2013;19:1577–86.

Taylor K, Sims A, Liang L, et al. Dynamic changes in gene expression in vivo predict prognosis of tamoxifen-treated patients with breast cancer. Breast Cancer Res. 2010;12:R39.

Teissier S, Ben J, Mori M, et al. New E6/P63 pathway, together with a strong E7/E2F mitotic pathway, modulates the transcriptome in cervical cancer cells. J Virol. 2007;81:9368–76.

Torti D, Trusolino L. Oncogene addiction as a foundational rationale for targeted anti-cancer therapy: promises and perils. EMBO Mol Med. 2011;3:623–36.

Tsoumpou I, Arbyn M, Kyrgiou M, et al. p16(INK4a) immunostaining in cytological and histological specimens from the uterine cervix: a systematic review and meta-analysis. Cancer Treat Rev. 2009;35:210–20.

Wang S, Ooi L, Hui K. Upregulation of Rac GTPase-activating protein 1 is significantly associated with the early recurrence of human hepatocellular carcinoma. Clin Cancer Res. 2011;17:6040–51.

Wentzensen N, Hampl M, Herkert M, et al. Identification of high-grade cervical dysplasia by the detection of p16INK4a in cell lysates obtained from cervical samples. Cancer. 2006;107:2307–13.

Whitlock E, Vesco K, Eder M, et al. Liquid-based cytology and human papillomavirus testing to screen for cervical cancer: a systematic review for the U.S. Preventive Services Task Force. Ann Intern Med. 2011;155:687–97.

Wright Jr T. Cervical cancer screening in the 21st century: is it time to retire the PAP smear? Clin Obstet Gynecol. 2007;50:313–23.

Xing C, Xie H, Zhou L, et al. Cyclin-dependent kinase inhibitor 3 is overexpressed in hepatocellular carcinoma and promotes tumor cell proliferation. Biochem Biophys Res Commun. 2012;420:29–35.

Zhai Y, Kuick R, Nan B, et al. Gene expression analysis of preinvasive and invasive cervical squamous cell carcinomas identifies HOXC10 as a key mediator of invasion. Cancer Res. 2007;67:10163–72.

HER2 as Biomarker for Endometrial Cancer 23

Diana P. English, Dana Marie Roque, Natalia Buza, and Alessandro D. Santin

Contents

D.P. English (✉) • A.D. Santin (✉)
Department of Obstetrics, Gynecology and Reproductive Sciences, Yale University School of Medicine, New Haven, CT, USA
e-mail: alessandro.santin@yale.edu

D.M. Roque
Division of Gynecologic Oncology, Greenebaum Cancer Center, University of Maryland-Baltimore, Baltimore, MD, USA
e-mail: droque@fpi.umaryland.edu

N. Buza
Department of Pathology, Yale University School of Medicine, New Haven, CT, USA
e-mail: natalia.buza@yale.edu

V.R. Preedy, V.B. Patel (eds.), *Biomarkers in Cancer, Biomarkers in Disease: Methods, Discoveries and Applications*,
DOI 10.1007/978-94-007-7681-4_26

Abstract

HER2 or ErbB2 is a member of the epidermal growth factor family and is a well-established biomarker that is overexpressed in a wide variety of tumor types including breast, ovarian, gastric, colorectal, pancreatic, and endometrial cancers. HER2 regulates signaling through several pathways (Ras/Raf/mitogen-activated protein kinase and phosphatidylinositol-3 kinase/protein kinase-B/mammalian target of rapamycin pathways) associated with cell survival and proliferation. In endometrial cancer there have been several studies linking the overexpression of HER2 and/or the amplification of the c-erbB2 gene with chemoresistance and overall poor survival. Immunotherapy with monoclonal antibodies targeting HER2 as well as the use of novel tyrosine kinase inhibitors targeting the erbB pathway may hold promise for patients harboring these biologically aggressive endometrial neoplasms.

List of Abbreviations

ADCC	Antibody-Dependent Cellular Cytotoxicity
CDC	Complement-Dependent Cytotoxicity
CISH	Chromogenic In Situ Hybridization
FISH	Fluorescence In Situ Hybridization
HER2	Human Epidermal Growth Factor Receptor
IHC	Immunohistochemistry
mCRPs	Membrane Complement Regulatory Proteins
NK	Natural Killer Cells
PBL	Peripheral Blood Lymphocytes
SISH	Silver-Enhanced In Situ Hybridization
T_c	Cytotoxic T Cells
T_{regs}	Regulatory T Cells
USC	Uterine Serous Carcinoma

Key Facts

Key Facts on HER2 in Endometrial Cancer

- HER2 or ErbB2 is a member of the epidermal growth factor family.
- Type I uterine cancers constitute 80 % of cases and consist of grades 1 and 2 endometrioid histologies; type II uterine cancers include grade 3 endometrioid, serous, carcinosarcoma, and clear cell histologies.
- HER2 overexpression results in constitutive activation and has been documented in a number of human cancers, including breast, esophageal, gastric, ovarian, and uterine cancers.
- HER2 amplification has been correlated with poor overall survival in some studies of uterine carcinoma.
- There has been a considerable interest in HER2-targeted therapy in endometrial cancer over the last decade, and studies are still ongoing in this field of research.

Definition of Words and Terms

Immunotherapy The prevention or treatment of disease with substances that stimulate the immune system.

Phenotype The set of observable characteristics of an individual resulting from the interaction of their genotype with the environment.

Antibody-Dependent Cellular Cytotoxicity A mechanism of cell-mediated immune defense whereby an effector immune cell actively lyses a target whose membrane-surface antigens have been bound by specific antibodies.

CDC Lysis of a target cell in the presence of complement system proteins.

Polymorphism Occurs when two or more clearly different phenotypes exist in the same population of a species or the occurrence of something in more than one form.

Microdissemination Widespread release of substances not capable of being seen with the naked eye throughout the body, for example, tumor microdissemination.

Monoclonal Antibody A type of protein made in the laboratory that can bind to substances in the body, for example, cancer cells.

Neoadjuvant Treatment given prior to mainstay of treatment to reduce disease burden, for example, chemotherapy done before surgery.

T_{regs} Regulatory T cells, formerly known as suppressor T cells, are a subpopulation of T cells which modulate the immune system and maintain tolerance to self-antigens.

Anthracyclines Anthracyclines are a class of drugs used in cancer chemotherapy derived from *Streptomyces* species. These compounds are used to treat many cancers, including leukemias, lymphomas, and breast, uterine, ovarian, and lung cancers.

Introduction

Receptor Family Characteristics and Biologic Pathway Crosstalk

HER2 (human epidermal growth factor receptor) is a 1,255 amino acid protein synonymous with metastatic lymph node gene 19 (MLN19), NGL, neu, or CD340. The protein is encoded by the gene *ErbB2*, located on chromosome 17q12, and is one of four members of the ErbB family including *ErbB1* (EGFR, epidermal growth factor receptor; HER1), *ErbB3* (HER3), and *ErbB4* (HER4).

These proteins share an extracellular binding domain, a single transmembrane-spanning portion, and a cytoplasmic tyrosine kinase domain. Unique among the family, HER2 is considered an orphan receptor as no direct ligand has been identified. Alternatively, HER2 tends to homo- or hetero-dimerize with other ErbB proteins leading to activation of numerous downstream and lateral pathways involving rat sarcoma/rapidly accelerated fibrosarcoma/mitogen-activated protein kinase (Ras/Raf/MAPK), phosphatidylinositol-3 kinase/protein kinase-B/mammalian target of rapamycin (PI3K/AKT/mTOR), and nuclear factor (NF)-κB, with subsequent effects on cell cycle control, proliferation, and invasion (Fig. 1).

HER2 overexpression results in constitutive activation; has been documented in a number of human cancers, including breast, esophageal, gastric, ovarian, and uterine cancers; and appears to have not only prognostic but therapeutic potential.

Uterine Cancer: Burden of Disease

Uterine cancer has become the most common gynecologic cancer in the developed world, with 49,560 new cases and 8,190 related deaths predicted to occur in the United States in 2013 (Siegel et al. 2012). Uterine cancers are commonly dichotomized into type I and type II variants (Bokhman 1983), which arise through distinct pathogenetic mechanisms (Table 1). Type I cancers constitute 80 % of cases (Felix et al. 2010) and consist of grades 1 and 2 endometrioid histologies; type II cancers include grade 3 endometrioid, serous, carcinosarcoma, and clear cell histologies. Uterine serous carcinomas (USC) account for 10 % of cases and a disproportionate number of deaths due to aggressive course and chemoresistance. While the 5-year overall survival for endometrioid cancers is 80 %, the rate for USC

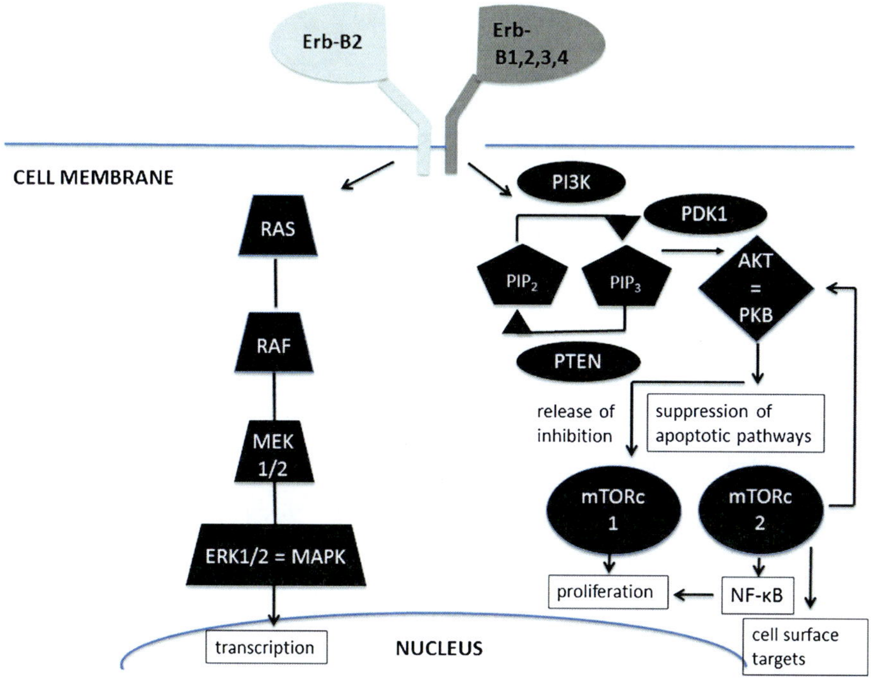

Fig. 1 HER2 signaling pathways. *RAS* rat sarcoma, *RAF* rapidly accelerated fibrosarcoma, *ERK* extracellular signal-regulated kinase, *MEK* mitogen-activated protein/extracellular signal-regulated kinase, *MAPK* mitogen-activated protein kinase, PIP_2 phosphatidylinositol 4,5-bisphosphate, PIP_3 phosphatidylinositol (3,4,5)-triphosphate, *PI3K* phosphatidylinositol 3-kinase, *PDK1* 3-phosphoinositide-dependent protein kinase-1, *PKB* protein kinase-B, *PTEN* phosphatase and tensin homologue, *mTORc* mammalian target of rapamycin complex, *NF-κB* nuclear factor kappa-light-chain-enhancer of activated B cells

Table 1 Genetic mechanisms and clinical associations of type I versus type II uterine cancer. The two types of uterine cancer are noted in the table with their corresponding characteristic mutational pattern and clinical history with regard to ER/PR receptor status, parity, and race. The references have also been included in the table (No copyright issues)

	Type I	Type II	Sources
Mutations and pathogenesis	K-Ras mutations	Aneuploidy	Lax et al. 1998; Sherman et al. 2000; Hecht et al. 2006
	PTEN mutations	TP53 mutations	
		HER2	
		E-cadherin	
ER/PR status	Positive	Negative	Grundker et al. 2008
Parity	Nulliparous	Parous	Wilson et al. 1990
Race	Lower frequency among black patients	Higher frequency among black patients	Wilson et al. 1990; Wright et al. 2009; Boruta et al. 2009

ER estrogen receptor, *PR* progesterone receptor

is only 54 %, due in part to greater propensity for extrauterine spread at time of initial diagnosis for type II cancers (Yoon et al. 2010).

Frequency of HER2 Overexpression and Prognostic Significance in Uterine Cancers

Frequency of Overexpression

HER2 overexpression is commonly tied to the development of a malignant phenotype, including correlation with depth of myometrial invasion, advanced stage (Diaz-Montes et al. 2006), and loss of progesterone receptor status. HER2/neu overexpression has been described in low-grade, low-stage tumors relative to normal endometrium and has been reported in 0–80 % of uterine cancers depending on analytic technique employed and histology (Santin et al. 2002; Buza et al. 2013, 2014).

In GOG-181B, in which 286 advanced or recurrent endometrial carcinomas were screened for HER2 overexpression, only 7 % of endometrioid tumors were HER2 amplified, compared to 38 % of clear cell and 28 % of serous cancers (Fleming et al. 2010). In GOG-177, 234 specimens representing advanced or recurrent endometrial cancer were available for immunohistochemistry and 182 for fluorescence in situ hybridization. Of these, 11 % of grade 3 endometrioid and 21 % of serous tumors overexpressed HER2 by FISH (Grushko et al. 2008). The proportion of overexpression was significantly higher in serous versus non-serous histologies (61 % vs. 41 %, $p = 0.03$). There was also correlation of amplification with grade: 3 % in grade 1, 2 % in grade 2, and 21 % in grade 3 cancers ($p = 0.003$). In other studies of endometrioid tumors, IHC positivity has ranged from 1 % to 47 %, with amplification rates of 0–38 %; IHC and amplification rates for clear cell carcinomas have been as high as 33–66 % and 22–38 %, respectively (Fleming et al. 2010).

Corresponding rates for carcinosarcoma may be as high as 75 % and 50 %, respectively (Saffari et al. 1995). In several analyses of carcinosarcomas, staining of 2+/3+ was present within the epithelial component in 22.5–56 % of cases but only 4–6 % within the sarcomatous component (Sawada et al. 2003). Endometrial stromal sarcomas, leiomyosarcomas, and adenosarcomas generally do not overexpress HER2 (Cheng et al. 2011), though EGFR may be strongly positive.

Impact on Survival

HER2 amplification has been correlated with poor overall survival in some studies of uterine carcinoma across a variety of histological subtypes yet not found to be prognostic in other studies of endometrioid, serous, or carcinosarcomatous histologies. Akin to breast cancer, a triple-negative phenotype (estrogen receptor, progesterone receptor, and HER2) has been associated with poor survival. In a retrospective study of early and advanced endometrial cancers including endometrioid, adenosquamous, serous, and carcinosarcomatous histology, the addition of adjuvant chemotherapy or radiation improved survival in those tumors that overexpressed HER2 but not in those that failed to exhibit overexpression (Saffari et al. 1995).

Racial Variation

Santin et al. (2005a) reported a 70 % HER2 overexpression rate (3+ by IHC) in uterine serous carcinoma tissue blocks from African-American patients with USC, in contrast to 24 % in tumors from Caucasian patients. Shorter survival was independently associated with HER2 expression, but not age or race. The authors concluded that HER2 expression may contribute significantly to racial disparities.

Polymorphisms

Recently, specific HER2 polymorphisms (e.g., +655 A/G) have been implicated in increased risk of breast, prostate, and gastric cancers. There is no evidence for a role in the pathogenesis of uterine cancers or any variation across subtype (Kitao et al. 2007); however, existing studies have been largely restricted to Japanese populations.

Techniques for Quantification

Immunohistochemistry

Immunohistochemistry (IHC) is a semiquantitative method for determination of protein expression. The technique is inexpensive and relatively quick to perform. Chromogenic results are not susceptible to degradation and may therefore be stored for reference over long periods of time. Unfortunately, interpretation may be highly subjective, and standardization of scoring systems is essential (Penault-Llorca et al. 2009). No specific guidelines exist for HER2 testing and scoring in endometrial cancer, and methodologies used in studies to date remain widely varied. Definitions of overexpression also differ between studies. Some clinicians and researchers apply the proposed guidelines put forth for breast cancers by the College of American Pathologists (CAP) and American Society for Clinical Oncology (ASCO) which were recently updated for 2013 (Wolff et al. 2013). In this scheme, an area of tumor consisting of >10 % of contiguous and homogeneous tumor cells is examined. The specimen is considered positive if IHC score is 3+ (complete, intense circumferential membrane staining). The specimen is considered negative if IHC score is 0 (no staining or faint membrane staining in $\leq$ 10 % of tumor cells) to 1+ (incomplete staining of >10 % of tumor cells). Testing is equivocal if IHC is 2+ (circumferential membrane staining that is incomplete

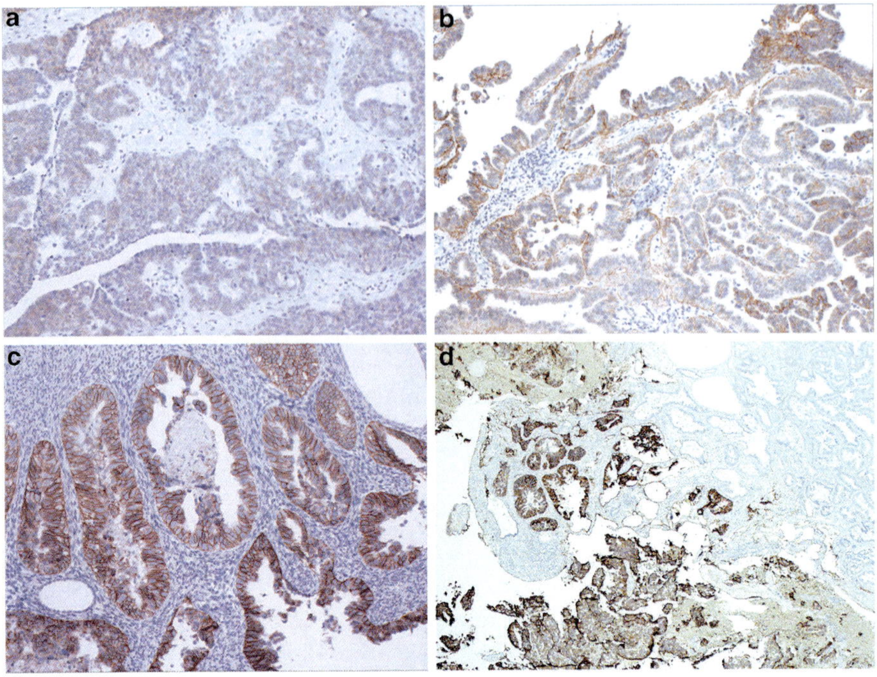

Fig. 2 HER2 expression by immunohistochemistry in endometrial serous carcinoma. (**a**) HER2 score 1+, negative: weak, incomplete membranous staining in majority of tumor cells. (**b**) HER2 score 2+, equivocal: weak to moderate membranous staining with a predominant lateral/basolateral pattern. (**c**) HER2 score 3+, positive: strong staining with a complete or lateral/basolateral membranous staining pattern. (**d**) Heterogeneous HER2 expression by immunohistochemistry in an endometrial serous carcinoma. Parts of the tumor show strong, complete membrane staining, while other areas (*right upper corner*) are completely negative

and/or weak/moderate and within >10 % of the invasive tumor or complete and circumferential membrane staining that is intense and within ≤10 % of the invasive tumor); in such instances, repeat testing on another sample or in situ hybridization (ISH, below) on the same sample is required (Fig. 2).

In Situ Hybridization

In situ hybridization is a technique for identification of the number of gene copies present. Fluorescence in situ hybridization (FISH) uses fluorescently labeled DNA probes to localize sequences of interest on cell blocks or formalin-fixed paraffin-embedded tissues sectioned to 4–5 μM. Because DNA is generally more stable than protein, results are more resilient to variations in processing. FISH interpretation is felt to be less subjective than IHC but requires fluorescence microscopy and is more time-consuming, though automated image analysis has been validated. The price of FISH testing may be more than twice that of IHC.

Chromogenic in situ hybridization (CISH) employs the same principles as FISH; however, nucleic acid probes are labeled by dye detectable by standard bright-field microscopy at less cost (Cayre et al. 2007). Dual-color CISH (dc-CISH) uses separate labels for HER2 and chromosome 17 centromere (CEP17). Silver-enhanced in situ hybridization (SISH) is a fully automated alternative to CISH interpretable by bright-field microscopy. SISH protocols can be completed in 6 h or less, compared to nearly 2 days required for FISH or CISH.

CAP/ASCO guidelines consider FISH/CISH testing positive if the single-probe average HER2 copy numbers are $\geq$6 signals/cell, the dual-probe HER2/CEP17 ratio is $\geq$2, or the dual-probe HER2/CEP17 ratio is $<$2, but the average HER2 copy number is $\geq$6 signals/cell (Wolff et al. 2013). SISH is scored similarly with no amplification if $<$6 copies are present in $>$50 % of tumor cells; high amplification requires $>$10 copies or large clusters in the nuclei of $>$50 % of tumor cells.

Concordance of IHC and FISH

In one study that examined IHC and FISH across 72 endometrial cancers, there were 2 cases of overexpression without altered copy number and 5 instances of amplification without overexpression (Rolitsky et al. 1999). Similar rates were identified in another study of 88 cases (Xu et al. 2010). Lower rates of concordance have been reported in other studies. Santin et al. 2005 identified heterogeneity of HER2 amplification in 27.3 % (3 of 11) cases with 2+ IHC but 100 % concordance among pure serous carcinomas that scored 0, 1+, or 3+ (Santin et al. 2005b).

Concordance Between IHC and FISH and Implications of Intratumoral Heterogeneity

In GOG-181B, single-agent trastuzumab produced no objective tumor responses in patients with advanced or recurrent HER2-positive endometrial cancers, though it was terminated prematurely due to slow accrual (Fleming et al. 2010). One explanation for the inconsistent biologic response of these tumors to targeted therapy and variable prognostic significance of HER2 overexpression lies in intratumoral heterogeneity.

In a study of 85 pure serous carcinomas and 23 mixed endometrial carcinomas with serous component identified over a 4-year period within a single institution, Buza and colleagues found that while 35 % exhibited HER2 overexpression and/or gene amplification, the rate of IHC heterogeneity in serous tumors was as high as 53 % in HER2-positive tumors (31 % of all serous tumors) (Buza et al. 2013; Buza and Hui 2013). Marked heterogeneity of HER2/neu gene amplification was also confirmed by FISH in a subset of these cases (Buza and Hui 2013). This mimics the experience in esophageal and gastric cancers and is generally higher than that described for breast cancers. Clinically meaningful testing will likely evolve to include composite scoring on multiple or large tumor sections (Buza et al. 2013).

In addition, loss of apical staining (lateral/basolateral staining pattern as opposed to complete circumferential staining) was also frequently observed, similar to gastric and esophageal adenocarcinomas (Buza et al. 2013).

Therapeutic Implications

Potential Applications to Prognosis, Other Diseases or Conditions

Several research groups have sought to evaluate potential biomarkers useful for predicting drug responsiveness and disease course. In breast cancer HER2 overexpression has been associated with both resistance to chemotherapeutic agents and also is predictive of a favorable response to other agents including trastuzumab (Herceptin) (Noguchi 2006). One study involving metastatic breast cancer patients treated with trastuzumab and paclitaxel found that high HER2 amplification index and high class III β-tubulin expression were predictive of a good response to therapy (Jung et al. 2012).

The prognostic impact of HER2 expression status and progesterone receptor expression in endometrial carcinoma patients with positive peritoneal washings has also been investigated. One study found that intraperitoneal microdissemination in association with HER2 tumor overexpression and the lack of progesterone receptor expression indicated the presence of a particularly aggressive tumor. There were 178 endometrioid and 22 papillary serous carcinoma patients in this study. Positive peritoneal washing and HER2 identified a group of patients with a higher probability of dying (Benevolo et al. 2007).

Yet another study demonstrated that HER2, as a single marker, plays a minor role in low-grade and low-stage endometrial cancer (the most common endometrial cancers) (Morrison et al. 2006). As such the use of a panel of biomarkers and tumor parameters instead of a single marker or parameter may be most appropriate for determining and planning adjuvant therapy.

In uterine serous carcinoma, both hormone receptor expression and HER2 expression have been recognized as prognostic variables. Hormone receptor expression in one study was defined as either estrogen or progesterone receptor positivity. In this study, overexpression of HER2 was correlated with lower overall survival, whereas hormone receptor expression was correlated on the other hand to higher overall survival (Togami et al. 2012).

Immunotherapy

Although several mechanisms of action have been attributed to anti-HER2 monoclonal antibodies, including inhibition of tumor proliferation and/or promotion of cell cycle arrest, strong investigational evidence suggests that engagement of Fc receptors on effector cells (i.e., mainly natural killer (NK) cells) represents the dominant component of the in vivo activity of these antibodies against tumors.

Humanized monoclonal antibodies (mAb) against HER2 induce tumor lysis through antibody-dependent cellular cytotoxicity (ADCC) or complement-dependent cytotoxicity (CDC) (Clynes et al. 2000). This notion is further supported by experimental studies comparing the in vitro and in vivo activities of IgG and $F(ab')_2$ fragments in a mixture of three monoclonal anti-HER2 antibodies. In these reports, the in vitro antiproliferative and proapoptotic effects of IgG and $F(ab')_2$ were similar, but only the IgGs had significant antitumor activity in vivo (Spiridon et al. 2004).

Clinical results have also shown that there is an improved response to trastuzumab in patients with a particular Fc polymorphism resulting in a higher NK affinity to IgG1, which again lends support to the view that ADCC inclusive of its mediators is critical for the in vivo efficacy of trastuzumab (Musolino et al. 2008). Clinical research has also since shown that patients responding to neoadjuvant trastuzumab showed a fourfold increase in antibody-dependent lytic activity from isolated peripheral blood mononuclear cells in contrast to patients without a response (Gennari et al. 2004).

Trastuzumab and Pertuzumab

As mentioned above, trastuzumab (Herceptin®, Genentech, CA, USA) is a humanized monoclonal IgG1 antibody that works both through recruitment of NK cells and initiation of ADCC as well as reducing signaling of downstream effectors, although all mechanisms of action have not been completely elucidated. In 2006, the FDA-approved trastuzumab as part of a regimen containing doxorubicin, cyclophosphamide, and paclitaxel for the adjuvant treatment of patients with early stage HER2-positive, node-positive breast cancer. Over the last decade, there has been significant interest in using anti-HER2 monoclonal antibodies for high HER2 expressing gynecologic malignancies.

Previous case reports of uterine serous and high-grade endometrioid tumors treated with trastuzumab have described clinical activity in these heavily pretreated patients with high HER2 expressing advanced stage endometrial carcinoma. The responses varied from complete response to stable disease with the longest period of stable disease being 11 months (Santin et al. 2008). However when evaluated as a single-agent, trastuzumab 4 mg/kg in week 1 then 2 mg/kg weekly until disease progression in stage III/IV or recurrent endometrial cancers at the phase II level in GOG-181B did not demonstrate significant clinical activity (Fleming et al. 2010). A multi-institutional phase II trial is underway to investigate whether the addition of trastuzumab to paclitaxel and carboplatin chemotherapy improves progression-free survival (PFS) when compared to paclitaxel and carboplatin alone in stages III and IV and recurrent USC patients overexpressing HER2 at 3+ level by IHC or positive by FISH (NCT01367002).

Trastuzumab binds to subdomain IV of the extracellular domain of HER2, whereas pertuzumab (Perjeta, Genentech, South San Francisco, CA, USA) is a humanized IgG1 mAb that binds to HER2 near the center of domain II, the dimerization domain, and thus inhibits HER heterodimerization. Pertuzumab compared to trastuzumab inhibits a broader array of downstream signal transduction pathways through reduction of lateral signal transduction. One preclinical study (El-Sahwi et al. 2010) investigated the sensitivity of USC cell lines to heterologous peripheral blood lymphocytes (PBLs) in the presence of pertuzumab (2.5 μg/mL), trastuzumab (2.5 μg/ml), and the combination of both in cell lines expressing high levels of HER2. Pertuzumab and trastuzumab were found to induce equally strong ADCC and CDC in FISH-positive uterine serous cell lines. Notably the combination of the two antibodies significantly increased ADCC also in low HER2 expressing USC cell lines (El-Sahwi et al. 2010).

Trastuzumab and pertuzumab combination may also enhance sensitivity to endocrine therapy in HER2-overexpressing uterine tumors as has been shown previously in ovarian cancer xenografts (Faratian et al. 2011).

Another area of blossoming research is the use of trastuzumab in cancers that are not growth inhibited by this drug. Data has emerged showing that long-term treatment with trastuzumab may facilitate responsiveness to alternate HER-targeted inhibitors such as gefitinib and cetuximab. Given the safety profile of trastuzumab along with the success of EFGR-targeted therapy in other solid tumors, this strategy may prove useful in all histological types of endometrial cancers (Wilken et al. 2010).

Trastuzumab Emtansine (T-DM1)

Trastuzumab emtansine (T-DM1, Genentech/Roche) is a novel antibody-drug conjugate that combines trastuzumab with targeted delivery of the antimicrotubule agent DM1. DM1 belongs to the maytansine class of chemotherapeutic agents, and on average 3–4 molecules of DM1 are conjugated to each trastuzumab molecule. T-DM1 is internalized by HER2 receptor-mediated endocytosis, and as such its action is specific to HER2-expressing cells. After internalization, T-DM1 is then degraded by lysosomes resulting in the release of free intracellular DM-1. DM-1 is a potent microtubule assembly inhibitor, and its activity leads to cell death as a result of G_2/M phase cell cycle arrest and apoptosis (Barok et al. 2011). T-DM1 also has the advantage of retaining the mechanism of action of trastuzumab in regard to reducing signaling in the HER2 pathway and initiation of ADCC. T-DM1 is the first antibody-drug conjugate receiving United States Food and Drug Administration approval for HER2-positive metastatic breast cancer following the results of the randomized phase III trial of T-DM1 versus lapatinib plus capecitabine in patients previously treated with taxane and trastuzumab (EMILIA). A total of 978 patients were treated in this study, and the median progression-free survival was 9.6 months in the T-DM1 arm compared with 6.4 months in the capecitabine/lapatinib arm (HR = 0.650, 95 % CI: 0.55–0.77; p <0.001). The objective response rate and overall survival were significantly higher in the T-DM1 group compared with the capecitabine/lapatinib group. Also T-DM1 was found to be much safer than the capecitabine/lapatinib combination. Overall T-DM1 appears to be well tolerated as a single agent given at 3.6 mg/kg every 3 weeks. This dosing differs from the 6 mg/kg every 3-week trastuzumab dosing. Based on this evidence, clinical trials exploring T-DM1 therapy in HER2-positive advanced/recurrent and/or refractory endometrial cancer are warranted.

Augmenting Targeted Immunotherapy

In vitro studies demonstrated that trastuzumab results in antibody-dependent cellular cytotoxicity (ADCC) in the range of 25–60 % against HER2-overexpressing uterine serous carcinoma, which can be augmented by several means including IL-2 administration, treatment with agonist monoclonal antibody for costimulatory receptors on NK cells, or the simultaneous administration of the heterodimerization inhibitor pertuzumab (Boyman et al. 2012). The cytokine interleukin (IL)-2 controls the growth and differentiation of a number of lymphocyte subsets, notably CD8+ cytotoxic T cells (T_c), NK cells, and CD4+ helper T regulatory cells (T_{regs}). High-dose recombinant IL-2 (aldesleukin, Proleukin®, Novartis, Switzerland) was approved by the Federal Drug Administration (FDA) as early as 1998 for treatment in metastatic melanoma and renal cell carcinoma. With IL-2 therapy comes certain common undesirable side effects including significant pulmonary and hepatic toxicities. Also IL-2 therapy may lead to parallel expansion of T_{regs} able to blunt antitumor immune responses, thereby limiting the beneficial effects of expanding tumor-reactive CD8+ T_c (Kohrt et al. 2012).

Although these side effects may limit somewhat IL-2 administration, there is literature showing improved anti-HER2 antibody therapy with the addition of IL-2. Research from El-Sawhi et al. 2010 showed enhanced cytotoxicity when pertuzumab was combined with low doses of IL-2 (mean ± SD: 46.9 ± 11 %; range, 22.4–74.2 %) versus pertuzumab alone (mean ± SD: 41.5 ± 12.8 %; range, 15.8–71.9 %) ($p = 0.04$) in preclinical experiments on uterine serous carcinoma.

Membrane Complement Regulatory Proteins

Tumors may escape immune surveillance through antigen evolution and upregulation of membrane complement regulatory proteins (mCRPs) that may inhibit complement-dependent pathways (Carter 2001). mCRPs' upregulation leads to inactivation of C4b/C3b, dissociation of C3/C5 convertases, and prevention of membrane-attack complex assembly (Gelderman et al. 2005). Recently, Bellone et al, have shown that uterine serous carcinoma overexpress CD46, CD55, and CD59 relative to normal endometrial cells; knockdown via siRNAs of CD55 and CD59 but not CD46 significantly sensitized uterine serous carcinoma to complement-dependent cytotoxicity and antibody-dependent cell-mediated cytotoxicity (Bellone et al. 2012). Similar results with anti-mCRP siRNAs have been reported in breast, ovarian, and lung cancer (Mamidi et al. 2013). As such the inhibition of mCRPs on type II endometrial cancers harboring c-erbB2 gene amplification may play a complementary role in improving the response rates of these aggressive tumors to trastuzumab-mediated CDC and ADCC (Bellone et al. 2012).

mTOR Inhibitors, Tyrosine Kinase Inhibitors, and Anti-HER2 Therapy

Blocking mTOR complex-1 induces upregulation of HER2 expression mediated by mTOR complex-2 in preclinical models (Lang et al. 2010). Trastuzumab-resistant HER2-positive breast cancer patients have derived clinical benefits from treatment with everolimus (mTOR inhibitor) in phase I and II trials (Andre et al. 2010). Thus, evaluation of mTOR inhibitors in combination with HER2-targeted therapy should be investigated in gynecologic cancer.

Lapatinib is a reversible dual inhibitor of both HER2 and EGFR and has shown efficacy in HER2-positive trastuzumab-resistant breast cancers and esophageal and gastric adenocarcinomas. Lapatinib's additive or synergistic effects with chemotherapy have also been demonstrated in these tumor types, and lapatinib has even been shown in preclinical models to be effective at restoring trastuzumab sensitivity (Ritter et al. 2007).

In GOG-229D, women with persistent/recurrent endometrial cancer following one or two prior regimens were treated with 1,500 mg of oral lapatinib daily until progression or severe toxicity. The majority of the patients had endometrioid adenocarcinoma (53.3 %), and 23.3 % of patients had uterine serous carcinoma. This study suggested that response in endometrial cancer patients may be correlated with a particular mutation in EGFR (E690K). However lapatinib may be of limited benefit in unselected endometrial cancer cases.

Pan-HER TKIs which inhibit epidermal growth factor family receptors and their downstream pathways have also proved beneficial in solid tumor clinical trials. Also new in therapeutic approaches for solid tumors is the targeting of heat shock protein 90 (hsp90) molecular chaperone. Hsp90 is essential for the stability and function of many oncogenic and signal-transduction proteins including HER2, AKT, and others involved in cell cycle regulation (Neckers 2007). Hsp90 inhibitors are thus currently under evaluation in early phase clinical trials as single-agent therapy or in combination with trastuzumab.

Radioimmunotherapy

Preclinical studies have recently shown the safe applicability of radioimmunotherapy in gynecologic cancer and other tumor types. A phase I trial evaluating lead-212 (^{212}Pb)-trastuzumab in patients with HER2-positive ovarian, pancreatic, colon, gastric, endometrial, or breast cancer patients documented to have peritoneal studding or positive washings (intraperitoneal disease) is ongoing. This represents a potential treatment approach for patients with metastatic endometrial cancer utilizing this lead isotope with a short path length specifically targeted to malignant cells by the trastuzumab antibody (http://www.clinicaltrials.gov/ct2/show/NCT01384253).

Anti-HER2 Vaccine

While trastuzumab is an effective immunotherapeutic agent against a variety of tumors overexpressing HER2, it potentially has limitations of eventual drug resistance and risk of cardiotoxicity, especially in patients on previous anthracycline-based regimens. As such interest naturally surfaced overtime in anti-HER2 vaccines. The vaccine stimulates a preexisting anti-HER2 immune response and as such has several advantages including fewer injections for patients but the most important being the possibility of establishing a memory immune response capable of preventing disease recurrence. Consistent with this view, several clinical trials are underway in patients with solid tumors overexpressing HER2.

Generally, toxicities reported with the HER2 vaccine have been commonly local reactions of erythema, induration, pruritus, and inflammation. The most frequent systemic toxicities were fatigue, headache, arthralgias, myalgias, chills, and bone and back pain.

HER2 vaccine-primed autologous T cells have also been studied in phase I clinical trials and have been shown to be feasible and well tolerated. As such this approach will form the basis of future trials utilizing HER2-primed T-cell therapy to several tumor types.

Mechanisms of Resistance to HER2-Targeted Therapy

HER2-targeted treatment is a biologic therapy that holds great potential in advanced and/or recurrent endometrial cancer patients. However there is a fraction of patients with HER2-overexpressing tumors who will not respond to initial anti-HER2 therapy (primary resistance), and those who respond may eventually lose the clinical benefit of this therapy (secondary resistance.) Mechanisms resulting in in vivo trastuzumab resistance are not fully understood.

It is important to first understand the suggested mechanisms of anti-HER2 monoclonal antibody therapy, and they include:

(I) The targeting of immune cells to HER2-positive tumor cells resulting in binding of immune cells to Fc domain of the antibody, thus effecting antibody-dependent cell-mediated cytotoxicity of HER2-positive tumor cells.
(II) Through the inhibition of proteolytic shedding via a possible steric or allosteric mechanism resulting in decreased HER2 kinase activity (Pupa et al. 1993).
(III) Through the internalization and degradation of HER2.

Most of the literature on trastuzumab resistance has focused on the mechanisms underlying secondary or acquired resistance. Primary resistance is overall less studied, but more research is ongoing in this area.

As it stands anti-HER2 therapy resistance may occur via varying mechanisms including secondary to proteolytic cleavage of full-length HER2 with the formation of the cell surface–associated fragment (p95HER2), a constitutively kinase-active

HER2 isoform lacking the trastuzumab-binding site. As p95HER2 lacks the trastuzumab-binding domain of the full-length HER2, it may also be an important mediator of primary trastuzumab resistance. Resistance to anti-HER2 therapy may also occur due to compensatory signaling by other cell surface receptors including EGFR/HER3 and other receptor tyrosine kinases suggesting that HER2 signaling may be a dispensable or redundant signaling pathway in some tumor cells. This theory is supported further by recent evidence that trastuzumab-mediated growth inhibition can be overcome by ectopic expression of EGFR in SKBR3 breast cancer cells (Dua et al. 2010).

Since tumor growth inhibition is dependent on the binding of anti-HER2 agents to commonly the extracellular domain of HER2, then any molecule or process that prevents this interaction with the HER2 receptor would hamper the effectiveness of HER2-targeted treatment. Previous studies have proposed that CD44 and/or MUC4 expression may be associated with the formation of a steric interference therefore reducing trastuzumab binding to cell surface HER2 (Palyi-Krekk et al. 2007). Besides these associations with extracellular matrix and cell surface proteoglycans, cytosolic regulators of HER2 such as cysteine protease calpain-1 have also been identified as vital moderators of primary trastuzumab resistance (Kulkarni et al. 2010).

The well-recognized protein synthesis regulator, eEF-2 kinase, has also been established to have a role in trastuzumab resistance. Cheng et al. 2010 have demonstrated that siRNA-mediated knockdown of eEF-2 kinase, a negative regulator of eukaryotic elongation factor-2, sensitizes breast cancer cells to trastuzumab (Cheng et al. 2010).

The activation of downstream effectors by other mechanisms may also lead to primary anti-HER2 therapy resistance. In vitro studies have identified phosphatidylinositol-3 kinase (PI3K) expression, low PTEN expression, AKT phosphorylation, and S6K phosphorylation as potential mediators of primary trastuzumab resistance.

Conclusions

Recent research has elucidated the distinct molecular pathways involved in the pathogenesis of the two types of endometrial carcinoma and subsequently laid the foundation for in vitro and in vivo studies aimed at identifying potential therapeutic targets. Based on several publications, HER2 appears to play an important role in the pathogenesis of uterine serous and other types of biologically aggressive endometrial cancers. HER2 protein expression/amplification thus has a potential crucial role as both a biomarker and as therapeutic option in these tumors. Targeting both HER2 and other gene targets downstream to HER2 provides a means of directing therapy in recurrent or advanced endometrial cancer. Further molecular profiling of endometrial cancer by next-generation sequencing technologies will facilitate the identification of clinically relevant gene amplifications/deletion and mutations which may potentially provide novel and/or improved therapeutic strategies in endometrial carcinoma. Parallel to the ongoing clinical studies, a detailed assessment of the HER2 testing methods will be necessary to identify the unique features of HER2 overexpression/amplification in endometrial cancer and correlate them with clinical response to therapy and prognosis.

Summary Points

- The chapter focuses on HER2 which is a key gene for cell survival and proliferation, and as a result HER2 amplification and protein expression may lead to a propensity for malignant formation.
- Uterine cancer is the most common gynecologic cancer in the developed world and is dichotomized into type I and type II variants.
- Clinicians and researchers evaluate HER2 expression in uterine cancer using the College of American Pathologists (CAP) and American Society for Clinical Oncology (ASCO) guidelines for determination of HER2 overexpression in breast cancers.
- Intratumoral heterogeneity may explain the inconsistent biologic response of HER2 expressing uterine tumors to targeted therapy.
- HER2-targeted treatment is a biologic therapy that holds great potential in advanced and/or recurrent endometrial cancer patients. However there is a fraction of patients with HER2-overexpressing tumors who will not respond to initial anti-HER2 therapy (primary resistance), and those who respond may eventually lose the clinical benefit of this therapy (secondary resistance).

References

Andre F, Campone M, O'Regan R, Manlius C, Massacesi C, Sahmoud T, Mukhopadhyay P, Soria JC, Naughton M, Hurvitz SA. Phase I study of everolimus plus weekly paclitaxel and trastuzumab in patients with metastatic breast cancer pretreated with trastuzumab. J Clin Oncol. 2010;28(34):5110–5.

Barok M, Tanner M, Koninki K, Isola J. Trastuzumab-DM1 causes tumour growth inhibition by mitotic catastrophe in trastuzumab-resistant breast cancer cells in vivo. Breast Cancer Res. 2011;13(2):R46.

Bellone S, Roque D, Cocco E, Gasparrini S, Bortolomai I, Buza N, Abu-Khalaf M, Silasi DA, Ratner E, Azodi M, Schwartz PE, Rutherford TJ, Pecorelli S, Santin AD. Downregulation of membrane complement inhibitors CD55 and CD59 by siRNA sensitises uterine serous carcinoma overexpressing Her2/neu to complement and antibody-dependent cell cytotoxicity in vitro: implications for trastuzumab-based immunotherapy. Br J Cancer. 2012;106(9):1543–50.

Benevolo M, Vocaturo A, Novelli F, Mariani L, Vocaturo G, Cianciulli AM, Marandino F, Perrone-Donnorso R, Giannarelli D, Natali PG, Mottolese M. Prognostic value of HER2 and progesterone receptor expression in endometrial carcinoma with positive peritoneal washing. Anticancer Res. 2007;27(4C):2839–44.

Bokhman JV. Two pathogenetic types of endometrial carcinoma. Gynecol Oncol. 1983;15 (1):10–7.

Boruta 2nd DM, Gehrig PA, Fader AN, Olawaiye AB. Management of women with uterine papillary serous cancer: a Society of Gynecologic Oncology (SGO) review. Gynecol Oncol. 2009;115(1):142–53.

Boyman O, Krieg C, Letourneau S, Webster K, Surh CD, Sprent J. Selectively expanding subsets of T cells in mice by injection of interleukin-2/antibody complexes: implications for transplantation tolerance. Transplant Proc. 2012;44(4):1032–4.

Buza N, Hui P. Marked heterogeneity of HER2/NEU gene amplification in endometrial serous carcinoma. Genes Chromosomes Cancer. 2013;52:1178–86.

Buza N, English DP, Santin AD, Hui P. Toward standard HER2 testing of endometrial serous carcinoma: 4-year experience at a large academic center and recommendations for clinical practice. Mod Pathol. 2013;26:1605–12.

Buza N, Roque DM, Santin AD. HER2/neu in endometrial cancer: a promising therapeutic target with diagnostic challenges. Arch Pathol Lab Med. 2014;138(3):343–50.

Carter P. Improving the efficacy of antibody-based cancer therapies. Nat Rev Cancer. 2001;1(2):118–29.

Cayre A, Mishellany F, Lagarde N, Penault-Llorca F. Comparison of different commercial kits for HER2 testing in breast cancer: looking for the accurate cutoff for amplification. Breast Cancer Res. 2007;9(5):R64.

Cheng Y, Li H, Ren X, Niu T, Hait WN, Yang J. Cytoprotective effect of the elongation factor-2 kinase-mediated autophagy in breast cancer cells subjected to growth factor inhibition. PLoS One. 2010;5(3):e9715.

Cheng X, Yang G, Schmeler KM, Coleman RL, Tu X, Liu J, Kavanagh JJ. Recurrence patterns and prognosis of endometrial stromal sarcoma and the potential of tyrosine kinase-inhibiting therapy. Gynecol Oncol. 2011;121(2):323–7.

Clynes RA, Towers TL, Presta LG, Ravetch JV. Inhibitory Fc receptors modulate in vivo cytotoxicity against tumor targets. Nat Med. 2000;6(4):443–6.

Diaz-Montes TP, Ji H, Smith Sehdev AE, Zahurak ML, Kurman RJ, Armstrong DK, Bristow RE. Clinical significance of Her-2/neu overexpression in uterine serous carcinoma. Gynecol Oncol. 2006;100(1):139–44.

Dua R, Zhang J, Nhonthachit P, Penuel E, Petropoulos C, Parry G. EGFR over-expression and activation in high HER2, ER negative breast cancer cell line induces trastuzumab resistance. Breast Cancer Res Treat. 2010;122(3):685–97.

El-Sahwi K, Bellone S, Cocco E, Cargnelutti M, Casagrande F, Bellone M, Abu-Khalaf M, Buza N, Tavassoli FA, Hui P, Silasi DA, Azodi M, Schwartz PE, Rutherford TJ, Pecorelli S, Santin AD. In vitro activity of pertuzumab in combination with trastuzumab in uterine serous papillary adenocarcinoma. Br J Cancer. 2010;102(1):134–43.

Faratian D, Zweemer AJ, Nagumo Y, Sims AH, Muir M, Dodds M, Mullen P, Um I, Kay C, Hasmann M, Harrison DJ, Langdon SP. Trastuzumab and pertuzumab produce changes in morphology and estrogen receptor signaling in ovarian cancer xenografts revealing new treatment strategies. Clin Cancer Res. 2011;17(13):4451–61.

Felix AS, Weissfeld JL, Stone RA, Bowser R, Chivukula M, Edwards RP, Linkov F. Factors associated with Type I and Type II endometrial cancer. Cancer Causes Control. 2010;21(11):1851–6.

Fleming GF, Sill MW, Darcy KM, McMeekin DS, Thigpen JT, Adler LM, Berek JS, Chapman JA, DiSilvestro PA, Horowitz IR, Fiorica JV. Phase II trial of trastuzumab in women with advanced or recurrent, HER2-positive endometrial carcinoma: a Gynecologic Oncology Group study. Gynecol Oncol. 2010;116(1):15–20.

Gelderman KA, Lam S, Gorter A. Inhibiting complement regulators in cancer immunotherapy with bispecific mAbs. Expert Opin Biol Ther. 2005;5(12):1593–601.

Gennari R, Menard S, Fagnoni F, Ponchio L, Scelsi M, Tagliabue E, Castiglioni F, Villani L, Magalotti C, Gibelli N, Oliviero B, Ballardini B, Da Prada G, Zambelli A, Costa A. Pilot study of the mechanism of action of preoperative trastuzumab in patients with primary operable breast tumors overexpressing HER2. Clin Cancer Res. 2004;10(17):5650–5.

Grundker C, Gunthert AR, Emons G. Hormonal heterogeneity of endometrial cancer. Adv Exp Med Biol. 2008;630:166–88.

Grushko TA, Filiaci VL, Mundt AJ, Ridderstrale K, Olopade OI, Fleming GF. An exploratory analysis of HER-2 amplification and overexpression in advanced endometrial carcinoma: a Gynecologic Oncology Group study. Gynecol Oncol. 2008;108(1):3–9.

Hecht JL, Mutter GL. Molecular and pathologic aspects of endometrial carcinogenesis. J Clin Oncol. 2006;24(29):4783–91.

Jung M, Koo JS, Moon YW, Park BW, Kim SI, Park S, Lee SH, Hong S, Rha SY, Chung HC, Kim JH, Sohn J. Overexpression of class III beta tubulin and amplified HER2 gene predict good response to paclitaxel and trastuzumab therapy. PLoS One. 2012;7(9):e45127.

Kitao K, Yoshida S, Kennedy S, Takemura N, Sugimoto M, Deguchi M, Ohara N, Maruo T. Epidermal growth factor receptor and human epidermal growth factor receptor 2 gene polymorphisms in endometrial cancer in a Japanese population. Reprod Sci. 2007;14(4): 349–57.

Kohrt HE, Houot R, Weiskopf K, Goldstein MJ, Scheeren F, Czerwinski D, Colevas AD, Weng WK, Clarke MF, Carlson RW, Stockdale FE, Mollick JA, Chen L, Levy R. Stimulation of natural killer cells with a CD137-specific antibody enhances trastuzumab efficacy in xenotransplant models of breast cancer. J Clin Invest. 2012;122(3):1066–75.

Kulkarni S, Reddy KB, Esteva FJ, Moore HC, Budd GT, Tubbs RR. Calpain regulates sensitivity to trastuzumab and survival in HER2-positive breast cancer. Oncogene. 2010;29(9):1339–50.

Lang SA, Hackl C, Moser C, Fichtner-Feigl S, Koehl GE, Schlitt HJ, Geissler EK, Stoeltzing O. Implication of RICTOR in the mTOR inhibitor-mediated induction of insulin-like growth factor-I receptor (IGF-IR) and human epidermal growth factor receptor-2 (Her2) expression in gastrointestinal cancer cells. Biochim Biophys Acta. 2010;1803(4):435–42.

Lax SF, Pizer ES, Ronnett BM, Kurman RJ. Comparison of estrogen and progesterone receptor, Ki-67, and p53 immunoreactivity in uterine endometrioid carcinoma and endometrioid carcinoma with squamous, mucinous, secretory, and ciliated cell differentiation. Hum Pathol. 1998;29(9):924–31.

Mamidi S, Cinci M, Hasmann M, Fehring V, Kirschfink M. Lipoplex mediated silencing of membrane regulators (CD46, CD55 and CD59) enhances complement-dependent anti-tumor activity of trastuzumab and pertuzumab. Mol Oncol. 2013;7(3):580–94.

Morrison C, Zanagnolo V, Ramirez N, Cohn DE, Kelbick N, Copeland L, Maxwell GL, Fowler JM. HER-2 is an independent prognostic factor in endometrial cancer: association with outcome in a large cohort of surgically staged patients. J Clin Oncol. 2006;24(15):2376–85.

Musolino A, Naldi N, Bortesi B, Pezzuolo D, Capelletti M, Missale G, Laccabue D, Zerbini A, Camisa R, Bisagni G, Neri TM, Ardizzoni A. Immunoglobulin G fragment C receptor polymorphisms and clinical efficacy of trastuzumab-based therapy in patients with HER-2/neu-positive metastatic breast cancer. J Clin Oncol. 2008;26(11):1789–96.

NCT01367002., N. C. T. E. o. c. p. w. o. w. t. H. i. u. s. c. h. c. g. c. s. https://clinicaltrials.gov/ct2/show/NCT01367002.

Neckers L. Heat shock protein 90: the cancer chaperone. J Biosci. 2007;32(3):517–30.

Noguchi S. Predictive factors for response to docetaxel in human breast cancers. Cancer Sci. 2006;97(9):813–20.

Palyi-Krekk Z, Barok M, Isola J, Tammi M, Szollosi J, Nagy P. Hyaluronan-induced masking of ErbB2 and CD44-enhanced trastuzumab internalisation in trastuzumab resistant breast cancer. Eur J Cancer. 2007;43(16):2423–33.

Penault-Llorca F, Bilous M, Dowsett M, Hanna W, Osamura RY, Ruschoff J, van de Vijver M. Emerging technologies for assessing HER2 amplification. Am J Clin Pathol. 2009;132(4): 539–48.

Pupa SM, Menard S, Morelli D, Pozzi B, De Palo G, Colnaghi MI. The extracellular domain of the c-erbB-2 oncoprotein is released from tumor cells by proteolytic cleavage. Oncogene. 1993;8(11):2917–23.

Ritter CA, Perez-Torres M, Rinehart C, Guix M, Dugger T, Engelman JA, Arteaga CL. Human breast cancer cells selected for resistance to trastuzumab in vivo overexpress epidermal growth factor receptor and ErbB ligands and remain dependent on the ErbB receptor network. Clin Cancer Res. 2007;13(16):4909–19.

Rolitsky CD, Theil KS, McGaughy VR, Copeland LJ, Niemann TH. HER-2/neu amplification and overexpression in endometrial carcinoma. Int J Gynecol Pathol. 1999;18(2):138–43.

Saffari B, Jones LA, el-Naggar A, Felix JC, George J, Press MF. Amplification and overexpression of HER-2/neu (c-erbB2) in endometrial cancers: correlation with overall survival. Cancer Res. 1995;55(23):5693–8.

Santin AD, Bellone S, Gokden M, Palmieri M, Dunn D, Agha J, Roman JJ, Hutchins L, Pecorelli S, O'Brien T, Cannon MJ, Parham GP. Overexpression of HER-2/neu in uterine serous papillary cancer. Clin Cancer Res. 2002;8(5):1271–9.

Santin AD, Bellone S, Siegel ER, Palmieri M, Thomas M, Cannon MJ, Kay HH, Roman JJ, Burnett A, Pecorelli S. Racial differences in the overexpression of epidermal growth factor type II receptor (HER2/neu): a major prognostic indicator in uterine serous papillary cancer. Am J Obstet Gynecol. 2005a;192(3):813–8.

Santin AD, Bellone S, Van Stedum S, Bushen W, De Las Casas LE, Korourian S, Tian E, Roman JJ, Burnett A, Pecorelli S. Determination of HER2/neu status in uterine serous papillary carcinoma: comparative analysis of immunohistochemistry and fluorescence in situ hybridization. Gynecol Oncol. 2005b;98(1):24–30.

Santin AD, Bellone S, Roman JJ, McKenney JK, Pecorelli S. Trastuzumab treatment in patients with advanced or recurrent endometrial carcinoma overexpressing HER2/neu. Int J Gynaecol Obstet. 2008;102(2):128–31.

Sawada M, Tsuda H, Kimura M, Okamoto S, Kita T, Kasamatsu T, Yamada T, Kikuchi Y, Honjo H, Matsubara O. Different expression patterns of KIT, EGFR, and HER-2 (c-erbB-2) oncoproteins between epithelial and mesenchymal components in uterine carcinosarcoma. Cancer Sci. 2003;94(11):986–91.

Sherman ME. Theories of endometrial carcinogenesis: a multidisciplinary approach. Mod Pathol. 2000;13(3):295–308.

Siegel R, Naishadham D, Jemal A. Cancer statistics, 2012. CA Cancer J Clin. 2012;62(1):10–29.

Spiridon CI, Guinn S, Vitetta ES. A comparison of the in vitro and in vivo activities of IgG and F (ab')2 fragments of a mixture of three monoclonal anti-Her-2 antibodies. Clin Cancer Res. 2004;10(10):3542–51.

Togami S, Sasajima Y, Oi T, Ishikawa M, Onda T, Ikeda S, Kato T, Tsuda H, Kasamatsu T. Clinicopathological and prognostic impact of human epidermal growth factor receptor type 2 (HER2) and hormone receptor expression in uterine papillary serous carcinoma. Cancer Sci. 2012;103(5):926–32.

Wilken JA, Webster KT, Maihle NJ. Trastuzumab sensitizes ovarian cancer cells to EGFR-targeted therapeutics. J Ovarian Res. 2010;3:7.

Wilson TO. Evaluation of unfavorable histologic subtypes in endometrial adenocarcinoma. Am J Obstet Gynecol. 1990;162(2):418–26.

Wolff AC, Hammond ME, Hicks DG, Dowsett M, McShane LM, Allison KH, Allred DC, Bartlett JM, Bilous M, Fitzgibbons P, Hanna W, Jenkins RB, Mangu PB, Paik S, Perez EA, Press MF, Spears PA, Vance GH, Viale G, Hayes DF. Recommendations for human epidermal growth factor receptor 2 testing in breast cancer: American Society of Clinical Oncology/College of American Pathologists Clinical Practice Guideline Update. J Clin Oncol. 2013;31(31):3997–4013.

Wright JD, Fiorelli J, Schiff PB, Burke WM, Kansler AL, Cohen CJ, et al. Racial disparities for uterine corpus tumors: changes in clinical characteristics and treatment over time. Cancer. 2009;115(6):1276–85.

Xu M, Schwartz P, Rutherford T, Azodi M, Santin A, Silasi D, Martel M, Hui P. HER-2/neu receptor gene status in endometrial carcinomas: a tissue microarray study. Histopathology. 2010;56(2):269–73.

Yoon JH, Yoo SC, Kim WY, Chang SJ, Chang KH, Ryu HS. Para-aortic lymphadenectomy in the management of preoperative grade 1 endometrial cancer confined to the uterine corpus. Ann Surg Oncol. 2010;17(12):3234–40.

Immunohistochemistry as Biomarker Platform in Endometrial Cancer

24

Joo-Hyun Nam, Jeong-Yeol Park, Min-Hyun Baek, Ji-Hyun Han, Woo-Suk Han, and A-Ra Ko

Contents

J.-H. Nam (✉) • J.-Y. Park • M.-H. Baek • J.-H. Han • W.-S. Han • A.-R. Ko
Department of Obstetrics and Gynecology, University of Ulsan College of Medicine, Asan Medical Center, Seoul, South Korea
e-mail: jhnam@amc.seoul.kr; catgut1-0@hanmail.net; baekminhyun@hotmail.com; gotogyn0130@gmail.com; bronx46@hotmail.com; finishi@naver.com

V.R. Preedy, V.B. Patel (eds.), *Biomarkers in Cancer, Biomarkers in Disease: Methods, Discoveries and Applications*,
DOI 10.1007/978-94-007-7681-4_42

Abstract

Endometrial cancer is the most common malignancy of the female genital tract in Western countries, and its incidence is rapidly increasing in Asia. The standard treatment for women with endometrial cancer is staging operation followed by adjuvant radiation therapy according to the risk factors for recurrence. These include tumor histology, differentiation grade, lymphovascular space invasion, myometrial invasion, lymph node metastasis, and disease stage. However, these factors are not accurate independent predictors of recurrence or prognosis in endometrial cancer. Therefore, several biomarkers have been investigated as potential predictive or prognostic factors, and immunohistochemical markers for endometrial cancer have been investigated extensively in the past decades. In this chapter, we review recent advances in the identification of immunohistochemical markers as predictive or prognostic markers in endometrial cancer.

List of Abbreviations

CEA	Carcinoembryonic Antigen
COX-2	Cyclooxygenase-2
EGF	Epidermal Growth Factor
FIGO	The International Federation of Obstetrics and Gynecology
GLUT	Glucose Transporter
HER-2	Human Epidermal Growth Factor
HIF-1 Alpha	Hypoxia-Induced Factor-1 Alpha
HNPCC	Hereditary Nonpolyposis Colorectal Cancer
IL	Interleukin
L1CAM	L1 Cell Adhesion Molecule
MLH	MutL Homolog
MMP	Matrix Metalloproteinases
MMR gene	Mismatch Repair Gene
MSH	MutS Homolog
MSI	Microsatellite Instability
mTOR	Mammalian Target of Rapamycin
Op 18	Oncoprotein 18
P53	Phosphoprotein p53
PD-ECGF	Platelet-Derived Endothelial Cell Growth Factor
PG	Prostaglandin
PIK3	Phosphatidylinositol 3-Kinase
PTEN	Phosphatase and Tensin Homolog

STMN 1	Stathmin 1
TGF-alpha	Transforming Growth Factor Alpha
VEGF	Vascular Endothelial Growth Factor

Key Facts of Endometrial Cancer

- Endometrial cancer is a malignancy of the endometrium of the uterus.
- It is the most common malignant tumor of the female genital tract in developed and Western countries.
- The incidence of endometrial cancer is rapidly increasing in Eastern countries because of the Westernized lifestyle.
- Unopposed estrogen exposure is the primary etiological factor in endometrial cancer.
- Endometrial cancer is usually diagnosed in perimenopausal women.
- Most endometrial cancers are diagnosed at an early stage because vaginal bleeding is present in most cases during the early course of the disease.
- The standard treatment of endometrial cancer is surgery, including hysterectomy.
- Adjuvant radiation therapy is recommended after surgery if there are risk factors for recurrence in the pathology report.
- The prognosis of early stage endometrial cancer is excellent, although curative treatment modalities for advanced endometrial cancer are lacking.

Definition of Words and Terms

Immunohistochemistry Histopathologic technique for the documentation and localization of immunoreactive proteins in cells or tissues using specific antibodies.

Biomarker Substances present in the blood, body fluids, or tissues of the human body or tumors that can be used in cancer diagnosis and in the prediction of treatment response and prognosis after treatment.

Predictive marker A molecular or clinical marker that can indicate disease status and predict the response to treatment in cancer patients.

Prognostic marker A molecular or clinical marker that can predict recurrence or survival after treatment in cancer patients.

Disease-free survival Time interval between the completion of cancer treatment and recurrence.

Overall survival Time interval between the completion of cancer treatment and death.

Introduction

Endometrial cancer is the most common malignancy of the female genital tract in developed countries (Bray et al. 2005). Its incidence differs among regions. In North America and Europe, it is the most common gynecologic cancer and the fourth most common cancer among women (Amant et al. 2005). The incidence of endometrial cancer is relatively low in Asian countries; however, it has become more prevalent in recent years and could become the most common gynecologic cancer in Asia in the near future (Ushijima 2009). Worldwide, endometrial cancer is the seventh most common cancer among women, with approximately 200,000 new cases diagnosed each year (Parkin et al. 2005).

Most endometrial cancers are diagnosed at an early stage because the disease presents with abnormal vaginal bleeding, which leads patients to seek medical help during the early course of the disease. The current standard treatment for endometrial cancer is staging operation followed by adjuvant radiation therapy according to the risk factors for recurrence (Wright et al. 2012). Several clinicopathologic factors have been suggested as predictive factors for recurrence or prognostic factors after treatment in patients with endometrial cancer, including tumor histology, differentiation grade, lymphovascular space invasion, myometrial invasion, lymph node metastasis, and disease stage (Colombo et al. 2013). However, none of these factors are sufficiently accurate for predicting the recurrence or prognosis of endometrial cancer. Therefore, many other biomarkers have been investigated as predictive or prognostic factors, and immunohistochemical markers, which have been extensively investigated in the past decades as biomarker platforms for endometrial cancer, have been adapted for the differential diagnosis and prediction of tumor behavior or prognosis after treatment in patients with endometrial cancer. Most studies and review articles have focused on the differential diagnosis of endometrial cancer using these markers. In this chapter, we review recent findings on the use of immunohistochemical markers as predictive or prognostic biomarkers in endometrial cancer.

p53

p53 is a guardian of the genome and gatekeeper of cells. However, mutations of this tumor suppressor gene are present in more than half of all human tumors, and p53 gene mutation is the most common genetic alteration in human cancer. The p53 gene, which is located on the short arm of chromosome 17, plays a role in the regulation of apoptosis and tumorigenesis. It encodes a short-lived protein that suppresses abnormal cell proliferation by inducing apoptosis and preventing cell division (Sakuragi et al. 2002). p53 mutations occur late in the development of type I endometrial cancer and early in the development of type II endometrial cancer and are an independent predictor of poor survival (Liu 2007; Fig. 1 and Table 1). p53 mutations are found in approximately 10–20 % of all endometrial cancers and occur mostly in high-grade tumors. Almost half of all grade 3 tumors

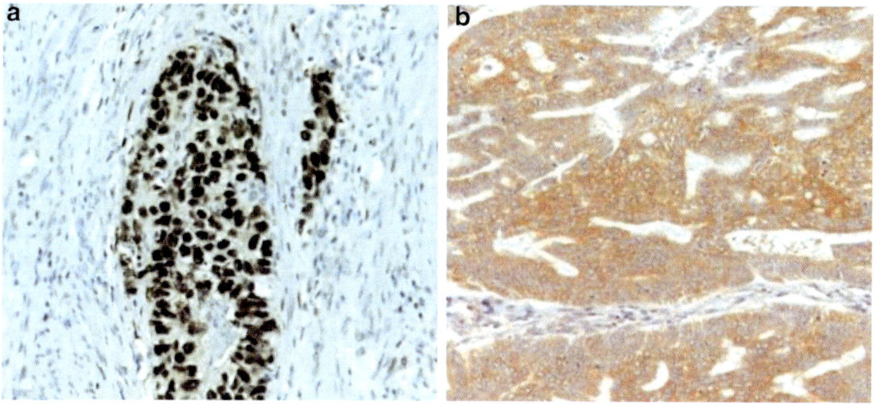

Fig. 1 Expression of p53/HIF-1α in endometrial cancer (**a** and **b** ×200. Provided by department of pathology, Asan Medical Center)

and rarely grade 2 tumors contain p53 mutations, which are not present in grade 1 endometrial cancer or endometrial hyperplasias. In addition, p53 mutations are more frequently observed in papillary serous and clear cell-type carcinoma (Salvesen and Akslen 2002).

HIF-1α

Overexpression of HIF-1α promotes angiogenesis and is associated with an unfavorable prognosis in endometrial cancer (Dousias et al. 2012; Table 1). HIF-1α positive tumors tend to be resistant to chemotherapy and radiotherapy (Koukourakis et al. 2000). The expression of HIF-1α increases gradually in correlation with the progression of endometrial cancer, and a similar trend is observed in its immediate downstream genes such as the GLUT I transporter and carbonic anhydrase 9 (Ozbudak et al. 2008). This phenomenon is associated with changes in microvascular density, a marker of angiogenesis, which indicates that the link between HIF-1α and angiogenesis is relevant to carcinogenesis (Espinosa et al. 2010). A positive correlation between HIF-1α expression and increased angiopoietin-1/2 and IL-8 production supports the important role of HIF-1α in angiogenesis in endometrial cancer (Fujimoto et al. 2006). The expression of HIF-1α is correlated with the development of type 1 endometrial cancers, although it is more common in type 2 endometrial cancers (Fig. 1). HIF-1α expression is associated with deep myometrial invasion, advanced clinical stage, high tumor grade, and adnexal or lymphovascular invasion in type 1 endometrial cancers (Pansare et al. 2007); however, its relationship with prognosis has not been investigated in detail. Studies investigating the relationship between HIF-1α and the prognosis of patients with endometrial cancer reported controversial results. While previous study showed that necrotic or perinecrotic HIF-1α

Table 1 Immunohistochemical markers in endometrial cancer

Immunohistochemical marker	Interpretation	References
p53	p53 mutations occur late in the development of type I endometrial cancer and early in the development of type II endometrial cancer and are an independent predictor of poor survival	Barbati (2000), Ben-Hur (1997), Feng (2005), Liu (2007), Salvesen and Akslen (2002)
HIF-1α	Overexpression of HIF-1α promotes angiogenesis and is associated with an unfavorable prognosis in endometrial cancer	Dousias et al. (2012), Espinosa et al. (2010)
PTEN	PTEN gene alterations are not associated with age, stage, depth of myometrial invasion, or histologic grade in endometrial cancer patients. However, PTEN-positive staining is positively associated with the survival of advanced endometrial carcinoma patients undergoing postoperative chemotherapy	Kanamori et al. (2002)
L1CAM	L1CAM expression was associated with an increase of distal or local recurrence and independently related to poor overall survival in FIGO stage I, type I endometrial cancers	Zeimet et al. (2013)
Steroid receptors	Estrogen receptor (ER) and progesterone receptor (PR) status in endometrial cancer is an independent prognostic marker	Salvesen et al. (2012)
Mismatch repair genes (microsatellite instability)	MSI-positive patients tend to show more progression and vascular invasion in endometrial cancer	Bilbao et al. (2010)
HER-2/neu (c-erbB-2) EGF, EGFR	c-erbB-2 overexpression correlated to poor clinical outcome and lower overall survival	Srijaipracharoen et al. (2010)
Stathmin	Stathmin-positive immunohistochemical staining identifies endometrial carcinomas with lymph node metastases and poor survival	Trovik et al. (2011)
mTOR	Phosphorylated nuclear mTOR was associated with tumor progression and poor survival in patients with endometrial endometrioid adenocarcinoma, among whom those with only nuclear phosphorylated mTOR expression had significantly poorer survival than those with only cytoplasmic p-mTOR expression	Yoshida et al. (2010)
PIK3CA	PIK3CA mutations are strongly associated with endometrioid histology and high-stage disease and a trend toward increased incidence of lymphovascular invasion. However, the association between *PIK3CA* mutations and tumor grade, stage, or depth of myometrial infiltration remains to be confirmed	Catasus et al. (2008), Konstantinova et al. (2010)

Ki-67	Higher values correlated to lower survival rates	Gassel et al. (1998), Pfisterer (1995), Strang (1996)
Bcl-2	Expression of Bcl-2 inversely correlated with depth of myometrial invasion	Sakuragi et al. (2002)
MMP	Immunostaining negativity might be correlated to a favorable prognosis	Egeblad and Werb (2002)
COX2	Higher COX-2 values correlated to higher FIGO grades of endometrial adenocarcinoma	Cao et al. (2002), Ferrandina et al. (2002)
	COX-2 positivity correlated to shorter disease-free survival	
VEGF	Possible association with higher histologic grade, greater depth of myometrial invasion, lymphovascular space invasion, lymph node metastasis, and shorter disease-free survival	Sanseverino et al. (2006), Hirai et al. (2001)
PD-ECGF	PD-ECGF is expressed in lymph nodes, peripheral lymphocytes, spleen, lung, liver, placenta, and the uterine endometrium. PD-ECGF has been implicated in the promotion of tumor growth based on its angiogenic potential	Fox et al. (1995), Moghaddam et al. (1995)
CEA	CEA is less frequently elevated in endometrial cancer than other gynecologic malignancy	Sheahan et al. (1990)
P16	Uterine serous carcinomas demonstrate usually diffuse strong intensity of P16 staining compare to patch weak-to-moderate staining of endometrioid carcinoma of the endometrium	Clarke and Gilks (2010), Salvesen et al. (2000)
	Loss of nuclear p16 protein expression was associated with aggressive endometrial carcinomas and high proliferative activity (Ki-67) and was found to represent a strong and independent prognostic indicator	
c-kit	Simple and complex hyperplastic endometrial tissues express diffuse cytoplasmic staining for c-kit, and the expression decreases with the progression of the lesion to malignancy	Yilmaz et al. (2012)

expression associated with p27kip expression is a prognostic factor of poor progression-free and overall survival in endometrial cancer, other study did not find such an association (Horree et al. 2008; Seeber et al. 2010). Therefore, larger well-designed studies are required to confirm that HIF-1α is an independent prognostic factor in endometrial cancer.

PTEN

Endometrial cancer is characterized by various genetic alterations, and mutations in the PTEN gene are among the most frequent changes associated with the disease (Tsikouras et al. 2013). The PTEN gene is located at q23 of chromosome 10 and acts as a tumor suppressor gene through the negative regulation of tyrosine kinase pathways. Up to 88 % of endometrial cancers and 55 % of precancerous endometrial lesions show PTEN gene alterations (Mutter 2001). Loss of heterozygosity and PTEN mutations leading to loss of expression result in abnormal cell growth and escape from apoptosis. Evidence of PTEN loss in precancerous lesions suggests that it is one of the early events in endometrial carcinogenesis. Estrogen promotes PTEN alterations, whereas progesterone reverses this effect, consistent with clinical observations of the effects of progesterone on the suppression and resolution of endometrial cancer and its precursors (Maxwell et al. 1998). PTEN gene alterations are not associated with age, stage, depth of myometrial invasion, or histologic grade in endometrial cancer patients. However, PTEN-positive staining is positively associated with the survival of advanced endometrial carcinoma patients undergoing postoperative chemotherapy (Kanamori et al. 2002; Table 1).

L1CAM

L1CAM, a 200–220 kDa membrane glycoprotein involved in neurogenesis, is a member of the immunoglobulin superfamily (Schafer and Altevogt 2010). It is encoded by a gene located on the X chromosome (Spatz et al. 2004). Although L1CAM expression is undetectable in the normal epithelium, it is overexpressed in various types of cancers. It is a key driver of epithelial-mesenchymal transition and tumor invasion (Kiefel et al. 2012). L1CAM is strongly expressed in serous and clear cell endometrial cancer, whereas it is not expressed in the normal endometrium or in most endometrioid adenocarcinomas of the uterus (Huszar et al. 2010). L1CAM is associated with advanced stage and high tumor grade and with deep myometrial invasion in stage I endometrial cancers (Zeimet et al. 2013). A recent international multicenter trial showed that L1CAM expression was associated with an increase of distal or local recurrence and independently related to poor overall survival in FIGO stage I, type I endometrial cancers (Zeimet et al. 2013; Table 1).

Steroid Receptors

Steroid hormones bind to nuclear receptors, promoting the transcription of genes and modulating gene expression. Steroid hormone imbalance can lead to cancer. Endometrial carcinogenesis is associated with overexposure to estrogen that is not counterbalanced by the differentiating effects of progesterone, androgens, and glucocorticoids. Previous retrospective studies showed that the estrogen receptor (ER) and progesterone receptor (PR) status in endometrial cancer is an independent prognostic marker (Salvesen et al. 2012; Fig. 2 and Table 1), and this might influence the choice of treatment for advanced disease with distant metastasis because of the association with a higher response rate (Kokka et al. 2010).

Recent study showed that double-negative hormone receptor status in endometrial cancer curettage specimens independently predicted lymph node metastasis and poor prognosis in aggressive phenotypes (Trovik et al. 2013).

Mismatch Repair Genes (Microsatellite Instability)

MSI is a phenomenon in which microsatellite repeat sequences in tumor tissues differ from those in nontumor tissues as a result of a deficient mismatch repair system. MSI was initially identified in association with mutations of MMR-associated genes including *hMLH1*, *hMSH2*, *hMSH6*, *PMS1*, and *PMS2* in germ cell lines derived from patients with hereditary nonpolyposis colorectal cancer (Lynch et al. 1996). MSI occurs in 20–30 % of endometrial cancers, and a major cause is epigenetic inactivation of *hMLH1* associated with promoter hypermethylation (Esteller et al. 1998). Inherited or somatically acquired mutations of *hMSH6*, although relatively uncommon in endometrial cancers in general, are

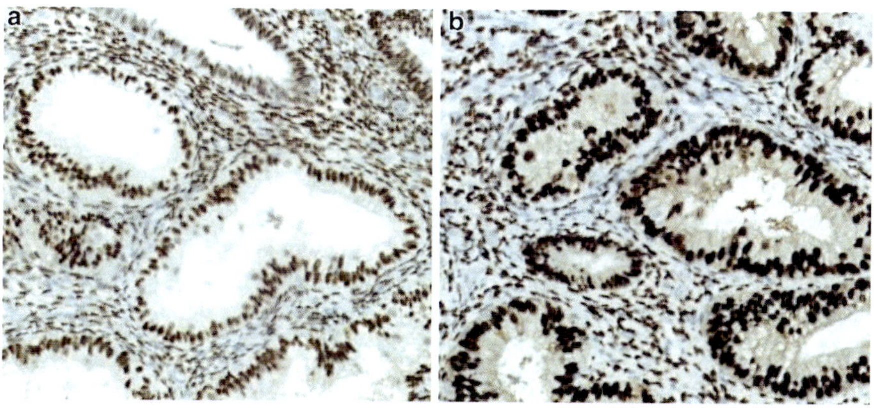

Fig. 2 Expression of ER/PR in endometrial cancer (**a** and **b** ×200. Provided by department of pathology, Asan Medical Center)

often seen in MSI endometrial cancer (Banno et al. 2013). MSI is more common in endometrioid cancer than in nonendometrioid cancer (Catasus et al. 1998). Analysis of *hMSH2* expression showed that 25 % of normal endometrial tissues were *hMSH2* negative and 75 % showed weak *hMSH2* immunoreactivity, whereas all malignancies of the uterine corpus showed strong nuclear immunoreactivity for human *hMSH2* (Friedrich 2000). In addition, expression of the *hMSH2* protein was statistically significantly upregulated in cells derived from tumors of the uterine corpus compared to normal endometrial tissues (Friedrich 2000). Hirai et al. (2008) showed that *hMSH6* is the most important MMR gene in endometrial cancer related to Lynch syndrome and that the Amsterdam Criteria II identifies only approximately half of the cases with germ cell mutations of MMR genes. In an analysis of 20 MSI-positive cases, Bilbao et al. (2010) identified a relationship between MSI and the progression and vascular invasion of endometrial cancer (Table 1). In addition, the 10-year disease-free survival was 53.8 % in MSI-positive patients, which was significantly lower than the 75.9 % survival rate in MSI-negative patients (Bilbao et al. 2010).

HER-2/neu, EGF, and EGFR

The epidermal growth factor system consists of four receptors, human epidermal growth factor receptor 1 (also called EGF receptor/EGFr/ErbB1), HER2 (also called ErbB2), HER3, and HER4 and numerous ligands or EGF-related peptide growth factors (Ejskjaer et al. 2007). HER1 and HER3 are downregulated, whereas HER4, AR, TGF-α, and HB-EGF are upregulated in endometrioid cancer compared to healthy premenopausal endometrium (Ejskjaer et al. 2007). The HER-2/neu (c-erbB-2) oncoprotein is a transmembrane glycoprotein that functions as a growth factor receptor involved in the regulation of cell growth and cell transformation (Kohlberger et al. 1996). HER-2/neu overexpression occurs in 9–30 % of endometrioid cancers and is frequently observed in nonendometrioid tumors (Slomovitz et al. 2004). Overexpression of the HER-2 protein is associated with reduced survival, although the clinical implications and predictive value for treatment response remain unclear. HER-2 is an important oncogene in high-grade and stage endometrial cancers, whereas it plays a minor role in the low-grade and stage tumors most commonly encountered in clinical practice (Morrison et al. 2006). Although several studies have examined the association of HER-2 overexpression with prognostic indicators such as clinical stage, histologic type, grade, and differentiation markers, as well as the clinical outcome of endometrial cancer patients, the results of these studies are not in agreement (Lukes et al. 1994; Pisani et al. 1995). Although HER-2/neu oncoprotein expression was not correlated with clinical stage, histologic stage, histologic grade, and depth of invasion, it was associated with poor overall survival in patients with endometrial cancer (Kohlberger et al. 1996). However, in a recent study, HER-2/neu expression was shown to be a poor indicator for both disease-free and overall survival (Srijaipracharoen et al. 2010; Table 1).

Stathmin

The oncoprotein STMN1 is a microtubule destabilizer that promotes cell proliferation, mobility, metastasis, and resistance to antimicrotubule therapy (Rubin and Atweh 2004). Studies have indicated that STMN1 is overexpressed in many human malignancies and therefore deserves the name of oncoprotein 18 (Op18). In primary tumors, it is preferentially expressed in advanced, invasive, and metastatic cancers. Stathmin-positive immunohistochemical staining identifies endometrial carcinomas with lymph node metastases and poor survival, as shown in a large prospective multicenter study (Trovik et al. 2011; Table 1). High STMN1 expression is associated with poor recurrence-free and overall survival in endometrial carcinomas, indicating a strong correlation between stathmin expression and cancer aggressiveness and identifying STMN1 as an independent prognostic indicator (Salvesen et al. 2009).

mTOR

The mammalian target of rapamycin (mTOR) is a serine/threonine kinase that is ubiquitously expressed in mammalian cells (Shaw and Cantley 2006). mTOR senses and integrates signals initiated by nutrient intake, growth factors, and other cellular stimuli to regulate downstream signaling and protein synthesis (Yuan et al. 2009). The loss of PTEN function and the consequent activation of the PI3K/AKT and mTOR signaling pathways occur in a large proportion of endometrioid-type endometrial carcinomas, suggesting a role for mTOR inhibition in this malignancy (Prat et al. 2007). In a recent study, mTOR expression was highly correlated with old age, menopausal status, and COX-2 expression, and the latter was the only independent factor associated with mTOR expression in multivariate analysis (No et al. 2009). However, no correlation was observed between mTOR expression and prognostic factors such as histologic type, grade, invasion of the myometrium, lymph node metastasis, stage, and survival (No et al. 2009). In another study, phosphorylated nuclear mTOR was associated with tumor progression and poor survival in patients with endometrial endometrioid adenocarcinoma (Fig. 3), among whom those with only nuclear phosphorylated mTOR expression had significantly poorer survival than those with only cytoplasmic p-mTOR expression (Yoshida et al. 2010; Table 1).

PIK3CA

The phosphatidylinositol 3-kinases (PI3Ks) are a family of lipid kinases that catalyze the production of phosphatidylinositol 3,4,5-triphosphate by phosphorylating its precursor, phosphatidylinositol 4,5-bisphosphate. PI3Ks are important regulators of cellular growth and proliferation, transformation, adhesion, apoptosis, survival, and motility (Cantley 2002). PI3Ks are composed of catalytic and regulatory subunits encoded by separate genes. *PI3KCA* mutations occur in 24–36 % of endometrioid cancers, and simultaneous mutation of *PTEN* is observed in 14–26 % of these cases (Oda et al. 2005). PIK3CA mutations are strongly associated with endometrioid histology and high-stage disease and a trend toward increased incidence of lymphovascular invasion (Catasus et al. 2008). However, the association between *PIK3CA* mutations and tumor grade, stage, or depth of myometrial infiltration remains to be confirmed (Konstantinova et al. 2010; Table 1). Nevertheless, PI3K activation is positively correlated with the aggressiveness of cancers (Salvesen et al. 2009). Rare mutations but not hotspot mutations in the *PIK3CA* gene are associated with aggressive endometrial cancers, as indicated by serous differentiation and the presence of metastasis, suggesting that further exploration of the molecular basis of rare mutations is necessary (Konstantinova et al. 2010).

Ki-67

Ki-67 is a nuclear antigen and a marker of cellular proliferation that is expressed in all stages of the cell cycle except G0 and can be detected by immunohistochemistry to estimate proliferative activity in tumors (Pansare et al. 2007). Ki-67 is a potential prognostic factor for survival in several human cancers, including endometrial cancer (Oreskovic et al. 2004). Type I endometrioid carcinomas are generally positive for hormone (estrogen and progesterone) receptor expression and negative for p53 overexpression, whereas type II papillary serous carcinomas are associated with p53 mutation and protein overexpression, absence of hormone receptors, and a very high Ki-67-defined cell proliferation rate (Lax and Kurman 1997). Ki-67 expression is a significant prognostic indicator in endometrial carcinoma patients (Fig. 3), and the independent prognostic value of the immunohistochemical

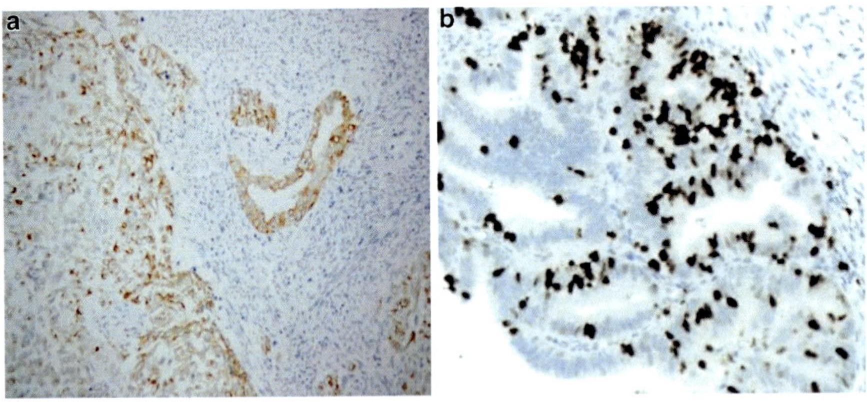

Fig. 3 Expression of p-mTOR/Ki-67 in endometrial cancer (**a** ×200 and **b** ×40. **a**, **b** reused figures from previously published articles under publisher's permission)

determination of proliferative activity using anti Ki-67 antibodies has been demonstrated (Gassel et al. 1998; Table 1). High Ki-67 values in tumors are correlated with low survival rates, and Ki-67 expression is associated with histologic grade, mitotic count, and previous estrogen therapy but not with disease stage (Nielsen and Nyholm 1993).

Bcl-2

Bcl-2 is a 25 kDa protein located within the inner membrane of mitochondria that plays a key role in the regulation of programmed cell death (Korsmeyer 1992). Bcl-2 protein expression has been reported in nonmalignant tissues such as the placenta, as well as in a number of malignant human neoplasms, including uterine, gastrointestinal, ovarian, breast, prostatic, esophageal, colorectal, and lung carcinomas. Abnormalities of the p53 tumor suppressor gene and the bcl-2 proto-oncogene, both of which are involved in the regulation of apoptosis, play an important role in tumorigenesis in several cancers (Sakuragi et al. 2002; Table 1). Apoptotic stimuli cause DNA damage and activation of the p53 tumor suppressor gene, which represses Bcl-2 expression (Miyashita et al. 1994). Furthermore, estrogen has been suggested to upregulate Bcl-2 expression in certain cell systems (Choi et al. 2001), and unopposed estrogen stimulation plays a role in the etiology of endometrial carcinoma. In the human endometrium, immunohistochemical analyses have shown that Bcl-2 expression is upregulated in the proliferative phase and downregulated in the secretory phase (Otsuki et al. 1994), which suggests that endometrial Bcl-2 expression is also regulated by estrogen and progesterone stimulation. Unopposed estrogen may induce sustained overexpression of Bcl-2 leading to increased Bcl-2 levels, which may deregulate the normal apoptotic cell death process and promote the survival of cells harboring mutations in oncogenes or tumor suppressor genes. This suggests that sustained Bcl-2 expression in endometrial gland cells has a pivotal role in the early stage of estrogen-dependent endometrial carcinogenesis (Sakuragi et al. 2002).

MMP

Matrix metalloproteinases are involved in the degradation of protein components of the extracellular matrix and therefore play an important role in tumor invasion and metastasis (Schropfer et al. 2010). The expression and activation of MMPs is increased in most human cancers compared to normal tissues (Curran et al. 2004). MMPs play a role in various physiological processes that require tissue remodeling such as wound healing, embryogenesis, angiogenesis, and ovulation (Page-McCaw et al. 2007). The physiological balance between the activation and inhibition of proteolysis is often disrupted in cancer (Sternlicht and Werb 2001); however, the mechanisms underlying the increased levels of MMPs in carcinoma tissues and the role and contribution of the tumor and stromal cell compartments are

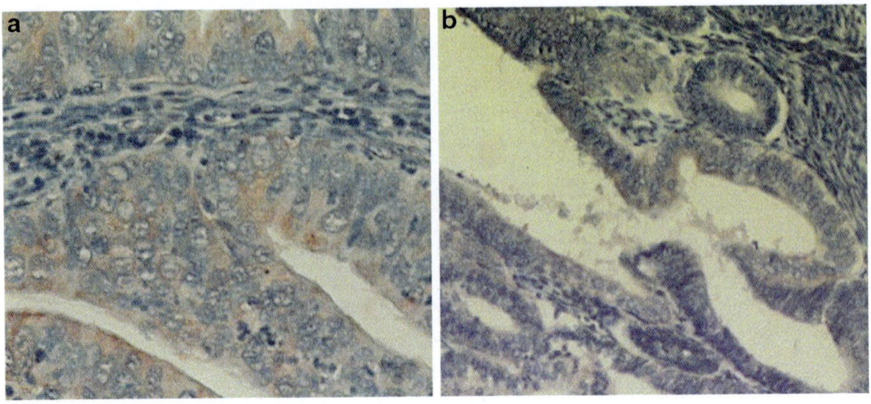

Fig. 4 Expression of MMP-2 and 9 in endometrial cancer (**a** and **b** ×40. **a**, **b** reused figures from previously published articles under publisher's permission)

poorly understood. Some investigators suggest an almost exclusive stromal origin of MMPs detected in cancer tissue (Egeblad and Werb 2002), whereas other studies have shown the constitutive expression of MMPs in several tumor cell lines in the absence of a stromal component (Giambernardi et al. 1998). Talvensaari-Mattila et al. (2005a) suggested that the immunoexpression of MMP2 is not associated with other prognostic factors in endometrial cancer (Talvensaari-Mattila et al. 2005a), and previous study showed that the immunoexpression of MMP2 and MMP9 are not predictive of survival or prognosis of endometrial cancer (Aglund et al. 2004; Talvensaari-Mattila et al. 2005a; Fig. 4). However, a positive correlation between MMP expression and survival has been suggested, despite the superiority of conventional clinicopathologic markers over MMP in predicting the clinical course of disease (Honkavuori et al. 2007; Table 1).

COX-2

Cyclooxygenase-1 (COX-1) and COX-2 are catalytic enzymes involved in prostaglandin synthesis. Prostaglandin E2 (PGE2) promotes the primary process of carcinogenesis and its further consolidation and progression by stimulating cell proliferation, inhibiting natural killer cell activity and inducing in situ immune downmodulation, neoangiogenesis, and the elevated expression of the antiapoptotic protein Bcl-2. COX enzyme overexpression has been associated with neoplasms at various sites, including the gastrointestinal tract, lung, and skin (Fosslien 2000). In recent years, there has been an emerging interest in the study of COX-2 in human gynecological neoplasms, and the clinical role of COX-2 inhibitors in this area is currently under investigation. COX-2 overexpression is mostly detected in adenocarcinoma cells (Landen et al. 2003). The presence of COX-2 in neoplastic cells in endometrial carcinomas with increasing FIGO grades (Cao et al. 2002; Ferrandina et al. 2002) and an association between COX-2 positivity and shorter disease-free survival (Ferrandina et al. 2002) have been reported (Table 1). Well-differentiated endometrial adenocarcinomas are characterized by minimal COX-2 staining, whereas moderately and poorly differentiated endometrial cancers show the strongest COX-2 expression, making a case for a possible role of COX-2 in tumor progression rather than tumor initiation (Cao et al. 2002).

VEGF and VEGFR

In solid tumors, including endometrial carcinomas, the induction of a vascular stroma is essential to grow beyond a minimal size. Vascular endothelial growth factor (VEGF) is a multifunctional cytokine that is an important regulator of tumor angiogenesis (Guidi et al. 1996). The most clinically significant member of the VEGF family is VEGF-A. VEGF is overexpressed in various gynecologic malignancies and is therefore an outstanding target of immunotherapy.

The role of VEGF and its receptors in endometrial carcinoma is not well understood. VEGF is an estrogen-responsive angiogenic factor, which indicates that it may play a significant role in endometrial cancer (Fujimoto et al. 1998; Fig. 5). Immunohistochemical detection of VEGF expression in tumor specimens has been correlated with high histologic grade (Sanseverino et al. 2006), increased depth of myometrial invasion, lymphovascular space invasion, lymph node metastasis, and shorter disease-free survival (Hirai et al. 2001; Table 1). VEGF-D and VEGFR-3 expression in endometrial carcinoma might predict myometrial invasion and lymph node metastasis (Guset et al. 2010). However, another study used immunohistochemistry to show that VEGF and the VEGF receptor are not useful prognostic factors in endometrial cancer (Frumovitz and Sood 2007). Therefore, the functional significance of the VEGF/VEGFR axis in endometrial cancer remains to be demonstrated (Talvensaari-Mattila et al. 2005b).

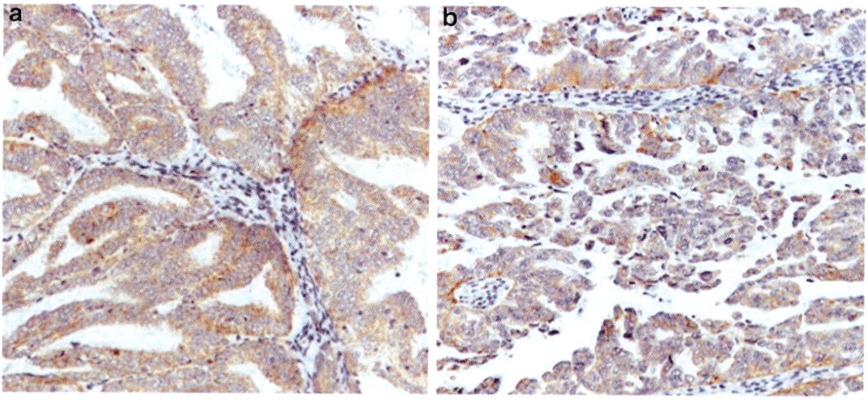

Fig. 5 Expression of VEGF in endometrial cancer (**a** in type I endometrial adenocarcinoma, **b** in type II endometrial adenocarcinoma. **a**, **b** reused figures from previously published articles under publisher's permission)

PD-ECGF

PD-ECGF was originally cloned as a novel angiogenic factor (45 kDa polypeptide) in human platelets (Ishikawa et al. 1989). Thereafter, PD-ECGF was shown to have an identical sequence to that of thymidine phosphorylase (TP) (Sumizawa et al. 1993). PD-ECGF/TP stimulates the chemotaxis of endothelial cells and induces angiogenesis upon activation of thymidine phosphorylase (Miyadera et al. 1995). PD-ECGF is expressed in lymph nodes, peripheral lymphocytes, the spleen, the lung, the liver, the placenta, and the uterine endometrium (Fox et al. 1995). PD-ECGF has been implicated in the promotion of tumor growth based on its angiogenic potential (Moghaddam et al. 1995; Table 1). Among solid tumors, PD-ECGF is expressed in malignant gliomas, thyroid tumors and cancers of the breast, esophagus, stomach, colon, pancreas, gall bladder, kidney, bladder, lung, ovary, and uterus (Moghaddam et al. 1995).

CEA

The carcinoembryonic antigen family comprises 29 genes of which 18 are expressed, with 7 belonging to the CEA subgroup, and 11 to the pregnancy-specific glycoprotein subgroup. CEA is an important tumor marker for colorectal and other carcinomas. The CEA subgroup members are cell membrane associated and show a complex expression pattern in normal and cancerous tissues, with CEA showing a selective epithelial expression (Liu et al. 2014). The expression of CEA family members is increased in endometrial adenocarcinoma (Thompson et al. 1993); however, the level of serum CEA or CEA immunoperoxidase staining is less frequently elevated in endometrial cancer than in other gynecologic malignancies (Sheahan et al. 1990; Table 1). Additional roles of CEA in gastrointestinal, mammary, bronchial, and ovarian carcinoma have been suggested.

P16

Since its discovery as a CDKI (cyclin-dependent kinase inhibitor) in 1993, the tumor suppressor p16 (INK4A/MTS-1/CDKN2A) has gained widespread importance in cancer. The frequent mutations and deletions of p16 in human cancer cell lines first suggested an important role for p16 in carcinogenesis (Liggett and Sidransky 1998). In endometrial carcinoma, uterine serous carcinomas show diffuse p16 staining (mean 95 % of cells) that is usually of strong intensity but is occasionally moderate (Table 1). Endometrioid carcinomas show patchy weak-to-moderate p16 staining (mean 38 % of cells) regardless of grade. Therefore, the distinction between serous and endometrioid carcinoma of the endometrium should be based on >90 % of tumor cells showing moderate-to-intense nuclear and cytoplasmic p16 positivity (Fig. 6). Certain endometrioid carcinomas show moderately intense p16 staining (Clarke and Gilks 2010). Loss of nuclear p16 protein

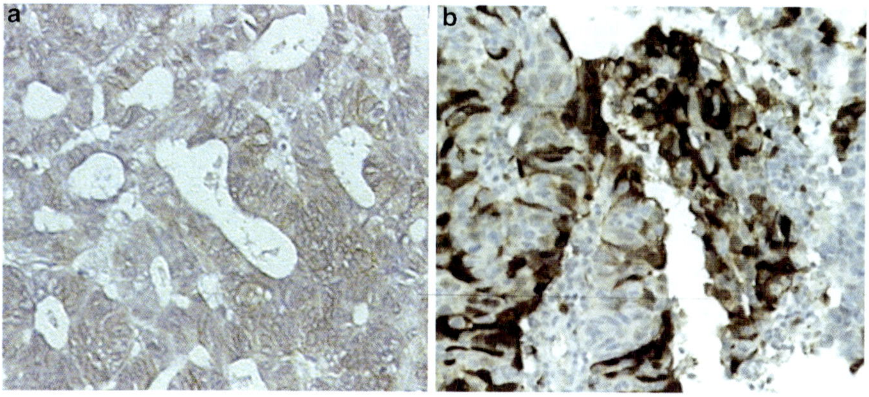

Fig. 6 Expression of c-kit/p16 in endometrial cancer (**a** ×400 and **b** ×200. **a** provided by department of pathology, Asan Medical Center. **b** reused figures from previously published articles under publisher's permission)

expression is associated with aggressive endometrial carcinomas and high proliferative activity (Ki-67), suggesting p16 as a strong and independent prognostic indicator; however, methylation of the promoter region is an uncommon mechanism of p16 inactivation in endometrial carcinoma (Salvesen et al. 2000; Table 1).

c-kit

The proto-oncogene c-kit, the cellular homolog of the oncogene v-Kit of HZ4 feline sarcoma virus, is located on chromosome 4 (4q11–12) in the human genome (Wang et al. 2003). c-Kit encodes a 145-kDa transmembrane tyrosine kinase receptor (CD117), and its ligand is stem cell factor (SCF) (McCulloch and Minden 1993). CD117 signaling plays a role in cell survival, proliferation, and differentiation. Overexpression of c-kit or mutation of CD117 has been implicated in a variety of malignant tumors. On the other hand, the downregulation of c-kit expression has been associated with the progression from endometrial hyperplasia to endometrial cancer (Yilmaz et al. 2012; Fig. 6 and Table 1). Immunostaining for c-kit was shown to be mostly focal and weak in the normal endometrium and mostly diffuse and strong in simple and complex endometrial hyperplasia. However, the application of c-kit immunohistochemistry in endometrial cancer is limited (Vandenput et al. 2011).

Potential Applications to Prognosis, Other Diseases, or Conditions

Most of the immunohistochemical markers of endometrial cancer reviewed in this chapter were extensively investigated in many other cancers. However, the clinical role or applicability of these markers differs according to the type of cancer.

Summary Points

- This chapter focuses on immunohistochemical markers that may play a role as predictive or prognostic biomarkers in endometrial cancer.
- Numerous prior studies have investigated immunohistochemical markers as predictors of tumor extent, tumor behavior, and prognosis after treatment in endometrial cancer.
- Several markers were reported to be predictive or prognostic markers in endometrial cancer; however, none of these can be used as a single reliable biomarker.
- L1CAM and stathmin are among the most promising immunohistochemical markers identified to date.
- L1CAM is a membrane glycoprotein involved in neurogenesis.
- In a large prospective clinical trial, L1CAM was associated with advanced stage, high tumor grade, and deep myometrial invasion in stage I endometrial cancer.
- L1CAM expression is associated with increased distal or local recurrence and is independently related to poor overall survival in FIGO stage I, type I endometrial cancers.
- Stathmin is an oncoprotein that functions as a microtubule destabilizer, promoting cell proliferation, mobility, metastasis, and resistance to antimicrotubule therapy.
- In a large prospective clinical trial, stathmin overexpression was associated with poor recurrence-free survival and overall survival in endometrial carcinomas.
- Further studies are required to identify powerful immunohistochemical markers that can be used as reliable predictive or prognostic biomarkers for endometrial cancer.

References

Aglund K, Rauvala M, Puistola U, Angstrom T, Turpeenniemi-Hujanen T, Zackrisson B, Stendahl U. Gelatinases A and B (MMP-2 and MMP-9) in endometrial cancer-MMP-9 correlates to the grade and the stage. Gynecol Oncol. 2004;94:699–704.

Amant F, Moerman P, Neven P, Timmerman D, Van Limbergen E, Vergote I. Endometrial cancer. Lancet. 2005;366:491–505.

Banno K, Nogami Y, Kisu I, Yanokura M, Umene K, Masuda K, Kobayashi Y, Yamagami W, Susumu N, Aoki D. Candidate biomarkers for genetic and clinicopathological diagnosis of endometrial cancer. Int J Mol Sci. 2013;14:12123–37.

Barbati A, Mariani L, Porpora MG, Anceschi M, Collini P, Lauro V, Cosmi EV. Serum evaluation of p53 protein in patients with gynaecological cancer. Anticancer Res. 2000;20(2A):1003–5.

Ben-Hur H, Berman V, Sandler B, Smimoff P, Gurevich P, Open M, Zusman I. Serological and immunohistochemical determinations of p53 protein in diagnosis of endometrial cancer: a comparative study. Eur J Gynaecol Oncol. 1997;18(5):400–6.

Bilbao C, Lara PC, Ramirez R, Henriquez-Hernandez LA, Rodriguez G, Falcon O, Leon L, Perucho M, Diaz-Chico BN, Diaz-Chico JC. Microsatellite instability predicts clinical outcome in radiation-treated endometrioid endometrial cancer. Int J Radiat Oncol Biol Phys. 2010;76:9–13.

Bray F, Loos AH, Oostindier M, Weiderpass E. Geographic and temporal variations in cancer of the corpus uteri: incidence and mortality in pre- and postmenopausal women in Europe. Int J Cancer. 2005;117:123–31.

Cantley LC. The phosphoinositide 3-kinase pathway. Science. 2002;296:1655–7.

Cao QJ, Einstein MH, Anderson PS, Runowicz CD, Balan R, Jones JG. Expression of COX-2, Ki-67, cyclin D1, and P21 in endometrial endometrioid carcinomas. Int J Gynecol Pathol. 2002;21:147–54.

Catasus L, Machin P, Matias-Guiu X, Prat J. Microsatellite instability in endometrial carcinomas: clinicopathologic correlations in a series of 42 cases. Hum Pathol. 1998;29: 1160–4.

Catasus L, Gallardo A, Cuatrecasas M, Prat J. PIK3CA mutations in the kinase domain (exon 20) of uterine endometrial adenocarcinomas are associated with adverse prognostic parameters. Mod Pathol. 2008;21:131–9.

Choi KC, Kang SK, Tai CJ, Auersperg N, Leung PC. Estradiol up-regulates antiapoptotic Bcl-2 messenger ribonucleic acid and protein in tumorigenic ovarian surface epithelium cells. Endocrinology. 2001;142:2351–60.

Clarke BA, Gilks CB. Endometrial carcinoma: controversies in histopathological assessment of grade and tumour cell type. J Clin Pathol. 2010;63:410–5.

Colombo N, Preti E, Landoni F, Carinelli S, Colombo A, Marini C, Sessa C, ESMO Guidelines Working Group. Endometrial cancer: ESMO Clinical Practice Guidelines for diagnosis, treatment and follow-up. Ann Oncol. 2013;24 Suppl 6:vi33–8.

Curran S, Dundas SR, Buxton J, Leeman MF, Ramsay R, Murray GI. Matrix metalloproteinase/ tissue inhibitors of matrix metalloproteinase phenotype identifies poor prognosis colorectal cancers. Clin Cancer Res. 2004;10:8229–34.

Dousias V, Vrekoussis T, Navrozoglou I, Paschopoulos M, Stefos T, Makrigiannakis A, Jeschke U. Hypoxia-induced factor-1alpha in endometrial carcinoma: a mini-review of current evidence. Histol Histopathol. 2012;27:1247–53.

Egeblad M, Werb Z. New functions for the matrix metalloproteinases in cancer progression. Nat Rev Cancer. 2002;2:161–74.

Ejskjaer K, Sorensen BS, Poulsen SS, Forman A, Nexo E, Mogensen O. Expression of the epidermal growth factor system in endometrioid endometrial cancer. Gynecol Oncol. 2007;104:158–67.

Espinosa I, Jose Carnicer M, Catasus L, Canet B, D'Angelo E, Zannoni GF, Prat J. Myometrial invasion and lymph node metastasis in endometrioid carcinomas: tumor-associated macrophages, microvessel density, and HIF1A have a crucial role. Am J Surg Pathol. 2010;34:1708–14.

Esteller M, Levine R, Baylin SB, Ellenson LH, Herman JG. MLH1 promoter hypermethylation is associated with the microsatellite instability phenotype in sporadic endometrial carcinomas. Oncogene. 1998;17:2413–7.

Feng YZ, Shiozawa T, Horiuchi A, Shih HC, Miyamoto T, Kashima H, Suzuki A, Nikaido T, Konishi I. Intratumoral heterogeneous expression of p53 correlates with p53 mutation, Ki-67, and cyclin A expression in endometrioid-type endometrial adenocarcinomas. Virchows Arch. 2005;447(5):816–22.

Ferrandina G, Legge F, Ranelletti FO, Zannoni GF, Maggiano N, Evangelisti A, Mancuso S, Scambia G, Lauriola L. Cyclooxygenase-2 expression in endometrial carcinoma: correlation with clinicopathologic parameters and clinical outcome. Cancer. 2002;95:801–7.

Fosslien E. Molecular pathology of cyclooxygenase-2 in neoplasia. Ann Clin Lab Sci. 2000;30:3–21.

Fox SB, Moghaddam A, Westwood M, Turley H, Bicknell R, Gatter KC, Harris AL. Platelet-derived endothelial cell growth factor/thymidine phosphorylase expression in normal tissues: an immunohistochemical study. J Pathol. 1995;176:183–90.

Friedrich M. Analysis of the DNA "mismatch-repair" enzyme human mut-S-homologon-2 in endometrial cancer on protein- and RNA-level. Eur J Gynaecol Oncol. 2000;21:273–7.

Frumovitz M, Sood AK. Vascular endothelial growth factor (VEGF) pathway as a therapeutic target in gynecologic malignancies. Gynecol Oncol. 2007;104:768–78.

Fujimoto J, Ichigo S, Sakaguchi H, Hirose R, Tamaya T. Expression of platelet-derived endothelial cell growth factor and its mRNA in uterine endometrium during the menstrual cycle. Mol Hum Reprod. 1998;4:509–13.

Fujimoto J, Sato E, Alam SM, Jahan I, Toyoki H, Hong BL, Sakaguchi H, Tamaya T. Plausible linkage of hypoxia-inducible factor (HIF) in uterine endometrial cancers. Oncology. 2006;71:95–101.

Gassel AM, Backe J, Krebs S, Schon S, Caffier H, Muller-Hermelink HK. Endometrial carcinoma: immunohistochemically detected proliferation index is a prognosticator of long-term outcome. J Clin Pathol. 1998;51:25–9.

Giambernardi TA, Grant GM, Taylor GP, Hay RJ, Maher VM, McCormick JJ, Klebe RJ. Overview of matrix metalloproteinase expression in cultured human cells. Matrix Biol. 1998;16:483–96.

Guidi AJ, Abu-Jawdeh G, Tognazzi K, Dvorak HF, Brown LF. Expression of vascular permeability factor (vascular endothelial growth factor) and its receptors in endometrial carcinoma. Cancer. 1996;78:454–60.

Guset G, Costi S, Lazar E, Dema A, Cornianu M, Vernic C, Paiusan L. Expression of vascular endothelial growth factor (VEGF) and assessment of microvascular density with CD34 as prognostic markers for endometrial carcinoma. Rom J Morphol Embryol. 2010;51:677–82.

Hirai M, Nakagawara A, Oosaki T, Hayashi Y, Hirono M, Yoshihara T. Expression of vascular endothelial growth factors (VEGF-A/VEGF-1 and VEGF-C/VEGF-2) in postmenopausal uterine endometrial carcinoma. Gynecol Oncol. 2001;80:181–8.

Hirai Y, Banno K, Suzuki M, Ichikawa Y, Udagawa Y, Sugano K, Miki Y. Molecular epidemiological and mutational analysis of DNA mismatch repair (MMR) genes in endometrial cancer patients with HNPCC-associated familial predisposition to cancer. Cancer Sci. 2008;99:1715–9.

Honkavuori M, Talvensaari-Mattila A, Soini Y, Turpeenniemi-Hujanen T, Santala M. MMP-2 expression associates with CA 125 and clinical course in endometrial carcinoma. Gynecol Oncol. 2007;104:217–21.

Horree N, Gort EH, van der Groep P, Heintz AP, Vooijs M, van Diest PJ. Hypoxia-inducible factor 1 alpha is essential for hypoxic p27 induction in endometrioid endometrial carcinoma. J Pathol. 2008;214:38–45.

Huszar M, Pfeifer M, Schirmer U, Kiefel H, Konecny GE, Ben-Arie A, Edler L, Munch M, Muller-Holzner E, Jerabek-Klestil S, et al. Up-regulation of L1CAM is linked to loss of hormone receptors and E-cadherin in aggressive subtypes of endometrial carcinomas. J Pathol. 2010;220:551–61.

Ishikawa F, Miyazono K, Hellman U, Drexler H, Wernstedt C, Hagiwara K, Usuki K, Takaku F, Risau W, Heldin C-H. Identification of angiogenic activity and the cloning and expression of platelet-derived endothelial cell growth factor. Nature. 1989;338:557–62.

Kanamori Y, Kigawa J, Itamochi H, Sultana H, Suzuki M, Ohwada M, Kamura T, Sugiyama T, Kikuchi Y, Kita T, et al. PTEN expression is associated with prognosis for patients with advanced endometrial carcinoma undergoing postoperative chemotherapy. Int J Cancer. 2002;100:686–9.

Kiefel H, Bondong S, Hazin J, Ridinger J, Schirmer U, Riedle S, Altevogt P. L1CAM: a major driver for tumor cell invasion and motility. Cell Adh Migr. 2012;6:374–84.

Kohlberger P, Loesch A, Koelbl H, Breitenecker G, Kainz C, Gitsch G. Prognostic value of immunohistochemically detected HER-2/neu oncoprotein in endometrial cancer. Cancer Lett. 1996;98:151–5.

Kokka F, Brockbank E, Oram D, Gallagher C, Bryant A. Hormonal therapy in advanced or recurrent endometrial cancer. Cochrane Database Syst Rev. 2010;CD007926

Konstantinova D, Kaneva R, Dimitrov R, Savov A, Ivanov S, Dyankova T, Kremensky I, Mitev V. Rare mutations in the PIK3CA gene contribute to aggressive endometrial cancer. DNA Cell Biol. 2010;29:65–70.

Korsmeyer SJ. Bcl-2 initiates a new category of oncogenes: regulators of cell death. Blood. 1992;80:879–86.

Koukourakis MI, Giatromanolaki A, Sivridis E, Fezoulidis I. Cancer vascularization: implications in radiotherapy? Int J Radiat Oncol Biol Phys. 2000;48:545–53.

Landen Jr CN, Mathur SP, Richardson MS, Creasman WT. Expression of cyclooxygenase-2 in cervical, endometrial, and ovarian malignancies. Am J Obstet Gynecol. 2003;188:1174–6.

Lax SF, Kurman RJ. A dualistic model for endometrial carcinogenesis based on immunohistochemical and molecular genetic analyses. Verh Dtsch Ges Pathol. 1997;81:228–32.

Liggett Jr WH, Sidransky D. Role of the p16 tumor suppressor gene in cancer. J Clin Oncol. 1998;16:1197–206.

Liu FS. Molecular carcinogenesis of endometrial cancer. Taiwan J Obstet Gynecol. 2007;46:26–32.

Liu T, Du X, Sheng X. Gene expression changes after ionizing radiation in endothelial cells derived from human endometrial cancer-preliminary outcomes. Arch Gynecol Obstet. 2014;289:1315–23.

Lukes AS, Kohler MF, Pieper CF, Kerns BJ, Bentley R, Rodriguez GC, Soper JT, Clarke-Pearson DL, Bast Jr RC, Berchuck A. Multivariable analysis of DNA ploidy, p53, and HER-2/neu as prognostic factors in endometrial cancer. Cancer. 1994;73:2380–5.

Lynch HT, Smyrk T, Lynch JF. Overview of natural history, pathology, molecular genetics and management of HNPCC (Lynch syndrome). Int J Cancer. 1996;69:38–43.

Maxwell GL, Risinger JI, Gumbs C, Shaw H, Bentley RC, Barrett JC, Berchuck A, Futreal PA. Mutation of the PTEN tumor suppressor gene in endometrial hyperplasias. Cancer Res. 1998;58:2500–3.

McCulloch E, Minden M. The cell surface receptor encoded by the proto-oncogene KIT and its ligand. In: Leukemia: advances in research and treatment. New York: Springer; 1993. p. 45–77.

Miyadera K, Sumizawa T, Haraguchi M, Yoshida H, Konstanty W, Yamada Y, S-i A. Role of thymidine phosphorylase activity in the angiogenic effect of platelet-derived endothelial cell growth factor/thymidine phosphorylase. Cancer Res. 1995;55:1687–90.

Miyashita T, Krajewski S, Krajewska M, Wang HG, Lin HK, Liebermann DA, Hoffman B, Reed JC. Tumor suppressor p53 is a regulator of bcl-2 and bax gene expression in vitro and in vivo. Oncogene. 1994;9:1799–805.

Moghaddam A, Zhang H-T, Fan T, Hu D-E, Lees VC, Turley H, Fox SB, Gatter KC, Harris AL, Bicknell R. Thymidine phosphorylase is angiogenic and promotes tumor growth. Proc Natl Acad Sci. 1995;92:998–1002.

Morrison C, Zanagnolo V, Ramirez N, Cohn DE, Kelbick N, Copeland L, Maxwell GL, Fowler JM. HER-2 is an independent prognostic factor in endometrial cancer: association with outcome in a large cohort of surgically staged patients. J Clin Oncol. 2006;24:2376–85.

Mutter GL. Pten, a protean tumor suppressor. Am J Pathol. 2001;158:1895–8.

Nielsen AL, Nyholm HC. Proliferative activity as revealed by Ki-67 in uterine adenocarcinoma of endometrioid type: comparison of tumours from patients with and without previous oestrogen therapy. J Pathol. 1993;171:199–205.

No JH, Jeon YT, Park IA, Kang D, Kim JW, Park NH, Kang SB, Song YS. Expression of mTOR protein and its clinical significance in endometrial cancer. Med Sci Monit. 2009;15:BR301–5.

Oda K, Stokoe D, Taketani Y, McCormick F. High frequency of coexistent mutations of PIK3CA and PTEN genes in endometrial carcinoma. Cancer Res. 2005;65:10669–73.

Oreskovic S, Babic D, Kalafatic D, Barisic D, Beketic-Oreskovic L. A significance of immunohistochemical determination of steroid receptors, cell proliferation factor Ki-67 and protein p53 in endometrial carcinoma. Gynecol Oncol. 2004;93:34–40.

Otsuki Y, Misaki O, Sugimoto O, Ito Y, Tsujimoto Y, Akao Y. Cyclic bcl-2 gene expression in human uterine endometrium during menstrual cycle. Lancet. 1994;344:28–9.

Ozbudak IH, Karaveli S, Simsek T, Erdogan G, Pestereli E. Neoangiogenesis and expression of hypoxia-inducible factor 1alpha, vascular endothelial growth factor, and glucose transporter-1 in endometrioid type endometrium adenocarcinomas. Gynecol Oncol. 2008;108:603–8.

Page-McCaw A, Ewald AJ, Werb Z. Matrix metalloproteinases and the regulation of tissue remodelling. Nat Rev Mol Cell Biol. 2007;8:221–33.

Pansare V, Munkarah AR, Schimp V, Haitham Arabi M, Saed GM, Morris RT, Ali-Fehmi R. Increased expression of hypoxia-inducible factor 1alpha in type I and type II endometrial carcinomas. Mod Pathol. 2007;20:35–43.

Parkin DM, Bray F, Ferlay J, Pisani P. Global cancer statistics, 2002. CA Cancer J Clin. 2005;55:74–108.

Pfisterer J, Kommoss F, Sauerbrei W, Rendl I, Kiechle M, Kleine W, Pfleiderer A. Prognostic value of DNA ploidy and S-phase fraction in stage I endometrial carcinoma. Gynecol Oncol 1995;58(2):149–56.

Pisani AL, Barbuto DA, Chen D, Ramos L, Lagasse LD, Karlan BY. HER-2/neu, p53, and DNA analyses as prognosticators for survival in endometrial carcinoma. Obstet Gynecol. 1995;85:729–34.

Prat J, Gallardo A, Cuatrecasas M, Catasus L. Endometrial carcinoma: pathology and genetics. Pathology. 2007;39:72–87.

Rubin CI, Atweh GF. The role of stathmin in the regulation of the cell cycle. J Cell Biochem. 2004;93:242–50.

Sakuragi N, Salah-eldin AE, Watari H, Itoh T, Inoue S, Moriuchi T, Fujimoto S. Bax, Bcl-2, and p53 expression in endometrial cancer. Gynecol Oncol. 2002;86:288–96.

Salvesen HB, Akslen LA. Molecular pathogenesis and prognostic factors in endometrial carcinoma. APMIS. 2002;110:673–89.

Salvesen HB, Das S, Akslen LA. Loss of nuclear p16 protein expression is not associated with promoter methylation but defines a subgroup of aggressive endometrial carcinomas with poor prognosis. Clin Cancer Res. 2000;6:153–9.

Salvesen HB, Carter SL, Mannelqvist M, Dutt A, Getz G, Stefansson IM, Raeder MB, Sos ML, Engelsen IB, Trovik J, et al. Integrated genomic profiling of endometrial carcinoma associates aggressive tumors with indicators of PI3 kinase activation. Proc Natl Acad Sci U S A. 2009;106:4834–9.

Salvesen HB, Haldorsen IS, Trovik J. Markers for individualised therapy in endometrial carcinoma. Lancet Oncol. 2012;13:e353–61.

Sanseverino F, Santopietro R, Torricelli M, D'Andrilli G, Russo G, Cevenini G, Bovicelli A, Leoncini L, Scambia G, Petraglia F. pRb2/p130 and VEGF expression in endometrial carcinoma in relation to angiogenesis and histopathologic tumor grade. Cancer Biol Ther. 2006;5:84–8.

Schafer MK, Altevogt P. L1CAM malfunction in the nervous system and human carcinomas. Cell Mol Life Sci. 2010;67:2425–37.

Schropfer A, Kammerer U, Kapp M, Dietl J, Feix S, Anacker J. Expression pattern of matrix metalloproteinases in human gynecological cancer cell lines. BMC Cancer. 2010;10:553.

Seeber LM, Horree N, van der Groep P, van der Wall E, Verheijen RH, van Diest PJ. Necrosis related HIF-1alpha expression predicts prognosis in patients with endometrioid endometrial carcinoma. BMC Cancer. 2010;10:307.

Shaw RJ, Cantley LC. Ras, PI(3)K and mTOR signalling controls tumour cell growth. Nature. 2006;441:424–30.

Sheahan K, O'brien M, Burke B, Dervan P, O'keane J, Gottlieb L, Zamcheck N. Differential reactivities of carcinoembryonic antigen (CEA) and CEA-related monoclonal and polyclonal antibodies in common epithelial malignancies. Am J Clin Pathol. 1990;94:157.

Slomovitz BM, Broaddus RR, Burke TW, Sneige N, Soliman PT, Wu W, Sun CC, Munsell MF, Gershenson DM, Lu KH. Her-2/neu overexpression and amplification in uterine papillary serous carcinoma. J Clin Oncol. 2004;22:3126–32.

Spatz A, Borg C, Feunteun J. X-chromosome genetics and human cancer. Nat Rev Cancer. 2004;4:617–29.

Srijaipracharoen S, Tangjitgamol S, Tanvanich S, Manusirivithaya S, Khunnarong J, Thavaramara T, Leelahakorn S, Pataradool K. Expression of ER, PR, and Her-2/neu in endometrial cancer: a clinicopathological study. Asian Pac J Cancer Prev. 2010;11:215–20.

Strang P, Nordstom B, Nilsson S, Bergstrom R, Tribukait B. Mutant p53 protein as a predictor of survival in endometrial carcinoma. Eur J Cancer. 1996;32A(4):598–602.

Sternlicht MD, Werb Z. How matrix metalloproteinases regulate cell behavior. Annu Rev Cell Dev Biol. 2001;17:463–516.

Sumizawa T, Furukawa T, Haraguchi M, Yoshimura A, Takeyasu A, Ishizawa M, Yamada Y, S-i A. Thymidine phosphorylase activity associated with platelet-derived endothelial cell growth factor. J Biochem. 1993;114:9–14.

Talvensaari-Mattila A, Santala M, Soini Y, Turpeenniemi-Hujanen T. Prognostic value of matrix metalloproteinase-2 (MMP-2) expression in endometrial endometrioid adenocarcinoma. Anticancer Res. 2005a;25:4101–5.

Talvensaari-Mattila A, Soini Y, Santala M. VEGF and its receptors (flt-1 and KDR/flk-1) as prognostic indicators in endometrial carcinoma. Tumor Biol. 2005b;26:81–7.

Thompson J, Mössinger S, Reichardt V, Engels U, Beauchemin N, Kommoss F, Von Kleist S, Zimmermann W. A polymerase-chain-reaction assay for the specific identification of transcripts encoded by individual carcinoembryonic antigen (CEA)-gene-family members. Int J Cancer. 1993;55:311–9.

Trovik J, Wik E, Stefansson IM, Marcickiewicz J, Tingulstad S, Staff AC, Njolstad TS, MoMaTec Study Group, Vandenput I, Amant F, et al. Stathmin overexpression identifies high-risk patients and lymph node metastasis in endometrial cancer. Clin Cancer Res. 2011;17:3368–77.

Trovik J, Wik E, Werner HM, Krakstad C, Helland H, Vandenput I, Njolstad TS, Stefansson IM, Marcickiewicz J, Tingulstad S, et al. Hormone receptor loss in endometrial carcinoma curettage predicts lymph node metastasis and poor outcome in prospective multicentre trial. Eur J Cancer. 2013;49:3431–41.

Tsikouras P, Bouchlariotou S, Vrachnis N, Dafopoulos A, Galazios G, Csorba R, von Tempelhoff GF. Endometrial cancer: molecular and therapeutic aspects. Eur J Obstet Gynecol Reprod Biol. 2013;169:1–9.

Ushijima K. Current status of gynecologic cancer in Japan. J Gynecol Oncol. 2009;20:67–71.

Vandenput I, Debiec-Rychter M, Capoen A, Verbist G, Vergote I, Moerman P, Amant F. Kit gene in endometrial carcinoma: an immunohistochemical and mutational analysis. Int J Gynecol Cancer. 2011;21:203–5.

Wang L, Felix JC, Lee JL, Tan PY, Tourgeman DE, O'Meara AT, Amezcua CA. The proto-oncogene c-kit is expressed in leiomyosarcomas of the uterus. Gynecol Oncol. 2003;90:402–6.

Wright JD, Barrena Medel NI, Sehouli J, Fujiwara K, Herzog TJ. Contemporary management of endometrial cancer. Lancet. 2012;379:1352–60.

Yilmaz E, Celik O, Simsek Y, Turkcuoglu I, Celik E, Gül M, Hascalik S, Aydin E. c-Kit proto-oncogene expression in endometrial hyperplasia and endometrial cancer. Arch Gynecol Obstet. 2012;286:197–200.

Yoshida Y, Kurokawa T, Horiuchi Y, Sawamura Y, Shinagawa A, Kotsuji F. Localisation of phosphorylated mTOR expression is critical to tumour progression and outcomes in patients with endometrial cancer. Eur J Cancer. 2010;46:3445–52.

Yuan R, Kay A, Berg WJ, Lebwohl D. Targeting tumorigenesis: development and use of mTOR inhibitors in cancer therapy. J Hematol Oncol. 2009;2:45.

Zeimet AG, Reimer D, Huszar M, Winterhoff B, Puistola U, Azim SA, Muller-Holzner E, Ben-Arie A, van Kempen LC, Petru E, et al. L1CAM in early-stage type I endometrial cancer: results of a large multicenter evaluation. J Natl Cancer Inst. 2013;105:1142–50.

Use of Visceral Adipocyte Biomarkers in Endometrial Cancer

25

Liz Y. Han and Yvonne G. Lin

Contents

Abstract

Repositories of visceral adipocytes, such as the omentum, have historically been regarded as accessory organs, providing insulation, mechanical, and/or nutritional support. However, the discovery of key adipokines and immune mediators within visceral adipocytes has precipitated revisiting and redefining the traditional function of the visceral adipose tissue, particularly as adipocytes relate to cancer development and progression. Parallel studies of the biology of adipocytes in obesity and cancer have also identified perturbations in cellular homeostasis with an imbalance of secreted adipokines tipped in favor of inflammation within the microenvironment as well as endoplasmic reticulum (ER) stress and its master regulator, the glucose-regulated protein-78 (GRP78). These proteins

L.Y. Han
Division of Gynecologic Oncology, Kaiser Permanente Northern California, Oakland, CA, USA
e-mail: Liz.Ye.Han@kp.org

Y.G. Lin (✉)
Division of Gynecologic Oncology, Department of Obstetrics-Gynecology, Norris Comprehensive Cancer Center, University of Southern California, Los Angeles, CA, USA
e-mail: YLINLIU@med.usc.edu; ylinliu@usc.edu

V.R. Preedy, V.B. Patel (eds.), *Biomarkers in Cancer, Biomarkers in Disease: Methods, Discoveries and Applications*,
DOI 10.1007/978-94-007-7681-4_28

are detectable in peripheral circulation and may provide insight into tumor biology and prognosis. Given the strong link between adiposity and endometrial cancer, evaluating these adipocyte-derived factors in the context may reveal a useful tool to aid clinical decisions. This chapter reviews several biomarker candidates emanating from adipocytes and the biological basis for their role in endometrial cancer.

List of Abbreviations

AMPK	AMP-Activated Protein Kinase
BMI	Body Mass Index
cAMP	Cyclic AMP
COX-2	Cyclooxygenase-2
CT	Computed Tomography
EAC	Endometrioid Adenocarcinoma
ER	Endoplasmic Reticulum
FABP4	Fatty Acid-Binding Protein 4
GPER	G protein-Coupled Estrogen Receptor
GRP78	Glucose-Regulated Protein 78
HMW	High Molecular Weight
IGF	Insulin Growth Factor
IGFBP	Insulin Growth Factor-Binding Protein
IRS	Insulin Receptor Substrate
JNK	c-Jun N-Terminal Kinase
LMW	Low Molecular Weight
MCP-1	Monocyte Chemotactic Protein-1
MMW	Medium Molecular Weight
mTOR	Mammalian Target of Rapamycin
NF-κB	Nuclear Factor κB
PPAR-α	Peroxisome Proliferator-Activated Receptor-α
PPAR-γ	Peroxisome Proliferator-Activated Receptor-γ
SOCS-3	Suppressors of Cytokine Signaling-3
STAT-3	Signal Transducer and Activator of Transcription-3
UCP1	Uncoupling Protein 1
UPR	Unfolded Protein Response
VEGF	Vascular Endothelial Growth Factor

Key Facts About Adipocytes and Endometrial Cancer

- Visceral adipocytes secrete and express proteins important in cancer, including endometrial cancer.
- Proteins expressed by adipocytes can be measured in the blood and the adipocytes.

- Levels of adipocyte-derived proteins can fluctuate in the presence or absence of cancer.
- Some of these adipocyte-derived proteins may play an antitumoral role, while others may encourage tumor growth; it is the net effects of these factors within the tumor environment that matter.
- Changes in levels of adipocyte-derived proteins may represent a means of monitoring the development and growth of cancers, such as endometrial cancer.

Definitions of Words and Terms

Adipokine Cytokine secreted by adipose tissues. May also be referred to as adipocytokine.

Visceral Adipocytes Fat cells within the abdominal cavity as opposed to subcutaneous adipocytes. A classic example of visceral adipocytes is the omentum.

Endoplasmic Reticulum An organelle within the eukaryotic cell largely responsible for protein production and processing into a usable form.

Adiponectin Most abundantly produced protein by the adipocytes with key functions involving insulin regulation, inflammation, and tumor progression.

Insulin Growth Factors A family of proteins important in cell growth, proliferation, and survival.

Leptin A protein made by adipocytes that regulates food intake relative to energy expenditure.

Monocytes A type of white blood cell that is activated in immunity and inflammation and can also produce cytokines.

Hypoxia A condition related to a low-oxygen state or perfusion.

Anthropometric Quantifiable and measureable parameters based on the human physicality.

Interleukins A superfamily of cytokines involved in infection and inflammation that are important for critical events in tumorigenesis.

Unfolded Protein Response The response within the cell due to an accumulation of misfolded or unfolded proteins within the endoplasmic reticulum. This response classically consists of the activation of 3 canonical pathways with the common goal of re-establishing cellular homeostasis.

Introduction

Epidemiological evidence has long associated obesity with cancer development; in fact, obesity has been identified as a key risk factor in several of the most prevalent human malignancies, including postmenopausal breast, colorectal, liver, and endometrial (Giovannucci et al. 2010; Schmandt et al. 2011). In addition to obesity's association with cancer development, being overweight and/or obese has increasingly been correlated with a greater risk of death in women with certain malignancies (e.g., breast and endometrial) (Calle et al. 2003; McTiernan et al. 2010). On the other hand, clinical and epidemiologic evidence suggest that intentional weight loss is associated with a 30–40 % reduction in cancer risk, particularly among women (McCawley et al. 2009; Renehan 2009). However, obesity represents a clinical diagnosis and provides no mechanistic insight into its contribution to cancer development.

Currently, standard anthropometric parameters such as weight (kilogram) and body mass index (BMI, kg/m^2) have been used to define obesity. Indeed, some investigators have postulated that every 5 kg/m^2 increase in BMI confers a 60 % increase in risk of developing endometrial cancerendometrial cancer (Mackintosh and Crosbie 2013). However, these measurements imperfectly represent the true composition of lean body mass, subcutaneous adipose tissue, and visceral adipose tissue, thereby prompting some investigators to propose other metrics, such as waist circumference and waist-to-hip ratio, to quantify obesity and even provide guidance for predicting risk for certain diseases (e.g., diabetes) (Giovannucci et al. 2010). More importantly, these measurements likely inaccurately reflect the biological contribution of each of these components to tumorigenesis and cancer progression. Therefore, a biochemical or mechanistic means of representing obesity is necessary to (1) understand obesity's contribution to cancer development and (2) provide a metric to monitor therapeutic efforts to mitigate the effects of obesity.

Adiposity represents a critical and increasingly appreciated contributor to human disease, including cancer. Furthermore, adipocytes from subcutaneous adipose tissue appear to be distinctly different biochemically and functionally from adipocytes from the viscera and adipocytes from the mesentery (Nieman et al. 2011, 2013). The omentum serves as a major repository of visceral adipocytes and has traditionally been regarded as a supportive organ for energy storage, immune surveillance, and insulation; however, increasing evidence now suggests that omental and visceral adipocytes are not innocent bystanders, but rather potentially direct mediators and contributors to tumorigenesis (Klopp et al. 2012; Matsuo et al. 2013; Nieman et al. 2013). Anthropometric parameters, such as BMI, have traditionally been used to represent adiposity. However, as the putative contribution of central adiposity has been increasingly recognized, alternative measures of abdominal adiposity (e.g., waist circumference, waist-to-height ratio, waist-to-hip ratio, and waist-to-thigh ratio) that reflect regional adipose distributions have been

Table 1 Adipocyte-associated factors implicated in tumorigenesis. Tumorigenesis is a process where the net effects of factors that promote (pro-tumorigenic) tumor growth outweigh the effects of those that block (anti-tumorigenic) tumor growth. This table outlines the key factors and their role discussed in this chapter (key abbreviations: *GRP* glucose-regulated protein, *IGF* insulin growth factor, *IL* interleukin, *MCP* monocyte chemoattractant protein, *MMP* matrix metalloproteinase, *TGF* tumor growth factor, *TNF* tumor necrosis factor)

Pro-tumorigenic	Anti-tumorigenic
Leptin	Adiponectin
Insulin	
Insulin growth factor-1 (IGF-1)	
Tumor necrosis factor-α (TNF-α)	
Interleukin-6 (IL-6)	
IL-8	
IL-1β	
Plasminogen activator inhibitor-1 (PAI-1, serpin-E1)	
Monocyte chemoattractant protein-1 (MCP-1)	
Tumor growth factor-β (TGF-β)	
Collagen VI	
Matrix metalloproteinase-11 (MMP-11)	
Glucose-regulated protein 78 (GRP78)	

proposed and investigated as possibly more accurate predictive indicators of adipocyte-mediated disease (Kahn et al. 2012).

Among gynecologic malignancies, endometrioid adenocarcinoma (EAC) carries the strongest association with obesity (McCawley et al. 2009; Renehan 2009). While the deleterious effects of obesity on endometrial cancer development have classically been ascribed to the presence of unopposed estrogen secreted by adipose tissue, recently, data implicate other novel tumorigenic mechanisms are likely to be at play (Klopp et al. 2012; Matsuo et al. 2013; McCawley et al. 2009). Furthermore, increased understanding of the biology of adipocytes and associated adipose tissue suggests both direct and indirect mechanisms in which adipocytes may either contribute to EAC development. The strong association of adiposity with EAC combined with better mechanistic understanding of the differential production and secretion of these adipokines makes examining these adipokines and other factors as potential biomarkers of endometrial cancer development and progression intriguing.

This chapter will first review the current body of knowledge on the role of adiposity in endometrial cancer development, while focusing on visceral adipocyte depots. The primary part of this chapter will focus on detectable and modifiable factors associated with visceral adipocytes and how these factors influence EAC cell proliferation and how they may serve as biomarkers for endometrial cancer development, progression, and recurrence (Table 1).

Adipose Tissue: Distribution, Composition, and Function

Three types of adipose tissue have been identified: brown, white, and, more recently, beige adipose tissue (Nieman et al. 2013; Wu et al. 2012). Brown adipose tissue is classically identified with human infants and is responsible for generating heat to protect against hypothermia by using the mitochondrial uncoupling protein (UCP1) present in the brown adipocyte mitochondria (Wu et al. 2012). On the other hand, white adipose tissue comprises the majority of adipose tissue found in human adults and is found in subcutaneous tissue, visceral adipose tissue, perinephric fat pad, postmenopausal mammary fat pad, and perivascular fat (Nieman et al. 2013). The classic primary functions of white adipocytes are fatty acid storage and mobilization with the ultimate goal to maintain energy homeostasis (Nieman et al. 2013). Beige adipocytes comprise the most recently identified class of adipocytes and possess the low basal levels of UCP1 gene expression characteristic of white adipocytes yet still maintain the ability to activate UCP1 expression in response to cyclic AMP (cAMP), which is characteristic of brown adipocytes (Wu et al. 2012).

In addition to functional differences among the three types of adipocytes, substantial population-based and biochemical data also show differences between the subcutaneous adipose repository and the omental adipose repository (Fox et al. 2007; Perez-Perez et al. 2009). Secondary analysis of computed tomographic (CT) volumetric imaging of subcutaneous and visceral adipose tissues from epidemiologic studies indicated that visceral adipose tissue more strongly correlated with adverse metabolic risks (Fox et al. 2007). Other gene expression data highlighted molecular differences between subcutaneous and visceral adipose tissue (Modesitt et al. 2012). Others have demonstrated proteomic differences between omental and subcutaneous adipose tissue further highlighting the disparate functions of these two adipose depots (Perez-Perez et al. 2009). Specifically, proteins involved in metabolism, inflammation, and cellular stress appear to be more upregulated in omental adipocytes than subcutaneous adipocytes (Perez-Perez et al. 2009).

The unifying theme across these studies appears to be the prominent role omental or visceral adipocytes play in cellular metabolic and pathogenic processes, including common tumorigenic pathways such as inflammation. Moreover, recent studies have described a mesenchymal progenitor population found within visceral adipocytes with potent tumorigenic properties including angiogenesis (Klopp et al. 2012; Zhang et al. 2009). While visceral adipocytes appear critical for the seamless progression of these pathways, dysregulation of these adipocytes can certainly contribute to disruption of the lipid and carbohydrate homeostasis within the adipocytes local environment, resulting in pathogenic processes such as endoplasmic reticular stress, mitochondrial damage, and excessive triacylglycerol accumulation due to upregulated fatty acid esterification (Nieman et al. 2013). This, in turn, can result in the increased production and secretion of pro-inflammatory adipokines and cytokines, as well as increased infiltration of inflammatory cells, such as lymphocytes and macrophages (Nieman et al. 2013; Soliman et al. 2006, 2011).

Potential Biomarkers from Visceral Adipocytes

Leptin

A vast body of literature has emerged about this 16-kDa non-glycosylated polypeptide since it was cloned and characterized in 1994 (Friedman and Halaas 1998). Fundamentally, leptin is a normophysiologic hormone primarily made in and secreted by adipocytes although it is also found elsewhere (e.g., ovaries, skeletal muscle, stomach, and placenta) (Friedman and Halaas 1998). Therefore, its level is directly proportional to obesity and functions centrally in the arcuate nucleus of the hypothalamus, providing negative-regulation food intake relative to total energy expenditure (Friedman and Halaas 1998). In obesity, over-production of leptin results in reduced leptin responsiveness or "leptin resistance" in the brain (Munzberg and Myers 2005).

Leptin is one of the most abundant proteins secreted by adipocytes with similar three-dimensional protein-folding properties as known cytokines (Kline et al. 1997; Zhang et al. 1997). In the body, it circulates bound to macromacules and acts via transmembrane receptors, for which there are at least five isoforms varied through posttranscriptional alternative splicing (Lee et al. 1996). Leptin receptor-b (OB-Rb) is the only receptor with signaling capability (White et al. 1997). Initial identification of leptin-mediated cellular signaling pathways was hypothesized to mirror that of cytokines due to their analogous structure with subsequent successful elucidation of its role in the activations of JAK/STAT, therefore making leptin a key player in the regulation of cellular transcription (Fruhbeck 2006; Fig. 1). OB-Rb lacks intrinsic enzymatic ability; however, when bound to its ligand, it transactivates JAK-2 which then autophosphorylates and activates signal transducer and activator of transcription-3 (STAT-3). One of the products of STAT-3-induced transcription is the suppressor of cytokine signaling (SOCS)-3, a key negative regulator of leptin signaling (Wunderlich et al. 2013). Furthermore, accumulation of SOCS-3 is an important factor in leptin resistance as SOCS-3 deficiency confers leptin sensitivity and abrogates diet-induced obesity (Mori et al. 2004).

Although leptin exerts its cellular influence mainly via activation of JAK/STAT pathways, the ERK members of the MAPK family are also downstream targets (Banks et al. 2000). Therefore, leptin plays a part in cellular proliferation and differentiation. Moreover, cross talk occurs between leptin and insulin when leptin phosphorylates insulin receptor substrate and transactivates PI3K pathway (Benomar et al. 2005; Hegyi et al. 2004).

In the setting of tumorigenesis, it has been postulated that leptin may have a localized pro-mitogenic, pro-survival, and pro-angiogenic effect (Hefetz-Sela and Scherer 2013). Production of leptin is also triggered by hypoxic conditions as its level rises in conjunction with adipose content in obesity. Research has demonstrated that in response to the local hypoxic environment, leptin-influenced PI3K/AKT and MAPK/ERK pathways activate HIF-1 and thereby initiate neovascularization. In short, since its discovery, the importance of leptin in cellular regulation is well established; hence, its potential utility as a biomarker in tumorigenesis should be recognized.

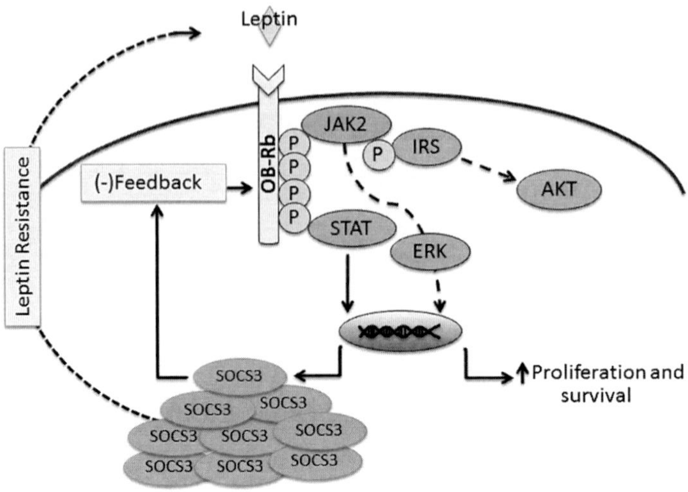

Fig. 1 Leptin influences cellular pathways. Leptin binds to its ligand and Ob-Rb and transactivates JAK-2 which then activates STAT-3 where one of its productions of transcription is SOCS-3, an important protein for negative regulation of leptin's downstream effects. Additionally, leptin influences cellular proliferation and survival via the ERK pathway

Studies in established endometrial cancer cell lines not only corroborate known knowledge of leptin function but also further our understanding of leptin in cellular metabolism. Leptin receptors are found in both normal endometrium (especially secretory phase) and endometrial cancers (Carino et al. 2008). Its signaling is vital for angiogenesis and inflammation necessary for endometrial cell adhesion, proliferation, survival, and migration (Carino et al. 2008); in fact, its influence on angiogenesis is more evident in malignant endometrial cell lines than that of benign. For example, in the endometrium, leptin stimulation yields an increase in cyclooxygenase-2 (COX-2) mRNA and prostaglandin E2 production that is mediated by JAK-2, MAPK, and PI3K pathways (Gao et al. 2009), thus providing a mechanism for ongoing inflammation within microenvironment. Moreover, leptin enables cell growth by actively decreasing cell population in G0/G1 phase while increasing cell population in S-phase (Catalano et al. 2009).

Clinically, leptin has been investigated as a potential biomarker for obesity-related cancers, including endometrial cancer. A great majority of recent publications addressing the relevance of leptin in endometrial cancers have been population-based studies with inconsistent findings (Karahanoglu et al. 2012; Zemlyak et al. 2012). When serum leptin levels are used together with adiponectin, this ratio appears to be predictive of increased risk of endometrial cancer development (Ashizawa et al. 2010; Nowosielski et al. 2012). Furthermore, even within the normal endometrium, a higher proliferation index, as measured by Ki-67, is positively correlated with a higher BMI and leptin levels (Villavicencio et al. 2010). These observations need to be clarified and best interrogated beyond protein levels.

Adiponectin

The primary adipokine secreted exclusively by visceral adipocytes is adiponectin which exists in various homomultimeric forms (Kadowaki and Yamauchi 2005). Within plasma, however, adiponectin is largely present in its full-length form; however, the various adiponectin multimers appear to have different target tissues with variable biological effects (Dalamaga et al. 2012; Kadowaki and Yamauchi 2005). Serum levels of this 30-kDa peptide are significantly, but inversely, correlated with obesity, type 2 diabetes, atherosclerotic disease, and other inflammatory states (Kadowaki and Yamauchi 2005; Soliman et al. 2011). Adiponectin is negatively regulated by TNF-α and IL-6, among other cytokines (Dalamaga et al. 2012).

At least three receptors have been identified for adiponectin: adipoR1, adipoR2, and T-cadherin (Dalamaga et al. 2012). Both adiponectin receptors (adipoR1 and adipoR2) have been identified in virtually all tissue, including benign endometrial tissue as well as endometrial cancer cells. However, AdipoR1 expression levels appear to prevail over AdipoR2 in endometrial cancer tissue (Dalamaga et al. 2012). After binding to its receptors, adiponectin activates important intracellular signaling pathways, including pathways common to inflammation and cancer proliferation such as AMP-activated protein kinase (AMPK), mammalian target of rapamycin (mTOR), nuclear factor κB (NF-κB), c-Jun N-terminal kinase (JNK), and STAT-3.

Evidence also supports adiponectin as an adipocyte-derived anti-angiogenic factor, likely via suppression of vascular endothelial growth factor (VEGF) through the NF-κB pathway (Cust et al. 2007). In addition to the effects of adiponectin on VEGF suppression, the adiponectin receptor, T-cadherin, has also been identified on tumor-associated endothelial cells and has been postulated to serve as a coreceptor or competitive receptor to adipoR1/R2 and its downstream effects (Dalamaga et al. 2012; Fig. 2).

Serum adiponectin levels have been correlated with several solid cancers, including endometrial cancer (Dalamaga et al. 2012). Whether levels of specific multimeric forms of adiponectin are more prognostic than levels of total adiponectin is unknown at present and represents an area for further study. Current epidemiologic studies generally do not distinguish among the different isoforms of adiponectin when estimating cancer risk. In the European Prospective Investigation into Cancer and Nutrition (EPIC) study, Cust and colleagues reported that lower plasma adiponectin levels were associated with elevated risk for endometrial cancer, independent of BMI and other anthropometric or biochemical risk factors (e.g., C-peptide, insulin growth factor) (Cust et al. 2007). On the other hand, however, analysis from the Nurses' Health Study (NHS) cohort did not show prediagnostic adiponectin to be predictive of endometrial cancer risk, again after controlling for confounders, such as BMI, parity, age at last birth, and diabetes (Soliman et al. 2011). Notable population differences existed between these two large prospective cohorts (e.g., younger age) that may account for these differing correlations. More recently, a nested case–control study within the Prostate, Lung, Colorectal, and Ovarian Cancer (PLCO) Screening Trial demonstrated that elevated

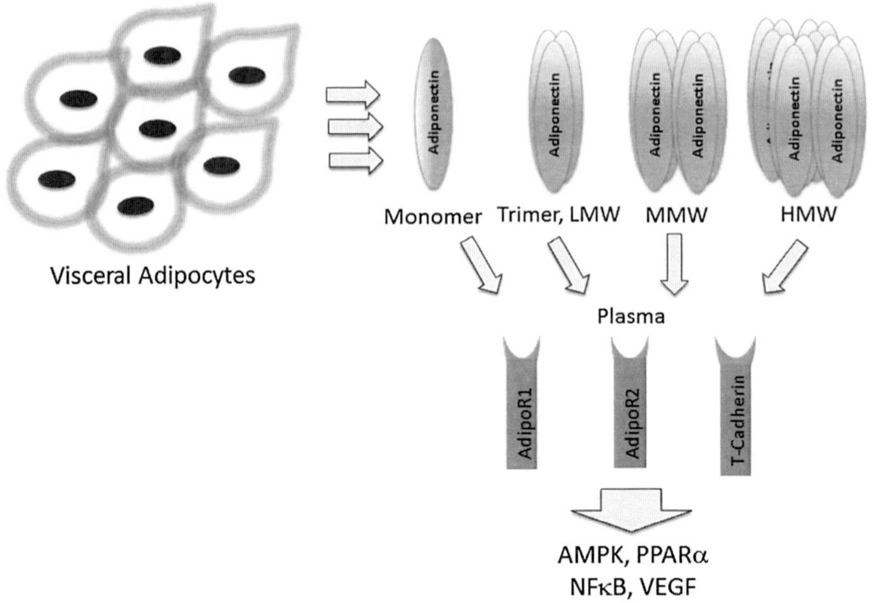

Fig. 2 Adiponectin influences downstream proliferation pathways. The adiponectin monomer exists within the adipocyte and is not detected in circulation. Trimeric (*LMW*) adiponectin is the primary form of adiponectin within circulation and may be responsible for anti-inflammatory properties. In contrast, hexameric (*MMW*) and multimeric (*HMW*) adiponectin may be more pro-inflammatory and have variable effects toward different target tissues

levels of circulating adiponectin were significantly associated with a nearly 50 % decreased risk of endometrial cancer (Luhn et al. 2013).

Further studies are sure to elucidate the relationship between adiponectin and endometrial cancer, and as the distinct roles of each adiponectin isoform are better understood, measuring the levels of specific adiponectin isoforms may evolve into a valuable biomarker and clinical predictor of endometrial cancer.

Insulin Growth Factor-1 (IGF-1) and IGF-2

The insulin-like growth factors engage in important function in regulating multiple cellular pathways paramount to tumor initiation and growth. The names are given because these growth factors share 62 % homology with proinsulin. There are two ligands within this family of growth factors: IGF-1 and IGF-2. These two growth factors have their corresponding transmembrane receptors, IGF-1R and IGF-2R. Additionally, there are at least six binding proteins (IGFBPs) that control its bioavailability (Bruchim and Werner 2013).

Because the structures of IGFs and their receptors are similar to insulin and insulin receptors, it is thought that both entities shared a common progenitor that regulated growth and metabolism with a certain level of cross talk between insulin, IGFs, and their receptors. As insulin resistance is a metabolic consequence of obesity and a

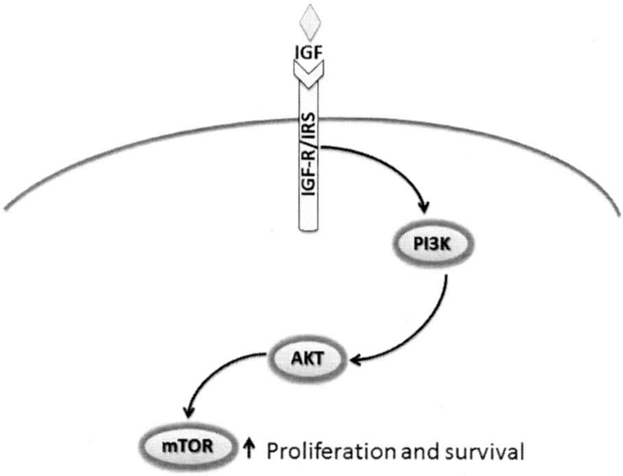

Fig. 3 IGF promotes cell survival. IGF promotes cellular survival by binding to their receptors and phosphorylating the insulin receptor substrate (*IRS*) and initiating a cascade of events via the activations of PI3K and AKT/mTOR pathways

well-recognized risk factor for endometrial cancer, chronic hyperinsulinemia increases IGF-1 production while reduces IGFBPs. Elevated IGF-1 and IGF-2, in turn, bind to their receptors and phosphorylate the insulin receptor substrate (IRS) and commence a cascade of signaling via activations of PI3K and AKT and finally mTOR which augments cellular proliferation and suppresses apoptosis (Bruchim and Werner 2013; Nieman et al. 2013; Fig. 3). Furthermore, in a hormone-enriched environment such as breast or endometrial cancer, functional cross talks between IGF-1 and estrogen result in tumor migration and proliferation via activation of the G-protein-coupled estrogen receptor (GPER) promoter sequence and upregulation of GPER mRNA and protein (De Marco et al. 2013).

Various independent investigators have examined the role of IGFs in endometrial cancer. IGF-1R mRNAs and protein were detected in 91.3 % of endometrial cancer tissues (Hirano et al. 2004). Two studies have found a positive association between plasma levels of IGF-2 and the risk of developing endometrial cancer and an inverse relationship between IGF-1 and endometrial cancer risk (Oh et al. 2004; Petridou et al. 2003), while another showed elevated circulating levels of IGF-1 and decreased levels of IGFBP-1 are associated with increased endometrial risk in the postmenopausal population. Although seemingly conflicting, due to cross talk between IGF-1 and IGF-2, it is now thought that most cellular activity is mediated through the interaction of IGF-1R, and hence, it serves as a viable target in oncology treatment (Sarfstein et al. 2011).

There are three ways to target IGF-1R: a tyrosine–kinase inhibitor that prevents the phosphorylation of IGF-1R, an antibody against IGF-1R, and an antibody that quenches circulating IGF ligands. To date, using a monoclonal antibody against IGF-1R has been the most developed approach, although monotherapies have yielded generally low objective response in early phase clinical trials; nonetheless, more promising results are seen when used with a conventional cytotoxic agent (Kindler et al. 2012). In endometrial cancers, however, there appears to be promising in vitro data to support targeting IGF-1R (Attias-Geva et al. 2011a, b; Bitelman et al. 2013).

For example, a fully humanized monoclonal antibody against IGF-1R, cixutumumab, was used in endometrioid endometrial cancer cell lines where it successfully blocked autophosphorylation of IGF-1R and halted downstream effectors of PI3K/MAPK pathways. Additionally, under microscopy, IGF-1R was found to localize within the cytoplasm. Further evidence also showed its role in augmenting apoptosis with increased activity of caspase 3 and PARP cleavage seen. To anticipate the drug's side effect of hyperglycemia, the authors also queried insulin receptor expression and IGF-1 activation of insulin receptor and found no significant change (Attias-Geva et al. 2011b).

An array of candidate biomarkers for IGF-1R targeting are under investigation, often times, as correlative studies associated with early phase clinical trials. Although still handicapped by technical limitations, circulating tumor cells offer an avenue of examining IGF-1R expression, and a positive association has been found in patients treated with prostate cancer (de Bono et al. 2007). Additionally, serum levels of IGFs or IGFBPs may also be predictive for IGF-1R targeting perhaps acting as a surrogate marker for tumoral expression of IGF-1R.

Interleukins (IL-6, IL-8, MCP-1)

Cytokines are of particular interest in tumors of adipose tissue because they often engage in a vicious cycle of unhindered bilateral stimulation between their effectors and the adipose microenvironment that result in localized inflammation, macrophage infiltration, and accelerated fibrosis and angiogenesis (Wagner et al. 2013). Within this adipose tissue microenvironment, there is a chronic low-grade systemic inflammation as a result of obesity and insulin resistance that can be characterized as a dysregulation between the pro-inflammatory adipokines such as IL-6, IL-8, and monocyte chemotactic protein-1 (MCP-1) and the anti-inflammatory adipokines such as adiponectin.

IL-6 is a pleiotropic cytokine of 185 amino acids arranged as two pairs of α-helices (Kamimura et al. 2003). It is made by preadipocytes, adipocytes, and macrophages with functions that include stimulation of lipolysis, inhibition of lipases, antagonizing insulin-related glucose uptake, and suppression of adiponectin release (Kamimura et al. 2003). Nearly 30 % of total IL-6 in obese patients can be traced to adipose; this particular cytokine is culpable in many of the malignant phenotypes seen in tumorigenesis (Fantuzzi 2005).

Specific etiology for IL-6 stimulation has been determined, and the local adipose milieu plays a unique role similar to the complexities of stromal interactions within tumor microenvironment. It is well known that adipose tissue, like that of the omentum, is in chronic inflammation as a result of baseline metabolic dysregulation with necrotic adipocytes being surrounded by macrophages which are activated via toll-like receptor 4, a stimulator of NF-κB with subsequent elevation in COX-2 and IL-6 transcription (Fig. 4). IL-6 when complexed with its receptor and co-activated by GP130 is known to phosphorylate JAK kinases with downstream effectors in STAT-3 (Ben-Jonathan et al. 2009). In return, there is an increase in SOCS transcription with its subsequent accumulation over extended time, playing a part in leptin and insulin resistance, albeit the exact

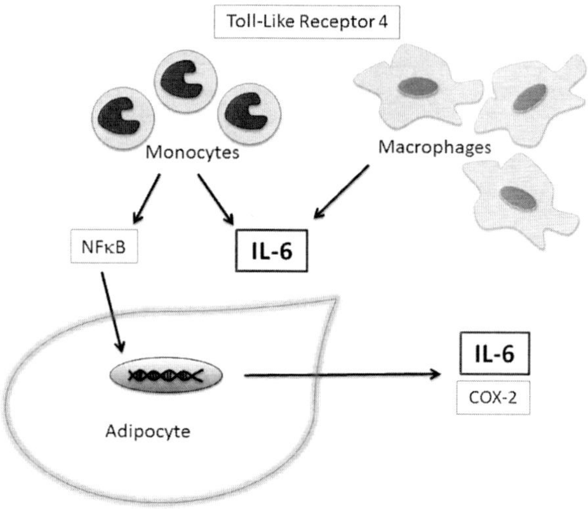

Fig. 4 Summary schema of IL-6 production in the adipocyte milieu. Monocytes and macrophages are activated in chronic inflammatory states such as obesity via toll-like receptor 4, a protein that also stimulates the production of NF-κB with subsequent increase in COX-2 and IL-6 transcription

mechanism is yet to be characterized (Wunderlich et al. 2013). Additionally, IL-6 also plays an integral part in monocyte-to-macrophage differentiation; thus, in the immediate peritumoral adipose tissue, it has been observed that there is an increased number of macrophages along with higher IL-6 expression. Peritumor adipose tissue is seen as atrophied with diminished expression of a major lipid storage mediator, perilipin-1, and phenotypically is seen to exhibit decreased adipocyte size, followed by infiltration of inflammatory cytokines such as IL-6, resulting in upregulation of fibrosis and angiogenesis (Wagner et al. 2013). Studies in ovarian cancer examining the role of tumor affinity for adiposity of the omentum reveal that cytokines such as IL-6 are responsible for "homing" of tumor cells to the omentum thereby providing rationale for the predilection of omental involvement in ovarian cancer (Nieman et al. 2011).

As key players in pro-inflammation, IL-6 and IL-8 are often found to be upregulated in the localized adipose milieu. IL-8 is a cytokine of 99 amino acids and secreted by activated macrophages and epithelial cells like adipocytes. In the presence of liposaccharide, an important cofactor in the high-fat-diet-induced metabolic dysregulation (Cani et al. 2007; Erridge et al. 2007), both IL-6 and IL-8 are found to be upregulated at the mRNA level by more than 10-fold from adipocytes differentiated from the white adipose tissue of patients undergoing surgery. Furthermore, this observation is abrogated when similar conditions were treated with the addition of siRNA against AMP-activated protein kinase (AMPK) subunit α (Grisouard et al. 2011). AMPK has been shown to influence adipokine secretion and affect lipid metabolism. Coculture of human ovarian cancer cell line with adipocytes demonstrates increased phosphorylation of AMPK through key enzyme regulators to increase β-oxidation facilitating ovarian cancer cells to feast on lipids acquired from the adipocytes (Nieman et al. 2011).

Recently, IL-8 has been further implicated in metabolic dysregulation (Hu et al. 2013). Almost 96 % of all high-grade serous ovarian cancers carry mutations in p53, and mutant p53 has been previously shown to promote lipid anabolism and result in tumor growth and progression by influencing sterol regulatory element-binding proteins (SREBPs) and guanidinoacetate *N*-methyltransferase (GAMT), key enzymes in fatty acid synthesis. Mutant p53 has now been demonstrated to interact with IL-8 secreted by adipocytes to regulate fatty acid-binding protein 4 (FABP4), a known protein that is upregulated in omental metastases of patients with ovarian cancer (Hu et al. 2013; Nieman et al. 2011). Additional experiments using FABP4 knockout mice inoculated with mouse ovarian cancer cells produced significantly lower tumor burden exhibiting reduction in microvessel density and tumor proliferation (Nieman et al. 2011).

MCP-1 is a cytokine that is of interest initially in the field of cardiovascular disease as it proved to be one of the main drivers of atherosclerosis (Gu et al. 1998). Furthermore, the association between chemocytokines and obesity in the pathogenesis of atherosclerosis is observed when murine models of obesity yielded confirmation that adipocytes overexpress MCP-1 which serves as a key regulator of monocyte infiltration in arterial intima (Takahashi et al. 2003). Finally, serum levels of adipokines, including MCP-1, have been found to be significantly elevated in morbidly obese patients and patients of cancers with a metastatic predilection for visceral fat stores, like colon cancer (Hillenbrand et al. 2012). Expanding adipocyte secretes MCP-1, and on a cellular level, pro-inflammatory cytokines such as IL-6 and MCP-1 localize in higher concentrations in the peritumoral adipose tissue (Wagner et al. 2012), thereby creating a microenvironment that is permissive to tumor progression and primed to achieve angiogenesis and stromal matrix remodeling (Low et al. 2001).

Glucose-Regulated Protein-78 (GRP78)

It is now well-recognized that adiposity also results in endoplasmic reticulum (ER) stress which, in turn, triggers the unfolded protein response (UPR) and other tumorigenic pathways, particularly relevant to EAC. The ER is a fundamental organelle critical for the proper folding and processing of proteins. However, in certain pathophysiologic conditions, including obesity (Sharma et al. 2008), the protein load within the ER exceeds the folding, processing, and transport. The consequence of this buildup of misfolded proteins has been termed ER stress which the cell attempts to mitigate by UPR activation to reduce translation while simultaneously increasing chaperone processing (Pfaffenbach and Lee 2011). The 78-kDa glucose-regulated protein (GRP78, BiP/HSPA5) is a molecular chaperone protein and member of the heat shock protein (HSP)-70 family and is widely regarded as the key regulator of ER stress (Pfaffenbach and Lee 2011; Wang et al. 2009). GRP78 overexpression is widely observed in several human cancers, including endometrial cancer, and is generally associated with worse clinical outcome, including diminished survival (Bifulco et al. 2012; Daneshmand et al. 2007; Lee 2007, 2009; Lin et al. 2010; Misra et al. 2011; Pfaffenbach and Lee 2011; Pootrakul et al. 2006; Uramoto et al. 2005; Wang et al. 2009; Westin et al. 2009; Zhang et al. 2006; Zhang and Zhang 2010). The chemoresistance associated with tumoral GRP78 overexpression has been shown in several cancer models; however, AKT-inhibition appears to mitigate some of platinum-resistance seen with GRP78 overexpression in EAC (Gray et al. 2013).

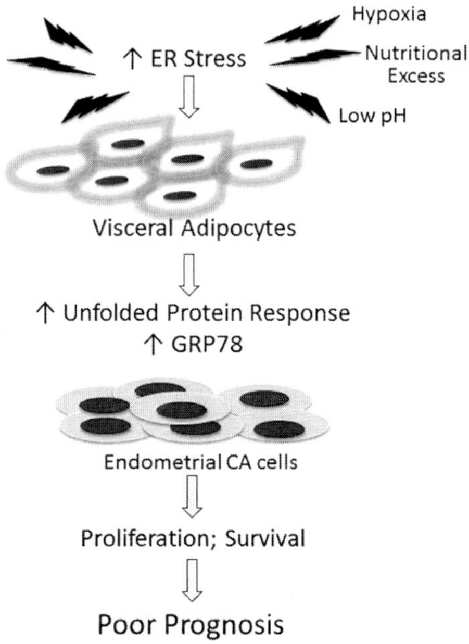

Fig. 5 Proposed relationship between visceral adipocyte GRP78, ER stress, and endometrial cancer prognosis. Hostile conditions such as hypoxia, nutritional excess, and low pH induce ER stress within the visceral adipocytes resulting in increased GRP78 and elevated unfolded protein response which have been shown to augment tumor proliferation and survival, thereby translating clinically to poor prognosis

In addition to UPR activation in tumor cells, visceral adipocytes have also been shown to exhibit ER stress and overexpress GRP78 in the setting of EAC (Matsuo et al. 2013). This is particularly intriguing given the close proximity of visceral adipocytes (e.g., omentum, mesenteric, and epiploic adipose tissue) to the uterus and the pelvis, and the possibility of paracrine-type cross talk among these tissues (Nieman et al. 2013). Recent experiments show that the extent of GRP78 expression within visceral adipocytes appears to correlate with worse clinicopathologic features, advanced stage disease, and even shorter survival (Matsuo et al. 2013). Of particular interest was the observation that GRP78 expression in visceral adipocytes appeared to be more predictive of survival and clinical outcome than GRP78 expression in the endometrial tumors themselves. These preliminary findings further implicate visceral adipocytes as, not simply innocent bystanders in EAC, but potentially contributing to the biology of EAC (Fig. 5). Further refinement of a tool to quantify the differential levels of adipocyte GRP78, either in visceral adipocytes or in peripheral circulation, may represent a novel biomarker with which to monitor or inform EAC management.

Potential Applications to Prognosis, Other Diseases, or Conditions

As cancer treatment becoming increasingly targeted, expectations from biomarkers range from diagnostic to prognostic as well as predictive. Indeed, for one biomarker to fulfill all these demands may be challenging and thus underscores the complexity and heterogeneity of a disease entity such as cancer. While obesity is now one of the premier public health concerns of developed countries, insights gained through its disease process can benefit not only cancer but also a vast array of pathophysiology related to insulin resistance and chronic inflammatory state.

Adipokines discussed in this chapter have been interrogated to determine their possible prognostic value in endometrial cancer. In general, these translational studies are limited by small sample size and heterogeneous population, thereby serving more for the purpose of hypothesis generating for future systematic examinations. Leptin has been shown to be a pro-inflammatory adipokine with central role in lipid metabolism. In a case–control study of 30 endometrial cancer patients and 30 healthy controls, preoperative serum levels of leptin was not found to be associated with traditional clinical prognostic factors such as stage, grade, histologic type, or lymph node metastasis (Karahanoglu et al. 2012). Adiponectin, an anti-inflammatory adipokine, has demonstrated to be independently and inversely associated with endometrial cancer (Soliman et al. 2006), although this observation is not uniformly seen in all cancer disease sites (Dalamaga et al. 2012). Further analyses using leptin/adiponectin ratio have been performed to characterize possible clinical relationship, and in ovarian cancer, leptin/adiponectin ratio correlated with overall survival such that patients with low leptin/adiponectin levels lived longer than their counterparts with high leptin/adiponectin; however, when adjusted for known clinical variables such as stage, grade, and age, this prognostic value failed to be significant (Diaz et al. 2013). Because insulin resistance appears to be a pivotal impetus driving tumorigenesis in endometrial cancer, IGF-1R expression has been studied in endometrial carcinoma and found to be overexpressed in patients with lymph node metastasis (Pengchong and Tao 2011).

The interplay between pro-inflammatory and anti-inflammatory adipokines extends beyond endometrial cancer, especially given some of the seminal research that fuels the advancement of our understanding of the balance between adipokines and their environment stemmed from studies in polycystic ovarian syndrome, diabetes, and atherosclerosis which share their root pathophysiology in insulin resistance and obesity. Furthermore, novel investigation in the active role of the omentum in attracting ovarian tumor cells has impactful implications in our knowledge of cancers known to have predilection for visceral adipose metastasis. This body of evidence, taken together, reinforces a necessity for future studies.

Summary Points

- Contrary to historical beliefs, adipose tissue likely plays an active role in endometrial cancer.
- Visceral adipocytes secrete factors that also promote cancer growth and progression.
- Secreted adipokines and adipocyte-associated factors dovetail with critical tumorigenic and angiogenic pathways.

- Adipocyte-derived factors are detectable in serum and in the adipose tissue and may serve as biomarkers for endometrial cancer development and progression.
- Further studies are warranted to better understand adipocyte biology and its clinical potential in endometrial cancer treatment.

References

Ashizawa N, Yahata T, Quan J, et al. Serum leptin-adiponectin ratio and endometrial cancer risk in postmenopausal female subjects. Gynecol Oncol. 2010;119:65–9.

Attias-Geva Z, Bentov I, Fishman A, et al. Insulin-like growth factor-I receptor inhibition by specific tyrosine kinase inhibitor NVP-AEW541 in endometrioid and serous papillary endometrial cancer cell lines. Gynecol Oncol. 2011a;121:383–9.

Attias-Geva Z, Bentov I, Ludwig DL, et al. Insulin-like growth factor-I receptor (IGF-IR) targeting with monoclonal antibody cixutumumab (IMC-A12) inhibits IGF-I action in endometrial cancer cells. Eur J Cancer. 2011b;47:1717–26.

Banks AS, Davis SM, Bates SH, et al. Activation of downstream signals by the long form of the leptin receptor. J Biol Chem. 2000;275:14563–72.

Ben-Jonathan N, Hugo ER, Brandebourg TD. Effects of bisphenol A on adipokine release from human adipose tissue: implications for the metabolic syndrome. Mol Cell Endocrinol. 2009;304:49–54.

Benomar Y, Roy AF, Aubourg A, et al. Cross down-regulation of leptin and insulin receptor expression and signalling in a human neuronal cell line. Biochem J. 2005;388:929–39.

Bifulco G, Miele C, Di Jeso B, et al. Endoplasmic reticulum stress is activated in endometrial adenocarcinoma. Gynecol Oncol. 2012;125:220–5.

Bitelman C, Sarfstein R, Sarig M, et al. IGF1R-directed targeted therapy enhances the cytotoxic effect of chemotherapy in endometrial cancer. Cancer Lett. 2013;335:153–9.

Bruchim I, Werner H. Targeting IGF-1 signaling pathways in gynecologic malignancies. Expert Opin Ther Targets. 2013;17:307–20.

Calle EE, Rodriguez C, Walker-Thurmond K, et al. Overweight, obesity, and mortality from cancer in a prospectively studied cohort of U.S. adults. N Engl J Med. 2003;348:1625–38.

Cani PD, Amar J, Iglesias MA, et al. Metabolic endotoxemia initiates obesity and insulin resistance. Diabetes. 2007;56:1761–72.

Carino C, Olawaiye AB, Cherfils S, et al. Leptin regulation of proangiogenic molecules in benign and cancerous endometrial cells. Int J Cancer. 2008;123:2782–90.

Catalano S, Giordano C, Rizza P, et al. Evidence that leptin through STAT and CREB signaling enhances cyclin D1 expression and promotes human endometrial cancer proliferation. J Cell Physiol. 2009;218:490–500.

Cust AE, Kaaks R, Friedenreich C, et al. Plasma adiponectin levels and endometrial cancer risk in pre- and postmenopausal women. J Clin Endocrinol Metab. 2007;92:255–63.

Dalamaga M, Diakopoulos KN, Mantzoros CS. The role of adiponectin in cancer: a review of current evidence. Endocr Rev. 2012;33:547–94.

Daneshmand S, Quek ML, Lin E, et al. Glucose-regulated protein GRP78 is up-regulated in prostate cancer and correlates with recurrence and survival. Hum Pathol. 2007;38:1547–52.

de Bono JS, Attard G, Adjei A, et al. Potential applications for circulating tumor cells expressing the insulin-like growth factor-I receptor. Clin Cancer Res. 2007;13:3611–16.

De Marco P, Bartella V, Vivacqua A, et al. Insulin-like growth factor-I regulates GPER expression and function in cancer cells. Oncogene. 2013;32:678–88.

Diaz ES, Karlan BY, Li AJ. Obesity-associated adipokines correlate with survival in epithelial ovarian cancer. Gynecol Oncol. 2013;129:353–7.

Erridge C, Attina T, Spickett CM, et al. A high-fat meal induces low-grade endotoxemia: evidence of a novel mechanism of postprandial inflammation. Am J Clin Nutr. 2007;86:1286–92.

Fantuzzi G. Adipose tissue, adipokines, and inflammation. J Allergy Clin Immunol. 2005;115:911–19; quiz 920.

Fox CS, Massaro JM, Hoffmann U, et al. Abdominal visceral and subcutaneous adipose tissue compartments: association with metabolic risk factors in the Framingham Heart Study. Circulation. 2007;116:39–48.

Friedman JM, Halaas JL. Leptin and the regulation of body weight in mammals. Nature. 1998;395:763–70.

Fruhbeck G. Intracellular signalling pathways activated by leptin. Biochem J. 2006;393:7–20.

Gao J, Tian J, Lv Y, et al. Leptin induces functional activation of cyclooxygenase-2 through JAK2/STAT3, MAPK/ERK, and PI3K/AKT pathways in human endometrial cancer cells. Cancer Sci. 2009;100:389–95.

Giovannucci E, Harlan DM, Archer MC, et al. Diabetes and cancer: a consensus report. CA Cancer J Clin. 2010;60:207–21.

Gray MJ, Mhawech-Fauceglia P, Yoo E, et al. AKT inhibition mitigates GRP78 (glucose-regulated protein) expression and contribution to chemoresistance in endometrial cancers. Int J Cancer. 2013;133:21–30.

Grisouard J, Dembinski K, Mayer D, et al. Targeting AMP-activated protein kinase in adipocytes to modulate obesity-related adipokine production associated with insulin resistance and breast cancer cell proliferation. Diabetol Metab Syndr. 2011;3:16.

Gu L, Okada Y, Clinton SK, et al. Absence of monocyte chemoattractant protein-1 reduces atherosclerosis in low density lipoprotein receptor-deficient mice. Mol Cell. 1998;2:275–81.

Hefetz-Sela S, Scherer PE. Adipocytes: impact on tumor growth and potential sites for therapeutic intervention. Pharmacol Ther. 2013;138:197–210.

Hegyi K, Fulop K, Kovacs K, et al. Leptin-induced signal transduction pathways. Cell Biol Int. 2004;28:159–69.

Hillenbrand A, Fassler J, Huber N, et al. Changed adipocytokine concentrations in colorectal tumor patients and morbidly obese patients compared to healthy controls. BMC Cancer. 2012;12:545.

Hirano S, Ito N, Takahashi S, et al. Clinical implications of insulin-like growth factors through the presence of their binding proteins and receptors expressed in gynecological cancers. Eur J Gynaecol Oncol. 2004;25:187–91.

Hu J, Liu Z, Wang X. Does TP53 mutation promote ovarian cancer metastasis to omentum by regulating lipid metabolism? Med Hypotheses. 2013;81:515–20.

Kadowaki T, Yamauchi T. Adiponectin and adiponectin receptors. Endocr Rev. 2005;26:439–51.

Kahn HS, Bullard KM, Barker LE, et al. Differences between adiposity indicators for predicting all-cause mortality in a representative sample of United States non-elderly adults. PLoS One. 2012;7:e50428.

Kamimura D, Ishihara K, Hirano T. IL-6 signal transduction and its physiological roles: the signal orchestration model. Rev Physiol Biochem Pharmacol. 2003;149:1–38.

Karahanoglu E, Adanir I, Boyraz G, et al. Preoperative serum leptin levels in patients with endometrial cancer and its correlation with prognostic variables. Eur J Gynaecol Oncol. 2012;33:278–80.

Kindler HL, Richards DA, Garbo LE, et al. A randomized, placebo-controlled phase 2 study of ganitumab (AMG 479) or conatumumab (AMG 655) in combination with gemcitabine in patients with metastatic pancreatic cancer. Ann Oncol. 2012;23:2834–42.

Kline AD, Becker GW, Churgay LM, et al. Leptin is a four-helix bundle: secondary structure by NMR. FEBS Lett. 1997;407:239–42.

Klopp AH, Zhang Y, Solley T, et al. Omental adipose tissue-derived stromal cells promote vascularization and growth of endometrial tumors. Clin Cancer Res. 2012;18:771–82.

Lee AS. GRP78 induction in cancer: therapeutic and prognostic implications. Cancer Res. 2007;67:3496–9.

Lee AS. The Par-4-GRP78 TRAIL, more twists and turns. Cancer Biol Ther. 2009;8:2103–5.
Lee GH, Proenca R, Montez JM, et al. Abnormal splicing of the leptin receptor in diabetic mice. Nature. 1996;379:632–5.
Lin CY, Chen WH, Liao CT, et al. Positive association of glucose-regulated protein 78 during oral cancer progression and the prognostic value in oral precancerous lesions. Head Neck. 2010;32:1028–39.
Low QE, Drugea IA, Duffner LA, et al. Wound healing in MIP-1alpha(−/−) and MCP-1(−/−) mice. Am J Pathol. 2001;159:457–63.
Luhn P, Dallal CM, Weiss JM, et al. Circulating adipokine levels and endometrial cancer risk in the prostate, lung, colorectal, and ovarian cancer screening trial. Cancer Epidemiol Biomarkers Prev. 2013;22:1304–12.
Mackintosh ML, Crosbie EJ. Obesity-driven endometrial cancer: is weight loss the answer? BJOG. 2013;120:791–4.
Matsuo K, Gray MJ, Yang DY, et al. The endoplasmic reticulum stress marker, glucose-regulated protein-78 (GRP78) in visceral adipocytes predicts endometrial cancer progression and patient survival. Gynecol Oncol. 2013;128:552–9.
McCawley GM, Ferriss JS, Geffel D, et al. Cancer in obese women: potential protective impact of bariatric surgery. J Am Coll Surg. 2009;208:1093–8.
McTiernan A, Irwin M, Vongruenigen V. Weight, physical activity, diet, and prognosis in breast and gynecologic cancers. J Clin Oncol. 2010;28:4074–80.
Misra UK, Payne S, Pizzo SV. Ligation of prostate cancer cell surface GRP78 activates a proproliferative and antiapoptotic feedback loop: a role for secreted prostate-specific antigen. J Biol Chem. 2011;286:1248–59.
Modesitt SC, Hsu JY, Chowbina SR, et al. Not all fat is equal: differential gene expression and potential therapeutic targets in subcutaneous adipose, visceral adipose, and endometrium of obese women with and without endometrial cancer. Int J Gynecol Cancer. 2012;22:732–41.
Mori H, Hanada R, Hanada T, et al. Socs3 deficiency in the brain elevates leptin sensitivity and confers resistance to diet-induced obesity. Nat Med. 2004;10:739–43.
Munzberg H, Myers Jr MG. Molecular and anatomical determinants of central leptin resistance. Nat Neurosci. 2005;8:566–70.
Nieman KM, Kenny HA, Penicka CV, et al. Adipocytes promote ovarian cancer metastasis and provide energy for rapid tumor growth. Nat Med. 2011;17:1498–503.
Nieman KM, Romero IL, Van Houten B, et al. Adipose tissue and adipocytes support tumorigenesis and metastasis. Biochim Biophys Acta. 2013;1831:1533–41.
Nowosielski K, Pozowski J, Ulman-Wlodarz I, et al. Adiponectin to leptin index as a marker of endometrial cancer in postmenopausal women with abnormal vaginal bleeding: an observational study. Neuro Endocrinol Lett. 2012;33:217–23.
Oh JC, Wu W, Tortolero-Luna G, et al. Increased plasma levels of insulin-like growth factor 2 and insulin-like growth factor binding protein 3 are associated with endometrial cancer risk. Cancer Epidemiol Biomarkers Prev. 2004;13:748–52.
Pengchong H, Tao H. Expression of IGF-1R, VEGF-C and D2-40 and their correlation with lymph node metastasis in endometrial adenocarcinoma. Eur J Gynaecol Oncol. 2011;32:660–4.
Perez-Perez R, Ortega-Delgado FJ, Garcia-Santos E, et al. Differential proteomics of omental and subcutaneous adipose tissue reflects their unalike biochemical and metabolic properties. J Proteome Res. 2009;8:1682–93.
Petridou E, Koukoulomatis P, Alexe DM, et al. Endometrial cancer and the IGF system: a case–control study in Greece. Oncology. 2003;64:341–5.
Pfaffenbach KT, Lee AS. The critical role of GRP78 in physiologic and pathologic stress. Curr Opin Cell Biol. 2011;23:150–6.
Pootrakul L, Datar RH, Shi SR, et al. Expression of stress response protein Grp78 is associated with the development of castration-resistant prostate cancer. Clin Cancer Res. 2006;12:5987–93.

Renehan AG. Bariatric surgery, weight reduction, and cancer prevention. Lancet Oncol. 2009;10:640–1.

Sarfstein R, Bruchim I, Fishman A, et al. The mechanism of action of the histone deacetylase inhibitor vorinostat involves interaction with the insulin-like growth factor signaling pathway. PLoS One. 2011;6:e24468.

Schmandt RE, Iglesias DA, Co NN, et al. Understanding obesity and endometrial cancer risk: opportunities for prevention. Am J Obstet Gynecol. 2011;205:518–25.

Sharma NK, Das SK, Mondal AK, et al. Endoplasmic reticulum stress markers are associated with obesity in nondiabetic subjects. J Clin Endocrinol Metab. 2008;93:4532–41.

Soliman PT, Wu D, Tortolero-Luna G, et al. Association between adiponectin, insulin resistance, and endometrial cancer. Cancer. 2006;106:2376–81.

Soliman PT, Cui X, Zhang Q, et al. Circulating adiponectin levels and risk of endometrial cancer: the prospective Nurses' Health Study. Am J Obstet Gynecol. 2011;204:167 e161–5.

Takahashi K, Mizuarai S, Araki H, et al. Adiposity elevates plasma MCP-1 levels leading to the increased CD11b-positive monocytes in mice. J Biol Chem. 2003;278:46654–60.

Uramoto H, Sugio K, Oyama T, et al. Expression of endoplasmic reticulum molecular chaperone Grp78 in human lung cancer and its clinical significance. Lung Cancer. 2005;49:55–62.

Villavicencio A, Aguilar G, Arguello G, et al. The effect of overweight and obesity on proliferation and activation of AKT and ERK in human endometria. Gynecol Oncol. 2010;117:96–102.

Wagner M, Bjerkvig R, Wiig H, et al. Inflamed tumor-associated adipose tissue is a depot for macrophages that stimulate tumor growth and angiogenesis. Angiogenesis. 2012;15:481–95.

Wagner M, Bjerkvig R, Wiig H, et al. Loss of adipocyte specification and necrosis augment tumor-associated inflammation. Adipocyte. 2013;2:176–83.

Wang M, Wey S, Zhang Y, et al. Role of the unfolded protein response regulator GRP78/BiP in development, cancer, and neurological disorders. Antioxid Redox Signal. 2009;11:2307–16.

Westin SN, Broaddus RR, Deng L, et al. Molecular clustering of endometrial carcinoma based on estrogen-induced gene expression. Cancer Biol Ther. 2009;8:2126–35.

White DW, Kuropatwinski KK, Devos R, et al. Leptin receptor (OB-R) signaling. Cytoplasmic domain mutational analysis and evidence for receptor homo-oligomerization. J Biol Chem. 1997;272:4065–71.

Wu J, Bostrom P, Sparks LM, et al. Beige adipocytes are a distinct type of thermogenic fat cell in mouse and human. Cell. 2012;150:366–76.

Wunderlich CM, Hovelmeyer N, Wunderlich FT. Mechanisms of chronic JAK-STAT3-SOCS3 signaling in obesity. JAKSTAT. 2013;2:e23878.

Zemlyak A, Zakhaleva J, Pearl M, et al. Expression of inflammatory cytokines by adipose tissue from patients with endometrial cancer. Eur J Gynaecol Oncol. 2012;33:363–6.

Zhang LH, Zhang X. Roles of GRP78 in physiology and cancer. J Cell Biochem. 2010;110:1299–305.

Zhang F, Basinski MB, Beals JM, et al. Crystal structure of the obese protein leptin-E100. Nature. 1997;387:206–9.

Zhang J, Jiang Y, Jia Z, et al. Association of elevated GRP78 expression with increased lymph node metastasis and poor prognosis in patients with gastric cancer. Clin Exp Metastasis. 2006;23:401–10.

Zhang Y, Daquinag A, Traktuev DO, et al. White adipose tissue cells are recruited by experimental tumors and promote cancer progression in mouse models. Cancer Res. 2009;69:5259–66.

Part VI

Colorectal

Colorectal Cancer Circulating Biomarkers

26

Rodrigo Barderas, Roi Villar-Vázquez, and J. Ignacio Casal

Contents

R. Barderas
Biochemistry and Molecular Biology I Department, Facultad de Ciencias Químicas, Universidad Complutense de Madrid, Madrid, Spain
e-mail: rodrigob@ucm.es

R. Villar-Vázquez • J.I. Casal (✉)
Department of Cellular and Molecular Medicine, Functional Proteomics Laboratory, Centro de Investigaciones Biológicas (CSIC), Madrid, Spain
e-mail: rvillar@cib.csic.es; icasal@cib.csic.es

V.R. Preedy, V.B. Patel (eds.), *Biomarkers in Cancer, Biomarkers in Disease: Methods, Discoveries and Applications*,
DOI 10.1007/978-94-007-7681-4_29

Abstract

Circulating CRC markers might become useful tools for the massive screening of people since they satisfy a high degree of accuracy, noninvasiveness, reproducibility, and economy. Within circulating biomarkers, we will focus on the detection of autoantibodies in serum from cancer patients and their target tumor-associated antigens (TAAs). Although the sensitivity, specificity, and predictive value of individual TAAs present low scores, the combination of multiple TAAs shows improved values to discriminate between CRC patients and controls. In this review, we outline the methodologies used to identify circulating autoantibodies and their target proteins and discuss the relevance of CRC autoantibodies for diagnosis at, particularly, early stages. An overview of the reported biomarkers is given, showing the large complexity of the autoantibody response in cancer. Different strategies to improve CRC diagnostic tests by combining autoantibodies from different studies will be discussed. Association of autoantibodies to prognosis, recurrence, and the survival of patients will be introduced. We conclude that there is a great potential for the use of autoantibodies as diagnostic CRC biomarkers in the near future.

List of Abbreviations

CEA	Carcinoembryonic antigen
CRC	Colorectal cancer
EMT	Epithelial to mesenchymal transition
HPLC	High-performance liquid chromatography
MSI	Microsatellite instability
NAPPA	Nucleic acid programmable protein arrays
PTMs	Posttranslational modifications
SEREX	Serological analysis of recombinant cDNA expression libraries
SERPA	Serological proteome analysis
TAA	Tumor-associated antigen

Key Facts of Circulating Biomarkers

- Tumor-associated antigens (TAAs) are self-proteins altered during tumor formation and progression.
- Cancer humoral responses take place against TAAs.
- Autoantibodies against TAAs can be used in colorectal cancer patients as circulating biomarkers.

- Immunoproteomics provide useful approaches for identifying autoantibodies and their reactive TAA targets.
- Circulating autoantibodies provide an effective, reliable, and reproducible tool in cancer patients for diagnosis, prognosis, recurrence, and therapy monitoring.
- Targets of circulating autoantibodies might be novel therapeutic targets for intervention.

Definitions of Words and Terms

Biomarker A biological marker usually a protein or glycoprotein that can be used as an indicator of a biological or pathological state or condition.

TAA Tumor-associated antigen which consists of an altered self-protein able to induce an immune response in cancer patients.

Autoantibody Immunoglobulin G produced in response to self-proteins altered during tumor formation or progression which can be used as a cancer biomarker.

ELISA Enzyme-linked immunosorbent assay which permits to detect the presence of an immune response to a specific TAA in a biological fluid (i.e., serum or plasma) by means of an enzyme immunoassay.

SEREX Acronym of serological analysis of recombinant cDNA expression libraries (SEREX) which is a technology based on the detection of tumor-associated antigens within recombinantly expressed tumor cDNA phage libraries by autologous antibodies.

SERPA Acronym of serological proteome analysis where proteins from tumoral samples are resolved by 2D gels to identify TAAs by immunostaining with sera from cancer patients and controls. TAAs are then identified in a subsequent step by LC–MS.

LC–MS Liquid chromatography coupled to mass spectrometry. High-performance liquid chromatography (LC) coupled to mass spectrometry (MS) to separate a peptide mixture in a liquid phase according to hydrophobic interactions provided by the C18 alkyl chains of the stationary phase of the chromatography column.

Protein Microarray A chip containing thousands to tens of thousands of different proteins attached to a support surface of glass slide or nitrocellulose membrane.

Phage Display This technique is used for the high-throughput screening of protein interactions and consists of libraries of millions of different M13 or T7 phages displaying in their surface proteins fused to the N- or C-terminal end, respectively, of proteins of the capsid of the phage.

ROC Curve Receiver-operating characteristic (ROC) curves illustrate the performance of a diagnostic test. It is obtained by plotting the fraction of true-positive cases among the actual number of positive patients versus the fraction of false-positive controls out of the total actual negative controls at various threshold settings.

PTM Posttranslational modification. After translation, proteins can be modified by the attachment of functional groups, including phosphorylation, acetylation, carbohydrate, lipid, etc.

CEA Carcinoembryonic antigen is a recommended clinical biomarker for colorectal cancer recurrence but not for screening.

Introduction

Colorectal cancer (CRC) is the major cause of cancer-associated mortality in developed countries (Duffy et al. 2007). CRC is mainly diagnosed at late stages, when patients have developed clinical symptoms and the tumor has already spread to adjacent lymph nodes or colonized other organs. At that point, 61 % of CRC tumors are so advanced that the 5-year survival rate of patients is only about 11 %, with 5-year survival rates of 91.1 % and 69.8 % for localized and regional stages, respectively (Surveillance, Epidemiology, and End Results Program (2011), National Cancer Institute, USA). If we could shift the diagnosis of CRC patients to early cancer stages, their final outcome would substantially improve.

A suitable biomarker for a screening test should demonstrate a high degree of accuracy, reproducibility, economy, and, more importantly, acceptance by the population. Actually, the current markers for CRC, CEA, CA19.9, and CA125 are not recommended for clinical screening (Levin et al. 2003; Locker et al. 2006; Duffy et al. 2007), because they can be altered in other diseases different from CRC and even in nonpathological states. Moreover, circulating CEA is only recommended to monitor therapy in advanced CRC and for prognostic information (Locker et al. 2006; Duffy et al. 2007).

Circulating biomarker molecules might consist of altered tumoral proteins, which are leaked to the blood. However, they are usually found at very low concentrations and exposed to degradation (Villanueva et al. 2006), making them questionable as diagnostic biomarkers and their actual discovery a challenge (Villanueva et al. 2006; Barderas et al. 2010; Casal and Barderas 2010). However, some cancer proteins are able to induce a humoral response in cancer patients, providing an effective, reliable, and noninvasive tool for cancer screening and preclinical diagnosis (Fig. 1; Anderson and LaBaer 2005; Murphy et al. 2012b).

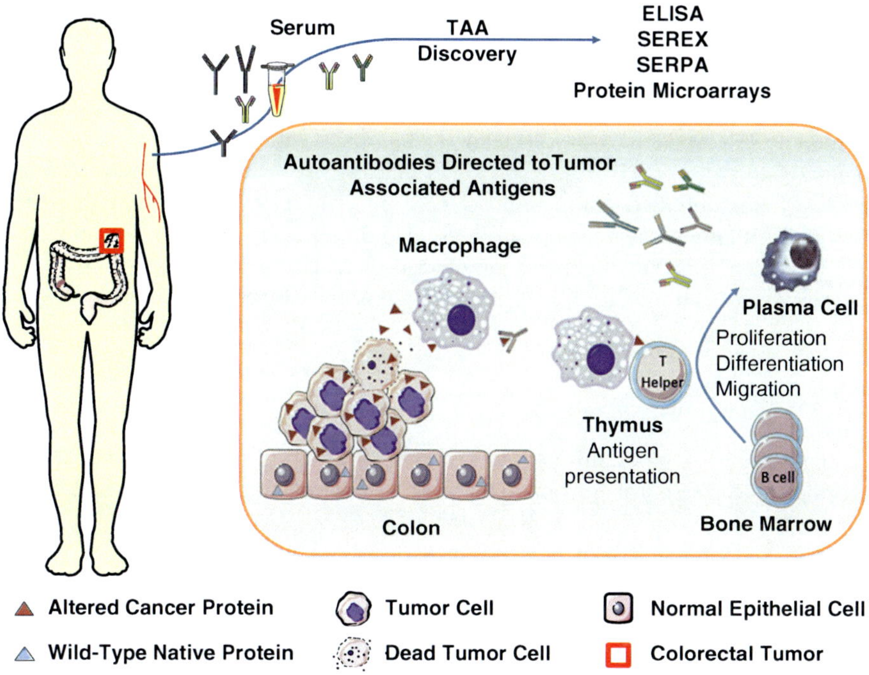

Fig. 1 Production of cancer autoantibodies against tumoral self-proteins. During tumor formation and progression, altered self-proteins and cellular debris are released from colorectal neoplastic tissue, which results in B-cell proliferation and antibody production when antigen-presenting cells present these proteins to the immune response

The molecular mechanisms of this humoral response to cancer proteins are rather uncharacterized. It might be due to the alterations of self-proteins during tumor formation and progression, punctual mutations, truncations, aberrant glycosylations, overexpression, or aberrant degradation (Anderson and LaBaer 2005; Murphy et al. 2012b).

Novel high-throughput proteomic approaches have accelerated the identification of circulating serum autoantibodies and their respective target proteins as potential cancer biomarkers. Antibodies are highly stable molecules with a long tradition of being used in immunoassays, thus facilitating their standardization. In the last years, the apparition of new techniques has delivered multiple studies related to the use of autoantibodies for cancer detection. In this review, we describe the features of circulating serum autoantibody biomarkers for CRC and outline the proteomic strategies employed to identify them since the first reports by Old's laboratory (Fig. 2). We will review the validation and optimization experiments required for use in clinical practice. CRC autoantibodies and their target proteins should facilitate the screening for early diagnosis, prognosis, and monitoring of therapy in CRC patients, as well as for the identification of novel therapeutic targets.

Strategies to Identify CRC Circulating Autoantibodies in Cancer Patients

The first reports identifying autoantibodies and cancer autoantigens were published in the late 1970s and early 1980s using an approach called autologous serological typing (Carey et al. 1976; Dippold et al. 1980; Fig. 2), where circulating autoantibodies were identified using tumoral cells in culture and sera from the same patients. Although researchers identified several melanoma tumor-associated antigens (TAAs), the heterogeneity of cancer patient's response complicated the antigen identification (Carey et al. 1976; Dippold et al. 1980).

SEREX and SERPA

From those early studies, different low- or medium-throughput technologies such as serological analysis of recombinant cDNA expression libraries (SEREX) or

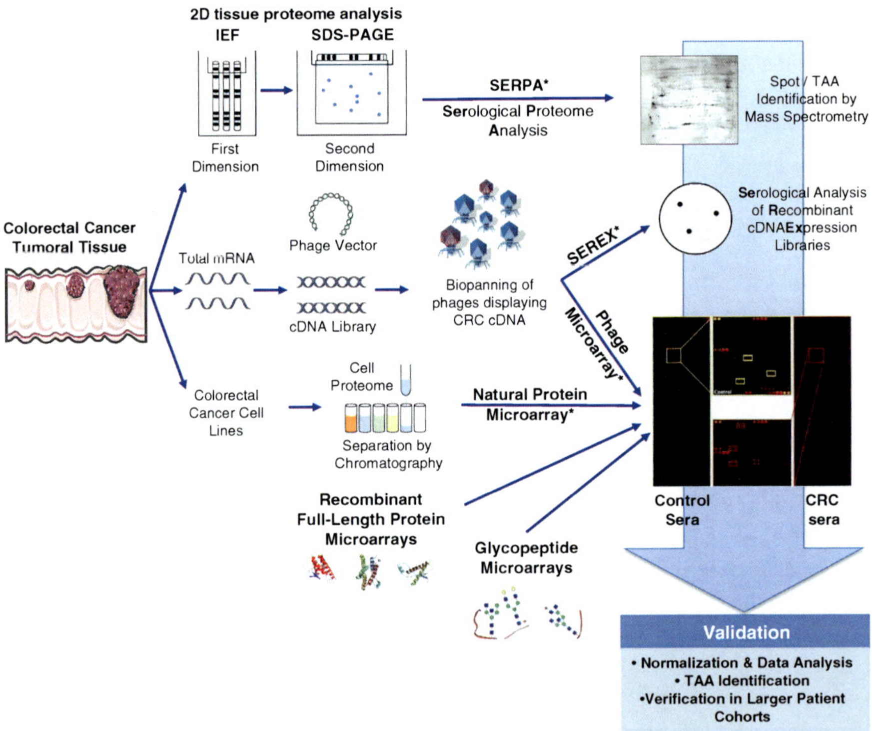

Fig. 2 Proteomic strategies used to identify CRC circulating autoantibodies. *, These strategies require a further step of identification of the TAA via sequencing (SEREX and phage microarrays) or LC–MS (SERPA and natural protein microarrays)

serological proteome analysis (SERPA) have been applied for the discovery of autoantibodies and their target TAAs as cancer diagnostic markers with different successes (Fig. 2; Sahin et al. 1995; Casal and Barderas 2010). SEREX involves the identification of TAAs using phage display expression libraries containing cDNA from tumoral tissues or cells, transferred onto membranes for screening with cancer sera. In SERPA, proteins from tumoral samples are separated in 2D gels to identify TAAs after transference to membranes for immunostaining with cancer sera and healthy controls (Klade et al. 2001).

A variant of SEREX, where phages are printed on a microarray format, has been also tested for autoantibody discovery in a high-throughput version (Wang et al. 2005; Chatterjee et al. 2006; Babel et al. 2011; Chatterjee et al. 2012). Here, TAA discovery takes advantage on the multiplexing analysis of both T7 phages and microarrays (Fig. 2). cDNA from a specific tumor is inserted in the genome of T7 phages, and cancer peptides and proteins are displayed on the surface of the capsid of the phage at the C-terminal end of 10B protein. Alternatively, a random peptide library can also be used instead of tumoral cDNA libraries (Mintz et al. 2003; Jiang et al. 2010). Then, several rounds of biopanning using sera from healthy individuals and cancer patients permit the enrichment of T7 phage libraries on phages displaying cancer-specific peptides or proteins. Finally, thousands of T7 phages are printed onto nitrocellulose microarrays to be screened with sera from cancer patients and controls, and TAAs can be (theoretically) identified after sequencing the cDNA inserted in the genome of the phage.

Although these techniques have permitted the identification of multiple TAAs, they present several problems. SEREX is technically demanding, is labor intensive, and presents several important bottlenecks in the construction of the phage libraries and the identification of the proteins displayed in the phages. In many occasions, it is impossible to identify peptides homologous to known proteins. This might be due to problems in the insertion of the cDNAs correctly in-frame or the cloning of noncoding regions. Despite this, SEREX has been probably the most commonly used technology for TAA discovery. SERPA is biased toward the identification of highly abundant proteins.

Recombinant Protein Microarrays

The low throughput of SEREX and SERPA and their limitations have pushed the field to look for alternatives in the screening of the humoral response against cancer (Fig. 2; Anderson and LaBaer 2005; Casal and Barderas 2010). To this end, high-content protein microarrays have been prepared with thousands of different probes printed on the surface of a chip. They have been used to identify substrates of kinases and small-molecule interactors and detect protein–protein interactions and also to track autoantibodies (Zhu et al. 2001; Zhu and Snyder 2001; Liotta et al. 2003). Protein microarrays provide the best tool to identify circulating cancer autoantibodies with high sensitivity and specificity in order to get the highest coverage of cancer patients. Recombinant proteins printed in the microarray are known beforehand, which facilitates their identification (Zhu and Snyder 2001). Proteins are expressed and purified before being printed at similar concentrations on the chip (Zhu et al. 2001), which increases the chance to discover circulating autoantibodies directed to low-abundant proteins (Babel et al. 2009; Barderas et al. 2010; Casal and Barderas 2010).

There are protein microarrays printed with proteins expressed in insect cells, which contain posttranslational modifications (PTMs) similar to those found in mammalian cells (Hudson et al. 2007; Babel et al. 2009). Commercially available protein arrays containing 9,500 human recombinant proteins expressed in *Sf9* insect cells (ProtoArray^{TM}, Invitrogen) have been used to identify TAAs in different cancer types (Hudson et al. 2007; Babel et al. 2009; Orenes-Pinero et al. 2010). However, in some cases, protein arrays express only fragments of many proteins, which change their conformation and folding and affect antibody recognition. Other alternatives consist of microarrays printed with the hEx1 human cDNA library, containing about 10,000 unique human proteins expressed in bacteria (Bussow et al. 1998, 2000). However, proteins expressed in bacteria lack most of the PTMs.

Importantly, a protein microarray technology is still being developed, and improvements are reported annually (Zhu and Snyder 2001; Liotta et al. 2003; Ramachandran et al. 2004; Chatterjee et al. 2006; Kung and Snyder 2006; Oishi et al. 2006; Hudson et al. 2007; Ran et al. 2008; Babel et al. 2009; Orenes-Pinero et al. 2010; Babel et al. 2011; Pedersen et al. 2011; Takulapalli et al. 2012; Festa et al. 2013). From the first commercially available human protein microarray consisting of 5,000 proteins in 2006, the number of proteins contained in the microarrays has grown up to 9,500 human full-length recombinant proteins in only one chip. Considering the advances performed in DNA microarrays, where microarrays covering the whole genome are available (Kronick 2004), we expect that the features in protein microarrays will keep growing up in the next years. Additionally, there is an alternative called NAPPA, where cDNAs codifying for the different proteins are printed on the surface of the chips and translated into proteins with rabbit reticulocyte lysates or a mammalian cancer cell milieu (Festa et al. 2013). Still, NAPPA technology has not been widely used, and its value remains to be demonstrated at a large scale in multiple laboratories.

Natural Protein Microarrays

In this case, protein extracts isolated from cancer cell lines are fractionated by liquid chromatography before being printed in the microarray slides (Qiu et al. 2004). The main advantage of this approach consists of the preservation of naturally occurring PTMs and other alterations observed in cancer proteins, which include alternative splicing, chimeras, or aberrant glycosylated proteins. This facilitates the display of relevant critical epitopes of the cancer patient's autoantibodies. Even though natural protein microarrays present advantages, the spots identified are complex mixtures of proteins, which complicate the actual identification of the target protein by mass spectrometry (Qiu et al. 2004). This technology only has been applied few times for the identification of cancer autoantibodies, including colon cancer (Nam et al. 2003; Qiu et al. 2004).

Glycopeptide Microarrays

This approach relies on the fact that malignant transformation of cells is accompanied by alterations in O-glycosylations able to induce a humoral immune response in cancer patients (Wandall et al. 2010). Glycopeptide microarrays are printed with peptides and O-glycosylated recombinant fragments purified by HPLC, which are obtained in vitro using recombinant ppGalNAc-transferases, Drosophila Core-1 b3GalT, human Core3 b3GnT6, and human ST6GalNAc-I (Wandall et al. 2010; Pedersen et al. 2011). These microarrays have been used to characterize humoral immune responses directed against aberrant glycosylated epitopes in colorectal cancer (Wandall et al. 2010).

Application of Circulating Autoantibodies to Colon Cancer Diagnostic Biomarker Discovery

SEREX and Phage Microarrays

The first report describing autoantibodies in CRC was published in 1998 by Old's group using SEREX (Scanlan et al. 1998). The authors identified 48 antigens, representing a broad spectrum of cellular components, with 31 clones as products of known genes and 17 representing novel gene products. The authors identified six clones that reacted exclusively with sera from colon cancer patients, with a frequency of recognition between 10 % and 27 %, indicating the great heterogeneity in the humoral immune response. Twenty out of 29 serum samples from colon cancer patients detected 1 or more of these clones.

The same group published 4 years later another SEREX study. Thirteen out of 77 antigens tested – p53, MAGEA3, SSX2, NY-ESO-1, HDAC5, MBD2, TRIP4, NYCO-45, KNSL6, HIP1R, Seb4D, KIAA1416, and LMNA – were serologically reactive with sera from CRC patients (Scanlan et al. 2002). In this study, 34 out of 74 colon cancer patients (46 %) were detected to have 1 or more of these 13 antigens. Several phage-displayed cDNA clones recognized in CRC patients showed no homology to sequences deposited in databases. This fact is a common problem of SEREX, which is observed in most of the published reports. The displayed peptide could mimic a conformational epitope or there could be other reasons (see above). Line and coworkers identified eight different serum-reactive cDNA clones with three potential targets C21ORF2, EPRS, and NAP1L1 not recognized by the sera of healthy individuals, but with frequencies of recognition between 4 and 17 % for the sera of CRC patients (Line et al. 2002). Ishikawa et al., also by SEREX, performed a screening of colon cancer cell lines with microsatellite instability (MSI) using the serum from a patient with MSI. The authors found 64 genes immunoreactive in colon cancer, with one of the identified antigens (CDX2) carrying a frameshift mutation in the repetitive G sequences (microsatellite) of its coding region, indicating that the immune response was also raised against TAAs generated by MSI (Ishikawa et al. 2003). Interestingly, the authors found galectin-4 among the immunoreactive clones as previously described (Scanlan et al. 1998). The frequency of recognition of this protein was low and not colon cancer specific, since it was also observed in renal, pancreatic, and esophageal cancer patient's sera and in 8 out of 38 healthy individuals (Ishikawa et al. 2003). Also by SEREX, it was found that HDAC3 autoantibodies were increased in CRC patients in comparison to controls. The authors found that the C-terminal region of HDAC3, with no homology to HDAC1 and HDAC2, contained the B-cell epitopes recognized by circulating autoantibodies (Shebzukhov et al. 2005).

In 2008, Ran et al. found six phages by SEREX technology able to classify CRC patients from healthy controls (Ran et al. 2008), with two of them showing partial homology to LGR6 and C6orf192 and the other four without obvious homology to any protein. Song et al. in 2011 identified BCP-20 (FBXO39) as a potential autoantigen, but with a prevalence of only 6 % in colon cancer patients (Song et al. 2011). Another study performed that year with a 12-mer random peptide library displayed in phages permitted the identification of a peptide motif (LYSNTL) with homology to ARD1A (Jiang et al. 2010). The authors found that the full-length recombinant protein elicited autoantibodies only in 14.7 % of CRC patients and 2 % of healthy controls (Jiang et al. 2010). Overexpression of ARD1A in CRC tumors was associated to poor prognosis for disease-free survival and shorter overall survival (Jiang et al. 2010). Chang et al. identified a five-phage classifier able to discriminate between CRC patients and controls. Phages were homologous to the uncharacterized protein hcg2038983, to TAS2R39, and to a peptide of the C-terminal constant region of the heavy chain of human IgG, which seems quite unusual, with two phages displaying peptides with no homology to any known protein (Chang et al. 2011). In 2011, Babel et al. by combining phage display and protein microarrays identified 43 phages showing higher immunoreactivity with CRC sera than control sera (Babel et al. 2011). Six phages displayed peptides with some homology to STK4/MST1, SULF1, NHSL1, SREBF2, GRN, and GTF2i amino acid sequences. Interestingly, the replacement of two phages for their corresponding recombinant proteins (STK4/MST1, SULF1) significantly improved the diagnostic ability of the predictor panel from an AUC of 0.78 % to 0.86 % and sensitivity from 72 % to 82.6 % while maintaining the specificity higher than 70 % (Babel et al. 2011).

SERPA and Natural Protein Microarrays

Hanash laboratory applied natural protein arrays printed with LoVo cells to the study of the humoral response in colon cancer (Nam et al. 2003). They identified the ubiquitin C-terminal hydrolase L3 (UCH-L3) as a protein target of autoantibodies in 19 out of 43 CRC patients' sera, without reactivity in lung cancer patients or healthy individuals' sera (Nam et al. 2003). The authors verified the reactivity of the UCH-L3 protein by immunostaining of 2D gels run with LoVo cell extracts. In 2007, SERPA was used on HCT116 colon cancer cell line. The authors only found HSP60 as a target, with increased autoantibody levels in 13 out of 25 CRC patients in comparison to 1 out of 15 healthy controls for a 52 % sensitivity and 93.3 % specificity (He et al. 2007). SERPA as well as natural protein microarrays presents the same disadvantage: the immunoreactive proteins need to be identified a posteriori by LC–MS. This is complicated by the complexity of the samples, due to the presence of several proteins in the 2D spots. This fact probably explains the low number of reports identifying immunoreactive proteins by these two approaches.

ELISA Approaches

The first report using ELISA plates coated with TAAs to identify colon cancer autoantibodies was published in 2005. The authors used Fas as a target of autoantibodies based on previous observations claiming that apoptosis and the expression of this receptor were altered during carcinogenesis in the human colon. Anti-Fas titers were significantly higher in patients with colorectal adenomas than in healthy controls and even higher in patients with adenocarcinomas (Reipert et al. 2005). Moreover, autoantibodies to Fas/CD95 showed also some specificity for early CRC detection using sera from 38 healthy controls, 38 patients with colorectal adenomas, and 21 patients with colorectal adenocarcinoma in an ELISA-based array (Reipert et al. 2005).

Kocer et al. found autoantibodies directed to MUC5AC in 45 % of polyp patients, 60 % of CRC patients, and 27.3 % of healthy individuals (Kocer et al. 2006). MUC5AC is a secreted mucin aberrantly expressed in colorectal polyps and carcinomas. In 2007, Chen et al. investigated the humoral immune response of Calnuc by ELISA (Chen et al. 2007). They found autoantibodies against Calnuc in 11.5 % of CRC patients' sera and only in 1.2 % of control sera (Chen et al. 2007). After testing Calnuc in combination with other previously described TAAs, c-myc, p53, G2/mitotic-specific cyclin-B1 (CCNB1), and G1/S-specific cyclin-D1 (CCND1), the ability to diagnose CRC increased up to 65.4 % sensitivity and 93.9 % specificity (Chen et al. 2007). In 2009, Liu et al. tested by ELISA five TAAs previously identified in other cancers with 46 CRC patients' sera and 58 healthy individual sera (Liu et al. 2009). Imp1, p62, Koc, p53, and c-myc, tested by ELISA, were permitted to discriminate CRC patients from controls with a sensitivity of 60.9 % and a specificity of 89.7 % (Liu et al. 2009). In 2011, two other different reports identified a humoral immune response against two proteins overexpressed in CRC tissue in comparison to normal mucosa – RPH3AL and SEC61β (Chen et al. 2011; Fan et al. 2011). Recently, Liu et al. in 2013 found autoantibodies against the IGF2 mRNA-binding protein (IMP2/p62) by ELISA in 23.4 % of CRC patients' sera in comparison to 4.8 % of patients' sera having colonic adenomas and 2.9 % of healthy individuals (Liu et al. 2013).

Protein and Glycopeptide Microarrays

Regarding protein microarrays, Babel et al. used a commercial ProtoArray v4.0 containing 8,000 human recombinant proteins with sera of metastatic CRC patients and controls (Babel et al. 2009). The authors found 43 protein targets of autoantibodies composing a diagnostic protein signature (Babel et al. 2009). Six TAAs (PIM1, MAPKAPK3, STK4, SRC, FGFR4, and ACVR2B) were validated with a different cohort of CRC sera. An AUC of 0.85 % with a specificity and sensitivity of 73.9 % and 83.3 %, respectively, was obtained with the combination of only two markers – ACVR2B and MAPKAPK3 (Babel et al. 2009). In addition, the same authors reanalyzed these recombinant TAAs (Babel et al. 2009) together with six validated phages displaying CRC-specific peptide TAAs (Babel et al. 2011) using a different set of 96 sera. Remarkably, a CRC predictor panel composed of three phages displaying peptides with homology to GRN, NHSL1, and SREBF2 and four full-length recombinant TAAs – PIM1, MAPKAPK3, FGFR4, and ACVR2B – correctly predicted the presence of cancer with a highly improved accuracy showing an AUC of 94 % for a sensitivity and specificity of 89.1 % and 90.0 %, respectively (Barderas et al. 2012). Later, Casal's group tested a variant version of the commercial ProtoArray v4.1 protein microarrays with a different nitrocellulose surface than ProtoArray v4.0, but containing the same number of human recombinant proteins (Barderas et al. 2013). After identifying 24 novel TAAs, the authors validated 3 TAAs (EDIL3, GTF2B, and HCK) with a different cohort of sera that correctly discriminate 50 CRC samples from 49 healthy individuals in combination with p53 for an AUC of 0.75 % and sensitivity and specificity of 82 % and 56 %, respectively (Barderas et al. 2013). In 2010, Kijanka et al. used high-density protein microarrays printed with the hEx1 human cDNA library with 43 CRC patient sera and 40 control sera. The authors identified a protein signature of 18 antigens associated to cancer and 4 to the absence of cancer, including p53, HMGB1, TRIM28, TCF3, LASS5, and ZNF346 (Kijanka et al. 2010), which was not further validated by other immunological approaches.

Interestingly, our group also proved that some TAAs can be used as potential therapeutic targets. In particular, blocking of FGFR4 with different small-molecule inhibitors and specific antibodies resulted in a significant reduction of tumor growth (Pelaez-Garcia et al. 2013). The silencing of this receptor in colon cancer cells reverted the epithelial to mesenchymal transition (EMT), producing a decrease in the tumorigenic properties of colon cancer cells (Pelaez-Garcia et al. 2013).

A glycopeptide array approach was also tested in 2011 for identifying aberrant glycopeptides as targets of an immune response in CRC patients (Pedersen et al. 2011). This approach allowed for the identification of a set of aberrant glycopeptides derived from MUC1 and MUC4 (Pedersen et al. 2011). The authors validated the immunogenicity of these glycopeptides using monoclonal antibodies and provided evidence of the expression of these aberrant glycosylated proteins in colon cancer cell lines (Pedersen et al. 2011). In addition, the same group also reported that MUC1-STn and MUC1-Core3 circulating IgG autoantibodies were able to discriminate CRC cases from controls with 8.2 % and 13.4 % sensitivity, respectively, at 95 % specificity in a cohort of 97 postmenopausal women with colorectal cancer and 97 postmenopausal women without any history of cancer (Pedersen et al. 2014).

Shortfalls and Limitations of Autoantibody Research

Interestingly, the use of protein microarrays provides the best results in terms of specificity, sensitivity, and predictive value of the identified TAAs for the discrimination of CRC patients and controls (Table 1). However, the poor matching between the identified TAAs by using different approaches, except for STK4 and MAPKAPK3, with galectin-4, p53, c-myc, p62, Koc, and Imp1 as cancer TAAs but nonspecific for CRC is worrisome. This poor coincidence is probably a consequence of multiple variables including the different sensitivities of the techniques and platforms, different repertoires of proteins printed in the microarrays, different expression systems for protein production, different tags fused to the proteins, or different PTMs in the proteins printed in microarrays with respect to the cancer forms.

Another problem is the absence of validation assays in many TAA discovery reports. Although an important number of autoantibodies have been identified in colon cancer patients, some reports used a small number of sera and nonmatching samples between CRC patient sera and control sera with regard to sex and age, and there is an absence of validation data using different sera cohorts. In this sense, only autoantibodies to MST1/STK4 and p53 have been reported in at least three different studies using different cohorts of serum samples (Table 1; Soussi 2000; Babel et al. 2009, 2011; Barderas et al. 2012), with p53 autoantibody frequency ranging between 20 % and 40 % in all cancer patients (Soussi 2000).

Early Responses

Early detection is critical in cancer diagnostics. Although different reports have claimed the utility of this approach for the early diagnosis of CRC (Barderas et al. 2010), few reports have tested autoantibody panels for early diagnosis. A predictor panel composed of a panel of 7 CRC-specific TAAs achieved an AUC of 90 % and a sensitivity of 88.2 % and specificity of 82.6 % for early stages (Duke's stage A and B) (Barderas et al. 2012). It has also been reported that humoral responses to p53 can appear in normal-risk individuals between 1.0 and 3.8 years before clinical diagnosis of CRC (Pedersen et al. 2013).

However, little is known about the exact moment when autoantibodies appear, their kinetics, and their evolution according to the progression of the disease. The answer to these questions is almost impossible to be performed using human samples due to the enormous difficulties to get preclinical samples. Even more, when the lesions are removed and the patient treated, the evolution of the autoantibodies cannot be monitored. In this sense, by using colon cancer murine models

Table 1 List of CRC-specific diagnostic and prognostic autoantibodies and their target TAAs. The study sample size, method used to identify and validate the autoantibodies and their target proteins, biomarker abbreviation, AUC, specificity, and sensitivity to discriminate CRC patients from controls are included. *np* not provided

References	Discovery method	TAA signature	Validation method	Number of sera (validation set)	Specificity (%)	Sensitivity (%)	AUC
(Scanlan et al. 1998)	SEREX	NY-CO8, NY-CO9, p53, NY-CO16, NY-CO38, NMDAr	Phage plaque assay	107	np	np	np
(Scanlan et al. 2002)	SEREX	MAGEA4, SSX2, NY-ESO-1, HDAC5, MBD2, TRIP4, KIAA1416, p53, NY-CO45, KNSL6, HIP15, SEB5D, LMNA	Phage plaque assay	149	np	Individual TAA sensitivity ranging from 2.7 to 14.8	–
(Line et al. 2002)	SEREX	C21ORF2, EPRS, NAP1L1, and other five unidentified phages	Seroblot	95	97.2, 95.7, 98.6, respectively	4.1, 16.6, 8.3, respectively	np
(Ishikawa et al. 2003)	SEREX	CDX2	Seroblot	np	np	np	np
(Shebzukhov et al. 2005)	SEREX	HDAC3	Phage plaque assay	498	99	5	na
(Ran et al. 2008)	SEREX	LGR6, C6orf192, and other four unidentified phages	Phage plaque assay	48	84	83	0.933
(Jiang et al. 2010)	SEREX	ARD1A	ELISA	398	98	14.7	np
(Song et al. 2011)	SEREX	BCP-20/FBXO39	ELISA	146	34	6	
(Chang et al. 2011)	SEREX	Hcg2038983, TAS2R39, and other three unidentified phages	ELISA	120	92	90	np
(Babel et al. 2011)	Phage microarrays	STK4, SULF1	ELISA	153	83	70	0.86

(Nam et al. 2003)	Natural protein microarrays	UCH-L3	Seroblot	97	97	44	np
(He et al. 2007)	SERPA	HSP60	ELISA	130	np	np	np
(Reipert et al. 2005)	Previous findings	Fas/CD95	ELISA	97	np	np	np
(Kocer et al. 2006)	Previous findings	MUC5AC	ELISA	72	73	54	np
(Chen et al. 2007)	Previous findings	Calnuc, c-myc, CCNB1, p53, CCND1	ELISA	447	94	65	np
(Liu et al. 2009)	Previous findings	Imp1, p62, Koc, p53, c-myc	ELISA miniarray	104	90	61	np
(Chen et al. 2011)	Previous findings	RPH3AL	Seroblot	147	73	84	0.84
(Fan et al. 2011)	Previous findings	SEC61B	Seroblot	158	75	79	0.795
(Liu et al. 2013)	Previous findings	IMP2/p62	ELISA	140	96	23	np
(Babel et al. 2009)	Recombinant protein microarray	MAPKAPK3, FGFR4, PIM1, ACVR2B, STK4, SRC	ELISA	94	73.9	83.3	0.85
(Barderas et al. 2012)	Recombinant and phage microarrays	PIM1, MAPKAPK3, MST1/STK4, FGFR4, ACVR2B, SRC and SULF1 full-length recombinant proteins, and SREBF2, GRN, GTF2i, and NHSL1 as peptides displayed in phages	ELISA	92	90	89	0.94
(Barderas et al. 2013)	Recombinant protein microarray	GTF2B, HCK, EDIL3, p53	ELISA	153	56	82	0.74

(continued)

Table 1 (continued)

References	Discovery method	TAA signature	Validation method	Number of sera (validation set)	Specificity (%)	Sensitivity (%)	AUC
(Kijanka et al. 2010)	Recombinant protein microarray	12 unspecified TAA among ITFG3, ZNF700, TSLCQ, LASS5, P53, ZNF768, SNP29, ZNF638, ICLN, ZNF346, STOM, TCF3, AOPJ75, VGLL4, HMGB1, TRIM28, HNRDL, BAC85857	np	83	80	87	np
(Pedersen et al. 2011)	Glycopeptide microarrays	MUC1 (STn), MUC4 (Tn-MUC4-1-TnMUC4-5)	Glycopeptide microarray	150	89	79.3	np
(Pedersen et al. 2013)	Previous findings	p53 (15-mer overlapping peptides covering the whole p53 sequence)	Glycopeptide microarray	194	95	31	0.687
(Syrigos et al. 1999)	Previous findings	Tropomyosin (TMS)	ELISA	Anti-TMS autoantibodies in CRC patients indicate a better outcome of the disease			
(Syrigos et al. 2000)	Previous findings	dsDNA	ELISA	Anti-dsDNA autoantibodies in CRC patients indicate a better outcome of the disease			
(Pedersen et al. 2013)	Glycopeptide microarrays/ previous findings	MUC4TR5	Glycopeptide microarray	Anti-MUC4TR5 autoantibodies indicate higher risk of death			
(Ochiai et al. 2012)	Previous findings	p53	ELISA	Seropositive CRC patients to p53 became seronegative after surgery indicating usefulness for therapy monitoring			

based on the use of azoxymethane/dextran sodium sulfate, our group recently demonstrated that (i) the autoantibodies were produced very early in the disease, even before the tumoral lesions might be detected by other techniques (histology), (ii) the autoantibody levels increased according to the progression of the disease, and (iii) the presence of autoantibodies was always associated to the presence of malignant lesions, since autoantibodies were not observed in those animals presenting nonmalignant lesions (Fig. 3; Barderas et al. 2013). A subset of human CRC TAAs, HCK, MST1/STK4, EDIL3, GTF2B, SRC, NY-ESO-1, MAPKAPK3, and p53 – identified through protein microarray or SEREX approaches (Soussi 2000; Scanlan et al. 2002; Babel et al. 2009, 2011; Barderas et al. 2013) – was tested using sera from these CRC murine models, which develop a cancer humoral response similar to that observed in human CRC patients (Barderas et al. 2013). This subset of human TAAs was able to discriminate mice carrying malignant lesions from controls (Barderas et al. 2013), showing a great potential to be included in CRC diagnostic tests. Indeed, we demonstrated the exquisite sensitivity of the humoral immune response to colon cancer for preclinical cancer diagnosis. Moreover, as autoantibody levels increase according to the progression of the disease, it might open its application to detect recurrences.

Optimization of a Diagnostic Test Based on Circulating Autoantibodies

Despite promising results, very few commercial kits using this technology have reached the market (Lam et al. 2011). Circulating autoantibodies need to be validated in a clinical context using independent and large patient's cohorts to verify their usefulness in terms of reproducibility, detection limit, and predictive value. Biomarker development consists of several phases including preclinical studies, clinical assay development and optimization, retrospective studies of stored specimens, prospective screening studies, and multicentered randomized clinical trials (Pepe et al. 2001). In addition, as mentioned above, other sources of optimization to improve the diagnostic ability of an autoantibody panel would include (i) the expression system to produce the TAA, (ii) the platform used for testing, and (iii) the number of TAAs to be included in the diagnostic test (Fig. 4).

Optimization of the TAA Expression and Purification

Peptides and proteins produced for the validation of the candidate biomarkers represent an important source of variability. Validation of the TAAs should be performed with purified proteins of the highest purity and quality, containing PTMs similar to the actual tumor target (Casal and Barderas 2010). Impurities, particularly after expression in *Escherichia coli*, might result in false-positive detection of cancer-specific autoantibodies due to the presence of bacteria in the intestinal microbiota. However, minor contaminants from insect cells have also been reported

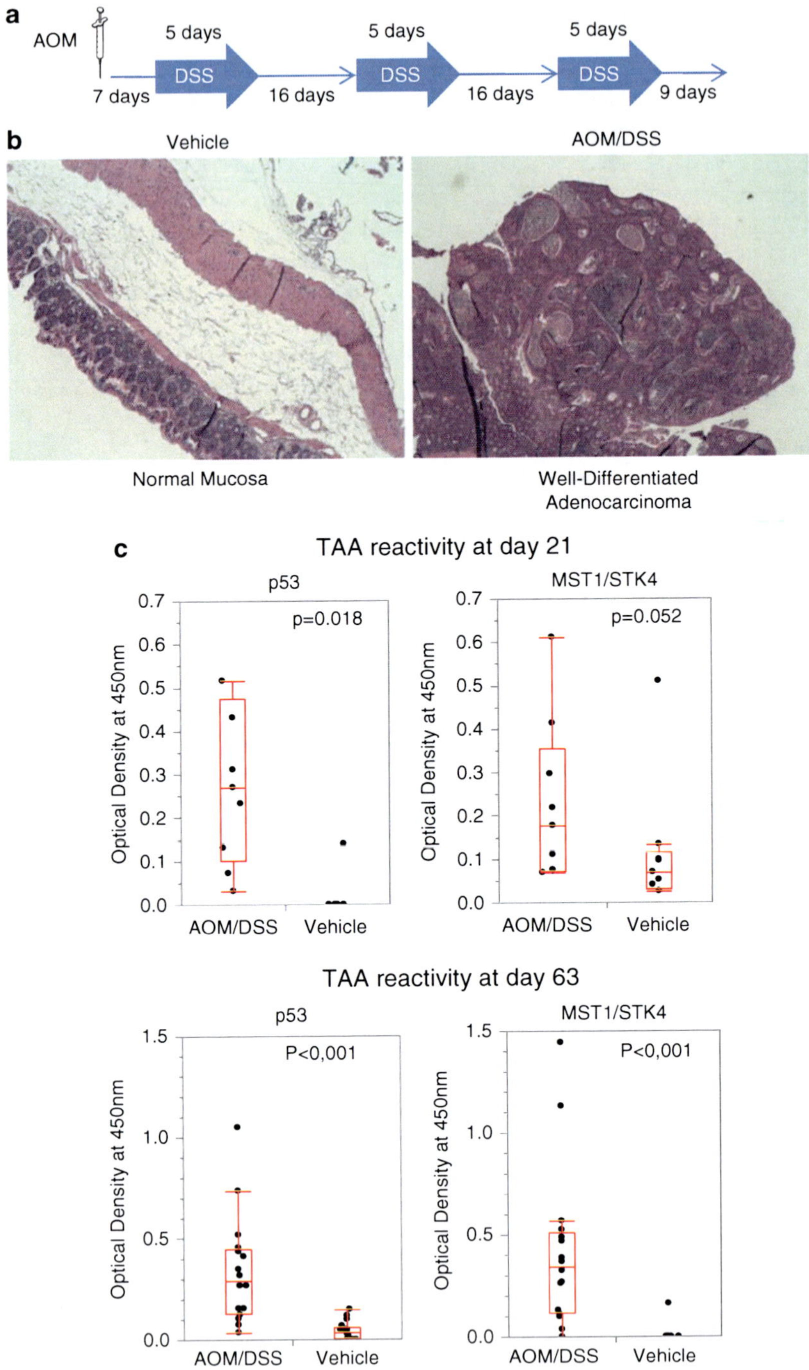

Fig. 3 (continued)

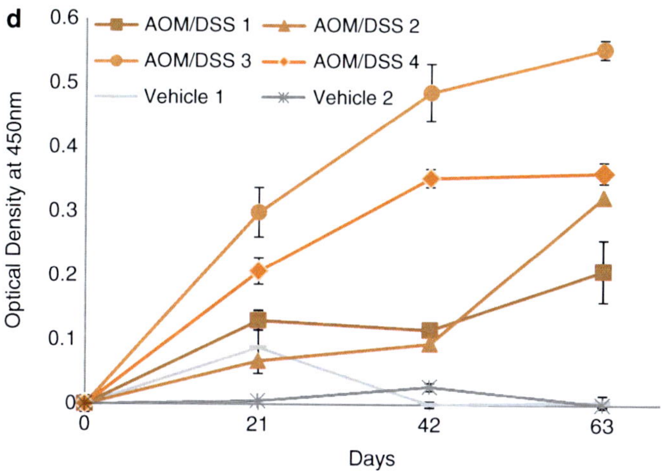

Fig. 3 Murine models mimic the humoral immune response observed in human CRC patients. (**a**) The protocol used to obtain chemically induced colitis-associated CRC in mice is outlined. AOM was injected intraperitoneally at a concentration of 10 mg/kg and DSS (2.5 %) supplied in drinking water. (**b**) Hematoxylin and eosin staining of distal colon tissue at the end of the protocol (day 63). Images are shown at 200× magnification. (**c**) Murine autoantibody levels to CRC-specific TAAs – p53 and MST1/STK4 – at day 21 and day 63 can be observed since day 21 and prior to the detection of neoplastic colon lesions by histological staining. (**d**) Autoantibody levels to p53 of four out of nine randomly selected AOM-/DSS-treated mice together with two out of nine vehicle-treated mice at indicated times to follow their levels according to the progression of the disease (Adapted from Barderas et al. 2013)

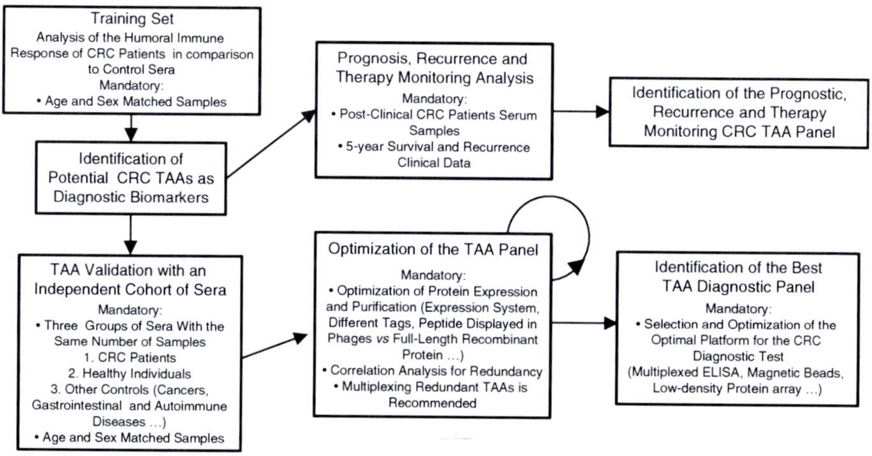

Fig. 4 Road map to identify and develop CRC diagnostic and prognostic tests. Steps considered as needed or mandatory are highlighted

to be reactive to immunoglobulins from cancer patients, which might affect the detection of cancer-specific autoantibodies (Schmetzer et al. 2005). The presence of different tags (GST, MBP, or 6xHis) fused to the selected TAAs in the N- or C-terminal end of the protein should also be tested since it could affect the binding of the autoantibodies to the protein. Moreover, optimization should include producing each antigen in *E. coli*, insect, and mammalian cells for testing autoantibody recognition. However, no comparative studies have been yet performed.

Optimization of the Platform for TAA Testing

The choice of the platform and/or the solid support used to probe the protein can also affect the final result. It has been recently published that autoantigens perform differently if the protein is coated (ELISA), immobilized on membranes (WB or protein microarrays), or highly unfolded as is the case for the hEx1 proteins (Murphy et al. 2012a). As each cancer patient can develop a different immune response to protein regions presented as discontinuous, conformational, or linear epitopes, diagnostic tests should contain multiple TAAs for a full coverage of cancer patients (Lam et al. 2011; Murphy et al. 2012a). The use of multiplexed immunoassays (magnetic beads or multiplexed ELISA) (Ling et al. 2007) or low-density protein microarrays (Liu et al. 2009) could be useful for the development of diagnostic tests.

Identification of the Minimum Number of TAAs to Be Included in a CRC Predictor Panel: Correlation Analyses

In order to overcome the heterogeneous response among patients, combinations of biomarkers are needed. Disease heterogeneity implies the use of biomarker panels. To avoid the overlap in reactivity with sera and to select the minimum number of TAAs for CRC diagnosis, it is convenient to calculate the redundancy of the markers and discern whether the information provided by each TAA is redundant or not, with the rest of TAAs to correctly classify patients and controls. Low correlation values indicate that reactivity between markers does not show association and they classify different subsets of CRC patients, whereas high correlation indicates that they are recognized by the same set of patients (Barderas et al. 2012). Globally, the final autoantibody panel would benefit if we find a combined classifier with their TAAs showing the lowest correlation to cover the largest number of different CRC patients (Barderas et al. 2012). On the other hand, we could test together those combinations of TAAs identifying the same groups of patients to simplify the diagnostic test (Barderas et al. 2012).

To identify redundancy, CRC-specific TAAs were tested with the same collection of sera, the ELISA values were plotted, and Pearson and Spearman correlation coefficients were performed for all combinations of TAAs (Barderas et al. 2012). An example of this correlation analysis was done for a panel of TAAs identified by

Table 2 Correlation study for CRC-specific TAAs identified through high-density protein microarray approaches. Correlation values were calculated for all pairs of TAAs identified through protein microarrays (Babel et al. 2009; Barderas et al. 2013) or phage microarrays (Babel et al. 2011). Markers showing redundancy are depicted in *green*, indicating that they should be tested together. In *yellow*, markers that show low levels of redundancy, indicating that those markers perform better if they are tested individually

	Protein Array (ProtoArray 4.1)				Phage Microarrays				Protein Array (ProtoArray 4.0)				
	EDIL3	GTF2b	HCK	p53	GRN	GTF2i	NHSL1	SREBF2	FGFR4	MAPKAPK3	PIM1	SRC	MST1/STK4
EDIL3	1	0.52	0.55	0.01	0.02	0.01	0.02	0.03	0.23	0.06	0.14	0.08	0.27
GTF2b		1	0.85	0.01	0	0.01	0	0	0.24	0.13	0.27	0.36	0.2
HCK			1	0.01	0	0.02	0.01	0.01	0.31	0.13	0.21	0.32	0.27
p53				1	0	0.01	0	0	0.06	0.19	0.15	0.05	0.07
GRN					1	0.64	0.88	0.86	0.05	0.07	0.01	0.01	0.03
GTF2i						1	0.67	0.65	0.02	0.02	0.02	0	0.03
NHSL1							1	0.83	0.04	0.05	0.02	0.01	0.04
SREBF2								1	0.06	0.08	0.02	0.01	0.04
FGFR4									1	0.38	0.34	0.44	0.16
MAPKAPK3										1	0.5	0.64	0.08
PIM1											1	0.42	0.12
SRC												1	0.1
MST1/STK4													1

protein and phage display protein microarray using 90 sera from CRC patient and healthy individual sera (Table 2; Babel et al. 2009, 2011; Barderas et al. 2012). Here, biomarker candidates discovered through the same platform showed correlation values higher than 0.4, indicating the necessity to combine TAAs with low correlation in the diagnostic TAA panel (Barderas et al. 2012). In summary, optimization steps are required for specificity and sensitivity improvements to get a reliable CRC diagnostic test (Fig. 4).

Potential Applications to Prognosis, Other Diseases, or Conditions

Prognostic markers indicate a survival outcome of patients. Although multiple reports have claimed that autoantibodies are useful not only for diagnosis but also for prognosis, survival, and recurrence, there are almost no reports showing correlation of circulating autoantibodies and prognosis of colorectal cancer. Babel et al. showed a protein signature able to differentiate between CRC patients suffering metastasis to liver and metastasis to lung (Babel et al. 2009). In addition, we also found, based on results with 96 colorectal cancer serum samples, that higher levels of circulating autoantibodies to MST1/STK4 were associated to a better prognosis (personal observations). In two other studies, sera from 55 patients with colon adenocarcinoma, 26 patients with benign surgical diseases, and 40 healthy individuals by ELISA were examined for autoantibodies to dsDNA and tropomyosin and its association to prognosis (Syrigos et al. 1999, 2000). The authors found that the presence of autoantibodies to both proteins was associated to a better outcome of the disease. Finally, in another recent study, an association of high levels of autoantibodies to the aberrant glycopeptide MUC4TR5 with a risk of death in CRC patients has been observed (Pedersen et al. 2013).

In any case, circulating autoantibodies have shown a strong prognostic power in other types of cancer. Using 120 cancer samples from benign ductal carcinoma in situ or invasive breast cancer, a signature of 5 TAAs (RBP-J kappa, HMGN1, PSRC, CIRBP, and ECHDC1) was able to discriminate patients with an AUC = 0.794. Higher autoantibody titers of RBP-J kappa were found in patients with a higher histotype grade and higher recurrence-free survival for those patients who were positive for the five-antibody signature (Mange et al. 2012). Similar results were found in pancreatic cancer (Bracci et al. 2012) and glioblastoma multiforme (Pallasch et al. 2005), where survival rates were higher in patients with higher levels of autoantibodies to CTDSP1 and NR2E3 and GLEA2 and PHF3 autoantigens, respectively. Finally, in prostate cancer patients, higher levels of autoantibodies to TARDBP, TLN1, PARK7, CALD1, and PISP1 were able to discriminate benign prostate hyperplasia patients from prostate cancer patients (O'Rourke et al. 2012).

More reports are necessary to clarify this question, since other reports claim that p53 autoantibodies negatively correlate with the survival of cancer patients (Lubin et al. 1995; Tang et al. 2001). Then, the correlation to overall patient survival of autoantibody levels against a specific TAA might depend on its nature and function in the tumoral tissue.

In addition, circulating biomarkers might be used to monitor the disease and detect recurrences by quantifying changes in autoantibody levels during treatment. However, there are few reports showing their usefulness to detect recurrences. In CRC, a decrease in the immune response to p53 in 78 % of p53-seropositive patients after surgery has been reported (Ochiai et al. 2012). In addition, a rapid and durable loss of p53 antibodies has also been observed in breast cancer after resection of tumors and treatment with neoadjuvant chemotherapy (Anderson et al. 2008). In ovarian cancer, Tainsky lab detected recurrences at 9.07 months prior to clinical recurrence (Chatterjee et al. 2012). They demonstrated that 3 out of 56 antigens displayed in phages and printed in microarrays correctly classified recurrent and nonrecurrent ovarian cancer patients (Chatterjee et al. 2012).

Perspectives and Concluding Remarks

The detection of CRC circulating autoantibodies holds great promise for CRC diagnosis. The combination of different TAAs has allowed the obtainment of assays with very high specificity and sensitivity. Their low invasiveness would facilitate their inclusion in a routine health check in contrast to other invasive screening methods, like colonoscopy. Moreover, the use for early clinical diagnosis would significantly improve the overall survival of CRC patients and save considerable amounts of money to the National Health Systems. However, there are some questions that still remain open. The first and most critical, which are the factors

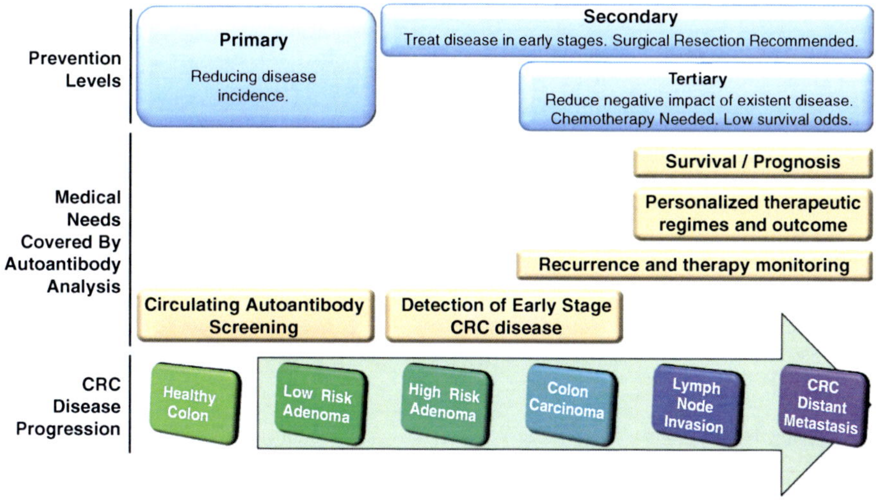

Fig. 5 Medical needs covered by CRC autoantibodies according to the stage of the disease

that induce this autoantibody response to cancer proteins? Second, which is the actual TAA repertoire generated for each tumor? The dispersion of identified TAAs among the different technologies and the little reproducibility among laboratories complicate the definition of clear guidelines for TAA acceptance. In this regard, the demonstration of a similar response in mouse cancer models supposes a strong support and provides a good tool for the testing of putative TAAs. Third and finally, validation is a fundamental issue that still continues to be neglected in many reports. A final support for the technology will come only from final clinical assays and application. In this regard, an initial product has been recently commercialized for lung cancer (Lam et al. 2011).

In addition to diagnostic power, the screening of the autoantibody response of CRC patients might be useful for prognostic or therapy monitoring purposes, but further studies are required (Fig. 5). The identification of new therapeutic targets for intervention is also a main strength of this strategy (Barderas et al. 2010; Dudas et al. 2010; Pelaez-Garcia et al. 2013).

Summary Points

- Colorectal cancer autoantibodies and their target proteins constitute a very promising alternative as a diagnostic test for the massive screening of populations to identify colon cancer-carrier individuals.
- A description of the methodologies used to identify circulating autoantibodies is given.
- Autoantibodies directed against tumor-associated antigens (TAAs) emerge early in the disease and follow its progression.

- Multiple reports have described a wide number of TAAs due to the heterogeneous response in cancer.
- Colorectal cancer murine models show similar humoral responses to that observed in humans, allowing its study in a more reproducible way and the possibility to compare predictive values of different autoantibodies identified elsewhere.
- Autoantibodies might be effective for identifying recurrence and monitoring therapy.
- Autoantibodies and their target proteins are useful for identifying potential therapeutic targets.

References

Anderson KS, LaBaer J. The sentinel within: exploiting the immune system for cancer biomarkers. J Proteome Res. 2005;4:1123–33.

Anderson KS, Ramachandran N, Wong J, et al. Application of protein microarrays for multiplexed detection of antibodies to tumor antigens in breast cancer. J Proteome Res. 2008;7:1490–9.

Babel I, Barderas R, Diaz-Uriarte R, et al. Identification of tumor-associated autoantigens for the diagnosis of colorectal cancer in serum using high density protein microarrays. Mol Cell Proteomics. 2009;8:2382–95.

Babel I, Barderas R, Diaz-Uriarte R, et al. Identification of MST1/STK4 and SULF1 proteins as autoantibody targets for the diagnosis of colorectal cancer by using phage microarrays. Mol Cell Proteomics. 2011;10:M110 001784.

Barderas R, Babel I, Casal JI. Colorectal cancer proteomics, molecular characterization and biomarker discovery. Proteomics Clin Appl. 2010;4:159–78.

Barderas R, Babel I, Diaz-Uriarte R, et al. An optimized predictor panel for colorectal cancer diagnosis based on the combination of tumor-associated antigens obtained from protein and phage microarrays. J Proteomics. 2012;75:4647–55.

Barderas R, Villar-Vazquez R, Fernandez-Acenero MJ, et al. Sporadic colon cancer murine models demonstrate the value of autoantibody detection for preclinical cancer diagnosis. Sci Rep. 2013;3:2938.

Bracci PM, Zhou M, Young S, et al. Serum autoantibodies to pancreatic cancer antigens as biomarkers of pancreatic cancer in a San Francisco Bay Area case–control study. Cancer. 2012;118:5384–94.

Bussow K, Cahill D, Nietfeld W, et al. A method for global protein expression and antibody screening on high-density filters of an arrayed cDNA library. Nucleic Acids Res. 1998;26:5007–8.

Bussow K, Nordhoff E, Lubbert C, et al. A human cDNA library for high-throughput protein expression screening. Genomics. 2000;65:1–8.

Carey TE, Takahashi T, Resnick LA, et al. Cell surface antigens of human malignant melanoma: mixed hemadsorption assays for humoral immunity to cultured autologous melanoma cells. Proc Natl Acad Sci U S A. 1976;73:3278–82.

Casal JI, Barderas R. Identification of cancer autoantigens in serum: toward diagnostic/prognostic testing? Mol Diagn Ther. 2010;14:149–54.

Chang WJ, Wu LL, Cao FA, et al. Development of autoantibody signatures as biomarkers for early detection of colorectal carcinoma. Clin Cancer Res. 2011;17:5715–24.

Chatterjee M, Mohapatra S, Ionan A, et al. Diagnostic markers of ovarian cancer by high-throughput antigen cloning and detection on arrays. Cancer Res. 2006;66:1181–90.

Chatterjee M, Dyson G, Levin NK, et al. Tumor autoantibodies as biomarkers for predicting ovarian cancer recurrence. Cancer Biomark. 2012;11:59–73.

Chen Y, Lin P, Qiu SM, et al. Autoantibodies to Ca^{2+} binding protein Calnuc is a potential marker in colon cancer detection. Int J Oncol. 2007;30:1137–44.

Chen JS, Kuo YB, Chou YP, et al. Detection of autoantibodies against Rabphilin-3A-like protein as a potential biomarker in patient's sera of colorectal cancer. Clin Chim Acta. 2011;412:1417–22.

Dippold WG, Lloyd KO, Li LT, et al. Cell surface antigens of human malignant melanoma: definition of six antigenic systems with mouse monoclonal antibodies. Proc Natl Acad Sci U S A. 1980;77:6114–8.

Dudas SP, Chatterjee M, Tainsky MA. Usage of cancer associated autoantibodies in the detection of disease. Cancer Biomark. 2010;6:257–70.

Duffy MJ, van Dalen A, Haglund C, et al. Tumour markers in colorectal cancer: European Group on Tumour Markers (EGTM) guidelines for clinical use. Eur J Cancer. 2007;43:1348–60.

Fan CW, Chan CC, Chen KT, et al. Identification of SEC61 beta and its autoantibody as biomarkers for colorectal cancer. Clin Chim Acta. 2011;412:887–93.

Festa F, Rollins SM, Vattem K, et al. Robust microarray production of freshly expressed proteins in a human milieu. Proteomics Clin Appl. 2013;7:372–7.

He YJ, Wu YZ, Mou ZR, et al. Proteomics-based identification of HSP60 as a tumor-associated antigen in colorectal cancer. Proteomics Clin Appl. 2007;1:336–42.

Hudson ME, Pozdnyakova I, Haines K, et al. Identification of differentially expressed proteins in ovarian cancer using high-density protein microarrays. Proc Natl Acad Sci U S A. 2007;104:17494–9.

Ishikawa T, Fujita T, Suzuki Y, et al. Tumor-specific immunological recognition of frameshift-mutated peptides in colon cancer with microsatellite instability. Cancer Res. 2003;63:5564–72.

Jiang BH, Ren TT, Dong B, et al. Peptide mimic isolated by autoantibody reveals human arrest defective 1 overexpression is associated with poor prognosis for colon cancer patients. Am J Pathol. 2010;177:1095–103.

Kijanka G, Hector S, Kay EW, et al. Human IgG antibody profiles differentiate between symptomatic patients with and without colorectal cancer. Gut. 2010;59:69–78.

Klade CS, Voss T, Krystek E, et al. Identification of tumor antigens in renal cell carcinoma by serological proteome analysis. Proteomics. 2001;1:890–8.

Kocer B, McKolanis J, Soran A. Humoral immune response to MUC5AC in patients with colorectal polyps and colorectal carcinoma. BMC Gastroenterol. 2006;6.

Kronick MN. Creation of the whole human genome microarray. Expert Rev Proteomics. 2004;1:19–28.

Kung LA, Snyder M. Proteome chips for whole-organism assays. Nat Rev Mol Cell Biol. 2006;7:617–22.

Lam S, Boyle P, Healey GF, et al. Early CDT-lung: an immunobiomarker test as an aid to early detection of lung cancer. Cancer Prev Res (Phila). 2011;4:1126–34.

Levin B, Brooks D, Smith RA, et al. Emerging technologies in screening for colorectal cancer: CT colonography, immunochemical fecal occult blood tests, and stool screening using molecular markers. CA Cancer J Clin. 2003;53:44–55.

Line A, Slucka Z, Stengrevics A, et al. Characterisation of tumour-associated antigens in colon cancer. Cancer Immunol Immunother. 2002;51:574–82.

Ling MM, Ricks C, Lea P. Multiplexing molecular diagnostics and immunoassays using emerging microarray technologies. Expert Rev Mol Diagn. 2007;7:87–98.

Liotta LA, Espina V, Mehta AI, et al. Protein microarrays: meeting analytical challenges for clinical applications. Cancer Cell. 2003;3:317–25.

Liu W, Wang P, Li Z, et al. Evaluation of tumour-associated antigen (TAA) miniarray in immunodiagnosis of colon cancer. Scand J Immunol. 2009;69:57–63.

Liu W, Li Z, Xu W, et al. Humoral autoimmune response to IGF2 mRNA-binding protein (IMP2/p62) and its tissue-specific expression in colon cancer. Scand J Immunol. 2013;77:255–60.

Locker GY, Hamilton S, Harris J, et al. ASCO 2006 update of recommendations for the use of tumor markers in gastrointestinal cancer. J Clin Oncol. 2006;24:5313–27.

Lubin R, Schlichtholz B, Teillaud JL, et al. p53 antibodies in patients with various types of cancer: assay, identification, and characterization. Clin Cancer Res. 1995;1:1463–9.

Mange A, Lacombe J, Bascoul-Mollevi C, et al. Serum autoantibody signature of ductal carcinoma in situ progression to invasive breast cancer. Clin Cancer Res. 2012;18:1992–2000.

Mintz PJ, Kim J, Do KA, et al. Fingerprinting the circulating repertoire of antibodies from cancer patients. Nat Biotechnol. 2003;21:57–63.

Murphy MA, O'Connell DJ, O'Kane SL, et al. Epitope presentation is an important determinant of the utility of antigens identified from protein arrays in the development of autoantibody diagnostic assays. J Proteomics. 2012a;75:4668–75.

Murphy MA, O'Leary JJ, Cahill DJ. Assessment of the humoral immune response to cancer. J Proteomics. 2012b;75:4573–9.

Nam MJ, Madoz-Gurpide J, Wang H, et al. Molecular profiling of the immune response in colon cancer using protein microarrays: occurrence of autoantibodies to ubiquitin C-terminal hydrolase L3. Proteomics. 2003;3:2108–15.

O'Rourke DJ, DiJohnson DA, Caiazzo RJ, et al. Autoantibody signatures as biomarkers to distinguish prostate cancer from benign prostatic hyperplasia in patients with increased serum prostate specific antigen. Clin Chim Acta. 2012;413:561–7.

Ochiai H, Ohishi T, Osumi K, et al. Reevaluation of serum p53 antibody as a tumor marker in colorectal cancer patients. Surg Today. 2012;42:164–8.

Oishi Y, Yunomura S, Kawahashi Y, et al. Escherichia coli proteome chips for detecting protein-protein interactions. Proteomics. 2006;6:6433–6.

Orenes-Pinero E, Barderas R, Rico D, et al. Serum and tissue profiling in bladder cancer combining protein and tissue arrays. J Proteome Res. 2010;9:164–73.

Pallasch CP, Struss AK, Munnia A, et al. Autoantibodies against GLEA2 and PHF3 in glioblastoma: tumor-associated autoantibodies correlated with prolonged survival. Int J Cancer. 2005;117:456–9.

Pedersen JW, Blixt O, Bennett EP, et al. Seromic profiling of colorectal cancer patients with novel glycopeptide microarray. Int J Cancer. 2011;128:1860–71.

Pedersen JW, Gentry-Maharaj A, Fourkala EO, et al. Early detection of cancer in the general population: a blinded case–control study of p53 autoantibodies in colorectal cancer. Br J Cancer. 2013;108:107–14.

Pedersen JW, Gentry-Maharaj A, Nostdal A, et al. Cancer associated auto-antibodies to MUC1 and MUC4 – A blinded case control study of colorectal cancer in UK Collaborative Trial of Ovarian Cancer Screening (UKCTOCS). Int J Cancer. 2014;134:2180–88.

Pelaez-Garcia A, Barderas R, Torres S, et al. FGFR4 role in epithelial-mesenchymal transition and its therapeutic value in colorectal cancer. PLoS One. 2013;8:e63695.

Pepe MS, Etzioni R, Feng Z, et al. Phases of biomarker development for early detection of cancer. J Natl Cancer Inst. 2001;93:1054–61.

Qiu J, Madoz-Gurpide J, Misek DE, et al. Development of natural protein microarrays for diagnosing cancer based on an antibody response to tumor antigens. J Proteome Res. 2004;3:261–7.

Ramachandran N, Hainsworth E, Bhullar B, et al. Self-assembling protein microarrays. Science. 2004;305:86–90.

Ran YL, Hu H, Zhou Z, et al. Profiling tumor-associated autoantibodies for the detection of colon cancer. Clin Cancer Res. 2008;14:2696–700.

Reipert BM, Tanneberger S, Pannetta A, et al. Increase in autoantibodies against Fas (CD95) during carcinogenesis in the human colon: a hope for the immunoprevention of cancer? Cancer Immunol Immunother. 2005;54:1038–42.

Sahin U, Tureci O, Schmitt H, et al. Human neoplasms elicit multiple specific immune responses in the autologous host. Proc Natl Acad Sci U S A. 1995;92:11810–3.

Scanlan MJ, Chen YT, Williamson B, et al. Characterization of human colon cancer antigens recognized by autologous antibodies. Int J Cancer. 1998;76:652–8.

Scanlan MJ, Welt S, Gordon CM, et al. Cancer-related serological recognition of human colon cancer: identification of potential diagnostic and immunotherapeutic targets. Cancer Res. 2002;62:4041–7.

Schmetzer O, Moldenhauer G, Riesenberg R, et al. Quality of recombinant protein determines the amount of autoreactivity detected against the tumor-associated epithelial cell adhesion molecule antigen: low frequency of antibodies against the natural protein. J Immunol. 2005;174:942–52.

Shebzukhov YV, Koroleva EP, Khlgatian SV, et al. Antibody response to a non-conserved C-terminal part of human histone deacetylase 3 in colon cancer patients. Int J Cancer. 2005;117:800–6.

Song MH, Ha JC, Lee SM, et al. Identification of BCP-20 (FBXO39) as a cancer/testis antigen from colon cancer patients by SEREX. Biochem Biophys Res Commun. 2011;408:195–201.

Soussi T. p53 antibodies in the sera of patients with various types of cancer: a review. Cancer Res. 2000;60:1777–88.

Syrigos KN, Charalampopoulos A, Pliarchopoulou K, et al. Prognostic significance of autoantibodies against tropomyosin in patients with colorectal adenocarcinoma. Hybridoma. 1999;18:543–6.

Syrigos KN, Charalambopoulos A, Pliarchopoulou K, et al. The prognostic significance of autoantibodies against dsDNA in patients with colorectal adenocarcinoma. Anticancer Res. 2000;20:4351–3.

Takulapalli BR, Qiu J, Magee DM, et al. High density diffusion-free nanowell arrays. J Proteome Res. 2012;11:4382–91.

Tang RP, Ko MC, Wang JY, et al. Humoral response to P53 in human colorectal tumors: a prospective study of 1,209 patients. Int J Cancer. 2001;94:859–63.

Villanueva J, Shaffer DR, Philip J, et al. Differential exoprotease activities confer tumor-specific serum peptidome patterns. J Clin Invest. 2006;116:271–84.

Wandall HH, Blixt O, Tarp MA, et al. Cancer biomarkers defined by autoantibody signatures to aberrant O-glycopeptide epitopes. Cancer Res. 2010;70:1306–13.

Wang X, Yu J, Sreekumar A, et al. Autoantibody signatures in prostate cancer. N Engl J Med. 2005;353:1224–35.

Zhu H, Snyder M. Protein arrays and microarrays. Curr Opin Chem Biol. 2001;5:40–5.

Zhu H, Bilgin M, Bangham R, et al. Global analysis of protein activities using proteome chips. Science. 2001;293:2101–5.

Biomarkers in Metastatic Colorectal Cancer 27

Predicting Prognosis and Therapeutic Response

Connie I. Diakos, Kellie A. Charles, Wei Chua, Viive M. Howell, and Stephen J. Clarke

Contents

C.I. Diakos • V.M. Howell • S.J. Clarke (✉)
Kolling Institute of Medical Research, Royal North Shore Hospital, University of Sydney, St Leonards, NSW, Australia
e-mail: connie.diakos@sydney.edu.au; viive.howell@sydney.edu.au; stephen.clarke@sydney.edu.au

K.A. Charles
School of Medical Sciences (Pharmacology), Sydney Medical School, University of Sydney, St Leonards, NSW, Australia
e-mail: kellie.charles@sydney.edu.au

W. Chua
Department of Medical Oncology, Liverpool Hospital, Liverpool, NSW, Australia
e-mail: wei.chua2@sswahs.health.nsw.gov.au

V.R. Preedy, V.B. Patel (eds.), *Biomarkers in Cancer, Biomarkers in Disease: Methods, Discoveries and Applications*,
DOI 10.1007/978-94-007-7681-4_1

Abstract
Significant advances in chemotherapeutics over the past decade have seen a doubling in the median survival time of patients with metastatic colorectal cancer. However, this comes at the cost of toxicity to the patient and financial burden to the community. Biomarkers to predict disease course and treatment response are therefore of major importance so as to allow for the judicious selection of treatment candidates and agents and doses. This review seeks to summarize the current markers available for the prediction of prognosis and treatment response in metastatic colorectal cancer.

List of Abbreviations

5-FU	5-fluorouracil
ASCO	American Society of Clinical Oncology
BMI	Body Mass Index
BSA	Body Surface Area
CRP	C-Reactive Protein
DACH	Diaminocyclohexane
DFS	Disease-Free Survival
DNA	Deoxyribonucleic Acid
DPD	Dihydropyrimidine Dehydrogenase
EGFR	Epithelial Growth Factor Receptor
ERCC-1	Excision Repair Cross-Complementing Group 1
GPS	Glasgow Prognosis Score
GST	Glutathione-S-Transferase
HIF-1α	Hypoxia-Inducible Factor 1α
KRAS	Kirsten Rat Sarcoma Viral Oncogene
LDH	Lactate Dehydrogenase
mAb	Monoclonal Antibody
MAPK	Mitogen-Activated Protein Kinase
mCRC	Metastatic Colorectal Cancer
MMR	Mismatch Repair
MSI	Microsatellite Instability
MSS	Microsatellite Stability
MTHFR	Methylenetetrahydrofolate Reductase
NF-κβ	Nuclear Factor-κβ
NLR	Neutrophil to Lymphocyte Ratio
NRAS	Neuroblastoma Ras
OS	Overall Survival
PD-ECGF	Platelet-Derived Endothelial Cell Growth Factor
PFS	Progression-Free Survival
PI3K	Phosphatidylinositol-3-kinase
PLR	Platelet to Lymphocyte Ratio
RCT	Randomized Controlled Trial
RNA	Ribonucleic Acid
RR	Response Rate

SNP	Single-Nucleotide Polymorphism
STAT3	Signal Transducers and Activators of Transcription 3
TCGA	The Cancer Genome Atlas
THBS2	Thrombospondin-2
Topo-1	Topoisomerase-1
TP	Thymidine Phosphorylase
TS	Thymidylate Synthase
UGT	Uridine-Diphosphoglucuronosyl Transferase
VEGF	Vascular Endothelial Growth Factor
WT	Wild Type
XPD	Xeroderma Pigmentosum Complementation Group D
XRCC-1	X-Ray Repair Cross-Complementing Protein 1

Key Facts of Biomarkers in Metastatic Colorectal Cancer

- Colorectal cancer (CRC) is the second most prevalent cancer worldwide and the third leading cause of cancer-related death.
- CRC is largely a disease of the elderly, with a median age of 69 years at diagnosis.
- When diagnosed in the early stages, CRC is one of the most curable of cancers. However, 20–25 % of patients already have metastatic disease at the time of diagnosis, i.e., cancer that has already spread beyond the bowel, which is generally incurable. A further 25 % of patients with early-stage disease will progress to metastatic disease following their surgery.
- Advances in chemotherapy and targeted agents over the past 10 years have seen a doubling of the median survival of patients with metastatic CRC (mCRC).
- The significant costs, both financial and in terms of side effects, make appropriate selection of treatment candidates vital.
- The personalization of cancer medicine through the use of biomarkers that predict disease course or response to therapy is a hallmark of modern medical oncology.
- Few biomarkers exist that accurately and consistently predict prognosis or treatment response, so continued research in this area is highly important.

Definitions of Words and Terms

Bevacizumab A monoclonal antibody against VEGF used in the treatment of metastatic colorectal cancer.

Biomarker Any entity that allows for individualized prediction of disease course or response to therapy.

Cetuximab A monoclonal antibody against EGFR used in the treatment of metastatic colorectal cancer.

Chemotherapy Chemical agents used in the systemic treatment of cancer.

Colorectal Cancer Cancer of the large bowel or rectum.

Epithelial Growth Factor Receptor (EGFR) A cell surface receptor frequently overexpressed in epithelial tumors.

Panitumumab A monoclonal antibody against EGFR used in the treatment of metastatic colorectal cancer.

Predictive Biomarker An entity that describes the impact of a treatment on outcome.

Prognostic Biomarker A factor relating to outcome that is independent of treatment.

Targeted Aagents/Targeted Antibodies Biological agents against specific molecular targets in a tumor.

Vascular Endothelial Growth Factor (VEGFR) A cell surface receptor linked to blood vessel formation in tumors and normal tissues.

Wild Type A gene that is unmutated.

Introduction

Colorectal cancer (CRC) is one of the most common of cancers and one of the leading causes of cancer mortality worldwide. Yet it is also one of the most treatable. While 40–50 % of patients develop or present with metastatic disease, significant advances in chemotherapeutics and targeted agents over the past decade have seen a doubling in the median overall survival of patients with metastatic CRC (mCRC) from 10 to more than 20 months. However, these improvements come at a cost, of a financial nature to government health budgets and of toxicities to the individual patient. Hence the selection of appropriate drugs and treatment candidates is paramount, especially in this new age of personalized medicine.

Predictive and prognostic biomarkers are vital in facilitating the ongoing personalization of treatment for mCRC. Predictive biomarkers pertain to the impact of specific treatments on outcome, described by response rates or survival. Prognostic biomarkers relate to outcomes that are independent of treatment. There are few biomarkers in routine clinical use currently for mCRC, including tumor-node-metastasis staging and histopathological features with their well-established prognostic role. However, these do not provide information of treatment response; to date, only *KRAS* mutation status has attained routine clinical use in mCRC, with the negative impact of *KRAS* mutations on treatment with epithelial growth factor receptor (EGFR) inhibitors now well established.

This review summarizes the advances made into the personalization of mCRC treatment by examining the evidence around existing biomarkers and discusses potential new markers for the prediction of disease course and treatment response.

Prognostic Biomarkers

Few prognostic markers exist for mCRC. Tumor staging and histopathological features are well established, but the majority of other entities examined have not been consistent in their utility between studies (summarized in Table 1).

Inflammation

Inflammation is a cardinal feature of malignancy, contributing to the development of cancers and playing a key role in cancer progression (Colotta et al. 2009;

Table 1 Prognostic factors in mCRC

Factor	Evidence	Utility	Reference
Patient age >85 years	Conclusive	Negative prognostic factor	Field et al. 2008
Obesity	Limited	Extremely obese patients have higher risk of local recurrence and cancer-specific mortality	Dignam et al. 2006
Smoking	Inconclusive	Heavy smokers have worse outcome	McCleary et al. 2010
Exercise	Limited	Lower risk of recurrence with more exercise	Meyerhardt et al. 2006
Glasgow prognosis score	Limited	Abnormal score associated with worse outcome after surgical resection and for inoperable CRC	McMillan 2013
Neutrophil/ lymphocyte ratio	Limited	High ratio correlates with worse PFS and OS in patients undergoing chemotherapy	Chua et al. 2011
MSI	Considerable	Positive prognostic factor in adjuvant setting; negative in metastatic setting	Popat et al. 2005; Tran et al. 2011
BRAF mutations	Considerable	Negative prognostic factor	Van Cutsem et al. 2011b; Samowitz et al. 2005
KRAS mutations	Insufficient	Negative prognostic factor	Andreyev et al. 2001
PIK3CA mutations	Insufficient	Negative prognostic marker for rectal cancer	Sartore-Bianchi et al. 2009

Hanahan and Weinberg 2011). In established cancers, inflammatory symptoms such as fevers, sweats, and weight loss occur commonly, and evidence exists that a systemic inflammatory response is predictive of worse outcomes in a number of malignancies, with earlier cancer recurrence and reduced cancer-specific survival (Clarke et al. 2011; Moore et al. 2010). Inflammation has also been shown to result in slower clearance of anticancer drugs and worse toxicities (Robertson et al. 2008; Kacevska et al. 2008).

Both local and systemic inflammations have demonstrated roles in prognosis (Roxburgh and McMillan 2010, 2012). Systemic inflammation appears to be mediated by the release of proinflammatory cytokines from the tumor itself, its supporting vasculature, and/or stroma (Charles et al. 2006). Chronic inflammation may be involved in the development and progression of cancers through a number of pathways, such as nuclear factor-κβ (NF-κβ) and signal transducers and activators of transcription 3 (STAT3) (Aggarwal et al. 2009).

Glasgow Prognosis Score (GPS)

Over the past decade, several markers of the systemic inflammatory response have been evaluated to determine utility as prognostic or predictive markers in CRC. These include plasma C-reactive protein (CRP), hypoalbuminemia, and the Glasgow prognosis score (GPS), comprising a three-point score based on CRP and serum albumin concentrations (McMillan 2013). The prognostic value of an abnormal baseline GPS in mCRC has been demonstrated, with utility in predicting survival in patients undergoing chemotherapy, as well as grade 2/3 toxicity from capecitabine chemotherapy.

Neutrophil to Lymphocyte Ratio (NLR)

Components of the full blood count have been evaluated as biomarkers, including white cell count, the platelet to lymphocyte ratio (PLR), and the neutrophil to lymphocyte ratio (NLR). An elevated pretreatment white cell count and NLR were independent predictors of worse survival in patients receiving chemotherapy for advanced CRC (Chua et al. 2011). Baseline NLR has been shown to negatively correlate with progression-free survival (PFS) and overall survival (OS) in patients undergoing chemotherapy, with normalization of the NLR after one cycle of chemotherapy reflective of an improvement in survival, versus poor survival if the NLR remained abnormal (Chua et al. 2011).

Patient-Related Factors

Age

CRC is largely a disease of the elderly, with a median age of 69 years at diagnosis and an increasing incidence with age. There is, however, little evidence to support age as either a prognostic or predictive factor in CRC. Most of the information on the treatment response of the elderly with CRC comes from pooled analyses in the adjuvant setting, where similar benefits have been demonstrated irrespective of age.

These findings suggest that age alone is not predictive of treatment response (Sargent et al. 2001; Goldberg et al. 2006).

Importantly, until recently, only very small numbers of patients aged ≥80 have been included in clinical trials, and those that have are a select group with good performance status and few comorbidities. Very advanced age could, however, be considered a negative prognostic factor for mCRC, as a recent retrospective study has demonstrated a large number of deaths occurring without disease recurrence, from competing causes of mortality (Field et al. 2008). With the growing interest in onco-geriatrics, two phase III studies targeting elderly patients with mCRC have been conducted, examining combination chemotherapy. Nonsignificant improvements in PFS were found with the addition of a second agent although reduced dosing regimens or large proportions of patients requiring dose reductions were a factor (Seymour et al. 2011b; Mitry et al. 2012).

The perception that elderly patients experience increased toxicities from chemotherapy is an important factor in decision-making by clinicians, and a number of scoring systems to assist in the prediction of toxicity risk have been developed (Aparicio et al. 2013; Extermann et al. 2012). The impact of age on toxicity has been examined, with conflicting results. In general, elderly patients experience increased severe toxicities with 5-fluorouracil (5-FU) (Sargent et al. 2001), but in combination regimens, severe toxicities occur at similar rates to younger patients, while lower-grade toxicities are more common (Goldberg et al. 2006; Mitry et al. 2012).

Obesity

While there is overwhelming evidence to support the association between obesity and the risk of developing CRC, there is conflicting evidence on the prognostic value of obesity in CRC. Very obese patients (body mass index [BMI] ≥35 kg/m^2) have demonstrated higher risk of cancer recurrence or death compared to those of normal weight, with no difference in risk of chemotherapy-related toxicities (Dignam et al. 2006). However, the reverse has also been found, with neither BMI nor weight change found to be associated with increased risk of cancer recurrence or death (Meyerhardt et al. 2008).

This conflicting evidence is perhaps due to the issue of drug dosing, as commonly the body surface area (BSA) is capped for obese patients, rather than dosing on actual body weight, thus leading to the possibility of underdosing in obese patients. It is well known that BSA is not predictive of drug handling in obese patients (Chambers et al. 2011). Indeed, nonrandomized evidence from three trials involving mCRC patients suggested worse outcomes when reduced dosing was given to obese patients (Chambers et al. 2011). The current recommendations from the American Society of Clinical Oncology (ASCO) are for full weight-based dosing of chemotherapy in obese patients with cancer, particularly when treatment is with curative intent (Griggs et al. 2012).

Lifestyle Factors

The prognostic or predictive value of factors such as diet, exercise, smoking, and alcohol consumption is not well established in mCRC, despite their role in the development of CRC being well known (Martinez 2005). Exercise is important for CRC patients, with more exercise undertaken leading to a lower risk of disease recurrence (Meyerhardt et al. 2006). Very heavy smokers have been shown to have a slightly worse outcome, but smoking in general appears to have negligible impact on outcome (McCleary et al. 2010). One explanation for the impact of lifestyle factors on cancer outcome is that a different biology of the tumor is induced, supported by preliminary data suggesting different genetic mutations caused by smoking and diabetes (Limsui et al. 2010).

Tumor-Related Factors

Microsatellite Instability

CRC is considered a genetic disease characterized by sequential genetic and epigenetic alterations marking its histological progression. Microsatellite instability (MSI) is a signature borne of inactivation of the DNA mismatch repair (MMR) system, seen in approximately 15 % of CRC tumors either due to epigenetic silencing of *MLH1* or germline mutation in one of the four MMR genes (Vilar and Gruber 2010). Tumors with high levels of MSI (MSI-H) exhibit a distinct phenotype, being more commonly right sided, poorly differentiated, mucin-containing, and occurring most commonly in females. These tumors are more common in early stage, i.e., stage II, CRC. Yet despite these normally adverse histological features, MSI-H tumors have a more favorable prognosis and lower risk of recurrence than MSI-low (MSI-L) or microsatellite-stable (MSS) tumors (Popat et al. 2005). In the metastatic setting, however, MSI is associated with poorer survival, driven by its association with *BRAF* mutation (Tran et al. 2011).

Epithelial Growth Factor Receptor

Overexpression of EGFR is a negative prognostic marker for mCRC, as activation of the EGFR pathway correlates with an aggressive phenotype, with greater proliferation and angiogenesis and reduced apoptosis. It is also associated with chemotherapy and radiotherapy resistance (reviewed in Markman et al. (2010)). EGFR is overexpressed in 50–70 % of CRCs.

KRAS and *BRAF* Mutations

Mutations in *KRAS* are the most commonly described in the *Ras/Raf/MAPK* pathway in CRC, with between a third to a half of patients with CRC carrying a *KRAS* mutation (De Mattos-Arruda et al. 2011). The prognostic significance of *KRAS* is unclear, with the large RASCAL2 collaborative trial suggesting that a mutation in codon 12 (glycine to valine) of the *KRAS* gene had a significant impact on survival in patients with Dukes C CRC (Andreyev et al. 2001), although this was not confirmed in a large adjuvant trial (PETACC-3) (Roth et al. 2012). Several monotherapy trials of EGFR monoclonal antibodies (mAbs) versus best supportive care have also failed to show *KRAS* status to be an important prognostic marker in patients receiving best supportive care alone (Karapetis et al. 2008; Amado et al. 2008).

BRAF codes for a downstream effector of *KRAS* in the *Ras/Raf/MAPK* pathway, with mutations identified in 10–15 % of CRC tumors (De Mattos-Arruda et al. 2011), the most common being the *BRAF V600E* mutation which accounts for 90 % of all *BRAF* mutations in CRC. *BRAF V600E* is usually mutually exclusive of *KRAS* mutations and is considered to be a poor prognostic marker in CRC with a more aggressive phenotype (Van Cutsem et al. 2011b; Samowitz et al. 2005), with evidence from several studies of a significantly higher cancer-specific mortality and worse OS in patients who are *KRAS* wild type (WT) with a *BRAF V600E* mutation, compared to those who are *BRAF V600E* WT (Rizzo et al. 2010; Van Cutsem et al. 2011b).

PIK3CA Mutations

A component of the PI3K/PTEN/AKT pathway, *PIK3CA* is responsible for producing PI3K, the catalytic component of the pathway. Mutations in *PIK3CA* occur in around 20 % of CRC tumors with *KRAS* mutations (Sartore-Bianchi et al. 2009). Loss-of-function mutations of the tumor suppressor *PTEN* can also activate the PI3K/AKT pathway, with *PTEN* loss occurring in around 20–40 % of CRC tumors (Laurent-Puig et al. 2009). The presence of *PIK3CA* mutations has been suggested to predict poor prognosis for mCRC patients (Sartore-Bianchi et al. 2009), and loss of *PTEN* expression has been associated with an aggressive phenotype in CRC (Sawai et al. 2008).

Vascular Endothelial Growth Factor

Fifty to seventy percent of CRCs express vascular endothelial growth factor (VEGF); however, its value as a prognostic marker is unclear, with conflicting results having been found among studies. VEGF tumor expression has been shown to have no significant prognostic utility (Jubb et al. 2006; Khorana et al. 2003), but it has been shown to correlate with increased microvessel density and poor prognosis (Manley et al. 2002). Similarly microvessel density has also shown contradictory results, with no prognostic value demonstrated in the Jubb study (Jubb et al. 2006). VEGF expression has been shown to be associated with increased median survival when expressed in tumor-associated macrophages/stroma (Khorana et al. 2003), giving rise to the possibility of a link with the causes and consequences of local inflammation. The VEGF ligands VEGF-A and -D have demonstrated prognostic value through studies showing that high expression correlates with tumor aggressiveness and shortened survival times (Kopetz et al. 2010; Moehler et al. 2008).

Predictive Biomarkers

Predictive biomarkers predict response to treatment, either in the form of outcome or toxicity. Measures used to describe these include response rates and survival.

Predicting Chemotherapeutic Response and Toxicity

Few biomarkers exist that predict chemotherapy utility or toxicity from therapy. The majority have generally demonstrated inconsistency of results, often due to technical issues of assay variability. Table 2 lists the chemotherapeutic agents used in the treatment of CRC, and Table 3 summarizes factors that have been assessed as prognostic or predictive of response.

Markers to Predict 5-FU Response and Toxicity

Mismatch repair deficiency is the single predictive marker of chemotherapy response to demonstrate consistent study results. In addition to having a more favorable prognosis and lower risk of recurrence, it has been reported that patients with MSI-H tumors may not benefit from 5-FU-based adjuvant chemotherapy due to a lack of sensitivity, with only MSS or MSI-L tumors benefitting (Des Guetz et al. 2009).

5-FU remains a key component in CRC treatment, both in the adjuvant and palliative settings. Its main mechanism of action is via inhibition of thymidylate synthase (TS), whose expression may be influenced by genetic variants of the *TYMS* gene. A significant inverse association between the number of 28-base pair tandem repeats in the *TYMS* promoter region and the severity of toxicity has been found, although the sensitivity and specificity is low (Schwab et al. 2008). Studies on TS expression and prognosis in CRC have shown high TS levels to be associated with

Table 2 Agents used in the treatment of mCRC and their biological targets

Agents	Target	Clinical place
5-fluorouracil/ capecitabine/S1	Inhibition of TS	Established, as single agent or combination regimens
Oxaliplatin	Nuclear DNA; intrastrand adduct formation	Established, in combination with 5-FU and leucovorin (FOLFOX) or capecitabine (CAPOX)
Irinotecan	Inhibition of topo-1	Established; combined regimen (FOLFIRI) and single-agent with cetuximab
Cetuximab	Chimeric IgG1 mAb against EGFR	Established in combination with irinotecan chemotherapy after prior treatment
Panitumumab	Fully human IgG2 mAb against EGFR	Established in combination with irinotecan chemotherapy after prior treatment
Bevacizumab	mAb against VEGF-A	Established as first-line treatment in combination with chemotherapy
Aflibercept	VEGF-A, -B, and placental growth factor inhibitor	Phase III RCT evidence of efficacy after previous treatment
Regorafenib	Multi-targeted tyrosine kinase inhibitor against VEGF	Phase III RCT evidence of efficacy after previous treatment
Valatinib	Oral VEGF inhibitor	Phase III RCT evidence of efficacy as first-line treatment in combination with chemotherapy

Table 3 Prognostic and predictive factors for chemotherapy in mCRC

Factor	Evidence	Utility	Reference
MSI	Considerable	Predicts lack of benefit from 5-FU	Des Guetz et al. 2009
TS polymorphisms	Insufficient	Predicts toxicity from 5-FU	Popat et al. 2006; Soong et al. 2008; Koopman et al. 2009b
DPD expression	Inconsistent	Low DPD predicts for greater 5-FU toxicity	Vallbohmer et al. 2007; Koopman et al. 2009c
TP expression	Conflicting	Evidence of both better and worse outcome and response to 5-FU	Soong et al. 2008; Meropol et al. 2006
MTHFR polymorphisms	Inconsistent	Potential predictive marker for 5-FU	Gusella et al. 2009; Ruzzo et al. 2007
ERCC-1 variant expression	Insufficient	Predictive of improved OS with *TT* or *CT* genotypes with oxaliplatin	Viguier et al. 2005; Moreno et al. 2006
XPD variant expression	Inconsistent	Improved RR, PFS, or OS with platinum drugs	Le Morvan et al. 2007
GSTP1 variant expression	Inconsistent	Prediction of oxaliplatin response	Stoehlmacher et al. 2002
GSTP1 variant	Conflicting	Prediction of oxaliplatin neurotoxicity	Lecomte et al. 2006; Ruzzo et al. 2007
Topo-1	Inconsistent	Low expression potentially negative predictor of irinotecan or oxaliplatin response	Braun et al. 2008; Koopman et al. 2009a
*UGT1A1*28* allele	Insufficient	Increased irinotecan-induced toxicity and perhaps improved response	Iyer et al. 2002; Hoskins et al. 2007
UGT locus	Insufficient	Potentially predictive of irinotecan-induced toxicity	Innocenti et al. 2004; Cecchin et al. 2009

poorer OS (Popat et al. 2004). Three large studies have examined TS expression in patients receiving 5-FU-based chemotherapy in the adjuvant setting, with no significant association between TS expression and outcome (Popat et al. 2006; Soong et al. 2008; Koopman et al. 2009b).

The enzymes dihydropyrimidine dehydrogenase (DPD), thymidine phosphorylase (TP), and methylenetetrahydrofolate reductase (MTHFR) have been examined for their predictive value for 5-FU chemotherapy. DPD is the rate-limiting enzyme in 5-FU metabolism, resulting in the formation of inactive dihydrofluorouracil that is eventually converted to fluoro-beta-alanine for hepatic excretion. Low DPD expression could cause a decrease in 5-FU catabolism and higher intracellular levels, resulting in increased neutropenia, stomatitis, and death (Wei et al. 1996). In patients with unexpectedly severe toxicity after 5-FU treatment, reduced DPD activity was seen in the peripheral mononuclear cells of at least 55 % of patients (van Kuilenburg et al. 2000). However, results have not been consistent. While low DPD levels have been associated with longer disease-free survival (DFS) or OS with fluoropyrimidine use in the metastatic setting (Vallbohmer et al. 2007; Koopman et al. 2009c), the reverse has also been found (Meropol et al. 2006).

TP is involved in the conversion of 5-FU to its active metabolite FdUMP and it is postulated that high levels result in better outcomes and responses. However, high TP levels may also confer a poorer outcome, given that TP is also known as platelet-derived endothelial cell growth factor (PD-ECGF), which has been associated with angiogenesis (Matsumura et al. 1998) and positively correlates with microvessel density (Matsuura et al. 1999). Not surprisingly, conflicting evidence exists regarding the utility of TP as a prognostic or predictive marker (Soong et al. 2008; Koopman et al. 2009b; Meropol et al. 2006).

MTHFR is the main enzyme involved in the conversion of 5,10-methylenetetrahydrofolate, as complex crucial in the activity of 5-FU; *MTHFR* polymorphisms responsible for 5,10-methylenetetrahydrofolate could therefore play an important role in the cytotoxicity of 5-FU. While numerous studies have examined this issue, the results have been inconsistent (Gusella et al. 2009; Chua et al. 2009; Capitain et al. 2008; Ruzzo et al. 2007).

Markers to Predict Oxaliplatin Response and Toxicity

Oxaliplatin ($PtCl_2$(1,2-diaminocyclohexane (DACH)]) exerts its cytotoxic effect primarily through formation of intrastrand DNA adducts, leading to inhibition of DNA replication and induction of apoptosis. Genetic variants such as single-nucleotide polymorphisms (SNPs) in genes involved in any of the DNA repair pathways may account for differences in individual responses or toxicity to oxaliplatin chemotherapy, but so far, no consistently useful biomarker has been found.

The excision repair cross-complementing group 1 (ERCC-1) and xeroderma pigmentosum complementation group D (XPD or ERCC-2) proteins are involved in the nuclear excision repair (NER) pathway. ERCC-1 SNPs or protein expression has failed to demonstrate clinical utility in prediction of outcome from oxaliplatin regimens in mCRC. The synonymous *ERCC1* variant Asn118Asn (C > T, rs11615) has shown improved RR or survival for mCRC patients with the *TT* (homozygous *mutant type*) or *CT* genotype when compared to patients with the *CC* genotype (homozygous *wild type*) (Viguier et al. 2005; Moreno et al. 2006), while other studies have found patients with the *T* allele to have worse survival or disease progression (Chua et al. 2009; Ruzzo et al. 2007; Stoehlmacher et al. 2004). An association between low *ERCC1* mRNA and protein expression with improved survival was seen in several small studies (Shirota et al. 2001; Kim et al. 2009) but not in two recent large randomized controlled trials (RCTs) (Koopman et al. 2009c; Braun et al. 2008). Similarly the *xeroderma pigmentosum* genes have failed to demonstrate consistency with the *ERCC2* missense variant Lys751Gln (rs13181) having demonstrated an association with improved RR, event-free survival, or PFS and OS with platinum drugs in some studies (Park et al. 2001; Le Morvan et al. 2007) but not in others (Moreno et al. 2006; Braun et al. 2008).

X-ray repair cross-complementing protein 1 (XRCC-1) is involved in DNA repair via the base-excision repair pathway. *XRCC1* polymorphisms have been investigated but generally not shown any association with outcome or toxicity (Chua et al. 2009; Ruzzo et al. 2007; Braun et al. 2008, 2009; Stoehlmacher et al. 2004). Similarly, detrimental effects of the missense variant Gln399Arg (rs25487) were seen on response rate (RR) in a large case–control study (Suh et al. 2006) but with improved prognosis for patients treated adjuvantly (Moreno et al. 2006).

Glutathione-S-transferase (GST) facilitates platinum-DACH binding to glutathione, with this new complex preventing platinum/DNA binding and thus rendering the platinum compound inactive (Kweekel et al. 2005). The missense variant Ile105Val (rs1695) in *GSTP1* has been investigated for its utility as a biomarker, given that it produces a variant GSTP1 protein that has demonstrated decreased ability to detoxify carcinogens (Kweekel et al. 2005); however, results have been inconsistent. A statistically significant reduction in the risk of death from advanced CRC has been shown for patients possessing the Ile105Val variant, with the greatest benefit being for those homozygous for Ile105Val (Stoehlmacher et al. 2002); however, subsequent studies failed to show a significant association between the Ile105Val variant or protein expression and survival or tumor response (Ruzzo et al. 2007; Braun et al. 2008; Kweekel et al. 2009). The influence of *GSTP1* variant on oxaliplatin-induced neurotoxicity has similarly been conflicting, with no influence on (Kweekel et al. 2009), increased (Ruzzo et al. 2007), and decreased (Lecomte et al. 2006) severe neuropathy all having been associated.

Markers to Predict Irinotecan Response and Toxicity

Irinotecan, a camptothecin analog, is converted to SN-38 in the liver, which inhibits the topoisomerase-1 (topo-1) enzyme and eventually inhibits DNA replication and transcription. Topo-1 is overexpressed in >40 % of CRCs (Paradiso et al. 2004), but its predictive value is inconclusive. Topo-1 was found to be predictive of outcome in a study of advanced CRC examining sequential versus combination chemotherapy, with patients with low levels of Topo-1 failing to derive a benefit from irinotecan or oxaliplatin combinations, while patients with high Topo-1 levels did better with combination rather than sequential treatment with longer median survival (Braun et al. 2008). However, validation of these results with the CAIRO study failed, with no correlation found between Topo-1 levels and OS (Koopman et al. 2009a).

Uridine-diphosphoglucuronosyl transferase (UGT) is the enzyme responsible for elimination of SN-38 by glucuronidation. It is encoded by the *UGT1A1* gene with its activity related to the number of TA repeats in the promoter region of each allele. Patients homozygous for the *UGT1A1*28* allele have been shown to have increased SN-38 concentrations due to decreased enzyme levels (Iyer et al. 1998), so the relationship between *UGT1A1*28* and irinotecan-induced toxicities has been investigated with inconsistent results. Patients with *UGT1A1*28/*28* genotype have demonstrated increased hematological toxicity requiring lower irinotecan starting doses, together with perhaps improved responses (Iyer et al. 2002; Liu et al. 2008; Hoskins et al. 2007); increased risk of grades 3–4 diarrhea has also been associated with the *UGT1A1*28* allele (Iyer et al. 2002; Ando et al. 2000). However, in the larger adjuvant PETACC3 and metastatic FOCUS studies, *UGT1A1*28* polymorphisms showed only weak or no association with toxicity (Roth et al. 2008; Braun et al. 2009). Similarly, *UGT1A1*28* polymorphisms have failed to demonstrate an association with treatment outcome or survival in mCRC (Liu et al. 2008). A significant racial association has been shown with the *UGT1A1*28* genotype, being more common in African-Americans than Caucasians, where high-grade adverse events and RR were significantly higher in Caucasians treated with modern combination chemotherapy regimens (Sanoff et al. 2009). UGT1A1 is part of a complex genomic locus (2q37) that encodes a number of uridine-diphosphoglucuronosyl transferases, and other members of this family have also shown potential utility in predicting neutropenia (Innocenti et al. 2004), such as *UGT1A7* (Cecchin et al. 2009). This suggests the entire *UGT* locus may be important, rather than just a single SNP.

Predicting Response to Targeted Agents

Targeted biological agents can exert a significant impact on a patient's prognosis, with the search for predictive biomarkers to aid selection of appropriate recipient patients the subject of considerable interest. The high costs associated with targeted agents have made the search for methods to improve their cost-effectiveness paramount. Most of the focus so far has been on tumor-related factors given the key influence they exert on response to biological agents. Table 4 summarizes factors assessed as predictive for targeted therapy benefit.

Predicting Response to EGFR Therapy

Belonging to the human epidermal growth factor receptor family, epithelial growth factor receptor (EGFR) is a receptor tyrosine kinase frequently overexpressed in epithelial tumors. Upon the binding of a ligand to the extracellular domain of EGFR, intracellular signaling is activated along one of several main pathways. The two major pathways are the RAS/RAF/mitogen-activated protein kinase (MAPK) pathway and the phosphatidylinositol 3-kinase/Akt (PI3K/Akt) pathway (Fig. 1).

There are two main routes of targeting EGFR therapeutically: these are the small-molecule tyrosine kinase inhibitors that target specific activating mutations in the intracellular domain of the receptor and have demonstrated utility in the treatment of non-small cell lung cancers and pancreatic cancers with these mutations and the mABs that are directed against the extracellular domain and overexpression of wild-type EGFR, with their established value in the treatment of mCRC and head and neck squamous cell carcinoma. In the case of mCRC,

Table 4 Predictive factors for targeted therapies in mCRC

Factor	Evidence	Utility	Reference
KRAS mutations	Conclusive	Negative predictive marker for EGFR mAbs	Van Cutsem et al. 2009; Linardou et al. 2008
BRAF mutations	Insufficient	Potential negative predictive marker for EGFR mAbs	Laurent-Puig et al. 2009
NRAS mutations	Insufficient	Potential negative predictive marker for EGFR mAbs	De Roock et al. 2010; De Mattos-Arruda et al. 2011
PTEN	Insufficient	Loss a potential negative predictive marker for cetuximab	De Mattos-Arruda et al. 2011
PI3KCA mutations (exon 20)	Insufficient	Potential negative predictive marker for cetuximab	De Roock et al. 2010
Epiregulin, amphiregulin	Insufficient	High expression may predict cetuximab response	Tabernero et al. 2010
VEGF-D	Insufficient	May predict bevacizumab resistance	Weickhardt et al. 2011
VEGF-A	Insufficient	Not predictive of bevacizumab response	Jubb et al. 2006
LDH	Insufficient	Predictive marker for valatinib response	Hecht et al. 2011; Van Cutsem et al. 2011a

two antibodies are approved for use: cetuximab, a chimeric IgG1 mAb, and panitumumab, a fully human IgG2 mAb. These agents interrupt the intracellular signaling cascade through binding to the extracellular ligand site of EGFR (Fig. 1).

KRAS Mutations

KRAS is an important component of the intracellular RAS/RAF/MAPK pathway which corresponds to ligand binding to the EGFR. Mutations in *KRAS* codons 12 and 13 occur in 35–45 % of CRC tumors (De Mattos-Arruda et al. 2011) and evidence from large clinical trials demonstrates that these mutations predict resistance to anti-EGFR mAbs in mCRC (Van Cutsem et al. 2009; Linardou et al. 2008). It is therefore mandatory to determine a patient's *KRAS* mutational status before starting therapy with an anti-EGFR mAb, with treatment limited to patients with wild-type (WT) tumors only. However, 40–60 % of mCRC patients with *KRAS* WT tumors fail to respond to anti-EGFR therapy (Linardou et al. 2008; Bardelli and Siena 2010), and those with initially response *KRAS* WT tumors inevitably acquire resistance. Hence the reasons for this high proportion of patients who fail to respond to anti-EGFR therapy need to be elucidated, and other downstream targets need to be considered as potential therapeutic targets (Weikhardt et al. 2010). There is emerging evidence to suggest that patients with a *KRAS* p.G13D mutation may derive benefit from cetuximab (Mao et al. 2013); this question is the subject of a current clinical trial (Segalov et al. 2013).

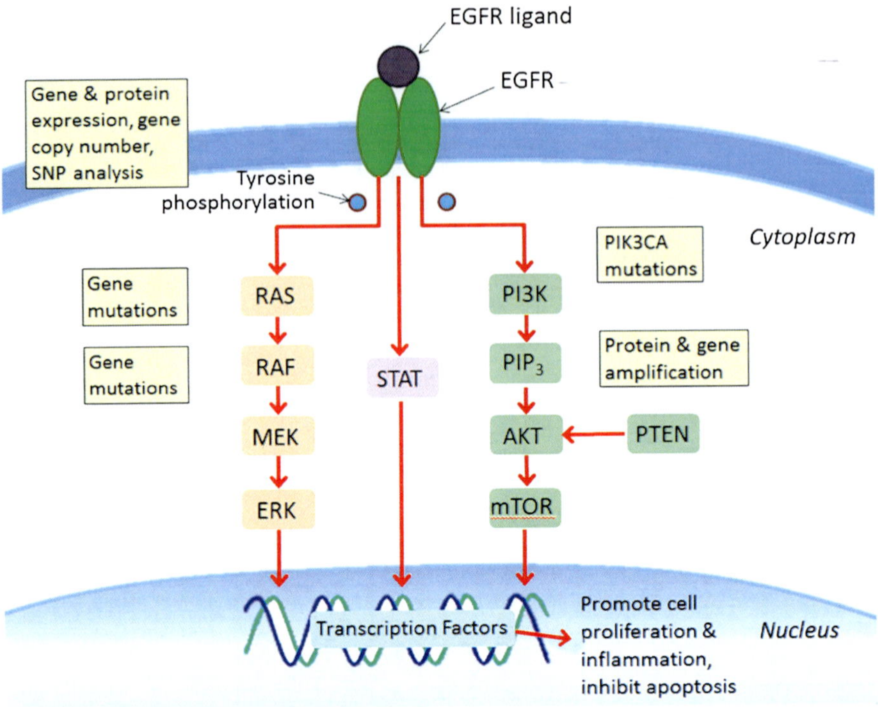

Fig. 1 EGFR signaling pathway with potential predictive markers. PIP_3, phosphatidylinositol (3,4,5)-triphosphate; PTEN, phosphatase and tensin homolog; SNP, single-nucleotide polymorphism

BRAF Mutations

BRAF is the principle downstream effector of KRAS and has been suggested as a predictive biomarker for cetuximab treatment. An association has been seen between *BRAF V600E* mutations and resistance to cetuximab in chemorefractory mCRC (Laurent-Puig et al. 2009), supported by randomized trial data of a lesser benefit from cetuximab in patients whose tumors harbored a *BRAF V600E* mutation (Bokemeyer et al. 2011; Van Cutsem et al. 2011b). Initial results from the PICCOLO study examining the value of panitumumab in combination with irinotecan chemotherapy have demonstrated that patients whose tumors have a *BRAF* mutation do not benefit from the addition of panitumumab and may in fact experience a detrimental effect (Seymour et al. 2011a).

NRAS Mutations

Neuroblastoma Ras gene (*NRAS*) is mutated in only 3–5 % of CRC tumors, usually mutually exclusive of *KRAS* mutation (De Roock et al. 2010; Downward 2003). At present, there is a paucity of evidence to warrant mutation testing in the clinical setting (Downward 2003). There is the suggestion of an association of *NRAS* mutations with a lower response to cetuximab and panitumumab from retrospective trial analyses (De Roock et al. 2010), and this is supported by emerging data from the PICCOLO study (Seymour et al. 2011a; De Mattos-Arruda et al. 2011).

PI3K/PTEN/Akt Pathway

Intracellular signaling can occur through the PI3K/PTEN/Akt pathway once EGFR is activated by its ligand binding. The value of PTEN loss and *PIK3CA* mutations as predictive biomarkers is uncertain due to inconsistency in study results (De Mattos-Arruda et al. 2011). Several studies have suggested they may be associated with resistance to anti-EGFR mAbs (Sartore-Bianchi et al. 2009), with the largest study, taken from retrospective analysis, showing negative outcome with cetuximab treatment if tumors have *PIK3CA* mutations in exon 20 but not exon 9 (De Roock et al. 2010). However, contradictory reports do also exist (De Mattos-Arruda et al. 2011).

EGFR Ligands

The EGFR ligands epiregulin and amphiregulin promote tumor growth and survival via an autocrine loop that signals through EGFR. High expression of these ligands may predict response to anti-EGFR mAbs, with the degree of response to cetuximab suggested to be proportional to the expression of tumor messenger RNA (mRNA) for epiregulin and amphiregulin (Khambata-Ford et al. 2007; Pentheroudakis et al. 2013). CRC patients with high epiregulin and amphiregulin mRNA expression and *KRAS* WT tumors have been shown to have a better response with cetuximab treatment (Tabernero et al. 2010). The utility of the EGFR ligand expression profiles and *KRAS* mutation status in improving patient selection for anti-EGFR mAb therapy needs further data to be fully established, however (De Mattos-Arruda et al. 2011).

Predicting Response to VEGF Inhibitors

Vascular endothelial growth factor (VEGF) is produced by tumor cells and tumor-associated stromal cells, together with a host of other cells such as leukocytes, platelets, and muscle cells. The VEGF family of circulating angiogenic molecules plays a critical role in the development of new blood vessels in the growing tumor, making VEGF an attractive target for anticancer therapies. VEGFRs are present on endothelial cells and tumor cells (Fig. 2).

The anti-VEGF agent in the clinic at present is the monoclonal antibody bevacizumab, targeting VEGF-A. The novel anti-angiogenic agent aflibercept, a VEGF-A, -B, and placental growth factor inhibitor, and the multi-targeted tyrosine kinase inhibitor regorafenib are anti-VEGF agents that have both demonstrated, in large phase III clinical trials (Van Cutsem et al. 2012; Grothey et al. 2013), significant improvements in OS and/or PFS in mCRC patients who have received previous treatment and are likely to become part of clinical practice in the near future.

There is currently no biomarker validated to predict response to anti-VEGF therapies (Jubb and Harris 2010). Research has so far focused on tissue and circulating VEGF isoforms, soluble receptors and VEGF polymorphisms, and

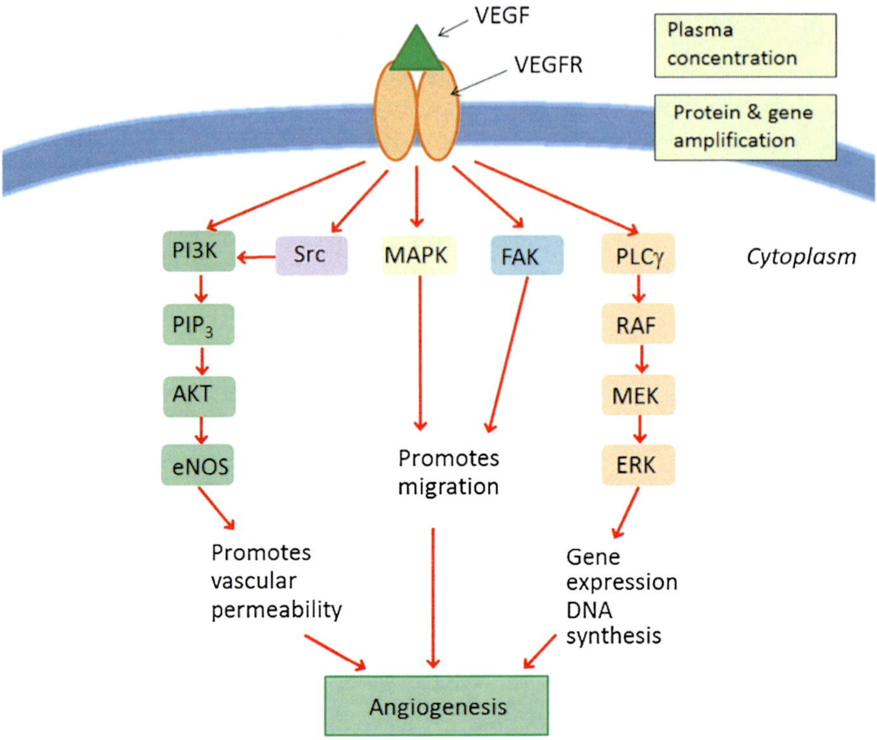

Fig. 2 VEGF signaling pathway. eNOS, endothelial nitric oxide synthase

other circulating molecules in the angiogenesis pathway. Retrospective analyses have demonstrated no predictive association between *KRAS* and *BRAF* mutations and clinical benefit of bevacizumab (Ince et al. 2005).

Tissue-Based Markers

While the prognostic role of VEGF expression in tumor tissue is uncertain, its predictive value is more clear-cut, with no association found between VEGF overexpression and response to bevacizumab (Jubb et al. 2006).

The thrombospondins are a family of negative regulators of angiogenesis and tumor growth that are present in the tumor microenvironment. While increased expression of the thrombospondin-2 gene (*THBS2*) has been associated with decreased tumor vascularity and a reduced frequency of distant metastases in CRC (Tokunaga et al. 1999), no association has been found with bevacizumab response (Jubb et al. 2006). Patients with higher THBS-2 expression did have an improved median survival with bevacizumab compared to those with low expression, but this did not remain significant when interaction with other potential predictors was probed (Jubb et al. 2006). The same study also examined the role of tumor microvessel density, again showing no value as a predictive marker of bevacizumab efficacy.

Given bevacizumab targets only VEGF-A, it has been hypothesized that overexpression of other VEGF ligands could present a mechanism of resistance. High tumor tissue expression of VEGF-D has been found to predict resistance to bevacizumab in a small study, with high expression predictive of shorter PFS (Weickhardt et al. 2011).

Circulating Markers

While circulating VEGF levels have been proposed to reflect VEGF-dependent tumor angiogenesis and therefore be predictive of bevacizumab benefit (Jubb and Harris 2010), no correlation has been found between pretreatment plasma levels of VEGF and bevacizumab response (Jubb et al. 2006). However, given that VEGF levels are dynamic, the change in VEGF level with treatment may be more useful as a predictive marker. This is an area that warrants consideration, as several studies in various settings and malignancies have shown acute increases in circulating VEGF after starting bevacizumab with or without chemotherapy (Willett et al. 2009; Baar et al. 2009), while others have shown a decrease when bevacizumab is given with 5-FU (Willett et al. 2009). The predictive value of selected polymorphisms that affect components of the VEGF pathway has also been demonstrated in small studies (Jubb and Harris 2010), indicating this to be an area worthwhile of larger-scale, prospective investigation.

Lactate dehydrogenase (LDH) has its expression regulated by hypoxia and hypoxia-inducible factor 1α (HIF-1α) and is critical for anaerobic metabolism. Its role as a prognostic factor in mCRC is recognized (Chibaudel et al. 2011), and it has been proposed that high serum LDH expression will identify tumors more dependent on abnormal angiogenesis and therefore more susceptible to anti-VEGF therapies. This has borne out in a study of valatinib, an oral VEGF inhibitor, and chemotherapy in two studies treating mCRC patients, with improved PFS seen in patients with high baseline LDH who received valatinib (Hecht et al. 2011; Van Cutsem et al. 2011a); however, no association has been found between LDH and bevacizumab effect in mCRC (Hurwitz et al. 2009).

Hypertension

Hypertension is a common side effect of anti-VEGF therapies and has been suggested as a potential predictive marker for survival benefit in bevacizumab treatment. Clinical trial evidence exists of its utility in a number of tumor types (Jubb and Harris 2010); however, a recent analysis of seven trials that included CRC failed to show predictive value of hypertension occurring within 60 days of commencing treatment in all but one study (Hurwitz et al. 2013). The pathogenesis of hypertension with anti-EGFR therapy is not fully understood; there are three main theories (Syrigos et al. 2011): (i) the nitric oxide and peripheral vascular resistance theory, (ii) the renal impairment theory, and (iii) the preeclampsia-like theory. It is a current standard clinical practice to treat hypertension as soon as it develops; however, there is a paucity of evidence to guide the optimal treatment strategy.

Technology-Facilitated Biomarkers

Genotyping

While testing for specific individual mutations is well established, the recent advent of next-generation sequencing has enabled simultaneous testing for hundreds of mutations. This presents the potential for developing gene signatures that offer prognostic or predictive significance. To date, these studies have been limited, with small patient numbers necessitated by costs and technical complications due to tumor heterogeneity and bioinformatics requirements for handling the large volumes of data produced (Van Schaeybroeck et al. 2011).

The Cancer Genome Atlas (TCGA) project has published the molecular profile of human CRC, determining 24 genes to be significantly mutated, with markers for disease aggression suggested through integrative analyses (Network 2012). The combination of gene expression profiling and established clinicopathological variables, such as tumor size and grade and lymph node involvement, presents the potential for greater individualization of patient care (Kheirelseid et al. 2013). A genetic signature for cetuximab treatment has been compared with a *KRAS* signature with significant overlap found for response to cetuximab treatment (Khambata-Ford et al. 2007), suggesting the *KRAS* genetic profile of a tumor may be important when predicting cetuximab response.

Epigenetics

CRC is considered a genetic disease with sequential genetic and epigenetic alterations occurring along the course of its histopathological progression. Microsatellite instability occurs either due to epigenetic silencing of the *MLH1* gene or germline mutation in one of the four MMR genes (Vilar and Gruber 2010). Evidence for epigenetic markers to predict treatment response however has been inconsistent. Markers such as CpG island methylation phenotype has been proposed as a marker of poor response to 5-FU treatment but with conflicting results among studies (Ogino et al. 2007; van Rijnsoever et al. 2003). CpG island promoter hypermethylation of the Werner syndrome gene (*WRN*) has been associated with longer survival of patients treated with irinotecan chemotherapy (Agrelo et al. 2006).

MicroRNA

MicroRNAs (miRNAs) are small (19–25-nucleotide) noncoding RNA molecules that regulate gene expression at the translational level, with involvement in a number of biological processes, including cancers. MiRNAs have demonstrated roles as both tumor suppressor genes and oncogenes, and their utility as biomarkers, being diagnostic, prognostic, and predictive, is under investigation. Serum, plasma, tissue, and feces are all sources of miRNA.

High expression of miR-21 in tumor tissue has been identified as a potential prognostic marker as well as a predictive marker for poor response to 5-FU chemotherapy in the adjuvant setting (Schetter et al. 2008). Low levels of let-7 g and miR-181b overexpression have been associated with a response to the fluoropyrimidine S-1 (Nakajima et al. 2006).

The circulation is an attractive source of potential biomarkers, given it is easily accessible and amenable to repeated measurements. Circulating miRNA studies have so far concentrated on determining miRNAs as potential diagnostic biomarkers; however, two studies have identified miRNAs, miR-144 and miR-221, prognostic for poor outcome (Cheng et al. 2011; Pu et al. 2010). No circulating miRNAs have yet been identified that predict treatment response or toxicity.

New Techniques

Proteomic analyses of blood and tumor tissue are recognized as having the potential to provide predictive or prognostic biomarkers, given that proteins are the actual effector molecules in cells; however, the results so far have been disappointing. Technical issues have been the main barrier to biomarker discovery, with more robust technologies needed (McHugh et al. 2009).

Other entities such as circulating tumor free DNA and circulating tumor cells (CTCs) are undergoing evaluation for their potential as biomarkers. To date, studies have largely focused on exploring their utility in early diagnostics, prognosis, and early detection of recurrence (Lecomte et al. 2010; Cohen et al. 2008). One small study found that the presence of CTCs after 3 months of first-line oxaliplatin, S-1, and panitumumab for mCRC predicted for significantly worse outcome (Kawahara et al. 2012; Neki et al. 2013), while another demonstrated prognostic and predictive value of CTC numbers before and during treatment (Cohen et al. 2008). Many of the tumor-associated molecular alterations detected in the CTCs are identical to those in the primary tumor, so the potential must exist for these entities providing a means of predicted treatment-related response and toxicity.

Potential Applications to Prognosis and Other Diseases or Conditions

The issue of biomarker research in mCRC for both prognosis and prediction of treatment response is one of considerable interest as we seek personalization of care in medical oncology. Throughout this chapter we have detailed that in many of the entities already examined, promise exists for utility as a biomarker, but validation in larger-scale studies or with more robust technologies is required before acceptance as a biomarker can be realized. This is an important issue for consideration in the design of future clinical trials, with attention to biomarker discovery, both now and with future technologies, a necessary inclusion.

Adequate biobanking of tissue and blood or plasma with comprehensive clinical data that is available to collaborative research groups is essential for cancer research, and provision needs to be made for this in the design of clinical trials. This will allow for the investigation of similar biological and pathological mechanisms in well-annotated samples across a variety of tumor types and provide for retrospective validation of potential biomarkers in multiple cohorts as technologies develop. Additionally, the results obtained from efforts made into CRC research in the realms of drug efficacy and mechanism of action will be useful for other cancers that also utilize the same drugs in their clinical treatment. One example of this is the use of bevacizumab in tumor types such as breast and ovarian cancer, with predictive biomarker research of interest here also.

Perhaps the most exciting area of research, as well as one of the most immature, is that of genetics. This holds the potential for the development of prognostic and predictive signatures of genes, presenting true personalization of medicine. With innovations in genomics and data handling technologies, this is within reach of the individual patient in the near future.

Summary Points

- This chapter focuses on means of predicting prognosis and response and toxicity to chemotherapy and targeted agents in metastatic colorectal cancer.
- With the high prevalence of colorectal cancer in what is a largely elderly population, the prediction of response to treatment and toxicity is important to help guide treatment populations, agents, and dosages and allow for early implementation of supportive treatments.
- Prognostic biomarkers, i.e., those that predict disease course, are useful in guiding appropriate treatment recipients.
- Predictive biomarkers that predict treatment response or toxicity are helpful in judicious drug and dosing selection.
- Few true prognostic or predictive biomarkers currently exist for metastatic colorectal cancer.

Acknowledgements Connie Diakos is supported by a Cancer Institute NSW and Northern Translational Cancer Research Unit (NTCRU) Clinical Research Fellowship. Kellie Charles is supported by a Cancer Institute NSW Career Development Fellowship.

References

Aggarwal BB, Vijayalekshmi RV, Sung B. Targeting inflammatory pathways for prevention and therapy of cancer: short-term friend, long-term foe. Clin Cancer Res. 2009;15:425–30.

Agrelo R, Cheng W-H, Setien F, et al. Epigenetic inactivation of the premature aging Werner syndrome gene in human cancer. Proc Natl Acad Sci U S A. 2006;103:8822–7.

Amado RG, Wolf M, Peeters M, et al. Wild-type *KRAS* is required for panitumumab efficacy in patients with metastatic colorectal cancer. J Clin Oncol. 2008;26:1626–34.

Ando Y, Saka H, Ando M, et al. Polymorphisms of UDP-glucuronosyltransferase gene and irinotecan toxicity: a pharmacogenetic analysis. Cancer Res. 2000;60:6921–6.

Andreyev HJN, Norman AR, Cunningham D, et al. Kirsten ras mutations in patients with colorectal cancer: the 'RASCAL II' study. Br J Cancer. 2001;85:692–6.

Aparicio T, Jouve J-L, Teillet L, et al. Geriatric factors predict chemotherapy feasibility: ancillary results of FFCD 2001–02 Phase III study in first-line chemotherapy for metastatic colorectal cancer in elderly patients. J Clin Oncol. 2013;31:1464–70.

Baar J, Silverman P, Lyons J, et al. A vasculature-targeting regimen of preoperative docetaxel with or without bevacizumab for locally advanced breast cancer: impact on angiogenic biomarkers. Clin Cancer Res. 2009;15:3583–90.

Bardelli A, Siena S. Molecular mechanisms of resistance to cetuximab and panitumumab in colorectal cancer. J Clin Oncol. 2010;28:1254–61.

Bokemeyer C, Bondarenko I, Hartmann JT, et al. Efficacy according to biomarker status of cetuximab plus FOLFOX-4 as first-line treatment for metastatic colorectal cancer: the OPUS study. Ann Oncol. 2011;22:1535–46.

Braun MS, Richman SD, Quirke P, et al. Predictive biomarkers of chemotherapy efficacy in colorectal cancer: results from the UK MRC FOCUS trial. J Clin Oncol. 2008;26:2690–8.

Braun MS, Richman SD, Thompson L, et al. Association of molecular markers with toxicity outcomes in a randomised trial of chemotherapy for advanced colorectal cancer: the FOCUS trial. J Clin Oncol. 2009;27:5519–28.

Capitain O, Boisdron-Celle M, Poirier A-L, et al. The influence of fluorouracil outcome parameters on tolerance and efficacy in patients with advanced colorectal cancer. Pharmacogenomics J. 2008;8:256–67.

Cecchin E, Innocenti F, D'Andrea M, et al. Predictive role of the *UGT1A1*, *UGT1A7*, and *UGT1a9* genetic variants and their haplotypes on the outcome of metastatic colorectal cancer patients treated with fluorouracil, leucovorin, and irinotecan. J Clin Oncol. 2009;27:2457–65.

Chambers P, Daniels SH, Thompson LC, et al. Chemotherapy dose reductions in obese patients with colorectal cancer. Ann Oncol. 2011;23:748–53.

Charles KA, Rivory LP, Brown SL, et al. Transcriptional repression of hepatic *cytochrome P450 3A4* gene in the presence of cancer. Clin Cancer Res. 2006;12:7492–7.

Cheng H, Zhang L, Cogdell DE, et al. Circulating plasma miR-141 is a novel biomarker for metastatic colon cancer and predicts poor prognosis. PLoS One. 2011;6:e17745.

Chibaudel B, Bonnetain F, Tournigand C, et al. Simplified prognostic model in patients with oxaliplatin-based or irinotecan-based first-line chemotherapy for metastatic colorectal cancer: a GERCOR study. Oncologist. 2011;16:1228–38.

Chua W, Goldstein D, Lee CK, et al. Molecular markers of response and toxicity to FOLFOX chemotherapy in metastatic colorectal cancer. Br J Cancer. 2009;101:998–1004.

Chua W, Charles KA, Baracos VE, et al. Neutrophil/lymphocyte ratio predicts chemotherapy outcomes in patients with advanced colorectal cancer. Br J Cancer. 2011;104:1288–95.

Clarke SJ, Chua W, Moore MM, et al. Use of inflammatory markers to guide cancer treatment. Clin Pharmacol Ther. 2011;90:475–8.

Cohen SJ, Punt CJA, Iannotti N, et al. Relationship of circulating tumour cells to tumour response, progress-free survival, and overall survival in patients with metastatic colorectal cancer. J Clin Oncol. 2008;26:3213–21.

Colotta F, Allavena P, Sica A, et al. Cancer-related inflammation, the seventh hallmark of cancer: links to genetic instability. Carcinogenesis. 2009;30:1073–81.

De Mattos-Arruda L, Dienstmann R, Tabernero J. Development of molecular biomarkers in individualised treatment of colorectal cancer. Clin Colorectal Cancer. 2011;10:279–89.

De Roock W, Claes B, Bernasconi D, et al. Effects of *KRAS*, *BRAF*, *NRAS*, and *PIK3CA* mutations on the efficacy of cetuximab plus chemotherapy in chemotherapy-refractory metastatic colorectal cancer: a retrospective consortium analysis. Lancet Oncol. 2010;11:753–62.

Des Guetz G, Schischmanoff O, Nicolas P, et al. Does microsatellite instability predict the efficacy of adjuvant chemotherapy in colorectal cancer? A systematic review with meta-analysis. Eur J Cancer. 2009;45:1890–6.

Dignam JJ, Polite BN, Yothers G, et al. Body mass index and outcomes in patients who receive adjuvant chemotherapy for colon cancer. J Natl Cancer Inst. 2006;98:1647–54.

Downward J. Targeting RAS signalling pathways in cancer therapy. Nat Rev Cancer. 2003;3:11–22.

Extermann M, Boler I, Reich RR, et al. Predicting the risk of chemotherapy toxicity in older patients: the chemotherapy risk assessment scale for high-age patients (CRASH) score. Cancer. 2012;118:3377–86.

Field KM, Kosnider S, Jefford M, et al. Chemotherapy dosing strategies in the obese, elderly, and thin patient: results of a nationwide survey. J Oncol Practice. 2008;4:108–13.

Goldberg RM, Tabah-Fisch I, Bleiberg H, et al. Pooled analysis of safety and efficacy of oxaliplatin plus fluorouracil/leucovorin administered bimonthly in elderly patients with colorectal cancer. J Clin Oncol. 2006;24:4085–91.

Griggs JJ, Mangu PB, Anderson H, et al. Appropriate chemotherapy dosing for obese adult patients with cancer: American Society of Clinical Society Clinical Practice Guideline. J Clin Oncol. 2012;30:1553–61.

Grothey AAG, Van Cutsem E, Sobrero A, et al. Regorafenib monotherapy for previously treated metastatic colorectal cancer (CORRECT): an international, multicentre, randomised, placebo-controlled phase III trial. Lancet. 2013;381:303–12.

Gusella M, Frigo AC, Bolzonella C, et al. Predictors of survival and toxicity in patients on adjuvant therapy with 5-fluorouracil for colorectal cancer. Br J Cancer. 2009;100:1549–57.

Hanahan D, Weinberg RA. Hallmarks of cancer: the next generation. Cell. 2011;144:646–74.

Hecht JR, Trarbach T, Hainsworth JD, et al. Randomised, placebo-controlled, phase III study of first-line oxaliplatin-based chemotherapy plus PTK787/ZK222584, an oral vascular endothelial growth factor receptor inhibitor, in patients with metastatic colorectal adenocarcinoma. J Clin Oncol. 2011;29:1997–2003.

Hoskins JM, Goldberg RM, Qu P, et al. UGT1A1*28 genotype and irinotecan-induced neutropaenia: dose matters. J Natl Cancer Inst. 2007;99:1290–5.

Hurwitz HI, Yi J, Ince W, et al. The clinical benefit of bevacizumab in metastatic colorectal cancer is independent of K-*ras* mutation status: analysis of a phase III study of bevacizumab with chemotherapy in previously untreated metastatic colorectal cancer. J Clin Oncol. 2009;14:22–8.

Hurwitz HI, Douglas PS, Middleton JP, et al. Analysis of early hypertension and clinical outcome with bevacizumab: results from seven Phase III studies. Oncologist. 2013;18:273–80.

Ince WL, Jubb AM, Holden SN, et al. Association of k-ras, b-raf, and p53 status with the treatment effect of bevacizumab. J Natl Cancer Inst. 2005;97:981–9.

Innocenti F, Undevia SD, Iyer L, et al. Genetic variants in the *UDP-glucuronosyltransferase 1A1* gene predict the risk of severe neutropenia of irinotecan. J Clin Oncol. 2004;22:1382–8.

Iyer L, King CDW, Peter F, Green MD, et al. Genetic predisposition to the metabolism of irinotecan (CPT-11). J Clin Invest. 1998;101:847–54.

Iyer L, Das S, Janisch L, et al. *UGT1A1*28* polymorphism as a determinant of irinotecan disposition and toxicity. Pharmacogenomics J. 2002;2:43–7.

Jubb AM, Harris AL. Biomarkers to predict the clinical efficacy of bevacizumab in cancer. Lancet Oncol. 2010;11:1172–83.

Jubb AM, Hurwitz HI, Bai W, et al. Impact of vascular endothelial growth factor-A expression, thrombospondin-2 expression, and microvessel density on the treatment effect of bevacizumab in metastatic colorectal cancer. J Clin Oncol. 2006;24:217–27.

Kacevska M, Robertson GR, Clarke SJ, et al. Inflammation and CYP3A4-mediated drug metabolism in advanced cancer: impact and implications for chemotherapeutic drug dosing. Expert Opin Drug Metab Toxicol. 2008;4:137–46.

Karapetis CS, Khambata-Ford S, Jonker DJ, et al. *K-ras* mutations and benefit from cetuximab in advanced colorectal cancer. N Engl J Med. 2008;359:1757–65.

Kawahara H, Watanabe K, Toyama Y, et al. Determination of circulating tumour cells for prediction of recurrent colorectal cancer progression. Hepatogastroenterology. 2012;59:2115–8.

Khambata-Ford S, Garrett CR, Meropol NJ, et al. Expression of epiregulin and amphiregulin and *K-ras* mutation status predict disease control in metastatic colorectal cancer patients treated with cetuximab. J Clin Oncol. 2007;25:3230–7.

Kheirelseid EAH, Miller N, Chang KH, et al. Clinical applications of gene expression in colorectal cancer. J Gastroint Oncol. 2013;4:144–57.

Khorana AA, Ryan CK, Cox C, et al. Vascular endothelial growth factor, CD68, and epidermal growth factor receptor expression and survival in patients with stage II and stage III colon carcinoma. Cancer. 2003;97:960–8.

Kim S-H, Kwon H-C, Oh SY, et al. Prognostic value of ERCC1, thymidylate synthase and glutathione S-transferase [pi] for 5-FU/oxaliplatin chemotherapy in advanced colorectal cancer. Am J Clin Oncol. 2009;32:38–43.

Koopman M, Krijin N, Richman SD, et al. Abstract 6003: The correlation between Topoisomerase-I (Topo1) expression and outcome of treatment with capecitabine and irinotecan in advanced colorectal cancer (ACC) patients (pts) treated in the CAIRO study of the Dutch Colorectal Cancer Group (DCCG). Eur J Cancer Suppl. 2009a;7:321.

Koopman M, Venderbosch S, Nagtegaal ID, et al. A review on the use of molecular markers of cytotoxic therapy for colorectal cancer, what have we learned? Eur J Cancer. 2009b;45:1935–49.

Koopman M, Venderbosch S, van Tinteren H, et al. Predictive and prognostic markers for the outcome of chemotherapy in advanced colorectal cancer, a retrospective analysis of the phase III randomised CAIRO study. Eur J Cancer. 2009c;45:1999–2006.

Kopetz S, Hoff PM, Morris JS, et al. Phase II trial of infusional fluorouracil, irinotecan, and bevacizumab for metastatic colorectal cancer: efficacy and circulating angiogenic biomarkers associated with therapeutic resistance. J Clin Oncol. 2010;28:453–9.

Kweekel DM, Gelderblom H, Guchelaar H-J. Pharmacology of oxaliplatin and the use of pharmacogenomics to individualise therapy. Cancer Treat Rev. 2005;31:90–105.

Kweekel DM, Gelderblom H, Antonini NF, et al. Glutathione-S-transferase pi (GSTP1) codon 105 polymorphism is not associated with oxaliplatin efficacy or toxicity in advanced colorectal cancer patients. Eur J Cancer. 2009;45:572–8.

Laurent-Puig P, Cayre A, Manceau G, et al. Analysis of *PTEN*, *BRAF* and *EGFR* status in determining benefit from cetuximab therapy in wild-type *KRAS* metastatic colon cancer. J Clin Oncol. 2009;27:5924–30.

Le Morvan V, Smith D, Laurand A, et al. Determination of *ERCC2* Lys751Gln and *GSTP1* Ile105Val gene polymorphisms in colorectal cancer patients: relationships with treatment outcome. Pharmacogenomics. 2007;8:1693–703.

Lecomte T, Landi B, Beaune P, et al. Glutathione *S*-transferase P1 polymorphism (Ile^{105}Val) predicts cumulative neuropathy in patients receiving oxaliplatin-based chemotherapy. Clin Cancer Res. 2006;12:3050–6.

Lecomte T, Ceze N, Dorval E, et al. Circulating free tumour DNA and colorectal cancer. Gastroenterol Clin Biol. 2010;34:662–81.

Limsui D, Vierkant RA, Tillmans LS, et al. Cigarette smoking and colorectal cancer risk by molecularly defined subtypes. J Natl Cancer Inst. 2010;102:1012–22.

Linardou H, Dahabreh IJ, Kanaloupiti D, et al. Assessment of somatic *k-RAS* mutations as a mechanism associated with resistance to EGFR-targeted agents: a systematic review and meta-analysis of studies in advanced non-small-cell lung cancer and metastatic colorectal cancer. Lancet Oncol. 2008;9:962–72.

Liu C-Y, Chen P-M, Chiou T-J, et al. UGT1A1*28 polymorphism predicts irinotecan-induced severe toxicities without affecting treatment outcome and survival in patients with metastatic colorectal carcinoma. Cancer. 2008;112:1932–40.

Manley PW, Martiny-Brown G, Schlaeppi J-M, et al. Therapies directed at vascular endothelial growth factor. Expert Opin Investig Drugs. 2002;11:1715–36.

Mao C, Huang Y-F, Yang Z-Y, et al. *KRAS* p.G13D mutation and codon 12 mutations are not created equal in predicting clinical outcomes of cetuximab in metastatic colorectal cancer. A systematic review and meta-analysis. Cancer. 2013;119:714–21.

Markman B, Ramos FJ, Capdevila J, et al. EGFR and KRAS in colorectal cancer. Adv Clin Chem. 2010;51:71–119.

Martinez ME. Primary prevention of colorectal cancer: lifestyle, nutrition, exercise. In: Tumour prevention and genetics III. Springer, Berlin Heidelberg; 2005. pp. 177–211.

Matsumura M, Chiba Y, Lu C, et al. Platelet-derived endothelial cell growth factor/thymidine phosphorylase expression correlated with tumour angiogenesis and macrophage infiltration in colorectal cancer. Cancer Lett. 1998;128:55–63.

Matsuura T, Kuratate I, Teramachi K, et al. Thymidylate phosphorylase expression is associated with both increase of intratumoural microvessels and decrease of apoptosis in human colorectal carcinomas. Cancer Res. 1999;59:5037–40.

McCleary NJ, Niedzwiecki D, Hollis D, et al. Impact of smoking on patients with stage III colon cancer. Cancer. 2010;116:957–66.

McHugh SM, O'Donnell J, Gillen P. Genomic and oncoproteomic advances in detection and treatment of colorectal cancer. World J Surg Oncol. 2009;7:36–44.

McMillan DC. The systemic inflammation-based Glasgow Prognosis Score: a decade of experience in patients with cancer. Cancer Treat Rev. 2013;39:534–40.

Meropol NJ, Gold PJ, Diasio RB, et al. Thymidylate phosphorylase expression is associated with response to capecitabine plus irinotecan in patients with metastatic colorectal cancer. J Clin Oncol. 2006;24:4069–77.

Meyerhardt JA, Giovannucci EL, Holmes MD, et al. Physical activity and survival after colorectal cancer diagnosis. J Clin Oncol. 2006;24:3527–34.

Meyerhardt JA, Niedzwiecki D, Hollis D, et al. Impact of body mass index and weight change after treatment on cancer recurrence and survival in patients with stage III colon cancer: findings from Cancer and Leukemia Group B 89803. J Clin Oncol. 2008;26:4109–15.

Mitry E, Venat-Bouvet L, Phelip J, et al. Randomised phase III in elderly patients comparing LV5FU2 with or without irinotecan for 1st-line treatment of metastatic colorectal cancer (FFCD 2001–02). Ann Oncol. 2012; 23: ix181. Abstract 529PD.

Moehler M, Frings C, Mueller A, et al. VEGF-D expression correlates with colorectal cancer aggressiveness and is downregulated by cetuximab. World J Gastroenterol. 2008;14:4156–67.

Moore MM, Chua W, Charles KA, et al. Inflammation and cancer: causes and consequences. Clin Pharmacol Ther. 2010;87:504–8.

Moreno V, Gemignani F, Landi S, et al. Polymorphisms in genes of nucleotide and base excision repair: risk and prognosis of colorectal cancer. Clin Cancer Res. 2006;12:2101–8.

Nakajima G, Hayashi K, Xi Y, et al. Non-coding microRNAs *hsa-let-7 g* and *hsa-miR-181b* are associated with chemoresponse to S-1 in colon cancer. Cancer Genomics Proteomics. 2006;3:317–24.

Neki K, Kawahara H, Watanabe K, et al. Usefulness of circulating tumour cells after preliminary chemotherapy for prediction of response to further anticancer therapy in patients with initially unresectable metastatic colorectal cancer. Anticancer Res. 2013;33:1769–72.

Network TCGA. Comprehensive molecular characterisation of human colon and rectal cancer. Nature. 2012;487:330–7.

Ogino S, Meyerhardt JA, Kawasaki T, et al. CpG island methylation, response to combination chemotherapy, and patient survival in advanced microsatellite stable colorectal carcinoma. Virchows Arch. 2007;450:529–37.

Paradiso A, Xu J, Mangia A, et al. Topoisomerase-1, thymidylate synthase primary tumour expression and clinical efficacy of 5-FU/CPT-11 chemotherapy in advanced colorectal cancer patients. Int J Cancer. 2004;111:252–8.

Park DJ, Stoehlmacher J, Zhang W, et al. A *Xeroderma Pigmentosum Group D* gene polymorphism predicts clinical outcome to platinum-based chemotherapy in patients with advanced colorectal cancer. Cancer Res. 2001;61:8654–8.

Pentheroudakis G, Kotoula V, De Roock W, et al. Biomarkers of benefit from cetuximab-based therapy in metastatic colorectal cancer: interaction of EGFR ligand expression with RAS/RAF, PIK3CA genotypes. BMC Cancer. 2013;13:49.

Popat S, Matakidou A, Houlston RS. Thymidylate synthase expression and prognosis in colorectal cancer: a systematic review and meta-analysis. J Clin Oncol. 2004;22:529–36.

Popat S, Hubner R, Houlston RS. Systematic review of microsatellite instability and colorectal cancer prognosis. J Clin Oncol. 2005;23:609–18.

Popat S, Chen Z, Zhao D, et al. A prospective, blinded analysis of thymidylate synthase and p53 expression as prognostic markers in the adjuvant treatment of colorectal cancer. Ann Oncol. 2006;17:1810–7.

Pu X-x, G-l H, H-q G, et al. Circulating miR-221 directly amplified from plasma is a potential diagnostic and prognostic marker of colorectal cancer and is correlated with p53 expression. J Gastroenterol Hepatol. 2010;25:1674–80.

Rizzo S, Bronte G, Fanale D, et al. Prognostic vs predictive molecular biomarkers in colorectal cancer: is KRAS and BRAF wild type status required for anti-EGFR therapy? Cancer Treat Rev. 2010;36:S56–61.

Robertson GR, Liddle C, Clarke SJ. Inflammation and altered drug clearance in cancer: transcriptional repression of a human CYP3A4 transgene in tumour-bearing mice. Clin Pharmacol Ther. 2008;83:804–7.

Roth AD, Yan P, Dietrich D, et al. Is UGT1A1*28 homozygosity the strongest predictor for severe hematotoxicity in patients treated with 5-fluorouracil (5-FU)-irinotecan (IRI)? Results of the PETACC 3 – EORTC 40993 -SAKK 60/00 trial comparing IRI/5-FU/folinic acid (FA) to 5-FU/FA in stage II- III colon cancer (COC) patients. J Clin Oncol. 2008; 26. Abstract 4036.

Roth AD, Delorenzi M, Tejpar S, et al. Integrated analysis of molecular and clinical prognostic factors in stage II/III colon cancer. J Natl Cancer Inst. 2012;104:1635–46.

Roxburgh CSD, McMillan DC. Role of systemic inflammatory response in predicting survival in patients with primary operable cancer. Future Oncol. 2010;6:149–63.

Roxburgh CS, McMillan DC. The role of the in situ local inflammatory response in predicting recurrence and survival in patients with primary operable colorectal cancer. Cancer Treat Rev. 2012;38:451–66.

Ruzzo A, Graziano F, Loupakis F, et al. Pharmacogenetic profiling in patients with advanced colorectal cancer treated with first-line FOLFOX-4 chemotherapy. J Clin Oncol. 2007;25:1247–54.

Samowitz WS, Sweeney C, Herrick J, et al. Poor survival associated with the *BRAF* V600E mutation in microsatellite-stable colon cancers. Cancer Res. 2005;65:6063–9.

Sanoff HK, Sargent DJ, Green EM, et al. Racial differences in advanced colorectal cancer outcomes and pharmacogenetics: a subgroup analysis of a large randomised controlled clinical trial. J Clin Oncol. 2009;27:4109–15.

Sargent DJ, Goldberg RM, Jacobson SD, et al. A pooled analysis of adjuvant chemotherapy for resected colon cancer in elderly patients. N Engl J Med. 2001;345:1091–7.

Sartore-Bianchi A, Martini M, Molinari F, et al. *PIK3CA* mutations in colorectal cancer are associated with clinical resistance to EGFR-targeted monoclonal antibodies. Cancer Res. 2009;69:1851–7.

Sawai H, Yasuda A, Ochi N, et al. Loss of PTEN expression is associated with colorectal cancer liver metastases and poor patient survival. BMC Gastroenterol. 2008;8:56.

Schetter AJ, Leung SY, Sohn JJ, et al. MicroRNA expression profiles associated with prognosis and therapeutic outcome in colon adenocarcinoma. JAMA. 2008;299:425–36.

Schwab M, Zanger UM, Mars C, et al. Role of genetic and nongenetic factors for fluorouracil treatment-related severe toxicity: a prospective clinical trial by the German 5-FU Toxicity Study Group. J Clin Oncol. 2008;26:2131–8.

Segalov E, Wilson K, Gebski V, et al. ICE CREAM: irinotecan cetuximab evaluation and the cetuximab response evaluation among patients with G13D mutation. Abstrct TPS3649. J Clin Oncol. 2013; 31.

Seymour MT, Brown SR, Richman S, et al. Addition of panitumumab to irinotecan: results of PICCOLO, a randomised controlled trial in advanced colorectal cancer (aCRC). J Clin Oncol. 2011a;29:a3523.

Seymour MT, Thompson LC, Wasan HS, et al. Chemotherapy options in elderly and frail patients with metastatic colorectal cancer (MRC FOCUS2): an open-label, randomised factorial trial. Lancet. 2011b;377:1749–59.

Shirota Y, Stoehlmacher J, Brabender J, et al. *ERCC1* and thymidylate synthase mRNA levels predict survival for colorectal cancer patients receiving combination oxaliplatin and fluorouracil chemotherapy. J Clin Oncol. 2001;19:4298–304.

Soong R, Shah N, Salto-Tellez M, et al. Prognostic significance of thymidylate synthase, dihydropyrimidine dehydrogenase and thymidine phosphorylase protein expression in colorectal cancer patients treated with or without 5-fluorouracil-based chemotherapy. Ann Oncol. 2008;19:915–9.

Stoehlmacher J, Park DJ, Zhang W, et al. Association between glutathione *S*-transferase P1, T1, and M1 genetic polymorphisms and survival of patients with metastatic colorectal cancer. J Natl Cancer Inst. 2002;94:936–42.

Stoehlmacher J, Park DJ, Zhang W, et al. A multivariate analysis of genome polymorphisms: prediction of clinical outcome to 5-FU/oxaliplatin combination chemotherapy in refractory colorectal cancer. Br J Cancer. 2004;91:344–54.

Suh KW, Kim JH, Kim DY, et al. Which gene is a dominant predictor of response during FOLFOX chemotherapy for the treatment of metastatic colorectal cancer, the MTHFR or XRCC1 gene? Ann Surg Oncol. 2006;13:1379–85.

Syrigos KN, Karapanagiotou E, Boura P, et al. Bevacizumab-induced hypertension. Pathogenesis and management. BioDrugs. 2011;25:159–69.

Tabernero J, Cervantes A, Rivera F, et al. Pharmacogenomic and pharmacoproteomic studies of cetuximab in metastatic colorectal cancer: biomarker analysis of a phase I dose-escalation study. J Clin Oncol. 2010;28:1181–9.

Tokunaga T, Nakamura M, Oshika Y, et al. Thrombospondin 2 expression is correlated with inhibition of angiogenesis and metastasis of colon cancer. Br J Cancer. 1999;79:354–9.

Tran B, Kopetz S, Tie J, et al. Impact of BRAF mutation and microsatellite instability on the pattern of metastatic spread and prognosis in metastatic colorectal cancer. Cancer. 2011;117:4623–32.

Vallbohmer D, Yang D, Kuramochi H, et al. DPD is a molecular determinant of capecitabine efficacy in colorectal cancer. Int J Oncol. 2007;31:413–8.

Van Cutsem E, Kohne C-H, Hitre E, et al. Cetuximab and chemotherapy as initial treatment for metastatic colorectal cancer. N Engl J Med. 2009;360:1408–17.

Van Cutsem E, Bajetta E, Valle J, et al. Randomised, placebo-controlled, phase III study of oxaliplatin, fluorouracil, and leucovorin with or without PTK787/ZK222584 in patients with previously treated metastatic colorectal adenocarcinoma. J Clin Oncol. 2011a;29:2004–10.

Van Cutsem E, Kohne C-H, Lang I, et al. Cetuximab plus irinotecan, fluorouracil, and leucovorin as first-line treatment for metastatic colorectal cancer: updated analysis of overall survival according to tumour *KRAS* and *BRAF* mutation status. J Clin Oncol. 2011b;29:2011–9.

Van Cutsem E, Tabernero J, Lakomy R, et al. Additional of aflibercept to fluorouracil, leucovorin, and irinotecan improves survival in a phase III randomised trial in patients with metastatic colorectal cancer previously treated with an oxaliplatin-based regimen. J Clin Oncol. 2012;30:3499–506.

van Kuilenburg ABP, Haasjes J, Richel DJ, et al. Clinical implications of dihydropyrimidine dehydrogenase (DPD) deficiency in patients with severe 5-fluorouracil-associated toxicity: identification of new mutations in the *DPD* gene. Clin Cancer Res. 2000;6:4705–12.

van Rijnsoever M, Elsaleh H, Joseph D, et al. CpG island methylator phenotype is an independent predictor of survival benefit from 5-fluorouracil in stage III colorectal cancer. Clin Cancer Res. 2003;9:2898–903.

Van Schaeybroeck S, Allen WL, Turkington RC, et al. Implementing prognostic and predictive biomarkers in CRC clinical trials. Nat Rev Clin Oncol. 2011;8:222–32.

Viguier J, Boige V, Miquel C, et al. *ERCC1* codon 118 polymorphism is a predictive factor for the tumour response to oxaliplatin/5-fluorouracil combination chemotherapy in patients with advanced colorectal cancer. Clin Cancer Res. 2005;11:6212–7.

Vilar E, Gruber SB. Microsatellite instability in colorectal cancer – the stable evidence. Nat Rev Clin Oncol. 2010;7:153–62.

Wei X, McLeod HL, McMurrough J, et al. Molecular basis of the human dihydropyrimidine dehydrogenase deficiency and 5-fluorouracil toxicity. J Clin Invest. 1996;98:610–5.

Weickhardt A, Williams D, Lee C, et al. Vascular endothelial growth factors (VEGF) and VEGF receptor expression as predictive biomarkers for benefit with bevacizumab in metastatic colorectal cancer (mCRC): analysis of the phase III MAX study. J Clin Oncol. 2011; 29. Abstract 3531.

Weikhardt AJ, Tebbutt NC, Mariadason JM. Strategies for overcoming inherent and acquired resistance to EGFR inhibitors by targeting downstream effectors in the *RAS/PI3K* pathway. Curr Cancer Drug Targets. 2010;10:824–33.

Willett CG, Duda DG, di Tomaso E, et al. Efficacy, safety, and biomarkers of neoadjuvant bevacizumab, radiation therapy, and fluorouracil in rectal cancer: a multidisciplinary phase II study. J Clin Oncol. 2009;27:3020–6.

Expression Profiling as Biomarkers in Colorectal Serrated Carcinoma

28

Mari Carmen Turpín Sevilla, José García Solano, Claudio Navarre, Miguel Pérez-Guillermo García, Ana Conesa, and Pablo Conesa Zamora

Contents

M.C.T. Sevilla
Department of Pathology (HGUSL) Cartagena, Spain; University Francisco of Vitoria, Madrid, Spain
e-mail: mc.turpin.prof@ufv.es

J.G. Solano • P.C. Zamora (✉)
Department of Pathology, Hospital General Universitario Santa Lucia (HGUSL), Cartagena, Spain

Facultad de Ciencias de la Salud, Catholic University of Murcia (UCAM), Murcia, Spain
e-mail: jose.garcia30@carm.es; pablo.conesa@carm.es

C. Navarre • A. Conesa
Genomics of Gene Expression Laboratory, Centro de Investigación Príncipe Felipe (CIPF), Valencia, Spain
e-mail: vickycoce@gmail.com

M.P.-G. García
Department of Pathology, Hospital General Universitario Santa Lucia (HGUSL), Cartagena, Spain
e-mail: miguel.perez-guillermo@carm.es

V.R. Preedy, V.B. Patel (eds.), *Biomarkers in Cancer, Biomarkers in Disease: Methods, Discoveries and Applications*,
DOI 10.1007/978-94-007-7681-4_4

Abstract

Serrated adenocarcinoma (SC) is a recently recognized colorectal cancer (CRC) subtype, accounting for 7.2–9.2 % of CRC. SC has a worse prognosis than conventional carcinoma (CC) probably due to specific features at the invasive front including high-grade tumor budding and cytoplasmic pseudofragments, infiltrating growth pattern, and a weak peritumoral lymphocyte response. SCs also have a different profile of mutations in KRAS or BRAF oncogenes, expression of DNA repair proteins, and MSI status. Histological and immunohistochemical protein expression criteria have been proposed for SC diagnosis. Molecular profile studies have revealed that in agreement with previous observations, SCs have several cellular functions differentially regulated, such as hypoxia-, cytoskeleton-, vesicle transport-, and apoptosis-related pathways, among others. Expressions of several genes that participate in these pathways, like ephrin receptor B2, hippocalcin, and fascin1, have been proposed as biomarkers for differential SC diagnosis. miRNA expression and methylome signatures seem to corroborate these functions. All these findings suggest that the correct SC diagnosis may have important clinical implications and that the identified pathways and molecular targets could be exploited in the interest of SC specific patient follow-up and treatment.

List of Abbreviations and Genes

Abbreviations

CC	Conventional Carcinoma
CIMP	CpG island Methylation Phenotype
CRC	Colorectal Carcinoma
CyPs	Cytoplasmic Pseudofragments
EMT	Epithelial-Mesenchymal Transition
HH	Hedgehog Signaling Pathway
IHC	Immunohistochemistry
LOH	Loss of Heterozygosity
miRNA	MicroRNA
MSI	Microsatellite Instability
MSI-H	High Microsatellite Instability
MSI-L	Low Microsatellite Instability
PLI	Peritumoral Lymphocytic Infiltrate

SA	Serrated Adenoma
SC	Serrated Carcinoma
SSA	Sessile Serrated Adenoma
TB	Tumor Budding
TGP	Tumor Growth Pattern
TILs	Tumor Infiltrating Lymphocytes
Genes	
APC	Adenomatous Polyposis Coli
EGFR	Epidermal Growth Factor Receptor
EPHB2	Ephrin Receptor B2
FSCN1	Fascin 1
HIF-1α	Hypoxia-Inducible Factor 1 α
HPCA	Hippocalcin
MGMT	*O*-6-Methylguanine-DNA Methyltransferase
MLH1	DNA Mismatch Repair Protein Mlh1
MSH2 and MSH6	DNA Mismatch Repair Protein MSH2 and MSH6
NAIP	Neuronal Apoptosis Inhibitory Protein
PTCH1	Patched
SMO	Smoothened
VEGF	Vascular Endothelial Growth Factor

Key Facts

- Serrated carcinoma (SC) is a recently recognized histological subtype accounting for 7.2–9.2 % of colorectal carcinoma (CRC).
- Clinicopathological studies have demonstrated that SC has worse prognosis than conventional carcinoma (CC), and therefore diagnostic markers are necessary for SC identification.
- Morphological, immunohistological, and molecular research have shown that, compared with CC, SC displays more conspicuous invasive properties.
- Molecular profiling studies using microarrays have identified several proteins that could be useful to distinguish SC from CC and from those CRCs showing high grade of microsatellite instability.
- Current information on biological functions altered in SC has provided possible therapeutic opportunities that can be used for a specific treatment in SC patients.

Definition of Words and Terms

Conventional carcinoma (CC) Colorectal carcinoma histological subtype characterized by the presence of single glands and complex glandular structures lined by cylindrical or cuboidal cells with basophilic or amphophilic cytoplasm. Nuclei are stratified and round to oval and mitotic figures are usually abundant. The so-called dirty necrosis usually occupies glandular lumina.

CpG island methylation phenotype (CIMP) A molecular process observed in cancer cells in which aberrant methylation of cytosines from CpG clusters causes gene expression silencing.

Epithelial-mesenchymal transition (EMT) A process of long-lasting morphological and molecular changes by which epithelial cells lose their cell polarity and cell-cell adhesion and gain migratory and invasive properties to become mesenchymal cells.

Microsatellite instability (MSI) A status of genetic hypermutability evidenced in repetitive DNA regions (microsatellites) that results from the impairment of DNA mismatch repair (MMR) proteins.

Serrated carcinoma (SC) Colorectal carcinoma histological subtype characterized by epithelial serrations, clear or eosinophilic cytoplasm, abundant cytoplasm, vesicular nuclei, absence of or less than 10 % necrosis of the total surface area, mucin production, and cell balls and papillary rods in mucinous areas of a tumor (Tuppurainen et al. 2005).

Tumor budding (TB) Isolated or small clusters of invasive carcinoma cells at the invasive front that penetrate a short distance into the subjacent stroma.

Introduction

Colorectal carcinoma (CRC) is one of the more frequent and more deathly tumors in Western countries. It is a complex disease that can be classified into different subtypes, each one with distinctive molecular, pathological, and clinical features, more than 90 % of the CRC being adenocarcinomas (Hamilton et al. 2010).

Approximately, 80 % of colorectal cancers (CRCs) are conventional carcinomas (CCs) (Fig. 1a) which developed through the so-called chromosomal instability or suppressor phenotype molecular pathway characterized by APC protein inactivation (Potter 1999; Hanahan and Weinberg 2000), although some CCs can develop from a non-APC-mutated lesion (Jass 2004). CC precursor lesions are a well-established series of polyps (tubular adenoma (TA), tubulovillous adenoma (TVA), and villous adenoma (VA)) characterized by microsatellite stability (MSS) and KRAS mutations (Noffsinger 2009).

In contrast, the molecular pathway and their precursor polyps behind the remaining 20 % of CRC are not fully identified. Serrated carcinoma (SC) is an entity recently recognized by the World Health Organization as a subtype accounting for 7.5–10 % of CRC which is associated with quicker development and worse

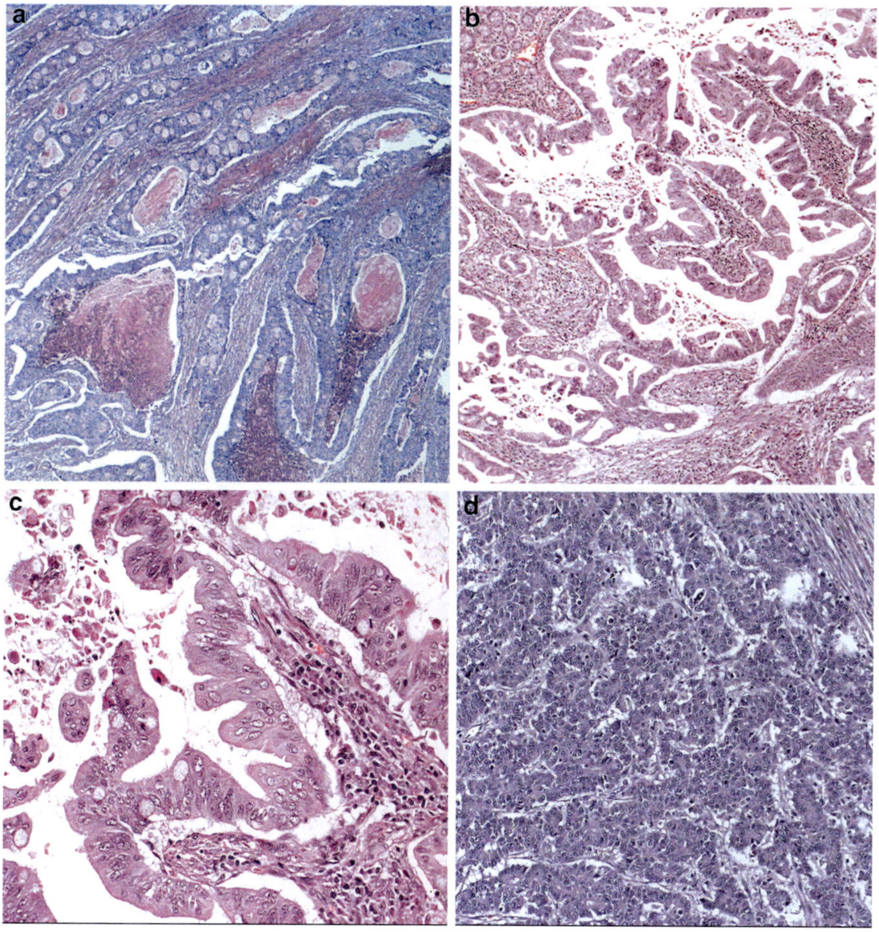

Fig. 1 Morphological differences between three different CRC histological subtypes. (**a**) Cribriform-comedo type conventional carcinoma showing dirty necrosis (HE 100×). (**b**) Serrated adenocarcinoma (HE 100×). (**c**) Typical serrated gland from a serrated adenocarcinoma (HE 400×). (**d**) Sporadic colorectal carcinoma with typical histological features of high level of microsatellite instability (HE 200×)

survival than CC (García-Solano et al. 2010). Based on its serrated "sawtooth" morphology (Fig. 1b) and the identification of residual adjacent serrated polyps in SC surgical specimens, it was assumed that SC was an end point of the serrated polyp pathological sequence which includes hyperplastic (HP), sessile serrated adenoma (SSA), traditional serrated adenoma (TSA), and mixed polyps. The molecular carcinogenic mechanisms involved in these polyps are not clearly discerned although microsatellite instability (MSI), BRAF mutation, and CpG island methylation phenotype (CIMP) seem to be implicated. In fact, three different serrated polyp pathways have been proposed: the BRAF mutated/high level of

CIMP (CIMP-H) MSI which is more frequently found in proximal colon, the BRAF mutated/CIMP-H/MSS which also used to be proximally located, and the KRAS mutated/low level of CIMP (CIMP-L)/MSS CRC which is often found in right colon (Leggett and Whitehall 2010). A Finnish research group was the first to describe serrated adenomas progressing toward an adenocarcinoma with serrated morphology, called "serrated adenocarcinoma" (Mäkinen et al. 2001), and in this work several histological criteria were proposed for SC diagnosis (Mäkinen et al. 2001) which were subsequently validated by the Spanish group (García-Solano et al. 2010). To date a total of 165 adenocarcinomas arising in serrated adenomas (SA) or large hyperplastic polyps have been described in different series (Jass and Smith 1992; Yao et al. 2000; Tuppurainen et al. 2005; García-Solano et al. 2010).

The aim of this chapter is to summarize the biological characteristics of SC in order to get a better understanding of SC/CC differences and how to apply this knowledge in diagnosis and in proposing possible molecular targets for SC.

Clinical and Pathological Aspects

No apparent significant differences in terms of age or sex of the patients have been observed between SC and CC. The average age of diagnosis in patients with SC was 69 years (range, 37–84; ±SD 10.1), while with CCs was 70.3 years (range, 35–96; ±SD 10.7) (García-Solano et al. 2010). In the studies from Finnish and Spanish populations, the location of the SCs is predominantly proximal (54.1 % and 52 %, respectively) (Tuppurainen et al. 2005; García-Solano et al. 2010) although the incidence of rectal SCs in the Finnish series was higher (33 %) (Tuppurainen et al. 2005) than in the Spanish one (15.3 %) (García-Solano et al. 2010). In the Spanish series, 16.4 % of males presented proximal SC, while in women this percentage reached 12.3 % (García-Solano et al. 2010), which contrasts with the results of the Finnish series in which proximal SCs were more frequent in women (18 %) (Tuppurainen et al. 2005).

It has been observed that SC presented, more often than CC, other synchronous CRCs (12.9 % vs. 3.0 %), and, in addition, these synchronous carcinomas were mostly SC (90.9 %), while all the synchronous CRCs found in a matched CC series had conventional histology (García-Solano et al. 2010). In the Spanish series of SCs, it could also be observed that the distant polyps in the surgical specimen were mainly of serrated histology, while the percentage of CC with distant serrated polyps was much lower (21.2 % vs. 8.4 %). This observation is even more striking when studying polyps adjacent to SC (51.8 % vs. 0 %) (García-Solano et al. 2010). All these findings are consistent with observations of Lazarus et al. (2005), in the sense that the lesions showing serrated adenomas indicated a significant risk for the development of both serrated adenomas and metachronous cancer, all these supporting the concept of colorectal carcinogenesis serrated route where SC would be one of its end points.

Table 1 Histological criteria for SC diagnosis proposed by Tuppurainen et al. (2005)

Predominant histological pattern (>50 % of tumor)	Cytological features	Tumor necrosis	In the case of mucinous pattern
Serrated gland	Broad eosinophilic cytoplasm	Absence or <10 %	Rigid pseudopapillae
Trabecular	Large vesicular nucleus		Cell balls within mucinous areas
Mucinous	Well- or moderate-conserved nuclear polarity		

Histologic Diagnosis

Histological criteria for the diagnosis of an SC were described by Mäkinen et al. (2001), in a number of SCs showing an adjacent SA to the invasive component. Later, the same group (Tuppurainen et al. 2005) refined and tested these criteria, and, more recently, García-Solano et al. (2010) proved these criteria (Table 1) to be valid in a different population as the Spanish one.

The three most important growth patterns observed in SC are: serrated, mucinous, and trabecular (Mäkinen 2007), and their histological features are described below.

- Serrated pattern: is the most common, accounting for about two-thirds of the SCs. It is often observed in well- and moderately differentiated SC (similar to the concept of differentiation applied to CCs) and as a focal pattern in mucinous and poorly differentiated SCs. This pattern consists of glands that show an irregular luminal "serrated" border constituted by projections to the lumen with or without basal membrane, but without a true fibrovascular core, i.e., there are no true papillae (Fig. 1c). The cells lining the glands show a clear or eosinophilic large cytoplasm, with a large and vesicular nucleus frequently displaying a nucleolus; nuclear polarity is quite conserved, the nucleus/cytoplasm (N/C) ratio is low, and dirty necrosis is not observed or, if present, is less than 10 % of the tumor. Often rounded glands can be observed without serrated luminal architecture, even with cribriform pattern, but with the aforementioned typical cytological features and absence of necrosis. These non-serrated glands usually represent a minor pattern accompanying the serrated component but on rare occasions may become the dominant pattern (García-Solano et al. 2010). Importantly, serrated architecture should not be confused with the pseudoserration pattern which is observed when cribriform glandular structures show central necrosis. Nuclear and cytoplasmic basophilia, loss of nuclear polarity, high N/C ratio, and presence of necrosis are suggestive indicators of a CC with pseudoserration (Mäkinen 2007).

In SCs with serrated pattern, mucinous areas representing less than 50 % of the tumor are more often than in the CCs.

– Mucinous pattern: is the second most common pattern, accounting for 24.7 % in the Spanish series, whereas this pattern appears in 17.6 % of CCs (García-Solano et al. 2010). In this SC type, mucin represents over 50 % of the tumor although there usually are areas showing the typical serrated pattern. In areas where large amount of mucus exists, pseudopapillae with rigid borders similar to pseudopapillary projections described in the serrated pattern and solid cell balls floating in the mucus whose cells show the cytologic features typical of SC can be observed.
– Poorly differentiated or trabecular pattern: the tumor grows as solid nests and cords with a solid pattern, trabecular or sometimes microglandular. It is composed of cells with the cytologic features of SC and absence of tumor necrosis, features that are not normally seen in the poorly differentiated CCs.

For the correct diagnosis of SC, all the criteria described in Table 1 must be met, or all but one, in most of the tumor (>50 %). It is important to stress that in order to diagnose an SC, it is not necessary to have an SA adjacent to the invasive carcinoma since García-Solano et al. (2010) demonstrated that there were no significant differences in the percentage of fulfillment in these criteria when comparing SC with and without adjacent SA.

The correct SC diagnosis would be based on the following criteria: serrated, mucinous, or trabecular pattern, typical SC cytology, absence of luminal "dirty" necrosis (or in less than 10 % of the tumor), rigid pseudopapillae, and cell balls floating in mucus in the case of SCs with a predominant mucinous pattern. In a surgical specimen, the existence of polyps with serrated morphology, serrated synchronous carcinomas, and areas of carcinoma with variable amounts of mucin are findings that often accompany the aforementioned histological criteria, but they are not necessary for diagnosis.

It is also worth mentioning that there is a group of CRCs (showing all but two) lacking two histological criteria for the diagnosis of SC, and they were considered as "doubtful SC." This group of tumors seems to be closer to SCs than to CCs, although further studies are needed to assess the potential biological implications and find out if they are genuine SCs or if they correspond to an intermediate group between the serrated route and the classical route of carcinogenesis. For practical purposes in daily practice, this group is diagnosed as CC.

It is important to note that there are special circumstances where the histological criteria for the diagnosis of SC have not been completely evaluated. These include its application in endoscopic biopsies, metastases, and in CRCs subjected to neoadjuvant therapy. In the first case, serrated pattern identification would be undoubtedly possible with the proviso that the biopsy includes sufficient number of malignant glands displaying the typical morphology and pathologist is acquainted with the histological features needed for its correct diagnosis. It also should be noticed that not all SCs display the typical cytological pattern over 100 % of the tumor surface. In the second case, serrated morphology is reproducible in metastasis, but may change the type of serrated pattern (serrated, mucinous, poorly differentiated) compared to the primary tumor. Finally, there are so far no data on the evaluation criteria in SC treated with neoadjuvant therapies. The cellular changes produced by neoadjuvant therapies could mask or mimic the histological criteria of SC, so it is not recommended to diagnose SC in these circumstances.

Prognosis

Mäkinen et al. (2001) and Laiho et al. (2007) suggested that SC had a different prognosis compared to CCs and that distal SCs even had a less favorable prognosis than CCs at this location. In a later study, it was shown that patients with SC show worse survival than a group of patients with CCs matched by age, sex, location, histological grade, and Dukes' stage, after 5 years of follow-up (García-Solano et al. 2010). In addition, patients with SC distal/rectal location had worse survival than patients with proximal SC and the rest of patients with CC, location being an independent predictor of worse survival in multivariate analysis (García-Solano et al. 2010).

Characterization of the Invasive Front in the SC

Histological Study

In agreement with clinical observations, it was shown in subsequent studies that, in comparison to CC, SC shows frequently adverse prognostic histological factors described for CRCs (Ueno et al. 2002; Prall et al. 2005; Shinto et al. 2005; Jass et al. 1987; Klintrup et al. 2005) such as tumor budding (TB), cytoplasmic pseudofragments (CyPs), infiltrative tumor growth pattern (TGP), and weak peritumoral lymphocytic infiltrate (PLI) (García-Solano et al. 2011a). Most of these factors, especially TB and CyPs, are morphological manifestations of the epithelial-mesenchymal transition (EMT). TB consists of isolated single cancer cell or a cluster of fewer than five cancer cells found in the stroma adjacent to the invasive front (Shinto et al. 2005). CyPs are rounded cytoplasm coreless fragments (>2 μm diameter) adjacent to the infiltrative edge showing IHQ-positive staining for cytokeratin (AE1/AE3) and no evidence of surrounding inflammatory cells (Shinto et al. 2005). These findings help explain why SCs have a worse prognosis than CCs.

Immunohistochemistry Study

In order to better characterize the active invasive front characteristic of SC proteins related to cell adhesion, GT formation and EMT were studied by immunohistochemistry. These proteins were β catenin from Wnt/β-catenin pathway, E-cadherin and P-cadherins, SMAD4 from the TGFβ, and mesenchymal markers such as laminin 5γ2 (García-Solano et al. 2011b). Nuclear expression of β-catenin in SC is much lower (21 %) than that observed in CCs (61 %). This lack of nuclear β-catenin suggests that the GT-forming route in the SCs must be different from the canonical pathway Wnt/β-catenin which was considered by Prall (2007) as one of the most important pathways in the formation of GT in the CRCs. It seems that SC displays more often loss of expression of E-cadherin and nuclear SMAD4 and increased expression of laminin 5γ2 in the invasive front than that of CC (García-Solano et al. 2011b). The loss of expression of E-cadherin and increased SMAD4 and laminin 5γ2 has been correlated with poor prognosis in CRCs (Morita et al. 1999; Masaki et al. 2001; Tanaka et al. 2008). Consequently, these data are consistent with a more active invasive front and the worse prognosis observed in patients with SC compared to patients with CC.

MSI Status and Oncogene Mutational Studies

Only two studies have examined the presence of mutation in KRAS and BRAF oncogenes, the microsatellite instability (MSI) status and the immunohistochemical expression of DNA repair proteins in SCs compared with CCs (Stefanius et al. 2011; García-Solano et al. 2012). In Table 2, the results of the two studies have been summarized. Both revealed that, in contrast to the assumed predominance of BRAF mutations in the serrated polyp pathway, KRAS mutations were even more frequent in SCs than in CCs. This finding suggests that the possible precursor polyp of SC might be a not very common serrated polyp with KRAS mutation, such as traditional serrated adenoma. Additionally, BRAF mutations and MSI-H status were also more common in SCs than in CCs (Stefanius et al. 2011;

Table 2 Results of the two independent studies evaluating the mutation occurrence in *KRAS* and *BRAF* oncogenes and the MSI status in SC and CC

	Stefanius et al. (2011)			García Solano et al. (2012)		
	SC	Non-serrated		SC	CC	
Reference	$n = 42$	$N = 59$	p value	$n = 89$	$n = 81$	p value
KRAS						
Mutated	19 (45.2)	16 (27.1)		38 (42.7)	26 (32.1)	
Native	23 (54.8)	43 (72.9)	0.059	50	55	0.092
BRAF						
Mutated	14 (33.3)	0 (0)		23 (25.8)	1 (1.2)	
Native	28 (66.7)	59 (100)	<0.0001	66	80	<0.0001
MSI status						
MSI-H	7 (18.9)	4 (7.1)		11 (12.4)	2 (2.5)	
MSI-L/MSS	30 (81.1)	52 (92.9)	0.164	78	79	0.014

SC Serrated carcinoma, *CC* conventional carcinoma, *MSI-H* high level of microsatellite instability, *MSI-L* low level of MSI, *MSS* microsatellite stability

García-Solano et al. 2012) MSI-H status in the SCs is associated with the MLH1 expression loss (Stefanius et al. 2011; García-Solano et al. 2012) caused by gene promoter methylation, while the few MLH1 CCs were associated with the loss of MSH2 expression (Stefanius et al. 2011). It was also observed that, compared to CCs, the loss of MGMT expression is a characteristic of SCs (García-Solano et al. 2012).

When the mutational status in SC considering its location was assessed, it was observed that proximally located SCs showed higher frequency of BRAF mutations, increased frequency of MSI-H, lower KRAS mutation occurrence, and less IHC loss of MGMT expression than SCs with distal location (García-Solano et al. 2012). These data support the opinion of Noffsinger (2009) and Mäkinen (2007) on the existence of two serrated carcinogenesis pathways: the proximal and distal serrated pathways.

The high frequency of mutations in the SCs (KRAS + BRAF) of up to 67 %, double those observed in CCs (33 %) (García-Solano et al. 2012), may have predictive implications as patients with SC carcinomas would not be candidates for anti-EGFR treatments. To the best of our knowledge, there are no reliable studies on the prognostic or predictive value of MSI status and KRAS/BRAF mutation in SC.

Relationship Between SC and Sporadic MSI-H CRCs

The sporadic MSI-H CRC, often has proximal location, is usually seen in older females and seems to be developed from an SSA (Bellizzi and Frankel 2009). It usually has a heterogeneous architecture since several tumor patterns are seen together: tubular, medullary-type, or poorly differentiated and mucinous areas and even signet-ring cells can be observed (Jenkins et al. 2007). Sporadic MSI-H CRC shares clinical, histological, and molecular features with proximally located SC which can also develop from serrated adenoma (probably SSA type), often contains mucus, a Crohn-like lymphoid infiltrate and tumor infiltrating lymphocytes (TILs) (García-Solano et al. 2012) with the loss of expression of nuclear β-catenin can be found (García-Solano et al. 2011b). In addition, compared with the CC, SC and MSI-H share some more common characteristics such as increased occurrence of mutations in BRAF, MSI-H status, CIMP phenotype and proximal colon location. Despite these common findings, MSI-H CRC and SC are not the same tumor type as in the former TB and CyPs are not common (Prall 2007; Wright and Stewart 2003), laminin 5γ2 expression is not generally seen (Shinto et al. 2006) and tend to have better prognosis than other CRCs (Popat et al. 2005). Compared to sporadic MSI-H CRC, KRAS mutations occur more frequently in SC and in a lower percentage in BRAF, and MSI-H is not very common (García-Solano et al. 2012).

Immunohistochemical markers identified in expression profiling studies from SC and CC comparison (fascin and hippocalcin) also showed to be useful in distinguishing SC from MSI-H CRC (Conesa-Zamora et al. 2013). Finally, it was observed that the application of MsPath, a histological score basically used for identification of CRC with MSI-H, is not effective in identifying SC showing MSI-H (García-Solano et al. 2013) (Fig. 1d).

Molecular Profiling Studies

Gene Expression Signatures in SC and CC

Microarray expression profiling provides an excellent tool for obtaining useful markers with diagnostic, prognostic, and predictive value. As previously stated, SCs present different clinical features than CCs. Microarray analysis has been used to determine which genes were differently expressed and which particular functions are behind SC morphology and clinical behavior. There are two published expression profile studies based in microarrays technologies: the first one analyzing Finnish patient samples using an Affymetrix platform (Laiho et al. 2007) and the other performed with Spanish patient samples onto an Agilent platform (Conesa-Zamora et al. 2013). Both studies revealed that proteins involved in hypoxia, membrane structure, and morphogenesis were differently expressed. These and other functions are summarized in Table 3 where the functions from the two articles are aggregated in gene ontology categories. The Spanish study also shown which KEGG pathways were enriched in SC samples and those included apoptosis (hsa04210); morphogenesis (Notch signaling pathway (hsa04330)); VEGF pathway (hsa04370); cytoskeleton organization in membrane junctions (gap junction (map04540), adherens junctions (hsa04520)); DNA repair and synthesis (pyrimidine metabolism (hsa00240), DNA replication (hsa03030), nonhomologous end joining (hsa03450), base excision repair (hsa03410), folate biosynthesis (hsa00790)); B-cell response (B-cell receptor signaling (hsa04662), Fc epsilon RI signaling (hsa04662), Fc gamma R-mediated phagocytosis (hsa04666)); growth factor receptor signaling (ErbB signaling pathway (hsa04012), mTOR signaling pathway (hsa04150)); and lipid and protein metabolism, whereas functions overexpressed in CCs were mainly associated with immune response either in xenograft rejection (allograft rejection (hsa05330), graft-versus-host disease (hsa05332)), or in autoimmune diseases (autoimmune thyroid disease (hsa05320), such as type I diabetes mellitus (hsa04940)) (Conesa-Zamora et al. 2013), which may be related with a recent report describing weaker tumoral lymphocytic infiltrate in SC compared to CC (García-Solano et al. 2011a). An overview by “Paintomics” of the CRC-related proteins and KEGG pathways which are differentially expressed between CC (in blue) and SC (in red) is shown in Fig. 2a (www.paintomics.org).

Concerning the differentially expressed genes between CC and SC, five genes have been validated by immunohistochemistry (Laiho et al. 2007; Conesa-Zamora et al. 2013; Table 4), and representative stainings are shown in Fig. 3. It is interesting to note that among the five validated proteins, three are participating in actin remodeling: patched, ephrin receptor B2 (Laiho et al. 2007), and fascin1 (Conesa-Zamora et al. 2013), which could be related for the characteristic

Table 3 Differentially represented functions between SC and CC

Main GO category		GO subcategories		
Description	GO number	Description	GO number	References
Morphogenesis	GO:0009653	Anatomical structure morphogenesis	GO:0009653	Laiho et al. (2007)
		Embryonic skeletal joint morphogenesis	GO:0060272	Conesa-Zamora et al. (2013)
Organogenesis	GO:0009887	Anatomical structure development	GO:0048856	Laiho et al. (2007)
		Mesenchymal to epithelial transition	GO:0060231	Conesa-Zamora et al. (2013)
		Nervous system development	GO: 0007399	Conesa-Zamora et al. (2013)
		Zygotic determination of dorsal/ventral axis	GO:0007352	Conesa-Zamora et al. (2013)
Integral_to_membrane	GO:0016021	Ion channel complex	GO:00354702	Laiho et al. (2007)
		Potassium ion transmembrane transporter activity	GO:0015079	Conesa-Zamora et al. (2013)
		Calcium channel inhibitor activity	GO:0019855	Conesa-Zamora et al. (2013)
Binding	GO:0005488	Receptor binding	GO:0005102	Laiho et al. (2007)
		Vitamin_D_receptor_binding	GO:0042809	Laiho et al. (2007)
		Positive regulation of transforming growth factor beta receptor signaling pathway	GO:0030511	Conesa-Zamora et al. (2013)
		Protein binding	GO:0005515	Conesa-Zamora et al. (2013)
		Clathrin binding	GO:0030276	Conesa-Zamora et al. (2013)
		Co-SMAD binding	GO:0070410	Conesa-Zamora et al. (2013)
		DNA binding	GO:0003677	Conesa-Zamora et al. (2013)
Catalytic activity	GO:0003824	Oxidoreductase activity	GO:0016667	Conesa-Zamora et al. (2013)
		Nucleoside-triphosphatase activity	GO:00016740	Laiho et al. (2007)
		Transferase activity	GO:0016740	Conesa-Zamora et al. (2013)
		Hydrolase activity	GO:0016787	Conesa-Zamora et al. (2013)
Trasporter activity	GO:005215	Transmembrane transporter activity	GO:0022857	Laiho et al. (2007)
		ATPase_activity, _coupled_to_transmembrane_movement_of_ions	GO:0042625	Laiho et al. (2007)
		Potassium/chloride symporter activity	GO:0015379	Conesa-Zamora et al. (2013)

(*continued*)

Table 3 (continued)

Main GO category		GO subcategories		
Description	GO number	Description	GO number	References
Enzyme regulator activity	GO:0030234	GTPase regulator activity	GO:0030695	Conesa-Zamora et al. (2013)
		RNA_polymerase_II_transcription_mediator_activity	GO:0016455	Laiho et al. (2007)
Molecular transducer activity	GO:0060089	Signaling receptor activity	GO:00004872	Conesa-Zamora et al. (2013)
		Vascular endothelial growth factor receptor activity	GO:0005021	Conesa-Zamora et al. (2013)
		Negative regulation of interleukin-12 biosynthetic process	GO:0045083	Conesa-Zamora et al. (2013)
		Intracellular transport	GO:0046907	Conesa-Zamora et al. (2013)
		Retrograde vesicle-mediated transport, Golgi to ER	GO:0006890	Conesa-Zamora et al. (2013)
		Late endosome to vacuole transport	GO:0045324	Conesa-Zamora et al. (2013)
Metabolic process	GO:0008152	Fatty acid metabolic process	GO:0006631	Conesa-Zamora et al. (2013)
		Vitamin D biosynthetic process	GO:0042368	Conesa-Zamora et al. (2013)
Regulation of gene expression	GO:0010468	DNA methylation during embryonic development	GO:0043045	Conesa-Zamora et al. (2013)

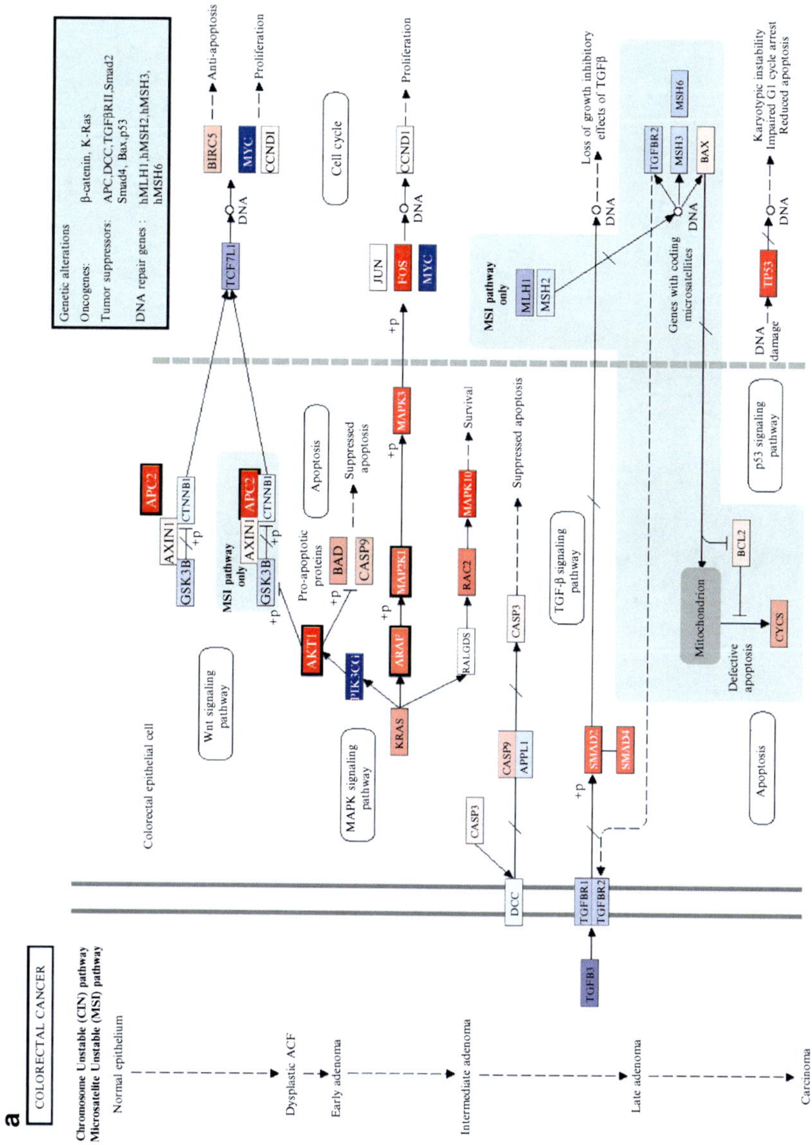

Fig. 2 (continued)

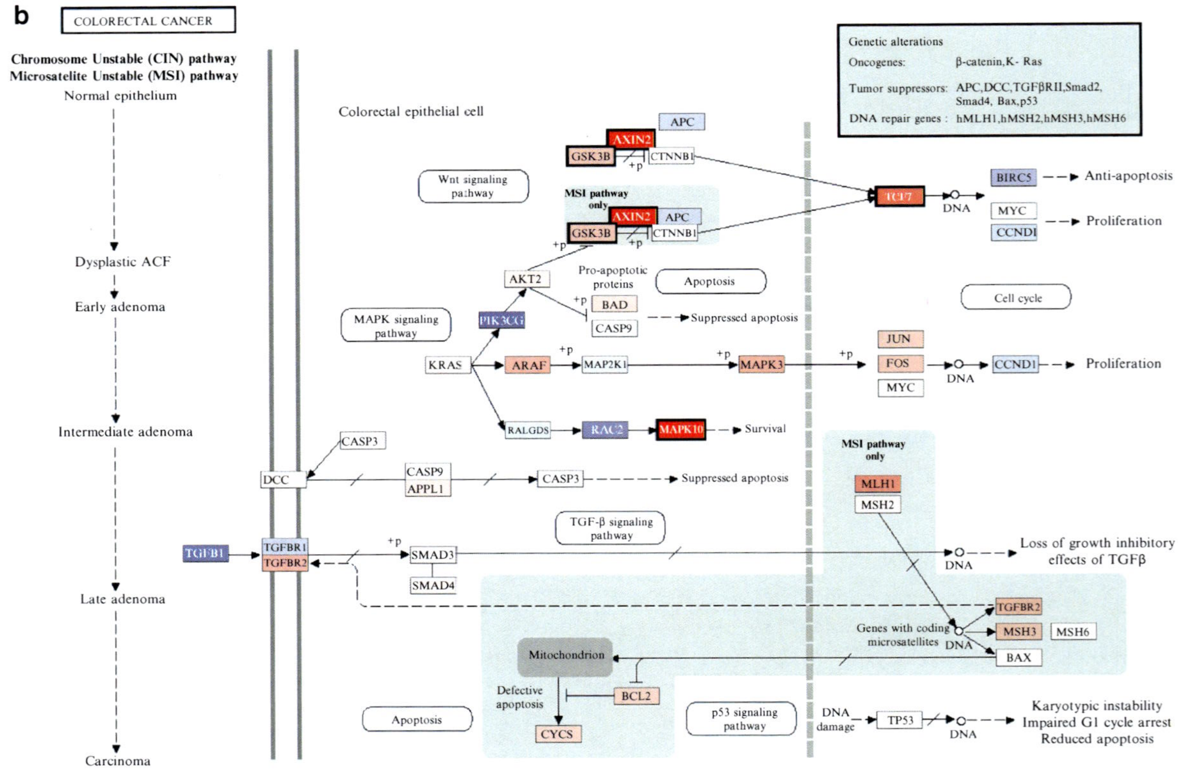

Fig. 2 Diagram showing differentially represented typical colorectal carcinoma pathways between different colorectal histological subtypes. Genes overexpressed in SC are shown in *red boxes*, whereas those in CC (**a**) or MSI-H CRC (**b**) are found in *blue*. The intensity of the color reflects the grade of differential expression (more information: www.paintomics.org)

Table 4 Differentially expressed genes between SC and CC

NM symbol	Gene	Function	SC versus CC expression	References
NM_017449	Ephrin receptor B2	Actin remodeling	Downregulated	Laiho et al. (2007)
NM_003088	Fascin1	Actin remodeling	Upregulated	Conesa-Zamora et al. (2013)
NM_181054	HIF-1α	Hypoxia	Upregulated	Laiho et al. (2007)
NM_002143	Hippocalcin	Antiapoptotosis	Upregulated	Conesa-Zamora et al. (2013)
NM_000264	Patched	Actin remodeling	Downregulated	Laiho et al. (2007)

serrated morphology. Moreover, fascin1 has been associated with filopodia formation and cell invasion which are consistent with the previous assessment of the conspicuous invasive front of SC. Patched (PTCH1) acts as receptor of Hedgehog (HH) signaling proteins (Chen and Struhl 1996) and interacts and suppresses Smoothened (SMO). Hedgehog signaling is important during the development for the patterning of the gastrointestinal tract (Oldakr et al. 2001). PTCH1 activation represses the activation of WNT and TGF signaling pathways, and it is considered as a tumor suppressor whose impairment has been related to several disorders such as holoprosencephaly (Ming et al. 2002) and Gorlin syndrome which is characterized by early-onset multiple basal cell carcinomas and increased rate of some other tumors such as medulloblastomas (Johnson et al. 1996). The PTCH1 staining pattern was more granular in CC than in SC, thus pointing *PTCH1* as a candidate gene for the development of SC (Laiho et al. 2007).

Ephrin receptor B2 EPHB2, also known as ELK-related tyrosine kinase or HEK5, is a member of EPHB receptor tyrosine kinases that are involved in formation and remodeling of dendritic spines and consequently are involved in the modification of brain synapses (Murai and Pasquale 2002). This spine modification is believed to be caused by actin remodeling, and it has been postulated that EPHB2 is associated with several actin-regulating proteins such as Cdc42 (Irie and Yamaguchi 2002). Battle et al. (2002) studied the EPHB2 participation in CRC and proposed that EPHB2 maintains the crypt-villus axis and that β-catenin and TCF control EPHB2 and EPHB3 expression. It was also described that in Ephb2/Ephb3 null mice, the proliferative and differentiated cell populations are abnormally mixed in the intestinal epithelium. By immunohistochemistry, EPHB2 expression was more often found in the CC when compared to serrated lesions (Laiho et al. 2007). It seems that EPHB2 loss could be due to LOH or promoter hypermethylation, and although this loss was not associated with SC tumor grade, it could be an important tumor suppressor (Laiho et al. 2007).

Fascin1 (FSCN1) is an actin-bundling protein that can cross-link actin filaments in vivo (Bryan and Kane 1982) and participates in the formation of microspikes, filopodia, membrane ruffles, and stress fibers (Yamashiro-Matsumura and Matsumura 1986). In *Drosophila*, the fascin1 homologue SNL has an actin-binding

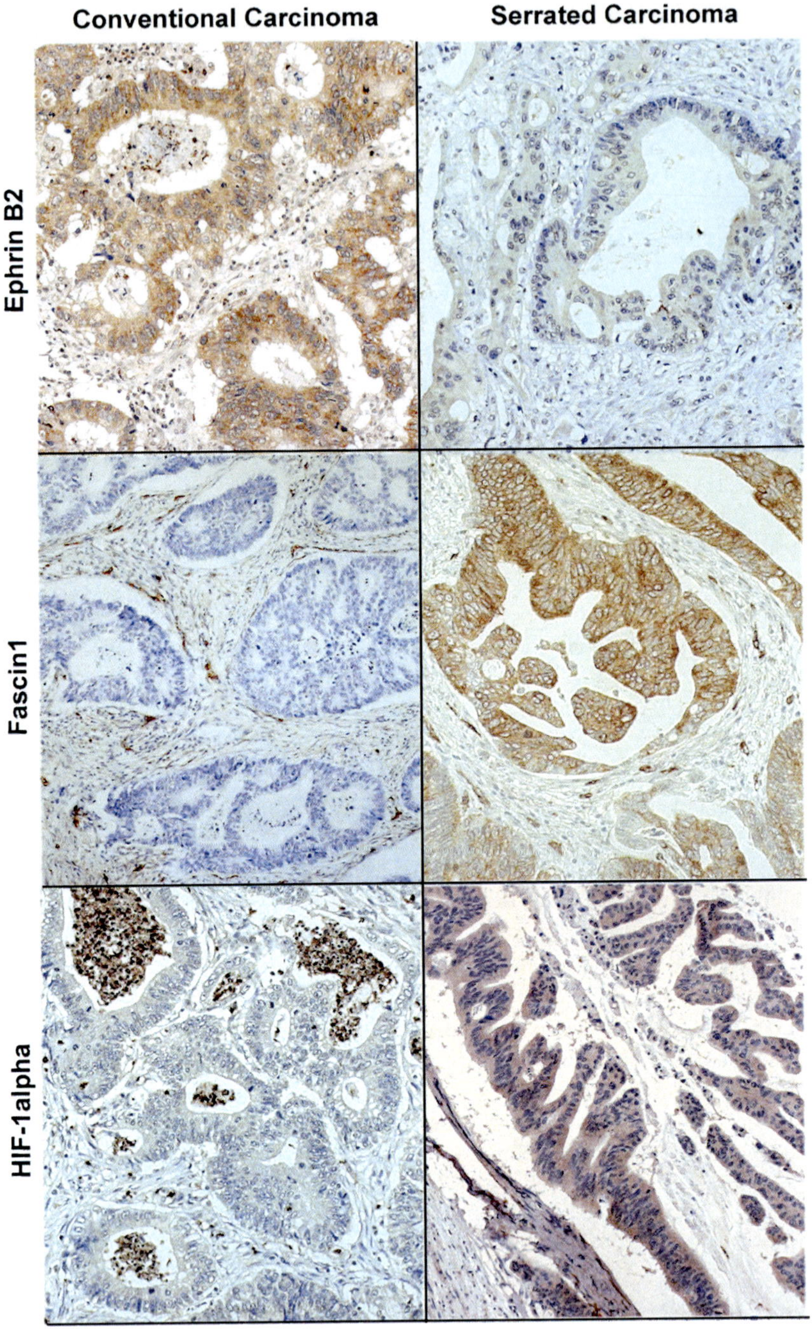

Fig. 3 (continued)

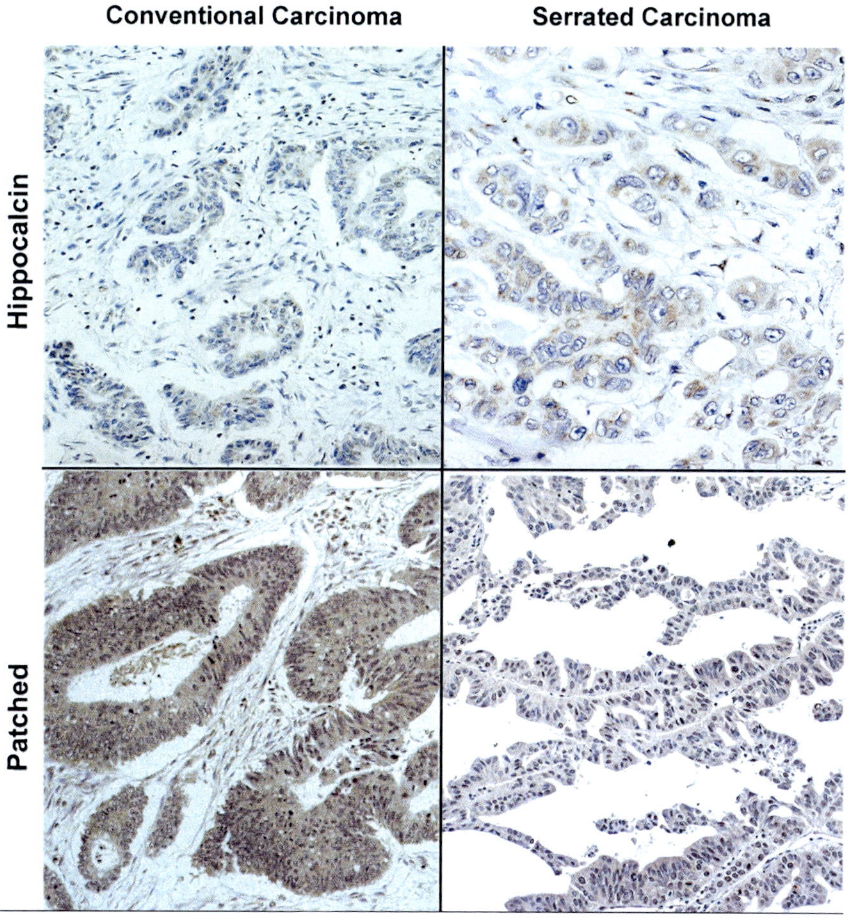

Fig. 3 Immunohistochemical markers obtained from expression profiling useful as potential diagnostic markers for SC identification. EPHB2, fascin1, HIF-1α, hippocalcin, patched in CC (*A*, *C*, *E*, *G*, *I*), and SC (*B*, *D*, *F*, *H*, *J*), respectively

domain (Ono et al. 1997) and has a role in cell migration and metastasis. Fascin1 expression seems to be regulated by several microRNAs, which can also participate in actin-mediated intracellular protein trafficking (Zhang et al. 2009), and its overexpression may play a role in the metastasis of multiple types of cancer by increasing cell motility (Jayo and Parsons 2010; Minn et al. 2005). In fact, fascin1 has also been related to poor survival in gastric (Kim et al. 2012) and colorectal cancers (Hashimoto et al. 2006). Fascin is more expressed in SC than CC (Conesa-Zamora et al. 2013) which is consistent with SC worse prognosis (García-Solano et al. 2010); the more "active" invasive front and the fully recognized histological manifestations of epithelial-mesenchymal transition (EMT) associated with SC such as tumor budding and cytoplasmic pseudofragments (García-Solano et al. 2011a) and less expression of E-cadherin epithelial marker and an increased of the stromal marker laminin 5γ2 (García-Solano et al. 2011b).

Another characteristic SC protein is the hypoxia-inducible factor 1 α (HIF-1α) (Laiho et al. 2007) that participates in angiogenesis, cell survival, and invasion (Harris 2002; Semenza 2003). HIF-1α is a transcription factor involved in the expression of genes facilitating hypoxia adaptation by triggering angiogenesis, cell survival, and invasion and plays an essential role in embryonic vascularization and pathophysiology of ischemic disease (Semenza et al. 1996). One of the most important HIF-1α targets is the vascular endothelial growth factor (VEGF) (Semenza 2000; Pagès and Pouysségur 2005) which participates in endothelial cell proliferation and induces permeabilization of blood vessel (Roskoski 2007). HIF-1α protein is subject to ubiquitination and proteasomal degradation at normoxia (Sutter et al. 2000) and acts as a transcriptional repressor of the MSH2 and MSH6 genes, thereby inhibiting DNA mismatch recognition and repair (Koshiji et al. 2005). HIF-1α is elevated in colon cancer cells during proliferation (Zhong et al. 1999) and was seen more frequently expressed by immunohistochemistry in SC than in CC (Laiho et al. 2007). The HIF-1α overexpression (Laiho et al. 2007) coupled with the differentially activated VEGF pathway observed between SC and CC (Conesa-Zamora et al. 2013) points HIF-1α and hypoxia as important facts in SC development.

Another gene that is differentially expressed in SC is hippocalcin (HPCA) (Conesa-Zamora et al. 2013) which is a neuronal Ca^{+2} binding protein found in the brain and retina. In rat, it is found in membrane and participate in the photosignal transduction in a calcium-sensitive manner (Kobayashi et al. 1992). It is an antiapoptotic protein that seems to protect neurons against Ca^{+2}-induced cell death through a caspase-3-dependent pathway for which it associates with the neuronal apoptosis inhibitory protein (NAIP) (Mercer et al. 2000; Karimpour et al. 2011). NAIP mutations are implicated in spinal muscular atrophy (Roy et al. 1995) that is caused by neuron apoptosis.

Hippocalcin and NAIP immunohistochemical expressions were correlated, thus suggesting a concerted action, and they were more often found in SC than in CC (Conesa-Zamora et al. 2013). Apoptotic evasion was one of the earliest feature characteristics of SC and has been suggested as the cause of its serrated morphology in which the transformed epithelium proliferates laterally adopting a sawtooth growth pattern (Hamilton et al. 2010; Mäkinen 2007), and consequently, it is not surprising that hippocalcin is more expressed in SC than in CC. Despite the fact that an aberrant expression of recoverin members has been reported in tumor cells (Miyagawa et al. 2003), no previous reports have described the presence of hippocalcin in CRC. It is important to note that several differentially expressed genes in SC are related to neural development and not only patched, Ephb2, and hippocalcin but also INSM1, a sensitive marker for neuroendocrine differentiation of human lung tumors (Lan and Breslin 2009), and the transcript THC2539939, which was found overexpressed in metastases of gastroenteropancreatic neuroendocrine tumors (Posorski et al. 2011), both also seen overexpressed in SC (Conesa-Zamora et al. 2013).

Performance Status of Molecular Markers for SC Diagnosis

The identification of reliable markers is not only useful for SC diagnosis but may also help to discern which type of adenoma is the precursor lesion of SC. In the report by Laiho et al. (2007), three markers (PATCH, HIF-1α, EphB2) were proposed for its value for SC diagnosis, the immunohistochemical expression of HIF-1α being the most discriminatory between SC and CC with percentages of positivity of 62.2 % and 21.7 %, respectively, for each tumor type. In a later microarray study, the positive expression of fascin1 was observed in 88.6 % of SC and in 14.3 % of CC (88.6 % sensitivity, 85.7 % specificity), thus demonstrating its important diagnostic value for SC diagnosis. Of note, the positivity for fascin1 or hippocalcin reaching a sensitivity of 100 % indicates that when both markers are negative, it is highly unlikely that a given tumor is an SC. It has been suggested that MGMT loss is typical of SC (García-Solano et al. 2012), and therefore it was observed that the addition of MGMT loss to fascin1 and hippocalcin positivity increases the specificity up to 94.3 % but with less sensitivity (54.3 %). A proposed diagnostic panel for SC diagnosis would be MGMT, fascin1, and hippocalcin.

Gene Expression Signatures in SC and MSI-H CRCs

An mRNA microarray study has compared the mRNA expression profile of 11 SCs and three sporadic CRCs fulfilling molecular and histological features of MSI-H (i.e., mucinous non-serrated morphology, signet-ring cell, medullar-like architecture, tumor infiltrating (TIL) and peritumoral lymphocytes, "Crohn-like" inflammatory response, poor differentiation, tumor heterogeneity, "pushing" tumor border, and positivity for BRAF mutations). This work revealed that many genes and functions were differentially expressed between SC and MSI-H CRC. Concerning the functions it was observed that MSI-H showed an upregulation of genes related to the immune response (KEGG pathways: antigen processing and presentation (map04612), Toll-like receptor signaling (map04620), chemokine signaling (map04062), and cytokine-cytokine receptor interaction (map04060)) (unpublished observations) which is concordant with the reported suboptimal peritumoral lymphocytic infiltration seen is SC (García-Solano et al. 2011a). An overview by "Paintomics" of the CRC-related proteins and KEGG pathways which are differentially expressed between MSI-H (in blue) and SC (in red) is shown in Fig. 2b (www.paintomics.org).

Serrated Carcinoma Methylome Studies

The global methylated DNA content seems to play an important role in CRC and is considered as a prognostic index (Frigola et al. 2005). Moreover, it has been demonstrated that CRC patients with hMLH1 methylation do not benefit from

5-fluorouracil treatment and those with MGMT methylation are better responders to alkylating agents (Ide et al. 2008).

Given that methylation is an early event in colorectal carcinogenesis, methylated markers could be detected in precursor lesions obtained by endoscopy, thus contributing to CRC early detection. As pointed previously, the serrated pathway is characterized by aberrant hypermethylation patterns in CpG islands (O'Brien et al. 2006). Moreover, it was recently observed that SC has more frequently methylation of MLH1 gene than non-serrated CRCs (Stefanius et al. 2011).

Most of the studies dealing with this issue have determined a limited panel of 4 or 5 loci (MINT1, MINT2, MINT12 o MLH1 y MINT31, p16), thus establishing CpG island methylation phenotype (CIMP) of high (3–4 methylated loci), low grade (1–2 methylated loci), and negative (O'Brien et al. 2006). However, the study of few loci ignoring other CpG sequences is an oversimplified vision of such a complex change of genomic scale. In fact, it was recently demonstrated that most methylations in cancer do not occur in CpG island but in 2 kb distant sequences termed CpG shores (Irizarry et al. 2009). High-throughput techniques (high-density CpG microarrays, next-generation sequencing of methylated-enriched, or whole bisulfite-treated genome sequences) investigating the SC methylome could shed light onto the differentially methylated functions of SC and solve the overlapping histological similarity between SC and sporadic MSI-H CRC that the CIMP testing cannot discern and render SC specific diagnostic markers. In this regard, a study is analyzing the SC methylome by means of a 450,000 CpG island microarray in 120 colorectal specimens from Spanish and Finnish patients encompassing SC, CC and MSI-H CRCs. The study has demonstrated an important degree of similarity in the biological functions differentially represented from mRNA expressions and methylome microarray platforms. Again, G-coupled receptor, ion channel, neural-related, and VEFG receptor activities were found differentially observed between SC and CC. Besides, in this study, new differentially methylated genes have been identified, which has been subsequently validated by methylation-specific PCR (MSP) (unpublished observations). Likewise, this study has confirmed what has been observed with mRNA expression microarrays, i.e., the molecular profiles of SC and MSI-H are not the same with functions affecting immune response differentially represented.

Future Developments

The clinicopathological and molecular characterization of SC has rendered distinct prognostic and biological information for this CRC subtype as well as useful markers with diagnostic value. However, to date there are no functional studies demonstrating these differential biological activities. The establishment of SC cell lines or the identification of previous existing CRC cell lines as SC (based on expression of discriminatory proteins) is mandatory to validate the findings reported and to evaluate possible therapeutic choices, one of which could be the use of macroketone-based agents for inhibiting fascin1 action on invasiveness. On the other hand, the integration of high-throughput data from different "omic" approaches (transcriptomic, genomic, methylomic) would allow us to define a more precise picture of SC. The identification, by next-generation sequencing, of a characteristic profile of somatic mutations or possible genetic susceptibility polymorphisms in SC would also complement this knowledge and help identify other possible therapeutical targets. Given the importance of early cancer detection and the absence of a clearly identified SC precursor polyp, the most useful knowledge that could be obtained from all these molecular studies would be the application of SC, CC, and MSI-H CRC typical markers in order to trace them along the different polyp pathogenic pathways. This approach will enable a more precise and individualized follow-up of patients with endoscopically removed polyps which could be performed based on the malignant potential of each adenoma type.

Conclusions

The SC is a subtype of CRC recognized in the fourth edition of the classification of tumors of the digestive tract of WHO. Its position as end point serrated carcinogenesis pathway has been demonstrated in several works (García-Solano et al. 2010; Mäkinen et al. 2001). Pathologists should be acquainted with the histological features of this subtype of tumor because its prognosis is worse than the rest of CRC, and it harbors a higher percentage of mutations in KRAS and BRAF oncogenes (67 %) which makes it more resistant to anti-EGFR therapies than CC. The different profile of protein expression at the invasive front and gene expression profiles in comparison with other non-serrated CRC can identify potential therapeutic targets for a specific treatment of SC.

Potential Applications to Prognosis, Other Diseases, or Conditions

The worse prognosis of SC compared to CC or MSI CRC makes the use of specific SC markers mandatory for an efficient follow-up and treatment schemes of CRC patients.

Fascin1 and hippocalcin can be used as diagnostic markers of SC especially for their high sensitivity and negative predictive value.

The characteristic high frequency of KRAS and BRAF mutation among SCs and the high expression of fascin1 and hypoxic markers, such as HIF-1α, suggest a resistance of SC against anti-EGFR therapies pointing that the use or macroketone-based or antiangiogenic agents could be useful for the treatment of this CRC type.

Summary Points

- Compared to CC and MSI-H CRC, SC has special clinical characteristics and an active invasive front that could be responsible for its worse prognosis.
- Tumor molecular profiles obtained from microarray studies have confirmed previous clinical-pathological observations, and several cellular functions characteristic of SC have been found.
- These studies have identified several proteins that could be useful to distinguish SC from CC and MSI-H CRC.
- Based on the proteins identified, there are experimental therapies like macroketones or antiangiogenesis therapy that might be used for a specific SC treatment.
- SC is different from MSI-H CRC in terms of morphology, immunohistochemical pattern, and molecular profile and should be considered as distinct end points of the serrated polyp pathological pathway.

References

Batlle E, Henderson JT, Beghtel H, et al. Beta-catenin and TCF mediate cell positioning in the intestinal epithelium by controlling the expression of EphB/EphrinB. Cell. 2002;111:251–63.

Bellizzi AM, Frankel WL. Colorectal cancer due to deficiency in DNA mismatch repair function: a review. Adv Anat Pathol. 2009;16:405–17.

Bryan J, Kane RE. Actin gelation in sea urchin egg extracts. Methods Cell Biol. 1982;25 Pt B:175–99.

Chen Y, Struhl G. Dual roles for Patched in sequestering and transducing hedgehog. Cell. 1996;87:553–63.

Conesa-Zamora P, García-Solano J, García-García F, et al. Expression profiling shows differential molecular pathways and provides potential new diagnostic biomarkers for colorectal serrated adenocarcinoma. Int J Cancer. 2013;132:297–307.

Frigola J, Solé X, Paz MF, et al. Differential DNA hypermethylation and hypomethylation signatures in colorectal cancer. Hum Mol Genet. 2005;14(2):319–26.

García-Solano J, Pérez-Guillermo M, Conesa-Zamora P, et al. Clinicopathologic study of 85 colorectal serrated adenocarcinomas: further insights into the full recognition of a new subset of colorectal carcinoma. Hum Pathol. 2010;41:1359–68.

García-Solano J, Conesa-Zamora P, Trujillo-Santos J, Mäkinen MJ, Pérez-Guillermo M. Tumour budding and other prognostic pathological features at invasive margins in serrated colorectal adenocarcinoma: a comparative study with conventional carcinoma. Histopathology. 2011a;59:1046–56.

García-Solano J, Conesa-Zamora P, Trujillo-Santos J, Torres-Moreno D, Mäkinen MJ, Pérez-Guillermo M. Immunohistochemical expression profile of β-catenin, E-cadherin, P-cadherin, laminin-5γ2 chain, and SMAD4 in colorectal serrated adenocarcinoma. Hum Pathol. 2011b;43:1094–102.

García-Solano J, Conesa-Zamora P, Carbonell P, et al. Colorectal Serrated Adenocarcinoma shows a different profile of oncogene mutations, MSI status and DNA repair protein expression compared to Conventional and Sporadic MSI-H carcinomas. Int J Cancer. 2012;131:1790–9.

García-Solano J, Conesa-Zamora P, Carbonell P, et al. Microsatellite pathologic score does not efficiently identify high microsatellite instability in colorectal serrated adenocarcinoma. Hum Pathol. 2013;44(5):759–65.

Hamilton SR, Bosman FT, Boffetta P, et al. Carcinoma of the colon and rectum. In: Bosman FT, Carneiro F, Hruban RH, Theise ND, editors. WHO classification of tumours of the digestive system. Lyon: International Agency for Research on Cancer (IARC); 2010. p. 134–46.

Hanahan D, Weinberg RA. The hallmarks of cancer. Cell. 2000;100:57–70.

Harris A. Hypoxia – a key regulatory factor in tumour growth. Nat Rev Cancer. 2002;2:38–47.

Hashimoto Y, Skacel M, Lavery IC, Mukherjee AL, Casey G, Adams JC. Prognostic significance of fascin expression in advanced colorectal cancer: an immunohistochemical study of colorectal adenomas and adenocarcinomas. BMC Cancer. 2006;6:241.

Ide T, Kitajima Y, Ohtaka K, Mitsuno M, Nakafusa Y, Miyazaki K. Expression of the hMLH1 gene is a possible predictor for the clinical response to 5-fluorouracil after a surgical resection in colorectal cancer. Oncol Rep. 2008;19(6):1571–6.

Irie F, Yamaguchi Y. EphB receptors regulate dendritic spine development via intersectin, Cdc42 and N-WASP. Nat Neurosci. 2002;5:1117–8.

Irizarry RA, Ladd-Acosta C, Wen B, Wu Z, Montano C, Onyango P, Cui H, Gabo K, Rongione M, Webster M, Ji H, Potash JB, Sabunciyan S, Feinberg AP. The human colon cancer methylome shows similar hypo- and hypermethylation at conserved tissue-specific CpG island shores. Nat Genet. 2009;41(2):178–86.

Jass JR. HNPCC and sporadic MSI-H colorectal cancer: a review of the morphological similarities and differences. Fam Cancer. 2004;3:93–100.

Jass JR, Love SB, Northover JMA. A new pronostic classification of rectal cancer. Lancet. 1987;1:1303–6.

Jass JR, Smith M. Sialic acid and epithelial differentiation in colorectal polyps and cancer – a morphological, mucin and lectin histochemical study. Pathology. 1992;24:233–42.

Jayo A, Parsons M. Fascin: a key regulator of cytoskeletal dynamics. Int J Biochem Cell Biol. 2010;42(10):1614–7.

Jenkins MA, Hayashi S, O'Shea AM, et al. Pathology features in Bethesda guidelines predict colorectal cancer microsatellite instability: A population-based study. Gastroenterology. 2007;133:48–56.

Johnson RL, Rothman AL, Xie J, et al. Human homolog of Patched, a candidate gene for the basal cell nevus syndrome. Science. 1996;272:1668–71.

Karimpour S, Davoodi J, Ghahremani MH. Integrity of ATP binding site is essential for effective inhibition of the intrinsic apoptosis pathway by NAIP. Biochem Biophys Res Commun. 2011;407(1):158–62.

Kim SJ, Kim DC, Kim MC, et al. Fascin expression is related to poor survival in gastric cancer. Pathol Int. 2012;62:777–84.

Klintrup K, Mäkinen JM, Kauppila S, et al. Inflammation and prognosis in colorectal cancer. Eur J Cancer. 2005;41:2645–54.

Kobayashi M, Takamatsu K, Saitoh S, Miura M, Noguchi T. Molecular cloning of hippocalcin, a novel calcium-binding protein of the recoverin family exclusively expressed in hippocampus. Biochem Biophys Res Commun. 1992;189:511–7.

Koshiji M, To KKW, Hammer S, Kumamoto K, Harris AL, Modrich P, Huang LE. HIF-1-alpha induces genetic instability by transcriptionally downregulating MutSalpha expression. Mol Cell. 2005;17:793–803.

Laiho P, Kokko A, Vanharanta S, et al. Serrated carcinomas form a subclass of colorectal cancer with distinct molecular basis. Oncogene. 2007;26:312–20.

Lan MS, Breslin MB. Structure, expression, and biological function of INSM1 transcription factor in neuroendocrine differentiation. FASEB J. 2009;23:2024–33.

Lazarus R, Junttila OE, Karttunen TJ, Mäkinen MJ. The risk of metachronous neoplasia in patients with serrated adenoma. Am J Clin Pathol. 2005;123:349–59.

Leggett B, Whitehall V. Role of the serrated pathway in colorectal cancer pathogenesis. Gastroenterology. 2010;138(6):2088–100.

Mäkinen MJ. Colorectal serrated adenocarcinoma. Histopathology. 2007;50:131–50.

Mäkinen MJ, George MC, Jervall P, Mäkelä J, Vihko P, Karttunen TJ. Colorectal carcinoma associated with serrated adenoma-prevalence, histological features, and prognosis. J Pathol. 2001;193:286–94.

Masaki T, Goto A, Sugiyama M, et al. Possible contribution of CD44 variant 6 and nuclear b-catenin expression to the formation of budding tumor cells in patients with T1 colorectal carcinoma. Cancer. 2001;92:2539–46.

Mercer EA, Korhonen L, Skoglösa Y, Olsson PA, Kukkonen JP, Lindholm D. NAIP interacts with hippocalcin and protects neurons against calcium-induced cell death through caspase-3-dependent and -independent pathways. EMBO J. 2000;19:3597–607.

Ming JE, Kaupas ME, Roessler E, et al. Mutations in PATCHED-1, the receptor for Sonic Hedgehog, are associated with holoprosencephaly. Hum Genet. 2002;110:297–301.

Minn AJ, Gupta GP, Siegel PM, et al. Genes that mediate breast cancer metastasis to lung. Nature. 2005;436:518–24.

Miyagawa Y, Ohguro H, Odagiri H, et al. Aberrantly expressed recoverin is functionally associated with G-protein-coupled receptor kinases in cancer cell lines. Biochem Biophys Res Commun. 2003;300:669–73.

Morita N, Uemura H, Tsumatani K, Cho C. E-cadherin and a-, b-, and g-catenin expression in prostate cancers: correlation with tumour invasion. Br J Cancer. 1999;79:1879–83.

Murai KK, Pasquale EB. Can Eph receptors stimulate the mind? Neuron. 2002;33:159–62.

Noffsinger AE. Serrated polyps and colorectal cancer: new pathway to malignancy. Annu Rev Pathol Mech Dis. 2009;4:343–64.

O'Brien MJ, Yang S, Mack C, et al. Comparison of microsatellite instability, CpG island methylation phenotype, BRAF and KRAS status in serrated polyps and traditional adenomas indicates separate pathways to distinct colorectal carcinoma end points. Am J Surg Pathol. 2006;30(12):1491–501.

Oldakr M, Grzela T, Lazarczyk M, Malejczyk J, Skopinski P. Clinical aspects of disrupted Hedgehog signaling. Int J Mol Med. 2001;8(4):445–52.

Ono S, Yamakita Y, Yamashiro S, et al. Identification of an actin binding region and a protein kinase C phosphorylation site on human fascin. J Biol Chem. 1997;272:2527–33.

Pagès G, Pouysségur J. Transcriptional regulation of the vascular endothelial growth factor gene–a concert of activating factors. Cardiovasc Res. 2005;65(3):564–73.

Popat S, Hubner R, Houlston RS. Systematic review of microsatellite instability and colorectal cancer prognosis. J Clin Oncol. 2005;23:609–18.

Posorski N, Kaemmerer D, Ernst G, et al. Localization of sporadic neuroendocrine tumors by gene expression analysis of their metastases. Clin Exp Metastasis. 2011;28:637–47.

Potter JD. Colorectal cancer: molecules and populations. J Natl Cancer Inst. 1999;91:916–32.

Prall F. Tumour budding in colorectal carcinoma. Histopathology. 2007;50:151–62.

Prall F, Nizze H, Barten M. Tumour budding as prognostic factor in stage I/II colorectal carcinoma. Histopathology. 2005;47:17–24.

Roskoski Jr R. Vascular endothelial growth factor (VEGF) signaling in tumor progression. Crit Rev Oncol Hematol. 2007;62:179–213.

Roy N, Mahadevan MS, McLean M, et al. The gene for neuronal apoptosis inhibitory protein is partially deleted in individuals with spinal muscular atrophy. Cell. 1995;80(1):167–78.

Semenza GL. HIF-1 and human disease: one highly involved factor. Genes Dev. 2000;14(16):1983–91

Semenza GL. Targeting HIF-1 for cancer therapy. Nat Rev Cancer. 2003;3(10):721–32.

Semenza GL. Transcriptional regulation by hypoxia-inducible factor 1 molecular mechanisms of oxygen homeostasis. Trends Cardiovasc Med. 1996;6:151–7.

Shinto E, Mochizuki H, Ueno H, Matsubara O, Jass JR. A novel classification of tumour budding in colorectal cancer based on the presence of cytoplasmic pseudo-fragments around budding foci. Histopathology. 2005;47:25–31.

Shinto E, Jass JR, Tsuda H, et al. Differential prognostic significance of morphologic invasive markers in colorectal cancer: tumor budding and cytoplasmic podia. Dis Colon Rectum. 2006;49:1422–30.

Stefanius K, Ylitalo L, Tuomisto A, et al. Frequent mutations of KRAS in addition to BRAF in colorectal serrated adenocarcinoma. Histopathology. 2011;58:679–92.

Sutter CH, Laughner E, Semenza GL. Hypoxia-inducible factor 1-alpha protein expression is controlled by oxygen-regulated ubiquitination that is disrupted by deletions and missense mutations. Proc Natl Acad Sci U S A. 2000;97:4748–53.

Tanaka T, Watanabe T, Kazama Y, et al. Loss of Smad4 protein expression and 18qLOH as molecular markers indicating lymph node metastasis in colorectal cancer – a study matched for tumor depth and pathology. J Surg Oncol. 2008;97:69–73.

Tuppurainen K, Mäkinen JM, Junttila O, et al. Morphology and microsatellite instability in sporadic serrated and non-serrated colorectal cancer. J Pathol. 2005;207:285–94.

Ueno H, Murphy J, Jass JR, Mochizuki H, Talbot IC. Tumour 'budding' as an index to estimate the potential of aggressiveness in rectal cancer. Histopathology. 2002;40:127–32.

Wright CL, Stewart ID. Histopathology and mismatch repair status of 458 consecutive colorectal carcinomas. Am J Surg Pathol. 2003;27:1393–406.

Yamashiro-Matsumura S, Matsumura F. Intracellular localization of the 55-kD actin-bundling protein in cultured cells: spatial relationships with actin, alpha-actinin, tropomyosin, and fimbrin. J Cell Biol. 1986;103(2):631–40.

Yao T, Nishiyama K, Oya M, Kouzuki T, Kajiwara M, Tsuneyoshi M. Multiple 'serrated adenocarcinomas' of the colon with a cell lineage common to metaplastic polyp and serrated adenoma: Case report of a new subtype of colonic adenocarcinoma with gastric differentiation. J Pathol. 2000;190:444–9.

Zhang J, Fonovic M, Suyama K, Bogyo M, Scott MP. Rab35 controls actin bundling by recruiting fascin as an effector protein. Science. 2009;325:1250–4.

Zhong H, De Marzo AM, Laughner E, et al. Overexpression of hypoxia-inducible factor 1alpha in common human cancers and their metastases. Cancer Res. 1999;59(22):5830–5.

Telomerase as Biomarker in Colorectal Cancer

29

Roberta Bertorelle and Anita De Rossi

Contents

Abstract

Colorectal cancer (CRC) is the third most commonly diagnosed cancer, with over one million new cases every year. Although improved treatments, increased awareness, and early detection have contributed to prolonged survival, CRC still represents an important cause of cancer-related deaths. CRC is a heterogeneous complex of diseases differing in molecular pathways and biological

R. Bertorelle
Immunology and Molecular Oncology Unit, Istituto Oncologico Veneto, IOV-IRCCS, Padova, Italy
e-mail: roberta.bertorelle@unipd.it

A. De Rossi (✉)
Department of Surgery, Oncology and Gastroenterology, Section of Oncology and Immunology, University of Padova, and Istituto Oncologico Veneto, IOV-IRCCS, Padova, Italy

Istituto Oncologico Veneto, Padova, Italy
e-mail: anita.derossi@unipd.it

V.R. Preedy, V.B. Patel (eds.), *Biomarkers in Cancer, Biomarkers in Disease: Methods, Discoveries and Applications*,
DOI 10.1007/978-94-007-7681-4_2

characteristics, arising through a multistep process; this molecular and biological heterogeneity also accounts for the great clinical variability of the disease. The management of CRC requires a multimodal approach, and many efforts have been made to identify molecular markers able to predict the outcome of CRC patients.

Telomerase is a ribonucleoprotein complex containing the catalytic protein telomerase reverse transcriptase (TERT) with telomere-specific reverse transcriptase activity which synthesizes telomere sequences utilizing an internal RNA template. The maintenance of telomere length by telomerase is critical to preserving the replicative potential of cancer cells. Several pieces of evidence suggest that TERT, besides its capacity to extend telomeres, is also involved in other cellular functions, including activation of proliferative signaling pathways and antiapoptotic activity, even by telomere-length-independent mechanisms. In view of its critical role in the oncogenetic process, telomerase may be a molecular marker of neoplastic disease.

The aim of this chapter is to analyze literature data in order to assess the role of telomerase expression and/or activity in the carcinogenesis of colorectal cancer and its value as a prognostic marker of disease progression. The potential use of circulating TERT as a biomarker for minimally invasive monitoring of the disease and response to therapy is also discussed.

List of Abbreviations

APC	Adenomatous Polyposis Coli
CIN	Chromosomal Instability
CRC	Colorectal Cancer
CRT	Chemoradiotherapy
DCC	Deleted in Colorectal Carcinoma
DFS	Disease-Free Survival
EGFR	Epidermal Growth Factor Receptor
FU	Fluorouracil
GAPDH	Glyceraldehyde-3-Phosphate Dehydrogenase
HIF	Hypoxia-Inducible Factor
HPRT1	Hypoxanthine Phosphoribosyltransferase 1
MAPK	Mitogen-Activated Protein Kinase
MMR	Mismatch Repair System
MSI	Microsatellite Instability
MSS	Microsatellite Stable
OS	Overall Survival
PCR	Polymerase Chain Reaction
TERT	Telomerase Reverse Transcriptase
TRAP	Telomere Repeat Amplification Protocol

Definition of Words and Terms

Adenoma-carcinoma sequence The continuous process of tumor initiation and progression from a single cell of colorectal mucosa to a small adenomatous polyp, which subsequently progresses to a larger lesion and then to a carcinoma.

Microsatellite One to six nucleotide repeated sequences, distributed throughout the genome and exhibiting length polymorphism.

Histological grading A score of the differentiation grade of neoplastic cells, measuring to what extent neoplastic cells differ from origin normal cells.

Histological staging A measure of the extent of a tumor.

Gene promoter DNA sequence located upstream of a gene, regulating transcription and thus the expression of that gene.

Promoter methylation A mechanism which, by the addition of a methyl (CH_3) group to a cytosine located in CpG sites of a gene promoter, can silence gene expression.

CpG islands DNA regions often localized in a gene promoter and characterized by high concentrations of cytosine located before a guanine molecule.

Telomere Specialized DNA structure located at the end of eukaryotic chromosomes, which protect them from end-to-end fusion and degradation.

Telomerase Ribonucleoprotein complex which extends telomeres at the end of eukaryotic chromosomes, thus preventing cell senescence and death.

TERT Telomerase reverse transcriptase, the catalytic protein of the telomerase complex, with telomere-specific reverse transcriptase activity which synthesizes telomere sequences de novo, using an internal RNA template (TR, telomerase RNA, or TERC, telomerase RNA component).

Introduction

Colorectal cancer (CRC) is the third most commonly diagnosed cancer in men and the second in women, with over 1.2 million new cancer cases and 608,700 deaths estimated to have occurred worldwide in 2008 (Jemal et al. 2011). Although improved treatments, increased awareness, and early detection have contributed to prolonged survival, CRC still represents an important cause of cancer-related deaths.

CRC is a heterogeneous complex of diseases differing in molecular pathways and biological characteristics, arising through a multistep process of which several genetic and epigenetic events have been characterized (Markowitz and Bertagnolli 2009). Molecular alterations accumulate with a stepwise change in morphology, from normal epithelium to carcinoma. Genetic instability plays a critical role in the oncogenetic process, and molecular heterogeneity accounts for the great clinical variability of the disease. There are at least two major pathways by means of which molecular events can lead to CRC; most CRCs (about 85 % of cases) are characterized by chromosomal instability (CIN) with allele imbalance at several chromosomal loci and chromosomal amplifications and translocations, whereas the other CRCs (about 15 % of cases) have a high-grade microsatellite instability (MSI) phenotype. The CIN pathway is characterized by alteration of the Adenomatous Polyposis Coli (*APC*) gene, which causes defective binding of APC protein to β-catenin resulting in elevated β-catenin levels and activation of proliferation signals by its translocation to the nucleus. APC deregulation may coexist with *KRAS* mutations, which constitutively activate the downstream mitogen-activated protein kinase (MAPK) pathway; loss of chromosome 18q, containing the *DCC* (deleted in colorectal carcinoma) gene; deletion of *SMAD2* and *SMAD4* genes involved in the TGF-β signaling pathway; and mutations on *TP53* gene, which influences a complex network of genes involved in cell cycle control, apoptosis, DNA repair, angiogenesis, and differentiation (Markowitz and Bertagnolli 2009; Winder and Lenz 2010). The MSI phenotype is generated by a deficient DNA mismatch repair system (MMR). Alterations of one of the seven known MMR genes (*MSH2*, *MLH1*, *MSH6*, *PMS1*, *PMS2*, *MSH3*, *MLH3*) cause unrepaired errors on nucleotide repeat sequences, known as microsatellites. Methylation of the promoter of MMR genes, in particular *MLH1*, is the most frequent mechanism in silencing MMR genes in sporadic CRC, which is frequently associated with the CpG island methylator phenotype (Pino and Chung 2010; Boland and Goel 2010).

The management of CRC requires a multimodal approach which must first take into account the location (i.e., colon vs. rectum) and stage of the disease (stage I, II, III, or IV) (Wilkes and Hartshorn 2012). Resection of the primary lesion is the treatment of choice for both colon and rectal cancers but is considered curative only for patients at stage I and for about 75 % of patients at stage II. After surgery, to reduce the risk of tumor recurrence, adjuvant chemotherapy with 5-fluorouracil (FU)-based regimens is considered the standard of care for patients with stage III CRC and for patients at stage II with poor prognostic features (Andrè et al. 2009). The benefit and improvement in disease-free survival (DFS) for patients with stage III CRC is well established, whereas for stage II patients adjuvant therapy offers little advantage over surgery (about 5 %), although this improvement in outcome is measurable. Therefore, for CRC patients at stage II, it is very important to identify those at high risk of recurrence in which the therapeutic approach could be improved (O'Connor et al. 2011), to avoid exposing patients to chemotherapy without benefit (Table 1).

Table 1 Key facts in colorectal cancer

Colorectal cancer (CRC) arises through a multistep process from adenoma to invasive carcinoma, for which several genetic events have been characterized
At least two molecular mechanisms of genetic instability underlie colorectal carcinogenesis: chromosomal instability (CIN) and microsatellite instability (MSI)
The management of CRC requires a multimodal approach which must first take into account the location (i.e., colon vs. rectum) and stage of the disease (stages I and II with cancer confined to wall of colon, stage III with regional lymph node metastases, stage IV with distant metastases)
Surgical resection and adjuvant chemotherapy are effective curative treatments, but the risk of recurrence cannot be accurately foreseen
Although pathologic tumor staging remains the key determinant of CRC prognosis, molecular heterogeneity accounts for the great clinical variability of the disease and highlights the need for prognostic markers capable of stratifying patients
Genetic alterations involved in the development of CRC have been identified in tumor tissues and proposed as potential markers of disease progression, but agreement on their prognostic value has not yet been reached. In particular for stage II tumors, it is very important to identify patients at high risk of recurrence who need to be treated with adjuvant chemotherapy
Tumor markers in plasma or serum have been studied for a minimally invasive detection of CRC in early stages and monitoring disease outcome and therapy response. Larger-scale studies are needed to confirm potential candidates

Factors for high risk of recurrence are mainly related to primary tumor characteristics, such as depth of tumor invasion (T4), grading (poorly differentiated tumors), lymphovascular invasion, or tumor presentation with perforation or obstruction, and inadequate lymph node sampling (<12) (Andrè et al. 2009). Nevertheless, identification of this subgroup of patients is still largely unsatisfactory (O'Connor et al. 2011), probably due to both the molecular characteristics of tumors and their intrinsic heterogeneity. Many efforts have been made to identify molecular markers capable of predicting the outcome of CRC patients, and several genetic and epigenetic alterations involved in the development of CRC have been proposed as prognostic markers of disease progression. *KRAS* and *TP53* gene mutations, involved in chromosome instability, and the MSI phenotype have been extensively studied for their prognostic and predictive roles. Although a predictive value of *KRAS* mutation status for response to epidermal growth factor receptor (EGFR)-targeted therapy has been defined in metastatic CRC (van Cutsem et al. 2009; Cunningham et al. 2010), agreement on the prognostic value of these markers in CRC stages I, II, and III has not yet been reached (Kim et al. 2007; Cunningham et al. 2010). MSI status has prognostic value in some studies (Sargent et al. 2010), but not in others (Bertorelle et al. 2013). Contrasting results are also reported about the predictive role of MSI in response to adjuvant therapy (Kim et al. 2007).

For locally advanced rectal cancer (stages II–III), an approach based on chemoradiotherapy prior to surgery (pCRT) is currently the standard treatment to reduce the risk of local recurrence and to increase the chances of sphincter preservation (NCCN Guidelines 2014). With this approach, outcomes are encouraging, with 5-year rates of local and distant recurrence ranging from 6 % to 9 % and 33 %

to 36 %, respectively. Approximately 40 % of patients show poor or no response to pCRT, while a complete pathologic response has been reported for up to 44 % of cases; for patients with pathologic response, less aggressive approaches have been advocated, such as the "wait-and-see" policy or transanal local excision (reviewed in Spolverato et al. 2011). Predicting tumor response to various combinations of treatments has important clinical implications, since it improves the selection of patients who have a greater likelihood of responding to treatment; patients with known resistant tumors can be spared from exposure to radiation or DNA-damaging drugs which are associated with adverse side effects. These considerations have prompted researchers to find biomarkers able to predict the tumor response. Within this framework, the identification of circulating biomarkers is important for minimally invasive monitoring of disease.

Telomere/Telomerase Interplay in Colorectal Cancers

Telomere/telomerase interplay is an important mechanism involved in the maintenance of chromosome stability and cellular replicative potential, and its dysfunction has emerged as playing a key role in carcinogenesis (Blackburn et al. 2006). Telomeres are specialized DNA structures located at the 3′ end of chromosomes; they are composed of (TTAGGG)n tandem repeats associated with a protein complex (TRF1, TRF2, Rap1, TIN2, TPP1, POT1), shelterin, and are essential in stabilizing chromosomes by protecting them from end-to-end fusion and DNA degradation (Palm and de Lange 2008). Telomeres are progressively shortened during each cell division by replication-dependent loss of sequences at DNA termini, due to the failure of DNA polymerase to replicate the 3′ end of chromosomes completely (Harley et al. 1990). When telomeres become critically short (the Hayflick limit), cells undergo replicative senescence and apoptosis (Fig. 1a); further erosion of telomeres may impair their function in protecting chromosome ends, resulting in genetic instability (Hackett and Greider 2002). Thus, telomere erosion has been proposed to play two conflicting roles: tumor suppression by inducing cell death and tumor promotion by inducing genetic instability, a key event in the initiation of carcinogenesis. However, cell division-associated telomere shortening prevents unlimited cell proliferation and, thus, tumor development/progression. To escape this proliferation barrier, cells must stabilize their telomeres. Most tumors maintain their ability to grow indefinitely by inappropriate expression of telomerase, a ribonucleoprotein complex containing an internal RNA component (TR) and a catalytic protein, telomerase reverse transcriptase (TERT), with telomere-specific reverse transcriptase activity (Fig. 1b). TERT, which synthesizes de novo telomere sequences using TR as template, is the rate-limiting component of the telomerase complex, and its expression is correlated with telomerase activity (Nakamura et al. 1997). While TR has broad tissue distribution and is constitutively present in normal and tumor cells, the expression of TERT is usually repressed in normal somatic cells and is essential for unlimited cell growth, thus playing a critical role in tumor formation and progression (Kim et al. 1994; Hanahan and Weinberg 2011).

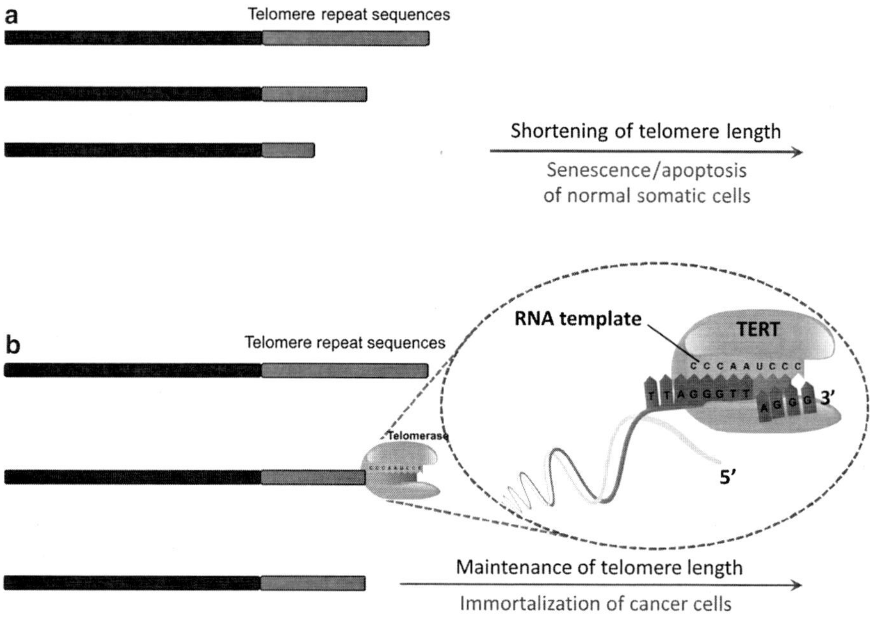

Fig. 1 Maintenance of telomere length by telomerase in cancer cells. (**a**) Telomeres are progressively shortened during each cell division due to the failure of DNA polymerase to replicate the 3′ end of chromosomes completely. When telomeres become critically short, normal somatic cells undergo replicative senescence and apoptosis. (**b**) Cancer cells maintain their ability to grow indefinitely by inappropriate expression of telomerase, a ribonucleoprotein complex containing a catalytic protein, telomerase reverse transcriptase (*TERT*), which synthesizes de novo telomere sequences using an internal RNA template

Regulation of telomerase operates at several biological levels: transcription, mRNA splicing, subcellular location of each component, and assembly of TR and TERT in an active ribonucleoprotein. Transcription of the *TERT* gene is probably the key determinant in regulating telomerase activity; notably, TERT transcription activity is specifically upregulated in cancer cells but silent in most normal cells. The *TERT* gene comprises about 35 Kb DNA and codes for an mRNA composed of 16 exons and 15 introns. At transcriptional level, more than 20 transcription factor-binding sites acting as activators or repressors have been identified within the *TERT* promoter. Cooperation of MYC and SP1 is required for full activation of the *TERT* promoter, while p53 protein, through its interaction with SP1, downregulates TERT. *TERT* is also directly activated by nuclear factor (NF)-kβ, hypoxia-inducible factor (HIF)-1, and ETS/MYC complex. The histone methyltransferase SMYD3 also directly contributes to inducible and constitutive TERT expression in normal and malignant human cells. TERT expression is suppressed by the oncosuppressor genes, WT127 and menin, and through the MAD/MYC and TGFβ/SMAD pathways. The cell cycle inhibitors p16INK4a and p27KIP1 have also been shown to downregulate TERT expression in cancer cells. Regulation of TERT transcription

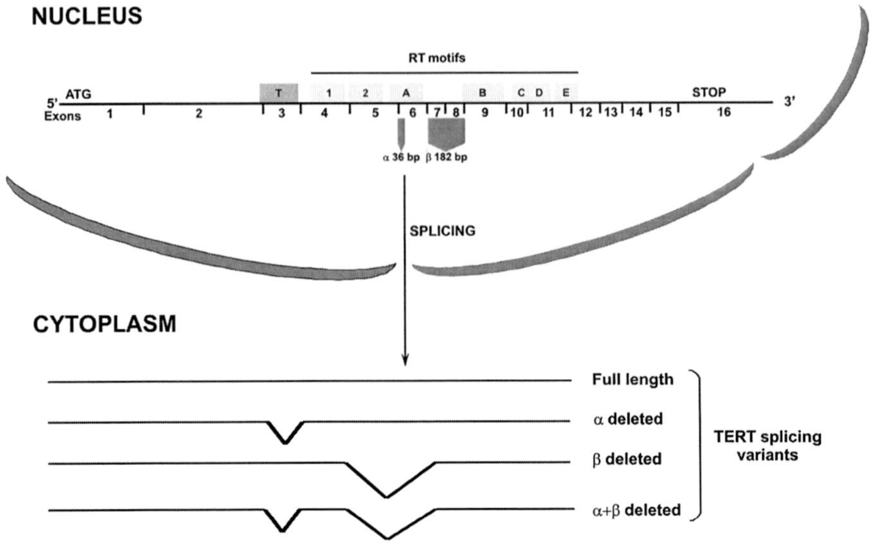

Fig. 2 ***TERT* genome and transcripts**. *TERT* gene comprises 16 exons and 15 introns, for about 35 Kb DNA. Reverse transcriptase (*RT*) motifs range from exon 3 to exon 12. At least 10 different splice variants of TERT mRNA are described. The most frequently studied variants involve the α splice site which produces a 36 bp deletion and the β splice site which results in a 183 bp deletion; mRNA variants lacking α and/or β regions translate truncated and dysfunctional protein products. Full-length mRNA encodes the functional TERT protein

may also involve DNA methylation, as the *TERT* promoter contains a cluster of CpG sites. At posttranscriptional level, modulation of telomerase may occur by alternative splicings; at least 10 different splice variants of TERT have been described. The most widely studied variants involve splicing at two main sites: the α splice site which produces a 36 bp deletion and the β site which results in a 183 bp deletion; mRNA variants lacking α and/or β regions translate truncated and dysfunctional protein products (Fig. 2). It has been proposed that some of these splicing products, such as isoform α, may exert a dominant negative function by competitive interaction with components of the telomerase complex. Telomerase activity is also controlled by posttranslational modifications of the TERT protein. Phosphorylation of the protein at critical sites by the PI3K/AKT kinase pathway seems to be crucial for telomerase activity (reviewed in Dolcetti and De Rossi 2012).

Several studies have demonstrated that telomeres are shorter in CRCs than in the adjacent mucosa (Hastie et al. 1990; Takagi et al. 1999; Gertler et al. 2004; Garcia-Aranda et al. 2006; Rampazzo et al. 2010). While telomere length in somatic cells primarily reflects cellular proliferation, in tumor cells, it reflects the balance between cellular proliferation with telomere loss and telomerase activity with de novo synthesis of telomere sequences. Evidence that telomeres are shorter in CRCs than in the adjacent mucosa, even in well-differentiated tumors, strongly supports the concept that telomere erosion is a critical initial event in colorectal

Table 2 Telomerase and colorectal cancers: outstanding questions in assessing TERT value as hallmark of disease and prognostic marker

Is TERT activation an initial or late event in colorectal carcinogenesis?
Are TERT mRNA levels correlated with telomerase activity?
Do levels of TERT expression/telomerase activity increase with disease progression?
Do levels of TERT expression/telomerase activity have prognostic value for disease-free survival and for overall survival?
Does TERT act as a circulating biomarker for monitoring disease and for monitoring therapy response?

carcinogenesis (Rampazzo et al. 2010; Roger et al. 2013). The activation of TERT and high levels of telomerase activity stabilize telomere length, thus preserving the replicative potential of cancer cells.

It should be noted that approximately 15 % of CRCs present MSI, while the *TP53* gene is the known major genetic alteration in CRCs with chromosomal instability and stable microsatellites (MSS) (Kim et al. 2007; Ogino et al. 2009). A study of a larger number of CRCs has demonstrated that both MSI and MSS tumors have shorter telomeres than those in the cells of adjacent mucosa, but MSI have shorter telomeres than MSS cancers (Rampazzo et al. 2010). The MSI pathway involves failure of the MMR system which maintains genetic stability not only by repairing DNA replication errors but also by preventing chromosomal recombinations; a deficiency of MMR helps cells overcome cellular crises caused by critical shortening of telomeres (Bechter et al. 2004). Thus, MSI cells may undergo more proliferative cycles and more pronounced shortening of telomeres before stabilizing than MSS cells. Of interest, the difference is particularly notable and significant when MSI tumors are compared to MSS tumors carrying the wild-type *TP53* gene. MSS tumors with the mutated p53 protein have slightly shorter telomeres than MSS tumors with the wild-type p53 (Rampazzo et al. 2010). In cells with mutated p53, telomeres may protract their shortening with cell proliferation. However, p53 is a well-known negative regulator of *TERT* promoter, and mutated p53 may also result in *TERT* activation, so that telomere stabilization may occur earlier than in MSI tumors.

While there is general agreement that telomere shortening is an early event in the carcinogenesis of both familial and sporadic CRC, its prognostic and predictive value is still largely controversial.

Telomerase as a Disease Marker

Several factors make TERT highly attractive as both a tumor marker and a target of new therapeutic strategies. First, it is repressed in somatic tissues and detected in more than 90 % of malignancies. Several questions listed in Table 2 are important in defining its value as a marker of CRC. Answers to these questions, first of all, require reliable methods to measure telomerase. Variations in the methods

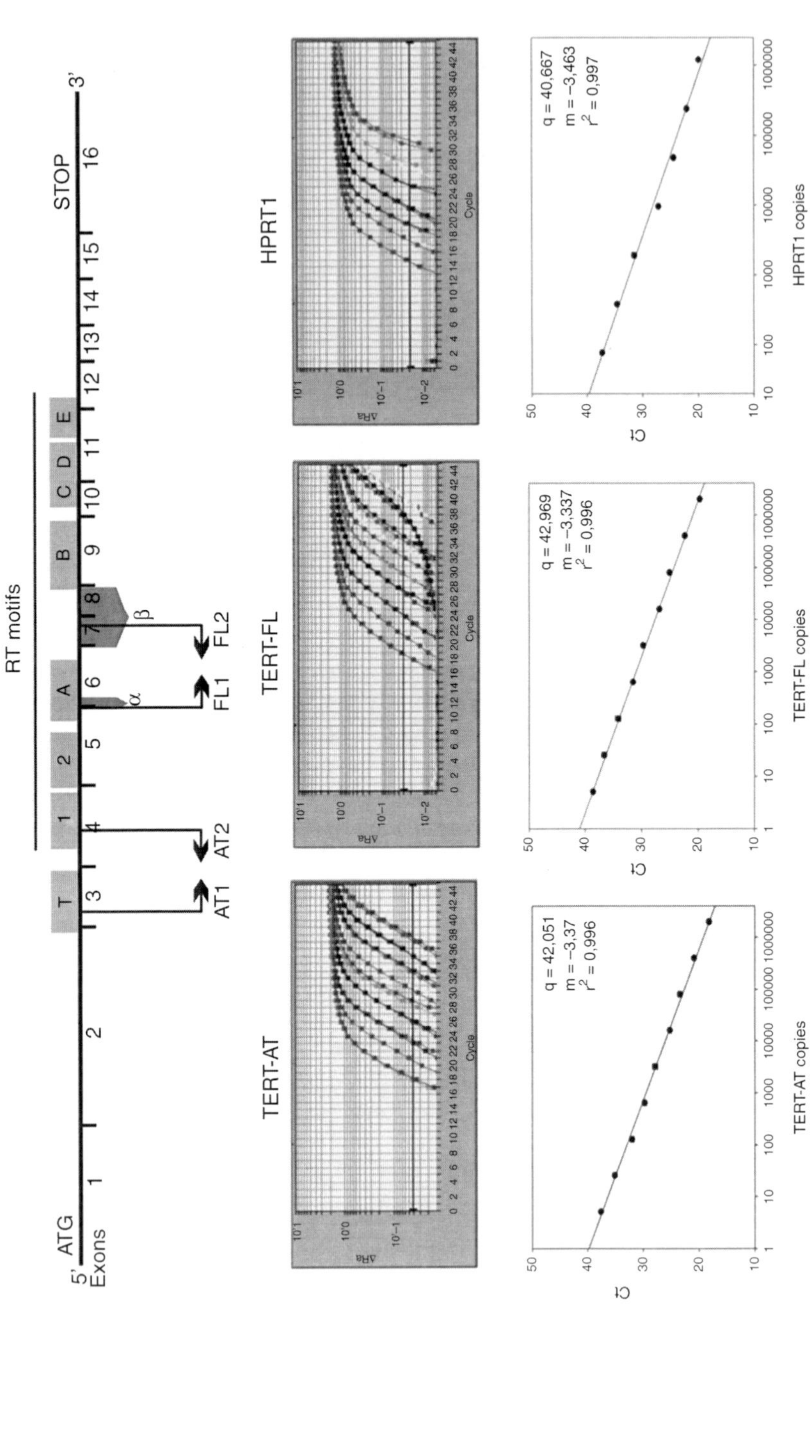

Fig. 3 (continued)

employed to measure this marker, i.e., TERT mRNA level or telomerase activity, may influence the results.

Two main strategies are used to estimate telomerase: (1) quantification of TERT mRNA levels and (2) quantification of telomerase activity. It has been estimated that the level of telomerase, even in telomerase-positive tumor cells, is relatively low, about 100 molecules per cell, so that its detection, as either mRNA or activity, requires methods based on amplification by polymerase chain reaction (PCR). Although there are no clinically approved telomerase assays, several promising approaches have recently been published (Zhou and Xing 2012).

To estimate the level of TERT mRNA, real-time PCR-based methods have recently been developed. The initially described TERT transcript has been shown to contain alternate splicing sites, and mRNA variants lacking α and/or β regions result in truncated and dysfunctional protein products. Thus, the best method to quantify TERT is to design primers which bind to the α and β sites and recognize the full-length mRNA which encodes the functional protein (Terrin et al. 2008). Primers which bind to conserved regions located upstream of the RT motifs recognize all TERT transcripts; this primer pair increases the sensitivity of the assay but lacks specificity about the quality of the transcript. RNA extracted from cancer cells should be retrotranscribed in vitro into cDNA and then amplified by real-time PCR by means of the specific *TERT* primer pairs and a standard reference curve, usually represented by serial dilution of a TERT amplicon or a plasmid coding TERT (Fig. 3). All data acquired by real-time PCR must be normalized using a housekeeping gene. The ideal housekeeping gene should not vary with disease progression. The glyceraldehyde-3-phosphate dehydrogenase (*GAPDH*) gene, often employed as housekeeping gene, is activated by HIF and thus expressed at higher levels in advanced diseases than in tumors at early stages. Other genes, such as hypoxanthine phosphoribosyltransferase 1(*HPRT1*) gene, which do not vary with tumor stage (de Kok et al. 2005), allow a more reliable estimate of TERT levels.

Fig. 3 Quantification of TERT transcripts. To quantify the mRNA of TERT, two sets of primers are designed. The forward primer AT1 and the reverse primer AT2 bind to nucleotide sequences located upstream of the RT motif 1 of the *TERT* gene. The forward primer FL1 and the reverse primer FL2 bind to nucleotide sequences located within the α and β splicing sites, respectively. While amplification with AT1 and AT2 primers allows the detection of all TERT transcripts (*TERT-AT*), amplification with FL1 and FL2 primers recognizes only mRNA containing the α and β sites (*TERT-FL*) and encoding the functional TERT protein. The standard reference curve to quantitate TERT-AT and TERT-FL transcripts is performed using serial fivefold dilutions of a TERT amplicon containing the sequences recognized by the AT1/AT2 and FL1/FL2 primer pairs. Each sample is run in triplicate; a threshold cycle (*Ct*) value for each triplicate is calculated and the mean values of the replicates, plotted against the standard TERT reference curve, are employed to calculate the copies of TERT transcripts in the sample. To normalize TERT transcripts for the amount and quality of RNA, *HPRT1* is employed as housekeeping gene. Representative standard reference curves of TERT-AT, TERT-FL, and HPRT1 are shown

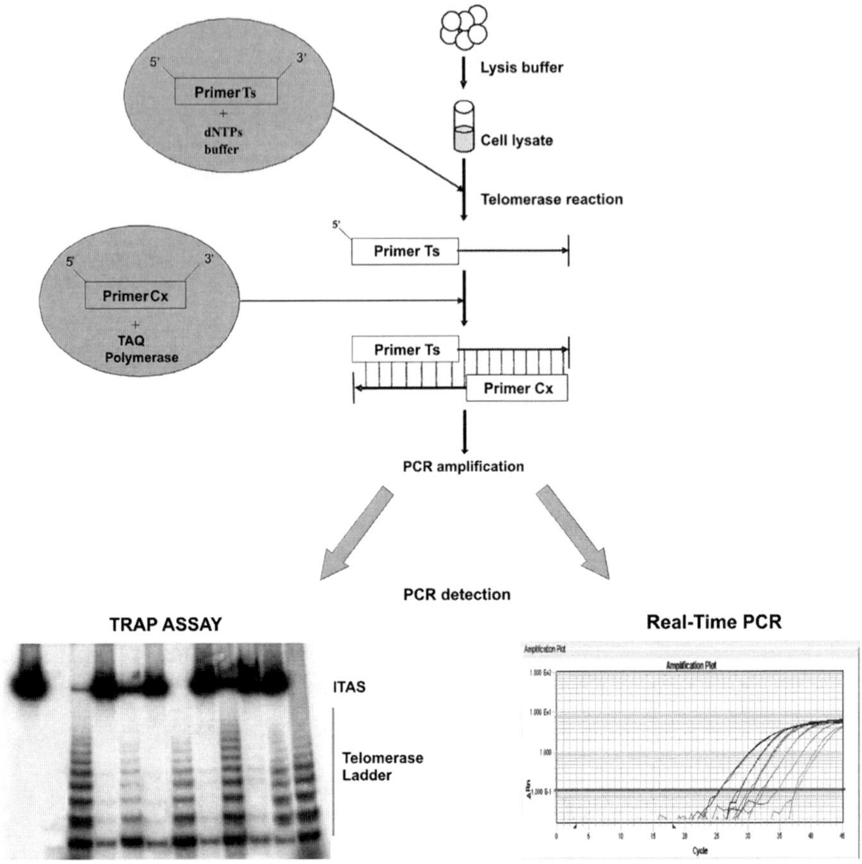

Fig. 4 **Quantification of telomerase activity**. To quantify telomerase activity, cellular extract is analyzed by a PCR-based telomere repeat amplification protocol (*TRAP*). Cellular samples are incubated with specific primers Ts and Cx and the telomerase products may be visualized by gel electrophoresis (telomerase ladder). Internal telomerase assay standard (*ITAS*) allows to semi-quantify telomerase activity. The products of telomerase activity may be quantified also by a real-time PCR assay

To quantify telomerase activity, a PCR-based telomere repeat amplification protocol (TRAP) assay has been developed. A synthetic non-telomere sequence is employed as substrate; the substrate is then elongated by the telomerase present in the sample and the product is analyzed by PCR. The addition of an internal control (e.g., ITAS, internal telomerase assay standard) allows semi-quantification of telomerase activity (Fig. 4). An important improvement in the quantification of telomerase activity is the development of real-time PCR-based assays (Fig. 4).

In colorectal cancer, a study by real-time PCR performed with *HPRT1* as housekeeping gene demonstrated that there is a good relationship between the levels of all TERT transcripts and the full-length TERT transcript

(Terrin et al. 2008). In addition, TERT mRNA levels were correlated with telomerase activity, estimated by TRAP assay (Terrin et al. 2008) and a real-time PCR assay (Rampazzo et al. 2012). A correlation between TERT mRNA levels estimated by real-time PCR and telomerase activity measured with a commercial TRAP-based assay (TRAPeze) has also been demonstrated (Naito et al. 2001).

Telomerase as a Marker of Disease Progression

Although telomeres are shorter in CRC than in the adjacent mucosa, there is general agreement that levels of telomerase expression and/or activity are higher in CRCs than in adjacent noncancerous mucosa (Enghelhart et al. 1997; Tatsumoto et al. 2000; Niiyama et al. 2001; Boldrini et al. 2002; Ghori et al. 2002; Maláska et al. 2004; Garcia-Aranda et al. 2006; Bautista et al. 2007; Terrin et al. 2008) (Table 3). The normal adjacent mucosa may have some detectable TERT mRNA and telomerase activity, mainly due to intestinal crypt basal cells (Tatsumoto et al. 2000; Terrin et al. 2008). These findings strongly support the fact that activation of telomerase is subsequent to telomere erosion, probably due to the high proliferation of preneoplastic lesions.

Only a few studies have analyzed telomerase expression in preneoplastic lesions. In a study performed on 50 adenomas, 6 mucosal carcinomas, and 10 invasive carcinomas, TERT mRNA level and telomerase activity increased with the adenoma-carcinoma sequence (Naito et al. 2001). A study performed on 36 CRCs, 8 adenomatous polyps, and 9 dysplastic polyps found that normal mucosa specimens and adenomas were negative for telomerase activity, whereas dysplastic polyps and CRCs were positive, telomerase activity being higher in the latter (Boldrini et al. 2002). Another study confirmed that both TERT mRNA level and telomerase activity were higher in CRCs than in adenomas (Niiyama et al. 2001).

Several studies have demonstrated that levels of TERT expression and/or telomerase activity increase with tumor progression (Table 3). Well-differentiated and moderately differentiated tumors had significantly lower TERT levels than poorly differentiated ones (Terrin et al. 2008; Bertorelle et al. 2013). Late-stage tumors (Dukes C and D) showed higher telomerase activity than early-stage tumors (Engelhardt et al. 1997; Ghori et al. 2002; Sanz-Casla et al. 2005). Telomerase activity tended to be higher in metastatic CRCs (Maláska et al. 2004). Moreover, it has been demonstrated that elongation of 3′OH of telomere by telomerase may increase the malignant potential of cancer cells (Kojima et al. 2011). Few studies found no correlation between levels of telomerase activity, assessed by the semi-quantitative TRAP assay, and tumor progression (Tatsumoto et al. 2000; Gertler et al. 2002; Garcia-Aranda 2006; Bautista et al. 2007) (Table 3).

Few studies have suggested that telomerase expression is related to tumor location, being higher in colon than in rectal cancer (Kawanishi-Tabata et al. 2002; Sanz-Casla et al. 2005), but other studies do not confirm this (Garcia-Aranda et al. 2006; Terrin et al. 2008; Bertorelle et al. 2013). Unlike telomere length, levels of telomerase expression/activity do not correlate with MSI status and

Table 3 Telomerase as marker of colorectal cancer

Reference	Cases	Method of measurement	Main findings
Engelhardt et al. (1997)	80 (50 CRCs, 20 polyps, 10 colitis) and 50 CRC patient-paired noncancerous mucosa specimens	Telomerase activity by TRAP assay	Telomerase activity
			Absent in normal tissues
			Higher in CRC than in nonneoplastic lesions
			Higher in late-stage than in early-stage tumors
Tatsumoto et al. (2000)	100 CRC and patient-paired adjacent noncancerous mucosa specimens	Telomerase activity by TRAP assay	Telomerase activity
			Higher in CRC than in adjacent noncancerous mucosa
			Some detectable in adjacent noncancerous mucosa derived from intestinal crypt basal cells
			Not correlated with CRC stage or grade
Niiyama et al. (2001)	140 CRC and patient-paired adjacent noncancerous mucosa specimens, 20 adenomas	TERT mRNA by competitive PCR and telomerase activity by TRAP assay	TERT mRNA and telomerase activity
			Higher in CRC than in adenomas
			Higher in adenomas than in normal mucosa
Naito et al. (2001)	66 (50 adenomas, 6 mucosal carcinomas, 10 invasive carcinomas) specimens	Telomerase activity by TRAP assay (TRAPeze assay)	Positive correlation between TERT mRNA and telomerase activity
		TERT mRNA by real-time PCR	TERT levels increase during adenoma-carcinoma sequence
Gertler et al. (2002)	57 CRC and patient-paired adjacent noncancerous mucosa specimens	TERT mRNA by real-time PCR	Both CRC and adjacent noncancerous mucosa were positive for TERT
			TERT levels lower in tumors than in noncancerous mucosa in most cases
			TERT levels not correlated with stage
Kawanishi-Tabata et al. (2002)	122 CRCs stage II (52 colon, 70 rectum)	Telomerase activity by TRAP assay	−80 % telomerase-positive CRC
			Higher percentage of telomerase-positive tumors in colon than in rectum
Ghori et al. (2002)	30 CRC and 20 adjacent noncancerous mucosa specimens	Telomerase activity by TRAP assay (TRAPeze assay)	Telomerase activity
			Higher in CRC than in adjacent noncancerous mucosa
			Correlated with Dukes stage

(*continued*)

Table 3 (continued)

Reference	Cases	Method of measurement	Main findings
Boldrini et al. (2002)	36 CRC and patient-paired noncancerous mucosa specimens, 8 adenomatous polyps, 9 dysplastic polyps	Telomerase activity	Telomerase activity
			Absent in normal mucosa and adenomas
			Higher in CRC than in dysplastic polyps
			Higher in late-stage than in early-stage tumors
Maláska et al. (2004)	41 CRC and paired noncancerous mucosa specimens	Telomerase activity and TERT level	Telomerase activity
			Present in 83 % of CRC
			Absent or at very low level in normal mucosa
			Higher in metastatic tumors
Boldrini et al. (2004)	43 CRCs	Telomerase activity and TERT level	TERT levels and telomerase activity higher in TP53 mutated tumors than in TP53 wild-type tumors
Sanz-Casla et al. (2005)	103 CRCs	Telomerase activity by TRAP assay	Telomerase activity increases with tumor progression (Dukes stage)
			Higher percentage of telomerase-positive tumors in colon than in rectum
Garcia-Aranda et al. (2006)	91 CRC and patient-paired adjacent noncancerous mucosa specimens	Telomerase activity by TRAP assay-based ELISA	Telomerase activity
			Present in 81 % of CRC
			Present at very low level in 15 % of normal samples
			Not correlated with tumor progression
			Not correlated with tumor location
Vidaurreta et al. (2007)	97 CRCs	Telomerase activity by TRAP assay-based ELISA	Telomerase activity
			Present both in MSI and MSS tumors
Bautista et al. (2007)	108 rectal cancer and paired adjacent noncancerous mucosa specimens	Telomerase activity by TRAP assay-based immunofluorescence assay	Telomerase activity
			Higher in rectal cancer than in normal mucosa
			Not correlated with tumor stage and grade

(*continued*)

Table 3 (continued)

Reference	Cases	Method of measurement	Main findings
Terrin et al. (2008)	85 CRC and 42 adjacent noncancerous mucosa specimens	TERT mRNA by real-time PCR	TERT levels
			Higher in CRC than in adjacent noncancerous mucosa
			Increase with tumor stage and grade
			Not correlated with MSI status
			Not correlated with tumor location
Kojima et al. (2011)	106 CRC and patient-paired adjacent noncancerous mucosa specimens	Telomerase activity by TRAP assay	Elongation of 3′OH of telomere by telomerase may increase malignant potential in cancer cells
Safont et al. (2011)	48 CRC and patient-paired adjacent noncancerous mucosa specimens, 48 plasma samples	TERT mRNA by real-time PCR	Relationship between TERT in CRC tumors and plasma
			Higher circulating TERT level in stage IV tumors
Bertorelle et al. (2013)	137 CRCs	TERT mRNA by real-time PCR	TERT levels
			Increase with tumor stage and grade
			Not correlated with MSI status
			Not correlated with tumor location

increase with disease progression in both MSI and MSS tumors (Vidaurreta et al. 2007; Bertorelle et al. 2013). The finding that TERT mRNA is higher in tumors bearing *TP53* mutations (Boldrini et al. 2004) may support the concept that high TERT expression is a marker of poor outcome and poor response to therapy (Fakhoury et al. 2007; Bertorelle et al. 2013).

Telomerase as a Prognostic Marker for Colorectal Cancers

Pathologic tumor staging remains a key determinant of CRC prognosis and treatment. Invasive cancers are confined within the wall of the colon (stages I and II), but if untreated, they spread to regional lymph nodes (stage III) and then metastasize to distant sites (stage IV). Although radical resection and adjuvant therapy are effective curative treatments, the risk of disease recurrence cannot be accurately foreseen, even in patients at the same tumor stage. Surgery is the primary treatment for patients in stages I–III, and adjuvant therapy provides additional survival benefits for patients in stage III. The controversial results obtained in different studies (Quasar Collaborative Group et al. 2007; Sargent et al. 2010) may reflect the molecular and biological heterogeneity of CRCs and highlight the need for strong prognostic markers capable of stratifying patients.

There are two main reasons why telomerase may be a useful prognostic factor: (1) the results of most studies agree that TERT expression and/or telomerase activity increases with tumor progression, and (2) several pieces of evidence suggest that TERT, besides its capability for extending telomeres, is also involved in other cellular functions, including activation of proliferative signaling pathways and antiapoptotic activity, even by telomere-length-independent mechanisms (Stewart et al. 2002; Rahman et al. 2005). Notably, high levels of telomerase confer resistance to several antineoplastic drugs (Tao et al. 2012; Shawi et al. 2013).

Several studies have addressed the prognostic value of telomerase expression in CRC. Table 4 lists the most significant studies addressing telomerase activity levels and prognosis. Differing results may partly be due to the different cohorts studied and assessment of different end points, disease-free survival (DFS) or overall survival (OS). Despite the varying methods used to measure the level of telomerase activity or TERT expression and the different end points (DFS or OS), most of the studies show that the high levels of telomerase are associated with poor prognosis. Most of the studies used a semiquantitative TRAP assay to evaluate telomerase activity (Tatsumoto et al. 2000; Kawanishi-Tabata et al. 2002; Sanz-Casla et al. 2005; Garcia-Aranda et al. 2006; Vidaurreta et al. 2007; Bautista et al. 2007; Kojima et al. 2011). Only a few studies, with different reference curves and housekeeping genes, employed real-time PCR to evaluate TERT mRNA levels (Gertler et al. 2002; Safont et al. 2011; Bertorelle et al. 2013).

High levels of TERT mRNA and/or telomerase activity are reported to be associated with a worse OS and this negative prognostic effect is also independent of pathologic stage (Gertler et al. 2002; Bertorelle et al. 2013). In particular, results obtained by quantification of TERT mRNA in 137 CRC patients with a median follow-up of 70 months strongly indicate that TERT is an independent prognostic indicator of OS; patients with high TERT levels (above the median) have an approximately double risk of death with respect to patients with low TERT levels (below the median) (Bertorelle et al. 2013). In addition, although it is clinically important to identify stage II CRC at high risk of recurrence, only two studies on telomerase have addressed this issue. In the first study, the positivity of telomerase activity, estimated by TRAP assay, was associated with better prognosis, and patients with telomerase-positive CRCs had longer DFS than patients with telomerase-negative tumors (Kawanishi-Tabata et al. 2002). In the second study, TERT levels, estimated by real-time PCR and previously found to be related to telomerase activity in CRCs (Terrin et al. 2008), significantly stratified stage II patients; in fact, such patients with high TERT levels had significantly worse

Table 4 The prognostic value of telomerase in colorectal cancer

Reference	Method of measurement	Cases	Prognostic value	Main findings
Tatsumoto et al. (2000)	Telomerase activity by TRAP assay: low, moderate, high levels	100	Telomerase activity has prognostic value DFS $p < 0.01$; OS $p < 0.01$	High telomerase activity and poor prognosis
Kawanishi-Tabata et al. (2002)	Telomerase activity by TRAP assay: positive vs. negative	122 stage II	Telomerase activity has prognostic value for: DFS $p < 0.05$; OS $p =$ n.s.	Positive telomerase activity and good prognosis for DFS
Gertler et al. (2002)	TERT mRNA by real-time PCR Ratio (TERT tumor/TERT normal mucosa) >0.57	57	TERT ratio has prognostic value OS $p < 0.05$	High telomerase activity and poor prognosis
Sanz-Casla et al. (2005)	Telomerase activity by TRAP assay	103	Telomerase activity has prognostic value DFS $p < 0.001$	High telomerase activity and poor prognosis
Garcia-Aranda et al. (2006)	Telomerase activity by TRAP assay-based ELISA (low, moderate, high levels)	91	Telomerase activity has no prognostic value for: DFS $p = 0.11$	No correlation with prognosis
Vidaurreta et al. (2007)	Telomerase activity by TRAP assay-based ELISA (low, moderate, high levels)	97	Telomerase activity has prognostic value OS $p = 0.04$	Positive telomerase activity and poor prognosis
Bautista et al. (2007)	Telomerase activity by TRAP assay-based immunofluorescence assay Telo index: (telo cancer-telo normal tissue)	108 rectal cancers	Telomerase activity has prognostic value for: DFS $p = 0.023$; OS $p = 0.011$	High telomerase index and poor prognosis
Safont et al. (2011)	TERT mRNA by real-time PCR TERT levels: tumor/normal (low <2, moderate <5, high >5)	48	TERT level has no prognostic value DFS $p =$ ns	No correlation with prognosis
Kojima K et al. (2011)	Telomerase activity by TRAP assay (TRAPeze kit)	106	Telomerase activity has prognostic value OS $p = 0.018$	Telomerase activated without 3′-OH shortened telomeres and poor prognosis
Bertorelle et al. (2013)	TERT mRNA by real-time PCR	137 50 stage II	TERT level has prognostic value OS $p < 0.009$ Stage II CRC OS $p = 0.008$ Stage II CRC DFS $p = 0.043$	High TERT level and poor prognosis

median OS and DFS values than those with low TERT levels (Bertorelle et al. 2013). Further studies with a prospective design and large sample sizes are required to define the prognostic role of telomerase properly in stage II CRC patients.

Telomerase as Circulating Marker

In recent years, great efforts have been made to identify noninvasive or minimally invasive tumor markers to detect CRC in its early stage and to monitor the disease outcome. Genomic mutations have been reported to be useful to detect either circulating tumor cells or tumor-derived DNA in serum and plasma (Hsieh et al. 2005). Expression of epithelial cell adhesion molecules has been used primarily to detect CRC cells in the hematopoietic milieu, and circulating cancer cells is a promising approach, although its diagnostic/prognostic role still needs to be established (Kin et al. 2013). Recently, the detection of cancer-related RNA molecules in plasma has been proposed as a marker of cancer onset and outcome (El-Hefnawy et al. 2004). Although plasma contains potent ribonucleases, extracellular RNA may survive in the blood because it is contained in apoptotic bodies/vesicles which are resistant to RNAse digestion (El-Hefnawy et al. 2004). Ongoing studies indicate that circulating microRNAs may be potential early detection biomarkers for CRC (Schetter et al. 2012). Within this framework, recent studies suggest that cell-free circulating TERT mRNA is a potential marker of disease. Transcripts of TERT have been detected in the plasma of patients with different type of tumors, i.e., breast cancer (Chen et al. 2000), hepatocellular carcinoma (Miura et al. 2005), lung cancer (Pelosi et al. 2006), prostate cancer (March-Villalba et al. 2012), and colorectal cancer (Lledó et al. 2004), but how TERT levels in plasma reflect those in tumors remains an open question. In a series of CRCs, from stage I to stage IV, plasma TERT mRNA levels were found to be related to those in tumors (Terrin et al. 2008). In addition, while 95 % of patients with tumors had detectable cell-free circulating TERT, aged-matched controls were negative in almost all cases; very low TERT levels were detected in few controls (Terrin et al. 2008). Larger-scale studies are needed to assess the cutoff value of TERT in order to estimate the sensitivity and specificity of this assay. However, the close association between tumor and plasma TERT levels makes this biomarker a potentially valuable tool in monitoring neoplastic disease as well as the response to therapy.

With this concern, recent research has focused on identifying new predictive factors of rectal tumor response to chemoradiotherapy prior to surgery (pCRT), and identification of circulating biomarkers is important for minimally invasive monitoring of patients. A study of rectal cancers in patients who underwent pCRT, and for whom baseline and paired post-pCRT plasma samples were available, demonstrated that baseline TERT levels did not predict the response to pCRT, but did significantly decrease in patients who had a complete pathologic response, while they remained unchanged or became higher in patients who did not respond to therapy (Pucciarelli et al. 2012). This finding strongly suggests that variation in TERT plasma levels is predictive of tumor response. Although the predictive value of TERT should be validated in larger studies, this finding supports the concept that plasma TERT reflects the telomerase expression in tumors.

Potential Applications

CRC is a heterogeneous complex of diseases differing in molecular pathways and biological characteristics, arising through a multistep process. The management of CRC requires a multimodal approach and many efforts have been made to identify molecular markers able to predict the outcome of CRC patients. Several genetic and epigenetic alterations involved in the development of CRC have been proposed as prognostic markers of disease progression, but agreement has not yet been reached. One limitation may be the fact that they are involved in a specific pathway of CRC and not in others. Besides molecular and biological heterogeneity, CRCs need telomerase activation to preserve the replicative potential. According to the majority of studies, activation of telomerase occurs during the adenoma-carcinoma sequence and increases during tumor progression.

Telomerase may therefore be a useful marker in monitoring and predicting the disease outcome. This may be particularly useful in stage II patients. Whereas adjuvant chemotherapy is standard care for stage III patients, the role of adjuvant therapy in stage II does remain controversial. High TERT levels represent a good prognostic marker for both OS and DFS in these patients. A caveat to the use of telomerase as a marker is the availability of simple and reliable assays to quantify telomerase expression and/or activity. This is important even because noncancerous cells may express low TERT levels and telomerase activity. In the case of colorectal mucosa, this may at least partly be due to intestinal crypt basal cells. Reliable assays will allow researchers to compare data and define useful cutoff values to discriminate patients at low and high risk of disease progression.

Recent studies indicate that circulating TERT levels reflect cancer TERT levels. While most CRC patients have plasma TERT, the few available data indicate that age-matched noncancer patients are negative or, in a few cases, have very low levels of circulating TERT. Furthermore, in patients with rectal cancer who received chemoradiotherapy prior to surgery, plasma levels of TERT decreased in patients with a complete pathologic response, while remained unchanged or increased in those who did not respond to therapy. These findings suggest that circulating TERT is a potential biomarker for minimally invasive monitoring of the disease as well as for response to therapy. However, many other studies are needed to confirm the reliability of TERT as a marker of neoplastic disease. A limitation to this approach is that the plasma levels of TERT may receive contributions by non-tumor sources, such as activated lymphocytes, and therefore additional studies with reliable quantitative assays are required to define the cutoff values of circulating TERT as marker of neoplastic disease.

Summary Points

- This chapter focuses on telomerase in colorectal cancers.
- Telomerase is a ribonucleoprotein complex containing a catalytic protein with reverse transcriptase activity (TERT, telomerase reverse transcriptase) which synthesizes telomere sequences using an internal RNA template. The activation of TERT and telomerase activity stabilizes telomere length, preserving the replicative potential of cancer cells.
- Two main strategies are used to estimate the expression of telomerase: (1) quantification of TERT mRNA levels and (2) quantification of telomerase activity. Several studies have shown that TERT mRNA levels correlate with telomerase activity in colorectal cancers.
- In colorectal carcinogenesis, telomerase is activated after erosion of telomere length.
- Levels of telomerase expression and/or activity are higher in cancers than in adjacent normal mucosa.
- Levels of telomerase expression and/or activity increase with the adenoma-carcinoma sequence.
- Levels of telomerase expression and/or activity increase with tumor progression.
- The majority of studies agree that telomerase has a prognostic value for overall survival (OS) and disease-free survival (DFS). However, a few studies do not confirm the prognostic role of telomerase, and cutoff values still represent an open question.
- Emerging studies report that circulating levels of TERT reflect cancer TERT levels and suggest that plasma TERT is a useful marker for minimally invasive monitoring of disease progression and/or response to therapy. Additional studies are required.

References

André T, Boni C, Navarro M, Tabernero J, Hickish T, Topham C, Bonetti A, Clingan P, Bridgewater J, Rivera F, de Gramont A. Improved overall survival with oxaliplatin, fluorouracil, and leucovorin as adjuvant treatment in stage II or III colon cancer in the MOSAIC trial. J Clin Oncol. 2009;27:3109–16.

Bautista CV, Felis CP, Espinet JM, García JB, Salas JV. Telomerase activity is a prognostic factor for recurrence and survival in rectal cancer. Dis Colon Rectum. 2007;50:611–20.

Bechter OE, Zou Y, Walker W, Wright WE, Shay JW. Telomeric recombination in mismatch repair deficient human colon cancer cells after telomerase inhibition. Cancer Res. 2004;64:3444–51.

Bertorelle R, Briarava M, Rampazzo E, Biasini L, Agostini M, Maretto I, Lonardi S, Friso ML, Mescoli C, Zagonel V, Nitti D, De Rossi A, Pucciarelli S. Telomerase is an independent prognostic marker of survival in patients with colorectal cancer. Br J Cancer. 2013;108:278–84.

Blackburn EH, Greider CW, Szostak JW. Telomeres and telomerase: the path from maize, Tetrahymena and yeast to human cancer and aging. Nat Med. 2006;12:1133–8.

Boland CR, Goel A. Microsatellite instability in colorectal cancer. Gastroenterology. 2010;138:2073–87.

Boldrini L, Faviana P, Gisfredi S, Zucconi Y, Di Quirico D, Donati V, Berti P, Spisni R, Galleri D, Materazzi G, Basolo F, Miccoli P, Pingitore R, Fontanini G. Evaluation of telomerase in the development and progression of colon cancer. Int J Mol Med. 2002;10:589–92.

Boldrini L, Faviana P, Gisfredi S, Donati V, Zucconi Y, Ursino S, Simi P, Baldinotti F, Berti P, Galleri D, Materazzi G, Basolo F, Miccoli P, Pingitore R, Fontanini G. Regulation of telomerase and its hTERT messenger in colorectal cancer. Oncol Rep. 2004;11:395–400.

Chen XQ, Bonnefoi H, Pelte MF, Lyautey J, Lederrey C, Movarekhi S, Schaeffer P, Mulcahy HE, Meyer P, Stroun M, Anker P. Telomerase RNA as a detection marker in the serum of breast cancer patients. Clin Cancer Res. 2000;6:3823–6.

Cunningham D, Atkin W, Lenz HJ, Lynch HT, Minsky B, Nordlinger B, Starling N. Colorectal cancer. Lancet. 2010;375:1030–47.

de Kok JB, Roelofs RW, Giesendorf BA. Normalization of gene expression measurements in tumor tissues: comparison of 13 endogenous control genes. Lab Invest. 2005;85:154–9.

Dolcetti R, De Rossi A. Telomere/telomerase interplay in virus-driven and virus-independent lymphomagenesis: pathogenic and clinical implications. Med Res Rev. 2012;32:233–53. Review.

El-Hefnawy T, Raja S, Kelly L, Bigbee WL, Kirkwood JM, Luketich JD, Godfrey TE. Characterization of amplifiable, circulating RNA in plasma and its potential as a tool for cancer diagnostics. Clin Chem. 2004;50:564–73.

Engelhardt M, Drullinsky P, Guillem J, Moore MA. Telomerase and telomere length in the development and progression of premalignant lesions to colorectal cancer. Clin Cancer Res. 1997;3:1931–41.

Fakhoury J, Nimmo GA, Autexier C. Harnessing telomerase in cancer therapeutics Anticancer Agents. Med Chem. 2007;7:475–83. Review.

Garcia-Aranda C, de Juan C, Diaz-Lopez A, Sanchez-Pernaute A, Torres AJ, Diaz-Rubio E, Balibrea JL, Benito M, Iniesta P. Correlation of telomere length, telomerase activity, and telomeric-repeat binding factor 1 expression in colorectal carcinoma. Prognostic indications. Cancer. 2006;106:541–51.

Gertler R, Rosenberg R, Stricker D, Werner M, Lassmann S, Ulm K, Nekarda H. Siewert JR Prognostic potential of the telomerase subunit human telomerase reverse transcriptase in tumor tissue and nontumorous mucosa from patients with colorectal carcinoma. Cancer. 2002;95:2103–11.

Gertler R, Rosemberg R, Stricker D, Friederichs J, Hoos A, Werner M, Ulm K, Holzmann B, Nekarda H, Siewert JR. Telomere length and human telomerase reverse transcriptase expression as markers for progression and prognosis of colorectal carcinoma. J Clin Oncol. 2004;22:1807–14.

Ghori A, Usselmann B, Ferryman S, Morris A, Fraser I. Telomerase expression of malignant epithelial cells correlates with Dukes' stage in colorectal cancer. Colorectal Dis. 2002;4:441–6.

Hackett JA, Greider CW. Balancing instability: dual roles for telomerase and telomere dysfunction in tumorigenesis. Oncogene. 2002;21:619–26. Review.

Hanahan D, Weinberg RA. Hallmarks of cancer: The next generation. Cell. 2011;144:646–74.

Harley CB, Futcher AB, Greider CW. Telomeres shorten during ageing of human fibroblasts. Nature. 1990;345:458–60.

Hastie ND, Dempster M, Dunlop MG, Thompson AM, Green DK, Allshire RC. Telomere reduction in human colorectal carcinoma and with ageing. Nature. 1990;346:866–8.

Hsieh JS, Lin SR, Chang MY, Chen FM, Lu CY, Huang TJ, Huang YS, Huang CJ, Wang JY. APC, K-ras, and p53 gene mutations in colorectal cancer patients: correlation to clinicopathologic features and postoperative surveillance. Am Surg. 2005;71:336–43.

Jemal A, Bray F, Center MM, Ferlay J, Ward E, Forman D. Global cancer statistics. CA Cancer J Clin. 2011;61:69–90.

Kawanishi-Tabata R, Lopez F, Fratantonio S, Kim N, Goldblum J, Tubbs R, Elson P, Lavery I, Bukowski RM, Ganapathi R, Ganapathi MK. Telomerase activity in stage II colorectal cancer. Cancer. 2002;95:1834–9.

Kim NW, Piatyszek MA, Prowse KR, Harley CB, West MD, Ho PL, Coviello GM, Wright WE, Weinrich SL, Shay JW. Specific association of human telomerase activity with immortal cells and cancer. Science. 1994;266:2011–5.

Kim GP, Colangelo LH, Paik S, O'Connell MJ, Kirsch IR, Allegra C, Wolmark N. Predictive value of microsatellite instability-high remains controversial. J Clin Oncol. 2007;25:4857–8.

Kin C, Kidess E, Poultsides GA, Visser BC, Jeffrey SS. Colorectal cancer diagnostics: biomarkers, cell-free DNA, circulating tumor cells and defining heterogeneous populations by single-cell analysis. Expert Rev Mol Diagn. 2013;13:581–99.

Kojima K, Hiyama E, Otani K, Ohtaki M, Fukuba I, Fukuda E, Sueda T, Hiyama K. Telomerase activation without shortening of telomeric 3′-overhang is a poor prognostic factor in human colorectal cancer. Cancer Sci. 2011;102:330–5.

Lledó SM, Garcia-Granero E, Dasí F, Ripoli R, García SA, Cervantes A, Aliño SF. Real time quantification in plasma of human telomerase reverse transcriptase (hTERT) mRNA in patients with colorectal cancer. Colorectal Dis. 2004;6:236–42.

Maláska J, Kunická Z, Borský M, Sklenicková M, Novotná M, Fajkusová L, Zaloudík J, Fajkus J. Telomerase as a diagnostic and predictive marker in colorectal carcinoma. Neoplasma. 2004;51:90–6.

March-Villalba JA, Martínez-Jabaloyas JM, Herrero MJ, Santamaria J, Aliño SF, Dasí F. Cell-free circulating plasma hTERT mRNA is a useful marker for prostate cancer diagnosis and is associated with poor prognosis tumor characteristics. PLoS One. 2012;7:e43470.

Markowitz SD, Bertagnolli MM. Molecular origins of cancer: molecular basis of colorectal cancer. N Engl J Med. 2009;361:2449–60.

Miura N, Maeda Y, Kanbe T, Yazama H, Takeda Y, Sato R, Tsukamoto T, Sato E, Marumoto A, Harada T, Sano A, Kishimoto Y, Hirooka Y, Murawaki Y, Hasegawa J, Shiota G. Serum human telomerase reverse transcriptase messenger RNA as a novel tumor marker for hepatocellular carcinoma. Clin Cancer Res. 2005;11:3205–9.

Naito Y, Takagi T, Handa O, Ishikawa T, Matsumoto N, Yoshida N, Kato H, Ando T, Takemura T, Itani K, Hisatomi H, Tsuchihashi Y, Yoshikawa T. Telomerase activity and expression of telomerase RNA component and catalytic subunits in precancerous and cancerous colorectal lesions. Tumour Biol. 2001;22:374–82.

Nakamura TM, Morin GB, Chapman KB, Weinrich SL, Andrews WH, Lingner J, Harley CB, Cech TR. Telomerase catalytic subunit homologs from fission yeast and human. Science. 1997;277:955–9.

National Comprehensive Cancer Network: NCCN guidelines version 3.2014-Rectal cancer

Niiyama H, Mizumoto K, Sato N, Nagai E, Mibu R, Fukui T, Kinoshita M, Tanaka M. Quantitative analysis of hTERT mRNA expression in colorectal cancer. Am J Gastroenterol. 2001;96:1895–900.

O'Connor ES, Greenblatt DY, LoConte NK, Gangnon RE, Liou JI, Heise CP. Smith MA Adjuvant chemotherapy for stage II colon cancer with poor prognostic features. J Clin Oncol. 2011;29:3381–8.

Ogino S, Nosho K, Kirkner GJ, Kawasaki T, Meyerhardt JA, Loda M, Giovannucci EL, Fuchs CS. CpG island methylator phenotype, microsatellite instability, BRAF mutation and clinical outcome in colon cancer. Gut. 2009;58:90–6.

Palm W, de Lange T. How shelterin protects mammalian telomeres. Annu Rev Genet. 2008;42:301–34. Review.

Pelosi G, Schianchi E, Dell'orto P, Veronesi G, Spaggiari L, Pasini F, Sozzi G, Brambilla E, Griso C, Viale G. Detecting cell-free circulating hTERT mRNA in the plasma may identify a subset of nonsmall cell lung cancer patients. Virchows Arch. 2006;448:7–15.

Pino MS, Chung DC. The chromosomal instability pathway in colon cancer. Gastroenterology. 2010;138:2059–72.

Pucciarelli S, Rampazzo E, Briarava M, Maretto I, Agostini M, Digito M, Keppel S, Friso ML, Lonardi S, De Paoli A, Mescoli C, Nitti D, De Rossi A. Telomere-specific reverse transcriptase (hTERT) and cell-free RNA in plasma as predictors of pathologic tumor response in rectal cancer patients receiving neoadjuvant chemoradiotherapy. Ann Surg Oncol. 2012;19:3089–96.

Quasar Collaborative Group, Gray R, Barnwell J, McConkey C, Hills RK, Williams NS, Kerr DJ. Adjuvant chemotherapy versus observation in patients with colorectal cancer: a randomised study. Lancet. 2007;370:2020–9.

Rahman R, Latonen L, Wiman KG. hTERT antagonizes p53-induced apoptosis independently of telomerase activity. Oncogene. 2005;24:1320–7.

Rampazzo E, Bertorelle R, Serra L, Terrin L, Candiotto C, Pucciarelli S, Del Bianco P, Nitti D, De Rossi A. Relationship between telomere shortening, genetic instability, and site of tumor origin in colorectal cancer. Br J Cancer. 2010;102:1300–5.

Rampazzo E, Bonaldi L, Trentin L, Visco C, Keppel S, Giunco S, Frezzato F, Facco M, Novella E, Giaretta I, Del Bianco P, Semenzato G, De Rossi A. Telomere length and telomerase levels delineate subgroups of B-cell chronic lymphocytic leukemia with different biological characteristics and clinical outcomes. Haematologica. 2012;97:56–63.

Roger L, Jones RE, Heppel NH, Williams GT, Sampson JR, Baird DM. Extensive telomere erosion in the initiation of colorectal adenomas and its association with chromosomal instability. J Natl Cancer Inst. 2013;105:1202–11.

Safont MJ, Gil M, Sirera R, Jantus-Lewintre E, Sanmartín E, Gallach S, Caballero C, Del Pozo N, Palomares E, Camps C. The prognostic value of hTERT expression levels in advanced-stage colorectal cancer patients: a comparison between tissue and serum expression. Clin Transl Oncol. 2011;13:396–400.

Sanz-Casla MT, Vidaurreta M, Sanchez-Rueda D, Maestro ML, Arroyo M, Cerdan FJ. Telomerase activity as prognostic factor in colorectal cancer. Onkologie. 2005;28:553–7.

Sargent DJ, Marsoni S, Monges G, Thibodeau SN, Labianca R, Hamilton SR, French AJ, Kabat B, Foster NR, Torri V, Ribic C, Grothey A, Moore M, Zaniboni A, Seitz JF, Sinicrope F, Gallinger S. Defective mismatch repair as a predictive marker for lack of efficacy of fluorouracil-based adjuvant therapy in colon cancer. J Clin Oncol. 2010;28:3219–26.

Schetter AJ, Okayama H, Harris CC. The role of microRNAs in colorectal cancer. Cancer J. 2012;18:244–52. Review.

Shawi M, Chu TW, Martinez-Marignac V, Yu Y, Gryaznov SM, Johnston JB, Lees-Miller SP, Assouline SE, Autexier C, Aloyz R. Telomerase contributes to fludarabine resistance in primary human leukemic lymphocytes. PLoS One. 2013;8:e70428.

Spolverato G, Pucciarelli S, Bertorelle R, De Rossi A, Nitti D. Predictive factors of the response of rectal cancer to neoadjuvant radiochemotherapy. Cancer. 2011;3:2176–94. Review.

Stewart SA, Hahn WC, O'Connor BF, Banner EN, Lundberg AS, Modha P, Mizuno H, Brooks MW, Fleming M, Zimonjic DB, Popescu NC, Weinberg RA. Telomerase contributes to tumorigenesis by a telomere length-independent mechanism. Proc Natl Acad Sci USA. 2002;99:12606–11.

Takagi S, Kinouchi Y, Hiwatashi N, Chida M, Nagashima F, Takahashi S, Negoro K, Shimosegawa T, Toyota T. Telomere shortening and the clinicopathologic characteristics of human colorectal carcinomas. Cancer. 1999;86:1431–6.

Tao SF, Zhang CS, Guo XL, Xu Y, Zhang SS, Song JR, Li R, Wu MC, Wei LX. Anti-tumor effect of 5-aza-2′-deoxycytidine by inhibiting telomerase activity in hepatocellular carcinoma cells. World J Gastroenterol. 2012;18:2334–43.

Tatsumoto N, Hiyama E, Murakami Y, Imamura Y, Shay JW, Matsuura Y, Yokoyama T. High telomerase activity is an independent prognostic indicator of poor outcome in colorectal cancer. Clin Cancer Res. 2000;6:2696–701.

Terrin L, Rampazzo E, Pucciarelli S, Agostini M, Bertorelle R, Esposito G, DelBianco P, Nitti D, De Rossi A. Relationship between tumor and plasma levels of hTERT mRNA in patients with colorectal cancer: implications for monitoring of neoplastic disease. Clin Cancer Res. 2008;14:7444–51.

van Cutsem E, Köhne CH, Hitre E, Zaluski J, Chang Chien CR, Makhson A, D'Haens G, Pintér T, Lim R, Bodoky G, Roh JK, Folprecht G, Ruff P, Stroh C, Tejpar S, Schlichting M, Nippgen J, Rougier P. Cetuximab and chemotherapy as initial treatment for metastatic colorectal cancer. N Engl J Med. 2009;360:1408–17.

Vidaurreta M, Maestro ML, Rafael S, Veganzones S, Sanz-Casla MT, Cerdán J, Arroyo M. Telomerase activity in colorectal cancer, prognostic factor and implications in the microsatellite instability pathway. World J Gastroenterol. 2007;13:3868–72.

Wilkes G, Hartshorn K. Clinical update: colon, rectal, and anal cancers. Semin Oncol Nurs. 2012;28:e1–e22.

Winder T, Lenz HJ. Beyond KRAS: a new approach in metastatic colorectal cancer. Lancet Oncol. 2010;11:706–7.

Zou X, Xing D. Assays for human telomerase activity: progress and prospects. Chem Soc Rev. 2012;41:4643–56.

Carcinoembryonic Antigen Family Cell Adhesion Molecules (CEACAM) as Colorectal Cancer Biomarkers

30

Marica Gemei, Claudia Corbo, Francesco Salvatore, and Luigi Del Vecchio

Contents

M. Gemei • C. Corbo
CEINGE-Biotecnologie avanzate, s.c.a r.l, Naples, Italy
e-mail: gemei@ceinge.unina.it; corbo@ceinge.unina.it

F. Salvatore (✉)
CEINGE-Biotecnologie avanzate, s.c.a r.l, Naples, Italy

Dipartimento di Medicina Molecolare e Biotecnologie Mediche, Università di Napoli "Federico II", Naples, Italy

IRCCS-SDN, Naples, Italy
e-mail: salvator@unina.it

L. Del Vecchio
CEINGE-Biotecnologie avanzate, s.c.a r.l, Naples, Italy

Dipartimento di Medicina Molecolare e Biotecnologie Mediche, Università di Napoli "Federico II", Naples, Italy
e-mail: luigi.delvecchio@unina.it

V.R. Preedy, V.B. Patel (eds.), *Biomarkers in Cancer, Biomarkers in Disease: Methods, Discoveries and Applications*,
DOI 10.1007/978-94-007-7681-4_30

Abstract

Each year, nearly one million people develop colorectal cancer, and 50 % of them are expected to die because of cancer within 5 years of diagnosis. Over the last two decades, significant advances in screening, surgery, adjuvant chemotherapy, and patient monitoring have improved the 5-year survival rate. Colorectal cancer is a molecularly heterogeneous disease, and the analysis of its molecular signatures and the identification of colorectal cancer biomarkers will lead to better screening approaches and personalized therapeutic plans. A biomarker is a substance that can be measured and used as an indicator of a biological and/or pathological state. In cancer pathology, biomarkers can be used to detect the disease, to predict prognosis or response to therapy, and to evaluate the efficacy of therapy thereby improving the patient's life expectancy and quality of life. The carcinoembryonic antigen (CEA) is the biomarker most frequently used in colorectal cancer. It is effective in the surveillance of colorectal cancer patients and in monitoring the efficacy of therapy, whereas it is less useful in colorectal screening. Recent studies indicate that also CEA-related proteins (CEACAMs) are promising potential colorectal cancer biomarkers. CEA and CEACAM proteins play important roles in cancer pathology, and the analysis of their functions will be useful for the identification of diagnostic and/or prognostic factors and therapeutic targets in colorectal and other cancers.

List of Abbreviations

CEA	Carcinoembyonic Antigen
CEACAM	Carcinoembryonic Antigen-Family Cell Adhesion Molecule
FOBT	Fecal Occult Blood Test
GPI	Glycosylphosphatidylinositol
Ig	Immunoglobulin
IgCAM	Ig-like Cell Adhesion Molecule
PCR	Polymerase Chain Reaction
TNM	Tumor Nodes Metastases

Key Facts of Colorectal Cancer

- The intestine is the main site of nutrient absorption; it is subdivided in small and large intestine. The latter comprises the right colon, transverse colon, left colon, sigma, and rectum.
- Colorectal cancer develops from uncontrolled growth of colorectal mucosa cells.
- Colorectal cancer is an epithelial cancer arising in almost 80 % of cases from nonmalignant lesions that turned into cancer within 5–10 years of their appearance.

- The rate of malignant transformation of polyps depends on their size.
- Genetic factors, such as Lynch syndrome and familial adenomatous polyposis, can increase the risk of developing colorectal cancer.
- Adequate screening for colorectal cancer considerably decreases the death rate of the disease.
- Surgery is the treatment of choice for colorectal cancer, but chemo-and radiotherapy could be useful as adjuvant therapies and also for nonoperable primary and metastatic colorectal cancers.
- Biologic drugs such as monoclonal antibodies (Bevacizumab and Cetuximab) can be successfully used to treat advanced cancers.

Definitions of Words and Terms

Glycosylation Glycosylation is a posttranslational modification that consists in the attachment of carbohydrates to proteins or other organic molecules.

Ig-like Fold This is a type of tertiary structure of proteins. It consists of a 2-layer sandwich of antiparallel β strands arranged in two β sheets consisting of about 80 amino acids.

β-Sheet Structure The β sheet is a type of secondary structure of proteins. Beta sheets are composed of beta strands connected laterally by hydrogen bonds.

Amino Acids These are organic compounds that form the backbone of proteins. They are made from aminic ($-NH^2$) and carboxylic acid ($-COOH$) groups, with a side chain specific to each amino acid.

Paralog A paralog is a pair of genes that derive from a duplication event and that reside within the same genome.

Microsatellite Instability Microsatellite instability (MSI) occurs when the DNA mismatch repair (MMR) system fails thereby allowing the accumulation of mutations that cause a condition of genetic hypermutability.

Loss of Heterozygosity Human somatic cells are diploid; this means that they bear a copy of the genome from the father and another from the mother. When a parental copy of a genome tract is lost, there is a loss of heterozygosity.

Orthologue Orthologues are homologous genes derived from a speciation event resulting in similar genes founded in different species.

Pseudogene Pseudogenes derive from the loss of protein-coding ability of genes that have accumulated multiple mutations and whose original product is not required for the survival of the organism.

Homologue Homologues are genes founded in different species that derive from a common ancestral gene following a speciation event or similar genes founded in the same species following a duplication and mutation event.

Phosphorylation Phosphorylation is a posttranslational modification of proteins that consists in the attachment of a phosphate (PO_4^{3-}) group.

Apoptosis Apoptosis is the sequence of events that determine a programmed cell death in the cells when they are damaged or senescent. Apoptosis leads to cell death without loss of cellular material in the surrounding environment, and consequently without generation of inflammation.

Anoikis Anoikis is a kind of programmed cell death that is induced when cells detach from the extracellular matrix to avoid their anchorage-independent growth.

CEACAM as Colorectal Cancer Biomarkers

Introduction

Colorectal cancer is a leading cause of cancer death in the industrialized world (Levy 2012). The 5-year survival rate is about 90 % when colorectal cancer is diagnosed at an early stage (American Cancer Society 2013), but most colorectal cancers are diagnosed when they are already in an advanced stage. Late diagnosis has been attributed mainly to the lack of noninvasive, cost-effective, and sensitive screening tests (Sepulveda 2013).

Colorectal Cancer Screening

The screening procedures recommended for average-risk individuals 50 years old or more are: an annual fecal occult blood test (FOBT) and flexible sigmoidoscopy and double-contrast barium enema or colonoscopy every 5 years (Levy 2012; Alberts et al. 2012; Hayat 2009). Flexible sigmoidoscopy together with a FOBT is a reliable screening test; double-contrast barium enema, although visualizing the entire colon, is not sufficiently sensitive to detect small lesions. Colonoscopy is the most sensitive test and is recommended every 10 years in people with an average risk of developing colorectal cancer (Levy 2012; Alberts and Grothey 2012; Hayat 2009). Risk factors are inflammatory bowel disease, familial adenomatous polyposis, hereditary nonpolyposis colorectal cancers, or a family history of cancer. People who present one or more of these risk factors are considered high-risk persons and are likely to follow more intense screening than average-risk individuals over 40 years old (Sepulveda 2013; Fleisher et al. 2002; Alberts and Grothey 2012).

Most colorectal cancers arise from nonmalignant polyps that become malignant within 10–12 years. Thus, this condition is amenable to early detection of precancerous lesions or early stage cancers. However, screening rates for colorectal cancer are low, and there is a need to increase the public's awareness to the importance of screening and to define effective screening programs.

Colorectal Cancer Staging

When cancer is diagnosed, it is also staged. "Cancer staging" is a standardized process by which clinicians describe the extent of the cancer. Colon cancer clinical staging goes from stage 0 to stage 4 (Fig. 1); each stage has peculiar characteristics although borderline cases are frequent. When patients undergo surgery, the process used to determine whether cancer has spread within the colon or to other parts of the body is called "pathologic staging" and is based on the results of the physical examination, biopsies, and imaging tests (Levy 2012; Sepulveda 2013). The most commonly used staging system for colorectal cancer is that of the American Joint Committee on Cancer (AJCC) known as the TNM system (Fig. 1, Table 1) (Levy 2012; Sepulveda 2013; Fleisher et al. 2002). Earlier staging systems for colorectal cancer are the Dukes and Astler-Coller systems (Table 1) (Sepulveda 2013). More recent is the TNM system, which describes three different aspects of colon cancer. The T parameter goes from 1 to 4 and describes how deep the primary tumor has grown into the wall of the intestine and whether it has invaded nearby areas. The N parameter goes from 1 to 2 and describes the extent of spread to nearby lymph

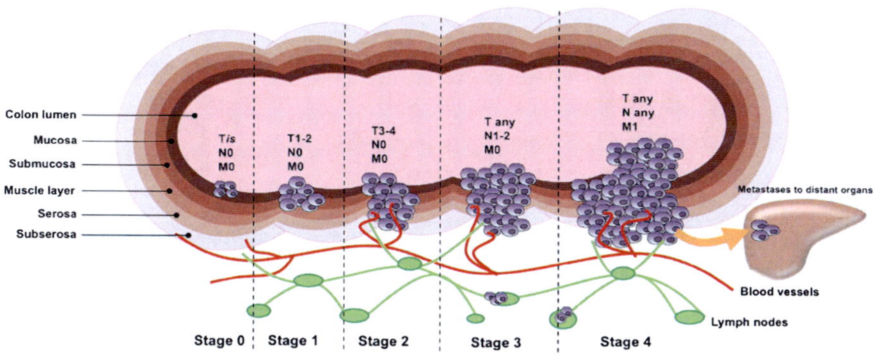

Fig. 1 Characteristics of colorectal cancer at different clinical/pathological stages. The clinical and pathological stages of colorectal cancers reflect their grade of severity in terms of cancer spreading to nearby and distant tissues and organs. Early stage disease (0–1) shows no or little invasion of the colon wall by tumor and no lymph node involvement or distant metastases; in the mid-stage (2), the invasion is more advanced and new vascularization is formed within the tumor, and cancer cell spreading through the bloodstream and lymphatic system promotes cancer diffusion; in more advanced stages (3–4), lymph node metastases can be observed, and distant metastases also appear

Table 1 Colorectal cancer pathologic staging. Characteristics of different colorectal cancer stages. Correlations between clinical stages and pathological stages. The correspondence between TNM, Dukes, and Astler-Coller staging systems is reported

Stage	TNM	Dukes	Astler-Coller	Characteristics
0	T*is*, N0, M0	–	–	Carcinoma in situ, intraepithelial or lamina propria invasion, no lymph node metastases, no distant metastases
I	T1, N0, M0	A	A, B1	Tumor invades the submucosa, no lymph node metastases, no distant metastases
	T2, N0, M0	B1	B2	Tumor invades the muscularis propria, no lymph node metastases, no distant metastases
II	T3, N0, M0	B2	B2	Tumor invades through the muscularis propria into the subserosa or into non-peritonealized, pericolic, or perirectal tissues, no lymph node metastases, no distant metastases
	T4, N0, M0	B2	B3	Tumor directly invades other organs or structures and/or perforates visceral peritoneum, no lymph node metastases, no distant metastases
III	T1–T2, N1–N2, M0	C1	C1–C2	Tumor invades the submucosa or the muscle layer, metastases are present in regional lymph nodes, no distant metastases
	T3–T4, N1–N2, M0	C2	C2–C3	Tumor invades the serosa of the colon wall, metastases are present in regional lymph nodes, no distant metastases
IV	Any T, any N, M1	D	D	Distant metastases

nodes. Finally, the M parameter goes from 0 to 1 and indicates whether the cancer has metastasized to other organs of the body, most frequently to the liver and lungs (Levy 2012). The information gathered from staging determines the stage of the disease; clinical and pathologic staging are complementary to each other (Fig. 1).

CEA and CEACAMs: Genetic and Molecular Structure

In the mid-1990s, CEA was identified as a tumor-associated antigen in human colon cancer (McClatchey 2002). Gold and Freedman identified this antigen in fetal colon and in adenocarcinoma but not in normal adult colon. Because of its expression in cancer and embryonic tissues, they called this antigen "carcinoembryonic antigen" (McClatchey 2002; Schwartz 2002; Sepulveda 2013). Subsequently, other studies showed that the expression of CEA is low in some normal tissues but 60-fold higher in cancer (Duffy 2001). CEA was also found to be higher in the serum of colorectal cancer patients than in healthy controls (McClatchey 2002; Schwartz 2002; Sepulveda 2013) (Table 2).

Table 2 CEA measurement in the management of colorectal cancer patients. CEA measurement in colorectal cancer screening, staging, treatment planning, postoperative surveillance, and therapy response. CEA is not recommended in screening, staging, and treatment planning, while it is useful in the detection of progressive and metastatic diseases as well as in the monitoring of therapy response

Screening	Staging	Treatment planning	Postoperative surveillance	Therapy response monitoring
CEA testing is not recommended	Preoperative elevated CEA levels (>5 mg/mL) seem to indicate an adverse outcome	Preoperative CEA levels are not recommended for adjuvant therapy planning	CEA levels should be tested every 3 months for 3 years after diagnosis if patients are candidates for surgery and systemic therapy	CEA is evaluated every 1–3 months for the entire duration of the treatment to monitor metastatic cancer during systemic therapy
			If CEA results elevated in two measurements, evaluation of metastatic disease should be conducted	If CEA elevation persists, current therapy needs to be reconsidered and, alternatives should be evaluated

CEA belongs to the immunoglobulin superfamily of cell adhesion molecules (IgCAMs) (Schwartz 2002). IgCAMs are highly glycosylated surface proteins whose function is fundamental in cell-cell adhesion, and they have recently been identified as important modulators of several physiopathological processes (Schwartz 2002; Weber 2007). The Ig fold shows small variations that allow the identification of the Ig variable (IgV) and Ig constant (IgC)-1 and (IgC)-2 domains (Kuespert et al. 2006; Schwartz 2002). The Ig fold is very common, and the Ig domain-encoding genes represent the most abundant portion in the whole human genome. Its structure is amenable to fine tuning, thereby enabling Ig-like proteins to be involved in various binding tasks.

The CEA Ig-like protein is characterized by seven extracellular Ig domains and a glycosylphosphatidylinositol (GPI) anchor. GPI-linked proteins are anchored to the cell membrane through an external anchor, which could explain why CEA is easily detected in a soluble form in the bloodstream (Fleisher et al. 2002; Weber 2007). The CEA protein is a primate-specific protein since it has no orthologues in non-primate species (Fleisher et al. 2002) (Fig. 2).

Together with its paralogs, CEA is a member of the family of CEA-related cell adhesion molecules (CEACAMs). In humans, CEACAMs comprise 23 genes located within a 1.2 Mb cluster along the long arm of chromosome 19. Eighteen are expressed, and 11 are pseudogenes (Schwartz 2002; Sepulveda 2013). CEACAMs comprise 6 transmembrane proteins, 4 GPI-linked proteins (CEACAM5–8), and 2 secreted proteins (CEACAM16 and CEACAM18) (Schwartz 2002; Sepulveda 2013) (Fig. 3).

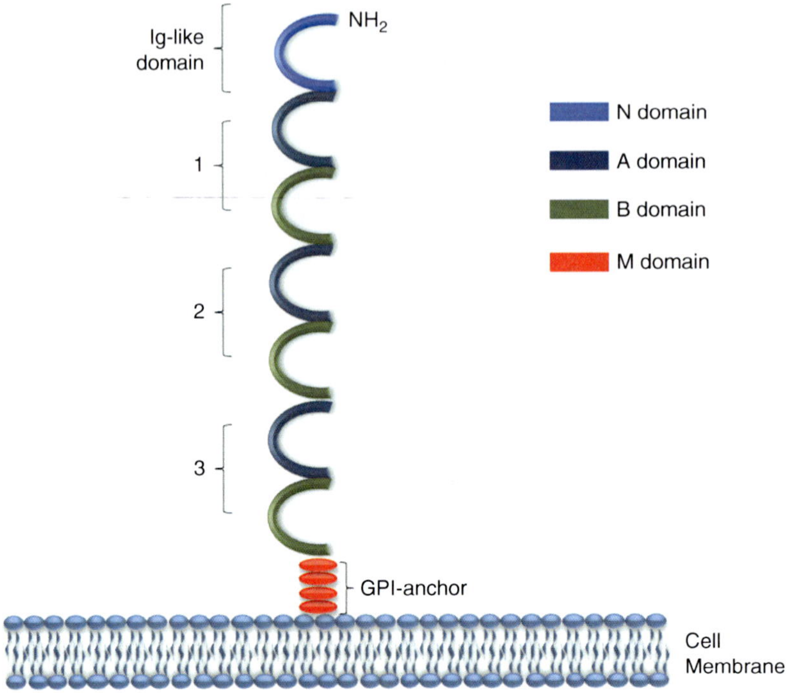

Fig. 2 CEACAM5 (CEA) protein structure. The CEACAM5 protein contains three Ig-like domains subdivided into sub-domains. Cysteine residues contained in A and B domains allow the formation of disulfide bonds which create the loops characteristic of the Ig-like fold. The mature protein is linked to the plasma cell membrane by a GPI anchor. The extracellular portion of the CEACAM5 protein is highly glycosylated at various points; the different glycosylation statuses change the size and immunogenicity of CEACAM5

Dysregulation of CEACAM Proteins and Their Involvement in Colorectal Cancer

CEA is abundantly expressed in the fetal gastrointestinal tract and other tissues, while it is generally downregulated in the adult, and residual CEA expression can be found in the apical part of the gastrointestinal epithelium and in such other mucosa as the lungs, sweat glands, urogenital tract, and nasopharynx (Schwartz 2002; Weber 2007; McClatchey 2002). High reexpression of CEA in the adult is often linked to epithelial carcinoma development. Other CEACAMs are also expressed in the gastrointestinal epithelia although their functions are still poorly explored. CEACAMs in cancer are involved in the prevention of anoikis, an adhesion-free form of apoptosis linked to the detachment of cells from the extra-cellular matrix, and in the blocking of intrinsic apoptosis pathways (Kuespert et al. 2006; Duxbury et al. 2004; Duxbury et al. 2004). Overexpression of CEA or CEACAM6 has been demonstrated to disrupt the ordered tissue architecture in

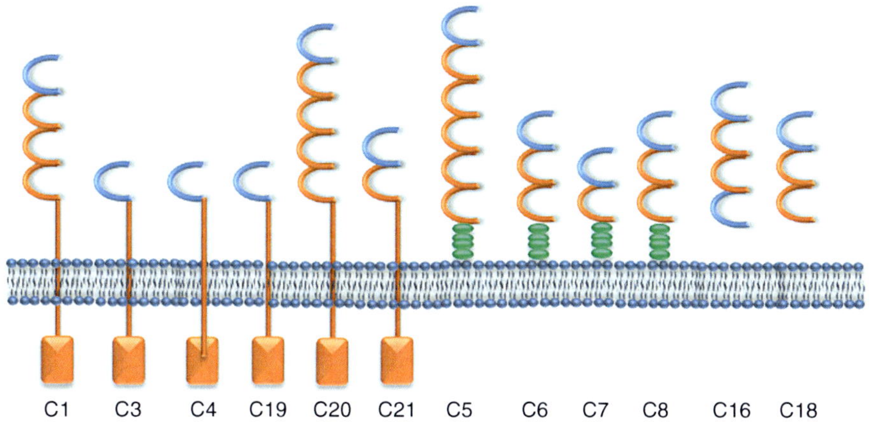

Fig. 3 Members of the CEACAM family. The CEACAM family is constituted by 12 members. Six are transmembrane CEACAMs (CEACAM1–4 and 19–21), four are GPI-linked proteins (CEACAM5–8, the GPI anchor is shown in *green*), and two CEACAMs are secreted (CEACAM16 and 18). They have different numbers of Ig-like loops in their structure which is composed of a constant (in *blue*) and a variable (in *orange*) part

3-D cultures of colon cell lines, thereby inhibiting the formation of glandular structures and enhancing their tumorigenicity in mice (Sepulveda 2013; Ilantzis et al. 2002; Chan et al. 2007), while in transgenic mice, CEACAM6 overexpression leads to uncontrolled proliferation of colonocytes and inhibits differentiation and anoikis (Sepulveda 2013; Ilantzis et al. 2002; Chan et al. 2007). In addition, transgenic mice expressing the human chromosomal region containing CEA and CEACAM6 displayed an abnormal colon structure with hyperplasia, severe dysplasia, and serrated adenomas, together with an increased tumor formation rate upon azoxymethane treatment (Ilantzis et al. 2002). Moreover, when normal myofibroblasts were transfected to express CEA or CEACAM6, they acquired the ability to grow in suspension (adherence-free growth), showed a reduced apoptosis rate, and acquired tumorigenic ability (Sepulveda 2013; Kuespert et al. 2006). CEA and CEACAM6 can modulate integrin clustering, thereby increasing cell adhesion to the extracellular matrix and creating a fibronectin shell around cancer cells (Kuespert et al. 2006; Fiori et al. 2012). This suggests that members of the CEACAM family play a role in tumorigenic transformation processes by promoting aberrant growth in human cells.

CEACAM6 has recently been investigated for its potential function in tumorigenesis (Sepulveda 2013; Blumenthal et al. 2005a; Duxbury et al. 2004a, b, e; Strickland et al. 2009). CEACAM6 expression, measured by immunohistochemistry, was found to be increased in colorectal malignancies, and its high expression was reported to be an independent prognostic factor for resectable colon cancers (Blumenthal et al. 2005a; Scholzel et al. 2000; Jantsheff et al. 2003; Zhao et al. 2011). CEACAM6 has been reported to be a differentiation marker in normal colonocytes, in which it plays a role in the maintenance of tissue architecture and in colonocyte differentiation. CEACAM6, in fact, is normally upregulated as colonocyte differentiation proceeds (Ilantzis et al. 1997; 2002).

CEACAM6 ectopic expression in rat myofibroblasts enabled the cells to form tumors in mouse (Screaton et al. 1997), whereas CEACAM6 overexpression in human cell lines such as Caco2 greatly reduced the latency time of tumor formation and resulted in larger tumors in mice (Ilantzis et al. 2002). CEACAM6 was identified in specific membrane rafts in which the cross-linking of its external domain was able to recruit and then to activate other molecules such as $\alpha 5\beta 1$ integrin whose involvement in cell-cell and cell-matrix interactions is relevant in cell differentiation, proliferation, and survival (Chan et al. 2007; Duxbury et al. 2004c; Ordonez et al. 2007). Taken together, these observations support the concept that CEACAM6 can contribute to colorectal tumorigenesis.

CEACAM7 has been described as a predictive marker for rectal cancer recurrence (Issues in surgical Research, Techniques, and Innovation 2011; Messick et al. 2010). Its use in the early monitoring of high-risk patients could result in timely adjuvant therapy and thus improve outcome. CEACAM7 mRNA levels were 21-fold lower in rectal cancers than in normal colon mucosa (Issues in surgical Research, Techniques, and Innovation 2011; Messick et al. 2010). CEACAM7 levels were relatively decreased in patients with cancer recurrences than in patients without recurrence (Issues in surgical Research, Techniques, and Innovation 2011; Messick et al. 2010).

CEACAM1 could exert a function opposite to that of CEA and CEACAM6. In fact, it has antitumor and proapoptotic factor functions (Sepulveda 2013; Fridman and Galon 2011). It is downregulated in about a quarter of human colorectal cancers (Sepulveda 2013; Fridman and Galon 2011). There are two CEACAM1 isoforms (short and long) whose expression varies depending on the location (Sepulveda 2013; Fridman and Galon 2011; Kuespert et al. 2006). Both are expressed weakly at the luminal surface of advanced colorectal cancer, while the long isoform is expressed at a higher level at the invasive front of tumors, and its expression is associated with lymph node metastasization, bloodstream spreading of cancer cells, and poor prognosis (Sepulveda 2013; Fridman and Galon 2011; Kuespert et al. 2006). In vitro experiments revealed that CEACAM1 is involved in promoting cancer cell invasion and migration. In particular, the long isoform is strongly reexpressed at the invasive front of colorectal cancers (Kuespert et al. 2006). Moreover, CEACAM1 expression is upregulated in response to interferon gamma in melanoma cells that survive lymphocyte-mediated injury (Kuespert et al. 2006; Fiori et al. 2012; Sepulveda 2013). Natural killer and T-cell attacks were inhibited by their interaction with CEACAM1; this specific promotion of immune escape could explain why CEACAM1 is sometimes overexpressed in human tumors (Kuespert et al. 2006; Fiori et al. 2012; Sepulveda 2013). CEACAM1 is also implicated in angiogenesis during the formation of tumor vasculature given its expression by tumor-associated vessels (Fiori et al. 2012). It exerts a proangiogenic effect by stimulating capillary-like tube formation in vitro, as well as by increasing vascularization in vivo in chicken embryos (Fiori et al. 2012). Specifically, CEACAM1 acts on the migratory abilities of endothelial cells and on the expression of the angiogenic factor CD105 (Fiori et al. 2012; Kuespert et al. 2006).

Potential of CEACAMs in the Targeting and Treatment of Cancer

The targeting potential of CEA has been demonstrated in mice. In fact, positron emission tomography and single-photon emission computed tomography with pre-targeted anti-CEA antibodies were able to identify human colon cancer in mouse lungs even when ^{18}F-fludeoxyglucose staining failed (Hayat 2009; Hammarström and Stigbrand 2002; Heine et al. 2011). In humans, pre-targeting with antibodies followed by radioisotope administration improved imaging resolution (Hayat 2009; Hammarström and Stigbrand 2002; Heine et al. 2011). Moreover, "CEA scan," a ^{99m}Tc-labeled anti-CEA F_{ab} fragment, has been approved by the US Food and Drug Administration for cancer imaging (Hayat 2009; Hammarström and Stigbrand 2002; Heine et al. 2011).

Encouraging results have been published supporting the role of CEA in colorectal cancer therapy. CEA inhibition in colorectal cancer cell lines has been linked to apoptosis induction and loss of metastatic potential in mice (Tiernan et al. 2013; Blumenthal et al. 2005b; Duxbury et al. 2004h; Strickland et al. 2009). CEA has also been used as a homing target for new experimental therapies, and promising effects have been observed with CEA-directed radiotherapy in human and mice, in immunotherapy with CEA-DNA vaccines, in treatment with CEA-stimulated dendritic and T-cells, and in gene therapy with viral vectors expressing CEA-binding domains (Sepulveda 2013; Barack 2006; Hammarström and Stigbrand 2002; Tiernan et al. 2013). However, these strategies need to be finely regulated because of the normal CEA expression in various adult tissues. In this context, other CEACAMs, for example, CEACAM6, showed promise as a therapeutic target for new therapies that have a low cytotoxicity (Duxbury et al. 2004a; Strickland et al. 2009). It has been proposed as a therapeutic target in colon cancer (Gemei et al. 2013), while, in pancreatic cancer, CEACAM6 has been evaluated in preclinical analysis with mice and nonhuman primates, using new monoclonal antibody and siRNA-based approaches (Strickland et al. 2009; Duxbury et al. 2004h).

CEA as a Biomarker in Colorectal Cancer

Few studies have been devoted to biomarkers in colorectal cancer (Bacolod and Barany 2011; Belov et al. 2010; Fleisher et al. 2002; Barak 2006). Hitherto, tumor markers have not been proved useful in detecting early colorectal cancer because of the lack of specificity, although they have been important in predicting recurrence and in the management of therapies (McClatchey 2002; Alberts and Grothey 2012; Fleisher et al. 2002).

In 1999, the College of American Pathologists released a consensus document on genetic, biologic, and molecular prognostic factors in colorectal cancer (McClatchey 2002; Fleisher et al. 2002; Compton et al. 2000). They include tumor grade, circumferential resection margin, tumor regression after adjuvant chemotherapy, histological type, tumor border configuration, microsatellite instability, and loss of heterozygosity. In this list of prognostic factors, the only biomarker mentioned is CEA, also known as CEACAM5 (McClatchey 2002; Fleisher et al. 2002; Newton et al. 2012).

CEA Expression in Colorectal Cancer

The concentration of CEA was found to be higher in patients with an advanced-stage colorectal cancer. In fact, serum levels of CEA were increased in 28 % of patients with Dukes' A disease, 45 % with Dukes' B disease, 75 % with Dukes' C disease, and 84 % with Dukes' D disease (Kuespert et al. 2006; Sepulveda 2013; Fleisher et al. 2002; Alberts and Grothey 2012; Levy 2012). In addition, several studies demonstrated that well-differentiated colorectal cancers produce a higher quantity of CEA than poorly differentiated cancers in terms of both tissue and serum CEA (Sepulveda 2013; Kuespert et al. 2006). With respect to tumor site, left-sided colorectal cancers generally produce more CEA than right-sided cancers. It is noteworthy that also bowel obstructions give rise to CEA concentrations above normal level (Kuespert et al. 2006), while smoking has been demonstrated to almost double CEA serum concentration in healthy subjects (Duffy 2001).

In addition, since CEA is metabolized and degraded in the Kupffer cells of the liver, some nonmalignant conditions of the liver can impair this clearance mechanism so that CEA could be elevated also in the serum of patients with liver pathologies (Kuespert et al. 2006; Fleisher et al. 2002).

CEA in Colorectal Cancer Screening and Prognosis

After its recognition as a cancer biomarker, CEA rapidly became the most widely used tumor marker worldwide and the most frequently analyzed marker in colorectal cancer patients even though its false-positive rate is unacceptably high, and so the use of CEA in colorectal cancer screening is controversial (Duffy 2001; McClatchey 2002; Fleisher et al. 2002; Sepulveda 2013; Kuespert et al. 2006; Sturgeon et al. 2008).

Baseline CEA can vary between countries and laboratories, but a value between 2.5 and 5 ng/mL is considered elevated. Using these values, about 50 % of colorectal cancer patients have normal levels of CEA, especially in the case of localized and poorly differentiated cancers, while in patients with true elevation of serum levels of CEA, hemodilution resulting from parenteral nutrition or transfusions could cause a false-negative result (McClatchey 2002; Fleisher et al. 2002; Sepulveda 2013; Kuespert et al. 2006). The main aim of colorectal cancer screening is to detect Dukes' A or B cancers; in fact, more advanced stages are unlikely to be easily and definitively treated. At an upper limit of 2.5 ng/mL, CEA has a sensitivity of 36 % and a specificity of 87 % in the detection of Dukes' A and B colorectal cancers (Chen et al. 2004). Thus, the positive predictive value of CEA is too low to be used in screening healthy subjects. In fact, the American Society of Clinical Oncology (ASCO) does not recommend CEA testing in colorectal cancer screening protocols even though it may occasionally identify colorectal cancer patients (Sepulveda 2013; Fleisher et al. 2002). Consequently, FOBT and colonoscopy are largely preferred for colorectal cancer screening. However, in symptomatic patients, who are likely to have a more advanced disease with respect to asymptomatic patients, a highly increased CEA level (five times or higher than normal level) is considered strongly suggestive of a cancer (Sepulveda 2013; Fleisher et al. 2002; Alberts and Grothey 2012; Levy 2012). ASCO also recommends CEA be tested preoperatively only for prognostic purposes. Of the seven studies that evaluated the prognostic impact of preoperative CEA levels, five reported that high CEA levels were associated with a poor prognosis, while the other two did not find a significant relationship between CEA levels and patient outcome (Duffy 2001). The finding of prognostic factors is particularly important in Dukes' B patients because approximately 40–50 % of these patients have an aggressive disease (Sepulveda 2013; Fleisher et al. 2002; Alberts and Grothey 2012; Levy 2012). To improve the prognostic value of CEA levels in Dukes' B patients, their analysis can be combined with CA-242 measurement. This combination was effective in predicting an adverse prognosis of more aggressive cancers (Sepulveda 2013; Fleisher et al. 2002; Duffy 2001). Differently, it remains to be established whether CEA levels are able to identify patients who would benefit from adjuvant chemotherapy. Furthermore, there are no sound data that CEA screening would improve survival (Barak 2006; Sepulveda 2013; Fleisher et al. 2002; Thirunavukarasu et al. 2011), and no reports have shown a benefit from the use of adjuvant therapy based only upon the increased preoperative CEA level (Barak 2006; Kuespert et al. 2006).

CEA in Colorectal Cancer Management

Although there is no formal prognostic algorithm that includes CEA, the College of American Pathologists and the American Joint Committee on Cancer consider it a class I prognostic factor. This means that it is a factor "definitively proven to be of prognostic import based on evidence from multiple statistically robust published trials and generally used in patient management" (Sepulveda 2013; Thirunavukarasu et al. 2011). In fact, even if CEA is not recommended for colorectal cancer screening, there is a general consensus that CEA is useful in the management of colorectal cancer patients, particularly in monitoring for recurrence and in assessing response to therapy (Alberts and Grothey 2012; Levy 2012; Sepulveda 2013; Fleisher et al. 2002). Serum CEA elevation frequently precedes the appearance of symptoms and clinical confirmation of disease progression by several months (Sepulveda 2013; Lee 1978). In the identification of recurrences in colorectal cancer patients, CEA had a sensitivity of about 80 % (range of 17–89 %) and a specificity around 70 % (range of 34–91 %) (Duffy 2001; Levy 2012). In particular, CEA testing was successful in the diagnosis of hepatic and retroperitoneal metastases, but not in identifying local, peritoneal, and lung involvement (Sepulveda 2013; Fleisher et al. 2002; Alberts and Grothey 2012; Levy 2012).

Moreover, persistent high levels of CEA are indicative of residual disease since, after curative surgery, CEA levels usually decrease to normal values (Sepulveda 2013; Alberts and Grothey 2012).

After curative resection, the 5-year overall recurrence rate in colorectal cancer patients was found to be about 40 % (including 12 % local relapses, 20 % liver metastases, 8 % pulmonary metastases, and 30 % other recurrences) (Sepulveda 2013; Alberts and Grothey 2012). CEA serum levels are commonly monitored after curative surgery to detect recurrent disease at an early stage. In the follow-up of colorectal cancer patients, CEA serum levels can detect a cancer relapse with a sensitivity ~80 % and a specificity ~70 % (Sepulveda 2013; Alberts and Grothey 2012; Fleisher et al. 2002; Levy 2012). Serial CEA level measurements are the most useful in the detection of liver metastases; indeed, they have a sensitivity close to 100 % (Duffy 2001; Levy 2012). A meta-analysis of 20 studies examining the performance of CEA in 4,285 patients after resection of the primary colorectal cancer demonstrated a sensitivity of 64 % and a specificity of 90 % for relapse detection (Sepulveda 2013).

Liver metastases is the most common complication of colorectal cancer (~60 % of colorectal cancer patients develop hepatic metastases), and hepatic resection is the only potential curative treatment of metastatic colorectal cancer. Unfortunately, 50–80 % of patients who undergo hepatic resection relapse (Sepulveda 2013; Alberts and Grothey 2012). For these patients, elevated CEA levels 1–3 months after hepatic resection correlate with an adverse prognosis (Sepulveda 2013; Alberts and Grothey 2012). A slow increase of serum CEA could indicate local recurrence, while a rapid increase probably indicates a hepatic metastasis (Sepulveda 2013; Alberts and Grothey 2012; Fleisher et al. 2002; Levy 2012).

Although CEA monitoring is the most cost-effective and sensitive method with which to diagnose recurrent disease in colorectal cancer patients, it is not clear what benefits arise from the routine assay of CEA in patients who undergo curative surgery (Sepulveda 2013; Alberts and Grothey 2012; Fleisher et al. 2002; Levy 2012). There are no prospective randomized trials that indicate benefits of serial CEA measuring in colorectal cancer patients, but the European Group on Tumor Markers suggests that the analysis of CEA levels could be useful to increase the interval between two radiological examinations, thus reducing their number and consequently the patient's exposure to radiation (Fleisher et al. 2002; Barak 2006). From a meta-analysis of two randomized and three comparative cohort studies, comprising 2005 patients, it emerged that the 5-year survival and overall survival were, respectively, 1.16 and 3.6 times higher in patients who underwent intensive monitoring of CEA (three times per year for at least 2 years) than in control patients, and patients intensively monitored underwent more than twice the number of curative re-resections versus control patients (Duffy 2001). Obviously, the value of CEA monitoring for the preclinical detection of hepatic metastases is valid only for patients who are willing and able to undergo liver resection for recurrent disease. In the monitoring of cancer recurrence, ASCO indicated that CEA levels should be tested in stage II and III patients every 2–3 months for 2 years after surgery (Alberts and Grothey 2012; Sepulveda 2013).

Although surgery is the preferred therapy for colorectal cancer, chemotherapy with 5-fluorouracil or levamisole is widely used in patients with advanced cancers. In these patients, CEA could be useful to evaluate therapy efficacy since it reflects disease status and can help clinicians to discontinue ineffective drugs in a timely fashion (Hayat 2009; Fleisher et al. 2002). It is important to note that transient elevation of CEA could be due also to chemotherapy (Brunner et al. 2009). Although there is no consensus about the use of CEA in the management of advanced colorectal cancer patients, the National Academy of Clinical Biochemistry, ASCO, and the European Group on Tumor Markers recommend its use in monitoring the efficacy of therapy (Sepulveda 2013; Fleisher et al. 2002). They recommend that CEA be measured before therapy and then at regular intervals of 2–3 months for at least 2 years thereafter. Two measures above baseline are indicative of progressive disease without any confirmatory analysis, but it has to be kept in mind that:

1. CEA elevation usually occurs in advanced-stage patients.
2. Not all patients with recurrent cancer exhibit CEA elevation.
3. CEA elevation may occur in conditions unrelated to cancer relapses.
4. Therapy could cause CEA elevation.

So, in conclusion, the National Academy of Clinical Biochemistry and the European Group on Tumor Markers do not recommend CEA testing in colorectal cancer screening, but CEA can be measured before surgery together with other parameters to complete staging and to determine the therapeutic plan (Fleisher et al. 2002; Hayat 2009; McClatchey 2002). Moreover, CEA levels should not be analyzed in the immediate postoperative period, but they can be evaluated in the follow-up of patients who would undergo hepatic resection in case of metastases. In addition, CEA can be measured to assess therapy efficacy and to detect progressive disease (Fleisher et al. 2002; Hayat 2009; McClatchey 2002; Sepulveda 2013).

CEACAM Proteins as Potential Biomarkers in Colorectal Cancer: CEACAM1, CEACAM6, and CEACAM7

Beside the widely recognized role of CEA in the management of colorectal cancer patients, other CEACAMs are being investigated as colorectal cancer biomarkers. CEACAM1 was found to be downregulated at transcriptional level in colon adenoma and carcinoma and overexpressed at protein level in colorectal cancer in which it correlates with clinical stage (Kuespert et al. 2006; Fridman and Galon 2011; Sepulveda 2013). It is not clear why CEACAM1 is reexpressed in colorectal cancer; however, multivariate analysis revealed that persistence of CEACAM1 is an independent risk factor for lymph node, hematogenous metastases and short survival (Kuespert et al. 2006; Fridman and Galon 2011; Sepulveda 2013).

Also CEACAM7 has been associated with recurrence risk in rectal cancer. A single institution colorectal cancer database and a frozen tissue biobank were queried for rectal cancer patients, and CEACAM7 messenger RNA was measured by real-time PCR in normal mucosa and cancer specimens (Messick et al. 2010). A comparison of CEACAM7 levels in normal tissue, tissue from disease-free survivors, and tissue from patients with cancer relapse showed that it was lower in rectal cancer with respect to normal mucosa, and it was also decreased in patients who relapsed with respect to disease-free survivors (Messick et al. 2010). Moreover, CEACAM7 expression was prognostic for rectal cancer recurrence and was statistically significant in stage II patients. In fact, it could be used to select stage II patients who would benefit from adjuvant chemotherapy (Messick et al. 2010; Issues in Surgical Research, Techniques, and Innovation 2011).

CEACAM6 overexpression is one of the first observable signs of transformation in colorectal tissue. It is one of the most highly expressed antigens in colorectal cancer, with an intensity of expression that parallels the severity of the lesion (Gemei et al. 2013; Blumenthal et al. 2007). In a multivariate analysis, CEACAM6 expression was found to be an independent prognostic factor for reduced overall survival (Jantsheff et al. 2003). Despite the paucity of data about the function of CEACAMs in colorectal cancer, it is clear that they are involved in colorectal pathology (Table 3).

Table 3 Roles of CEACAMs in colorectal pathology. CEACAMs play several roles in colorectal pathology, and emerging studies revealed their utility as therapeutic targets and prognostic factors and in the development of new cancer imaging and surveillance tools

CEACAM	Condition	Role – potential use	Reference
CEACAMs	Colorectal cancer	Cancer imaging	Hayat (2009); Heine et al. (2011)
CEACAM5 (CEA)	Colorectal cancer	Cancer surveillance, therapy efficacy monitoring, therapeutic target, cancer imaging	Duffy (2001); Sepulveda (2013); Fleisher et al. (2002); Hammarström and Stigbrand (2002); Hayat (2009); Barak (2006)
CEACAM1	Rectal cancer	Prognostic factor	Fiori et al. (2012)
	Colitis	Regulation of Th1 response	Iijima (2004)
	Colorectal cancer	Promotion of invasion and migration	Ieda (2011)
CEACAM6	Crohn disease	Receptor for invasive *Escherichia coli*	Barnich and Darfeuille-Michaud (2010)
	Colorectal cancer	Therapeutic target	Gemei et al. (2013)
	Colorectal cancer	Prognostic factor	Jantsheff et al. (2003); Zhao et al. (2011)

Potential Applications to Prognosis of Other Diseases and Conditions

Almost all CEACAM proteins are dysregulated in cancer, so they can be useful to assess the efficacy of new diagnostic/prognostic protocols, and they may also have potential as therapeutic targets in different types of cancer. In particular, CEA is overexpressed in several epithelial cancers and is currently used to monitor disease status after therapy in patients overexpressing it (Sepulveda 2013; Tiernan et al. 2013).

The CEACAM1 protein is reduced in colon cancer and also in endometrium, breast, and prostate cancers in which it seems to act as a tumor suppressor (Kuespert et al. 2006; Fiori et al. 2012). However, the function of CEACAM1 in various cancers remains to be established. In fact, it is a marker of metastasization and cancer progression in non-small cell lung cancer and lung adenocarcinomas as well as in malignant melanoma. In lung adenocarcinomas, CEACAM1 was reexpressed in 81 % of patients, and its expression was significantly correlated with primary tumors, lymph nodes, and hematogenous metastases (Fiori et al. 2012). Moreover, overall survival was reduced in CEACAM1-positive patients (Fiori et al. 2012; Sepulveda 2013). In a 10-year follow-up study, 100 primary cutaneous melanomas, 11 distant metastases, and 6 sentinel lymph nodes were immunohistochemically evaluated for CEACAM1 expression (Utikal et al. 2012). The results revealed a strong correlation between CEACAM1 expression in primary tumors and subsequent development of metastases. In fact, 70 % of CEACAM1-positive patients developed distant metastases versus only 10 % of CEACAM1-negative patients. The expression of CEACAM1 was highest at the invasive front of melanomas, and in multivariate analysis, its expression was found to be an independent factor of risk for metastases with a predictive value superior to that of tumor thickness (Kuespert et al. 2006; Fiori et al. 2012). These findings were confirmed by a study in which CEA and CEACAM1 expression was evaluated in such preneoplastic lesions as spreading melanoma and dysplastic and benign nevi. In these samples, similarly, also CEA expression was higher in dysplastic nevi and in spreading melanomas with respect to benign nevi.

In prostate cancer, CEACAM1 is involved in the transition between noninvasive, nonvascularized, and invasive and vascularized tumors (Fiori et al. 2012). In breast cancer, the CEACAM1 protein is expressed in an apical membrane pattern in benign and premalignant lesions, while it moves to a bilateral membrane and cytoplasmic localization at early stages of malignant transformation (Fiori et al. 2012). Cytoplasmic expression of CEACAM1 in gastric and intestinal carcinomas indicates a worse prognosis (Fiori et al. 2012). Besides its function in angiogenesis, CEACAM1 promotes endocytosis of the insulin-receptor complex and so plays a role in the regulation of insulin action (Kuespert et al. 2006). In fact, in transgenic CEACAM1-lacking mice, impaired insulin clearance by hepatocytes in the liver induced hyperinsulinemia (Kuespert et al. 2006).

CEACAM6 is overexpressed in several cancers: breast, lung, pancreatic, prostate, endometrial, and colon cancers. Its expression frequently parallels cancer stage

(Blumenthal et al. 2005a; Cameron et al. 2012; Duxbury et al. 2004f; Scholzel et al. 2000; Gemei et al. 2013). In pancreatic cancer, it enhances cell invasiveness and resistance to anoikis and apoptosis (Blumenthal et al. 2005b; Duxbury et al. 2004g). In pancreatic cancer, CEACAM6 has been successfully used as a therapeutic target in preclinical studies (Duxbury et al. 2004h; Strickland et al. 2009). In breast cancer, CEACAM6 overexpression promotes migration and invasion of drug-resistant estrogen-deprived breast cells (Lewis-Wambi et al. 2008).

In conclusion, the expression of CEACAMs is dysregulated in almost 50 % of human cancers. Their dysregulation is a marker of malignant transformation, and their expression is often a prognostic factor for a worse outcome (Kuespert et al. 2006; Sepulveda 2013; Tiernan et al. 2013).

Summary Points

1. CEACAM proteins play important roles in colorectal cancer, and their functions and possible role as biomarkers are currently being investigated.
2. CEACAM5 and CEACAM6 function as tumor suppressors, and their dysregulated expression enhances cell proliferation and inhibits apoptosis and differentiation while disrupting colon architecture.
3. CEACAM7 is a putative predictive marker for rectal cancer recurrence.
4. CEACAM1 has an antitumor function, and it is downregulated in a quarter of human colorectal cancers.
5. Preliminary studies indicate that CEACAM6 has prognostic importance in colorectal cancer; moreover, it is a promising therapeutic target in several human cancers.
6. The use of CEA measurement in colorectal cancer screening is controversial, but its role as a prognostic factor and in therapy efficacy evaluation is well established.
7. CEACAMs play different roles in several human cancers and are promising therapeutic targets as well as diagnostic, predictive, and prognostic biomarkers.

Acknowledgments The original experiments by the authors cited in this paper were supported by grants L.502/94 2006 from the Ministero della Salute and L.5/95 (to L. D. V.), grant POR Campania FSE 2007/2013 (CREME) from the Regione Campania (to F. S.), and grant RF-2010-2318372 from the Ministry of Health (to F. S.).

References

Alberts SR, Grothey A. Gastrointestinal tract cancers. In: Casciato MC, editor. Manual of clinical oncology. Philadelphia: Lippincott Williams & Wilkins; 2012. p. 246–70.

American Cancer Society. Colorectal cancer early detection. American Cancer Society; 2013. http://www.cancer.org/acs/groups/cid/documents/webcontent/003170-pdf.pdf. Accessed 28 Oct 2013.

Bacolod MD, Barany F. Molecular profiling of colon tumors: the search for clinically relevant biomarkers of progression, prognosis, therapeutics, and predisposition. Ann Surg Oncol. 2011;18:3694–700.

Barak V. Tumor biology: tumor markers, tumor targeting and translational cancer research. Basel Karger Publishers; 2006.

Barnich N, Darfeuille-Michaud A. Abnormal CEACAM6 expression in Crohn disease patients favors gut colonization and inflammation by adherent-invasive *E. coli*. Virulence. 2010;1:281–2.

Belov L, Zhou J, Christopherson RI. Cell surface markers in colorectal cancer prognosis. Int J Mol Sci. 2010;12:78–113.

Blumenthal RD, Hansen HJ, Goldenberg DM. Inhibition of adhesion, invasion, and metastasis by antibodies targeting CEACAM6 (NCA-90) and CEACAM5 (Carcinoembryonic Antigen). Cancer Res. 2005a;65:8809–17.

Blumenthal RD, Osorio L, Hayes MK, et al. Carcinoembryonic antigen antibody inhibits lung metastasis and augments chemotherapy in a human colonic carcinoma xenograft. Cancer Immunol Immunother. 2005b;54:315–27.

Blumenthal RD, Leon E, Hansen HJ, et al. Expression patterns of CEACAM5 and CEACAM6 in primary and metastatic cancers. BMC Cancer. 2007;7:2.

Brünner N, Duffy MJ, Haglund C, Holten-Andersen M, Nielsen HJ. Tumor markers in colorectal malignancy. American Association for Clinical Chemistry; 2009. http://www.aacc.org/members/nacb/LMPG/OnlineGuide/PublishedGuidelines/major/Documents/TumorMarkersMajor10.pdf#page=27.

Cameron S, de Long LM, Hazar-Rethinam M, et al. Focal overexpression of CEACAM6 contributes to enhanced tumourigenesis in head and neck cancer via suppression of apoptosis. Mol Cancer. 2012;11:74.

Chan CH, Camacho-Leal P, Stanners CP. Colorectal hyperplasia and dysplasia due to human carcinoembryonic antigen (CEA) family member expression in transgenic mice. PLoS One. 2007;2:e1353.

Chen Y, Zheng S, Yu J, Hu X. Artificial neural networks analysis of surface-enhanced laser desorption/Ionization mass spectra of serum protein pattern distinguishes colorectal cancer from healthy population. Clin Cancer Res. 2004;10:1162–203.

Compton CC, Fielding LP, Burgart LJ, et al. Prognostic factors in colorectal cancer. College of American Pathologists Consensus Statement 1999. Arch Pathol Lab Med. 2000;124:979–94.

Duffy MJ. Carcinoembryonic antigen as a marker for colorectal cancer: is it clinically useful? Clin Chem. 2001;47:624–30.

Duxbury MS, Ito H, Ashley SW, et al. CEACAM6 as a novel target for indirect type 1 immunotoxin-based therapy in pancreatic adenocarcinoma. Biochem Biophys Res Commun. 2004a;317:837–43.

Duxbury MS, Ito H, Ashley SW, et al. CEACAM6 cross-linking induces caveolin-1-dependent, Src-mediated focal adhesion kinase phosphorylation in BxPC3 pancreatic adenocarcinoma cells. J Biol Chem. 2004b;279:23176–82.

Duxbury MS, Ito H, Ashley SW, et al. c-Src-dependent cross-talk between CEACAM6 and alphavbeta3 integrin enhances pancreatic adenocarcinoma cell adhesion to extracellular matrix components. Biochem Biophys Res Commun. 2004c;317:133–41.

Duxbury MS, Ito H, Benoit E, et al. A novel role for carcinoembryonic antigen-related cell adhesion molecule 6 as a determinant of gemcitabine chemoresistance in pancreatic adenocarcinoma cells. Cancer Res. 2004d;64:3987–93.

Duxbury MS, Ito H, Benoit E, et al. CEACAM6 is a determinant of pancreatic adenocarcinoma cellular invasiveness. Br J Cancer. 2004e;91:1384–90.

Duxbury MS, Ito H, Benoit E, et al. Overexpression of CEACAM6 promotes insulin-like growth factor I-induced pancreatic adenocarcinoma cellular invasiveness. Oncogene. 2004f;23:5834–42.

Duxbury MS, Ito H, Zinner MJ, et al. CEACAM6 gene silencing impairs anoikis resistance and in vivo metastatic ability of pancreatic adenocarcinoma cells. Oncogene. 2004g;23:465–73.

Duxbury MS, Matros E, Ito H, et al. Systemic siRNA-mediated gene silencing: a new approach to targeted therapy of cancer. Ann Surg. 2004h;240:667–74. discussion 675–6.

Fiori V, Magnani M, Cianfriglia M. The expression and modulation of CEACAM1 and tumor cell transformation. Ann Ist Super Sanita. 2012;48:161–71.

Fleisher M, Dnistrian AM, Sturgeon CM, Lamerz R, Wittliff JL. Practice guidelines and recommendations for the use of tumor markers in the clinic. In: Diamandis EP, Fritsche HA, Lilja H, Chan DW, Schwartz MK, editors. Tumor markers: physiology, pathobiology, technology, and clinical applications. Washington, DC: AACC Press; 2002. p. 47–75.

Fridman WH, Galon J. Infiltration in human cancer: prognostic significance and disease control. In: Dranoff G, editor. Cancer immunology and immunotherapy, Current topics in microbiology and immunology. Berlin: Springer; 2011. p. 20.

Gemei M, Mirabelli P, Di Noto R, et al. CD66c is a novel marker for colorectal cancer stem cell isolation, and its silencing halts tumor growth in vivo. Cancer. 2013;119:729–38.

Hammarström S, Stigbrand T. Gastric cancer. In: Diamandis EP, Fritsche HA, Lilja H, Chan DW, Schwartz MK, editors. Tumor markers: physiology, pathobiology, technology, and clinical applications. Washington, DC: AACC Press; 2002. p. 375–7.

Hayat MA. Methods of cancer diagnosis, therapy, and prognosis, volume 4: colorectal cancer. Dordrecht: Springer; 2009.

Heine M, Nollau P, Masslo C, et al. Investigations on the usefulness of CEACAMs as potential imaging targets for molecular imaging purposes. PLoS One. 2011;6:e28030.

Ieda J, Yokoyama S, Tamura K, Takifuji K, Hotta T, Matsuda K, Oku Y, Nasu T, Kiriyama S, Yamamoto N, Nakamura Y, Shively JE, Yamaue H. Re-expression of CEACAM1 long cytoplasmic domain isoform is associated with invasion and migration of colorectal cancer. Int J Cancer. 2011;129(6):1351–61. doi:10.1002/ijc.26072. Epub 2011 May 25.

Iijima H, Neurath MF, Nagaishi T, Glickman JN, Nieuwenhuis EE, Nakajima A, Chen D, Fuss IJ, Utku N, Lewicki DN, Becker C, Gallagher TM, Holmes KV, Blumberg RS. Specific regulation of T helper cell 1-mediated murine colitis by CEACAM1. J Exp Med. 2004;199(4):471–82.

Ilantzis C, DeMarte L, Screaton RA, et al. Deregulated expression of the human tumor marker CEA and CEA family member CEACAM6 disrupts tissue architecture and blocks colonocyte differentiation. Neoplasia. 2002;4:151–63.

Issues in surgical research, techniques, and innovation: 2011 edition. Scholarly Editions; 2011.

Jantscheff P, Terracciano L, Lowy A, et al. Expression of CEACAM6 in resectable colorectal cancer: a factor of independent prognostic significance. J Clin Oncol. 2003;21:3638–46.

Kuespert K, Pils S, Hauck CR. CEACAMs: their role in physiology and pathophysiology. Curr Opin Cell Biol. 2006;18:565–71.

Lee YTN. Carcinoembryonic antigen in patients with breast or colon cancer. West J Med. 1978;129:374–80.

Levy M. Follow up and recurrence of colorectal cancer, colorectal cancer – from prevention to patient care. In: Ettarh R, editor. Colon cancer from prevention to patient care. Rijeka: InTech; 2012. p. 363–78.

Lewis-Wambi JS, Cunliffe HE, Kim HR, et al. Overexpression of CEACAM6 promotes migration and invasion of oestrogen-deprived breast cancer cells. Eur J Cancer. 2008;44:1770–9.

McClatchey KD. Clinical laboratory medicine. Philadelphia: Lippincott Williams & Wilkins; 2002. p. 490–4.

Messick CA, Sanchez J, Dejulius KL, et al. CEACAM-7: a predictive marker for rectal cancer recurrence. Surgery. 2010;147:713–19.

Newton KF, Newman W, Hill J. Review of biomarkers in colorectal cancer. Colorectal Dis. 2012;14:3–17.

Ordonez C, Zhai AB, Camacho-Leal P, et al. GPI-anchored CEA family glycoproteins CEA and CEACAM6 mediate their biological effects through enhanced integrin alpha5beta1-fibronectin interaction. J Cell Physiol. 2007;210:757–65.

Schölzel S, Zimmermann W, Schwarzkopf G, et al. Carcinoembryonic antigen family members CEACAM6 and CEACAM7 are differentially expressed in normal tissues and oppositely deregulated in hyperplastic colorectal polyps and early adenomas. Am J Pathol. 2000;156:595–605.

Schwartz MK. Tumor markers for colorectal cancer. In: Diamandis EP, Fritsche HA, Lilja H, Chan DW, Schwartz MK, editors. Tumor markers: physiology, pathobiology, technology, and clinical applications. Washington, DC: AACC Press; 2002. p. 254–6.

Screaton RA, Penn LZ, Stanners CP. Carcinoembryonic antigen, a human tumor marker, cooperates with Myc and Bcl-2 in cellular transformation. J Cell Biol. 1997;137:939–52.

Sepulveda JL. Serological markers of digestive tract cancers. In: Sepulveda AR, Lynch JP, editors. Molecular pathology of neoplastic gastrointestinal diseases. New York: Springer; 2013.

Strickland LA, Ross J, Williams S, et al. Preclinical evaluation of carcinoembryonic cell adhesion molecule (CEACAM) 6 as potential therapy target for pancreatic adenocarcinoma. J Pathol. 2009;218:380–90.

Sturgeon CM, Duffy MJ, Stenman UH, et al. National academy of clinical biochemistry laboratory medicine practice guidelines for use of tumor markers in testicular, prostate, colorectal, breast, and ovarian cancers. Clin Chem. 2008;54:e11–79.

Thirunavukarasu P, Sukumar S, Sathaiah M, et al. C-stage in colon cancer: implications of carcinoembryonic antigen biomarker in staging, prognosis, and management. J Natl Cancer Inst. 2011;103:689–97.

Tiernan JP, Perry SL, Verghese ET, et al. Carcinoembryonic antigen is the preferred biomarker for in vivo colorectal cancer targeting. Br J Cancer. 2013;108:662–7.

Utikal J, Becker JC, Ugurel S. Diagnostic and prognostic biomarkers in melanoma: current state of play. In: Murphy MJ, editor. Diagnostic and prognostic biomarkers and therapeutic targets in Melanoma. New York: Humana Press; 2012. p. 9–17.

Weber GF. Colorectal cancer. In: Weber GF, editor. Molecular mechanisms of cancer. Dordrecht: Springer; 2007. p. 453–61.

Zhao ZS, Li L, Wang HJ, et al. Expression and prognostic significance of CEACAM6, ITGB1, and CYR61 in peripheral blood of patients with gastric cancer. J Surg Oncol. 2011;104:525–9.

Part VII

Head and Neck

Human Papillomavirus (HPV) Biomarkers in Head and Neck: Squamous Cell Carcinoma (HNSCC)

31

Arunkumar Anandharaj, Oleksandr Ekshyyan, Tara Moore-Medlin, Vikas Mehta, and Cherie-Ann O. Nathan

Contents

Abstract

Head and cell neck squamous carcinomas are a heterogeneous group of neoplasms evolved through multistep carcinogenesis, which is commonly attributed to the abuse of tobacco and alcohol. The epidemiological and molecular evidences from recent decades show the human papillomavirus (HPV) to be causative in a subset of HNSCC. Anatomically, HPV exhibits a predilection

A. Anandharaj • O. Ekshyyan • T. Moore-Medlin • V. Mehta • C.-A.O. Nathan (✉)
Department of Otolaryngology, Head and Neck Surgery, LSU Health Shreveport, Shreveport, LA, USA
e-mail: aanan1@lsuhsc.edu; oekshy@lsuhsc.edu; tmoor5@lsuhsc.edu; vmeht2@lsuhsc.edu; cnatha@lsuhsc.edu

V.R. Preedy, V.B. Patel (eds.), *Biomarkers in Cancer, Biomarkers in Disease: Methods, Discoveries and Applications*,
DOI 10.1007/978-94-007-7681-4_31

for the oral cavity and oropharyngeal and laryngeal regions of the head and neck. HPV-positive and HPV-negative tumors differ in many facets that include histology, differentiation, risk factors, and prognosis. At present, no guidelines are available to choose an appropriate biomarker for the clinical assessment of HPV in HNSCC malignancies. Currently, p16 immunohistochemistry is used as a potential surrogate marker, but its use as a predictive marker is still questionable. Taking the present scenario into consideration, we present in this chapter a list of biomolecules that have higher possibility for use as biomarkers. A randomized clinical trial is required for validation of each biomolecule before designating it as a biomarker that can be subsumed for routine analysis.

List of Abbreviations

APC	Adenomatous Polyposis Coli
ATP	Adenosine Triphosphate
BER	Base Excision Repair
CDC	Centers for Disease Control and Prevention
CH1	Cysteine/Histidine-Rich 1
CI	Confidence Interval
DNA	Deoxyribonucleic Acid
EGFR	Epidermal Growth Factor Receptor
FDA	Food and Drug Administration
HLA	Human Leukocyte Antigen
HNSCC	Head and Neck Squamous Cell Carcinoma
HPV	Human Papillomavirus
hTERT	Human Telomerase Reverse Transcriptase
ISH	In Situ Hybridization
KRT14	Human Keratin 14
LCR	Long Control Region
MCM7	Minimicrosome Protein 7
MDM2	Mouse Double Minute 2 Homolog
MHC	Major Histocompatibility Complex
mMU	Milli-Merk Units
MPG	Multiplex Human Papillomavirus Genotyping
OPSCC	Oropharyngeal Squamous Cell Carcinoma
OR	Odds Ratio
OSCC	Oral Squamous Cell Carcinoma
PDCD4	Programmed Cell Death Protein 4
PSCC	Pharyngeal Squamous Cell Carcinoma
Rb	Retinoblastoma
RNA	Ribonucleic Acid
RTOG	Radiation Therapy Oncology Group
RT-qPCR	Reverse Transcription Quantitative Polymerase Chain Reaction
SSB	Single-Strand Break
TGF	Transforming Growth Factor

TGFBR3	TGF Beta-Receptor 3
TIL	Tumor-Infiltrating Lymphocytes
VLP	Viruslike Particles
XRCC1	X-ray Repair Cross-Complementing Protein 1

Key Facts

- Human papillomavirus (HPV) is the principal causative agent for the development of a subgroup of head and neck cancers.
- The combined activity of E6 and E7 proteins is responsible for the oncogenic property of the HPV virus.
- Both the viral proteins are retained and continuously expressed throughout the development of the disease.
- At present p16 is used as a biomarker for identification of HPV infection, but it is not adequately reliable.
- In this book chapter, we have discussed other possible factors that could be used as biomarkers for HPV-induced HNSCC.

Definition for Words

Biomarker Any quantifiable or measurable biological substance that can be used to identify or predict the state of a disease.

Cis Elements It is a short sequence of DNA present upstream to the promoter in the LCR region of HPV viruses responsible for the regulation of viral gene expression.

Clinical Outcome It is defined as any change in the health condition of a subject as a result of undergoing treatment.

Clinicopathology Assessing the status of disease with the help of laboratory results.

DNA Repair It is defined as the property of the cell to fix the damages in its genetic materials caused by replicative errors, drugs, or radiation.

Good Prognosis An expected clinical improvement especially an increase in the chance of recovery from the disease.

HPV Prevalence Presence of HPV-positive cases at a specified time in a specific population.

Malignant Phenotype The capability of a tumor to invade nearby tissues.

Neoplasm An uncontrolled progressive cell growth especially attributed to tumor.

Transgenic Mouse A mouse whose genome is altered with a foreign gene, often used in laboratory settings as models for studying human disease.

Tumor Suppressor Any gene or protein that prevents the cell transformation from normal to malignant phenotype.

Introduction

Head and neck cancer includes cancers that originate in the oral cavity, oropharynx, hypopharynx, nasopharynx, and larynx. About 40,000 new cases of head and neck cancer are diagnosed every year in North America, and there are 650,000 new cases worldwide. It is ranked as the sixth most common malignancy worldwide (Jemal et al. 2003). Traditionally, alcohol and tobacco abuse are the major risk factors for head and neck squamous cell carcinoma (HNSCC). The possible association of HPV in HNSCC was first reported by Syrjanen et al. in 1983, when they detected HPV proteins in oral squamous cell carcinoma (OSCC) by immunohistochemistry (IHC) (Syrjanen et al. 1983). Since then, efforts have been made to understand the role of HPV in head and neck cancer. It is now recognized as one of the major causes of oropharyngeal cancer, which includes the soft palate, the tonsil, and the base of the tongue. To date, over 100 different types of HPV are identified and classified either by their specificity for host tissue (cutaneous or mucosal) or by their association with cancer (high risk, intermediate, and low risk) (zur Hausen 1996; de Villiers et al. 2004; Munoz et al. 2003; Table 1). HNSCCs are predominantly associated with mucosal high-risk HPV types, HPV16 and HPV18, in addition to other high-risk types of HPV which are less common. HPV16 is the most prevalent genotype accounting for 87 % of the oropharyngeal, 68 % of oral, and 69 % of laryngeal carcinomas associated with HPV (Dayyani et al. 2010). Most of the patients with HPV tend to be younger in age with no history of tobacco or alcohol abuse. Evidence-based studies have reported that HPV-associated HNSCC is a sexually transmitted disease. A strong association has been observed between the sexual behavior and the risk of oropharyngeal cancer (Gillison 2008). HPV prevalence in OSCC is higher in Asia (33 %), while Europe and North America have similar levels (16 %). Comparable levels of HPV prevalence were seen for OPSCC in North America (47 %) and Asia (46.3 %). Again Asia is found to possess higher HPV prevalence in the larynx followed by Europe (21.3 %) and North America (13.8 %) (Kreimer et al. 2005). In contrast, a multi-continent study conducted by IARC on oropharyngeal cancer, oral, and HPV showed no significant difference in HPV prevalence between Asia, Africa, Europe, and North and South America (Kreimer et al. 2005; Table 2).

Table 1 Overall HPV types, causes and classification. This table shows the types of human papillomavirus classified into different categories based on their biological property. HPV types associated with the head and cancer are indicated with a superscript alphabet

Classification	HPV types	Association with HNSCC
Undetermined	7, 30[a], 32[b], 34, 55, 57[bc], 67, 69, 71, 74, 77	[a]Laryngeal carcinoma
		[b]Oral cavity cancer
Low risk	1, 2, 3, 4, 5, 6, 8, 9, 10, 11, 12, 13[d], 14, 15, 17, 19, 20, 21, 22, 23, 24, 25, 27, 28, 29, 36, 37, 38, 40, 41[e], 42, 43, 44[b], 46, 47, 48[e], 49, 50, 54, 60, 61, 62, 63, 64, 65, 70, 72[f], 75, 76, 82	[c]Oral and inverted maxillary sinus papilloma
		[d]Oral and epithelial hyperplasia
		[e]Cutaneous squamous cell carcinoma
Probably high	26, 53[b], 81[b]	[f]Oral papilloma in HIV patients
High risk	16[abg], 18[abg], 31[ab], 33[abg], 35[bg], 39, 45[ag], 51[a], 52[a], 56[b], 58[b], 59, 66, 68, 73[f]	[g]Oropharyngeal carcinoma

Table 2 HPV prevalence in HNSCC by geographic location and site of origin (Kreimer et al. 2005). This table shows that HPV prevalence is heterogeneous over different geographic locations. The difference in the heterogeneity is lesser in oropharynx and may be an indication of HPV preference to oropharynx over other anatomical sites

	Overall HPV prevalence (%)	HPV16 prevalence (%)
Oral cavity		
Europe	16.0	10.8
North America	16.1	10.1
Asia	33.0	22.3
Others	18.1	14.9
Oropharynx		
Europe	28.2	23.8
North America	47.0	42.1
Asia	46.3	35.2
Others	36.6	33.7
Larynx		
Europe	21.3	13.8
North America	13.8	10.1
Asia	38.2	26.5
Others	48.5	45.5

In the past 20 years, limited improvements have been achieved in treatment outcomes despite multidisciplinary approaches and advances in chemotherapy, radiotherapy, and surgical techniques. Often, treatment failures occur due to locoregional recurrence, metastasis, and second primaries. In this regard, the search for proteins, DNA, or RNA that can be used to predict or detect tumors at an early stage becomes important. Subsequently, these candidates should be validated through randomized clinical trials to confirm their role as a stable clinical endpoint (Atkinson et al. 2001). Such candidates, which can be used for tumor detection, for disease prognosis, or as a monitor response to therapeutic intervention, are called biomarkers. Biomarkers can be identified and derived from several types of biological tissues, including biopsies from primary tumors and margins or bodily fluids such as blood, saliva, and urine.

HPV Biology

Human papillomaviruses are double-stranded DNA viruses that are capable of inducing hyperproliferation of the epithelium and promote either premalignant or malignant lesion of infected epithelium. The genomic organization of HPV viruses is well conserved and coded for eight different proteins that are transcribed from a single DNA strand (Fig. 1). The viral early (E) genes transcribe proteins required for its DNA replication, the late (L) region encodes for structural proteins L1 and L2, and a noncoding part is denoted as long control region (LCR) that has cis elements necessary for the replication and transcription of viral DNA. Molecular studies now provide a clear overall picture of HPV biology (Abeloff et al. 2009; Harrison et al. 2009).

The E1 and E2 proteins serve as factors that are responsible for identifying the origin of viral replication. The E1 is an ATP-dependent helicase that enables the DNA to unwind during viral replication. The E2 functions as an associate to E1 and also as a transcriptional repressor for HPV E6 and E7 proteins. Variable expression of E6 and E7 is frequently observed as a consequence of disrupted E2 expression during viral integration to the host genome, which is a major reason for tumorigenesis.

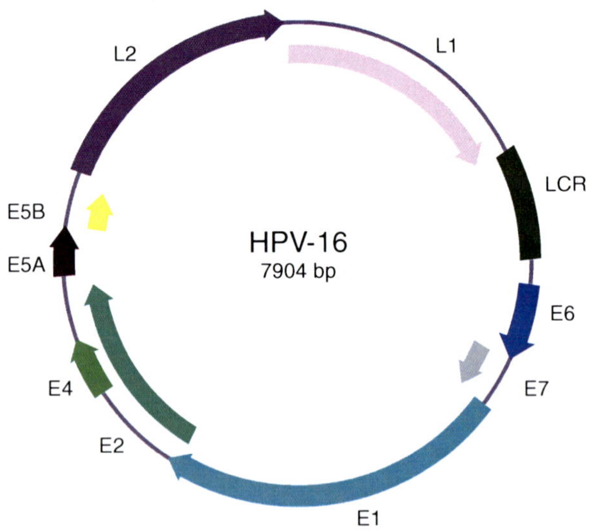

Fig. 1 HPV genome map. Human papillomavirus (*HPV*) is a double-stranded DNA virus of approximately 8,000 bp in length. Various translational open-reading frames are denoted by *arrow* marks embedded in the *circle*. These include early (*E*) and late (*L*) genes. The early genes are expressed throughout the viral life cycle, and the late genes encode viral capsid proteins

E4 is involved in the later stages of the viral life cycle by modulating the viral genome expression and viral replication. It also facilitates the viral proteins' interaction with the host cell's cytokeratin network by establishing G2 arrest of the cell cycle. The E5 being an integral membrane protein is involved both in the early and late stages of the viral life cycle. It mediates cellular transformation through the EGFR pathway by phosphorylation thereby preventing the receptor from degradation. Additionally, E5 represses MHC class I molecules on the infected cell favoring HPV to modulate and bypass the host immune response (Harrison et al. 2009).

Particularly, noteworthy progress was made in defining the role of oncoproteins E6 and E7 in the cell cycle and etiopathology of HPV. These proteins act as negative regulators of host cell cycle machinery, specifically retinoblastoma protein (p105Rb) and tumor suppressor protein p53, which is essential to facilitate a stable maintenance of viral episomes. The E6 protein forms a complex with a ubiquitin ligase E6-AP and targets p53 favoring a proteosomal-mediated degradation. Simultaneously, E6 activates the catalytic subunit of human telomerase reverse transcriptase (hTERT) required for the immortalization of the host cell. The E7 protein blocks the pRb protein rendering the latter unavailable for the E2F transcription factor, which normally effectuates an S-phase arrest of the cell cycle. This leads to the constitutive activation of cell cycles producing high copies of the viral episomes. Thus both E6 and E7 are required for viral transformation and cellular proliferation (Klingelhutz et al. 1996; Munger et al. 2001).

In general, head and neck cancers maintain a high viral load when HPV DNA is present in the episomal state. The first and foremost biomarker for HPV detection is the presence of viral DNA in tumor samples. PCR-based methods with specific primers or in situ hybridization techniques employing specific probes targeting the HPV E6/E7/L1 DNA can be used to detect HPV DNA. PCR-based testing of HPV has been used for more than 20 years because of its advantage in providing genotype-specific information. In the clinical setting, detection of HPV DNA is commonly conducted using PCR amplification with consensus sequence primers MY09/MY11 and GP5+/GP6+ (Fig. 2). These primers amplify DNA fragments in the L1 region encoding the hypervariable V loop of the major capsid protein generating a fragment size approximately 450 and 150 bp (McLemore et al. 2010). Several types of PCR-based detection for HPV have evolved over the past decade. A recent PCR-based study showed HPV16 prevalence varied significantly by anatomic site with a higher prevalence observed in the oropharynx (35 %) as compared to the hypopharynx (29 %), larynx (5 %), and oral cavity (3 %; $P < 0.0001$) (Salazar et al. 2014; Table 3). A similar study employing a PCR-based approach found that 57 % of tonsillar tumors were positive for HPV16 which represented a significant increase from 1993–1999 to 2006–2011, indicating an increase in total HPV-positive cancers from 25 % to 62 % ($P < 0.002$) (Nichols et al. 2013). RT-qPCR analyses conducted on 150 oral squamous cell carcinoma tissues revealed the presence of HPV in 81.3 % of the samples (Gao et al. 2013). Multiplex human papillomavirus genotyping (MPG) is a PCR assay that detects HPV DNA by utilizing a broad-spectrum general primer. Overall, 35 % of head and

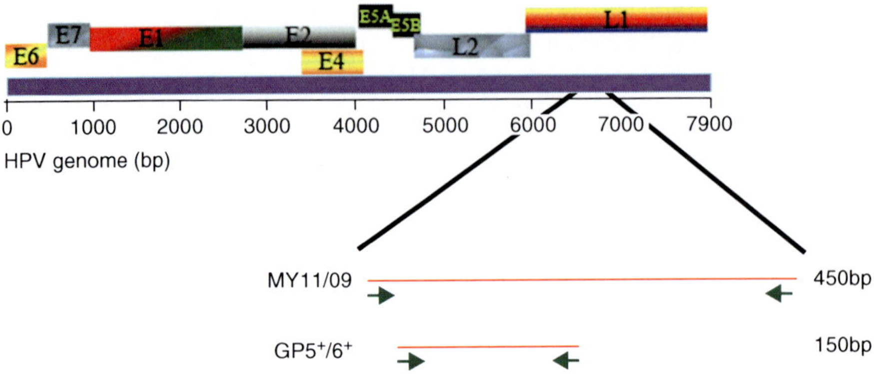

Fig. 2 PCR-based amplification of HPV genome. The regions amplified by traditional PCR with MY09/MY11 and GP5+/6+ primer pairs are indicated in *red lines*. The *arrow heads* represent the annealing position of the respective primers used in nested PCR

Table 3 The type-specific prevalence of HPV in HNSCCs (Kreimer et al. 2005). Types of human papillomavirus predominantly found in head and neck cancer. Variations that are found in the prevalence of HPV infection are shown based on the anatomic subsite

HPV type	Prevalence in HNSCC (%)		
	Oral cavity	Oropharynx	Larynx
6	3.1	2.5	5.1
11	1.6	0.7	0.5
16	16	30.9	16.6
18	8	1	3.9
31	0.2	0	0.3
32	0.2	0	0
33	0.8	1.1	0.9
35	0.1	0.4	0
39	0	0	0
44	0.1	0	0
45	0	0.2	0.2
51	0	0	0.3
52	0	0	0.2
53	0.2	0	0
56	0.1	0	0
57	0.3	0	0
58	0.1	0	0
59	0	0.2	0
68	0.1	0	0
73	0	0	0
81	0.2	0	0
82	0	0	0

neck tumors are reported to be HPV positive as detected by PCR methods (Chaturvedi et al. 2007).

Several studies have been carried out with the objective of identifying oral HPV by noninvasive methods. PCR was employed to identify HPV16 E6 and E7 and HPV18 E7 DNA in salivary rinses from patients with HNSCC. Saliva from 17 of 92 patients (18.5 %) showed positivity for HPV16, while only 8 of 740 healthy volunteer samples were positive for HPV16 ($P < 0.0001$) (Zhao et al. 2005). A similar study conducted by D'Souza et al. (2005) found the prevalence of oral HPV in the study population ranged from 44 % to 52 % with many of the subjects having a concurrent HPV infection by more than one type. PCR amplification with consensus sequence primers MY09/MY11 and GP5+/GP6+ is 90.2 % sensitive in identifying HPV DNA, but sensitivity is highly variable depending on the quality of DNA and the tissue samples used for the study. Another limitation is that these primers may miss HPV sequences that are integrated into the host genome and have lost the capsid-encoding sequences.

In spite of all the limitations in sensitivity, HPV L1 PCR is the preferred method to detect the presence of HPV because it can be performed in any molecular diagnostic laboratory and is economically advantageous compared to in situ hybridization (ISH) (Fig. 3; Agoston et al. 2010). However, ISH is a widely utilized technique for HPV identification due to its biological and practical considerations. It can be performed using specific probes to identify either DNA (DNA-ISH) or RNA (RNA-ISH). Often large variations in HPV prevalence between ISH- and PCR-based methods are reported, which are solely due to the inability of PCR methods to accurately discern the biologically active from trivial forms of virus. In a RTOG 0129 study, a large-scale analysis of patients with oropharyngeal cancers, ISH showed that 64 % of tumors were positive for HPV (Ang et al. 2010). Another study corroborated this finding with very high prevalence of HPV (69 %) in oropharyngeal cancers as detected by ISH (Singhi and Westra 2010). One aspect of ISH that is superior to other techniques is that it offers the precise location of HPV sequences in tumor cells since a punctuate pattern of hybridization signals within the nuclei of tumor cells shows integration of HPV DNA into the host genome (Westra 2009). Although PCR and ISH are extensively used on clinical specimens, the histologic findings suggest that there are limitations to ISH. Based on reports published thus far, PCR methods (39.9 %) consistently report higher prevalence rates than ISH methods (32.9 %).

In terms of HPV status as a prognostic biomarker, a meta-analysis of 42 studies to examine the difference in the survival outcomes between HPV-positive and HPV-negative HNSCC demonstrated that HPV-positive cases had a 54 % better overall survival compared to HPV-negative patients (hazard ratio [HR] = 0.46; 95 % CI 0.37–0.57). The pooled analysis from multivariate estimates demonstrated a 72 % reduction in disease-specific mortality (HR = 0.28; 95 % CI 0.19–0.40), and pooled HR of multivariate estimates for progression-free survival was 0.40 (95 % CI 0.29–0.56) (O'Rorke et al. 2012).

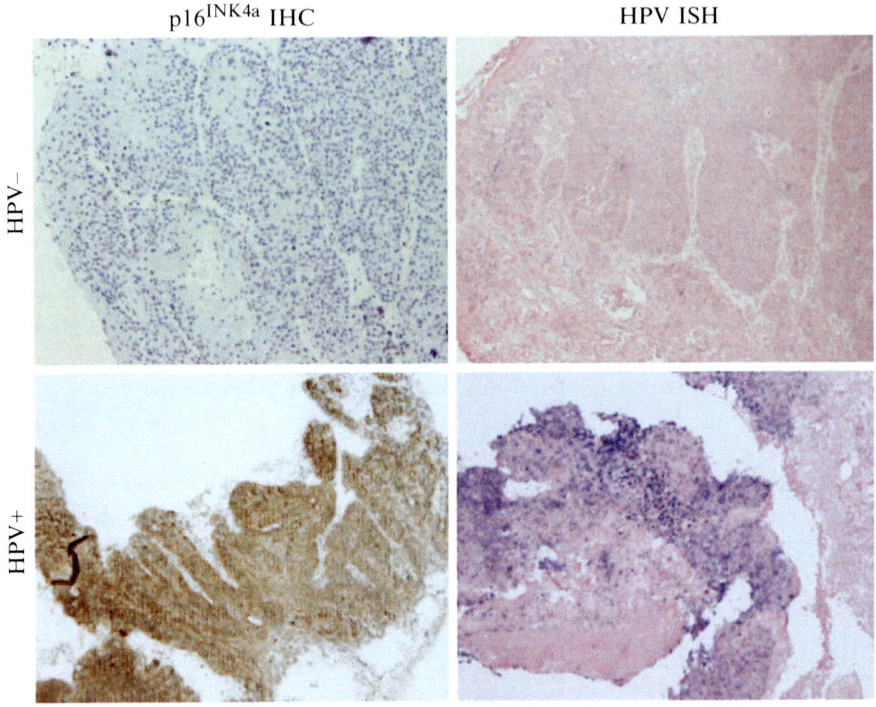

Fig. 3 p16INK4a immunohistochemistry (*IHC*) and HPV in situ hybridization (high-risk probe) in oropharyngeal tissues. p16INK4a IHC results in *pale* to *dark blue* staining of nuclei in negative cells and *brown* staining in positive cells (basal and parabasal epithelium). HPV ISH positivity displays as *dark blue* staining of epithelial cell nuclei which can then be further classified as episomal or integrated (100× magnification)

p16

In HPV-positive head and neck cancers, functional inactivation of Rb protein by the viral protein E7 is believed to contribute to p16 overexpression that can be readily detected by IHC. For this reason p16 IHC is often used as a surrogate marker for detecting HPV-associated lesions of the head and neck. p16 is a highly sensitive marker for HPV infection demonstrating a sensitivity rate close to 100 %. Therefore, p16 immunostaining is a sound first-line assay for eliminating HPV-negative cases from additional analysis (Westra 2009). It has been widely observed in head and neck cancer that HPV- and p16-positive patients respond better to chemoradiotherapy. Therefore, the mechanisms between the HPV and p16 association have been demonstrated through the utilization of in vitro studies. When both p16 and HPV are present, an augmented therapeutic response to radiotherapy is consistently observed in vitro. A recent study concluded that radiosensitization of HPV-positive HNSCC is not a result of enhanced apoptosis or permanent G1 cell cycle arrest. Conversely, the cancer cells exhibited an extensive G2 arrest with a prominent residual DNA double-strand breaks. The compromised DNA double-strand break repair capacity is responsible for enhanced radiosentivity in HPV- and p16-positive head and neck tumors (Rieckmann et al. 2013). A five-year follow-up study comparing accelerated radiotherapy to conventional radiotherapy showed the former is better in regard to outcome. Though regression was found in both HPV-positive and HPV-negative tumors, accelerated radiotherapy was advantageous for HPV-positive tumors that are also positive for p16. The locoregional control and disease-specific overall survival were well correlated with the levels of p16 (Bussu et al. 2013).

However, a follow-up study conducted on 54 patients with a median survival rate of 20.3 months concluded that p16 overexpression did not show a difference in survival data when considered alone ($P = 0.4295$). On the contrary, though statistically not significant, the combination of HPV positivity and p16 overexpression resulted in better overall survival time ($P = 0.2985$) (Hoffmann et al. 2012). Although p16 has been documented as a predictive marker of survival in head and neck cancer patients who receive radiotherapy, it is still unknown whether p16 levels can predict treatment outcome in patients receiving radiotherapy without surgery. Moreover loss of p16 expression may arise due to epigenetic changes, Rb degradation-mediated silencing, promoter hypermethylation, or homozygous deletion. Additionally, p16 upregulation may also occur due to the alternative mechanism of cell cycle disruption. It is important to consider data that show p16 is not a predictive marker in HNSCC (Fountzilas et al. 2009). However, current data suggest that p16 testing has not been standardized at a national level, resulting in up to 30 % discordance between local and national testing. These discrepancies in the reliability of p16 as a biomarker can best be resolved with central confirmation through randomized clinical trials (Thomas et al. 2005). Such contradictions are important in fully understanding the role of p16 in HNSCC.

p53

p53 aberrations are predominant in HNSCC. HPV-positive tumors are more likely to express wild-type p53, which is significantly associated with better prognosis (Perez-Ordonez et al. 2006). FISH analyses of oropharyngeal cancer specimens showed wild-type p53 in 9/10 cases that are HPV positive. In all nine cases, nuclear accumulation of p53 was found in over 30 % of cells (Hafkamp et al. 2003). Several studies were carried out so far with an objective either to liberate or stabilize p53 from inhibition by E6. The process of liberation is generally accomplished by two methods: (i) siRNA suppression of E6/E7 RNA and (ii) proteasomal inhibitors such as bortezomib and MG132. These approaches successfully liberated p53, and cell death was induced by negative regulation of E6 and cell cycle arrest in HPV-positive cancer (Li and Johnson 2013). Alternative molecular mechanisms that underlie this stabilization and/or overexpression have been explored and identified that high-risk HPV E6 inactivates p53 through two distinct mechanisms: (i) a 100KD E6-associated protein (E6AP) cooperates with E6 to transfer ubiquitin to p53 resulting in proteosomal degradation and (ii) E6 binds to the CH1 domain of P300 to block P300-mediated p53 acetylation that is required for the stabilization and transcriptional activity of p53. Disrupting the association of E6-P300 is an attractive target in the p53 stabilization approach. CH1iB is a small molecule that is designed to inhibit the CH1 domain necessary for E6 docking to P300, which in turn reactivates p53 and potentiates the antitumor activity (Xie et al. 2014).

MDM2

Human *MDM2* is a gene responsible for the rapid degradation of p53 protein, leading to cell proliferation and perpetuated cell cycle (Vogelstein et al. 2000). *MDM2* plays an important role in the regulation of p53, and overexpression of this gene is seen in most cancers (Freedman and Levine 1999). A case-control study including 325 patients and 325 matched controls was conducted to test the association between HPV16 L1 and two promoter variants of MDM2, viz., *MDM2*-rs2279744 GT or GG and TT. The results indicated that GT/GG genotype and HPV16 L1 seropositivity are associated with an increased oral cancer risk (OR 2.81 [95 % CI 1.67–4.74]), and the TT genotype patients with HPV16 L1 seropositivity had an OR of 5.57 (95 % CI 2.93–10.6). Similar results were observed for another type of promoter variant *MDM2*-rs937283 (AA and AG/GG) polymorphism. *MDM2* genotypes had a significant or near-significant effect on the association between HPV16 serology and the risk of OSCC ($P_{int} = 0.060$ for *MDM2*-rs2279744, $P_{int} = 0.009$ for *MDM2*-rs937283, and $P_{int} = 0.005$ for the combined *MDM2* genotypes). Additionally, the study revealed that *MDM2* polymorphism is found commonly in patients designated as never smokers and never drinkers – a property commonly found in HPV-associated head and neck cancer (Chen et al. 2010).

p21

In patients with HNSCC, the presence of oral HPV is an indicator for favorable recovery from the disease. Clinically, these tumors are poorly differentiated and easily metastasize to local lymph nodes (Hafkamp et al. 2003). The highest prevalence of oncogenic HPV is observed in tonsillar carcinomas. Seventy-seven tonsillar carcinoma specimens were selected to assess the expression of key cell cycle regulators, such as p21, for which HPV status was already known. The study determined that p21 is significantly overexpressed in most samples, and expression had a strong correlation with HPV positivity ($P = 0.008$). Additionally, this study also revealed that no or low expression of p21 is one of the strongest indicators of cancer-specific death (Hafkamp et al. 2009). A study analyzing 75 hypopharynx specimens found a 5-year disease-free survival rate of 60 % for p21-positive patients. When considering positivity for both p21 and high-risk HPV types, the survival rate increased to 79.5 %. No statistically significant difference in p21 expression was found between HPV-positive and HPV-negative specimens (Ernoux-Neufcoeur et al. 2011). Despite the fact that p21 is a downstream effector of p53, its overexpression in HPV tumors is not understood, even though it favors a good prognosis.

MCM7

The first transgenic animal model of HPV-induced head and neck cancer was developed by Strati et al. (2006). In this model the expression of the HPV16 oncogenes E6 and E7 is driven by a 2-kb fragment of human keratin 14 (KRT14) promoter or enhancer targeting stratified epithelium. Under the control of KRT14 promoter, E6 and E7 are capable of inducing a variety of intense phenotypes such as cellular hyperproliferation and epidermal hyperplasia in the murine epidermis. Using this model, minichromosome maintenance protein 7 (MCM7) was identified as a biomarker capable of characterizing HPV-positive and HPV-negative HNSCC. The expression of MCM7 is more abundant in HPV transgenic mice than in non-transgenic control, which exhibits similarities to HPV16 E7 by inactivating pRb family proteins and increasing E2F transcriptional activity (Strati et al. 2006). In a similar study, E7 inhibition of pocket proteins was mimicked in transgenic knockout mouse models $Rb^{f/f}p107^{-/-}$ and $Rb^{f/f}p130^{-/-}$. MCM7 staining was robust in basal cells with additional staining in parabasal cells, while only epithelial staining was noticed in the non-transgenic model (Shin et al. 2006). Few studies show E6 is involved in the regulation of MCM7 to a lesser extent by cooperating with E6AP. MCM7, as part of replication licensing factor, is recruited to cellular DNA replication origins (*ori*). It is responsible to check *ori* and fires only once in each round of cell cycle. The association of E6 and E6AP allows ubiquitin to bind MCM7 rendering it to proteosomal degradation causing pronounced cell cycle arrest (Blow 1993; Kuhne and Banks 1998; Thommes et al. 1997).

XRCC1

Highly efficient DNA repair capacity leads to tolerance in DNA damage, resulting in resistance to radiotherapy. X-ray repair cross-complementing protein 1 (XRCC1) is involved in base excision repair (BER) and single-strand break (SSB) repair by forming a complex with DNA ligase III. XRCC1 is a component of the scaffold protein complex that executes the BER/SSB repair mechanism (Weaver et al. 2005). Single nucleotide polymorphisms (SNPs) present in XRCC1 are associated with cancer susceptibility to radiation therapy. XRCC1 staining was carried out to further discriminate within the HPV category. Higher expression of XRCC1 by IHC in HPV-positive cases was associated with poor survival (5-year OS of 35 %), and lower expression was associated with better survival (5-year OS of 100 %; $P = 0.001$). This makes XRCC1 IHC staining a potentially useful, prognostic biomarker in HPV-associated HNSCC (Ang et al. 2011).

MHC Class I

Alterations in major histocompatibility complex (MHC) class I molecules are consistently observed in tumors; simultaneous downregulation of these genes (HLA-A, HLA-B, HLA-C) is a frequent feature in many tumor types (Campoli and Ferrone 2008), and overexpression of E and G is associated with tumor progression (Yie et al. 2007). A cohort of 175 HNSCC patients was selected for a study that included 138 HPV-positive and 37 HPV-negative cases. Among HPV-positive tonsillar squamous cell carcinoma (TSCC) with good clinical outcome, a majority (79 % and 68 %) of the tumors had a weak or absent intensity of HLA-A, HLA-B, and HLA-C staining for HCA-2 and HC-10, respectively, compared with 38 % of the tumors among HPV-positive TSCC cases with a poor clinical outcome (OR 6.0; 95 % CI, 2.2 to 16.3; $P = 0.001$ and OR 3.7; 95 % CI, 1.4 to 9.8; $P = 0.01$). Therefore, a significant negative correlation between HLA expression and positive prognosis for HPV-positive TSCC was determined. In contrast, there was a positive correlation between high expression of MHC class I and positive prognosis for patients with HPV-negative TSCC (HCA-2: OR 0.05; 95 % CI, 0.001 to 0.46; $P = 0.002$. HC-10: OR 0.07; 95 % CI 0.001 to 0.7; $P = 0.008$). E6 and E7 antigens are easy targets to elicit an immune response against HPV-induced tumors. Tumor-infiltrating lymphocytes (TIL) which are $CD8^+$ have been linked to better prognosis in other HPV-induced cancers (Nedergaard et al. 2007). TILs are predominantly accompanied by infiltrating T-regulatory cells (Tregs), and $Foxp3^+$ Tregs are associated with tumor progression (Talmadge et al. 2007). TIL was evaluated as a potential biomarker in a study that included 31 HPV-negative patients and 109 HPV-positive tonsil cancer patients. The results showed that those patients who had a significantly higher number of $CD8^+$ TILs in the tumor had a better clinical outcome than those who had a fewer number of $CD8^+$ TILs ($P < 0.001$). With respect to HPV, positive tonsil cancer cases had a higher number of $Foxp3^+$ Tregs than the negative cases ($P < 0.001$). However, no differences were observed between patients with good versus poor clinical outcome. Hence, the presence of CD8+ cells was associated with better clinical outcome in TSCC patients and thus may serve as a potential biomarker in tonsillar cancer (Nasman et al. 2012).

miRNA

miRNAs are a naturally occurring small, noncoding RNA strands 19–25 nucleotides long that mature from a 70- to 100-nucleotide-long hairpin pre-miRNA. It is involved in the regulation of gene expression and terminal differentiation and plays a critical role in carcinogenesis. miRNAs are tissue specific, and their differential expression helps to clearly distinguish between normal and cancer cells (Bartel 2004). RT-qPCR confirmed differential regulation of miRNA expression and gene expression analysis performed in tumor and adjacent normal tissues of same-paired samples with exhibited loss of putative mRNA targets such as adenomatous polyposis coli (APC), programmed cell death protein 4 (PDCD4), and TGF beta-receptor 3 (TGFBR3) in the tumor samples (Ramdas et al. 2009). To date, only limited information about miRNAs in HPV-positive head and neck cancer is available. A miRNA expression profile was created by comparing nine HPV-positive and 10 HPV-negative tonsil carcinoma samples, which showed that 36 miRNA were differentially expressed between the two groups of samples ($P < 0.01$). The miR-15a, miR-16, miR-143, miR-145, and miR-106-363 cluster appear to be controlled by HPV. Specifically, miR-106-363 is the most consistently and significantly upregulated molecule among the HPV-positive tonsillar carcinoma (Lajer et al. 2012). A similar miRNA profiling study conducted using oropharyngeal cancer samples of 88 patients analyzed a correlation between expression of candidate miRNAs and clinical outcome such as overall survival (OS), disease-free survival (DFS), and distant relapse-free survival (DM). When miR-107 and miR-151 were upregulated and miR-492 was downregulated, this scenario was significantly associated with worse OS ($P < 0.0001$). For DFS, when miR-107, miR-151, miR-182, and miR-361 were upregulated and miR-20b downregulated, the patients had a statistically significant higher risk of recurrence ($P < 0.0001$). Finally, in regard to DM, upregulation of miR-151, miR-361, and miR-324-5p and downregulation of miR-492 and miR-152 were associated with distant metastases ($P < 0.0088$). miR-107 is implicated in mammalian development and cellular metabolism, while miR-151 is associated with tumor invasion and metastasis. miR-182 is implicated in zinc homeostasis, while miR-152 is a well-characterized tumor suppressor miRNA. Collectively, the results indicated that miR-151 is significantly associated in all three clinical outcome measures (OS, DM, and DFS) of oropharyngeal cancer independent of p16 status (Hui et al. 2013). A similar study carried out in biopsies obtained from 51 patients, either with OSCC or PSCC (pharyngeal squamous cell carcinoma), uncovered that 114 miRNAs were differentially expressed between OSCC and normal oral epithelium, whereas 38 miRNAs were differentially expressed in PSCC compared with normal pharyngeal epithelium. HPV infection is more significantly associated with alterations in miR-127-3p and miR-363 levels in oral and pharyngeal SCCs (Lajer et al. 2011). The identification of miRNAs associated with different HPV-mediated cancers is important, as they may be useful as general and HPV-specific tumor markers.

CL1A Antibodies

HPV entry into cells automatically triggers an immune response that is invariably not connected to the initiation of cancer. Antibodies produced against viral proteins are present in the serum several years before the cancer is clinically detectable. Detection of antibodies for HPV proteins such as L1, E6, and E7 can serve as biomarkers in predicting the risk of HNSCC. Results from a hospital-based study for tonsillar carcinoma identified 8.9 % seroprevalence for HPV16 E6 and E7 while only 0.1 % for healthy control subjects. The data showed more than a 300-fold increased risk for the development of tonsillar carcinoma (Ribeiro et al. 2011). Similarly, a case-controlled study with 486 HNSCC cases and 550 control subjects revealed HPV16 L1 seropositivity for 29 % of patients and 11 % for controls. HPV16 seropositivity was associated with a highly significant 4.1-fold (95 % CI 2.9–5.8) increased risk for HNSCC. Increased risk of HPV-associated head and neck cancer correlated with the titer levels. With a medium titer value ($\leq 39 < 253$ mMu), there was a 3.8-fold (95 % CI; 2.3–5.8) overall risk for HNSCC, and with a high titer value ($\geq$253mMu), the overall risk level was 19.2-fold (95 % CI; 8.1–45.6) (Furniss et al. 2007). A single-nested case-control study exhibited that HPV16 seropositivity individuals had a twofold increase in risk for HNSCC (OR 2.1, 95 % CI; 1.4–3.2), a 14-fold increase for oropharyngeal cancer (OR 14.4, 95 % CI; 3.6–58.1), threefold increase in risk for tongue cancer (OR 2.8, 95 % CI; 1.2–6.6), and twofold increase for laryngeal cancer (OR 2.1, 95 % CI; 1.0–5.6) (Gillison et al. 2012). A factor to consider is that the serological assay is not site specific, and an infection outside the head and neck would account for increased estimate of HPV prevalence. Additionally, antibodies evoked by distant and past infection may die out over time, which would account for reduced HPV prevalence.

Vaccines

HPV-associated HNSCC can be prevented by vaccines which were shown to induce HPV-specific immune responses. HPV vaccines are classified as either prophylactic or therapeutic. Prophylactic vaccines became feasible when the L1 major viral capsid protein of HPV16 was demonstrated to self-assemble into viruslike particles (VLP) in yeast. These VLPs are capable of inducing high titer serum antibodies, protecting against papillomavirus infection, and preventing the formation of viral-induced mucosal papilloma. The success of prophylactic vaccine depends on the timing of administration. It is critical that prophylactic vaccines be administered before possible exposure to HPV infection. Therapeutic vaccines are capable of generating a cellular immune response to viral oncoproteins E6 and E7. While other viral early and late proteins are expressed only during productive viral infection, E6 and E7 are extraneous proteins which possess more epitopes that can readily elicit an immune response (IARC 2007).

At present two prophylactic HPV vaccines approved by the FDA and CDC are commercially available: one is the bivalent vaccine Cervarix® from GlaxoSmithKline that offers protection against HPV16 and HPV18 and the other is a quadrivalent vaccine Gardasil® from Merck that offers protection against HPV6, HPV11, HPV16, and HPV18. These vaccines were developed to prevent infection against specific types, though follow-up data show that these vaccines also confer some protection against other high-risk HPV types phylogenetically related to types 16 and 18. The extended protection is presumed to have conferred by the generation of cross-neutralizing antibodies. At present several efforts are underway to generate a second-generation vaccine that aims to extend cross protection and reduce cost simultaneously preserving the efficacy (Harrison et al. 2009; Syrjanen 2010). These vaccines showed very high efficacy (97–98 %) in the prevention of high-risk HPV16/18 cancers in naïve individuals (Psyrri et al. 2012). Therapeutic vaccines targeting HPV16 E7 and p16INK4a peptide are being evaluated in several clinical trials (Psyrri et al. 2012).

Conclusion

Over the course of the last two decades, a clear association has already been established for the role of high-risk HPV in the oncogenesis of oropharyngeal SCC. Laboratory and clinical observations firmly indicate that HPV-associated OSCC is a distinct entity from tobacco-related oral cancer with significantly different molecular characteristics and tumor behavior. While the incidence of tobacco-induced HNSCC has been decreasing in the USA, the incidence of HPV-associated head and neck cancer has been gradually increasing over the last three decades. Collectively tumor HPV status is a strong and independent prognostic factor for survival among patients with oropharyngeal cancer (Ang et al. 2010). Since HPV-associated head and neck cancer has favorable prognosis, distinct etiology treatment de-escalation and novel HPV-targeted approaches to therapy must be thoroughly evaluated to minimize severe side effects of the conventional treatment options. Our success in identifying reliable HPV-related biomarkers, especially for screening purposes, has been limited to date with potential candidates still to be explored in HPV-associated HNSCC.

Summary Points

- Increased incidence of HPV-positive HNSCC is prominently seen in young adults especially in developed countries including the USA, Sweden, the UK, and the Netherlands.
- Epidemiological studies over the past two decades show that HPV positivity in head and neck cancer is on the rise, which represent distinct clinicopathological features.
- Better survival and prognosis have been noticed consistently and observed in HPV-positive over HPV-negative cases of HNSCC irrespective of the treatment regimen.
- p16 immunohistochemistry could serve as a potential biomarker, but its usefulness is still unproven. Additional predictive markers are needed besides a p16 status.
- Therefore, this chapter focuses on candidate biomarkers for HPV-positive head and neck squamous cell carcinoma that have previously shown through experimental data to be potentially useful in daily clinical practice.

References

Abeloff MD, Armitage J, Niederhuber JE, Kastan MB, et al. Abeloff's clinical oncology. 4th ed. Philadelphia: Elsevier; 2009.

Agoston ES, Robinson SJ, Mehra KK, et al. Polymerase chain reaction detection of HPV in squamous carcinoma of the oropharynx. Am J Clin Pathol. 2010;134:36–41.

Ang KK, Harris J, Wheeler R, et al. Human papillomavirus and survival of patients with oropharyngeal cancer. N Engl J Med. 2010;363:24–35.

Ang MK, Patel MR, Yin XY, et al. High XRCC1 protein expression is associated with poorer survival in patients with head and neck squamous cell carcinoma. Clin Cancer Res. 2011;17:6542–52.

Atkinson AJ, Colburn WA, DeGruttola VG, et al. Biomarkers and surrogate endpoints: preferred definitions and conceptual framework. Clin Pharmacol Ther. 2001;69:89–95.

Bartel DP. MicroRNAs: genomics, biogenesis, mechanism, and function. Cell. 2004;116:281–97.

Blow JJ. Preventing re-replication of DNA in a single cell cycle: evidence for a replication licensing factor. J Cell Biol. 1993;122:993–1002.

Bussu F, Sali M, Gallus R, et al. HPV infection in squamous cell carcinomas arising from different mucosal sites of the head and neck region. Is p16 immunohistochemistry a reliable surrogate marker? Br J Cancer. 2013;108:1157–62.

Campoli M, Ferrone S. HLA antigen changes in malignant cells: epigenetic mechanisms and biologic significance. Oncogene. 2008;27:5869–85.

Chaturvedi AK, Engels EA, Anderson WF, et al. Incidence trends for human papillomavirus-related (HPV-R) and unrelated (HPV-U) head and neck squamous cell carcinomas (HNSCC) in the United States (US). J Clin Oncol. 2007;25:6001.

Chen X, Sturgis EM, Lei D, et al. Human papillomavirus seropositivity synergizes with MDM2 variants to increase the risk of oral squamous cell carcinoma. Cancer Res. 2010;70:7199–208.

D'Souza G, Sugar E, Ruby W, et al. Analysis of the effect of DNA purification on detection of human papillomavirus in oral rinse samples by PCR. J Clin Microbiol. 2005;43:5526–35.

Dayyani F, Etzel CJ, Liu M, et al. Meta-analysis of the impact of human papillomavirus (HPV) on cancer risk and overall survival in head and neck squamous cell carcinomas (HNSCC). Head Neck Oncol. 2010;2:15.

de Villiers EM, Fauquet C, Broker TR, et al. Classification of papillomaviruses. Virology. 2004;324:17–27.

Ernoux-Neufcoeur P, Arafa M, Decaestecker C, et al. Combined analysis of HPV DNA, p16, p21 and p53 to predict prognosis in patients with stage IV hypopharyngeal carcinoma. J Cancer Res Clin Oncol. 2011;137:173–81.

Fountzilas G, Kalogera-Fountzila A, Lambaki S, et al. MMP9 but not EGFR, MET, ERCC1, P16, and P-53 is associated with response to concomitant radiotherapy, cetuximab, and weekly cisplatin in patients with locally advanced head and neck cancer. J Oncol. 2009;2009:305908.

Freedman DA, Levine AJ. Regulation of the p53 protein by the MDM2 oncoprotein – thirty-eighth G.H.A. Clowes Memorial Award Lecture. Cancer Res. 1999;59:1–7.

Furniss CS, McClean MD, Smith JF, et al. Human papillomavirus 16 and head and neck squamous cell carcinoma. Int J Cancer. 2007;120:2386–92.

Gao G, Chernock RD, Gay HA, et al. A novel RT-PCR method for quantification of human papillomavirus transcripts in archived tissues and its application in oropharyngeal cancer prognosis. Int J Cancer. 2013;132:882–90.

Gillison ML. Human papillomavirus-related diseases: oropharynx cancers and potential implications for adolescent HPV vaccination. J Adolesc Health. 2008;43:S52–60.

Gillison ML, Alemany L, Snijders PJ, et al. Human papillomavirus and diseases of the upper airway: head and neck cancer and respiratory papillomatosis. Vaccine. 2012;30:F34–54.

Hafkamp HC, Speel EJ, Haesevoets A, et al. A subset of head and neck squamous cell carcinomas exhibits integration of HPV 16/18 DNA and overexpression of p16INK4A and p53 in the absence of mutations in p53 exons 5–8. Int J Cancer. 2003;107:394–400.

Hafkamp HC, Mooren JJ, Claessen SM, et al. P21 Cip1/WAF1 expression is strongly associated with HPV-positive tonsillar carcinoma and a favorable prognosis. Mod Pathol. 2009;22:686–98.

Harrison LBS, Roy B, Waun Ki Hong, editors. Head and neck cancer: a multidisciplinary approach. 3rd ed. Philadelphia: Lippincott Williams & Wilkins; 2009.

Hoffmann M, Tribius S, Quabius ES, et al. HPV DNA, E6*I-mRNA expression and p16INK4A immunohistochemistry in head and neck cancer – how valid is p16INK4A as surrogate marker? Cancer Lett. 2012;323:88–96.

Hui AB, Lin A, Xu W, et al. Potentially prognostic miRNAs in HPV-associated oropharyngeal carcinoma. Clin Cancer Res. 2013;19:2154–62.

IARC. IARC monographs on the evaluation of carcinogenic risks to humans human papillomaviruses. Lyon: IARC; 2007.

Jemal A, Murray T, Samuels A, et al. Cancer statistics, 2003. CA Cancer J Clin. 2003;53:5–26.

Klingelhutz AJ, Foster SA, McDougall JK. Telomerase activation by the E6 gene product of human papillomavirus type 16. Nature. 1996;380:79–82.

Kreimer AR, Clifford GM, Boyle P, et al. Human papillomavirus types in head and neck squamous cell carcinomas worldwide: a systematic review. Cancer Epidemiol Biomarkers Prev. 2005;14:467–75.

Kuhne C, Banks L. E3-ubiquitin ligase/E6-AP links multicopy maintenance protein 7 to the ubiquitination pathway by a novel motif, the L2G box. J Biol Chem. 1998;273:34302–9.

Lajer CB, Nielsen FC, Friis-Hansen L, et al. Different miRNA signatures of oral and pharyngeal squamous cell carcinomas: a prospective translational study. Br J Cancer. 2011;104:830–40.

Lajer CB, Garnaes E, Friis-Hansen L, et al. The role of miRNAs in human papilloma virus (HPV)-associated cancers: bridging between HPV-related head and neck cancer and cervical cancer. Br J Cancer. 2012;106:1526–34.

Li C, Johnson DE. Liberation of functional p53 by proteasome inhibition in human papilloma virus-positive head and neck squamous cell carcinoma cells promotes apoptosis and cell cycle arrest. Cell Cycle. 2013;12:923–34.

McLemore MS, Haigentz Jr M, Smith RV, et al. Head and neck squamous cell carcinomas in HIV-positive patients: a preliminary investigation of viral associations. Head Neck Pathol. 2010;4:97–105.

Munger K, Basile JR, Duensing S, et al. Biological activities and molecular targets of the human papillomavirus E7 oncoprotein. Oncogene. 2001;20:7888–98.

Munoz N, Bosch FX, de Sanjose S, et al. Epidemiologic classification of human papillomavirus types associated with cervical cancer. N Engl J Med. 2003;348:518–27.

Nasman A, Romanitan M, Nordfors C, et al. Tumor infiltrating CD8+ and Foxp3+ lymphocytes correlate to clinical outcome and human papillomavirus (HPV) status in tonsillar cancer. PLoS One. 2012;7:e38711.

Nedergaard BS, Ladekarl M, Thomsen HF, et al. Low density of CD3+, CD4+ and CD8+ cells is associated with increased risk of relapse in squamous cell cervical cancer. Br J Cancer. 2007;97:1135–8.

Nichols AC, Palma DA, Dhaliwal SS, et al. The epidemic of human papillomavirus and oropharyngeal cancer in a Canadian population. Curr Oncol. 2013;20:212–19.

O'Rorke MA, Ellison MV, Murray LJ, et al. Human papillomavirus related head and neck cancer survival: a systematic review and meta-analysis. Oral Oncol. 2012;48:1191–201.

Perez-Ordonez B, Beauchemin M, Jordan RC. Molecular biology of squamous cell carcinoma of the head and neck. J Clin Pathol. 2006;59:445–53.

Psyrri A, Sasaki C, Vassilakopoulou M, et al. Future directions in research, treatment and prevention of HPV-related squamous cell carcinoma of the head and neck. Head Neck Pathol. 2012;6:S121–8.

Ramdas L, Giri U, Ashorn CL, et al. miRNA expression profiles in head and neck squamous cell carcinoma and adjacent normal tissue. Head Neck. 2009;31:642–54.

Ribeiro KB, Levi JE, Pawlita M, et al. Low human papillomavirus prevalence in head and neck cancer: results from two large case–control studies in high-incidence regions. Int J Epidemiol. 2011;40:489–502.

Rieckmann T, Tribius S, Grob TJ, et al. HNSCC cell lines positive for HPV and p16 possess higher cellular radiosensitivity due to an impaired DSB repair capacity. Radiother Oncol. 2013;107:242–6.

Salazar CR, Smith RV, Garg MK, et al. Human papillomavirus-associated head and neck squamous cell carcinoma survival: a comparison by tumor site and initial treatment. Head Neck Pathol. 2014;8:77–87.

Shin MK, Pitot HC, Lambert PF. Pocket proteins suppress head and neck cancer. Cancer Res. 2006;72:1280–9.

Singhi AD, Westra WH. Comparison of human papillomavirus in situ hybridization and p16 immunohistochemistry in the detection of human papillomavirus-associated head and neck cancer based on a prospective clinical experience. Cancer. 2010;116:2166–73.

Strati K, Pitot HC, Lambert PF. Identification of biomarkers that distinguish human papillomavirus (HPV)-positive versus HPV-negative head and neck cancers in a mouse model. Proc Natl Acad Sci U S A. 2006;103:14152–7.

Syrjanen S. The role of human papillomavirus infection in head and neck cancers. Ann Oncol. 2010;21:vii243–5.

Syrjanen KJ, Pyrhonen S, Syrjanen SM, et al. Immunohistochemical demonstration of human papilloma virus (HPV) antigens in oral squamous cell lesions. Br J Oral Surg. 1983;21:147–53.

Talmadge JE, Donkor M, Scholar E. Inflammatory cell infiltration of tumors: Jekyll or Hyde. Cancer Metastasis Rev. 2007;26:373–400.

Thomas GR, Nadiminti H, Regalado J. Molecular predictors of clinical outcome in patients with head and neck squamous cell carcinoma. Int J Exp Pathol. 2005;86:347–63.

Thommes P, Kubota Y, Takisawa H, et al. The RLF-M component of the replication licensing system forms complexes containing all six MCM/P1 polypeptides. EMBO J. 1997;16:3312–19.

Vogelstein B, Lane D, Levine AJ. Surfing the p53 network. Nature. 2000;408:307–10.

Weaver DA, Crawford EL, Warner KA, et al. ABCC5, ERCC2, XPA and XRCC1 transcript abundance levels correlate with cisplatin chemoresistance in non-small cell lung cancer cell lines. Mol Cancer. 2005;4:18.

Westra WH. The changing face of head and neck cancer in the 21st century: the impact of HPV on the epidemiology and pathology of oral cancer. Head Neck Pathol. 2009;3:78–81.

Xie X, Piao L, Cavey GS, et al. Phosphorylation of Nanog is essential to regulate Bmi1 and promote tumorigenesis. Oncogene. 2014;33:2040–52.

Yie SM, Yang H, Ye SR, et al. Expression of HLA-G is associated with prognosis in esophageal squamous cell carcinoma. Am J Clin Pathol. 2007;128:1002–9.

Zhao M, Rosenbaum E, Carvalho AL, et al. Feasibility of quantitative PCR-based saliva rinse screening of HPV for head and neck cancer. Int J Cancer. 2005;117:605–10.

zur Hausen H. Papillomavirus infections – a major cause of human cancers. Biochim Biophys Acta. 1996;1288:F55–78.

Biomarkers in NeoMark European Project for Oral Cancers

32

Tito Poli, Chiara Copelli, Davide Lanfranco, Dario Salvi, Konstantinos Exarchos, Marco Picone, Diego Ardigò, Sebastian Steger, Manuel José Rolo da Fonseca, Marco De Fazio, Elena Martinelli, and Enrico Sesenna

Contents

T. Poli (✉) • C. Copelli • D. Lanfranco • E. Martinelli • E. Sesenna
Maxillofacial Surgery, University-Hospital of Parma, Parma, Italy
e-mail: tito.poli@unipr.it; chiaracopelli@hotmail.it; lanfranco82@yahoo.it; martinel.ele@virgilio.it; enrico.sesenna@unipr.it

D. Salvi
Life Supporting Technologies, ETSI Telecomunicación, Universidad Politécnica de Madrid, Madrid, Spain
e-mail: dsalvi@lst.tfo.upm.es; dario.salvi.work@gmail.com

K. Exarchos
University of Ioannina, Ioannina, Greece
e-mail: kexarcho@gmail.com

M. Picone
Department of Information Engineering, University of Parma, MultiMed s.r.l., Cremona, Italy
e-mail: marco.picone@unipr.it

D. Ardigò
MultiMed s.r.l., Cremona, Italy
e-mail: diego.ardigo@multi-med.it

S. Steger
Fraunhofer Institute for Computer Graphics (IGD) Cognitive Computing and Medical Imaging (A7), Darmstadt, Germany
e-mail: sebastian.steger@igd.fraunhofer.de

V.R. Preedy, V.B. Patel (eds.), *Biomarkers in Cancer, Biomarkers in Disease: Methods, Discoveries and Applications*,
DOI 10.1007/978-94-007-7681-4_12

Abstract

Oral cavity cancers are the seventh tumor by diffusion worldwide with more than 90 % being diagnosed as oral squamous cell carcinomas (OSCCs). According to the latest WHO statistics, OSCC accounts for 5 % of the cancer deaths worldwide, being the eighth more lethal cancer entity. Early identification of cancer relapses would have the potentiality to improve the disease control and the patient survival.

NeoMark is a European co-funded research project (Seventh Framework Program, Information and Communication Technologies: EU-FP7-ICT-2007-2-22483-NeoMark) that has the objective to identify relevant biomarkers of OSCC recurrence. It integrates high-throughput gene expression analysis in tumor cells and IT-assisted imaging with traditional staging and follow-up protocols to improve the recurrence risk stratification and to obtain the earlier identification of locoregional relapses.

The architecture of the project is based on the following key points:

- Creation of a web application tool: a unified interface that helps the storage and management of all information
- NeoMark database: the heterogeneous NeoMark data (demographics and risk factors; clinical, pathological, and immunohistochemical parameters; filtered and cleaned genomic and imaging data) are stored in a single database – the

M.J.R. da Fonseca
Link Consulting – Tecnologias De Informaçao S.A., Lisbon, Portugal
e-mail: manuel.fonseca@link.pt

M. De Fazio
STMicroelectronics, Agrate Brianza (MI), Italy
e-mail: marco.de-fazio@st.com

Integrated Health Record Repository (IHRR) – on a central NeoMark server. The server contains the *marker definition functional environment (MDFE)*, a data analysis module. Based on the heterogeneous input data, it estimates the likelihood of a relapse and identifies OSCC risk factors.

- Imaging biomarker extraction: several biomarkers are obtained from medical images such as CT and MRI scans (size, amount of necrosis from tumor and lymph nodes, etc.). To extract those features, a custom software tool – called the NeoMark Image Processing Tool – has specifically been developed.
- Genomic data cleaning and filtering: extraction of genomic data and filtering of genes with low data quality and of those with high number of missing values.

The NeoMark system was trained and initially validated in a multicenter pilot study (three European clinical centers involved: two in Italy and one in Spain) basing on 86 patients affected by OSCC with a minimum follow-up of 12 months.

The clinicians recognized the usefulness of the disease bioprofile (or disease-specific profile) identified by NeoMark to evaluate the risk of disease reoccurrence of a patient at diagnosis, to stratify patients affected by OSCC at baseline according to the risk of recurrence, and to reserve a "tailored therapy" to each case.

List of Abbreviations

DBN	Dynamic Bayesian Network
FE	Feature Extraction
ICT	Information and Communication Technologies
IHRR	Integrated Health Record Repository
MDFE	Marker Definition Functional Environment
OSCC	Oral Squamous Cell Carcinomas
PCR	Polymerase Chain Reaction
RECIST	Response Evaluation Criteria in Solid Tumors
ROI	Region(s) of Interest
RT-PCR	Real-Time PCR
SW	Software
WHO	World Health Organization

Key Facts

- Oral squamous cell carcinoma (OSCC): it accounts for 5 % of the cancer deaths worldwide, being the eighth more lethal cancer entity.
- Tumor relapse that afflicts 25–50 % of the surgically treated OSCC patients represents the main cause of failure and death.
- Early identification of OSCC relapses can improve patient survival and quality of life.

- The state of the art in OSCC patient classification is mainly based on TNM staging that relates on the dimensional characteristics of the tumor and on the presence, number, and site of neck lymph nodes metastases.
- TNM staging system is nowadays considered not sufficiently precise to stratify patients by risk of relapse because it doesn't consider the biological variability of the tumor and the host-neoplasia complex and multilevel relationships.
- The main research field in OSCC is represented by the possibility to reveal the real weight of each biomarker (clinical, pathological, immunohistochemical, radiological, and genetic factors) in the comprehensive risk prediction score by integrating it in a multilevel evaluation system.

Definition of Words and Terms

Risk Factor A variable associated with an increased risk of disease.

Prognostic Factor A situation or condition or a characteristic of a patient that can be used to estimate the chance of recovery from a disease or the chance of the disease recurring.

OSCC (Oral Squamous Cell Carcinoma) Carcinoma developed from squamous epithelium of the oral cavity, having cuboid cells and characterized by keratinization. Initially local and superficial, the lesion may later invade and metastasize.

TNM Staging Is a cancer staging system that describes the extent of a person's cancer using the size and extension of the primary tumor (T), its lymphatic involvement (N), and the presence of metastases (M) to classify the progression of cancer. TNM is developed and maintained by the Union for the International Cancer Control (UICC) to achieve consensus on one globally recognized standard for classifying the extent of spread of cancer.

RT-PCR A highly sensitive technique for the detection and quantitation of mRNA (messenger RNA). The technique consists of two parts: the synthesis of cDNA (complementary DNA) from RNA by reverse transcription (RT) and the amplification of a specific cDNA by the polymerase chain reaction (PCR).

Microarray A tool used to sift through and analyze the information contained within a genome. A microarray consists of different nucleic acid probes that are chemically attached to a substrate, which can be a microchip, a glass slide, or a microsphere-sized bead.

Local Recurrence Cancer that has recurred at or near the same place as the original (primary) tumor, usually after a period of time during which the cancer could not be detected.

Regional Recurrence Cancer that recurs at the lymph nodes.

Distant Recurrence Cancer that recurs to another area of the body.

Biomarker A measurable characteristic that reflects the severity or presence of some disease state. More generally, a biomarker is anything that can be used as an indicator of a particular disease state or some other physiological state of an organism.

Gene Signature The group of genes in a type of cell whose combined expression pattern is uniquely a characteristic of a medical or other condition.

Targeted Therapy Is a medical model that proposes the customization of therapy – with medical decisions, practices, and/or products being tailored to the individual patient.

Introduction

Oral cavity cancers are the seventh tumor by diffusion worldwide with more than 90 % being diagnosed as oral squamous cell carcinomas (OSCCs). Late diagnosis and the aggressive nature of the disease are the main causes of tumor relapse, which afflict 25–50 % of the surgically treated OSCC patients over a period of 5 years. Tumor recurrence leads to severe aesthetic and functional consequences, incites invasive and disabling surgical interventions, and may cause death in a significant percentage of cases (25–50 %). According to the latest WHO statistics, OSCC accounts for 5 % of the cancer deaths worldwide, being the eighth more lethal cancer entity. Early identification of cancer relapses would have the potentiality to improve patient survival and to lower the additional probability of the patients to develop a second tumor lesion, providing the bases for the adoption of more personalized and effective treatment regimens, a better definition of the follow-up strategies, a more rationalized posttreatment follow-up, and a more targeted adjuvant therapy. Although different clinical markers, pathological and immunohistochemical parameters, and biomolecular prognostic factors (TNM staging, grading, plasma markers, etc.) have been reported during the years, none of them showed sufficient accuracy in discriminating relapsing versus non-relapsing patients, and, hence, personalized patient care still remains a distant vision. Presently, OSCC patients must undergo frequent and expensive clinical evaluations, performed by different physicians (pathologists, radiologists, surgeons, oncologists) not always working in the same hospital with possible negative effects on patient treatment. Moreover, the current scenario implies that clinical relevant parameters (which may alert for tumor recurrence and may direct the individual patient treatment and follow-up) are often overlooked or not detected with standardized diagnostic tests performed routinely, no tumor genomic information of each single patient are usually collected, and data are not analyzed in an integrated way to find clinical relapse-predicting correlations. Currently standardized treatment modalities and follow-up approaches are therefore uniform and do not distinguish patients at low risk for relapse from those at high risk, until some clinical signs of disease are detectable. Accordingly, the impact on the patients' quality of life and on the cost of care is high: management of low-risk patients requires unnecessary high resources, while high-risk patients may present themselves with relapsing tumors and need high-cost clinical management, including additional surgical treatments.

The most classical method to predict OSCC recurrence is the TNM staging, which is based mainly on the dimensional characteristics of the tumor and on the presence, number, and site of neck nodes metastasis. Unfortunately, its inadequacy is today recognized because of the uncertain behavior of squamous cancer, which can be sometimes very aggressive and others can metastasize slowly after surgery. This uncertainty in progression has led researchers to seek a larger number of markers (clinical, histopathological, immunohistochemical, radiological, and genetic factors), but to date none provides sufficiently reliable predictions of tumor aggressiveness. Given the multilevel nature of cancer (genes, cells, tissues, organs, systems, and the whole body), integration of the heterogeneous data from different sources may represent the key to understand the biological behavior of OSCCs.

Trying to achieve this target, the NeoMark European research project, submitted for assessment in the call FP7 (Seventh Framework Program) – ICT (Information and Communication Technologies) – 2007–2, was finally selected and co-funded by the EC (European Community, Brussels, Belgium).

The project started from the need of researchers and clinicians in the field of oncology to improve the representation of biological processes related to the onset, growth, and dissemination of human cancer.

The approach chosen by NeoMark has been to address this need through in silico representation, modeling, and prediction of biological phenomena linked to the disease evolution (the so-called Virtual Physiological Human approach or VPH in short).

In fact, the application of the VPH principles to clinical research and practice still presents a number of interesting, unaddressed challenges – linked to the need for multilevel, multiscale modeling – for which cancer biology is a particularly good candidate, since the disease ranges from molecular aberrations, to cellular modifications, to systemic influences and consequences.

The main challenge in disease biology representation is exactly the incapability of current research approaches to represent this multiscale biology of the disease.

Accordingly, the primary objective of the project has been to provide a proof of concept that integration of multiscale clinical, imaging, and genomic data from a sufficient sample of patients diagnosed with OSCC can provide reliable indications on the evolution of the disease at diagnosis and can predict with a sufficient accuracy the onset of a reoccurrence and the time of this onset.

For these purposes, an innovative strategy to identify the relevant biomarkers of cancer reoccurrence was tested in NeoMark, integrating high-throughput gene expression analysis in tumor cells and IT-assisted imaging with traditional staging and follow-up protocols to improve the reoccurrence risk stratification and to obtain the earlier identification of relapses.

The idea behind NeoMark is that by analyzing a sufficient amount of heterogeneous data (clinical, histopathological, immunohistochemical, radiological, and genomic) in patients affected by OSCC before treatment and at the time of remission, a set of relevant biomarkers appearing only in the presence of the disease might be identified. The reoccurrence of the same biomarker phenotype during post-remission follow-up may precede the clinical manifestation of the relapse, thus allowing earlier intervention. Therefore, the project has two main objectives: (1) to identify prognostic factors at baseline associated with a higher risk of disease reoccurrence and (2) to extract a bioprofile of reoccurrence that could identify the presence of relapse earlier than what is provided by traditional clinical evaluation.

Whereas different reports are present in literature on data integration and creation of standardized prognostic algorithms for bladder and breast cancer, nothing is available so far for head and neck cancer. The NeoMark project was conceived to fill this gap (Schmidt 2009; Pillai 2011; Fascina 2007).

In the next paragraphs, the authors describe the NeoMark protocol and methodology, analyzing the results obtained and its hypothetical impact in the clinical practice.

Study Population and Data Collection

Study Population

The study population included 213 patients affected by OSCC treated and followed in the NeoMark cancer clinics according to standard state-of-the-art therapeutic and follow-up approaches as recommended by clinical guidelines. All the patients with diagnosis of the disease during the enrollment period were screened and entered the selection procedure. To obtain the baseline data, tumor and blood samples were collected from all the screened patients and imaging examinations (CT, MRI) were performed. All the patients with histologically proven OSCC and considered apt to undergo first-line treatment were managed, following the usual procedures and protocols. Patients with a complete remission of the disease from a clinical and laboratory point of view were be selected for the follow-up phase. In the patients selected for the follow-up phase, specimens were been collected periodically through dedicated NeoMark tools, as described later. During follow-up period (a minimum of 12 months), a group of patients developed a clinically, pathologically, and radiologically proven reoccurrence of OSCC, whereas another group remained disease-free. Figure 1 illustrates in brief the concept and design of the NeoMark pilot study.

Data Collection

For each patient affected by OSCC enrolled in one of the three clinical centers (Maxillofacial Surgery Unit, University Hospital of Parma, Italy; Centro

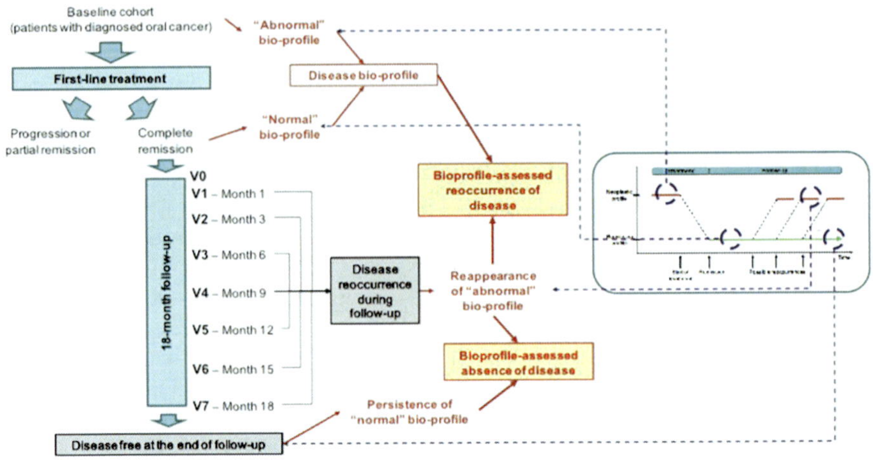

Fig. 1 The NeoMark pilot study. The scheme shows the starting point and the evolution of the project. For all the patients of the baseline cohort, a bioprofile was be identified. After treatment, only patients with complete remission of the disease were be included in the study. During the postoperative follow-up, a new bioprofile was created and compared to the starting one. Changes in the bioprofile can early detect reoccurrence of the disease

Oncológico MD Anderson, Madrid, Spain; Department of Otolaryngology–Head and Neck Surgery, Istituti Fisioterapici Ospitalieri–Istituto Regina Elena, Rome, Italy), the collection of heterogeneous data (clinical, pathological, imaging, and genomic) was conducted, following well-defined protocols. The gathering of all data at baseline and during follow-up is illustrated in Fig. 2.

The NeoMark System Overview

The aim of the NeoMark system was been to integrate a significant and relevant set of functionalities in a single, unified, service-oriented system in order to achieve great flexibility and usability and to satisfy the versatile user requirements and in particular the integration of heterogeneous input data for each enrolled patient.

The designed architecture and its modules are depicted in Fig. 3. Most of the user interaction is done via the web interface in order to increase the usability, reduce the learning curve, and maximize the platform adoption. The physicians can manage patient records, enter clinical data, and view all the collected features and the extracted results coming from the NeoMark engine. The clinicians have the opportunity to upload genomic data, and researchers can view anonymous statistics, which could serve as a basis for future research on oral cancer. The uploading of imaging and genomic data is performed using dedicated stand-alone tools able to easily and efficiently process a huge amount of data and upload into the system only

Activity	Baseline (V-1)	Remission (V0)	Months after remission							Relapse (VR) (at any time)
			1 (V1)	3 (V2)	6 (V3)	9 (V4)	12 (V5)	15 (V6)	18 (V7)	
Clinical evaluation	X	X	X	X	X	X	X	X	X	X
Laboratory measurements	X	X	-	X	X	X	X	X	X	X
Histology	X	-	-	-	-	-	-	-	-	if applicable
Imaging	X	X	-	-	X	-	X	-	X	X
Turner specimen collection	X	-	-	-	-	-	-	-	-	if applicable
Whole-blood specimen collection	X	X	X	X	X	X	X	X	X	X
Turnor expression profile	X	-	-	-	-	-	-	-	-	if specimen available
Whole-blood expression profile	X	X	If R	If R	If R	If R	If R	If R	X	X
Biomarker profile validation	X	X	X	X	X	X	X	X	X	X

Fig. 2 The scheme for collection of NeoMark data. The scheme shows the steps and times of collection of the different samples and data necessary for the creation of the bioprofile

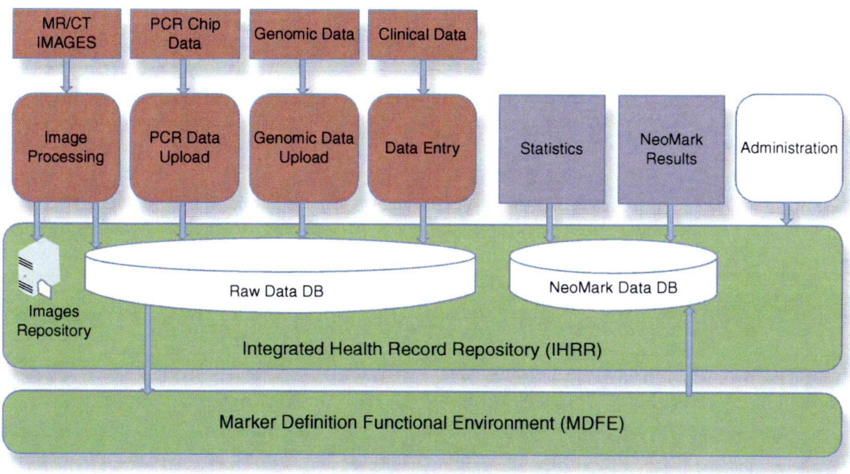

Fig. 3 NeoMark system overview and logical architecture. The image depicts the overall NeoMark logical architecture by grouping its components into several layers and also identifying the several data sources: Integrated NeoMark Health Repository (it includes the images repository and NeoMark databases), NeoMark applications (it enumerates all necessary tools to input and extract data from the health data repository), and marker definition functional environment

the relevant information. Heterogeneous NeoMark data (demographics and risk factors; clinical, pathological, and immunohistochemical parameters; filtered and cleaned genomic and imaging data) are stored in a single database – the Integrated Health Record Repository (IHRR) – on a central NeoMark server. The participating hospitals are connected to the very same NeoMark server, allowing the data-driven training algorithm to incorporate patient data from all participating hospitals at the same time and enabling users to perform interhospital comparisons of patient data.

The NeoMark server contains the *marker definition functional environment (MDFE)*, a data analysis module which is the core of the system. Based on the heterogeneous input data, this module estimates the likelihood of a relapse and identifies OSCC risk factors (Exarchos 2012; Gerds 2008).

In order to protect the patient's right of privacy, none of the sensitive data (e.g., the name) that allow to uniquely identify the patient are stored on the central NeoMark server. Only a unique NeoMark ID can identify a patient. Those IDs are connected to the patients via individual databases that are located within each hospital.

Genomic Data Cleaning and Filtering

The genomic data management system is shown in Fig. 4. Blood samples and tumor samples are traditionally analyzed during the experiments with a standard microarray scanner which produces as output a feature extraction (FE) file. This file

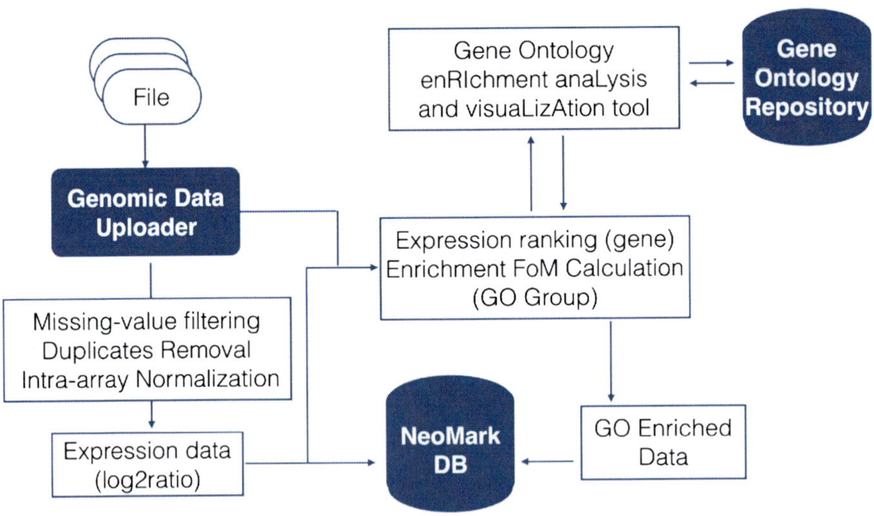

Fig. 4 Genomic data management. This figure presents NeoMark's genomic data input process, starting with the genome data uploader tool and highlighting the major building blocks and data processing procedures, such as the gene grouping through the use of the gene ontology repository

format is a tab-delimited text document that contains all the data such as the log2-ratio value as well as (very) raw intensity data, background information, metadata on the experiment and on the scanning settings, annotation data to identify genes, etc.

In order to integrate this data into the project database, the expression values of each sample is been extracted from the FE file and uploaded into the data matrix after being associated to the correct patient or sample. The relevant information that are extracted and stored in the database are feature name, probe name, gene name, systematic name, description, and log2 ratio. In order to achieve this pre-filtering task, a dedicated stand-alone tool was been developed to analyze both control and duplicate features, to filter genes with low data quality and those with high number of missing values. The output of application is a cleaned and lighter file (in terms of MBytes) that contains only the relevant fields for the analysis. The new file is eventually associated to the specific patient's sample and is uploaded through the web interface of the NeoMark system into the central database, while the original copy of the FE file is kept in the local hospital repository.

On the server side, the storage of the extracted genomic data is organized and structured using two different kinds of tables. The first one contains only the cleaned and relevant information with the log2-ratio value plus the normalized one calculated using the records that are already stored in the database. The second table is designed to store genomic data expression following the group ontology. In particular it contains a collection of information provided by the gene ontology analyses of a single FE file obtained using the Gorilla web application based on the approach presented by Eden, 2009; http://cbl-gorilla.cs.technion.ac.il.

The RT-PCR Tool

In NeoMark a portable, real-time, low-cost RT-PCR tool was been developed (Fig. 5). The device serves as a lab-on-a-chip alternative to microarrays for examining patient's RNA extracted from tumor specimens and/or lymphocytes.

The tool can analyze several types of biological contents including enzymes, primers, targets, and DNA and RNA.

The device is composed of a core silicon chip containing heaters and thermal sensors, a cooling fan, and an optical system that detects the fluorescence intensity of the monitored reaction. As fluorescent dyes, commercial FAMTM or VIC® fluorophores can be used. The practitioner, after preparing the chips with a genetic material, operates an SW tool that controls the device, clears and filters data, and sends it to the NeoMark central database.

The idea behind the tool is to use it to assess the presence of the biomarkers identified by NeoMark. The qPCR, in fact, can measure the expression value of a set of predefined genes (up to 20) and to gather their expression value in relation with a housekeeping gene.

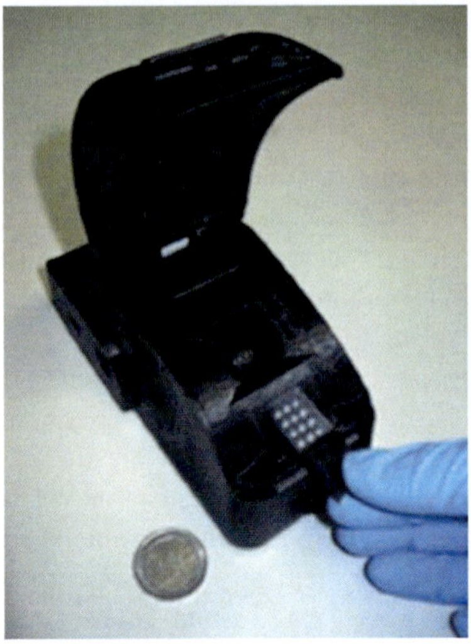

Fig. 5 The NeoMark RT-PCR tool (Source: NeoMark). The NeoMark RT-PCR tool is a portable, real-time, low-cost RT-PCR that can work as an alternative to microarrays for examining patient's RNA extracted from tumor specimens and/or lymphocytes. The device is composed of a core silicon chip containing heaters and thermal sensors, a cooling fan, and an optical system that detects the fluorescence intensity of the monitored reaction. Reused with permission from STMicroelectronics

Imaging Biomarker Extraction

Further biomarkers for disease reoccurrence prediction have been obtained from medical images such as CT and MRI scans. The imaging biomarkers include geometric (e.g., size) as well as texture-based features (e.g., amount of necrosis) from the primary tumor and relevant lymph nodes.

To extract those features, a radiologist used a custom software tool – called the NeoMark Image Processing Tool – which has specifically been developed for that purpose (Fig. 6). The remainder of this section will describes how the imaging biomarkers are extracted by the radiologist using the NeoMark Image Processing Tool.

Imaging Protocol

For each patient, the following set of head and neck medical images is acquired at baseline (i.e., upon diagnosis, before treatment) and every 6 months during remission: high-resolution CT with and without contrast agent; MRI T2, coronal, TSE, fat suppression; MRI T1 + T2, axial, TSE; and MRT T1, axial + coronal + sagittal, fat suppression, contrast enhanced.

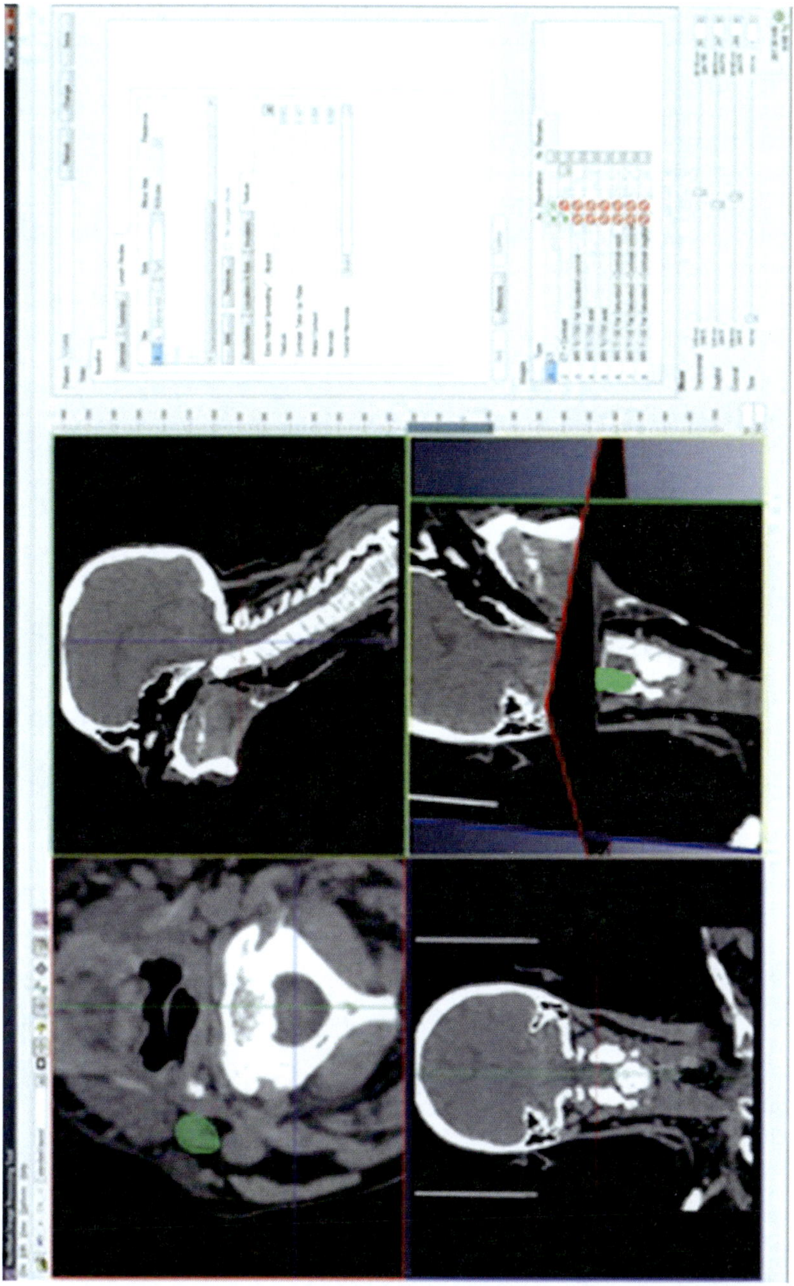

Fig. 6 **Screenshot of the NeoMark Image Processing Tool**. The figure shows the screenshot of the NeoMark Image Processing Tool, through which imaging biomarkers, such as geometric and texture-based features from primary tumor and lymph nodes, can be extracted

ROI Definition

At baseline, the targets from which image features are extracted are the primary tumor and all enlarged or otherwise suspicious lymph nodes. Since the tumor and maybe some of the lymph nodes are dissected, features in the follow-up images can only be extracted from the remaining lymph nodes.

For each target, a 3D model is created (Fig. 7). For lymph nodes, this is done on the contrast-enhanced CT image with a semiautomatic radial ray-based segmentation approach (Fig. 8). The radiologist only places a single click in the approximate center of the structure. Due to the large shape variability, low image contrast, and the unknown heterogeneous surrounding tissue, the segmentation of a tumor is very challenging and thus an interactive approach is used. Upon a click in the approximate center of the tumor, the system provides an initial proposal of the 3D contour which can then be interactively adapted by the user (Steger, Erdt 2009; Steger and Franco 2011).

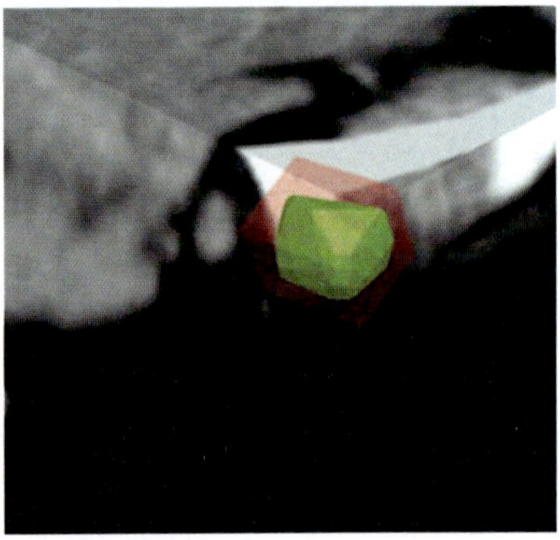

Fig. 7 3D model of a lymph node. The figure shows the tridimensional reconstruction of a lymph node. It allows a better detection of its tridimensional characteristics (e.g., size, form, location, etc.)

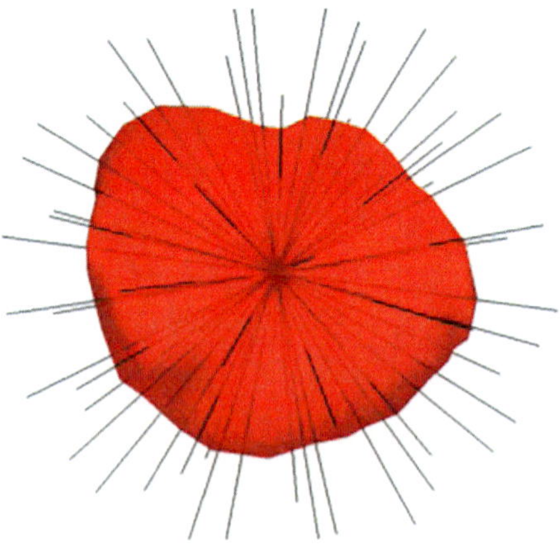

Fig. 8 Radial ray-based segmentation of lymph nodes. The tridimensional reconstruction of lymph nodes is done on the contrast-enhanced CT image with a semiautomatic radial ray-based segmentation approach

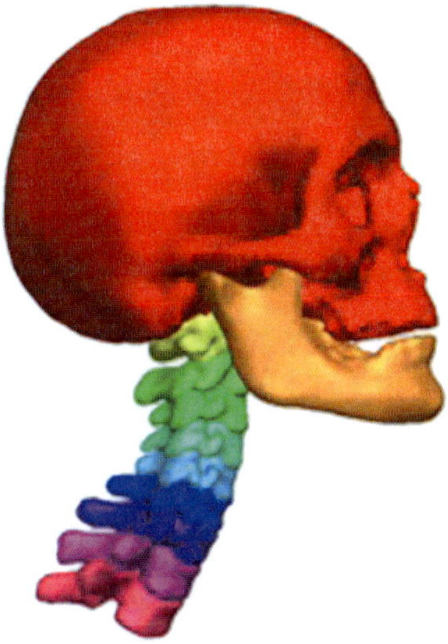

Fig. 9 Articulated atlas for the segmentation of the skeleton. The segmentation of the skeleton is done, extracting on the CT image the different bones through an anatomical atlas present in the software

Image Fusion

To be able to jointly extract features from more than one imaging modality and multiple points in time, all input images need to be aligned properly, resulting in a single multimodal/multi-temporal fusion image. This alignment process is carried out fully automatically using image intensity-based rigid registration of the head as the first step.

Whereas rigid registration is sufficient in the head, deformation due to different neck positions may be present in the neck area. Thus, fully automatic deformable image registration based on the skeleton is performed as the second step. An articulated atlas is used to extract individual bones in the CT image (Fig. 9) (Steger and Sakas 2012; Steger and Kirschner 2012). For each of the bones, a single rigid transformation is successively found based on the maximization of an image similarity metric. Finally, those transformations are propagated into the surrounding soft tissue, resulting in a dense deformation field (Fig. 10).

To increase the alignment accuracy in the ROIs, a local rigid registration for those image regions is deployed eventually.

Feature Extraction

For each ROI given by the 3D model, a set of geometric and texture-based image features is extracted automatically.

The geometric features consist of the volume, the 3D longest and shortest diameter, as well as derived measurements such as the aspect ratio. According to

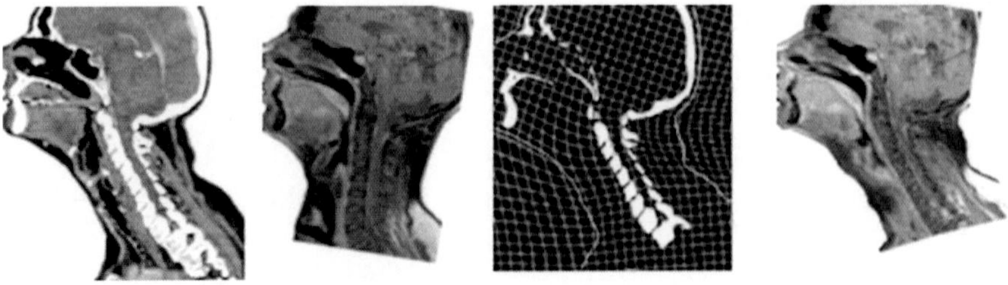

Fig. 10 **Skeleton-based deformable registration of CT/MR images**. After segmentation, for each bone, a single rigid transformation is successively found based on the maximization of an image similarity metric. Finally, those transformations are propagated into the surrounding soft tissue, resulting in a dense deformation field

this, automatic 3D assessment of the size is less prone to inter- and intra-observer variability than the standard assessment using the RECIST criteria. Texture-based features include the contrast take-up rate, the texture homogeneity, and the amount of necrosis and water content (Steger and Keil 2010; Steger and Wesarg 2012; Steger 2011; Steger and Bozoglu 2013).

Additionally, the radiologist manually defines further clinically relevant properties such as infiltration of the surrounding tissue and site and extracapsular spreading.

Upon confirmation by the user, the NeoMark Image Processing Tool uploads those biomarkers to the NeoMark environment for the integration with the clinical and genomic data.

Further Functionality

Besides the imaging biomarkers extraction, the NeoMark Image Processing Tool allows to extract annotated image slices of interest which can then be viewed with a web browser by the doctors, e.g., during the tumor board. Furthermore, an image search is implemented, enabling to obtain cases with specific features (e.g., all images with a tumor of size larger than 3 cm). This can, for example, facilitate the comparison of cases.

The NeoMark Web Application Tool

As mentioned earlier, NeoMark provides a unified interface that allows a doctor to manage his/her patients through an easy-to-understand and user-friendly web interface.

The interface provides a set of tools to help the doctor store and manage all information, including some intelligent tools to categorize each patient accordingly with his/her risk of relapse, TNM staging, or simply any risk factor.

The Data Entry Tool

One of the main functionalities provided by NeoMark is the ability to store all clinical, pathological, and imaging information down on a central server, accessible to any authorized personnel. This enables the clinicians to enter data structured into well-known and useful blocks of information that will then be automatically processed by the NeoMark "intelligent" algorithms to classify the each patient according to his/her risk of relapse.

The tool also enables the clinician to understand at which stage a patient is in and quickly browse through all his patient's visits in order to access specific data.

The Annotations Tools

In most cases, the clinicians also use a set of simple tools to describe the visible points of the disease. This information could then be viewed by the radiologist or can later be used by the doctor to check on the imaging results.

To achieve this, a set of interactive diagrams are made available to the doctors, and through them the doctor can then mark the areas where the disease symptoms are located.

Reports and Patient Stratification

One functionality which was considered by the physicians as extremely useful was the reporting tool. This enabled the physician to quickly segment his patients and identify which ones have the higher recurrence risk.

The application included a set of reports that, based on a well-defined criteria and rules, will allow the physician to filter and group patients. The reports included were:

- Patient stratification by risk of recurrence
- Patient list by TNM staging
- Patient list by risk factors
- Patient list by T-localization
- Patient list by surgical procedure
- Patient list by tumor imaging parameters
- Patient list by follow-up

NeoMark Data Analysis

The primary aim of the data mining performed within NeoMark is to identify the factors that influence significantly the progression of oral cancer and subsequently formulate a decision support system that is able to predict potential disease relapses

Table 1 **Best-performing classification schemes.** For each type of data employed in this work (i.e., clinical, imaging, tissue genomic, and blood genomic), the best-performing classification schemes have been selected. A classification scheme consists of a feature selection technique coupled with a classification algorithm. The selection has been performed based on the following performance metrics, accuracy, sensitivity, specificity, and AUC; the selected schemes have yielded quite high values for all these metrics. (Pillai 2011; Schmidt 2009; Murphy 2002; Guarino 2009; Smith 2007)

Data	Feature selection	Classification algorithm	Accuracy (%)	Sensitivity (%)	Specificity (%)	AUC
Clinical	Wrapper	Decision trees	83.3	73.7	93	0.84
Imaging	Wrapper	Naïve Bayes	90.9	88.6	93.2	0.89
Tissue genomic	Literature∪ current work	Artificial neural networks	91.23	94.7	87.7	0.96
Blood genomic	No feature selection	Artificial neural networks	95.8	100	91.7	1

during remission. In order to analyze the multiscale and multiparametric data collected within NeoMark, we have a twofold approach was devised, namely, baseline data analysis and disease evolution monitoring. The former approach employs baseline information (i.e., clinical, imaging, and genomic) in order to assess the probability of a patient to suffer a local relapse. The latter approach involves the analysis of time-varying information (i.e., blood gene expression) collected at predefined intervals over the follow-up period in order to model the temporal progression of the disease.

For the baseline data analysis, a wide range of classification schemes have been exploited and evaluated involving the state-of-the-art classification algorithms coupled with feature selection techniques (Pillai 2011; Schmidt 2009; Murphy 2002; Guarino 2009; Smith 2007). Each source of data was been initially analyzed independently in order to evaluate its discriminating potential; afterwards a consensus decision was procured. The best-performing classification schemes based on each source of data are shown in Table 1.

For the case of tissue genomic data, the set that yielded the best results consisted of the genes identified within NeoMark combined with a set of 28 genes identified in the literature. The combination of the decisions from the individual schemes using a majority voting algorithm resulted in complete discrimination.

The disease evolution monitoring encompasses a dynamic Bayesian network (DBN) which is fed with gene expression information from the circulating blood. DBN is able to analyze snapshots of information in consecutive time slices in order to model the evolution of the disease over time. By providing as input to the DBN data solely from the baseline visit, we achieve accuracy of 86 %; the provision of data from the first follow-up visit as well leads to perfect discrimination (Murphy 2002).

NeoMark Data Validation and Results

The NeoMark system was validated in a pilot study which involved 86 OSCC patients fully compliant with the selection criteria, completely investigated with all data uploaded in the system, surgically treated (with more than 12 months of follow-up), and recruited in the three clinical centers in Italy and Spain. The results are shown in Tables 2 and 3.

The clinical, pathological, and imaging data obtained were largely supported by literature findings. Analyzing the genomic expression in tissue and the blood, a strong concordance with previous studies in particular regarding the altered expression of SOD2 and RPRM was observed. They are in fact both tissue genomic factors associated with a higher risk of lymphatic metastases. A special attention was devoted on the modifications of the blood genomic expression in patients with and without recurrences. The altered expression of genes shown in Table 1 was present in relapsers.

These data become more significant when correlated to the site of the tumor in accordance with the previous studies that reported the importance of the anatomic location of the tumor in terms either of prognosis or risk of relapse. In fact some sites such as the tongue and floor of the mouth generally have poorer prognosis due to the frequent presence of cervical metastases and have to be considered in the risk assessment.

We noted that almost all the clinical and imaging markers identified by NeoMark are reported in literature (Table 2). Genomic markers however are different (Table 3). The inclusion of genes present in literature led to an increase in accuracy from 80 % to 91.23 %. We must however note that research on OSCC genomic factors is still ongoing in particular through retrospective studies on tissue samples which are available in tumor banks. Also the inclusion criteria adopted in the different published studies are less strict than NeoMark, so increasing the variability of results. We can therefore propose NeoMark as a new approach and data analysis tool for further research.

The NeoMark system has proved to be effective for the management of patients' data and for the optimization of the follow-up activities. The immediate value of the tools – as perceived by using physicians – refers but is not limited to the possibility to access through a unique repository all available information regarding each patient and also to improve some diagnostic referrals (especially imaging) through data comparison and integration.

NeoMark has also demonstrated that it is possible to integrate clinical, imaging, and genomic data to obtain predictions regarding disease evolution in patients with OSCC and that the identified prognostic factors are in line with most recent research findings and can be reduced to a limited but well-performing number, easily checked by physicians through simple diagnostic exams.

In particular, the clinicians recognized the usefulness of the disease-specific bioprofile identified by NeoMark to evaluate the risk of disease recurrence in each

Table 2 Prognostic factors extracted from literature (in red the factors also identified by NeoMark). The table shows the prognostic factors of oral squamous cell cancer extracted from literature. They include clinical, pathological, radiological, and genetic factors (Rogers 2008; Woolgar 2006, 2009; Warner 2004; Wang 2009; Ye 2008; Giles 2004; liao 2011; Liu 2009, 2010; Pusapati 2010; Reis 2011; Chen 2008; Bisdas 2009; Gil 2009). Those in red are factors identified also by NeoMark

Clinical and histopathological factors	Imaging factors	Genetic factors
Smoke	Site	LOC401010
Alcohol	Number of Lymphnodes	FKBPL
Familiarity	Shape Deviation	SMARCC2
Substance exposition	Number Lymphnodes > 3 cm	CIDEB
Eating habits	Side	CLDN1
Mechanical trauma	Cluster	ANP32A
Precancerous lesions	Central necrosis	GALNT6
pT stage	Minor axis >10mm	PRKAR2A
pN stage	Carotid infiltration	EST
M stage	Bone infiltration	HP1-BP74
Surgical margins	Extranodal spreading	CLDN1
Tumor thickness	Contrast takup rate	AP1G2
Depth invasion	Cuteneous invasion	PKD2
Tumor maxDiameter	Watercontent	GTF2H4
D240 stain	Necrosis	C1orf144
Martinez Gimeno score	Texture	LOC644276
Anneroth score		NP285481
Perineural invasion		LIG3
Degree cell keratinisation		LOC492303
Grade differentiation		A_24_P170365
Lymphovascular invasion		ZNF205
Lymphoplasmacytic reaction		CRYAA
HPV DNA		LOC389786
Num mitosesHPF		C17orf71
Nuclear pleomorphism		KIAA1033
Basaloid features		KIAA0140
cyclinD1 stain		THC2280373
Ki67 stain		BF368414
P53 stain		ENST0000034433
EGFR stain		BQ333643
P16ink4a stain		A_32_P133402
		C21orf87
		A_24_P101503

single case at baseline to stratify patients affected by OSCC according to the risk of recurrence and so the possibility to reserve them a "tailored" therapy and follow-up.

Regarding the Disease Evolution Bioprofile, the physicians agree that the approach is correct and is aligned with the more recent research trends. The hypothesis that the presence of tumor could induce perturbation of homeostasis not only locally but also systemically was only recently proposed, and so NeoMark provides additional evidence. However, this hypothesis has to be confirmed with more analyses.

Table 3 Prognostic factors extracted after NeoMark data integration plus the best-performing genes extracted from literature (Rogers 2008; Warner 2004; Wang 2009; Ye 2008; Giles 2004; Liao 2011; Liu 2009, 2010; Pusapati 2010; Reis 2011; Peng 2011; Saintigny 2011; Chen 2008). In the table are listed the prognostic factors used to create the bioprofile. They include factors extracted from literature and factors, especially genetic, identified by the NeoMark algorithm (in blue the genes which were not listed in literature selection)

Source of data	Feature/Marker included in bio-profile		
Clinical	N staging	Perineural invasion	Smoke
	Lymphoplasmacytic reaction	Number of mitoses per HPF	p53 stain
	Surgical margins	Tumor thickness	
Imaging	Extra Tumor Spreading	Number of Lymph Nodes	Site
	Texture	Extra Nodal Spreading	Side
Tissue genomic	PHACTR1	SOD2	C17orf71
	RPRM	CRYAA	ZNF205
	AMDHD1	SLC5A12	C21orf87
Blood genomic	A_24_P221960	THC2410448	THC2399272
	A_24_P230388	AL566369	BM683433
	A_32_P57247	CN391963	OXCT2
	A_24_P942151	X58809	
Additional Literature genes	LOC492303	ENST00000344339	KIAA1033
	CLDN1	LOC644276	LOC389786
	FKBPL	C1orf144	PKD2
	A_32_P133402	CRYAA	

Additionally, NeoMark proved that it is possible to realize and use a real-time PCR device to analyze tissue and blood RNA, obtaining results even more precise than what is currently achieved by standard laboratory equipment. The RT-PCR device and associated protocol may constitute a real breakthrough in clinical practice for early diagnosis or reoccurrence of oral cancer. As such NeoMark can be seen as a pioneering platform, demonstrating that the NeoMark approach can be extended to other cancers.

Potential Applications to Prognosis, Other Diseases, or Conditions

NeoMark research is oriented to find a tool and to experience a methodology for assisting physicians in a more effective care of a particular family of tumors, whose numbers are increasing and which have not been extensively studied and investigated so far.

NeoMark can bring to research a better understanding of the correlations between biological factors (either patient or cancer specific) that are characteristic for oral cancer and fostering reoccurrences.

Therefore, the NeoMark follow-up scheme adopted in the project; the NeoMark data acquisition and analysis system, including advanced image feature extraction and analysis and interpretation tools; and the NeoMark lab-on-chip diagnostic device are expected to bring significant contributions to clinical knowledge, to the early diagnosis of oral cancer relapses, and to the simplification of the diagnostic procedures.

The NeoMark research created a system helping clinicians in their decisions for treatments and intervention methodologies, based on the availability of aggregated and complete data, showing trends of oral cancer in relation to specific biomarkers and imaging aspects, currently not possible due to the lack of integration and to the enormous number of genetic data to be processed.

Summary Points

- NeoMark is a European Commission co-funded research project, under the Seventh Framework Program, Objective ICT-2007.5.3: Virtual Physiological Human. The objective of the study is to identify relevant biomarkers of cancer reoccurrence and to stratify patients by the risk of relapse.
- NeoMark starts from the need of researchers and clinicians in the field of oncology to improve the representation of biological processes related to the onset, growth, dissemination, and relapse of human cancer.
- The project involves clinical research institutions with specific expertise in data integration and analysis, medical image processing, modeling, and gene expressions processing and industrial companies expert in the realization of medical devices for biomarker analysis and in the development of market solutions.
- A specific software is developed to extract, integrate, process, relate, analyze, aggregate, and present to clinicians different possible sets of medical information (clinical, pathological, imaging, biomolecular, genomic) in order to identify the most relevant factors characterizing the disease and the risks of relapses.
- For each patient included in the study, a personal and disease bioprofile useful to evaluate the risk of disease reoccurrence at baseline, to calculate the risk of recurrence, and to plan a "tailored" therapy and follow-up was identified.

References

Bisdas S, et al. Outcome prediction after surgery and chemioradiation of squamous cell carcinoma in the oral cavity, oropharynx and hypopharynx: use of baseline perfusion CT microcirculatory parameters vs tumor volume. Int J Radiat Oncol Biol Phys. 2009;73(5):1313–8. Epub 2008 Oct 27.

Chen C, et al. Gene expression profiling identifies genes predictive of oral squamous cell carcinoma. Cancer Epidemiol Biomarkers Prev. 2008;17(8):2152–62.

Eden E, Navon R, Steinfeld I, Lipson D, Yakhin Z. GOrilla: a tool for discovery and visualization of enriched GO terms in ranked gene lists. BMC Bioinf. 2009;10:48. doi:10.1186/1471-2105-10-48.

Exarchos KP, Goletsis Y, Fotiadis DI. A multiscale and multiparametric approach for modeling the progression of oral cancer. BMC Med Inform Decis Mak. 2012;12:136.

Fascina PA, et al. Evaluation of mathematical models for breast cancer risk assessment in routine clinical use. Eur J Cancer Prev. 2007;16(3):216–24.

Gene Ontology enRIchment anaLysis and visuaLizAtion tool. http://cbl-gorilla.cs.technion.ac.il.

Gerds TA, et al. The performance of risk prediction models. Biom J. 2008;50(4):457–79. Review.

Gil Z, et al. Lymph node density is a significant predictor of outcome in patients with oral cancer. Cancer. 2009;115(24):5700–10.

Giles CW, et al. Molecular classification of oral cancer by cDNA microarrays identifies overexpressed genes correlated with nodal metastasis. Int J Cancer. 2004;110:857–68.

Guarino N, Oberle D, Staab S. What is an ontology? In: Handbook on ontologies, International handbooks on information systems. Berlin/Heidelberg: Springer; 2009. p. 1–17.

Liao CT, Lee LY, Huang SF, Chen IH, Kang CJ, Lin CY, Fan KH, Wang HM, Ng SH, Yen TC. Outcome analysis of patients with oral cavity cancer and extracapsular spread in neck lymph nodes. Int J Radiat Oncol Biol Phys. 2011 Nov 15;81(4):930–7.

Liu X, Yu J, Jiang L, Wang A, Shi F, Ye H, Zhou X. MicroRNA-222 regulates cell invasion by targeting matrix metalloproteinase 1 (MMP1) and manganese superoxide dismutase 2 (SOD2) in tongue squamous cell carcinoma cell lines. Cancer Genomics Proteomics. 2009;6(3):131–9.

Liu X, Wang A, Lo Muzio L, Kolokythas A, Sheng S, Rubini C, Ye H, Shi F, Yu T, Crowe DL, Zhou X. Deregulation of manganese superoxide dismutase (SOD2) expression and lymph node metastasis in tongue squamous cell carcinoma. BMC Cancer. 2010;10:365.

Murphy KP. Dynamic Bayesian networks: representation, inference and learning. In: Computer science division. Berkeley: University of California; 2002.

Peng C-H, Liao C-T, Peng S-C, Chen Y-J, Cheng A-J, et al. A novel molecular signature identified by systems genetics approach predicts prognosis in oral squamous cell carcinoma. PLoS One. 2011;6(8):e23452. doi:10.1371/journal.pone.0023452.

Pillai R, et al. Do standardised prognostic algorithms reflect local practice? Application of EORTC risk tables for non-muscle invasive (pTa/pT1) bladder cancer recurrence and progression in a local cohort. Sci World J. 2011;11:751–9.

Pusapati RV, Weaks RL, Rounbehler RJ, McArthur MJ, Johnson DG. E2F2 suppresses Myc-induced proliferation and tumorigenesis. Mol Carcinog. 2010;49(2):152–6.

Reis PP, Waldron L, Perez-Ordonex B, Pintilie M, Naranjo Galloni N, Xuan Y, Cervigne NK, Warner GC, Makitie AA, Simpson C, et al. A gene signature in histologically normal surgical margins is predictive of oral carcinoma recurrence. BMC Cancer. 2011;11:437.doi:10.1186/1471-2407-11-437, Epub http://www.biomedcentral.com/1471-2407/11/437.

Rogers SN, et al. Survival following primary surgery for oral cancer. Oral Oncol. 2009;45(3):201–11. Epub 2008 July 31.

Saintigny P, et al. Gene expression profiling predicts the development of oral cancer. Cancer Prev Res (Phila). 2011;4(2):218–29.

Schmidt M, et al. Long-term outcome prediction by clinicopathological risk classification algorithms in node-negative breast cancer–comparison between Adjuvant!, St Gallen, and a novel risk algorithm used in the prospective randomized Node-Negative-Breast Cancer-3 (NNBC-3) trial. Ann Oncol. 2009;20(2):258–64. Epub 2008 Sept 29.

Smith B, Ashburner M, Rosse C, Bard J, Bug W, Ceusters W, Goldberg LJ, Eilbeck K, Ireland A, Mungall CJ, the OBI Consortium, Leontis N, Rocca-Serra P, Ruttenberg A, Sansone S-A, Scheuermann RH, Shah N, Whetzel PL, Lewis S. The OBO foundry: coordinated evolution of ontologies to support biomedical data integration. Nat Biotechnol. 2007;25(11):1251–5.

Steger S. Local rigid registration for multimodal texture feature extraction from medical images. In: SPIE medical imaging, Orlando; 2011.

Steger S, Keil M. Automated initialization and region of interest detection for successful head registration of truncated CT/MR head&neck images. In: Information technology and applications in biomedicine (ITAB), 2010 10th IEEE international conference on, Corfu; 2010.

Steger S, Wesarg S. Automated skeleton based multi-modal deformable registration of head&neck datasets. In: Ayache N, Delingette H, Golland P, Mori K, editors. Medical image computing and computer-assisted intervention – MICCAI 2012, Nice, vol. 7511. Berlin/Heidelberg: Springer; 2012. p. 66–73.

Steger S, Erdt M, Chiari G, Sakas G. Feature extraction from medical images for an oral cancer reoccurrence prediction. In: World congress on medical physics and biomedical engineering. Munich; 2009.

Steger S, Franco F, Sverzellati N, Chiari G, Colomer R. 3D assessment of lymph nodes vs. RECIST 1.1. Acad Radiol. 2011;18(3):391–4.

Steger S, Sakas G. FIST: fast interactive segmentation of tumors. In: Abdominal imaging. Computational and clinical applications, Toronto; 2012.

Steger S, Kirschner M, Wesarg S. Articulated atlas for segmentation of the skeleton from head&neck CT datasets. In: Biomedical imaging (ISBI), 2012 9th IEEE international symposium on, Barcelona; 2012.

Steger S, Bozoglu N, Kuijper A, Wesarg S. On the segmentation of cervical lymph nodes from CT images using radial rays. IEEE Trans Med Imaging. 2013;32(5):888–900.

Wang Z, Zhang B, Jiang L, Zeng X, Chen Y, Feng X, Guo Y, Chen Q. RACK1, an excellent predictor for poor clinical outcome in oral squamous carcinoma, similar to Ki67. Eur J Cancer. 2009;45(3):490–6.

Warner GC, et al. Molecular classification of oral cancer by cDNA microarrays identifies overexpressed genes correlated with nodal metastasis. Int J Cancer. 2004;110(6):857–68.

Woolgar JA. Histopathological prognostic factors in oral and oropharyngeal squamous cell carcinoma. Oral Oncol. 2006;42(3):229–39. Epub 2005 Sept 16. Review.

Woolgar JA, et al. Determinants of outcome following surgery for oral squamous cell carcinoma. Future Oncol. 2009;5(1):51–61. Review.

Ye H, Wang A, Lee BS, Yu T, Sheng S, Peng T, Hu S, Crowe DL, Zhou X. Proteomic based identification of manganese superoxide dismutase 2 (SOD2) as a metastasis marker for oral squamous cell carcinoma. Cancer Genomics Proteomics. 2008;5(2):85–94.

Telomerase as Biomarker for Oral Cancer 33

Shigeori Takenaka and Shinobu Sato

Contents

Abstract

Telomerase is a ribonucleoprotein enzyme that extends telomere DNA located in the chromosomal termini. Telomerase is known to specifically express in cancer cells, and telomerase activity was found in more than 80 % of cancer patients. Therefore, telomerase may represent a promising cancer biomarker and therapeutic target. The telomerase repeat amplification protocol (TRAP) assay is a polymerase chain reaction (PCR)-based method to detect telomerase activity. In this assay, the telomerase substrate (TS) primer is elongated and its extended DNA is amplified by PCR. Telomerase activity is evaluated by a ladder of bands differing by 6 bp after gel electrophoresis of the PCR products. Recently, non-PCR-based methods to detect telomerase activity have been reported by many researchers. Electrochemical telomerase assay (ECTA), which was developed by Takenaka's group, is a simple and rapid PCR-free method to detect

S. Takenaka (✉) • S. Sato
Department of Applied Chemistry, Research Center for Bio-microsensing Technology, Kyushu Institute of Technology, Kitakyushu, Fukuoka, Japan
e-mail: shige@che.kyutech.ac.jp; tshige@iki.bbiq.jp; shinobu@che.kyutech.ac.jp

V.R. Preedy, V.B. Patel (eds.), *Biomarkers in Cancer, Biomarkers in Disease: Methods, Discoveries and Applications*,
DOI 10.1007/978-94-007-7681-4_8

telomerase activity. ECTA consists of a TS primer-immobilized electrode and ferrocenylnaphthalene diimide derivative as a tetraplex binder. Takenaka's group compared the efficacy of ECTA and TRAP methods in detecting telomerase activity in oral cancer screening. Telomerase activity was observed in 90 % and 30 % of oral cancer tissues and exfoliative cells using the TRAP method, respectively, whereas the ECTA method detected telomerase activity in 90 % and 85 % of oral cancer tissues and exfoliative cells, respectively. These findings suggested that the ECTA method is useful for oral cancer screening because exfoliative cells can be easily obtained by scraping the inside of the mouth. Because telomerase activity is specific to cancer cells, ligands that inhibit telomerase activity may show promise as anticancer drugs. ECTA has also been used to estimate the inhibitory activity of telomerase ligands in cancer cells by determining TS primer elongation in a concentration-dependent manner. The ECTA method was used to screen for the telomerase inhibitory activity of 10 ligands and demonstrated not only the inhibitory activity of the ligands but also their mechanisms of action. The drugs having non-elongating capability directly inhibited telomerase. On the other hand, another set of drugs that can elongate at a 24-mer expansion indirectly inhibited telomerase access by binding and stabilizing the tetraplex structures.

List of Abbreviations

Ca9-22	Human Gingival Squamous Cell Carcinoma Cell Lines
ECTA	Electrochemical Telomerase Assay
EtBr	Ethidium Bromide
FND	Ferrocenylnaphthalene Diimide
HSC-2	Human Oral Squamous Cell Carcinoma Cell Lines
HSC-3	Human Tongue Squamous Cell Carcinoma Cell Lines
hTERT	Human Telomerase Reverse Transcriptase
IC_{50}	Half maximal (50 %) Inhibitory Concentration
Inhibitor III	Hexameric Phosphorothioate Oligonucleotide, 5′-d(TTAGGG)-3′
Inhibitor V	2,6-bis[3-(*N*-piperidino)propionamido]anthracene-9,10-dione
PCR	Polymerase Chain Reaction
PIPER	*N*,*N*′-bis [2-(1-piperidino)ethyl]-3,4,9,10-tetracarboxylic diimide
Q	Charge Quantity
SAS	Human Tongue Squamous Cell Carcinoma Cell Line
SPR	Surface Plasmon Resonance
SWV	Square Wave Voltammetry
TBM	3,3′,5,5′-Tetramethylbenzidine
TER	Telomerase RNA Component
TERT	Telomerase Reverse Transcriptase
TMPyP4	5,10,15,20-tetra-(*N*-methyl-4-pyridyl)porphine
TND	Tri Naphthalene Diimide
TRAP	Telomerase Repeat Amplification protocol
TS	Primer Telomerase Substrate Primer

Key Facts of Hemodialysis

- Telomerase: A ribonucleoprotein that consists of protein and RNA components known as TERT and TER, respectively, and elongates telomeres by adding (TTAGGG) repeat sequences to their ends. Telomerase was first reported in the ciliate *Tetrahymena* by C. W. Greider and E. Blackburn in 1985.
- Telomere DNA: The terminal ends of chromosomes consist of telomere repeat sequences of TTAGGG, which are associated with telomere-binding proteins. This structure protects chromosome ends from being recognized as DNA double-strand breaks by the DNA repair machinery. Telomere DNA has been found to form different types of G-quadruplex structures in vitro depending on the medium conditions, such as the basket, chair, and hybrid. Recently, it has been suggested that telomere DNA exists as tetraplex structure in vivo.
- Ferrocenylnaphthalene diimide (FND): FND is a naphthalene diimide derivative composed of ferrocene moieties at the termini of its amide substituents. FND was first synthesized by S. Takenaka's group as an electrochemically active ligand having a preference for double-stranded DNA with threading intercalation. Some FND derivatives exhibit a higher preference for tetraplex DNA than for double-stranded DNA, which is used for electrochemical detection of tetraplex DNA.
- Electrochemical telomerase assay (ECTA): ECTA is performed using a telomerase substrate (TS) primer-immobilized electrode. The immobilized TS primer is elongated with TTAGGG repeats if telomerase is present in the sample solution. Elongation of the TS primer is detected by the electrochemical signal of FND, which increases with the increased extension of the TTAGGG repeats.

Definitions of Words and Terms

Oral cancer Oral cancer affects 640,000 people in the world every year and has a particularly high incidence in South Asia. Oral cancer is difficult to diagnose at an early stage. Patients with advanced carcinoma show significant decrease in quality of life even after surgery.

Telomerase repeat amplification protocol (TRAP) assay The TRAP assay is a detection method for telomerase activity and was reported by Kim et al. in 1994. Telomerase elongates telomeres by adding TTAGGG repeat units to their ends. Elongation of the telomerase substrate (TS) primer is used to estimate telomerase activity and is determined by the number or intensity of ladders in gel electrophoresis after PCR amplification. The TS and telomeric repeat (CX) sequences are used as forward and reverse primers in the PCR amplification, respectively.

Differential pulse voltammetry (DPV) and square wave voltammetry (SWV) DPV and SWV are techniques to diminish capacitive charging current by applying the potential in a stepwise manner when the reduction or oxidation current based on electroactive species in electrolyte is measured at the varied potential. DPV and SWV are different from other techniques that apply potential and correct the subsequent current.

Chronocoulometry (CC) CC is a technique used to measure the amount of charge in an electrochemically active species in an electrolyte. Absolute amount of the species is estimated based on the proportion between molecular weight and charge amount and is obtained from the temporal integration of charge amount.

DNAzyme DNAzyme is DNA carrying a catalytic activity such as site-specific DNA cleavage.

Telomerase inhibitor Telomerase inhibitors are molecules that inhibit the elongation of telomere DNA by telomerase either directly or indirectly. Telomerase is expressed in cancer cells, and therefore, telomerase inhibitors are expected to induce cancer cell death. Telomerase inhibitors can bind directly to telomerase to inhibit its activity or indirectly inhibit telomerase by binding tetraplex DNA to prevent telomerase access. Tetraplex DNA stabilizers, which bind to and stabilize tetraplex structures, are good candidates for anticancer drugs.

Introduction

Cancer is caused by the deregulation of biological functions in living cells. Telomerase is a ribonucleoprotein enzyme that elongates telomere DNA located at chromosomal termini. The association of telomere DNA and telomerase with cancer was proposed in 1973 by A. M. Olovnikov (1973). Telomerase was first reported in the ciliate *Tetrahymena* by C. W. Greider and E. Blackburn in 1985 (Greider and Blackburn 1985), and the elongation of telomere DNA by telomerase was reported by Greider in 1989 (Greider and Blackburn 1989). Since 1990, many studies have reported the connection between cancer and telomerase.

Aging and cancer cause the shortening of telomere DNA by triggering several stress-induced imbalances in the body (Fig. 1). Telomere DNA commonly exists as a D-loop structure to protect the chromosomal termini. Telomere DNA shortening prevents D-loop formation and causes DNA uncapping. DNA uncapping leads to exposing single-stranded DNA termini and subsequently end-to-end fusion of chromosomes or oncogene activation and causes genomic instability, which may contribute to cell death or carcinogenesis (Greider 1999). Generally, cell death is induced in normal cells by apoptosis. However, genomic instability can lead to inappropriate telomerase activation, resulting in cell immortalization and subsequent canceration.

Telomerase consists of a telomerase RNA component (TER); telomerase reverse transcriptase (TERT); catalytic core components, such as p65; and accessory factors including p75, p19, p45, p50, and Teb1 (Fig. 1). Electronic microscopic

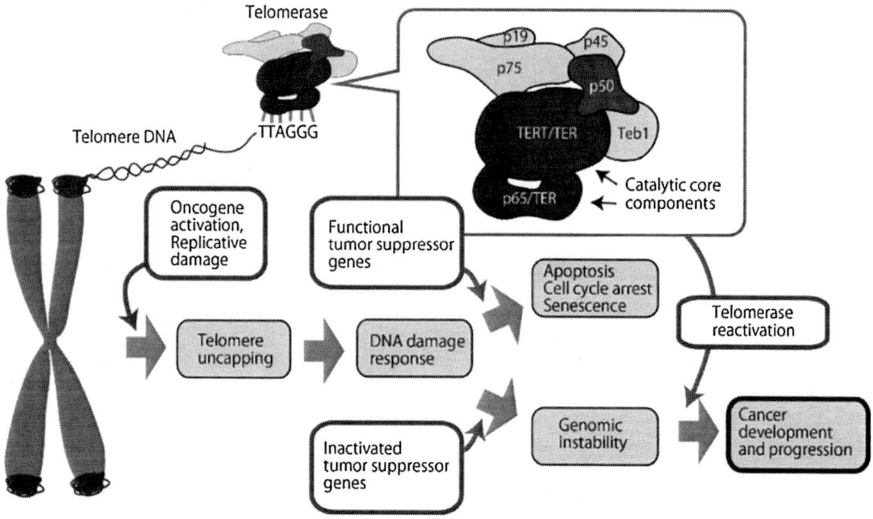

Fig. 1 Relationship between telomerase and telomere DNA in cancer development. The end of chromosomes are organized into telomere DNA, which consists of 2–30 kb of noncoding double-stranded TTAGGG repeats extended by 50–150-nucleotide overhangs of single-stranded TTAGGG repeats. Telomerase is a two-component enzyme composed of a catalytic protein subunit (*TERT*) and RNA template (*TER*) with accessory factors including Teb1, p75, p19, p45, and p50

images have revealed that these components are intricately combined like a jigsaw puzzle (Jiang et al. 2013). Telomerase components also contribute to TER stabilization through complexation. Teb1 forms a complex with telomere DNA to help elongate telomere DNA, and the p75-p19-p45 complex enhances telomerase activity. p50 binds the TER, Teb1, and the p75-p19-p45 complex. The TERT structure of *Tribolium castaneum* was realized by X-ray structural analysis (Gillis et al. 2008). The telomerase complex consists of dimers of human TERT units and the TER complex. Telomerase is thought to function as a dimer; however, this is still a matter of debate (Sauerwald et al. 2013). Current knowledge of telomere DNA elongation by telomerase has shown that extranuclear TERT is transported to the nucleus and forms a complex with TER (Hukezalie and Wong 2013). The D-Loop structure formed by telomere DNA at chromosomal termini is displaced (collapsed?), and the TER–TERT complex elongates the telomere termini by the addition of 6-bp TTAGGG repeats. A tetraplex structure is formed when the elongation reaction reaches four 6-bp TTAGGG repeats. Stabilization of tetraplex DNA at chromosomal termini inhibits the elongation reaction of telomerase. Therefore, ligands that stabilize the tetraplex structure are expected to inhibit telomerase activity and, therefore, may represent potential anticancer drugs.

Methods to detect telomerase activity have mainly analyzed the expression of the *hTERT* gene, the active component of telomerase (Hiyama and Hiyama 2003), or its catalytic activity by telomerase repeat amplification protocol (TRAP)

Table 1 Utility of telomerase as a diagnostic marker by TRAP assay

	Cancer patients	Normal individuals
	Telomerase positive (%)	
Biopsy		
Head and neck	25/26 (96.2)	9/41 (22.0)
Lung	86/128 (67.2)	0/10
Esophagus	52/54 (96.3)	33/48 (68.8)
Stomach	23/29 (79.3)	10/28 (35.7)
Colon	110/126 (87.3)	57/148 (38.5)
Liver	53/86 (61.6)	17/58 (29.3)
Bile duct	20/26 (76.9)	0/10
Bladder	46/54 (85.2)	30/56 (53.6)
Prostate	101/134 (75.4)	14/120 (11.7)
Uterus	138/164 (84.1)	58/158 (36.7)
Skin	130/159 (81.8)	14/58 (24.1)
Washing/brushing		
Head and neck	110/195 (56.4)	70/321 (21.8)
Brushing/bronchial alveolar lavage	123/188 (65.4)	16/211 (7.6)
Washing/urine	166/229 (72.5)	6/153 (3.9)
Cervical scraping	105/273 (38.5)	36/189 (19.0)

assay (Kim et al. 1994). The TRAP assay has been used to evaluate telomerase activity in many tumor types (Hiyama and Hiyama 2003) and to screen telomerase inhibitors (Cian et al. 2007). The TRAP assay uses the telomerase substrate (TS) primer (5′-AAT CCG TCG AGC AGA GTT-3′) as a telomerase substrate. Telomerase elongates the TS primer by adding TTAGGG repeats to the 3′-terminal. Extended products are amplified by polymerase chain reaction (PCR) using the CX primer and resolved by electrophoresis. The CX primer comprises a partially complementary sequence to the TTAGGG repeat so as not to increase the melting temperature or stability of the DNA duplex. A ladder of bands differing by 6 bp is obtained by the partial hybridization of the CX primer with the PCR products. Telomerase activity is estimated by the number of ladders and their intensities. Telomerase activity has been detected in many human cancers using the TRAP assay, with an expression rate of 85 % in most tumor tissues (Table 1; Hiyama and Hiyama 2003). Therefore, telomerase is expected to be a useful marker for cancer diagnosis. However, the cancer detection rate of the washing/brushing sample (38.5–72.5 %) was inferior to that of the biopsy sample (61.6–96.3 %). The low detection rate in the washing/brushing sample was due to contamination by foreign substances in the sample, which inhibited PCR. Telomerase activity has been detected in invasive samples such as saliva (Zhong et al. 2005; Mutirangura et al. 1996; Mao et al. 1996; Thongprasom et al. 1998) and urine (Sanchini 2005).

Oral cancer occurs at a high rate in southern Asia and is difficult to discriminate from other diseases of the oral mucosa, such as oral leukoplakia or oral lichen planus. Precancerous lesions of the oral mucosa require continuous monitoring because of their high probability for cancer progression. Telomerase activity and *hTERT* gene expression analysis have been achieved in human oral squamous cell carcinoma cell lines such as HSC-2 cells and human tongue squamous cell carcinoma cell lines such as HSC-3 and have shown high levels of telomerase activity and *hTERT* gene expression in these cell lines (Fujimoto et al. 2001). Furthermore, telomerase activity was detected even in 0.6-μl culture cell extracts (Fujimoto et al. 2001). Telomerase activity was tested in oral cancer patients by TRAP assay soon after it was developed by Kim et al. (Mutirangura et al. 1996; Mao et al. 1996). Mutirangura et al. reported that telomerase activity was observed in 88 % of oral cancers and in 38 % of oral leukoplakias, a precancerous lesion. Telomerase activity was also detected in oral lichen planus (Thongprasom et al. 1998). However, precancerous lesions were benign and none of the leukoplakia samples progressed to cancer. Therefore, the development of rapid and simple methods is important to quantitatively monitor the progression of precancerous lesions. The TRAP assay can determine the presence or absence of telomerase activity but not the degree of activity. This is due to the PCR step, which amplifies the elongated TS primer. Therefore, research efforts have focused on the development of PCR-free methods to detect telomerase activity.

Recent Developments in Detection Methods for Telomerase Activity

TRAP assay is a detection method for telomerase activity and includes a PCR amplification step. Contaminated clinical samples inhibit PCR, resulting in a lack of ladders in the gel electrophoresis. These samples may be considered negative even when telomerase activity is present (Kulla and Katz 2008). Therefore, many research groups have investigated non-PCR-based methods to alternatively detect telomerase activity (Kulla and Katz 2008; Zhou and Xing 2012). Detection methods for telomerase activity are summarized below from a standpoint of practical realization. Direct assay of telomerase activity was achieved using the radiation ^{32}P-α-dGTP marker (20 μCi; 3,000 Ci/mmol; Cian et al. 2007). Because ^{32}P-α-dGTP is incorporated into the elongated TS primer, ladders differing by 6 bp are observed on gel electrophoresis without PCR amplification. This direct assay was used to evaluate the telomerase inhibitory activity of a drug without the issue of drug-related PCR inhibition (Cian et al. 2007).

Willner's group developed several detection methods for telomerase activity (Pavlov et al. 2004; Xiao et al. 2004). In one method, the telomerase elongation reaction was achieved using a TS primer-immobilized electrode in the presence of biotinylated UTP. The addition of dNTP results in the incorporation of biotin into thymine residues in the elongated TS primer. The TS primer is treated with alkaline phosphatase-modified streptavidin, and telomerase activity is monitored by the electrochemical response induced by the hydrolysis of 5-bromo-4-chloro-3-indolylphosphate (Pavlov et al. 2004). The telomerase detection method developed by Willner's group amplifies the elongated TS primer directly or indirectly

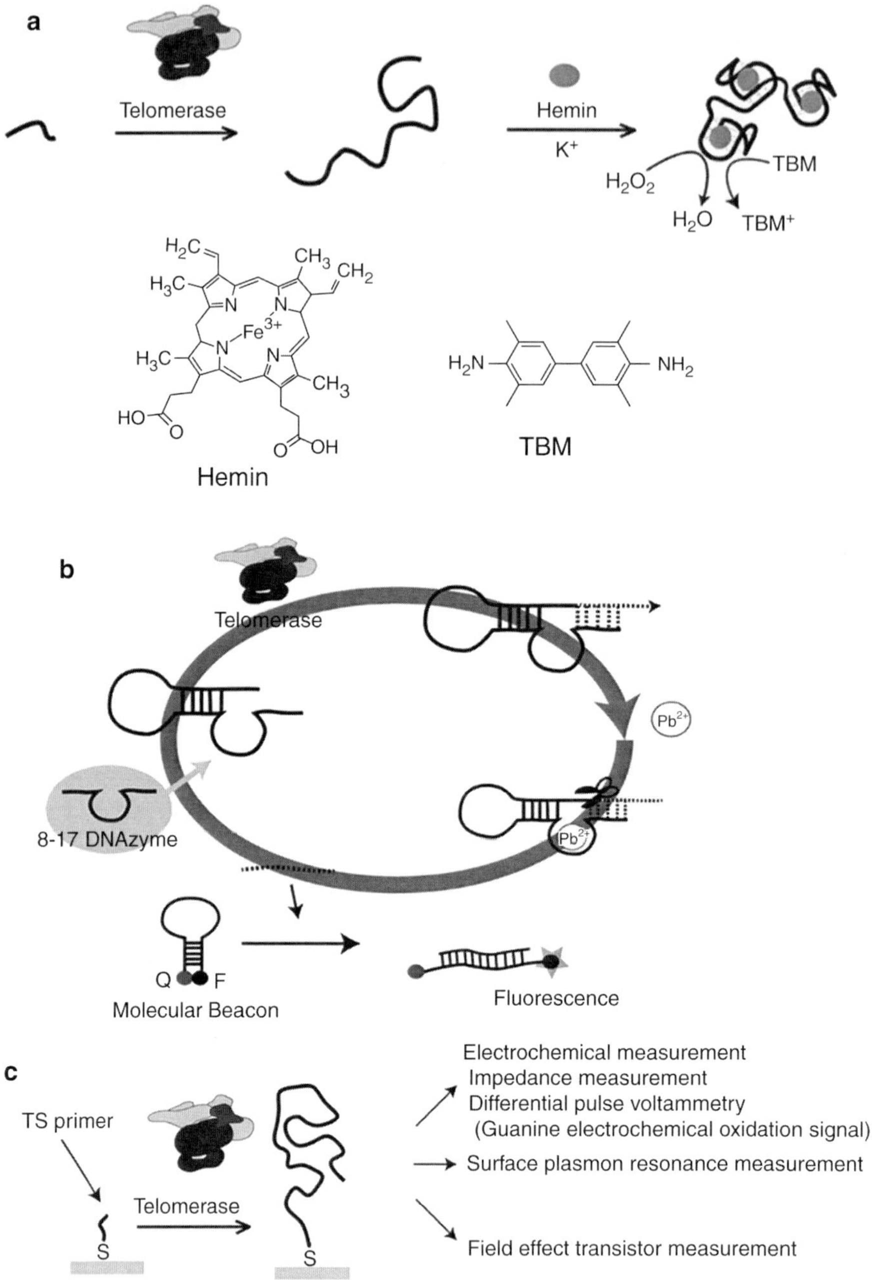

Fig. 2 Principle of non-PCR-based telomerase detection methods. (**a**) Hemin-catalyzed telomerase detection. The elongated telomerase substrate (*TS*) primer forms a tetraplex structure with bound hemin, and this complex acts as DNAzyme to generate TMB+ from TMB and H_2O_2. Telomerase activity is estimated by measuring the absorbance of TMB^+ at 650 nm.

on modified catalytic sites. Quach et al. reported fluorometric telomerase detection using SYBR Green to detect tetraplex DNA (Quach et al. 2013). Willner's group also developed a telomerase detection method that uses a TS primer carrying quantum dots conjugated with a complementary telomere DNA fragment and doxorubicin (Raichlin et al. 2011). The complementary telomere DNA fragment hybridizes with the elongated TS primer, and elongated telomere DNA is detected by the fluorescence quenching of quantum dots induced by the binding of the DNA duplex with doxorubicin. Using this method, telomerase activity was quantitated in over 270–2,700 cancer cells/μL, with a detection limit of 270 cells/μL.

Hemin–G-quadruplex DNAzyme units have been used to detect telomerase activity (Freeman et al. 2010). DNA elongated by telomerase forms a tetraplex structure in the presence of potassium ions and binds to hemin to generate TBM^+. Hemin, which acts as a tetraplex DNA binder, catalyzes the conversion of TMB and H_2O_2 to TMB+ (Fig. 2a). TMB+ is quantitated by determining its absorbance at 650 nm. TMB+ generation is dependent on the level of telomerase activity and, therefore, can be used to assess telomerase activity. This method is capable of quantitating telomerase activity in 200–3,000 cancer cells within 1.5 h.

8–17 DNAzyme, a hammerhead DNAzyme, has also been used to detect telomerase activity (Santoro and Joyce 1997). Wang et al. introduced the Pb^{II}-dependent 8–17 DNAzyme to the TS primer and developed a detection method by combining this modified primer with the molecular beacon system as shown in Fig. 2b (Wang et al. 2013). In this system, the hammerhead-like loop structure, which is formed by telomerase elongation of the TS primer, is cleaved by Pb^{2+}, and the cleaved fragments are fluorometrically detected by the molecular beacon. This method permits telomerase detection in 0.1–1.0 μg lysate containing misplaced proteins within 1 h. Tian et al. also reported the successful detection of telomerase activity using this system, with a detection limit of 200 cancer cells (Tian et al. 2013).

Many detection methods for telomerase activity have used TS primer-immobilized substrates. These methods are summarized in Fig. 2c. Zheng et al. monitored TS primer elongation by immobilizing it on a silicon nanowire to create a field-effect transistor system (Zheng et al. 2005). Maesawa et al. used a surface plasmon resonance (SPR) technique to analyze the elongation kinetics of the immobilized TS primer in various cell culture lysates and found that the elongation rate was dependent on cell type (Maesawa et al. 2003). Eskiocak et al.

Fig. 2 (continued) (**b**) DNAzyme-based probes for telomerase detection. Telomerase elongation of the TS primer carrying 8–17 DNAzyme forms a hammerhead DNAzyme structure. Cleavage of the telomere DNA fragment from the hammerhead DNAzyme by Pb^{2+} results in its hybridization with the molecular beacon to produce fluorescence. Telomerase activity is estimated by the fluorescence intensity. (**c**) Principle of telomerase detection methods using a TS primer-immobilized electrode. Elongation of the immobilized TS primer by telomerase is determined by electrochemical, surface plasmon resonance, and field-effect transistor measurements

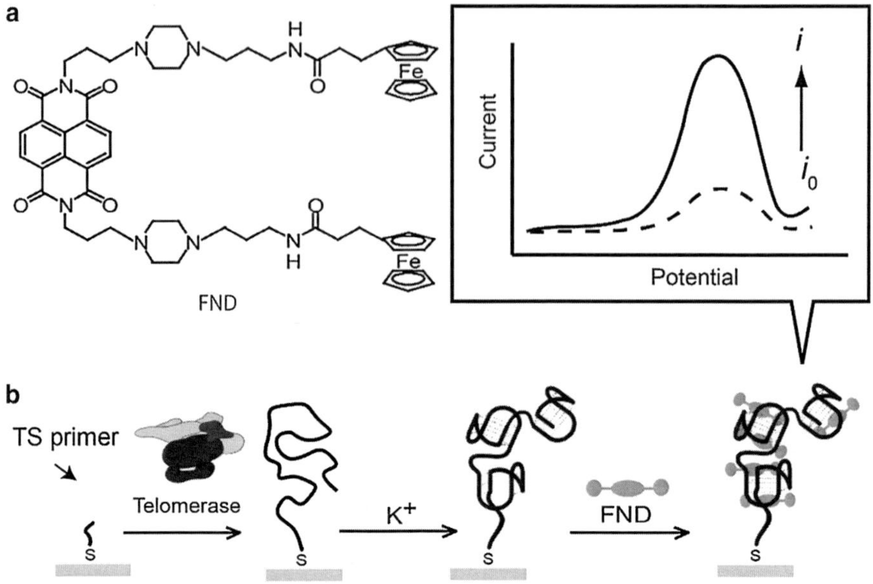

Fig. 3 Principle of electrochemical telomerase assay (*ECTA*) using *FND*. (**a**) Chemical structure of ferrocenylnaphthalene diimide (*FND*). (B) Electrochemical telomerase assay (*ECTA*) using *FND*. The TS primer immobilized on the electrode is elongated by telomerase, and *FND* binds to the product to give rise to a current. The data are standardized with Δi, defined as $(i/i_0-1) \times 100$ %, where i_0 and i refer to the current before and after elongation, respectively

monitored telomerase activity electrochemically based on the oxidation current of guanine bases using a TS primer-immobilized electrode (Eskiocak et al. 2007). This method showed a detection limit of 100 ng/μL cancer cell lysate. Impedance change in the TS primer-immobilized electrode was used to detect telomerase activity in 10^3–10^5 cancer cells (Yang et al. 2011). Telomerase detection based on SPR is superior in terms of label-free detection.

Electrochemical techniques also offer label-free detection coupled with high sensitivity. Takenaka's group developed an electrochemical telomerase assay (ECTA) using ferrocenylnaphthalene diimide (FND), an electrochemically active tetraplex ligand (Sato et al. 2005, Sato et al. 2012; Mori et al. 2013). The principle of the ECTA method is shown in Fig. 3. Elongation of the immobilized TS primer is electrochemically detected as concentrated FND bound to tetraplex DNA, which is formed using the square wave voltammetry (SWV) technique in the presence of potassium ions. This method including the telomerase elongation step can be performed within 30 min (Sato 2005; Mori et al. 2013).

Takenaka's group also developed another method to quantitate telomerase activity based on the chronocoulometric technique (Steel et al. 1998). This method can be used for the detailed analysis of telomerase activity due to its ability to quantify DNA elongation by telomerase (Sato and Takenaka 2012).

Oral Cancer Screening Using ECTA

Many researchers, including Takenaka's group, have increased the amount of DNA immobilized on the electrode to improve hybridization detection. This method has been applied to hybridization assays using 20–40-mer DNA probe-immobilized electrodes (Drummond et al. 2003; Luo and Hsing 2009) for the analysis of *p53* point mutations (Boon et al. 2000; Umek et al. 2001; Miyahara et al. 2002; Weng et al. 2008) and hypermethylation of specific genes (Sato et al. 2006; Kato et al. 2008; Sato et al. 2012) and has shown high detection limits (Takenaka et al. 2000; Xiao et al. 2006). Takenaka's group applied this method to detect elongated TS primer in clinical oral cancer samples (Mori et al. 2013). When the TS primer-immobilized electrode was immersed with sample solution and incubated at 37 °C for 30 min, elongated TS primer was formed on the electrode. The quantity of DNA elongated with TTAGGG repeating units in the sample solution was estimated electrochemically by FND bound to the tetraplex structure in electrolyte containing 0.1 M KCl. Telomerase activity was estimated by the increase in current after incubation of sample solution in the presence of 20 μM FND in 0.1 M KCl using the SWV technique (Sato 2005; Mori et al. 2013). Naphthalene diimide derivatives specifically bind double-stranded DNA through threading intercalation (Yen et al. 1982). Takenaka's group found that FND does not bind to double-stranded DNA but binds to tetraplex DNA with high affinity depending on its substituent structure (Sato 2005). FND binds tetraplex DNA through stacking interactions with the G-tetrad plane as has been described for similar derivatives (Cuenca et al. 2008). This electrochemical FND-based telomerase assay has been named ECTA by Takenaka's group.

Takenaka's group compared the ability of TRAP and ECTA methods to detect telomerase activity in HSC-2 cells, HSC-3 cells, and Ca9-22 cells, a series of human gingival squamous cell carcinoma cell lines, and SAS cells, a human tongue squamous cell carcinoma cell line. The TRAP method detected telomerase activity in the four cell lines in over 200 cells. In contrast with the TRAP method, the ECTA method detected telomerase activity in the four cell lines in over 10 cells. These results indicate that the ECTA method is a highly sensitive telomerase detection method and is 20 times more sensitive than the TRAP method. Furthermore, telomerase activity was correlated with the gene expression level of *hTERT*, telomerase catalytic factor, in the four cell lines. Takenaka's group also evaluated telomerase activity in oral tissues and exfoliative cells from oral cancer patients and normal individuals using the ECTA and TRAP methods. A telomerase-positive decision was obtained in 90 % (+ decision, 50 %; ± decision, 40 %) of oral cancer tissues and 30 % (positive decision, 10 %; ambiguous decision, 20 %) of oral exfoliative cells with the TRAP method (Fig. 4a). These findings were in agreement with a previous report (Hiyama and Hiyama 2003) and suggested that telomerase activity in oral exfoliative cells is difficult to detect with the TRAP method. The telomerase activity in oral tissue and exfoliative cell samples was also tested using the ECTA method, which evaluated the change in current before and after sample treatment. The results are summarized in Fig. 4b. ECTA showed a current increase

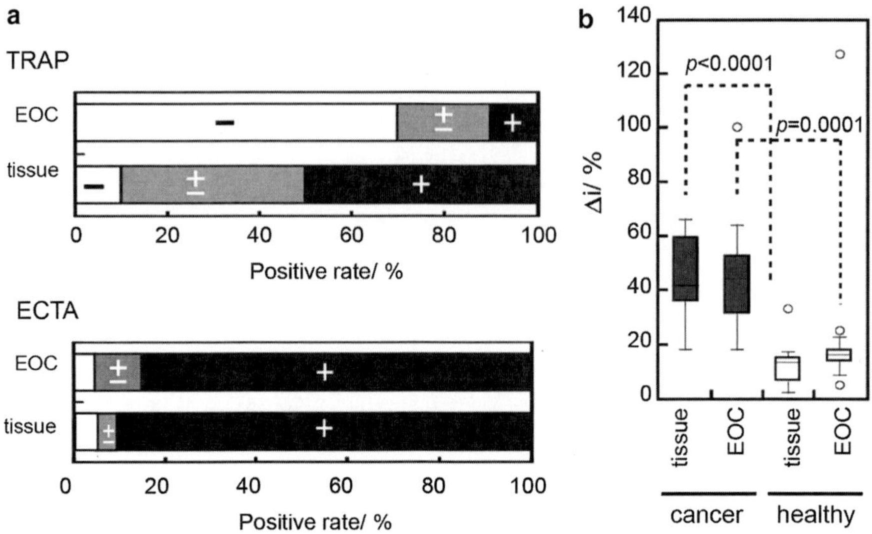

Fig. 4 Comparison of telomerase repeat amplification protocol (*TRAP*) and electrochemical telomerase assay (*ECTA*) methods. (**a**) Comparison of telomerase repeat amplification protocol (*TRAP*) and electrochemical telomerase assay (*ECTA*) methods to detect telomerase activity in tissues and exfoliative oral cells (*EOC*) from oral cancer patients and healthy individuals. In the TRAP assay, more than five clear ladders were considered positive (+), 1–4 ladders were considered ambiguous (±), and no ladder was considered negative (−). In ECTA, current increase $> 30\ \%\ \Delta i$ was considered positive (+), current increase between 20 % and 30 % was considered ambiguous (±), and current increase < 20 % was considered negative (−). (**b**) Box plots for telomerase activity expressed as current increase in Δi for 20 oral cancer patients (*filled boxes*) and 10 healthy volunteers (*open boxes*)

greater than 34 % and 30 % in the tissues and oral exfoliative cells of oral cancer patients, respectively, whereas the current increase was less than 15 % and 18 % in the tissues and oral exfoliative cells of normal individuals, respectively. Therefore, the ECTA method was able to discriminate between cancer patients and normal individuals regardless of the specimen type. Positive telomerase rates were observed in tissue and oral exfoliative cells whether the threshold was set to 30 %, 90 %, or 85 %, (Fig. 4a). These results showed that ECTA method is superior to the TRAP method. In particular, the positive rate in oral exfoliative cells was dramatically improved with the ECTA method compared with the TRAP method. Together, these findings demonstrated that ECTA is a highly sensitive electrochemical PCR-free technique.

Telomerase activity using the ECTA method was compared with T criterion to assess the stage of cancer progression. Telomerase activity was tested in T1 (<2 cm in size) and T2 (>2 cm in size) tumors. The positive rate of telomerase activity for T1 tumors was 10 % higher than that of T2 tumors. This result is reasonable when considering that cancer progression is expected to influence the protein expression of telomerase. In a blind test of 31 cancer patients and 25 normal individuals, the right diagnosis ratio was 84 % when the threshold was set to 30 %. Because the ECTA method has a higher detection ratio for T1 tumors, this method is suitable for the screening of early stage oral cancer.

Telomerase Inhibition Assay Using ECTA

Telomerase elongation of telomere DNA at chromosomal termini leads to cell immortalization and canceration. Therefore, anticancer drugs have been developed to inhibit telomerase function, such as tetraplex DNA stabilizers (Cian et al. 2007) or antisense targeting of telomerase RNA (Mergny et al. 2002). Drug-related inhibition of telomerase activity is commonly evaluated using the PCR-based TRAP method. However, anti-telomerase drugs may inhibit PCR itself; therefore, this methodology may not be suitable for drug screening of telomere inhibitory activity. ECTA, which is a PCR-free detection method, is suitable for screening the telomerase inhibitory activity of drug candidates. Because FND also binds to tetraplex DNA, precise evaluation of telomerase reaction is not possible if the inhibitory compound does not bind strongly enough to tetraplex DNA so that it is not removed upon washing in the proper buffer solution. Therefore, FND was replaced by hexaammineruthenium (III) complex, which is known to bind with one ligand per three DNA phosphate anions (Steel et al. 1998), to evaluate the inhibitory activity of anti-telomerase compounds (Sato and Takenaka 2012). The principle behind the ECTA telomerase assay using hexaammineruthenium (III) chloride is summarized in Fig. 5. An initial chronocoulometric analysis of the TS primer-immobilized electrode in the absence or presence of hexaammineruthenium (III) complex is performed to determine the charge quantity (Q) of hexaammineruthenium (III) complex using the Cottrell equation. This analysis is done to determine the immobilization density of TS primer on the electrode. The TS primer-immobilized electrode is treated with cancer cell lysate in the presence of various drug concentrations at 37 °C for 30 min. After washing the electrode, chronocoulometric measurement is performed in the presence of the hexaammineruthenium (III) complex. Increased Q in this process indicates DNA elongation on the electrode.

The telomerase inhibitory activity of 10 compounds was evaluated using the ECTA assay based on chronocoulometry with hexaammineruthenium (III) chloride: TMPyP4 (Han et al. 1999), PIPER (Fedoroff et al. 1998), 3′-azido-3′-deoxythymidine triphosphate (AZT; Arion et al. 1998), 5′-d(TTAGGG)-3′ (Inhibitor III; Mergny et al. 2002), 2,6-bis[3-(*N*-piperidino)propionamido]anthracene-9,10-dione (Inhibitor V; Perry et al. 1998), ethidium bromide (EtBr), guanidine thiocyanate (Chomczynski and Sacchi 1987), FND3 (Sato and Takenaka 2008), FND7 (Sato et al. 2005), and tri naphthalene diimide (TND). The results are summarized in Fig. 6a. The increase in Q percentage was compared for a 10-μL lysate of 2.5 HeLa cervical cancer cells/μL in the presence of 2.5 μM of each reagent. Under these conditions, elongated DNA around $(TTAGGG)_{11}$ was observed in the absence of the compounds. Elongated DNAs of $(TTAGGG)_{10}$,

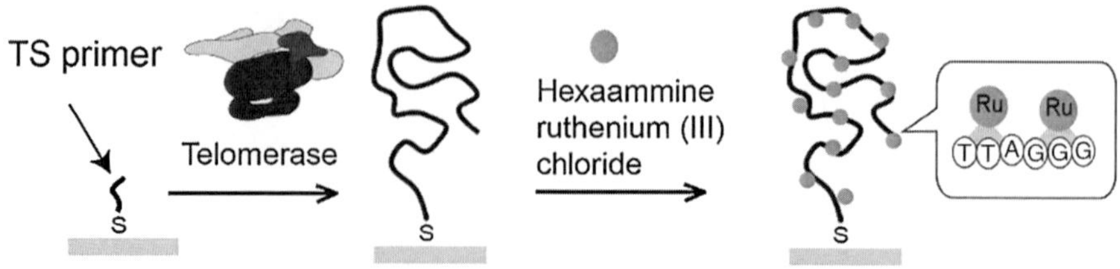

Fig. 5 Principle of electrochemical telomerase assay (*ECTA*) using hexaammineruthenium (III) chloride. Electrochemical telomerase assay based on chronocoulometry with hexaammineruthenium (III) chloride. This system estimates telomerase activity from the elongation of the telomerase substrate (*TS*) primer

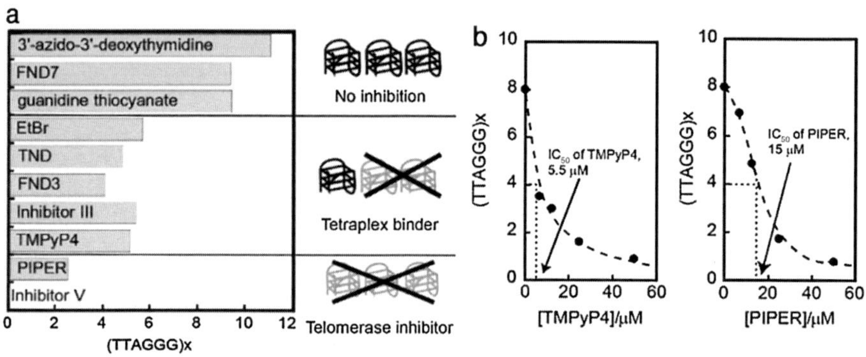

Fig. 6 Telomerase inhibition assay using the electrochemical telomerase assay (*ECTA*) method. (**a**) Telomerase inhibition assay using the electrochemical telomerase assay (*ECTA*) method. 3′-azido-3′-deoxythymidine triphosphate, *FND7*, guanidine thiocyanate, ethidium bromide (*EtBr*), *TND*, *FND3*, Inhibitor III, *TMPyP4*, *PIPER*, and *Inhibitor V* at a concentration of 2.5 μM were incubated with 25-cell extracts at 37 °C for 30 min. Immobilization density of the telomerase substrate (TS) primer was 4×10^{10} molecules/cm^2. (**b**) Telomerase inhibition assay using the *ECTA* method. *TMPyP4* and *PIPER* at concentrations of 6.8, 13, 25, and 50 μM were incubated in the presence of 100-cell extracts at 37 °C for 30 min. Immobilization density of the TS primer was 4×10^{10} molecules/cm^2

$(TTAGGG)_{10}$, and $(TTAGGG)_{11}$ were observed in the presence of FND7, guanidine thiocyanate, and AZT, respectively, suggesting a lack of telomerase inhibitory activity. $(TTAGGG)_4$, which is long enough to form one unit of tetraplex structure, was observed in the presence of TND, FND3, EtBr, TMPyP4, and Inhibitor III. This finding suggested that these compounds bind and stabilize the tetraplex DNA structure to prevent telomerase access. In the case of PIPER and Inhibitor V, $(TTAGGG)_3$ and $(TTAGGG)_0$ were obtained, respectively. Therefore, these compounds directly inhibit telomerase binding rather than indirectly inhibiting telomerase by binding to telomere DNA. These results suggested that the ECTA method not only estimates the telomerase inhibitory activity of compounds but also their mechanism of inhibition by providing the DNA length after the elongation reaction in the presence of the compound. The compound concentration required to inhibit telomerase activity 50 % (IC_{50} value) was also estimated from the plot of the inhibitory activity against the compound concentration. The IC_{50} values for TMPyP4 and PIPER were estimated to be 5.5 μM and 15 μM, respectively, using a modified ECTA method (Fig. 6b) and were in agreement with the values of 8.9 μM and >20 μM obtained from the TRAP assay.

Conclusion

Although cancer development is a complicated process, telomerase is undoubtedly an important factor in this process. As an enzyme, telomerase RNA is not very stable; therefore, its functional analysis was delayed. However, the analysis of telomerase and its telomere DNA substrates and the structure of chromosomal termini have increased precipitously since 2000. After 2000, high-ordered structures of telomere DNA have been reported and include a variety of tetraplex structures, such as basket type (Wang and Patel 1993) and hybrid type (Xu et al. 2006). Ligands capable of specifically binding to telomere tetraplex structures represent potential anticancer drugs (Cian 2008). Although tetraplex binders were initially investigated as anticancer drugs, they also show promise as analytical reagents to detect telomere DNA and telomerase activity and to visualize the fluorescently labeled tetraplex structure of chromosomal DNA in a cell. Anti-telomerase drugs will not only allow for the mechanistic analysis of cancer development but also cancer repression. Telomerase is expected to be an excellent tumor marker, and therefore, rapid and simple screening methods for telomerase activity in clinical samples should facilitate cancer diagnosis.

Summary Points

- Since 85 % of telomerase activity was observed in cancer tissue using TRAP assay, telomerase is expected as useful cancer marker.
- Some of the cancer drug exhibits by inhibition of telomerase activity and is expected as new anticancer drug. TRAP assay known as screening method of telomerase activity provides evaluation of telomerase inhibitory ability of drug. However, telomerase inhibition ability of drug showing PCR inhibition is difficult to evaluate, and thus, development of PCR-free telomerase assay is required.
- Novel telomerase screening methods have been developed that do not require PCR and gel electrophoresis based on the DNAzyme and TS primer-immobilized methods. These methods have improved the positive rate of sample brushing/washing.
- Oral cancer screening using PCR-free ECTA assay with FND as the tetraplex DNA binder has shown telomerase-positive rates of 90 % and 85 % in lysates of cancerous tissue and exfoliated oral cells, respectively, and an accuracy rate of 84 % for 56 unknown clinical samples in a blind test.

- ECTA using hexaammineruthenium (III) chloride is useful for the high-throughput screening of telomerase inhibitors and the study of their inhibition mechanisms.

References

Arion D, Kaushik N, McCormick S, et al. Phenotypic mechanism of HIV-1 resistance to 3′-azido-3′-deoxythymidine (AZT): increased polymerization processivity and enhanced sensitivity to pyrophosphate of the mutant viral reverse transcriptase. Biochemistry. 1998;37:15908–17.

Boon EM, Ceres DM, Drummond TG, et al. Mutation detection by electrocatalysis at DNA-modified electrodes. Nat Biotechnol. 2000;18:1096–100.

Chomczynski P, Sacchi N. Single-step method of RNA isolation by acid guanidinium thiocyanate-phenol-chloroform extraction. Anal Biochem. 1987;162:156–9.

Cian AD, Cristofari G, Reichenbach P, et al. Reevaluation of telomerase inhibition by quadruplex ligands and their mechanisms of action. Proc Natl Acad Sci U S A. 2007;104:17347–52.

Cuenca F, Greciano O, Gunaratnam M, et al. Tri- and tetra-substituted naphthalene diimides as potent G-quadruplex ligands. Bioorg Med Chem Lett. 2008;18:1668–73.

Drummond TG, Hill MG, Barton JK. Electrochemical DNA sensors. Nat Biotechnol. 2003;21:1192–9.

Eskiocak U, Ozkan-Ariksoysal D, Ozsoz M, et al. Label-free detection of telomerase activity using guanine electrochemical oxidation signal. Anal Chem. 2007;79:8807–11.

Fedoroff OY, Salazar M, Han H, et al. NMR-Based model of a telomerase-inhibiting compound bound to G-quadruplex DNA. Biochemistry. 1998;37:12367–74.

Freeman R, Sharon E, Teller C, Henning A, Tzfati Y, Willner I, et al. DNAzyme-like activity of hemin-telomeric G-quadruplexes for the optical analysis of telomerase and its inhibitors. Chembiochem. 2010;11:2362–7.

Fujimoto R, Kamata N, Yokoyama K, et al. Expression of telomerase components in oral keratinocytes and squamous cell carcinomas. Oral Oncol. 2001;37:132–40.

Gillis AJ, Schuller AP, Skordalakes E. Structure of the tribolium castaneum telomerase catalytic subunit TERT. Nature. 2008;455:633–7.

Greider CW, Telomeres Do D-Loop-T-Loop. Cell. 1999;97:419–22.

Greider CW, Blackburn EH. Identification of a specific telomere terminal transferase activity in Tetrahymena extracts. Cell. 1985;43:405–13.

Greider CW, Blackburn EH. A telomeric sequence in the RNA of Tetrahymena telomerase required for telomere repeat synthesis. Nature. 1989;337:331–7.

Han FX, Wheelhouse RT, Hurley LH. Interactions of TMPyP4 and TMPyP2 with quadruplex DNA. Structural basis for the differential effects on telomerase inhibition. J Am Chem Soc. 1999;121:3562–9.

Hiyama E, Hiyama K. Telomerase as tumor marker. Cancer Lett. 2003;194:221–33.

Hukezalie KR, Wong JMY. Structure–function relationship and biogenesis regulation of the human telomerase holoenzyme. FEBS J. 2013;280:3194–204.

Jiang J, Miracco EJ, Hong K, Ecket B, et al. The architecture of Tetrahymena telomerase holoenzyme. Nature. 2013;496:187–92.

Kato D, Sekioka N, Ueda A, et al. A nanocarbon film electrode as a platform for exploring DNA methylation. J Am Chem Soc. 2008;130:3716–7.

Kim NW, Piatyszek MA, Prowse KR, et al. Specific association of human telomerase activity with immortal cells and cancer. Science. 1994;266:2011–5.

Kulla E, Katz E. Biosensor techniques used for determination of telomerase activity in cancer cells. Sensors. 2008;8:347–69.

Luo X, Hsing IM. Electrochemical techniques on sequence-specific PCR amplicon detection for point-of-care applications. Analyst. 2009;134:1957–64.

Maesawa C, Inaba T, Sato H, et al. A rapid biosensor chip assay for measuring of telomerase activity using surface plasmon resonance. Nucleic Acids Res. 2003;31:E4–4.

Mao L, El-Naggar AK, Fan YH, et al. Telomerase activity in head and neck squamous cell carcinoma and adjacent tissues. Can Res Suppl. 1996;56:5600–4.

Mergny JL, Riou JF, Mailliet P, Teulade-Fichou MP, Gilson E. Natural and pharmacological regulation of telomerase. Nucleic Acid Res. 2002;30:839–65.

Miyahara H, Yamashita K, Kanai M, et al. Electrochemical analysis of single nucleotide polymorphisms of p53 gene. Talanta. 2002;56:829–35.

Mori K, Sato S, Kodama M, et al. Oral cancer diagnosis via a ferrocenylnaphthalene diimide-based electrochemical telomerase assay. Clin Chem. 2013;59:289–95.

Mutirangura A, Supiyaphun P, Trirekapan S, et al. Telomerase activity in oral leukoplakia and head and neck squamous cell carcinoma. Can Res Suppl. 1996;56:3530–3.

Olovnikov AM. A theory of marginotomy. The incomplete copying of template margin in enzymic synthesis of polynucleotides and biological significance of the phenomenon. J Theor Biol. 1973;41:181–90.

Pavlov V, Willner I, Dishon A, et al. Amplified detection of telomerase activity using electrochemical and quartz crystal microbalance measurements. Biosens Bioelectron. 2004;20:1011–21.

Perry PJ, Gowan SM, Reszka AP, et al. 1,4- and 2,6-disubstituted amidoanthracene-9,10-dione derivatives as inhibitors of human telomerase. J Med Chem. 1998;41:3253–60.

Quach QH, Jung J, Kim H, et al. A simple, fast and highly sensitive assay for the detection of telomerase activity. Chem Commun. 2013;49:6596–8.

Raichlin S, Sharon E, Freeman R, Tzfati Y, Willner I. Electron-transfer quenching of nucleic acid-functionalized CdSe/ZnS quantum dots by doxorubicin: a versatile system for the optical detection of DNA, aptamer-substrate complexes and telomerase activity. Biosens Bioelectron. 2011;26:4681–9.

Sanchini MA, Gunelli R, Nanni O, et al. Relevance of urine telomerase in the diagnosis of bladder cancer. JAMA. 2005;294:2052–6.

Santoro SW, Joyce GF. A general purpose RNA-cleaving DNA enzyme. Proc Natl Acad Sci U S A. 1997;94:4262–6.

Sato S, Takenaka S. Linker effect of ferrocenylnaphthalene diimide ligands in the interaction with double stranded DNA. J Organomet Chem. 2008;693:1177–85.

Sato S, Takenaka S. PCR-free telomerase assay using chronocoulometry coupled with hexaammineruthenium(III) chloride. Anal Chem. 2012;84:1772–5.

Sato S, Kondo H, Nojima T, et al. Electrochemical telomerase assay with ferrocenylnaphthalene diimide as a tetraplex DNA-specific binder. Anal Chem. 2005a;77:7304–9.

Sato S, Nojima T, Waki M, et al. Supramolecular complex formation by beta-cyclodextrin and ferrocenylnaphthalene diimide-intercalated double stranded DNA and improved electrochemical gene detection. Molecules. 2005b;10:693–707.

Sato S, Hokazono K, Irie T, et al. Ferrocenylnaphthalene diimide-based electrochemical detection of methylated gene. Anal Chim Acta. 2006;578:82–7.

Sato S, Tsueda M, Kanezaki Y, et al. Detection of an aberrant methylation of CDH4 gene in PCR product by ferrocenylnaphthalene diimide-based electrochemical hybridization assay. Anal Chim Acta. 2012;715:42–8.

Sauerwald A, Sandin S, Cristofari G, et al. Structure of active dimeric human telomerase. Nat Struct Mol Biol. 2013;20:454–61.

Steel AB, Herne TM, Tarlov MJ. Electrochemical quantitation of DNA immobilized on gold. Anal Chem. 1998;70:4670–7.

Takenaka S, Yamashita K, Takagi M, et al. DNA sensing on a DNA probe-modified electrode using ferrocenylnaphthalene diimide as the electrochemically active ligand. Anal Chem. 2000;72:1334–41.

Thongprasom K, Mutirangura A, Cheerat S. Telomerase activity in oral lichen planus. J Oral Pathol Med. 1998;27:395–8.

Tian T, Peng S, Xiao H, et al. Highly sensitive detection of telomerase based on a DNAzyme strategy. Chem Commun. 2013;49:2652–4.

Umek RM, Lin SW, Vielmetter J, et al. Electronic detection of nucleic acids: a versatile platform for molecular diagnostics. J Mol Diagn. 2001;3:74–84.

Wang Y, Patel DJ. Solution structure of the human telomeric repeat d[AG3(T2AG3)3] G-tetraplex. Structure. 1993;1:263–82.

Wang H, Donovan MJ, Meng L, et al. DNAzyme-based probes for telomerase detection in early-stage cancer diagnosis. Chemistry. 2013;19:4633–9.

Weng J, Zhang J, Li H, et al. Label-free DNA sensor by boron-doped diamond electrode using an ac impedimetric approach. Anal Chem. 2008;80:7075–83.

Xiao Y, Lubin AA, Baker BR, et al. Single-step electronic detection of femtomolar DNA by target-induced strand displacement in an electrode-bound duplex. Proc Natl Acad Sci U S A. 2006;103:16677–80.

Xiao Y, Pavlov V, Gill R, Bourenko T, Willner I. Lighting up biochemiluminescence by the surface self-assembly of DNA-hemin complexes. Chem Bio Chem. 2004;5:374–9.

Xu Y, Noguchi Y, Sugiyama H. The new models of the human telomere d[AGGG(TTAGGG)3] in K+ solution. Bioorg Med Chem. 2006;14:5584–91.

Yang W, Zhu X, Liu Q, et al. Label-free detection of telomerase activity in HeLa cells using electrochemical impedance spectroscopy. Chem Commun. 2011;47:3129–31.

Yen SF, Gabbay EJ, Wilson WD. Interaction of aromatic imides with deoxyribonucleic acid. Spectrophotometric and viscometric studies. Biochemistry. 1982;21:2070–6.

Zheng G, Patolsky F, Cui Y, et al. Multiplexed electrical detection of cancer markers with nanowire sensor arrays. Nat Biotechnol. 2005;23:1294–301.

Zhong LP, Chen GF, Xu ZF, et al. Detection of telomerase activity in saliva from oral squamous cell carcinoma patients. Int J Oral Maxillofac Surg. 2005;34:566–70.

Zhou X, Xing D. Assays for human telomerase activity: progress and prospects. Chem Soc Rev. 2012;41:4643–56.

Matrix Metalloproteinase Family as Molecular Biomarkers in Oral Squamous Cell Carcinoma

34

Thian-Sze Wong, Wei Gao, and Zeng-Hong Li

Contents

Abstract

Oral squamous cell carcinoma (OSCC) is one of the most common head and neck malignancies. Affected by the nonspecific symptoms, the OSCC patients are usually diagnosed in the advanced stages. To improve the treatment outcome and survival of OSCC, identification of the reliable biomarkers for early detection and prognosis

T.-S. Wong (✉) • W. Gao
Department of Surgery, Queen Mary Hospital, The University of Hong Kong, Pokfulam, Hong Kong
e-mail: thiansze@gmail.com; thiansze@graduate.hku.hk; gaoweiwayne@gmail.com

Z.-H. Li
Department of Surgery, The University of Hong Kong, Pokfulam, Hong Kong
e-mail: john19850920@gmail.com

V.R. Preedy, V.B. Patel (eds.), *Biomarkers in Cancer, Biomarkers in Disease: Methods, Discoveries and Applications*,
DOI 10.1007/978-94-007-7681-4_10

prediction is necessary. Matrix metalloproteinases (MMPs) function in degradation of ECM, generation of active peptides, and activation of specific growth factors, resulting in forming an environment promoting tumor progression, invasion, and metastasis. MMPs can be applied as potential cancer biomarkers for early detection, risk assessment, prognostic analysis, and evaluation of response to treatment in OSCC. Moreover, the detection of MMPs in blood and saliva is a feasible mean to monitor OSCC in a noninvasive manner. Among all of the MMPs, MMP-9 probably appears to be the most promising biomarker with most of the documented cases. However, an updated meta-analysis is needed to confirm the advantages of MMP-9 over other MMPs in monitoring OSCC. Furthermore, an observation that MMP-11 in combination with Ets-1 or vascular endothelial growth factor (VEGF) leads to more accurate prediction in comparison with MMP-11 alone warrants further studies on the use of combined biomarkers in OSCC management.

List of Abbreviations

BL	Basal Lamina
ECM	Extracellular Matrix
EGF	Epidermal Growth Factor
ELISA	Enzyme-Linked Immunosorbant Assay
ER-a	Estrogen Receptor-a
ER-b	Estrogen Receptor-b
FGF-2	Fibroblast Growth Factor-2
HPV	Human Papillomavirus
MMPs	Matrix Metalloproteinases
MT-MMPs	Membrane-Type MMPs
OSCC	Oral Squamous Cell Carcinoma
OTSCC	Oral Tongue Squamous Cell Carcinoma
TGF-β	Transforming Growth Factor-β
VEGF	Vascular Endothelial Growth Factor

Key Facts

Key Facts of Oral Squamous Cell Carcinoma (OSCC)

Approximately 90 % oral cancers are squamous cell carcinomas.
OSCC is one of the most common head and neck cancers.
Surgery, radiotherapy, and chemotherapy are the common treatment strategies.
Migration and invasion are often observed in OSCC.
OSCC has a high recurrence rate.

Key Facts of Matrix Metalloproteinases (MMPs)

MMPs are a family of endopeptidases capable of degrading extracellular matrix components.
The human MMPs family is composed of at least 28 members.

MMPs are classified into six groups: collagenases, gelatinases, stromelysins, matrilysins, membrane-type MMPs, and other MMPs.
The expression levels of MMPs were higher in tumor samples from patients with OSCC compared with normal controls.
MMPs can be detected in tissue, blood, as well as saliva from patients with OSCC.
MMPs are potential biomarkers for OSCC.

Definitions of Words and Terms

Extracellular Matrix (ECM) ECM consists of a variety of macromolecules including collagen, fibronectin, laminin, and proteoglycans and plays a crucial role in regulating cell functions and establishing a specific microenvironment.

ECM Remodeling The degradation of ECM by multiple proteolytic enzymes such as cysteine proteases, aspartic proteases, serine proteases, as well as MMPs. It occurs in both normal physiological situations and pathological conditions.

Human Papillomavirus (HPV) HPV is a circular double-stranded DNA virus with approximately 7,900 base pairs in size and is one of the most critical risk factors of cancer.

Zymography Zymography is a technique to evaluate the activity of matrix metalloproteinase by detecting the degradation of their preferential substrates.

Oral Dysplasia Oral dysplasia is defined as the development of cytologic atypia in cells of oral cavity and is visualized as leukoplakia.

Oral Lichen Planus Oral lichen planus is a T cell-mediated chronic mucocutaneous disease affecting oral mucosa. Reticular and erosive/ulcerative forms are the most common forms of oral lichen planus.

Oral Precancerous Lesions Oral precancerous lesions refer to morphologically altered oral tissues with high risk of tumor transformation. Common oral precancerous lesions include oral lichen planus, leukoplakia, erythroplakia, oral submucous fibrosis, and actinic cheilitis.

Introduction

Oral Squamous Cell Carcinoma (OSCC)

OSCC is one of the most common cancer types in head and neck malignancies. According to the guideline of American Joint Committee on Cancer and the Union for International Cancer Control, the involved regions of OSCC include lip, anterior two-thirds of the tongue (oral tongue), buccal mucosa, floor of mouth, hard palate, lower and upper alveolus and gingiva, and the retromolar trigone (Scully and Bagan 2009). Among these, the tongue is the most common place where the tumor located. It's estimated that there are 13,590 new patients (male 9,900 and female 3,690 respectively) suffering from oral tongue squamous cell carcinoma (OTSCC) in the United States in 2013, accounting for 0.8 % of the total new cancer cases. It also accounts for about 0.4 % estimated cancer-related death (Siegel et al. 2013). The definite cause of OSCC is not yet determined, but some risk factors are believed to be implicated in this disease: (1) tobacco and alcohol consumption, (2) betel quid usage, and (3) human papillomavirus (HPV) infection (Scully and Bagan 2009). In addition, the presence of precancerous lesions, such as leukoplakia, oral lichen planus, and oral submucous fibrosis, is also associated with the greater risk of malignant transformation.

Currently, the diagnosis of OSCC depends on the clinical manifestation and histological analysis. However, in the early stage, OSCC usually presents with atypical and painless signs, such as ulcer, exophytic mass, and deep infiltration with varying degrees of induration. It rarely draws the patients' attentions until the cancer develops to the advanced stage and becomes visually detectable (Rusthoven et al. 2008). Moreover, the diagnostic routine with visual inspection may have difficulty to find out the latent or hidden tumors, leading to false-negative results. Due to the rich lymphatic network and highly vascularized structure, regional migration and invasion are common. The common treatment strategies for OSCC include surgery, radiotherapy, and chemotherapy. In most of the cases, surgery is the primary choice, and radiotherapy and chemotherapy would be applied to improve locoregional control after surgery. Primary radiotherapy or chemotherapy is used for the unresectable OSCC or for the early stage disease to avoid functional and cosmetic defects. Again, due to the late diagnosis, the overall OSCC prognosis is unsatisfied with a high recurrence rate (Rusthoven et al. 2008). To improve the treatment outcome for OSCC patients, identification of the reliable biomarkers for early detection and prognosis prediction is necessary.

Matrix Metalloproteinases (MMPs)

MMPs are a family of zinc-dependent endopeptidases that have the capacity to degrade extracellular matrix (ECM) components (Tallant et al. 2010). The structures of MMPs comprise an N-terminal signal peptide that targets the protein to plasma membrane or secretory pathway, a propeptide domain, a catalytic domain, and a hemopexin-like domain (Fig. 1) (Parks et al. 2004). The propeptide contains a cysteine residue that binds to zinc ion of the catalytic site through its side-chain thiol group, thus maintaining proMMPs in a catalytically inactive state (Kohrmann et al. 2009). Proteolytic removal of the propeptide domain *via* other activated MMPs or serine proteinases outside the cell leads to activation of proMMPs. The catalytic domain consists of a zinc ion in the active site that is essential for the catalytic processes of MMPs (Parks et al. 2004). The catalytic zinc ion is ligated to

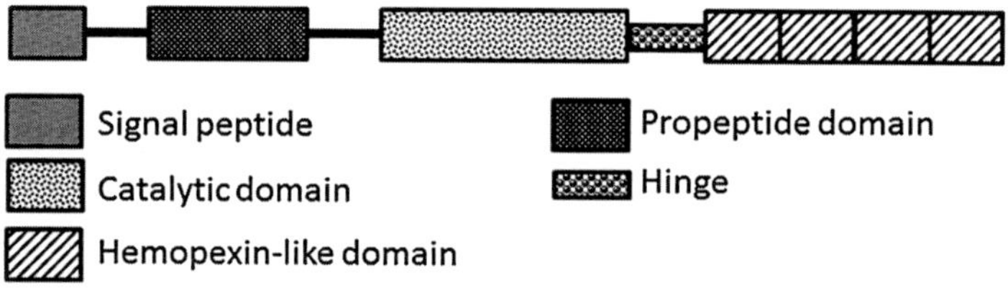

Fig. 1 Domain structure of matrix metalloproteinase. The structures of MMPs comprise an N-terminal signal peptide that targets the protein to plasma membrane or secretory pathway, a propeptide domain, a catalytic domain, a hinge, and a hemopexin-like domain

three histidine residues, which are conserved among all MMPs. The highly conserved hemopexin-like domain shares sequence similarity to plasma protein hemopexin and participates in substrate recognition and interaction with tissue inhibitors of metalloproteinases (Massova et al. 1998). Depending on substrate specificity for ECM components and structural characteristics, MMPs are classified into 6 groups: collagenases, gelatinases, stromelysins, matrilysins, metalloelastases, membrane-type MMPs, and other MMPs that do not belong to any of the previous (Table 1) (Groblewska et al. 2012).

The ECM is composed of collagen, fibronectin, laminin, and proteoglycans of connective tissue and functions as barriers preventing the spread of tumor cells (Roy et al. 2009). MMPs promote tumor invasion and metastasis by degradation of ECM, which permits cancer cells to invade the surrounding tissue or nearby blood vessels. Furthermore, degradation of ECM by MMPs produces biologically active peptides, such as a peptide harboring epidermal growth factor (EGF)-like motifs that participates in EGFR signaling and a peptide involved in integrin signaling and insulin-like growth factor which stimulates tumor progression (Hua et al. 2011). In addition, MMPs activate the bioavailability of growth factors including vascular endothelial growth factor (VEGF), fibroblast growth factor-2 (FGF-2), and transforming growth factor-β (TGF-β), thus promoting cell proliferation and angiogenesis (Shuman Moss et al. 2012). MMPs thereby function in forming an environment facilitating tumor progression by generating biologically active peptides and activating specific growth factors (Fig. 2).

MMPs as Biomarkers in OSCC

In OSCC, a series of in vitro studies revealed that the MMP family members were related to OSCC development in diverse stages, including carcinogenesis, growth, and aggressive behaviors (Table 2). Moreover, MMP level in tissue (Table 3), blood, and salivary (Table 4) of patients with OSCC can be applied as potential cancer biomarkers for early detection, risk assessment, prognostic analysis, and evaluation of response to treatment. MMPs were found to be overexpressed in tissue, blood, and salivary of patients with OSCC, and the overexpression could be detected and quantified using various methods including immunohistochemistry,

Table 1 Classification of MMP Family

Subtype	Name	Former name	Encoding gene	Chromosome
Collagenases	MMP-1	Collagenase-1	MMP-1	11q21-q22
	MMP-8	Collagenase-2	MMP-8	11q21-q22
	MMP-13	Collagenase-3	MMP-13	11q22.3
Gelatinases	MMP-2	Gelatinase A	MMP-2	16q13-q21
	MMP-9	Gelatinase B	MMP-9	20q12-q13
Stromelysins	MMP-3	Stromelysin-1	MMP-3	11q22.3
	MMP-10	Stromelysin-2	MMP-10	11q22.3
	MMP-11	Stromelysin-3	MMP-11	22q11.23
Matrilysins	MMP-7	Matrilysin	MMP-7	11q21-q22
	MMP-26	Endometase	MMP-26	11p15
Membrane-type (MT) MMPs	MMP-14	MT1-MMP	MMP-14	14q11-q12
	MMP-15	MT2-MMP	MMP-15	16q13
	MMP-16	MT3-MMP	MMP-16	8q21
	MMP-17	MT4-MMP	MMP-17	12q24.3
	MMP-24	MT5-MMP	MMP-24	20q11.2
	MMP-25	MT6-MMP	MMP-25	16p13.3
Metalloelastases	MMP-12	MME	MMP-12	11q22.3
Others	ILF3	–	MMP-4	19p13.2
	MMP-19	–	MMP-19	12q14
	MMP-20	Enamelysin	MMP-20	11q22.3
	MMP-21	–	MMP-21	10q26.3
	MMP-23	CA-MMP	MMP-23B	1p36.3
	MMP-27	–	MMP-27	11q24
	MMP-28	Epilysin	MMP-28	17q21.1

The classification of the MMPs has multiple criteria. Depending on substrate specificity for extracellular matrix (ECM) components and structural characteristics, MMPs are classified into seven groups above. *MME* (macrophage metalloelastase)

reverse transcriptase-polymerase chain reaction, in situ hybridization, zymography, and enzyme-linked immunosorbant assay (ELISA). In the following sections, we focused on the MMPs which demonstrated potential clinical utility by documented studies in OSCC.

Collagenases

Collagen is the major component of the ECM and the basement membrane. It has a fibrillar organization and a triple-helical structure formed by three polypeptide chains, making it hard to be degraded by proteolysis. In light of this property, the basement membrane is an effective barrier to prevent the invasion and migration of abnormal cells. Before the tumor cells invade or migrate to the distant sites, production of substrates including MMPs to degrade this barrier mainly composed by collagens is therefore essential.

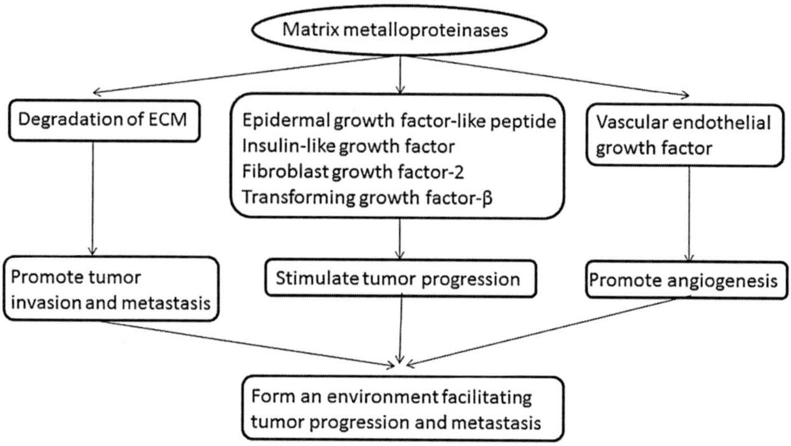

Fig. 2 Biological functions of matrix metalloproteinases in tumor progression and metastasis. MMPs promote tumor invasion and metastasis by degradation of ECM. Furthermore, degradation of ECM by MMPs produces growth factors such as a peptide harboring epidermal growth factor-like motifs, insulin-like growth factor, fibroblast growth factor-2, and transforming growth factor-β, which stimulate tumor progression. In addition, MMPs activate the bioavailability of vascular endothelial growth factor, thus promoting angiogenesis

Table 2 The MMP family members involved in OSCC development

	MMP family members
Promoting the precancerous lesion to the OSCC	MMP-1, MMP-2, MMP-9
Inhibiting proliferation of OSCC	MMP-8
Promoting the migration of OSCC to the lymph node	MMP-1, MMP-8
Enhancing invasion of OSCC	MMP-1, MMP-8, MMP-13
Enhancing angiogenesis of OSCC	MMP-13

A series of in vitro studies revealed that the MMP family members were related to OSCC development in diverse stages, including carcinogenesis, growth, and aggressive behaviors. *OSCC* oral squamous cell carcinoma

The collagenases contribute to the initiation of fibrillar collagens (type I, II, III, V, and IX) degradation. They cleave the collagens into triple-helical fragments, which are further broken down by the other MMPs family members (Massova et al. 1998). The collagenases contain three members: MMP-1 (collagenase-1), MMP-8 (collagenase-2), and MMP-13 (collagenase-3). MMP-1 is also known as interstitial collagenase and fibroblast collagenase for the degradation of the ECM-interstitial collagens types I, II, and III; MMP-8, also named neutrophil collagenase, is considered as the most effective collagenase to initiate type I collagen degradation; MMP-13 plays an important role in the degradation of the type II collagen (Tallant et al. 2010). The whole OSCC development progress is in a stepwise manner and could broadly divide into two stages: (1) before breaking down the basement membrane (from precancerous disease, to epithelial dysplasia, and then to

Table 3 Tissue MMP levels act as biomarkers in OSCC

	MMP family members
Cancerization from oral preneoplastic lesion	MMP-7, MMP-9, MMP-11
OSCC identification	MMP-2, MMP-9
Advanced tumor stage	MMP-2, MMP-3, MMP-9
Lymph node metastasis	MMP-1, MMP-2, MMP-3, MMP-9
Aggressive invasion	MMP-1, MMP-3, MMP-7, MMP-13, MMP-14
Poor differentiation	MMP-1, MMP-2, MMP-3, MMP-7, MMP-9, MMP-26
Cisplatin resistance	MMP-13
Poor prognosis	MMP-2, MMP-8, MMP-9, MMP-14

The diagnostic and prognostic value of MMP family members in OTSCC was firstly studied through the traditional histological analysis in tissue samples. Besides distinguishing the OTSCC patients, MMPs could also applied to evaluate the specific situation and the treatment effect, as well as accessing the prognosis of OSCC. *OTSCC* oral tongue squamous cell carcinoma

Table 4 Plasma, serum, or saliva MMP levels serve as biomarkers in OSCC

	Plasma/ Serum	Saliva
OSCC identification	MMP-2, MMP-9	MMP-1, MMP-3, MMP-2, MMP-9
Advanced tumor stage	MMP-2, MMP-9	MMP-1, MMP-3
Lymph node metastasis	MMP-2	–
Poor differentiation	MMP-2, MMP-9	–

Compared to the traditional histological analysis in tissue, plasma/serum sample analysis and salivary analysis have the advantages of noninvasiveness and revealing local alteration of the oral environment and systemic change simultaneously. Part of the MMP family members were validated to be able to act as OSCC biomarkers in the noninvasive test

carcinoma in situ) and (2) after breaking down the basement membrane (from the early stage to the advanced stage of carcinoma, with an increasing invasiveness).

All the three collagenases have been documented to contribute in all the stages of OSCC progression. The MMP-1 mRNA was overexpressed in the oral dysplasia (Jordan et al. 2004). MMP-1 dysregulation promoted the progression from the precancerous lesion to the OSCC (Nishizawa et al. 2007). Moreover, MMP-1 expression was correlated with the histopathological grading of OSCC. The expression of MMP-1 protein in epithelium was significantly elevated with the increase in histopathological grade (George et al. 2010). However, for MMP-8, contradictory reports were noted. Korpi et al. suggested that high MMP-8 expression had a protective function to the patients with OTSCC. Tongue carcinoma patients with high MMP-8 expression had a better prognosis (Korpi et al. 2008). MMP-8 can cleave the estrogen receptor-a (ER-a) and estrogen receptor-b (ER-b) and thus activated the estrogen-related pathway, which consequently decreased the proliferation rate of the cancer cells (Korpi et al. 2008).

Clinical studies demonstrated that MMP-1 mRNA was involved in the tissue remodeling and cell-ECM adhesion, facilitating the tumor cells to migrate into the lymph nodes (Nagata et al. 2003). Moreover, MMP-1 overexpression was an early marker for predicting lymph node metastasis of OTSCC (Zhang et al. 2011). MMP-13 was positively related to the invasion depth and tumor size (Mäkinen et al. 2012). Further, overexpression of MMP-1 and MMP-13 was linked to the aggressive behavior of OSCC, leading to adjacent bone invasion in OSCC patients (Lim et al. 2012; Mäkinen et al. 2012; Erdem et al. 2007). In addition, enhanced angiogenesis was closely correlated with an aggressive tumor development and a poor prognosis of the patients. MMP-13 was able to promote angiogenesis in OSCC. Its overexpression could enhance the capillary tube formation, and immunochemistry test on tumor tissues revealed that high MMP-13 expression was related to the larger number of blood vessels. FAK and ERK signaling pathways were involved in the mechanisms by which MMP-13 promoted angiogenesis. Moreover, MMP-13 upregulated VEGF-A secretion, which was also positively correlated with the vessel formation (Kudo et al. 2012).

MMPs are also implicated in the response of OSCC to the treatment. Chemotherapy is one of the common treatment selections for advanced OSCC. It is usually adopted as part of the chemoradiotherapy, which is believed to have an improved effect compared with the exclusive radiotherapy. However, not all the patients can benefit from the chemotherapy due to the chemoresistance, while they have to suffer from the adverse effect of the chemical drugs. Therefore, effective biomarkers are needed to predict the patient's response to chemotherapy, in order to decide whether the chemotherapy should be adopted. In head and neck squamous cell carcinoma cell lines, MMP-13 was identified as predictive biomarkers for the resistance of cisplatin, which is one of the most common chemotherapeutic reagents treating advanced OSCC (Ansell et al. 2009). The higher the MMP-13 expressed, the higher survival rate the HNSCC cells showed under the cisplatin treatment. Therefore, for an OSCC patient with MMP-13 overexpression, cisplatin treatment was probably not suitable.

Detection of genetic polymorphism in MMPs provides another approach to evaluate the risk of OSCC. Genetic polymorphism is defined as "the occurrence in the same population of two or more alleles at one locus, each with appreciable frequency" (Cavalli-Sforza 1973). With the technical advances in molecular diagnosis, detection of genetic polymorphism in MMP is easy to conduct. It was found that gene polymorphism in MMP-1 was an effective biomarker for the susceptibility of OSCC. For example, the 2G allele of MMP-1 promoter region played a key role in the early onset of OSCC. Using age of 45 years old as a cutoff point, the 2G allele was closely associated with a significantly higher risk of OSCC in the patients younger than 45 years old (Nishizawa et al. 2007). Normal individuals with MMP-1-1607 1G/2G polymorphism showed an evaluated risk for OSCC compared with the 1G allele carriers (Vairaktaris et al. 2007).

With the emerging understanding on the molecular mechanisms of collagenase expression, it is recognized that there are a number of upstream regulators for collagenase overexpression in OSCC. For instance, the E1AF (Shindoh et al. 1996), c-Met (Lim et al. 2012), and S100A14 (Sapkota et al. 2011) were proved to promote the OSCC cell invasion and migration by stimulating MMP-1 expression.

CXCR4 enhanced the migration and invasion of oral tongue squamous cell carcinoma cell line by promoting MMP-13 overexpression (Yu et al. 2011). Endostatin could inhibit the activation of MMP-13 and thus suppressed the tumor cell invasion (Nyberg et al. 2003).

Upregulation of collagenase is also controlled by external factors' exposure including environmental carcinogen and natural cancer-preventive agents. Betel quid chewing is a common habit existing in China and South Asia, which has been proved as a risk factor to OSCC by the International Agency for Research on Cancer (IARC 2004). Although the definite carcinogenic mechanism of betel quid usage is still unknown, MMPs are proved to play an important role in it. MMP-1 was highly expressed among the OSCC patients with history of betel quid usage (Lee et al. 2008). The OSCC cell lines survived from the cytotoxic betel quid extract showed higher MMP-1 mRNA and protein levels, as well as a significant acceleration of motility compared with their parental controls, which would lead to worse prognosis and higher recurrence rate (Lee et al. 2008). Additionally, the betel quid extract could increase the expression of MMP-8 in the OSCC cells, which enhanced the migration and invasion of the tumor cells (Liu et al. 2007). The intake of green vegetable was suggested to be good for suppressing the invasiveness of cancer cells as the antitumor components were targeting collagenase. In the antitumor effect test of the isothiocyanate in cruciferous vegetables, the secret form of MMP-1 and MMP-2 was inhibited by sulforaphane, leading to proliferation suppression in various oral cell lines (Jee et al. 2011).

Gelatinases

Gelatinases comprise two members: gelatinase A (MMP-2, 72 kDa) and gelatinase B (MMP-9, 92 kDa). Both MMP-2 and MMP-9 contain a gelatin-binding domain, similar to the motif in fibronectin (Parks et al. 2004). This domain distinguishes MMP-2 and MMP-9 from other MMPs and is involved in the interaction with gelatin or gelatin-like substrates. The substrates of gelatinases include type IV, V, VII, X, XI, and XIV collagens, gelatin, elastin, proteoglycan, and fibronectin (Kerkelä and Saarialho-Kere 2003). Cleavage of the prodomain of inactive zymogens results in the activation of latent gelatinases. Inactive proMMP-2 is activated by thrombin, plasmin, and other MMPs including MMP-1, MMP-7, MMP-13, MMP-14, MMP-15, MMP-16, MMP-24, and MMP-25. Inactive proMMP-9 is activated by MMP-2, MMP-3, MMP-7, MMP-10, MMP-13, and MMP-26, trypsin-2, plasmin, and chymotrypsin-like proteinase (Vilen et al. 2013). MMP-2 was expressed in cells around carcinoma islands and in some fibroblast-like cells of tumoral stroma. MMP-9 was expressed in tumor cells and macrophages.

The mechanisms underlying the regulation of MMP-2 and MMP-9 have been demonstrated by several studies. TGF-β1 elevated the expression of MMP-2 and enhanced MMP-2 activation. Moreover, ERK1/2 and p38 MAPK were involved in the regulation of MMP-2 activity (Munshi et al. 2004). Additionally, MMP-2 and MMP-9 expression were activated by scatter factor, also known as hepatocyte growth factor, in OSCC cell line (Bennett et al. 2000). In addition, exocyst complex component Sec8 regulated the secretion of MMP-2 and MMP-9 (Yamamoto et al. 2013). Expression of Sec8 was elevated in OSCC cell lines. Sec8 participated in the regulation of actin dynamics during cellular migration. Knockout of Sec8 resulted in decreased secretion of proMMP-2 and proMMP-9 in OSCC cell lines.

MMP-2 and MMP-9 were useful markers for judging transformation potency from oral dysplasia or lichen planus to OSCC. Malignant development of oral dysplasia can be predicted through identifying specific architectural and cytological alterations of oral dysplasia (Tamamura et al. 2013). Only certain oral dysplasia will inevitably develop into cancer. Alterations in type IV collagen, the major structural component of basal lamina (BL), were associated with progression from a preneoplastic state to malignant. MMP-2 and MMP-9 degrade BL type IV collagen and other extracellular matrix protein. Normal oral mucosa, oral dysplasia, and carcinoma in situ maintained continuous collagen chain expression patterns in the BLs, while OSCC displayed varying degrees of collagen α(IV) chain loss. In the meantime, expression levels of MMP-2 and MMP-9 were increased in OSCC than in normal oral mucosa or oral dysplasia. OSCC with higher degree exhibited enhanced MMP-2 and MMP-9 expression, especially along the tumor advancing front. Furthermore, MMP-2 and MMP-9 expressed in the areas corresponding to collagen α(IV) chain loss in OSCC. Taken together, these results suggested that the degradation of collagen α(IV) chain was consistent with elevated expression levels of MMP-2 and MMP-9, which contributed to progression from oral dysplasia to OSCC. Moreover, the expression of MMP-9 in oral dysplasia progressed to OSCC was higher than those that did not, implicating the prediction value of MMP-9 in malignant progression of oral dysplasia (Jordan et al. 2004). Oral lichen planus is a chronic inflammatory disease of oral mucosa and about 1–4 % cases will transform into oral cancer (Chen et al. 2008). Depending on clinical behavior and histological changes, lichen planus is classified into nonatrophic form and atrophic form. Expression levels of MMP-2 and MMP-9 in OSCC from oral lichen planus were higher than those in nonatrophic oral lichen planus or normal oral mucosa. Moreover, expression level of MMP-9 was elevated in atrophic oral lichen planus in comparison with nonatrophic oral lichen planus, indicating that atrophic form is more likely to transform into tumor than nonatrophic form, and MMP-9 may be a potential marker for predicting cancerization from lichen planus.

MMP-2 and MMP-9 were correlated with lymph node metastasis, clinical stage, differentiation degree, survival rate, recurrence, and risk in OSCC. Tumor tissues from patients with OSCC displayed higher tissue mRNA level of MMP-2 and MMP-9 in comparison with adjacent normal tissues (Singh et al. 2010). Patients with OSCC also exhibited elevated plasma pro, active, and total MMP-2 and MMP-9 levels from zymography and ELISA in comparison with healthy volunteers. The receiver operating characteristic curve analysis from both zymography and ELISA showed that plasma MMP-2 and MMP-9 levels could significantly distinguish OSCC patients from healthy controls. In addition, proMMP-9 and active MMP-9 levels derived from zymography were associated with differentiation, stage, and infiltration. ProMMP-2 and active MMP-2 levels from zymography were related to differentiation and lymph node metastasis. Additionally, plasma MMP-2 protein level determined by ELISA was positively correlated with lymph node metastasis, tumor stage, and differentiation degree by the multivariate analysis (Singh et al. 2010). Although MMP-2 and MMP-9 were not correlated with survival rate of all patients with OSCC, MMP-9 was associated with survival rate of patients without lymph node metastasis. In this subgroup of patients, the survival of patients with MMP-9 negative was longer than that of patients with MMP-9 positive (de Vicente et al. 2005). Patients with MMP-9-positive margins exhibited a decreased recurrence-free survival than those with MMP-9-negative ones by Kaplan-Meier analysis. In multivariate analysis, MMP-9 was negatively correlated with recurrence-free survival (Ogbureke et al. 2012). In addition, the -1562 C-to-T polymorphism in MMP-9 promoter was correlated with OSCC risk only in younger areca chewers (Tu et al. 2007). In a similar study, patients with initial (I and II) stages of OSCC displayed higher detection frequency for the high expression T allele in the -1562 C-to-T polymorphism in the MMP-9 gene promoter than that of control (Vairaktaris et al. 2008).

Besides the studies on tissue and plasma samples, MMP-2 and MMP-9 were also applied in the salivary analysis. Saliva is secreted by salivary glands, the oral, and oropharyngeal mucosa, playing a crucial role in the OTSCC pathogenesis. Furthermore, serum is another important resource of saliva, which means that the similar components are shared in these two substrates. Theoretically, analysis of the saliva can reveal the local alteration of the oral environment, as well as the systemic change which can be detected by the serum evaluation. Finally, compared to serum, saliva has a lower background and inhibitory substances (Zimmermann et al. 2007). With these advantages, the salivary analysis played a more and more important role in the OSCC screening, diagnosis, and follow-up after treatment. The concentration of MMP-2 and MMP-9 was significantly increased in saliva of patients with oral cancer compared with normal control (Shpitzer et al. 2007).

However, contradictory results were reported by some studies. High-grade tumor had lower expression level of MMP-2 than low-grade tumor in patients with OSCC (Barros et al. 2011). Similarity, expression of MMP-2 was not correlated with invasion depth of the early OSCC, tumor-free survival rate, cervical lymph node metastasis, or tumor cell differentiation in patients with OSCC (Kim et al. 2006). MMP-9 was not related to lymph node metastasis or distal metastasis, although it was correlated with clinical stage or tumor size in OSCC (Lin et al. 2012).

Moreover, some studies demonstrated that MMP-9 was a better diagnostic and prognostic marker than MMP-2 in OSCC. MMP-9 was more useful for predicting malignant progression from oral lichen planus than MMP-2 (Chen et al. 2008). MMP-9 was more reliable for OSCC grading than MMP-2 (Mohtasham et al. 2013). Expression level of MMP-9 and activated form of MMP-9 were associated with metastasis, while MMP-2 was not significantly related to metastasis (Hong et al. 2000). The expression levels of MMP-2 and MMP-9 were determined at histologically negative margins of OSCCs with tumor recurrence. MMP-9 was preferred predictor for tumor recurrence than MMP-2 (Ogbureke et al. 2012).

Stromelysins

Stromelysins are composed of three MMPs: stromelysins-1 (MMP-3), stromelysins-2 (MMP-10), and stromelysin-3 (MMP-11) (Groblewska et al. 2012). In OSCC, MMP-3 was expressed by epithelial cancer cells and stromal cells around the tumor nests (Kusukawa et al. 1995). MMP-3 was present inside the tumor and in the invasive front. The substrates of MMP-3 include collagen type II, IV, IX, X, and XI, fibronectin, gelatins, elastin, proteoglycanase, E-cadherin, and osteopontin (Tadbir et al. 2012). Trypsin-2 activated MMP-3 by proteolytic cleavage of its propeptide domain. MMP-10 was expressed only by epithelial cells but not by stromal cells and expressed in both tumor and the invasive front. MMP-11 was present in stromal fibroblast cells around tumor islands as well as the stroma near the invasive front (Soni et al. 2003). MMP-11 was localized to perinuclear region and cytoplasm of epithelial tumor cells. MMP-11 was activated by furin-dependent proteolytic cleavage inside the cells and was secreted in an active form, which makes it different from other MMPs (Soni et al. 2003).

Tissue MMP-3 expression was associated with tumor stage, invasive mode, differentiation, and lymph node metastasis (Kusukawa et al. 1995). Tissue MMP-3 expression was higher in stage II OSCC tumors than that in stage I tumors. The well-differentiated OSCC displayed a higher expression of MMP-3 compared with moderately differentiated OSCC. Stronger expression of MMP-3 was observed in more invasive tumor. Tumors with lymph node metastasis showed increased expression level of MMP-3 in comparison with those without lymph node metastasis. However, serum MMP-3 expression was not correlated with clinicopathological features including tumor stage, lymph node or distant metastasis, and histological grade (Tadbir et al. 2012).

MMP-11 was associated with OSCC progression from precancerous lesions. The precancerous lesions with histologic evidence of hyperplasia or dysplasia may transform into OSCC with a rate of 5–10 % over a period of 10 years (Soni et al. 2003). Hyperplastic and dysplastic lesions exhibited increased expression level of MMP-11 compared with normal oral tissues. In addition, the expression level of MMP-11 was correlated with the expression of angiogenesis marker MVD in precancerous lesions, implicating a role of MMP-11 in angiogenesis during oral cancer progression.

MMP-11 in combination with Ets-1 or VEGF represented the most significant predictor in OSCC progression. VEGF could increase blood vessel permeability and enhance endothelial cell proliferation and migration, thus facilitating angiogenesis (Arora et al. 2005). It could promote metastasis by activating proteolytic enzymes that degrade tumor marginal extracellular matrix. The transcription factor Ets-1 was regulated by VEGF and could activate the expression of extracellular matrix proteases (Arora et al. 2005). A combination between MMP-11 and Ets-1 was the most accurate biomarker for predicting transformation from normal oral epithelium to precancerous stage, while concomitant expression of MMP-11 and VEGF represented the most significant biomarker for judging malignant transition from precancerous stage (Arora et al. 2005).

Matrilysins

There are two members in this subgroup: MMP-7 (matrilysin) and MMP-26 (endometase). Compared with other MMPs, hinge region and hemopexin domain are absent in the matrilysins, making MMP-7 and MMP-26 have the smallest structure among the 23 human MMP family members.

MMP-7, also named as the small putative uterine metalloproteinase (PUMP) at the beginning, was well known for its contribution in the epithelium repair (Dunsmore et al. 1998). This MMP was highly expressed in many epithelial tumors and acted as an important promoter in the cancerogenesis especially in the early stage of cancer (Fingleton et al. 1999). On the other hand, however, MMP-7 hindered the tumor angiogenesis by producing angiostatin, resulting in the subsequent suppression in tumor progression (Patterson and Sang 1997). Although MMP-7 showed a dual role in human cancers, all the current publications elucidated positive associations between MMP-7 and OSCC. As early as the oral precancerous lesions and carcinoma in situ, detection of MMP-7 by immunochemistry could be used to determine the cell proliferation center, and MMP-7 was involved in the malignant transformation process of oral epithelia (Tilakaratne et al. 2009). After this early period, the value of MMP-7 acted as a biomarker linked to the evaluation of invasiveness, metastasis, and the subsequent prognosis in OSCC cases. The high expression level of MMP-7 was positively associated with the invasive status in OSCC (Li and Cui 2013), as well as the poor differentiation of the cancer cells (Barros et al. 2011). On the contrary, it was not a satisfactory biomarker to predict lymph node metastasis (de Amorim et al. 2010; Li and Cui 2013).

MMP-26 is firstly detected in the fetal, placenta, and uterus (de Coignac et al. 2000; Marchenko et al. 2001). It was distinguished from other MMPs by the structure including an unusual cysteine-switch propeptide sequence and a threonine residue adjacent to the Zn-binding site. Similar to MMP-7, MMP-26 was positively related to the histopathological grade in OSCC (Barros et al. 2011), whereas it was not useful in recognition of metastasis (de Amorim et al. 2010).

Membrane-Type MMPs

Membrane-type MMPs (MT-MMPs) exist on the surface of invasive tumor cells depending on the exclusive transmembrane domain (Sato et al. 1994), which has a glycosylphosphatidylinositol anchor for binding (Kojima et al. 2000). Besides this domain and a cytoplasmic tail at the C-terminus, the membrane-type MMPs share the similar domain structure with other MMPs. There are totally 6 members: MT1-MMP (MMP-14), MT2-MMP (MMP-15), MT3-MMP (MMP-16), MT4-MMP (MMP-17), MT5-MMP (MMP-24), and MT6-MMP (MMP-25). They contribute richly to activation of other MMPs and the cell-matrix interaction. For instance, the MT1-MMP, MT2-MMP, and MT3-MMP could transform the proMMP-2 into the proteolytic enzymes. The MT1-MMP was able to activate the proMMP13 (Kerkela and Saarialho-Kere 2003).

Similar to a variety of human cancers, MT-MMP overexpression was found in OSCC. However, only MMP-14 was considered as an effective biomarker (Shimada et al. 2000). Firstly, MMP-14 was used to predict the possibility of metastasis in OSCC. In the tumor tissues especially the cases with lymph node metastasis, MMP-14 significantly overexpressed (Kurahara et al. 1999). Moreover, it was positively associated with the proMMP-2 activation ratio (Shimada et al. 2000), suggesting its key role in initiation of MMP-2-related pathway in OSCC cell migration and invasion. In view of this, high MMP-14 expression level could predict an aggressive status and a poor prognosis of OSCC.

Detection of MMP-14 also assisted in OSCC risk assessment in susceptibility and pathological evaluation. In a study including 363 OSCC patients and 506 healthy controls, single nucleotide polymorphisms and haplotypes of MMP-14 were proved to be associated with the risk and pathological development of OSCC. Cases with MMP-14 + 7,096 TC/CC genotypes showed a lower potential to be confirmed as OSCC, whereas the +6,727 C: +6,767 G: +7,096 T: +8,153 G haplotype and diplotype showed the opposite pattern. Furthermore, the cases owning this diplotype with at least one CGTG were more likely to suffer from a poor clinicopathological status. This correlation was also revealed between the MMP-14 + 6,767 GA/AA genotypes and clinical characters of OSCC (Weng et al. 2012).

Potential Application to Prognosis, Other Diseases or Conditions

The initial studies on MMPs in pathological conditions almost focused in the field of malignancy. However, other than playing critical roles in the tumor progression, nowadays increasing evidence indicates that MMPs are also implicated in a variety of diseases, including cardiovascular disease, bacterial infection, arthritis, lung injury, periodontal diseases, and Alzheimer's disease.

Due to their capacity of ECM degradation and processing a series of molecules that are related to different events such as cell growth, adhesion, neovascularization, and inflammation, forced MMP expression and activation are more likely to show potent effect on the disease states which refer to structural remodeling, angiogenesis, and inflammatory molecular recruitments. For instance, MMPs play multiple roles since the initial stage of plaque forming in atherosclerosis. Evaluated expression of MMP-1, MMP-8, MMP-13, MMP-2, MMP-9, MMP-3, MMP-10, and MMP-11 was detected in the plaque by immunostaining, zymography, and in situ hybridization studies. Furthermore, MMP-2 and MMP-9 enhanced the migration and proliferation of vascular smooth muscle cells, leading to the plaque growth as well as the vascular wall remodeling. MMP-3 was contributory in the intraplaque angiogenesis. One of the most prevalent and fatal consequence of atherosclerotic development is plaque rupture due to the structural instability, which can further trigger a series of life-threatening diseases such as the myocardial infarction, stroke, and abdominal aneurysms. Most of the MMPs involved in the atherosclerosis were positively correlated with the plaque rupture, indicating an unfavorable prognosis of patients. Despite most of these effects led to a fatal ending, MMP-1 and MMP-3 played protective roles by promoting the plaque cap stability (Sbardella et al. 2012). Such dual roles of MMPs may be explained by the theory that ECM degradation and molecular recruitment in diverse degrees and in diverse stages can differently influence the cardiovascular diseases, either beneficially or detrimentally.

Inflammation is another MMP-involved pathological condition. Generally, inflammation could be divided into two major groups: infection and noninfective inflammation. The notion that the overexpression of diverse MMP members such as MMP-1, MMP-2, MMP-7, MMP-8, MMP-9, MMP-10, MMP-13, and MMP-14 is positively related to the stage and severity of infection is supported by in vitro and in vivo tests. Tissue degradation by MMP-related effects also played a crucial role in preventing the dissemination of bacteria. For instance, activation of MMP-7 enabled the α-defensins in the Paneth cells of the small intestinal crypts to defeat the *Salmonella enterica* serovar Typhimurium and *Escherichia coli* in the gastrointestinal infection. Additionally, MMP-12 participated in the macrophage-related intracellular antibacterial activity (Vanlaere and Libert 2009).

Since MMPs play such key roles in the multiple stages in multiple diseases, it is not surprising to find increasing interest in the application of MMP and their inhibitors on the pathological conditions, especially the pharmacologic roles. In the experimental system, a variety of MMP inhibitors have been suggested to be beneficial to diverse diseases. For instance, CMT-3 and regasepin-1 can impede the gram-negative bacteria-induced infection moving towards to adverse ending such as mortality due to endotoxic shock (Vanlaere and Libert 2009). However, the MMP inhibitors failed to reach the utility as valid therapeutic approaches in the clinical trials. The reasons are multiple. Firstly, the MMPs are involved in multiple normal organic processes such as growth and wound healing, as well as the pathological progression. A long-term challenge of MMP inhibitors can disrupt both the normal organic function and the self-response for diseases, leading to adverse side effects such as musculoskeletal dysfunction. Secondly, diverse MMPs exert different effects (either beneficial or detrimental) on the lesions, and individual MMP may play different roles in diverse stages of diseases (Fingleton 2007). Due to the lack of highly specific MMP inhibitors and consensus in the timing of MMP inhibitor administration, an overall advantage of MMP manipulation has not yet been proved in the clinical settings. It is no doubt that regulation of MMPs is meaningful in the pathological conditions. The question that researchers now should resolve is to elucidate that the regulation of a particular MMP positively influences a particular disease.

Summary Points

- Affected by the nonspecific symptoms, the OSCC patients are usually diagnosed in the advanced stage.
- To improve the treatment outcome and survival of OSCC, identification of the reliable biomarkers for early detection and prognosis prediction is necessary.

- MMPs function in degradation of ECM, generation of active peptides, and activation of specific growth factors, resulting in forming an environment promoting tumor progression, invasion, and metastasis.
- MMPs can be applied as potential cancer biomarkers for early detection, risk assessment, prognostic analysis, and evaluation of response to treatment in OSCC.
- MMP-1, MMP-2, MMP-9, and MMP-11 were useful markers for judging transformation potency from oral dysplasia or lichen planus to OSCC.
- MMP-1, MMP-2, MMP-3, MMP-9, and MMP-14 were correlated with lymph node metastasis.
- Among all of the MMPs, MMP-9 probably appears to be the most promising biomarker with most of the documented cases.
- Further studies on combined biomarkers of MMPs in OSCC are warranted.

References

Ansell A, Jerhammar F, Ceder R, et al. Matrix metalloproteinase-7 and -13 expression associate to cisplatin resistance in head and neck cancer cell lines. Oral Oncol. 2009;45:866–71.

Arora S, Kaur J, Sharma C, et al. Stromelysin 3, Ets-1, and vascular endothelial growth factor expression in oral precancerous and cancerous lesions: correlation with microvessel density, progression, and prognosis. Clin Cancer Res. 2005;11:2272–84.

Barros S, Henriques Á, Pereira K, et al. Immunohistochemical expression of matrix metalloproteinases in squamous cell carcinoma of the tongue and lower lip. Arch Oral Biol. 2011;56:752–60.

Bennett J, Morgan M, Whawell S, et al. Metalloproteinase expression in normal and malignant oral keratinocytes: stimulation of MMP-2 and -9 by scatter factor. Eur J Oral Sci. 2000;108:281–91.

Cavalli-Sforza L. Analytic review: some current problems of human population genetics. Am J Hum Genet. 1973;25:82–104.

Chen Y, Zhang W, Geng N, et al. MMPs, TIMP-2, and TGF-beta1 in the cancerization of oral lichen planus. Head Neck. 2008;30:1237–45.

De Amorim R, da Silveira E, Queiroz L, et al. Matrilysins may not predict the metastatic potential in squamous cell carcinoma of the tongue. Acta Odontol Scand. 2010;68:228–31.

De Coignac A, Elson G, Delneste Y, et al. Cloning of MMP-26. A novel matrilysin-like proteinase. Eur J Biochem. 2000;267:3323–9.

De Vicente J, Fresno M, Villalain L, et al. Expression and clinical significance of matrix metalloproteinase-2 and matrix metalloproteinase-9 in oral squamous cell carcinoma. Oral Oncol. 2005;41:283–93.

Dunsmore S, Saarialho-Kere U, Roby J, et al. Matrilysin expression and function in airway epithelium. J Clin Invest. 1998;102:1321–31.

Erdem N, Carlson E, Gerard D, et al. Characterization of 3 oral squamous cell carcinoma cell lines with different invasion and/or metastatic potentials. J Oral Maxillofac Surg. 2007;65:1725–33.

Fingleton B. Matrix metalloproteinases as valid clinical targets. Curr Pharm Des. 2007;13:333–46.

Fingleton B, Heppner Goss K, Crawford H, et al. Matrilysin in early stage intestinal tumorigenesis. APMIS. 1999;107:102–10.

George A, Ranganathan K, Rao U. Expression of MMP-1 in histopathological different grades of oral squamous cell carcinoma and in normal buccal mucosa – an immunohistochemical study. Cancer Biomark. 2010;7:275–83.

Groblewska M, Siewko M, Mroczko B, et al. The role of matrix metalloproteinases (MMPs) and their inhibitors (TIMPs) in the development of esophageal cancer. Folia Histochem Cytobiol. 2012;50:12–9.

Hong S, Hong S, Lee J, et al. Expression of matrix metalloproteinase-2 and -9 in oral squamous cell carcinomas with regard to the metastatic potential. Oral Oncol. 2000;36:207–13.

Hua H, Li M, Luo T, et al. Matrix metalloproteinases in tumorigenesis: an evolving paradigm. Cell Mol Life Sci. 2011;68:3853–68.

IARC Working Group on the Evaluation of Carcinogenic Risks to Humans. Betel-quid and areca-nut chewing and some areca-nut derived nitrosamines. IARC Monogr Eval Carcinog Risks Hum. 2004;85:1–334.

Jee H, Lee K, Kim J, et al. Sulforaphane inhibits oral carcinoma cell migration and invasion in vitro. Phytother Res. 2011;25:1623–8.

Jordan R, Macabeo-Ong M, Shiboski C, et al. Overexpression of matrix metalloproteinase-1 and -9 mRNA is associated with progression of oral dysplasia to cancer. Clin Cancer Res. 2004;10:6460–5.

Kerkela E, Saarialho-Kere U. Matrix metalloproteinases in tumor progression: focus on basal and squamous cell skin cancer. Exp Dermatol. 2003;12:109–25.

Kim SH, Cho NH, Kim K, et al. Correlations of oral tongue cancer invasion with matrix metalloproteinases (MMPs) and vascular endothelial growth factor (VEGF) expression. J Surg Oncol. 2006;93:330–7.

Kohrmann A, Kammerer U, Kapp M, et al. Expression of matrix metalloproteinases (MMPs) in primary human breast cancer and breast cancer cell lines: new findings and review of the literature. BMC Cancer. 2009;9:188.

Kojima S, Itoh Y, Matsumoto S, et al. Membrane-type 6 matrix metalloproteinase (MT6-MMP, MMP-25) is the second glycosyl-phosphatidyl inositol (GPI)-anchored MMP. FEBS Lett. 2000;480:142–6.

Korpi J, Kervinen V, Mäklin H, et al. Collagenase-2 (matrix metalloproteinase-8) plays a protective role in tongue cancer. Br J Cancer. 2008;98:766–75.

Kudo Y, Iizuka S, Yoshida M, et al. Matrix metalloproteinase-13 (MMP-13) directly and indirectly promotes tumor angiogenesis. J Biol Chem. 2012;287:38716–28.

Kurahara S, Shinohara M, Ikebe T, et al. Expression of MMPS, MT-MMP, and TIMPs in squamous cell carcinoma of the oral cavity: correlations with tumor invasion and metastasis. Head Neck. 1999;21:627–38.

Kusukawa J, Sasaguri Y, Morimatsu M, et al. Expression of matrix metalloproteinase-3 in stage I and II squamous cell carcinoma of the oral cavity. J Oral Maxillofac Surg. 1995;53:530–4.

Lee C, Liu S, Lin M, et al. Upregulation of matrix metalloproteinase-1 (MMP-1) expression in oral carcinomas of betel quid (BQ) users: roles of BQ ingredients in the acceleration of tumor cell motility through MMP-1. Arch Oral Biol. 2008;53:810–8.

Li T, Cui J. COX-2, MMP-7 expression in oral lichen planus and oral squamous cell carcinoma. Asian Pac J Trop Med. 2013;6:640–3.

Lim Y, Han J, Kang H, et al. Overexpression of c-Met promotes invasion and metastasis of small oral tongue carcinoma. Oral Oncol. 2012;48:1114–9.

Lin C, Tseng S, Yang S, et al. Role of lipocalin 2 and its complex with matrix metalloproteinase-9 in oral cancer. Oral Dis. 2012;18:734–40.

Liu S, Liu Y, Huang W, et al. Up-regulation of matrix metalloproteinase-8 by betel quid extract and arecoline and its role in 2D motility. Oral Oncol. 2007;43:1026–33.

Mäkinen L, Häyry V, Atula T, et al. Prognostic significance of matrix metalloproteinase-2, -8, -9, and -13 in oral tongue cancer. J Oral Pathol Med. 2012;41:394–9.

Marchenko G, Ratnikov B, Rozanov D, et al. Characterization of matrix metalloproteinase-26, a novel metalloproteinase widely expressed in cancer cells of epithelial origin. Biochem J. 2001;356:705–18.

Massova I, Kotra L, Fridman R, et al. Matrix metalloproteinases: structures, evolution, and diversification. FASEB J. 1998;12:1075–95.

Mohtasham N, Babakoohi S, Shiva A, et al. Immunohistochemical study of p53, Ki-67, MMP-2 and MMP-9 expression at invasive front of squamous cell and verrucous carcinoma in oral cavity. Pathol Res Pract. 2013;209:110–4.

Munshi H, Wu Y, Mukhopadhyay S, et al. Differential regulation of membrane type 1-matrix metalloproteinase activity by ERK 1/2- and p38 MAPK-modulated tissue inhibitor of metalloproteinases 2 expression controls transforming growth factor-beta1-induced pericellular collagenolysis. J Biol Chem. 2004;279:39042–50.

Nagata M, Fujita H, Ida H, et al. Identification of potential biomarkers of lymph node metastasis in oral squamous cell carcinoma by cDNA microarray analysis. Int J Cancer. 2003;106:683–9.

Nishizawa R, Nagata M, Noman A, et al. The 2G allele of promoter region of matrix metalloproteinase-1 as an essential pre-condition for the early onset of oral squamous cell carcinoma. BMC Cancer. 2007;7:187.

Nyberg P, Heikkilä P, Sorsa T, et al. Endostatin inhibits human tongue carcinoma cell invasion and intravasation and blocks the activation of matrix metalloprotease-2, -9, and -13. J Biol Chem. 2003;278:22404–11.

Ogbureke K, Weinberger P, Looney S, et al. Expressions of matrix metalloproteinase-9 (MMP-9), dentin sialophosphoprotein (DSPP), and osteopontin (OPN) at histologically negative surgical margins may predict recurrence of oral squamous cell carcinoma. Oncotarget. 2012;3:286–98.

Parks W, Wilson C, Lopez-Boado Y. Matrix metalloproteinases as modulators of inflammation and innate immunity. Nat Rev Immunol. 2004;4:617–29.

Patterson B, Sang Q. Angiostatin-converting enzyme activities of human matrilysin (MMP-7) and gelatinase B/type IV collagenase (MMP-9). J Biol Chem. 1997;272:28823–5.

Roy R, Yang J, Moses M. Matrix metalloproteinases as novel biomarkers and potential therapeutic targets in human cancer. J Clin Oncol. 2009;27:5287–97.

Rusthoven K, Ballonoff A, Raben D, et al. Poor prognosis in patients with stage I and II oral tongue squamous cell carcinoma. Cancer. 2008;112:345–51.

Sapkota D, Bruland O, Costea D, et al. S100A14 regulates the invasive potential of oral squamous cell carcinoma derived cell-lines in vitro by modulating expression of matrix metalloproteinases, MMP1 and MMP9. Eur J Cancer. 2011;47:600–10.

Sato H, Takino T, Okada Y, et al. A matrix metalloproteinase expressed on the surface of invasive tumour cells. Nature. 1994;370:61–5.

Sbardella D, Fasciglione G, Gioia M, et al. Human matrix metalloproteinases: an ubiquitarian class of enzymes involved in several pathological processes. Mol Aspects Med. 2012;33:119–208.

Scully C, Bagan J. Oral squamous cell carcinoma: overview of current understanding of aetiopathogenesis and clinical implications. Oral Dis. 2009;15:388–99.

Shimada T, Nakamura H, Yamashita K, et al. Enhanced production and activation of progelatinase A mediated by membrane-type 1 matrix metalloproteinase in human oral squamous cell carcinomas: implications for lymph node metastasis. Clin Exp Metastasis. 2000;18:179–88.

Shindoh M, Higashino F, Kaya M, et al. Correlated expression of matrix metalloproteinases and ets family transcription factor E1A-F in invasive oral squamous-cell-carcinoma-derived cell lines. Am J Pathol. 1996;148:693–700.

Shpitzer T, Bahar G, Feinmesser R, et al. A comprehensive salivary analysis for oral cancer diagnosis. J Cancer Res Clin Oncol. 2007;133:613–7.

Shuman Moss LA, Jensen-Taubman S, Stetler-Stevenson WG. Matrix metalloproteinases: changing roles in tumor progression and metastasis. Am J Pathol. 2012;181:1895–9.

Siegel R, Ward E, Brawley Q, et al. Cancer statistics, 2011: the impact of eliminating socioeconomic and racial disparities on premature cancer deaths. CA. 2013;63:11–30.

Singh R, Haridas N, Patel J, et al. Matrix metalloproteinases and their inhibitors: correlation with invasion and metastasis in oral cancer. Indian J Clin Biochem. 2010;25:250–9.

Soni S, Mathur M, Shukla NK, et al. Stromelysin-3 expression is an early event in human oral tumorigenesis. Int J Cancer. 2003;107:309–16.

Tadbir A, Purshahidi S, Ebrahimi H, et al. Serum level of MMP-3 in patients with oral squamous cell carcinoma–lack of association with clinico-pathological features. Asian Pac J Cancer Prev. 2012;13:4545–8.

Tallant C, Marrero A, Gomis-Rüth F. Matrix metalloproteinases: fold and function of their catalytic domains. Biochim Biophys Acta. 2010;1803:20–8.

Tamamura R, Nagatsuka H, Siar C, et al. Comparative analysis of basal lamina type IV collagen α chains, matrix metalloproteinases-2 and -9 expressions in oral dysplasia and invasive carcinoma. Acta Histochem. 2013;115:113–9.

Tilakaratne W, Kobayashi T, Ida-Yonemochi H, et al. Matrix metalloproteinase 7 and perlecan in oral epithelial dysplasia and carcinoma in situ: an aid for histopathologic recognition of their cell proliferation centers. J Oral Pathol Med. 2009;38:348–55.

Tu H, Wu C, Kao S, et al. Functional -1562 C-to-T polymorphism in matrix metalloproteinase-9 (MMP-9) promoter is associated with the risk for oral squamous cell carcinoma in younger male areca users. J Oral Pathol Med. 2007;36:409–14.

Vairaktaris E, Yapijakis C, Derka S, et al. Association of matrix metalloproteinase-1 (-1607 1G/2G) polymorphism with increased risk for oral squamous cell carcinoma. Anticancer Res. 2007;27:459–64.

Vairaktaris E, Vassiliou S, Nkenke E, et al. A metalloproteinase-9 polymorphism which affects its expression is associated with increased risk for oral squamous cell carcinoma. Eur J Surg Oncol. 2008;34:450–5.

Vanlaere I, Libert C. Matrix metalloproteinases as drug targets in infections caused by gram-negative bacteria and in septic shock. Clin Microbiol Rev. 2009;22:224–39.

Vilen ST, Salo T, Sorsa T, et al. Fluctuating roles of matrix metalloproteinase-9 in oral squamous cell carcinoma. Sci World J. 2013;2013:920595.

Weng C, Chen M, Lin C, et al. Single nucleotide polymorphisms and haplotypes of MMP-14 are associated with the risk and pathological development of oral cancer. Ann Surg Oncol. 2012;19:S319–27.

Yamamoto A, Kasamatsu A, Ishige S, et al. Exocyst complex component Sec8: a presumed component in the progression of human oral squamous-cell carcinoma by secretion of matrix metalloproteinases. J Cancer Res Clin Oncol. 2013;139:533–42.

Yu T, Wu Y, Helman J, et al. CXCR4 promotes oral squamous cell carcinoma migration and invasion through inducing expression of MMP-9 and MMP-13 via the ERK signaling pathway. Mol Cancer Res. 2011;9:161–72.

Zhang Z, Pan J, Li L, et al. Survey of risk factors contributed to lymphatic metastasis in patients with oral tongue cancer by immunohistochemistry. J Oral Pathol Med. 2011;40:127–34.

Zimmermann B, Park N, Wong D. Genomic targets in saliva. Ann N Y Acad Sci. 2007;1098:184–91.

Tissue Microarray for Biomarkers Studies in Salivary Gland Tumors

35

Tissue Microarray and Salivary Gland Tumors

Pablo Agustin Vargas, Felipe Paiva Fonseca, Oslei Paes de Almeida, and Paul M. Speight

Contents

P.A. Vargas (✉)
Piracicaba Dental School, Department of Oral Diagnosis (Pathology), State University of Campinas, Areão, Piracicaba, São Paulo, Brazil

Department of Oral Pathology and Oral Biology, School of Dentistry, Faculty of Health Sciences, University of Pretoria, Pretoria, South Africa
e-mail: pavargas@fop.unicamp.br

F.P. Fonseca
Piracicaba Dental School, Department of Oral Diagnosis (Pathology), State University of Campinas, Areão, Piracicaba, São Paulo, Brazil

School of Clinical Dentistry, Department of Oral and Maxillofacial Pathology, The University of Sheffield, Claremont Crescent, Sheffield, UK
e-mail: felipepfonseca@hotmail.com

O.P. de Almeida
Piracicaba Dental School, Department of Oral Diagnosis (Pathology), State University of Campinas, Areão, Piracicaba, São Paulo, Brazil
e-mail: oslei@fop.unicamp.br

P.M. Speight
School of Clinical Dentistry, Department of Oral and Maxillofacial Pathology, The University of Sheffield, Claremont Crescent, Sheffield, UK
e-mail: p.speight@sheffield.ac.uk

V.R. Preedy, V.B. Patel (eds.), *Biomarkers in Cancer, Biomarkers in Disease: Methods, Discoveries and Applications*,
DOI 10.1007/978-94-007-7681-4_40

Abstract

Tissue microarray (TMA) modern methodology was first described by Wan et al. in 1987, being further adapted by Kononen et al. in 1998 after which the technique became quickly and widely accepted and described in the scientific literature worldwide. Its development took place at a time which demanded maximum results in a minimum period of time that followed the onset of other important methodological approaches like cDNA microarray and proteomics. Hence, with this new technique intended to be used in association with paraffin-embedded neoplastic or nonneoplastic human tissues, the biomarkers recently described with the use of cDNA microarray and proteomics could be clinicopathologically validated on a large-scale basis. The main advantage of TMA methodology is related to its ability of aggregating hundreds of tumor samples from different cases in a single paraffin block. Despite its possible limitations with regard to tissue representation, numerous validation studies have demonstrated its statistical equivalence with conventional tissue sections, further supporting its use in the study of molecular biomarkers at a DNA, RNA, or protein level. Because of the scarce knowledge currently available regarding the molecular pathogenesis of salivary gland tumors, the use of a high-throughput technology like TMA in the investigation of such group of tumors becomes extremely interesting. As a consequence, we have witnessed an increase in the number of studies looking for new potentially useful biomarkers using TMA sections for better understanding of the etiopathogenesis of salivary gland tumors. In this chapter the authors aim to describe the laboratory and scientific advantages that TMA methodology has brought in recent decades, describing its most important characteristics and potential limitations, especially related to the study of biomarkers in the highly morphologically heterogeneous group of salivary gland tumors.

List of Abbreviations

CD34	Cluster of Differentiation 34
cDNA	Complementary Deoxyribonucleic Acid
Mcm2	Minichromosome Maintenance Complex Component 2
PCR	Polymerase Chain Reaction
PLUNC	Palate, Lung, and Nasal Epithelium Clone
RNA	Ribonucleic Acid
TMA	Tissue Microarray

Key Facts of Salivary Gland Tumors

- Salivary gland tumors are an uncommon group of human neoplasms that accounts for approximately 3 % of all head and neck tumors.
- The World Health Organization currently classifies salivary gland tumors in 34 different benign and malignant microscopic subtypes.

- Salivary gland tumors are characterized by a heterogeneous clinical behavior and a broad microscopic diversity.
- Little is known about salivary gland tumor molecular pathogenesis, and the use of new laboratorial techniques like tissue microarray may favor their better understanding.

Key Facts of Tissue Microarray

- Tissue microarray represents a reliable, cost-effective, and a high-throughput methodology for molecular study of many human conditions.
- The use of tissue microarray methodology has already been validated in tumors from almost all anatomic sites, including the salivary glands.
- Because of the high morphological heterogeneity of salivary gland tumors, especially pleomorphic adenomas, larger cores (1.0 mm or greater) arranged in duplicate seem to be preferable than the most often used 0.6 mm diameter cores in other solid neoplasms like prostatic cancer.
- Tissue microarrays have been used for investigating different biomarkers in salivary gland tumors since 2004, and immunohistochemistry and in situ hybridization are the most used reactions associated with TMA studies.
- Because of the ability to arrange hundreds of different tumors in a single block and to correlate the results obtained with the use of immunohistochemical or in situ hybridization reactions to the clinic parameters of the cases, tissue microarray methods represent an excellent auxiliary for prognostic analysis of new potential biomarkers in salivary gland tumors.

Definition of Words and Terms

Tissue Microarray Laboratory method where cores of tissue as small as 0.6 mm diameter are taken from original paraffin-preserved tissue blocks to be included in a single paraffin block that allows the simultaneous study of hundreds of different cases

cDNA Microarray Technology which enables the researcher to evaluate the pattern of transcription of a large number of genes simultaneously, identifying specific genes with higher or lower transcriptional activity in a given tumor

Proteomics Large-scale comprehensive study of a specific group of proteins, including description of their abundances, variations, and modifications, along with informations related to their interaction with partners and networks, in order to understand cellular processes

In Situ Hybridization Laboratory methodology that uses a specific DNA or RNA strand as a probe to identify a given DNA or RNA sequence in histologic tissues

Immunohistochemistry Technique that uses antibodies and chromogen substances to identify a given antigen in a histological section

TMA Design Number and size of cores used in a given TMA block

TMA Layout Disposal and position of the cores in a given TMA block

Introduction

In the last few decades, significant improvements have been seen in the understanding of innumerous human pathological conditions, in most cases because of the discovery of new proteins and a better comprehension of the function of different group of genes, both related to the control of intracellular signaling pathways or extracellular matrix modulations. As a consequence of this great development, a number of new clinical approaches have been developed, including the use of monoclonal antibodies for the inhibition of specific molecules known to play important roles in various human neoplasms. Many other therapeutic protocols are currently undergoing laboratory investigations prior to being clinically tested.

This evolution in the better understanding of biological and biomedical events that are leading to an improvement in the clinical management of human diseases has been preceded by an important development in laboratory tools and techniques that allowed the genetic and molecular studies to be performed in a larger scale and in a shorter time. Throughout the 1980s the emergence of cDNA microarrays, PCR, and proteomics permitted rapid and broad screening to be done, and new molecular biomarkers potentially related to important disease steps could be more easily investigated (Torhorst et al. 2001; Karlsson et al. 2009).

Although tissue samples represent an important research resource, laboratory methods for the use of histological specimens have not experienced many further developments since the introduction of immunohistochemistry, which is often expensive and time consuming for acquiring significant results (Taylor 2011). It was only in the last years of the 1990s that the microarray principles previously used in genetic studies were broadly accepted and more widely used with paraffin-preserved histological tissues. Although the methodology and concepts currently well established and accepted for TMA studies have only been recently proposed, the first attempt to arrange small samples of hundreds of different cases in a single paraffin block that could be studied simultaneously in a much smaller space of time leading to a more favorable laboratory workflow was performed in the 1980s by Wan et al. (1987). These authors adapted the original description of the "multitumor (sausage) tissue block" described 1 year before that inserted hundreds of tissue cores in the receptor paraffin block in a non-orderly way, not allowing the researcher to identify each case after its construction (Battifora 1986). However, the technique was still difficult to reproduce and highly complex and was not widely accepted, until Kononen's more simple and reproducible method, described in 1998, was seen as a good research alternative for large-scale investigations involving paraffin-embedded tissues (Kononen et al. 1998). Thereafter, the number of studies using TMA technology as an auxiliary tool for identification and validation of new potential biomarkers in many human neoplastic and nonneoplastic conditions has seen a huge increase. It is important to highlight that despite some attempts to validate TMA technology for diagnostic purposes (van Zwieten 2013), its use is currently accepted for research only.

Despite the improvements in TMA methodology which have established the technique in a distinguished position with an increased number of studies using it, some possible limitations are still being intensely debated, and TMA remains a questionable approach for an important part of the scientific community. The possible lack of adequate tissue representation of TMA cores is the most frequently questioned feature of the technique. According to its main critics, this deficiency is even more important in highly heterogeneous tissues, since the use of histological cores as small as 0.6 mm of diameter would not be enough to adequately represent a whole section of a morphologically and genetically heterogeneous human neoplasm. As a consequence, many studies have been carried out in recent years with the purpose of validating the use of TMA as a research tool for many human neoplastic and nonneoplastic lesions. The great majority of these studies have shown significant similarity of the results obtained with TMA cylinders and conventional slides of whole tissue section (Kallioniemi et al. 2001; Goldstine et al. 2002; Chen et al. 2007; Boone et al. 2008; Toberer et al. 2013).

Among the various groups of human neoplasias, salivary gland tumors are well recognized because of their highly heterogeneous microscopic morphology, which is even more present in specific subtypes such as pleomorphic adenomas. Salivary gland tumors account for approximately 3 % of all head and neck neoplasms and represent a challenge for clinic oncology, since surgical approaches still represent the main therapeutic modality for treating these neoplasms (Fonseca et al. 2012). Although benign salivary gland tumors do not represent a significant risk for patients' survival due to their indolent clinical behavior with low levels of malignant transformation and long time of evolution, their malignant counterparts are commonly associated with local and regional recurrences and in a significant number of cases with distant metastases, decreasing patients' survival rates and increasing their therapeutic morbidities. In contrast to the discovery of new molecules used as therapeutic targets for treating innumerous other human malignancies that significantly improved the chemotherapeutic approaches in theses lesions, only few developments have been described for salivary gland tumors, and consequently, chemotherapy protocols are used primarily as a palliative approach in cases where surgery cannot be performed or in disseminated disease, most of the time with unsatisfactory results.

Hence, the search for new biomarkers that might correlate with tumor progression and behavior in this group of neoplasms becomes extremely important for the improvement of chemotherapeutic protocols and for the development of new therapeutic interventions. There is therefore a need to correlate the expression of new markers with clinicopathologic parameters in large-scale studies. In this context TMA techniques would represent an excellent methodology for getting results in large samples of tumors. Moreover, despite concerns about the validity of TMAs, recent studies have shown good results for the identification of new biomarkers in these neoplasms (Fonseca et al. 2014; Schneider et al. 2013).

Tissue Microarray Principles: Advantages and Disadvantages

The growing number of studies looking for new molecular markers possibly related to human cancer onset and progression in the last decades demanded the development of new methodological approaches capable of analyzing innumerous genes and proteins simultaneously with the purpose of getting relevant results in a shorter time and with minimum waste of laboratory resources. In this context, progressions in human DNA sequencing and the development of cDNA microarrays and proteomics deserve special distinction, due to their ability of identifying new potential molecular targets among thousands of genes and proteins (Simon and Sauter 2002; van de Rijn and Gilks 2004; Karlsson et al. 2009).

Because of the necessity of validating these potential new molecular candidates, what is usually performed by correlating their expression patterns with microscopic and clinicopathological features, this new methodological requirement found a broad and rich available field in the use of paraffin-preserved histological tissues. Hence, in the last years of the 1980s, the TMA technology was described with the main purpose of making possible to carry out in situ analyses of thousands of different tissue specimens simultaneously either at the DNA, RNA or protein levels, in a same recipient TMA block, accelerating the study of new molecular markers in a histopathologic basis and further preserving unique and precious research materials (Torhorst et al. 2001; Simon and Sauter 2002; Chen et al. 2007; Karlsson et al. 2009; Eckel-Passow et al. 2010).

A number of TMA facilities ranging from manual equipment to totally automated kits are currently commercially available (Figs. 1 and 2); however, they all share the same principles of construction. In summary, the TMA technique uses tissue cores usually ranging from 0.6 to 2.0 mm diameter acquired from different primary tumor blocks and arrayed into a single recipient paraffin block (Fig. 3). Histologic sections from the resulting TMA blocks can then be used for simultaneous analyses of any given molecular marker. Each recipient block may contain up to a hundred or more tissue cores allowing many tumors to be sampled and examined in a single histological section. The tissue cores are positioned in the recipient block with the help of an *x*-*y* axis locator, which permits each core to be placed in a previously determined site making it possible to localize them according to a predetermined "map" so that the subsequent quantitative analyses can be performed adequately (Kallioniemi et al. 2001; Voduc et al. 2008; Parsons and Grabsch 2009).

TMA blocks can be classified according to the original material used to receive the cylinders. Paraffin TMA blocks are by far the most used sources for TMA constructions, but they can also be made of tumors preserved in resin or even with frozen tissues (the so-called cryo-arrays). TMA can also be classified according to

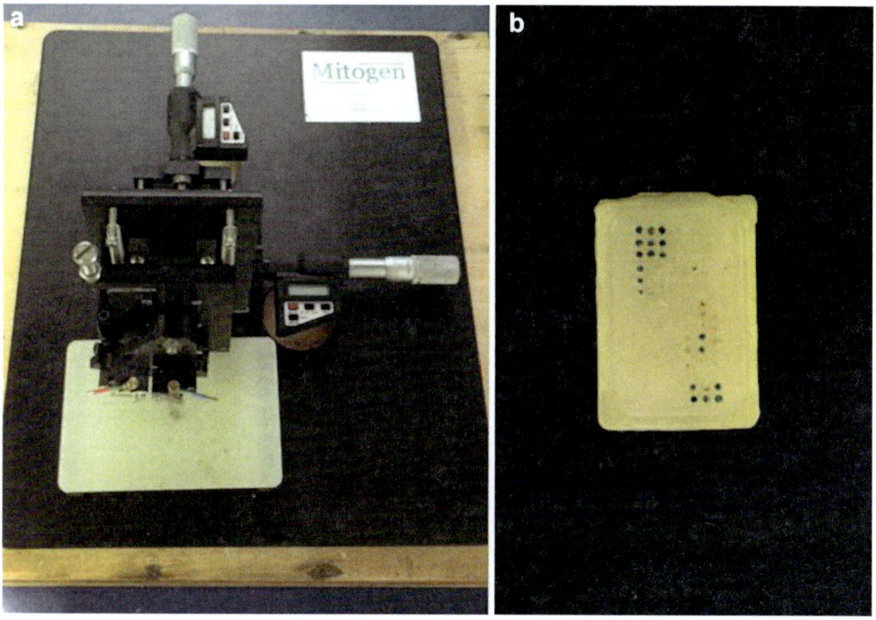

Fig. 1 A large number of TMA kits or machines are commercially available, ranging from totally manual appliances to completely automated facilities. (**a**) Original TMA arrayers use an *x-y* axis locator to accurately insert the cores at predetermined sites in the (**b**) recipient paraffin block

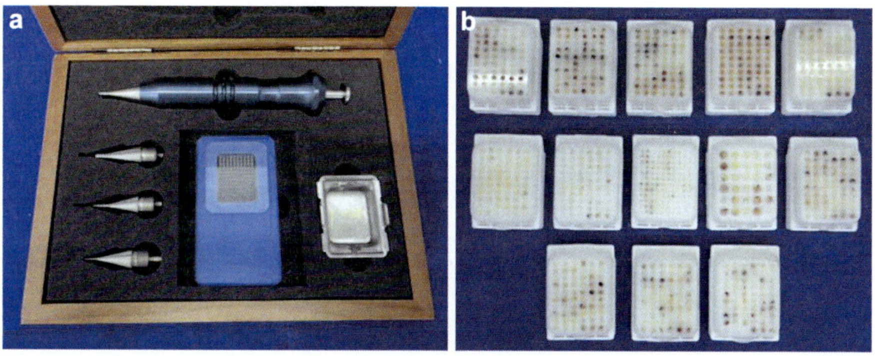

Fig. 2 More recently, many variations in TMA arrayers have been developed. (**a**) Sakura TMA Labtek kit® is a manual TMA arrayer that requires only a small laboratory space and is designed to be used with (**b**) ready-to-use TMA paraffin blocks

their designs, which are usually related to their main objective of construction. In this classification the *multi-tumor TMAs* composed of samples from multiple histological tumor types or organ sites, which can be used to screen different tumor types for the expression of a molecular target of interest, can be found. *Tumor progression TMAs* can be used to study molecular alterations in different

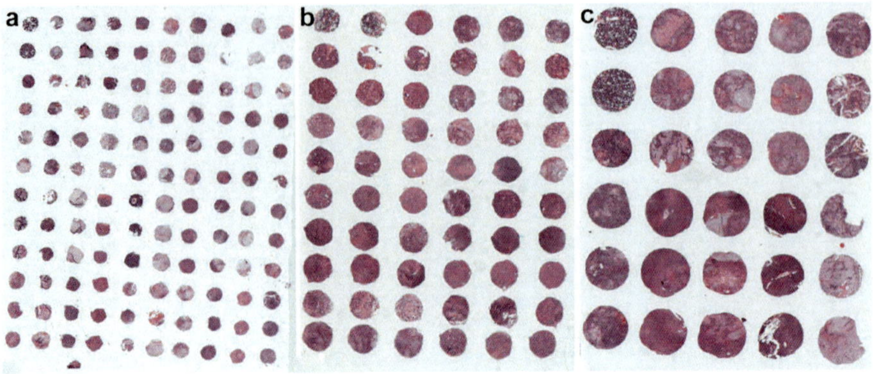

Fig. 3 Salivary gland tumor TMA sections obtained from a TMA block constructed using a manual arrayer and ready-to-use TMA paraffin blocks suitable to receive as many as 30, 60, or 120 cores of 3.0, 2.0, or 1.0 mm diameter, respectively (Hematoxilin and eosin)

stages of tumor progression within a given organ or tumor type, such as the brain, breast, urinary bladder, kidney, prostate, and others. *Patient outcome TMAs* contain tumor samples from patients for whom clinical follow-up data are available, such as data on tumor recurrence, therapy response, time to metastasize, or patient survival. Finally, TMAs can also be classified according to the type of acquisition of the tissue cores, which can be done in a *targeted* fashion when the authors aim to compare the periphery and the central areas of a given tumor or when a specific location of the neoplasm is intended to be studied or in a *random* fashion TMA, usually used to evaluate the expression pattern of a given marker in the tissue (Simon and Sauter 2002; Parsons and Grabsch 2009).

The layout of TMA blocks can also show a broad variability among different laboratories, which reveals the lack of standardization in TMA constructions worldwide (Fig. 4). Some authors have proposed the use of a peripheral "wall" of protection in the TMAs made of cores of undesired histological tissues to overcome the usual antibody precipitations found in the periphery of tissue sections submitted to immunohistochemical reactions. Because high-density TMAs may pose difficulties for finding specific cores during the analysis of the reactions, some authors proposed the use of different cores or gaps for orientation that could be used by the researcher to more easily find specific cores. On the other hand, some authors suggested the use of asymmetrically built TMAs to better identify the position of TMA cores, so that they would not have problems with possible orientation, especially if cores are lost during the reactions. In summary, TMA layout must be chosen according to the users preferences, and the option of choice must be that which the researcher feels easiest to use (Simon and Sauter 2002; Parsons and Grabsch 2009).

TMA use has a number of advantages, it permits the concomitant use of a large number of cases in one single paraffin block, it has been shown to significantly

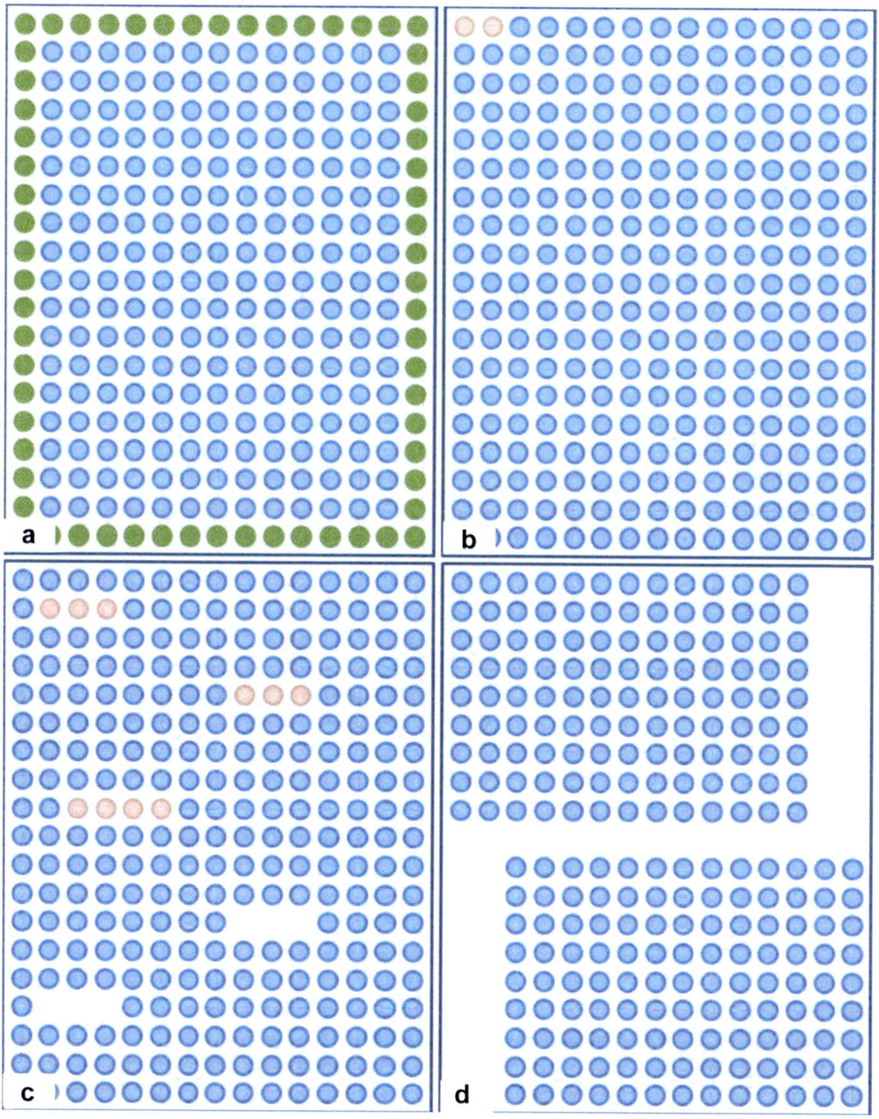

Fig. 4 The arrangement of cores in a tissue microarray block can be done following different layouts depending on the preferences of each laboratory. (**a**) A peripheral wall of protection can be included in the TMA block using non-interesting tissues to overcome frequent antibody precipitation in the periphery of the slides. (**b**) The inclusion of positive and negative controls in the *left upper corner* of the TMA block might be useful to ensure proper orientation of the slides for immunohistochemical quantitative analysis. (**c**) Insertion of different tissue cores or removal of a number of them in the middle of the TMA block can also be useful for orientation and identification of specific cases in the slides. (**d**) TMA blocks asymmetrically built may also assist with orientation and the identification of each case in the sections

reduce the experimental expenses (more cost-effective approach) and handling time (less time-consuming approach), and because the reactions are done in one single slide, the reagent concentrations, incubation times, temperature, wash conditions, and antigen retrieval are the same for all specimens, standardizing the reactions carried out. The use of small cores usually allows the authors to arrange the same case in different TMAs, and each final block is suitable for being used in many different projects; so, TMA use also favors the preservation of important tissues at the same time that permits its maximum usage. All these advantages improve the laboratory workflow and may have been responsible for the large increase in the number of studies using TMA (Kallioniemi et al. 2001; El-Mansi and Williams 2006; Voduc et al. 2008; Karlsson et al. 2009).

However, as with any other laboratory technique, a number of potential disadvantages of TMA approach are frequently raised by different authors, although most of them have been proved to be overcome with variations in the technique depending on the purposes of each study. The use of tissues from different sources and, therefore, fixed and preserved in different conditions but assembled in the same block is one of the criticisms of the use of TMAs containing large numbers of cases. The extensive time for building TMA blocks and the necessity of technical skills for creating it and for performing the histological sections are also often cited. Overall however the possible lack of representation of the whole tumor by the simple use of tiny cores is by far the main concern about the use of TMAs (Kallioniemi et al. 2001; Camp et al. 2008). A large number of studies have been conducted with the purpose of evaluating the most adequate TMA assembly in order to obtain a valid methodology for each kind of neoplastic or nonneoplastic tissues. In the majority of them, cores as small as 0.6 mm arranged in duplicate have been shown to be representative of the tumor as seen in whole conventional tissue sections. In cases of highly heterogeneous tumors, some authors have proposed the use of increased sized cores or a larger number of cores, which would also overcome the frequent loss of cores observed after immunohistochemical or in situ hybridization reactions. However, the use of cylinders larger than 2.0 mm and in more than triplicate has not shown any additional advantages with regard to tissue representation, and the damage caused to the original donor tissue may not support such excessive use. However, it has also been proposed that the best TMA arrangement must depend on the markers and tumors used, so there would not be one single TMA design ideal for all the different studies (Eckel-Passow et al. 2010).

Ironically, the ability to sample large numbers of different cases in a single TMA block might cause a potential problem for researchers not familiar with the technique, since the application of simultaneous studies can result in an ocean of data, which has to be organized and analyzed. Fortunately, the technology of digital analyses for immunohistochemical and other molecular reactions carried out in histologic sections has improved significantly and can now be used in association with TMA slides, so that this possible pitfall can be easily surpassed by using new software and algorithms designed to perform multiple quantitative analyses, overcoming this time-consuming step (van de Rijn and Gilks 2004; Camp et al. 2008). Moreover, the laborious first steps of building TMA blocks have also been decreased by the development of new automated tissue microarrays, giving rise to the now so-called next-generation tissue microarray (Ng-TMA) (Zlobec et al. 2013).

Because of its advantages, TMA technology has been applied an almost indescribable number of human pathological conditions, especially in the study of benign and malignant neoplasms from different anatomical sites. Not by coincidence the TMA approach has been used more often in morphologically homogeneous tumors like lymphomas and carcinomas (Glimelius et al. 2012; Nelhubel et al. 2013). Among head and neck neoplasms, squamous cell carcinoma is by far the most common malignant entity diagnosed and, therefore, the subtype more frequently studied. TMA methodology has been applied in many studies of head and neck squamous cell carcinoma (Radhakrishnan et al. 2008; Nelhubel et al. 2013). On the other hand, salivary gland tumors comprise a group of heterogeneous lesions with complex clinicopathological characteristics and distinct biological behavior (Vargas et al. 2002; Fonseca et al 2012). According to the World Health Organization (Barnes et al. 2005), the global annual incidence, when all salivary gland tumors are considered, varies from 0.4 to 13.5 cases per 100,000 inhabitants, which accounts for only 0.3 % of all malignancies in the United States. However, reports from numerous regions of the world have shown differences in the incidence and frequency of tumor types, indicating a geographic variation in the frequency of these neoplasias (Fonseca et al. 2012).

Tissue Microarray Employment in Studies of Salivary Gland Tumors

Salivary gland tumors consist of a group of heterogeneous lesions with complex clinicopathologic features and biological behavior that corresponds to approximately 3 % of all head and neck neoplasms. According to the World Health Organization, the global annual incidence of all salivary gland tumors varies from 0.4 to 13.5 cases per 100,000 inhabitants, accounting for only 0.3 % of all malignancies in the United States (Barners et al. 2005). However, reports from various regions of the world have shown differences in the incidence of these tumors, revealing a geographic variation in the frequency of tumor subtypes (Ito et al. 2005; Fonseca et al. 2012).

Salivary gland tumors are well known because of their broad microscopic diversity that causes significant difficulty to their accurate microscopic classification, a matter of constant discussion among pathologists. An important consequence of such difficult classification of salivary gland tumors is evidenced in their poor molecular understanding. In contrast to many other human cancers that have revealed significant improvements in the understanding of their molecular mechanisms, salivary gland tumors remain to be further investigated, and the use of TMA technology to acquire new knowledge about these tumors may represent a useful auxiliary tool (Figs. 5 and 6). However, the morphological diversity of salivary gland tumors, especially in some histopathological subtypes like pleomorphic adenoma, has raised many doubts about the real utility of TMA in these cases.

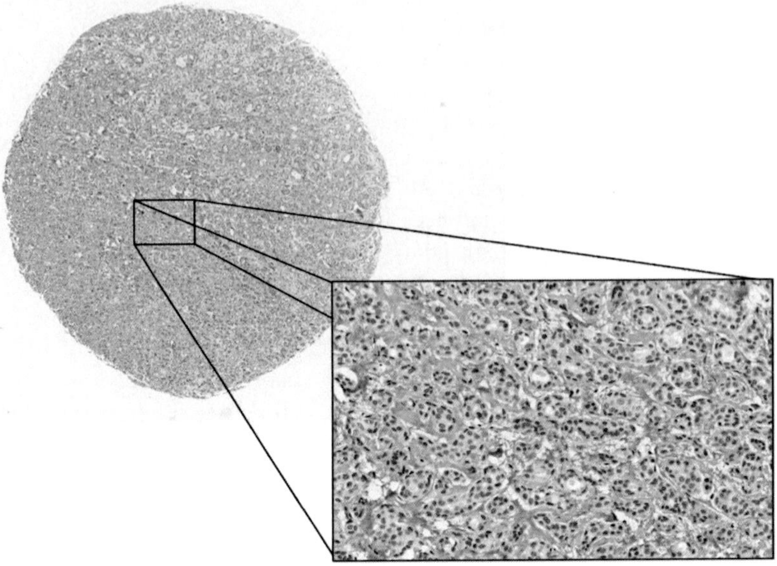

Fig. 5 Different molecular reactions can be performed in TMA histological sections including immunohistochemistry, in situ hybridization, and DNA ploidy analysis. The quality of the immunohistochemical reactions done in TMA sections of salivary gland tumors is comparable to those in conventional whole-section slides and has recently been demonstrated to be a valid methodology for immunohistochemical study of this group of neoplasias. MCM2 nuclear staining (in adenoid cystic carcinoma) has been investigated in salivary gland tumors with the auxiliary of TMA technology

Consequently, only a few studies have performed molecular analysis of salivary gland tumors with the use of TMAs (Williams et al. 2010; Yamazaki et al. 2010; Clauditz et al. 2011).

Considering the challenges imposed by salivary gland tumors' morphological heterogeneity for building TMA blocks, a review paper detailing the use of the technique specifically in the context of salivary gland tumors has recently been published and some guidelines suggested (Fonseca et al. 2013). Regarding solely the histologic aspects of the tumors, it seemed to be possible to acquire adequately representative samples of all neoplastic subtypes studied, including the most heterogeneous ones, using cores of 1.0, 2.0, or 3.0 mm of diameter. However, the authors highlighted the problems faced by trying to arrange highly cystic tumors in TMAs, resulting in very small amounts of neoplastic tissue to be studied, suggesting that TMA should not be used for these cases (Fonseca et al. 2013). However, it was only more recently that an attempt to validate TMA for molecular analysis of salivary gland tumors has been performed. Analyzing 82 cases of pleomorphic adenoma and using four different biomarkers directed to specific features and components of the neoplastic cells and stroma (the proliferative marker Ki67, the myoepithelial cell marker p63, the epithelial luminal cell marker cytokeratin 7, and the stromal vascular

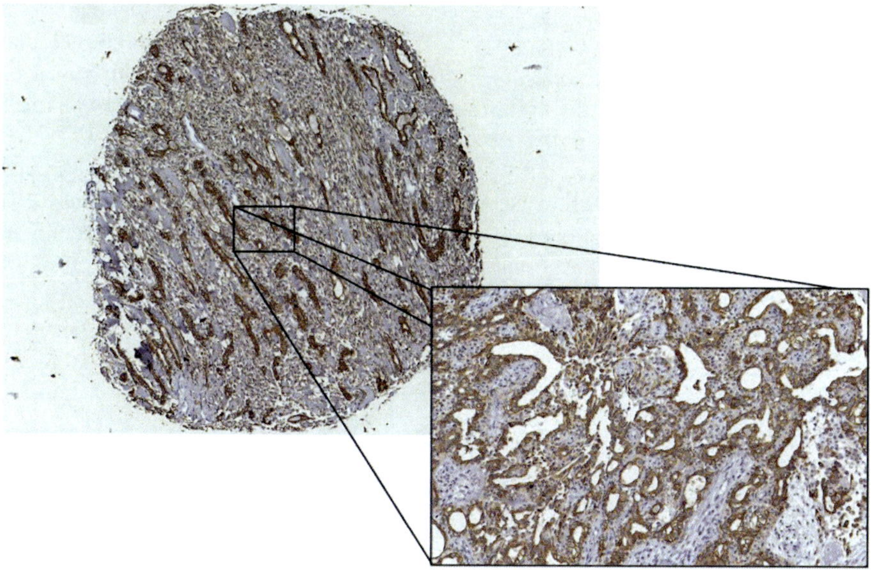

Fig. 6 Luminal epithelial cells of a pleomorphic adenoma can be well characterized using TMA cores by cytokeratin 7 immunoreactions

marker CD34), the authors suggested that no significant difference could be found by comparing the immunoexpression of all markers using TMA sections containing 2.0 mm cores arranged in duplicate and the conventional whole section slides (Fonseca et al. 2014). They concluded that TMA is therefore a reliable methodology for immunohistochemical study of salivary gland pleomorphic adenoma.

Although specific guidelines for building TMAs of salivary gland tumors and its validation have only been described recently, this methodological modality had already been used several years for investigation of salivary gland tumors. TMAs were first used in 2004 by a Japanese group (Iwafuchi et al. 2004) that attempted to examine how the anatomical components of the normal salivary glands would be associated with morphological subtypes of tumors. The authors used a broad immunohistochemical panel in association with TMA blocks containing 4 cores of 0.6 mm diameter. They showed that salivary gland tumors could be well characterized by using markers toward only three components, myoepithelial, luminal, and basal cells. In the following year, two manuscripts were released by the same German group using for the first time in situ hybridization technique in association with TMA sections of salivary gland tumors. In both cases the authors also used 0.6 mm cores to show that different levels of KIT expression could be found in different subtypes of adenoid cystic carcinoma, and that, there was frequent copy number gain of 22q13 gene in this same tumor type, irrespective of its histological variant (Freier et al. 2005a, b).

Further studies were conducted in the following years using TMAs designed in different fashions. Vargas et al. (2008a) first used 1.0 mm cores for study of salivary gland tumors. The authors arranged the cores in triplicate to evaluate the expression pattern of the proliferation markers Mcm-2, Ki-67, and geminin and suggested that Mcm-2 would be a suitable marker for the differential diagnosis of this group of tumors. In the same year, the authors also investigated the immunohistochemical expression pattern of a recently described group of proteins, the BPFI (PLUNC) family, in salivary gland tumors, also using 1.0 mm cores arranged in triplicate, revealing the presence of an intense expression of PLUNC proteins in mucous cells and mucin plugs of mucoepidermoid carcinoma and papillary cystadenocarcinoma, once again suggesting such biomarkers as new tools for differential diagnosis of salivary gland tumors (Vargas et al. 2008b).

TMA methodology has also been useful for correlating biomarker expression to clinicopathological features of patients affected by salivary gland tumors. Yamazaki et al. (2010) demonstrated in their study, using 2.0 mm cores arranged in duplicate, that geminin protein could predict salivary gland carcinoma aggressiveness, whereas Williams et al. (2010) suggested that HER-2 gene amplification and high protein expression could be a useful target for future therapies of such tumors. Marques et al. (2012) used TMA-based research to suggest that estrogen receptor β (ERβ) could be involved in tumor progression and development of adenoid cystic carcinomas, corroborating the indication for ER antagonists in the clinical control of this malignancy.

In conclusion, the results obtained from these TMA-based studies conducted in recent years and the recently described guidelines and validation approach of TMA for salivary gland tumors strongly suggest that this already proven high-throughput methodology may be of significant value in the study of different biomarker expressions in this heterogeneous group of human neoplasms.

Potential Application of Tissue Microarray to Prognosis, Other Diseases or Conditions

TMA methods have been widely used for studying different biomarkers in a diverse range of human pathological entities. Benign and malignant solid neoplasms are by far the most targeted entities, and validation studies have already been conducted and have proven TMA to be a reliable technique for molecular assessment of tumors from kidney (Eckel-Passow et al. 2010), prostate (Datta et al. 2007), breast (Alkushi 2009), esophagus (Boone et al. 2008), ovary (Rosen et al. 2004), bladder (Nocito et al. 2001), vulva (Fons et al. 2009), colon (Chen et al. 2007), cervix (El-Mansi and Williams 2006), lung (Karlsson et al. 2009), endometrium (Fons et al. 2007), and others. Similarly, TMA has also been used together with immunohistochemistry in the study of nonneoplastic human diseases (Goldstine et al. 2002; Toberer et al. 2013).

As mentioned before, the potential use of hundreds of different tumors simultaneously arranged in a single TMA block is the main advantage of this method, which allows the easy study of the prognostic potential of a given biomarker, which can be analyzed in a large, statistically representative cohort of cases. Hence, TMA technology has been frequently used to determine the potential prognostic value of innumerous new and well-recognized markers (Kallioniemi et al. 2001; Boos et al. 2013; Nowak et al. 2013).

Using differently designed TMAs, the well-known proliferative marker Ki67 has been widely evidenced to be correlated with poor prognosis in patients affected by kidney, endometrial, lung, breast, melanoma, and other cancers, whereas the expression of the cell cycle regulator p53 has been proved to be significantly correlated with inferior survival rates and poorer prognoses in breast, ovarian, and prostate cancers in studies using TMA sections (Landstein et al. 2010; Tennstedt et al. 2012; Skirnisdottir and Seidal 2013; Gayed et al. 2013; Lee et al. 2014). In addition, the immunohistochemical expression of the hormonal receptors, progesterone, estrogen, and HER-2, important for therapeutic purposes in breast cancer, has also been evaluated and correlated with prognosis in TMA-based studies (Bhargava et al. 2004; Madeira et al. 2013).

Summary Points

- Modern tissue microarray technique has been created in the late 1980s following the development of new high-throughput laboratory methodologies like cDNA microarray and proteomics.
- Tissue microarray principles were important to give rise to a new laboratory approach that would allow the evaluation of the increasing number of new molecular makers in clinical and histologic studies.
- The main advantage of tissue microarray methodology is related to its ability of aggregating tissue samples of hundreds of different cases in a single paraffin block, leading to preservation of the original tissues, reduction of the amount of antibodies and other laboratory reagents, and reduction of execution time.
- Some potential limitations of TMA are frequently raised, including the variable quality of the tissues inserted in the TMA, the technical skills required for arranging and cutting TMA blocks, and the most relevant its capacity to adequately represent heterogeneous neoplasms.
- Numerous validation studies in the last few years have demonstrated that tissue microarrays are a valid approach for the molecular study of many human neoplastic and nonneoplastic conditions.
- Salivary gland tumors are a highly morphologically heterogeneous group of neoplasms that correspond to approximately 3–10 % of head and neck neoplasms whose molecular etiopathogenesis remains poorly understood.
- Tissue microarray techniques have only recently been validated in the study of pleomorphic adenoma, the most morphologically heterogeneous of the salivary gland tumors.
- An increased number of studies have been conducted in the recent years using tissue microarray for the investigation of different biomarkers in salivary gland tumors.

References

Alkushi A. Validation of tissue microarray biomarker expression of breast carcinomas in Saudi women. Hematol Oncol Stem Cell Ther. 2009;2:394–8.

Barnes L, Eveson JW, Reichart PA, et al. World health organization classification of tumours. Pathology and genetics of head and neck tumours. 1st ed. Lyon: IARC Press; 2005.

Battifora H. The multitumor (sausage) tissue block: novel method for immunohistochemical antibody testing. Lab Invest. 1986;55:244–8.

Bhargava R, Lal P, Chen B. Feasibility of using tissue microarrays for the assessment of HER-2 gene amplification by fluorescence in situ hybridization in breast carcinoma. Diagn Mol Pathol. 2004;13:213–16.

Boone J, van Hillegersberg R, van Diest PJ, et al. Validation of tissue microarray technology in squamous cell carcinoma of the esophagus. Virchows Arch. 2008;452:507–14.

Boos LA, Dettmer M, Schmitt A, et al. Diagnostic and prognostic implications of the PAX8–PPARγ translocation in thyroid carcinomas – a TMA-based study of 226 cases. Histopathology. 2013;63:234–41.

Camp RL, Neumeister V, Rimm DL. A decade of tissue microarrays: progress in the discovery and validation of cancer biomarkers. J Clin Oncol. 2008;26:5630–7.

Chen WC, Lin MS, Zhang BF, et al. Survey of molecular profiling during human colon cancer development and progression by immunohistochemical staining on tissue microarray. World J Gastroenterol. 2007;13:699–708.

Clauditz TS, Reiff M, Gravert L, et al. Human epidermal growth factor receptor 2 (HER2) in salivary gland carcinomas. Pathology. 2011;43:459–64.

Datta MW, True LD, Nelson PS, et al. The role of tissue microarrays in prostate cancer biomarker discovery. Adv Anat Pathol. 2007;14:408–18.

Eckel-Passow JE, Lohse CM, Sheinin Y, et al. Tissue microarrays: one size does not fit all. Diag Pathol. 2010;5:48.

El-Mansi MT, Williams ARW. Validation of tissue microarray technology using cervical adenocarcinoma and its precursors as a model system. Int J Gynecol Cancer. 2006;16:1225–33.

El-Mansi MT, Williams AR. Evaluation of PTEN expression in cervical adenocarcinoma by tissue microarray. Int J Gynecol Cancer. 2006;16(3):1254–60.

Fons G, Hasibuan SM, van der Velden J, et al. Validation of tissue microarray technology in endometrioid cancer of the endometrium. J Clin Pathol. 2007;60:500–3.

Fons G, van der Velden J, Burger M, et al. Validation of tissue microarray technology in vulvar cancer. Int J Gynecol Pathol. 2009;28:76–82.

Fonseca FP, Carvalho MV, Almeida OP, et al. Clinicopathologic analysis of 493 cases of salivary gland tumors in a Southern Brazilian population. Oral Surg Oral Med Oral Pathol Oral Radiol. 2012;114:230–9.

Fonseca FP, Rangel ALC, Almeida OP, et al. Tissue microarray construction for salivary gland tumors study. Med Oral Patol Oral Cir Bucal. 2013;18:e1–6.

Fonseca FP, Andrade BAB, Rangel ALCA, et al. Tissue microarray is a reliable method for immunohistochemical analysis of pleomorphic adenoma. Oral Surg Oral Med Oral Pathol Oral Radiol. 2014;117:81–8.

Freier K, Flechtenmacher C, Walch A, et al. Differential KIT expression in histological subtypes of adenoid cystic carcinoma (ACC) of the salivary gland. Oral Oncol. 2005a;41:934–9.

Freier K, Flechtenmacher C, Walchd A, et al. Copy number gains on 22q13 in adenoid cystic carcinoma of the salivary gland revealed by comparative genomic hybridization and tissue microarray analysis. Cancer Gen Cytogen. 2005b;159:89–95.

Gayed BA, Youssef RF, Bagrodia A, et al. Ki67 is an independent predictor of oncological outcomes in patients with localized clear-cell renal cell carcinoma. BJU Int. 2014;113(4):668–73.

Glimelius I, Qvarnström F, Simonsson M, et al. Tissue microarray and digital image analysis: a methodological study with special reference to the microenvironment in Hodgkin lymphoma. Histopathology. 2012;61:26–32.

Goldstine J, Seligson DB, Beizai P, et al. Tissue microarrays in the study of non-neoplastic disease of the nervous system. J Neuropathol Exp Neurol. 2002;61:653–62.

Ito FA, Ito K, Vargas PA, et al. Salivary gland tumors in a Brazilian population: a retrospective study of 496 cases. Int J Oral Maxillofac Surg. 2005;34:533–6.

Iwafuchi H, Mori N, Takahashi T, et al. Phenotypic composition of salivary gland tumors: an application of principle component analysis to tissue microarray data. Mod Pathol. 2004;17:803–10.

Kallioniemi O, Wagner U, Kononen J, et al. Tissue microarray technology for high-throughput molecular profiling of cancer. Human Mol Gen. 2001;10:657–62.

Karlsson C, Bodin L, Piehl-Aulin K, et al. Tissue microarray validation: a methodologic study with special reference to lung cancer. Cancer Epidemiol Biomarkers Prev. 2009;18:2014–21.

Kononen J, Bubendorf L, Kallioniemi A, et al. Tissue microarrays for high-throughput molecular profiling of tumor specimens. Nat Med. 1998;4:844–7.

Ladstein RG, Bachmann IM, Straume O, et al. Ki67 expression is superior to mitotic count and novel proliferation markers PHH3, MCM4 and mitosin as a prognostic factor in thick cutaneous melanoma. BMC Cancer. 2010;10:140.

Lee HE, Han N, Kim MA, et al. DNA damage response-related proteins in gastric cancer: ATM, Chk2 and p53 expression and their prognostic value. Pathobiology. 2014;81:25–35.

Madeira M, Mattar A, Logullo AF, et al. Estrogen receptor alpha/beta ratio and estrogen receptor beta as predictors of endocrine therapy responsiveness – a randomized neoadjuvant trial comparison between anastrozole and tamoxifen for the treatment of postmenopausal breast cancer. BMC Cancer. 2013;13:425.

Marques YMFS, Giudice FS, Freitas VM, et al. Oestrogen receptor b in adenoid cystic carcinoma of salivary glands. Histopathology. 2012;60:609–16.

Nelhűbel GA, Károly B, Szabó B, et al. The prognostic role of claudins in head and neck squamous cell carcinomas. Pathol Oncol Res. 2014;20(1):99–106.

Nocito A, Bubendorf L, Tinner EM, et al. Microarrays of bladder cancer tissue are highly representative of proliferation index and histological grade. J Pathol. 2001;194:349–57.

Nowak M, Svensson MA, Carlsson J, et al. Prognostic significance of phospho-histone H3 in prostate carcinoma. World J Urol. 2014;32(3):703–7.

Parsons M, Grabsch H. How to make tissue microarrays. Diagn Histopathol. 2009;15:142–50.

Radhakrishnan R, Solomon M, Satyamoorthy K, et al. Tissue microarray – a high-throughput molecular analysis in head and neck cancer. J Oral Pathol Med. 2008;37:166–76.

Rosen DG, Huang X, Deavers MT, et al. Validation of tissue microarray technology in ovarian carcinoma. Modern Pathol. 2004;17:790–7.

Schneider S, Kloimstein P, Pammer J, et al. New diagnostic markers in salivary gland tumors. Eur Arch Otorhinolaryngol. 2014;271(7):1999–2007.

Simon R, Sauter G. Tissue microarrays for miniaturized high-throughput molecular profiling of tumors. Exp Hematol. 2002;30:1365–72.

Skirnisdottir I, Seidal T. Association of p21, p21 p27 and p21 p53 status to histological subtypes and prognosis in low-stage epithelial ovarian cancer. Cancer Genomics Proteomics. 2013;10:27–34.

Taylor CR. From microscopy to whole slide digital images: a century and a half of image analysis. Appl Immunohistochem Mol Morphol. 2011;19:491–3.

Tennstedt P, Köster P, Brüchmann A, et al. The impact of the number of cores on tissue microarray studies investigating prostate cancer biomarkers. Int J Oncol. 2012;40:261–8.

Toberer F, Sykora J, Göttel D, et al. Apoptotic signal molecules in skin biopsies of cutaneous lupus erythematosus: analysis using tissue microarray. Exp Dermatol. 2013;22:656–9.

Torhorst J, Bucher C, Kononen J, et al. Tissue microarray for rapid linking of molecular changes to clinical endpoints. Am J Pathol. 2001;159:2249–56.

van de Rijn M, Gilks CB. Applications of microarrays to histopathology. Histopathology. 2004;44:97–108.

van Zwieten A. Tissue microarray technology and findings for diagnostic immunohistochemistry. Pathology. 2013;45:71–9.

Vargas PA, Gerhard R, Araújo Filho VJF, et al. Salivary gland tumors in a Brazilian population: a retrospective study of 124 cases. Rev Hosp Clín Fac Med S Paulo. 2002;57(6):271–6.

Vargas PA, Cheng Y, Barrett AW, et al. Expression of Mcm-2, Ki-67 and geminin in benign and malignant salivary gland tumours. J Oral Pathol Med. 2008a;37:309–18.

Vargas PA, Speight PM, Bingle CD, et al. Expression of PLUNC family members in benign and malignant salivary gland tumours. Oral Dis. 2008b;14:613–19.

Voduc D, Kenney C, Nielsen TO. Tissue microarrays in clinical oncology. Semin Radiat Oncol. 2008;18:89–97.

Wan WH, Fortuna MB, Furmanski P. A rapid and efficient method for testing immunohistochemical reactivity of monoclonal antibodies against multiple tissue samples simultaneously. J Immunol Methods. 1987;103:121–9.

Williams MD, Roberts DB, Kies MS, et al. Genetic and expression analysis of HER-2 and EGFR genes in salivary duct carcinoma: empirical and therapeutic significance. Clin Cancer Res. 2010;16:2266–74.

Yamazaki M, Fujii S, Murata Y, et al. High expression level of geminin predicts a poor clinical outcome in salivary gland carcinomas. Histopathology. 2010;56:883–92.

Zlobec I, Koelzer VH, Dawson H, et al. Next-generation tissue microarray (ngTMA) increases the quality of biomarker studies: an example using CD3, CD8, and CD45RO in the tumor microenvironment of six different solid tumor types. J Transl Med. 2013;11:104.

FGFR4 as a Biomarker in Squamous Cell Cancers of Mouth and Oropharynx

36

Roberta Lelis Dutra, Marcelo dos Santos, Suzanny Oliveira Mendes, Gabriela Tonini Peterle, Iúri Drumond Louro, and Adriana Madeira Álvares da Silva Conforti

Contents

R.L. Dutra
Department of Pathology, University of Sao Paulo, Laboratório de Citogenômica, LIM 03, São Paulo, SP, Brazil
e-mail: lelis.roberta@gmail.com

M. dos Santos
Department of Medicine, Federal University of Rio Grande do Norte (UFRN) – Campus Caicó, Caicó, RN, Brazil
e-mail: marcelo.catg@gmail.com

S.O. Mendes • G.T. Peterle
Programa de Pós-graduação em Biotecnologia, Núcleo de Genética Humana e Molecular, Federal University of Espirito Santo (UFES), Vitória, ES, Brazil
e-mail: suzannymendes@gmail.com; gabi-1989@hotmail.com

I.D. Louro
Department of Biology, Federal University of Espirito Santo (UFES), Human and Molecular Genetics Center, Vitória, ES, Brazil
e-mail: iurilouro@yahoo.com

A.M.Á. da Silva Conforti (✉)
Department of Biology, Federal University of Espirito Santo – Center of Agrarian Sciences (CCA/UFES), Alegre, ES, Brazil
e-mail: adriana.biomol@gmail.com

V.R. Preedy, V.B. Patel (eds.), *Biomarkers in Cancer, Biomarkers in Disease: Methods, Discoveries and Applications*,
DOI 10.1007/978-94-007-7681-4_41

Abstract

Head and neck squamous cell carcinoma (HNSCC) is a malignancy associated with severe mortality despite advances in therapy, and it ranks among the top ten most common cancers worldwide, with a large incidence variation according to sex and geographical location. At the moment, no biomarkers are currently available for HNSCC patients; prognosis depends largely on the stage at presentation, with the most important prognostic factor. Fibroblast growth factor receptors (FGFRs) and ligand binding are among the many molecules that are involved in the tumorigenesis process. These receptors, including FGFR4, belong to the receptor tyrosine kinase family leads to cell growth, mitosis, and differentiation. Mutations and amplifications in FGFR4 have been linked to aggressive tumor progression, and metastasis is associated with poor prognosis in HNSCC. In this review, we summarize the FGF/FGFR complex, signalization mechanisms, and the molecular implications of FGFR4 as potential biomarker for HNSCC.

List of Abbreviations

AKT	Serina/Treonina Kinase, Also Known as Protein Kinase B (PKB)
CAMs	Cell Adhesion Molecules
CHD	CAM Homology Domain
CNV	Copy Number Variation
EGFR	Epidermal Growth Factor Receptor
FGF	Fibroblast Growth Factor
FGFR	Fibroblast Growth Factor Receptor
HER2 (ErbB2)	Human Epidermal Growth Factor Receptor 2
HNSCC	Head and Neck Squamous Cell Carcinoma
HRAS	Harvey Rat Sarcoma Viral Oncogene Homologue
HSPGs	Heparin and Heparan Sulfate Proteoglycans
Ig	Immunoglobulin
KRAS	Kirsten Rat Sarcoma Viral Oncogene Homologue
MAPK	Mitogen-Activated Protein Kinases
MHC	Major Histocompatibility Complex
NCAMs	Neural Cell Adhesion Molecules
PLCγ	Phopholipase C – gamma
RTK	Receptor Tyrosine Kinase
SNP	Single Nucleotide Polymorphism
STAT	Signal Transducer and Activator of Transcription

Key Facts

- Head and neck squamous cell carcinoma is among the most common cancers in the world population.
- Fibroblast growth factors are biomarkers for cancer etiology, mainly in HNSCC, responsible for promoting the cell proliferation and, thus, presenting a mitogenic activity.
- Approximately 22 FGFs with mitogenic activity are observed in a variety of organisms, including humans.
- The family of fibroblast growth factor receptor comprises five transmembrane receptors (FGFR1 to FGFR4) which require the binding of many cell-surface proteins (cell adhesion molecules), leading to intracellular signaling.
- Several transmembrane receptors, including FGFRs, present a region with tyrosine kinase activity, promotion of cellular signaling, mainly during embryogenesis and adult tissue homeostasis.
- The presence of polymorphism Gly388Arg can interfere on the signaling pathway via FGFR4, resulting in poor prognosis or not, depending on the specific tumor.
- Mutations and amplifications may change the FGFR4 signaling pathway, resulting in excessive proliferation, as well as carcinogenesis.
- FGFR4 can be considered as an important biomarker and target for cancer treatment.

Definitions of Words and Terms

Acidic Box Region rich in acidic amino acids present between two immunoglobulin (Ig)-like domains.

Cell Adhesion Molecules (CAMs) Proteins located on the cell surface involved in binding with other cells or with the extracellular matrix (ECM) in the process called cell adhesion. Cell adhesion molecules help cells stick to each other and to their surroundings.

C-terminus Region (Also known as the carboxyl-terminus, carboxy-terminus, C-terminal tail, C-terminal end, or COOH-terminus) is the end of an amino acid chain (protein or polypeptide), terminated by a free carboxyl group (–COOH). When the protein is translated from messenger RNA, it is created from N-terminus to C-terminus.

Epigenetic Mechanisms They are changes in gene expression or cellular phenotype, caused by modifications to the genome that do not involve changes to the nucleotide sequence. Examples are DNA methylation and histone modification, both of which serve to regulate gene expression without altering the underlying DNA sequence.

Heparan Sulfate Proteoglycan (HSPG) Molecules Heparan sulfate (HS) is a linear polysaccharide that occurs as a proteoglycan (PG) in which HS molecules chains are attached in close proximity to the cell surface. It is in this form that HS binds to a variety of protein ligands and regulates a wide variety of biological processes, including angiogenesis, blood coagulation, and tumor metastasis.

Immunoglobulin-Like Domains The immunoglobulin domain is a type of protein domain that consists of a two-layered sandwich of between 7 and 9 antiparallel β-strands arranged in two β-sheets, with approximately 80 amino acids. Immunoglobulin-like domains are involved in protein–protein and protein–ligand interactions, and some examples include antibodies and receptor tyrosine kinases.

Isoforms A protein isoform is a different form of the same protein that can be produced from closely related genes or by alternative splicing.

Major Histocompatibility Complex (MHC) The major histocompatibility complex (MHC) is a set of cell-surface molecules that mediates interactions among other kinds of cells and determines compatibility of donors for organ transplant as well as one's susceptibility to an autoimmune disease via cross-reacting immunization.

Monoclonal Antibody Monoclonal antibodies are monospecific antibodies that are the same because they are made by identical immune cells that are all clones of a unique parent cell and that bind to the same epitope, in contrast to polyclonal antibodies, made from several different immune cells.

N-Cadherin This protein is a calcium-dependent cell–cell adhesion glycoprotein comprising five extracellular cadherin repeats, a transmembrane region, and a highly conserved cytoplasmic tail.

Sprouty (SPRY) Sprouty (SPRY) proteins represent a major class of ligand-inducible inhibitors of RTK-dependent signaling pathways.

Tyrosine Kinase Activity A tyrosine kinase is an enzyme that transfers a phosphate group from ATP to a protein in a cell. The process of activation occurs from the phosphorylation of proteins by kinases, an important mechanism in communicating signals within a cell (signal transduction).

Introduction

In the year 2012, over half a million new cases of head and neck squamous cell carcinoma (HNSCC) were diagnosed, representing the sixth most common cancer type in the world, with a 5-year survival rate of around 50 %. In North America, the head and neck cancers account for 2–3 % of all newly cases (Haddad and Shin 2008).

Most head and neck cancers are squamous cell carcinomas (SCCs), including carcinomas of the oral cavity, pharynx, and larynx, and they vary according to their degree of differentiation to well, moderate, and poor carcinomas (Azad et al. 2012).

Although some anatomic subsites appear to have better prognosis, this may be more related to earlier symptoms, leading to diagnosis at an earlier stage. Between 33 % and 50 % of head and neck cancers are early diagnosed at stages I and II (Argiris et al. 2008).

The major risk factors associated with the HNSCC are smoking or tobacco chewing, alcohol consumption, the use of smokeless tobacco products (synergistic effect), and genetic predisposition. Recently, the human papilloma virus (HPV) was documented as a cause of specific subsets of head and neck SCCs (D'Souza et al. 2007).

The treatment of HNSCC is heavily based on radiotherapy in combination with surgery and/or cytostatic drugs. However, radio- and/or chemotherapy resistance and tumor recurrences are important clinical problems in the management of HNSCC. With this, the identification of predictive factors of treatment response is critically important.

Deeper understanding of the molecular biology of HNSCC can provide new insights into its development and progression; it also provides various biomarkers with a potential application for cancer screening and monitoring of the response to therapy.

The fibroblast growth factor receptor (FGFR) family comprises structurally related tyrosine kinase receptors (FGFR1–FGFR4) involved in signaling via interactions with fibroblast growth factors (FGFs), playing an important role in a wide range of biological processes, including differentiation, proliferation, cell motility, and angiogenesis . Most FGFs have mitogenic activity in a variety of systems, including cell growth, differentiation, and migration. The proliferative capacity of FGFs is a function of FGFRs, to which they bind and through which they signal (Powers et al. 2000).

Deregulation in FGF/FGFR signaling has been implicated in human malignant diseases. Functional studies demonstrated that FGFR4 interferes in signaling events, leading to normal cell adhesiveness and corresponding invasive properties of pituitary tumors. Although the molecular basis of this function is still a matter of intense research, FGFR4 seems to play a role in a broader range of human cancers (Ezzat et al. 2002).

Receptor Tyrosine Kinases

Receptor tyrosine kinases (RTKs) are transmembrane proteins which function as growth factor receptors. This RTK superfamily consists of multiple families, such as the epidermal growth factor receptor (EGFR) and the vascular endothelial growth factor receptor (VEGFR), which includes the fibroblast growth factor receptor (FGFR) family (Manning et al. 2002).

Normally, RTKs play a role in developmental signaling and adult homeostasis. However, activation of RTKs during carcinogenesis leads to the proliferative and antiapoptotic process called "addiction to oncogenic RTKs," or simply "oncogenic addiction" (Krause and Van Etten 2005; Weinstein and Joe 2006).

In the carcinogenesis process, epigenetic changes and genetic alterations lead to the heterogeneity of cancer cells, which results in the evolution of subclones with more malignant phenotypes, as well as the accumulation of genetic alterations in cancer cells, such as single nucleotide polymorphisms (SNPs) and copy number variations (CNVs) (Katoh 2007).

Fibroblast growth factor receptor 4 (FGFR4) belongs to the tyrosine kinase receptor family. Although FGFR4 does not present an essential function during embryogenesis and adult life, the cellular signaling by tyrosine kinase appear to be involved in several metabolic pathways, as well as in the mitogenic effect (Gutierrez et al. 2006).

Previous studies have shown a reduced autophosphorylation and tyrosine kinase activity of FGFR4 compared to other FGFRs (Shaoul et al. 1995). In the absence of a clear mitogenic effect of FGFR4, the potential FGFR4 ligands can influence on regulated signaling system.

FGF/FGFR Complex

Fibroblast growth factors (FGFs) and their receptors (FGFR) have important roles in cell behavior, such as proliferation, differentiation, migration, survival, embryogenesis, and angiogenesis in adults. Alterations in the FGF/FGFR signaling pathway have been associated with many developmental disorders, especially cancer (Brooks et al. 2012).

Since the discovery of the first FGF, approximately 22 distinct FGFs have been identified in a variety of organisms from nematode and drosophila to mouse and human. FGF family genes can vary in size from 17 to 34 kDa with a conserved sequence of 120 amino acids (Ornitz and Itoh 2001).

Binding of FGF ligand to cells has been described by several authors, but Moscatelli et al. (1987), was the first to observe that each cell type expresses low- and high-affinity receptors for FGF. FGFR family members are divided into two main classes: low-affinity FGFRs, which require the binding of heparan sulfate proteoglycan molecules on the cell surface for the attachment of its ligands, and high-affinity FGFRs. High-affinity receptors are the ones that mediate biological responses to FGFs (Coughlin et al. 1988; Mohammadi et al. 2005).

In contrast to the multiple FGF molecules, there are only five FGFRs, although receptor diversity is increased by alternative splicing of FGFR1, FGFR2, and FGFR3, generating receptor isoforms with dramatically altered FGF binding specificity (Brooks et al. 2012).

Like all tyrosine kinase receptors, FGFR1–FGFR4 are transmembrane proteins, composed of an extracellular ligand-binding domain, a single transmembrane domain, and a cytoplasmic domain containing the catalytic protein tyrosine kinase core as well as additional regulatory sequences (Eswarakumar et al. 2005). The extracellular FGFR ligand-binding domain is composed of three extracellular

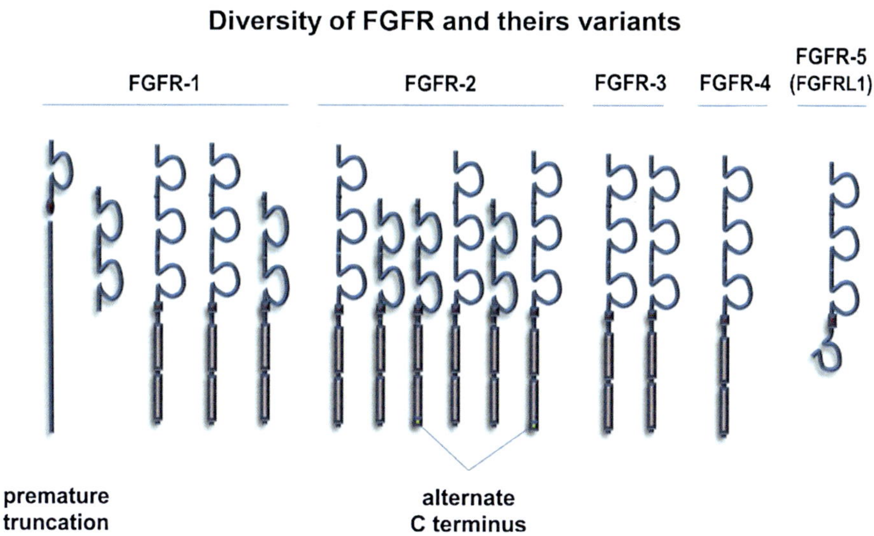

Fig. 1 Representative view of FGFRs showing the diversity created by alternative splice variants. The alternate C-terminus variants are designated C1 and C3. The open square in the extracellular domain represents the acid box region. The last receptor (*FGFR5*) has an intracellular domain without tyrosine kinase activity (Modified from Powers et al. 2000)

immunoglobulin-like domains – designated IgI, IgII, and IgIII – a single-pass transmembrane domain, and an intracellular dimerized tyrosine kinase domain. IgI and IgII are separated by a stretch of acidic residues, known as the acid box (Powers et al. 2000).

Through the use of splice variants, a variety of different receptor types are possible to create, dramatically increasing FGF binding selectivity (Ornitz and Itoh 2001). The diversity of the FGF receptors is shown in the Fig. 1.

Different exon usage produces transcripts that result in the translation of proteins that can be prematurely truncated and lack Ig-like domains or utilize different exon coding regions for the same Ig-like domain. One of the most important mechanisms involves the alternative splicing of the IgIII domain and can be observed in FGFRs 1–3 but not in FGFR4, creating IIIb and IIIc variants with differing ligand-binding specificities that are expressed in a tissue-specific manner (Eswarakumar et al. 2005). The case of FGF7, known to bind FGFR2 (IIIb) but not to the closely related FGFR2 (IIIc), is used to explain the high level of ligand specificity (Korc and Friesel 2009).

A fifth receptor FGFR5 (also known as FGFRL1) can bind FGFs with high affinity, but lacks the intracellular tyrosine kinase domain, and therefore the role of this receptor is poorly understood (Turner and Grose 2010).

Two other members of the FGFR family were reported in literature and the sequences are designated as FGFR6 and HrFGFR. The first one was identified during cloning and sequencing studies of primate major histocompatibility complex (MHC) proteins that were found to contain sequences related to the FGFR gene family, yielding the characterization of PERB1 or FGFR6 (Leelayuwat et al. 1996). This new receptor revealed 80 % homology at the amino acid level to the immunoglobulin-like domain I of FGFR3 and is more closely related to FGFR3 and FGFR5 than FGFR1, FGFR2, and FGFR4.

The second is named HrFGFR and it was isolated from a cDNA library, showing a 50 % and 40 % homology at the ligand-binding domain and overall amino acid sequence, respectively, in comparison to that of the four classic FGFRs. Owing to the isolation of a second HrFGFR lacking the acid box and the immunoglobulin-like domain I, it has been suggested that the HrFGFR gene may be transcribed into two different mRNAs by alternative splicing (Kamei et al. 2000).

The FGF receptor–ligand system is considered highly complex by the existence of an increasing number of proteins that interact directly with FGF and/or FGFR either to produce intracellular signals directly or to modulate FGFR signal output (Ornitz et al. 1992). Some of the noncanonical FGF ligands can activate FGFR signaling in the absence of FGFs (e.g., NCAMs, N-cadherin), whereas other FGFs that reside mainly in the extracellular matrix can form complexes with heparin and heparan sulfate proteoglycans (HSPGs), considered coreceptors for pathway signaling (Polanska et al. 2009).

These proteins are responsible for carrying FGFs within the extracellular matrix, an important step in the interaction of these growth factors with their specific cellular receptors; however, there is controversy regarding the exact manner by which this occurs, although it is thought to involve the induction of receptor dimerization and to be heparin dependent (Korc and Friesel 2009; Powers et al. 2000).

The initial models for the role of heparin/heparan sulfate (HS) in FGF signaling were based on the assumption that this complex interacts with FGF only, where it (i) stabilizes and protects FGFs from thermal, proteolytic, or pH-dependent degradation (Saksela et al. 1988), (ii) functions as storage reservoirs where FGF can be freed to interact with FGFR (Folkman et al. 1988), or (iii) facilitates FGF–FGFR binding by limiting the conformation of FGF ligand (Eswarakumar et al. 2005). However, other authors verified that heparin promotes FGF signaling by simultaneously interacting with FGF and FGFR, thereby facilitating the formation of a ternary complex (Mohammadi et al. 2005).

FGF ligands and FGFRs have been found to interact with a variety of proteins and glycolipids that are unrelated to the classic form of FGF/FGFR/HSPG ligand–receptor system. Some of these proteins include integrins, which are classic receptors for extracellular matrix proteins, which interact with FGFR and FGF ligand; NCAMs, L1, and cadherins, which can interact with FGFR, as well as present noncanonical FGF ligands to the receptor (Polanska et al. 2009; Sanchez-Heras et al. 2006).

Otherwise, FGFR4 is implicated in signaling cascades with regard to cell–matrix adhesion and angiogenesis. Abnormal expression of FGFR4 has been suggested as a potential mechanism in the progression of cancers, including the upregulation of a urokinase-type plasminogen activator (uPA), a proteolytic enzyme, required for cell migration and the association with NCAM in cell adhesion to the extracellular matrix.

FGF/FGFR Signaling

FGFR signaling is primarily triggered by the binding of receptors to FGF ligands. Dimerization of FGF/FGFR/HPSG complex leads to a conformational change in FGFR structure, resulting in the formation of various complexes to initiate downstream signal transduction including the activation of PLCc, MAPK, AKT, and STAT cascades (Fig. 2).

Ligand-induced dimerization of these molecules leads to the successful activation of several intracellular receptor domain tyrosine residues, through FGFR sequential transphosphorylation (Acevedo et al. 2009).

The biological process outcomes of FGF/FGFR activation are dependent on a complex network of signaling and transcriptional events regulated by multiple factors. The specific modulated biological response can be proliferative, apoptotic, or migratory, depending on the interplay between these factors. This process involves specific signal transduction molecules, feedback loops, cross talk with other signaling networks, and the activation or repression of target genes. In this manner, the MAPK signaling cascade is implicated in cell growth and

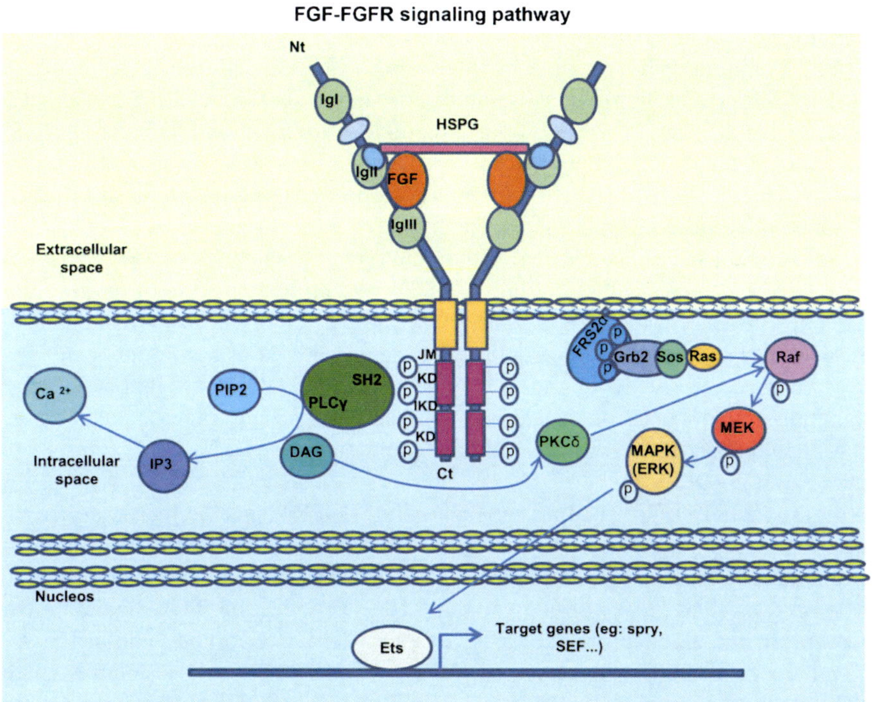

Fig. 2 FGF–FGFR signaling pathway showing several proteins participating on the intracellular activation process (Reprinted from Developmental Biology, 287, Bernard Thisse, Christine Thisse, Functions and regulations of fibroblast growth factor signaling during embryonic development, 390–402, Copyright (2005), with permission from Elsevier)

differentiation, the PI3K/Akt signaling cascade is involved in cell survival and cell fate determination, while the PI3K and PKC signaling cascades have a function in cell polarity control (Korc and Friesel 2009).

FGFRs, like other receptor tyrosine kinases, transmit extracellular signals to various cytoplasmic signal transduction pathways through tyrosine autophosphorylation. Activation of FGFRs by tyrosine phosphorylation leads to signal transduction through multiple pathways, including phospholipase Cγ (PLCγ), phosphatidylinositol 3-kinase (PI3K), mitogen-activated protein kinases (MAPK), protein kinase C (PKC), and signal transducers and activators of transcription (STATs) (Hart et al. 2001).

FGF signaling induced by proteins such as MAPK phosphatase 3 (MKP3) and similar expression to FGF (Sef) may cause receptor dephosphorylation. Other molecules have been identified that can attenuate signaling, such as cell-surface molecules NCAM and N-cadherin and the sprouty-related enabled/vasodilator-stimulated phosphoprotein homology 1 domain-containing protein (Turner and Grose 2010).

FGF/FGFR signaling is also tightly regulated by feedback mechanisms that occur at many points in the signaling pathway, such as FGF-induced Sprouty (SPRY) proteins, which in turn are important negative regulators that bind to growth factor receptor-bound protein 2 (GRB2), thereby disrupting downstream signaling (Lo et al. 2004).

SPRY inhibits FGF signaling by interfering with extracellular signal-regulated kinase (ERK) activation either by binding to and sequestering the growth factor receptor-bound protein 2 (Grb2) or by binding to Raf1 and preventing Raf1 activation. This downregulation seems to correlate with an aggressive tumor phenotype. The mechanisms for SPRY regulation appear to be tumor-type specific and include both epigenetic and nonepigenetic mechanisms (Mason et al. 2006).

Sef is a transmembrane protein with homology to the interleukin (IL)-17 receptor family and binds to FGFR1 and FGFR2, preventing activation of the receptor tyrosine kinase (Kovalenko et al. 2003). Sef protein activity is also downregulated in several tumor types of epithelial origin, including breast, thyroid, prostate, and ovarian cancers. Owing to the downregulation of feedback inhibitors of FGF signaling in tumor cells, as well as an increased expression of FGF ligands, tumors may show enhanced growth, progression, and metastasis (Darby et al. 2006; Korc and Friesel 2009).

In the absence of a potential signalization of FGFR4, specific ligands relied on an expressed chimeric receptor where the FGF-binding domain was of FGFR4 origin and the intracellular domain was of FGFR1 origin (Ornitz et al. 1996).

Moreover, FGF receptor 4 may not necessarily require FGF ligand. First, heparin, in the absence of FGF, may activate FGFR4 (Gao and Goldfarb 1995; Cavallaro et al. 2001). Second, FGFR4 was found function in a complex with NCAM, independently of FGF (Cavallaro et al. 2001). Detection of N-linked glycosylation on an overexpressed extracellular domain of human FGFR4 (Tuominen et al. 2001) suggested that the function of this receptor might be regulated by glycosylation, similar to the other FGFRs. However, *N*-glycosylation of native FGFR4 has not been analyzed yet.

FGFR Mutations/Amplifications

Recent studies have shown that FGFR-activating mutations and overexpression are closely associated with the development and progression of tumors in humans, as well as the persistent and excessive activation of the FGFR signaling pathway, resulting in carcinogenic functions in cells, such as excessive proliferation and apoptosis evasion (Greulich and Pollock 2011). For example, FGFR-activating mutations in bladder cancer, endometrial carcinomas, multiple myeloma, and rhabdomyosarcomas lead to the development and progression of tumors, resulting in poor prognosis, angiogenesis, invasion, and metastasis (Greulich and Pollock 2011; Liang et al. 2012).

In vivo and in vitro studies using FGFR gene knockout and pharmacological inhibition have provided further confirmation that FGFR is an important biomarker and target for cancer treatment (Brooks et al. 2012). Several major pharmaceutical companies and research institutions have designed various types of nonselective and selective FGFR inhibitors, some of which have entered antitumor clinical trials and have shown promising clinical effects and application prospects (Liang et al. 2012).

Although the molecular basis of this event is still a matter of intense research, FGFR4 plays a role in a broader range of human cancers. A single nucleotide polymorphism (SNP) in exon 9 (substitution of a glycine residue for an arginine – Gly388Arg in FGFR4) has been responsible for a positive correlation with prognostic parameters in several human cancers, including breast, colon, lung, prostate, and head and neck cancers (Bange et al. 2002; Ezzat et al. 2002; Streit et al. 2004).

Some researchers have reported that the allele showed a significantly higher risk of developing cancer, proposing the Gly388 allele as a risk allele for head and neck cancer (Ansell et al. 2009).

For the HNSCC, Streit et al. (2004) reported that in, expression of Gly388 FGFR4 had no impact on disease progression. Other studies also showed that the presence of at least one Arg allele was significantly correlated with reduced overall survival and an increased mortality risk of 2.2 and that FGFR4 Arg388 allele also was strongly associated with poor prognosis. This can be explained by the fact that indeed other factors, for example, genetic alterations in receptor tyrosine kinases, are key players in the progressive course of the disease.

Although the presence of FGFR4 Arg388 allele has been shown to indicate a poor prognosis in several tumors, the mechanism by which it affects cancer progression remains unclear (da Costa Andrade et al. 2007).

Dutra et al. (2012) verified the association of the presence of Arg388 allele with lymphatic embolization and with disease-related premature death. In addition, the authors observed which FGFR4 low expression was related with lymph node positivity and premature relapse of disease, as well as disease-related death in squamous cell carcinoma of the mouth and oropharynx.

Low FGFR4 expression in the presence of Arg388 allele is associated with worse survival in patients with oral and oropharyngeal squamous cell carcinoma. Thus, not only mutations in FGFR could influence the signaling cascade and lead to poor cancer prognosis but that FGFR4 expression alone has no impact on disease progression in HNSCC (Dutra et al. 2012).

Nevertheless, FGFR4 Arg388 has not been considered an oncogene per se, but rather collaborates with oncogenes involved in cell motility and invasiveness (Seitzer et al. 2010).

This might be related to signaling cascades that control cell–matrix adhesion and angiogenesis. Although some mechanisms have been described in the literature, the influence of Gly388Arg polymorphism in tumor aggressiveness may differ in specific tumors.

In animal model, low protein expression, even in the presence of FGFR4 Arg388 polymorphism, was related to increased pathway activity. This may be explained by the activation of alternative proteins in the signaling cascade or other cascades (Seitzer et al. 2010). This propose, has been reported that the presence of polymorphism Gly388Arg is associated with increased cancer risk and progression of pituitary tumors through recruitment of STAT3 signaling cascade. Activation of this cascade can result in deregulation of cell proliferation and apoptosis, leading to tumor progression. Signaling hyperactivation by specific mutations depends on their resistance to negative feedback loops (Chandarlapaty et al. 2011).

In addition, several ubiquitylation proteins bind directly to RTKs, altering receptor activation. RTK ubiquitylation may promote receptor degradation, creating an important negative feedback mechanism (Lemmon and Schlessinger 2010).

Potential Applications to Prognosis, Other Diseases, or Conditions

FGFRs have been identified as part of the most commonly mutated kinase genes in human cancers, presenting mutations in FGFR2 and FGFR3 as the most prevalent (Turner and Grose 2010). For example, activating and oncogenic FGFR2 mutations located in the extracellular and kinase receptor domains have been described in 12 % of endometrial carcinomas, causing sensitivity to FGFR inhibition (Dutt et al. 2008). In contrast, mutations in FGFR3 present in bladder cancer and FGFR2 mutations in endometrial cancer are mutually exclusive with mutations in HRAS and KRAS, respectively. In addition, mutations in the FGFR4 kinase domain have been found in the childhood soft tissue sarcoma rhabdomyosarcoma, causing autophosphorylation and constitutive signaling (Brooks et al. 2012; Taylor et al. 2009).

Several studies have examined the role of FGFR4 in carcinogenesis, providing evidences for the complexity of FGF/FGFR signaling pathways in different tumor types (Olson et al. 1988; Ezzat et al. 2002).

FGFR Targeting Cancer Therapeutics

FGFR-targeted therapeutics using small-molecule compounds is an active topic in the field of clinical oncology because FGF signaling is involved in various aspects of cancer biology such as proliferation, anti-apoptosis, drug resistance, angiogenesis, and invasion (Heinzle et al. 2011; Ota et al. 2009).

Several small-molecule compounds fitting into the ATP-binding pockets of the tyrosine kinase domain have been developed for cancer therapeutics, targeting specific receptors (Katoh and Nakagama 2013). Thus, FGFR-targeted drugs exert direct as well as indirect anticancer effects, because FGFRs and endothelial cells are involved in tumorigenesis and vasculogenesis, respectively (Daniele et al. 2012).

The activity of most of these agents against FGFRs is still unknown. Although the broader specificity of these compounds could add to its efficacy, the inhibition of several tyrosine kinases will likely result in increased side effects, which may limit the ability to achieve doses required for effective FGFR inhibition.

Deregulation in FGF/FGFR signaling has been implicated in human malignant diseases. In normal cells, RTK activity (FGF/FGFR/HSPG) is strictly regulated, but dysregulation or constitutive RTK activation has been found in a wide range of cancers. The deregulated activation occurs by gain-of-function mutations, gene rearrangement, gene amplification, and overexpression or abnormal autocrine, endocrine, or paracrine stimulation of both receptor and ligand, and, in some cases, it has been shown to correlate with the development and progression of numerous human cancers. Since RTKs have been implicated in many aspects of the malignant phenotype, they are emerging as promising therapeutic targets (Ezzat et al. 2002; Jeffers et al. 2002; Lopez-Knowles et al. 2006).

However, the cancer therapy targeting RTKs will be successful only if the targeted RTK is a major regulator of cancer cell survival (Takeuchi and Ito 2011).

Cancer cells contain multiple genetic and epigenetic abnormalities and their survival and/or proliferation can often be impaired by the inactivation of a single oncogene.

Recently, an explanation for the molecular targeted therapy phenomenon, called "oncogene addiction," was proposed. Evidences for the concept of oncogene addiction come from the increasing number of examples of the therapeutic efficacy of antibodies or small molecules that target specific oncogenes (Weinstein and Joe 2006).

Many targeted molecular cancer therapeutics, including antibodies or small molecules, have been approved in different countries and for different target receptors (Table 1). One example for target growth factor receptors is the overexpression of HER2 (ErbB2) that occurs in approximately 25 % of breast cancer patients and is associated with shorter survival. Other receptor with RTK activity is the epidermal growth factor receptor (EGFR), widely upregulated in solid tumors and mediates many characteristics of malignant phenotype, including proliferation, protection from apoptosis, and tumor cell motility (Nahta et al. 2006).

Thus, these findings led to the development of antibodies that target HER2 and EGFR, and the validity of both growth factor receptors as therapeutic targets is illustrated by the successes of trastuzumab and cetuximab and the oncogenic role of aberrant signaling from RTK, which has become an attractive therapeutic target (Laird and Cherrington 2003; Takeuchi and Ito 2011).

Although studies have associated the Gly388Arg polymorphism with prognosis in several tumors, their effects in response to radiotherapy still remains unclear (Farnebo et al. 2013).

Table 1 Examples of targeted molecular cancer therapeutics received marketing (Reproduced with permission from Biol. Pharm. Bull. Vol. 34 No. 12. Copyright (2011) The Pharmaceutical Society of Japan)

Drug type	Drug	Disease indication	Primary molecular target
Antibody	Trastuzumab (Herceptin)	Breast cancer	HER2
	Bevacizumab (Avastin)	Metastatic colorectal carcinoma	VEGFR
	Cetuximab (Erbitux)	EGFR-expressing metastatic colorectal cancer	EGFR
	Panitumumab (Vectibix)	Wild-type KRAS-expressing metastatic colorectal cancer	EGFR
Small molecule	Imatinib (Gleevec)	CML, GIST	BCR-ABL, c-KIT, PDGFR
	Gefitinib (Iressa)	Metastatic non-small cell lung cancer	EGFR
	Erlotinib (Tarceva)	Metastatic non-small cell lung cancer	EGFR
	Sorafenib (Nexavar)	Renal cell cancer	VEGFR, c-RAF, PDGFR
	Sunitinib (Sutent)	Gleevec-resistant CML	BCR-ABL, SRC
	Nilotinib (Tasigna)	Gleevec-resistant CML	BCR-ABL
	Dasatinib (Sprycel)	Gleevec-resistant CML	BCR-ABL, SRC
	Lapatinib (Tykerb)	HER2-positive breast cancer	EGFR, HER2

A few studies with cell lines of squamous cell carcinoma related to the presence of the mutations in FGFR4 with increased sensitivity to treatment with sensitivity to chemotherapy (Ansell et al. 2009; Farnebo et al. 2009; Marme et al. 2012). In addition, the presence of Arg388 allele was associated with resistance to adjuvant therapy in breast cancer (Thussbas et al. 2006).

These findings have important therapeutic implications, because inhibition of one intracellular pathway may lead to the activation of parallel signaling pathways, thereby decreasing the effectiveness of single-agent-targeted therapies.

Summary Points

- Head and neck squamous cell carcinoma (HNSCC) is among the most common cancers worldwide, representing the sixth most common cancer type in the world. However, there are a few specific biomarkers available for HNSCC patients.
- In the year 2012, over half a million new cases of head and neck squamous cell carcinoma (HNSCC) were diagnosed,
- Considered one of the main biomarker for the HNSCC, FGF and FGFR complex is an important mediator of cellular processes such as proliferation, differentiation, survival, and motility, occurring mainly during embryonic development.

- The four signaling FGFR1–FGFR4 are transmembrane proteins, composed of an extracellular ligand-binding domain, a single transmembrane domain, and a cytoplasmic tyrosine kinase domain.
- Fibroblast growth factor receptors (FGFRs) form a subfamily of the receptor tyrosine kinase (RTK) superfamily, and they are encoded by four genes (FGFR1, FGFR2, FGFR3, and FGFR4). They are involved in the regulation of organ development, cell proliferation and migration, angiogenesis, and other processes.
- FGFR signaling is primarily triggered by the binding of FGF/FGFR/HPSG complex causing a conformational alteration in the FGFR structure, resulting in the activation of many proteins, such as PLCc, MAPK, AKT, and STAT cascade. Alterations in FGFR4 (mutations/amplifications) have an important role in the broader range of human cancers.
- A specific polymorphism in FGFR4 (Gly388Arg) has been responsible for the poor prognosis in several human cancers, including head and neck cancers. However, the influence of Gly388Arg polymorphism in tumor aggressiveness may differ in specific tumors.
- The study of specific biomarkers allows the development molecular targeted therapy and which has become an attractive therapeutic target.

References

Acevedo VD, Ittmann M, Spencer DM. Paths of FGFR-driven tumorigenesis. Cell Cycle. 2009;8(4):580–8.

Ansell A, Farnebo L, Grenman R, et al. Polymorphism of FGFR4 in cancer development and sensitivity to cisplatin and radiation in head and neck cancer. Oral Oncol. 2009;45:23–9.

Argiris A, Karamouzis MV, Raben D, Ferris RL. Head and neck cancer. Lancet. 2008;371:1695–709.

Azad AK, Bairati I, Samson E, Cheng D, Mirshams M, Qiu X, Savas S, Waldron J, Wang C, Goldstein D, Xu W, Meyer F, Liu G. Validation of genetic sequence variants as prognostic factors in early-stage head and neck squamous cell cancer survival. Clin Cancer Res. 2012;18(1):196–206.

Bange J, Prechtl D, Cheburkin Y, Specht K, Harbeck N, et al. Cancer progression and tumor cell motility are associated with the FGFR4 Arg(388) allele. Cancer Res. 2002;62:840–7.

Brooks AN, Kilgour E, Smith PD. Molecular pathways: fibroblast growth factor signaling: a new therapeutic opportunity in cancer. Clin Cancer Res. 2012;18(7):1855–62.

Cavallaro U, Niedermeyer J, Fuxa M, Christofori G. N-CAM modulates tumour-cell adhesion to matrix by inducing FGF-receptor signalling. Nat Cell Biol. 2001;3(7):650–7.

Chandarlapaty S, Sawai A, Scaltriti M, Rodrik-Outmezguine V, Grbovic-Huezo O, et al. AKT inhibition relieves feedback suppression of receptor tyrosine kinase expression and activity. Cancer Cell. 2011;19:58–71.

Clarke JM, Hurwitz HI. Understanding and targeting resistance to anti-angiogenic therapies. J Gastrointest Oncol. 2013;4(3):253–63.

Coughlin SR, Barr PJ, Cousens LS, Fretto LJ, Williams LT. Acidic and basic fibroblast growth factors stimulate tyrosine kinase activity in vivo. J Biol Chem. 1988;263(2):988–93.

D'Souza G, Kreimer AR, Viscidi R, Pawlita M, Fakhry C, Koch WM, et al. Case–control study of human papillomavirus and oropharyngeal cancer. N Engl J Med. 2007;356:1944–56.

da Costa Andrade VC, Parise Jr O, Hors CP, et al. The fibroblast growth factor receptor 4 (FGFR4) Arg388 allele correlates with survival in head and neck squamous cell carcinoma. Exp Mol Pathol. 2007;82:53–7.

Daniele G, Corral J, Molife LR, de Bono JS. FGF receptor inhibitors: role in cancer therapy. Curr Oncol Rep. 2012;14:111–9.

Darby S, Sahadevan K, Khan MM, Robson CN, Leung HY, Gnanapragasam VJ. Loss of Sef (similar expression to FGF) expression is associated with high grade and metastatic prostate cancer. Oncogene. 2006;25:4122–7.

Dutra RL, de Carvalho MB, Dos Santos M, Mercante AM, Gazito D, de Cicco R, Group G, Tajara EH, Louro ID, da Silva AM. FGFR4 profile as a prognostic marker in squamous cell carcinoma of the mouth and oropharynx. PLoS One. 2012;7(11):e50747.

Dutt A, Salvesen HB, Chen TH, Ramos AH, Onofrio RC, Hatton C, et al. Drug-sensitive FGFR2 mutations in endometrial carcinoma. Proc Natl Acad Sci U S A. 2008;105(25):8713–7.

Eswarakumar VP, Lax I, Schlessinger J. Cellular signaling by fibroblast growth factor receptors. Cytokine Growth Factor Rev. 2005;16:139–49.

Ezzat S, Zheng L, Zhu XF, Wu GE, Asa SL. Targeted expression of a human pituitary tumor-derived isoform of FGF receptor-4 recapitulates pituitary tumorigenesis. J Clin Invest. 2002;109:69–78.

Farnebo L, Jedlinski A, Ansell A, et al. Proteins and single nucleotide polymorphisms involved in apoptosis, growth control, and DNA repair predict cisplatin sensitivity in head and neck cancer cell lines. Int J Mol Med. 2009;24:549–56.

Farnebo L, Tiefenbock K, Ansell A, Thunell LK, Garvin S, Roberg K. Strong expression of survivin is associated with positive response to radiotherapy and improved overall survival in head and neck squamous cell carcinoma patients. Int J Cancer. 2013;133:1994–2003.

Folkman J, Klagsbrun M, Sasse J, Wadzinski M, Ingber D, Vlodavsky I. A heparin-binding angiogenic protein–basic fibroblast growth factor–is stored within basement membrane. Am J Pathol. 1988;130(2):393–400.

Gao G, Goldfarb M. Heparin can activate a receptor tyrosine kinase. EMBO J. 1995;14(10): 2183–90.

Greulich H, Pollock PM. Targeting mutant fibroblast growth factor receptors in cancer. Trends Mol Med. 2011;17:283–92.

Gutierrez A, Ratliff EP, Andres AM, Huang X, McKeehan WL, Davis RA. Bile acids decrease hepatic paraoxonase 1 expression and plasma high-density lipoprotein levels via FXR-mediated signaling of FGFR4. Arterioscler Thromb Vasc Biol. 2006;26(2):301–6.

Haddad RI, Shin DM. Recent advances in head and neck cancer. N Engl J Med. 2008;359(11): 1143–54.

Hart KC, Robertson SC, Donoghue DJ. Identification of tyrosine residues in constitutively activated fibroblast growth factor receptor 3 involved in mitogenesis, Stat activation, and phosphatidylinositol 3-kinase activation. Mol Biol Cell. 2001;12:931–42.

Heinzle C, Sutterlüty H, Grusch M, Grasl-Kraupp B, Berger W, Marian B. Targeting fibroblast-growth-factor-receptor-dependent signaling for cancer therapy. Expert Opin Ther Targets. 2011;15:829–46.

Jeffers ML, LaRochelle WJ, Lichenstein HS. Fibroblast growth factors in cancer: therapeutic possibilities. Expert Opin Ther Targets. 2002;6(4):469–82.

Kamei S, Yajima I, Yamamoto H, Kobayashi A, Makabe KW, Yamazaki H, Hayashi SI, Kunisada T. Characterization of a novel member of the FGFR family, HrFGFR, in Halocynthia roretzi. Biochem Biophys Res Commun. 2000;275(2):503–8.

Katoh M. Dysregulation of stem cell signaling network due to germline mutation, SNP, Helicobacter pylori infection, epigenetic change and genetic alteration in gastric cancer. Cancer Biol Ther. 2007;6(6):832–9.

Katoh M, Nakagama H. FGF receptors: cancer biology and therapeutics. Med Res Rev. 2013. doi:10.1002/med.21288.

Korc M, Friesel RE. The role of fibroblast growth factors in tumor growth. Curr Cancer Drug Targets. 2009;9(5):639–51.

Kovalenko D, Yang X, Nadeau RJ, Harkins LK, Friesel R. Sef inhibits fibroblast growth factor signaling by inhibiting FGFR1 tyrosine phosphorylation and subsequent ERK activation. J Biol Chem. 2003;278(16):14087–91.

Krause DS, Van Etten RA. Tyrosine kinases as targets for cancer therapy. N Engl J Med. 2005;353:172–87.

Laird AD, Cherrington JM. Small molecule tyrosine kinase inhibitors: clinical development of anticancer agents. Expert Opin Investig Drugs. 2003;12(1):51–64.

Leelayuwat C, Abraham LJ, Pinelli M, Townend DC, Wilks AF, Dawkins RL. The primate MHC contains sequences related to the fibroblast growth factor receptor gene family. Tissue Antigens. 1996;48(1):59–64.

Lemmon MA, Schlessinger J. Cell signaling by receptor tyrosine kinases. Cell. 2010;141:1117–34.

Liang G, Liu Z, Wu J, Cai Y, Li X. Anticancer molecules targeting fibroblast growth factor receptors. Trends Pharmacol Sci. 2012;33:531–41.

Lo TL, Yusoff P, Fong CW, Guo K, McCaw BJ, Phillips WA, Yang H, Wong ES, Leong HF, Zeng Q, Putti TC, Guy GR. The ras/mitogen-activated protein kinase pathway inhibitor and likely tumor suppressor proteins, sprouty 1 and sprouty 2 are deregulated in breast cancer. Cancer Res. 2004;64:6127–36.

López-Knowles E, Hernández S, Malats N, Kogevinas M, Lloreta J, Carrato A, Tardón A, Serra C, Real FX. PIK3CA mutations are an early genetic alteration associated with FGFR3 mutations in superficial papillary bladder tumors. Cancer Res. 2006;66(15):7401–4.

Manning G, Whyte DB, Martinez R, Hunter T, Sudarsanam S. The protein kinase complement of the human genome. Science. 2002;298:1912–34.

Marmé F, Hielscher T, Hug S, Bondong S, Zeillinger R, Castillo-Tong DC, Sehouli J, Braicu I, Vergote I, Isabella C, Mahner S, Ferschke I, Rom J, Sohn C, Schneeweiss A, Altevogt P. Fibroblast growth factor receptor 4 gene (FGFR4) 388Arg allele predicts prolonged survival and platinum sensitivity in advanced ovarian cancer. Int J Cancer. 2012;131(4):E586–91.

Mason JM, Morrison DJ, Basson MA, Licht JD. Sprouty proteins: multifaceted negative- feedback regulators of receptor tyrosine kinase signaling. Trends Cell Biol. 2006;16:45–54.

Mohammadi M, Olsen SK, Ibrahimi OA. Structural basis for fibroblast growth factor receptor activation. Cytokine Growth Factor Rev. 2005;16(2):107–37.

Moscatelli D. High and low affinity binding sites for basic fibroblast growth factor on cultured cells: absence of a role for low affinity binding in the stimulation of plasminogen activator production by bovine capillary endothelial cells. J Cell Physiol. 1987;131(1):123–30.

Nahta R, Yu D, Hung MC, Hortobagyi GN, Esteva FJ. Mechanisms of disease: understanding resistance to HER2-targeted therapy in human breast cancer. Nat Clin Pract Oncol. 2006;3(5):269–80.

Olson DC, Deng C, Hanahan D. Fibroblast growth factor receptor 4, implicated in progression of islet cell carcinogenesis by its expression profile, does not contribute functionally. Cell Growth Differ. 1988;9:557–64.

Ornitz DM, Itoh N. Fibroblast growth factors. Genome Biol. 2001;2(3):REVIEWS3005.

Ornitz DM, Yayon A, Flanagan JG, Svahn CM, Levi E, Leder P. Heparin is required for cell-free binding of basic fibroblast growth factor to a soluble receptor and for mitogenesis in whole cells. Mol Cell Biol. 1992;12(1):240–7.

Ornitz DM, Xu J, Colvin JS, McEwen DG, MacArthur CA, Coulier F, Gao G, Goldfarb M. Receptor specificity of the fibroblast growth factor family. J Biol Chem. 1996;271(25): 15292–7.

Ota S, Zhou ZQ, Link JM, Hurlin PJ. The role of senescence and prosurvival signaling in controlling the oncogenic activity of FGFR2 mutants associated with cancer and birth defects. Hum Mol Genet. 2009;18:2609–21.

Polanska UM, Fernig DG, Kinnunen T. Extracellular interactome of the FGF receptor-ligand system: complexities and the relative simplicity of the worm. Dev Dyn. 2009;238(2):277–93.

Powers CJ, McLeskey SW, Wellstein A. Review Fibroblast growth factors, their receptors and signaling. Endocr Relat Cancer. 2000;7(3):165–97.

Saksela O, Moscatelli D, Sommer A, Rifkin DB. Endothelial cell-derived heparan sulfate binds basic fibroblast growth factor and protects it from proteolytic degradation. J Cell Biol. 1988;107(2):743–51.

Sanchez-Heras E, Howell FV, Williams G, Doherty P. The fibroblast growth factor receptor acid box is essential for interactions with N-cadherin and all of the major isoforms of neural cell adhesion molecule. J Biol Chem. 2006;281(46):35208–16.

Seitzer N, Mayr T, Streit S, Ullrich A. A single nucleotide change in the mouse genome accelerates breast cancer progression. Cancer Res. 2010;70:802–12.

Shaoul E, Reich-Slotky R, Berman B, Ron D. Fibroblast growth factor receptors display both common and distinct signaling pathways. Oncogene. 1995;10(8):1553–61.

Streit S, Bange J, Fichtner A, Ihrler S, Issing W, et al. Involvement of the FGFR4 Arg388 allele in head and neck squamous cell carcinoma. Int J Cancer. 2004;111:213–7.

Takeuchi K, Ito F. Receptor tyrosine kinases and targeted cancer therapeutics. Biol Pharm Bull. 2011;34(12):1774–80.

Taylor 6th JG, Cheuk AT, Tsang PS, Chung JY, Song YK, Desai K, et al. Identification of FGFR4-activating mutations in human rhabdomyosarcomas that promote metastasis in xenotransplanted models. J Clin Invest. 2009;119:3395–407.

Thisse B, Thisse C. Functions and regulations of fibroblast growth factor signaling during embryonic development. Dev Biol. 2005;287(2):390–402. Epub 2005 Oct 10.

Thussbas C, Nahrig J, Streit S, Bange J, Kriner M, et al. FGFR4 Arg388 allele is associated with resistance to adjuvant therapy in primary breast cancer. J Clin Oncol. 2006;24:3747–55.

Tuominen H, Heikinheimo P, Loo BM, Kataja K, Oker-Blom C, Uutela M, Jalkanen M, Goldman A. Expression and glycosylation studies of human FGF receptor 4. Protein Expr Purif. 2001;21(2):275–85.

Turner N, Grose R. Fibroblast growth factor signalling: from development to cancer. Nat Rev Cancer. 2010;10:116–29.

Vainikka S, Joukov V, Wennström S, Bergman M, Pelicci PG, Alitalo K. Signal transduction by fibroblast growth factor receptor-4 (FGFR-4). Comparison with FGFR-1. J Biol Chem. 1994;269(28):18320–6.

Weinstein IB, Joe AK. Mechanisms of disease: oncogene addiction – a rationale for molecular targeting in cancer therapy. Nat Clin Pract Oncol. 2006;3:448–57.

DNA Methylation as a Biomarker in Nasopharyngeal Carcinoma

37

Feryel Ksiâa and Mounir Trimeche

Contents

Abstract

Nasopharyngeal carcinoma (NPC) is a malignancy with remarkable ethnic and geographic distribution. Initially, point mutations and chromosomal deletions were considered to be the major events involved in the inactivation of tumor-suppressor genes in NPC. The discovery that many tumor-suppressor genes can also be inactivated by hypermethylation of the CpG islands in their promoter region clearly indicates that epigenetic events also play an important role as alternative mechanisms in NPC carcinogenesis.

In this chapter, we update current information on methylated genes associated with the development and progression of NPC. Promoter

F. Ksiâa • M. Trimeche (✉)
Department of Pathology, University Hospital Farhat Hached, Sousse, Tunisia
e-mail: feryel_ksia@yahoo.fr; m_trimech@yahoo.fr

V.R. Preedy, V.B. Patel (eds.), *Biomarkers in Cancer, Biomarkers in Disease: Methods, Discoveries and Applications*,
DOI 10.1007/978-94-007-7681-4_43

hypermethylation of critical genes could be potential biomarkers and therapeutic targets for NPC.

Several genes have been investigated for methylation in the promoter region in NPC. These methylated genes are involved in critical pathways, such as DNA repair, cell cycle regulation, and invasion/metastasis.

The role of hypermethylated genes in the deregulation of critical pathways in NPC is now well known. Besides their role on the pathogenesis of NPC, results from many investigations have provided additional information on the potential role of hypermethylated genes as predictive biomarkers in the development and progression of NPC.

List of Abbreviations

CDH1	Epithelial E-Cadherin
CGH	Comparative Genomic Hybridization
DAB2	Human Disabled-2
DAP-kinase	Death-Associated Protein Kinase
DLC-1	Deleted in Liver Cancer-1
DLEC1	Deleted in Lung and Esophageal Cancer 1
DNMT	DNA Methyltransferase
EBV	Epstein–Barr Virus
GSTP1	Glutathione S-Transferase P1
HIN-1	High in Normal-1
HLA	Histocompatibility Leukocyte Antigens
IARC	International Agency for Research on Cancer
LARS2	Leucyl-tRNA Synthetase 2, Mitochondrial
LOH	Loss of Heterozygosity
MGMT	O^6-Methylguanine-DNA Methyltransferase
MSP	Methylation-Specific PCR
NPC	Nasopharyngeal Carcinoma
PCR	Polymerase Chain Reaction
RARβ2	Retinoic Acid Receptor β2
RASSF1A	Ras Association Domain Family 1A
TFPI-2	Tissue Factor Pathway Inhibitor-2
TIMP-3	Tissue Inhibitor of Metalloproteinase-3
TSG	Tumor-Suppressor Genes
TSLC1	Tumor Suppressor in Lung Cancer 1
WHO	World Health Organization

Key Facts of Methylation

The following are the key facts of DNA methylation including the location and the mechanism of this main epigenetic change, its role in the control of gene expression during embryogenesis, its implication in cancer development, and its importance as a potential biomarker in human cancers:

- DNA methylation is a biological process consisting in the addition of a methyl (CH_3) group at the carbon 5 position of cytosines (C) located 5′ of guanidines (G).
- This process often occurs in cytosine–guanine-rich regions of DNA (CpG islands), which are common in the promoter regions of genes.
- DNA methylation involves an enzymatic reaction catalyzed by a group of enzymes known as DNA methyltransferases (DNMT1, DNM3a, and DNMT3b).
- DNA methylation is one of the main epigenetic modifications implicated in the control of gene expression during the embryonic development of organisms.
- The presence of aberrant methylation in the promoter region of genes is associated with the suppression of gene expression in several types of cancer and in developmental disorders.
- DNA methylation is a reversible mechanism, making it an interesting therapeutic target.
- Several methods have been developed to investigate DNA methylation in tumors as well as in body fluids.
- The detection of DNA methylation has emerged as a potential biomarker for several types of cancer and a promising therapeutic target.

Definitions of Words and Terms

Undifferentiated Carcinoma A term used to describe poorly differentiated malignant epithelial tumor that does not have specialized structures. Undifferentiated cancer cells often grow and spread quickly.

Gene Polymorphism Difference in DNA sequence among individuals. Genetic variations occurring in more than 1 % of a population would be considered useful polymorphisms for genetic analysis.

Familial Predisposition Individuals with a family history of cancer in a first-degree or second-degree relative may have a genetic predisposition to developing the disease. Familial predisposition is an inherited risk of developing a cancer. Having a familial predisposition for a disease does not mean that you will get that disease, but your risk may be higher than that of the general population.

Risk Factor A risk factor is a condition that is known to increase susceptibility to a disease or outcome. Risk factors are usually determined through epidemiological studies, which track diseases or health events through a given population. Examples of risk factors are tobacco smoking, which can increase your risk of getting nasopharyngeal carcinoma.

Endemic Population A disease that is prevalent in a certain population or people or region. Diseases in endemic population are not always present at high levels.

They can be relatively rare, but the defining feature of a regional endemic disease is that it can always be found in the population that lives there.

Epigenetic Epigenetic changes modify the physical structure of DNA and may indirectly influence the expression of the genome. One example of an epigenetic change is DNA methylation – the addition of a methyl group – of the DNA molecule, which prevents certain genes from being expressed. For instance, an epigenetic change that silences genes could lead to uncontrolled cellular growth or to an increase in DNA damage, which, in turn, increases cancer risk.

Cancer Biomarker A distinctive biological indicator used for cancer. A handful of cancer biomarkers are currently used routinely for population screening, disease diagnosis, prognosis, monitoring of therapy, and prediction of therapeutic response. Although it is highly desirable to have biomarkers suitable for population screening and early diagnosis, none of the current biomarkers has adequate sensitivity, specificity, and predictive value for population screening.

Apoptosis It refers to the death of a cell resulting from a normal series of genetically programmed events, when a cell is no longer needed. Apoptosis is a natural process that removes cells that have become unhealthy. Apoptosis is important in understanding cancer, because cancer cells have developed ways to avoid apoptosis. Newer treatments are being studied that interfere with the cancer cell's ability to avoid apoptosis.

Tumor-Suppressor Genes Genes that regulate the growth of cells. When these genes are functioning properly, they can prevent and inhibit the growth of tumors. When tumor-suppressor genes are altered or inactivated (by genetic or epigenetic alterations), they lose the ability to make a protein that controls cell growth. Cells can then grow uncontrolled and develop into a cancer.

Noninvasive Screening Tests Procedures that does not require insertion of an instrument or device through the skin or a body orifice for diagnosis or treatment.

Tumor Aggressiveness It is the ability of cancer cells to spread in the body.

Introduction

Nasopharyngeal carcinoma (NPC) is a highly invasive and metastatic malignant tumor with remarkable racial and geographic distribution. In 2002, according to the data of the International Agency for Research on Cancer (IARC), 80,000 cases of NPC were newly diagnosed worldwide (Parkin et al. 2005).

NPC is very different from other head and neck cancers not only because of its geographic distribution but also because of its specific multifactorial etiology. Epstein–Barr virus (EBV) infection, intake of salted-preserved foods, tobacco and alcohol consumption, and inherited susceptibilities such as gene polymorphisms or familial predisposition are major factors associated with the development of NPC.

Approximately 80 % of patients with NPC are diagnosed at an advanced tumor stage. The delay in the disease discovery is mainly due to the deep-cited location and nonspecific symptoms of the tumor. With the introduction of new treatment modalities, survival has steadily improved over recent decades. However, cancer relapse is still the leading cause of cancer-related deaths in patients with NPC.

The early detection, prognosis, and monitoring of therapy are especially important parameters for NPC because of the high propensity for spreading to more sites. Knowledge about new biomarkers in NPC is important in improving optimal patient treatment. In this context, the epigenetic alterations, especially methylation of DNA, emerge as a promising track.

Regional Variation in the Incidence of NPC

There are remarkable regional variations in the incidence of NPC worldwide. In southern China and Southeast Asia, the NPC is the most common malignant tumor with an incidence rate ranging from 20 to 50/100,000 people per year. Hong Kong detains the highest NPC incidence. NPC is the major cause of cancer morbidity and mortality in these endemic regions. Moderately higher incidence of NPC is reported in some other population groups also such as Eskimos in the Arctic, Arabs in North Africa, and few other population groups of Southeast Asia. Conversely, the estimated incidence of NPC is lower than 1/100,000 people per year in most part of the world (Chang and Adami 2006).

In areas of low to moderate risk for NPC, a bimodal age distribution is always depicted. The first peak in incidence is observed in adolescents of each sex (10–19 years) and the second peak, higher than the first one, in the age group 50–59 years. This relatively high frequency of NPC among young population seems to be a characteristic feature of areas of moderate incidence of NPC.

Another important characteristic of NPC epidemiology is sex distribution. In virtually all of the populations studied, the rates are higher among males than females. In most populations, the male/female ratio is 2–3:1.

Histology of NPC

Arising in the epithelial lining of the nasopharynx, NPC comprises the vast majority of nasopharyngeal cancers in both high- and low-incidence populations. The World Health Organization (WHO) histopathological classification of NPC (Chan et al. 2005) has been adopted by several investigators. It comprises three histological types, (1) keratinizing squamous-cell carcinoma (type 1) and nonkeratinizing carcinoma. The nonkeratinizing group can further be separated into differentiated carcinoma (type 2) and undifferentiated carcinoma (type 3) group (Fig. 1).

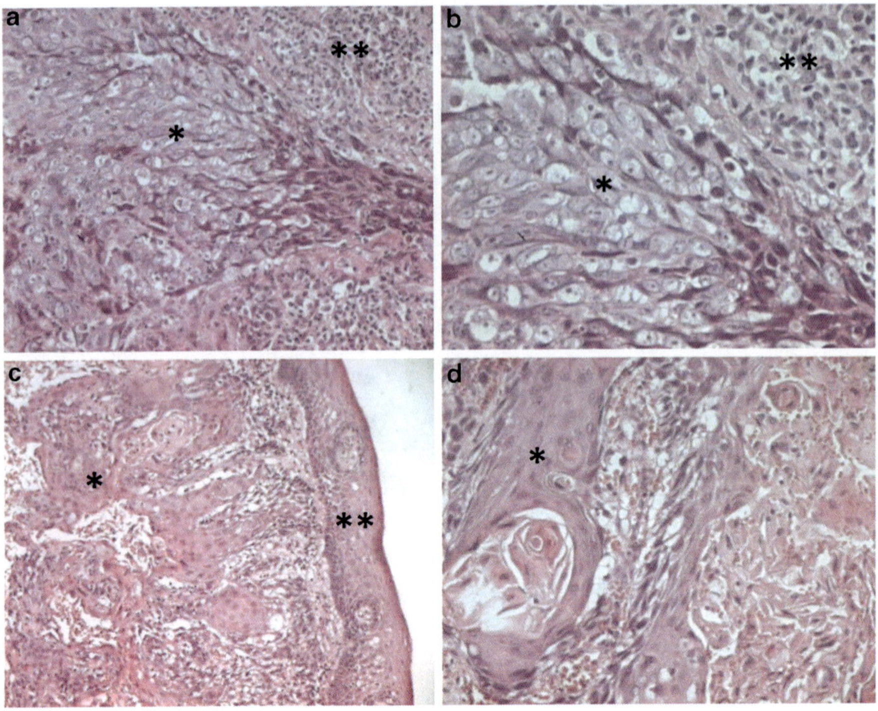

Fig. 1 **Histology of nasopharyngeal carcinoma.** (**a**, **b**) Undifferentiated carcinoma featuring cohesive sheet of tumor cells (*asterisk*) with plentiful intermixed lymphocytes (*double asterisks*) (hematoxylin and eosin staining, original magnification: **a** ×200 and **b** ×400). (**c**, **d**) Keratinizing squamous-cell carcinoma showing cohesive tumor cells with well-defined cell borders (hematoxylin and eosin, original magnification: **c** ×200, **d** ×400)

The proportions of the histological types of NPC appear to vary with geographical location and race. However, undifferentiated carcinoma or type 3 is the major histopathological type of NPC. In the low-risk areas of Japan, type 1 NPC accounts for 12 % of cases, whereas undifferentiated carcinoma or type 3 predominates in high-risk areas and takes up 92 % of all cases.

Types 2 and 3 NPC are Epstein–Barr virus (EBV) associated and have better prognoses than type 1; EBV infection is generally absent in type1 (Wei et al. 2011).

Etiological Factors in NPC

It is believed that a number of etiological environmental factors along with genetic/host factors might be responsible for the causation of NPC. At least three etiological factors are strongly suspected in NPC carcinogenesis: the ubiquitous EBV infection, genetically determined susceptibility, and associated environmental factors. Figure 2 summarizes the main factors related to the development of nasopharyngeal carcinoma.

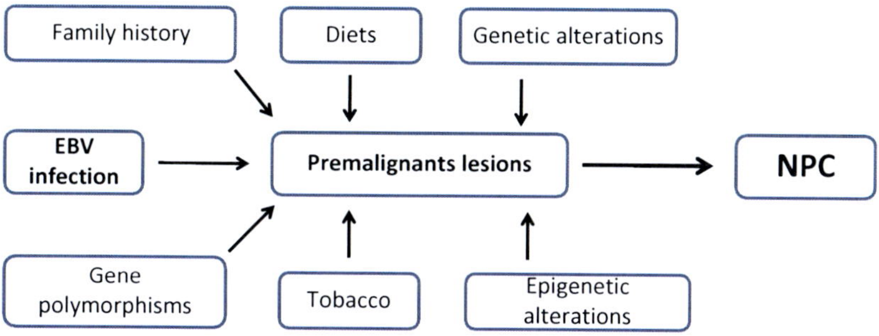

Fig. 2 Proposed causal factors of nasopharyngeal carcinoma. The interaction between host factors, such as inherited susceptibilities, and environmental factors, including Epstein–Barr virus (EBV), diet, and tobacco, initiates the progression from normal to premalignant disease stages. These factors combined with genetic and epigenetic alterations lead to the development of nasopharyngeal carcinoma (NPC)

EBV is a member of the large herpesvirus family and distributed ubiquitously. It is found throughout all human populations, with a prevalence of over 90 % in adult. Initially, the association between NPC and EBV was revealed by results of seroepidemiological studies from different parts of the world. It was confirmed subsequently by the demonstration of the persistence of EBV DNA and/or antigens in NPC tumor cells (Frappier 2012; Fig. 3). EBV is intimately related to NPC and elicits the formation of antibodies that are useful for diagnosis and follow-up study. Numerous studies have reported that antibodies to EBV antigens can be used in the early detection of NPC. Serological assays are being utilized in mass screening of high-risk populations for NPC. The serology value of EBV was also observed for the early detection of NPC relapse (Han et al. 2012; Chan et al. 2013).

From the viewpoint of genetic susceptibilities, a growing number of reports have confirmed an association between the histocompatibility leukocyte antigens (HLA) gene polymorphism and increased risk for NPC. Simons et al. (1978) were the first to describe the association of HLA antigens with NPC in southern Chinese and demonstrated that HLA antigens play a role in determining both susceptibility for NPC and survival after diagnosis. Later, several studies have supported the strong genetic etiology of NPC (Li et al. 2009). Studies are in progress in different laboratories to elucidate the exact location and function of these genes.

Although most NPCs are sporadic cases, the familial clustering of NPC has been also demonstrated worldwide. Such clustering can result from shared genetic susceptibility and/or shared environmental risk factors. The excess risk was generally four- to tenfold among individuals with a first-degree relative with NPC, compared with those without a family history (Bei et al. 2012).

Some dietary habits are reported to be associated with the increased risk for NPC. Salted fish and smoking have been suspected as possible etiological factors in the development of NPC. In Asian countries, intake of salted fish and other preserved foods is particularly high in families of lower socioeconomic status

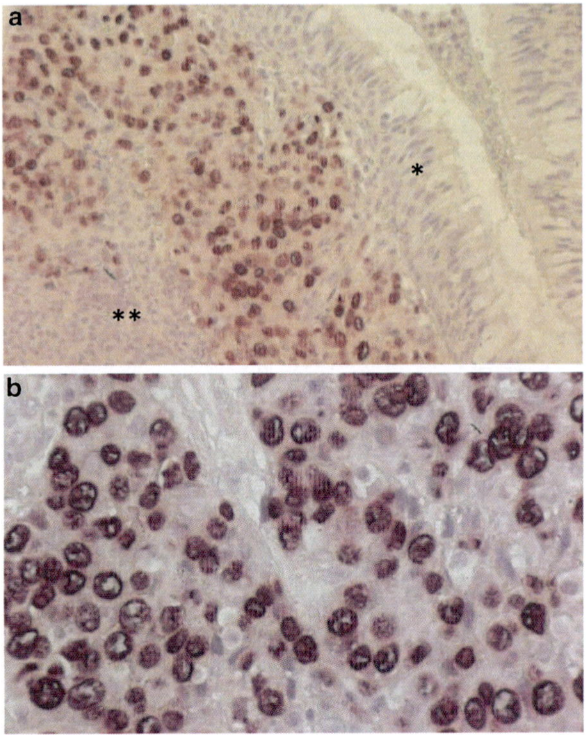

Fig. 3 Detection of Epstein–Barr virus by chromogenic in situ hybridization (CISH) for Epstein–Barr virus-encoded RNA (EBER) in nasopharyngeal carcinoma. *Dark blue/black* positive staining for EBER in the nuclei of almost all tumor cells, whereas the normal epithelial cells (*asterisk*) and stromal lymphocytes (*double asterisk*) remain negative (original magnification, **a** ×100, **b** ×400)

(Jia et al. 2010). Furthermore, several studies have shown that childhood exposure and increasing duration and frequency of consumption of salt preserved foods are independently associated with elevated risk for NPC. In contrast, consumption of fresh fruits and/or vegetables, especially during childhood, is associated with a lower risk for NPC. The noticeable protective effect of fruits and vegetables may be attributed to antioxidant effects, prevention of nitrosamine formation, and other anticarcinogenic properties (Polesel et al. 2013). It has been also reported that persons who have smoked cigarettes for many years have a higher risk for NPC, particularly for the well-differentiated subtype (Xu et al. 2012).

Genetic Alterations in NPC

The viral causative, genetic, and environmental factors, either acting alone or in combination, would lead to multiple genetic and epigenetic alterations. The development of NPC involves accumulation of genetic changes leading to the evolution of clonal cell population that possesses growth advantages over other cells.

NPC exhibits numerous genetic abnormalities, namely, chromosomal deletions, gene amplifications, and mutations. By comparative genomic hybridization (CGH) analyses, a large number of primary NPC have been examined for a gain and loss of genetic material in the genome, including gain at chromosomes 12p, 1q, 3q, 8q, 5p, and 7q as well as loss at chromosomes 3p, 11q, 13q, 14q, 16q, 16p, 1p, 9q, and 22q.

Among these allelic loss, 3p and 9q detain the highest frequencies and were detected in almost 95–100 % of primary NPC biopsies and in 75 % of precancerous lesions (Li et al. 2006). It is well known that the 3p chromosomal arm contains some important tumor-suppressor genes (TSGs). Thus, loss of heterozygosity (LOH) on 3p in premalignant lesions indicates that this alteration could be an early and critical molecular event in the carcinogenesis of NPC. Despite the many efforts provided, the sequence in which these genetic alterations participate in the evolution of NPC has not been established as clearly as in other cancers such as colon cancer (Chen et al. 2012).

Besides genetic deletion and mutation, it has been identified a second mechanism, termed epigenetic alterations, potentially responsible for NPC carcinogenesis.

Role of DNA Methylation in NPC

Epigenetic and DNA Methylation

The term epigenetic designs an inheritable change in the pattern of gene expression without a change in DNA sequence. The methylation of DNA is an important epigenetic modification that has physiologic effects on embryogenesis, cellular development, differentiation, senescence, and aging. Three well definite DNA methyltransferases (DNMTs), DNMT1, DNMT3a, and DNMT3b, are responsible for DNA methylation. These enzymes act by adding a methyl group to the carbon 5 position of a cytosine already present in the DNA strand and therefore transform the cytosine residues to 5-methylcytosine forms (Robertson 2005). DNA methyltransferases use *S*-adenosylmethionine as the methyl donor. Approximately 3–5 % of the cytosine residues in genomic DNA are of the 5-methylcytosine forms and are principally scattered in selected regions, called CpG islands. CpG islands of many tissue-specific genes are methylated, except in the tissue in which they are expressed, while unmethylated CpG islands are associated with housekeeping genes.

Nevertheless, aberrant and/or excessive DNA methylation can lead to neoplastic transformation. Indeed, several reports have demonstrated that hypermethylation in particular genes, namely, in TSGs, can be one of the main driving forces in carcinogenesis. The presence of 5-methylcytosines into the promoter region of genes prevents transcription factors from binding, by steric hindrance, and consequently reduces and even inhibits gene transcription (Fig. 4).

Several studies investigating methylation profile in various tumors have shown that the hypermethylation of a specific gene depends on tumor type (Esteller 2002). For example, hypermethylation of *p14* (*ARF*) and *APC* is most prevalent in gastric and colon cancers, whereas that of *GSTP1* is characteristic of steroid-related tumors such as the breast, liver, and prostate. Other genes, such as

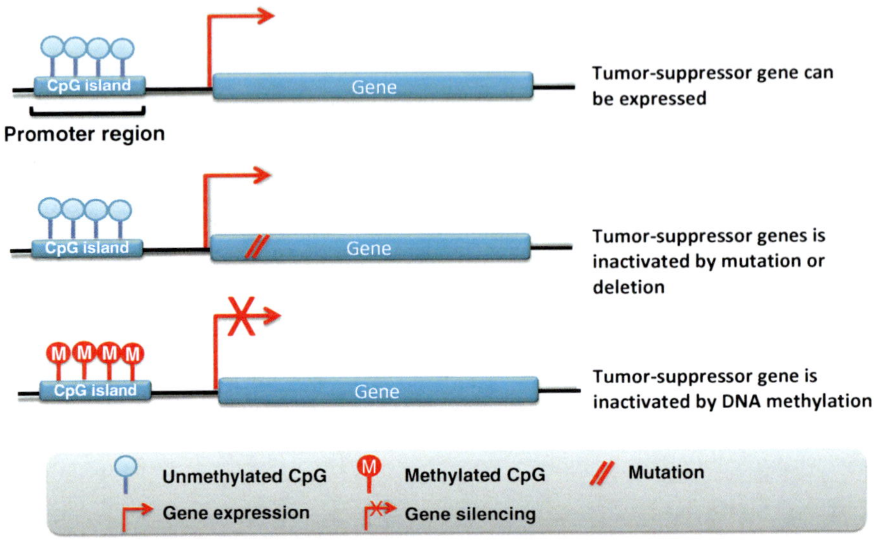

Fig. 4 A mechanism for gene silencing. Different mechanisms by which tumor-suppressor genes could be inactivated in the tumor

p16 (*INK4A*) and *O^6-methylguanine-DNA methyltransferase* (*MGMT*), are less exclusive and are hypermethylated across many tumor types.

Hypermethylated Genes in NPC

In primary NPC tissues, many TSGs exhibit high frequencies of methylation. Moreover, NPC has its own unique and specific methylation profile, slightly different to that described for other cancers. Indeed, results from numerous investigations in NPC have shown aberrant methylation at CpG islands in a growing list of genes, including the human *Ras association domain family 1A (RASSF1A)*; *retinoic acid receptor β2 (RARβ2)*; cell cycle regulator *p16 (INK4A)*, *p15 (INK4b)*, and *p14 (ARF) genes*; the DNA repair *MGMT*; the apoptosis-related and potential metastasis inhibitor (*DAP-kinase*); and the detoxifying (*GSTP1*) genes and others. These genes belong to different pathways in cells. Epigenetic inactivation of them may affect all of the molecular pathways involved in cell immortalization and transformation.

Methylation-specific PCR (MSP) was the main methodology applied to access data about DNA methylation in the promoter genes. MSP is a powerful and sensitive technique used to detect hypermethylation based on primer annealing during PCR. However, such a qualitative technique is only able to detect methylation present in more than one CpG in the primer set and is susceptible to false-positive results (Cottrell 2004).

The Human *Ras Association Domain Family (RASSF)* Genes

RASSF1, a critical tumor-suppressor gene, has been initially isolated from the lung tumor-suppressor locus *3p21.3*. *RASSF1* gene encodes more than seven isoforms, including *RASSF1A*, *RASSF1B*, and *RASSF1C*, which are derived from alternative mRNA splicing and promoter usage (Van der Weyden and Adams 2007). RASSF1A protein is involved in the Ras signaling pathway mediating the apoptotic effects of oncogenic Ras. RASSF1A protein structure also suggests that it may participate in the DNA damage response (Donninger et al. 2007).

RASSF1A is commonly inactivated through its promoter methylation (Dammann et al. 2005; Chow et al. 2004). Indeed, high frequency of promoter hypermethylation of *RASSF1A* has been reported in primary NPCs and varied from 67 % to 91 % (Fendri et al. 2009; Lo et al. 2001; Challouf et al. 2012). These data suggest that promoter hypermethylation of *RASSF1A* has a critical role in NPC carcinogenesis. Interestingly, aberrant methylation of *RASSF1A* correlates with lymph node metastasis in NPC (Fendri et al. 2009).

Because of its consistently frequent promoter hypermethylation in NPC and its correlation with clinicopathological parameters of tumor aggressiveness, *RASSF1* may be a useful cancer biomarker for the identification of the aggressive NPC that may benefit from different therapeutic modalities.

Similarly, *RASSF2A*, an isoform of *RASSF2*, has been reported to be inactivated by its promoter methylation in 61 % of NPC and correlates with lymph node metastasis (Zhang et al. 2007).

The Retinoic Acid Receptor β2 (RARβ2) Gene

Retinoids are known to possess antiproliferative, differentiative, immunomodulatory, and apoptosis-inducing properties. The regulation of cell growth and differentiation of normal, premalignant, and malignant cells by retinoids are thought to result from the direct and indirect effects of retinoids on gene expression. These effects are mediated by the nuclear receptors, including retinoic acid receptor β2 (*RARβ2*) located at 3p24 (Mark et al. 2006).

It has been suggested that methylation of *RARβ2* may block or interfere with the retinoid signaling pathways in NPC. Studies performed in primary NPC have reported high frequency of promoter hypermethylation for *RARβ2*, varying from 81 % to 88 % (Kwong et al. 2002; Fendri et al. 2009). Hypermethylation of the *RARβ2* promoter has been correlated with lymph node metastasis in NPC (Fendri et al. 2009; Challouf et al. 2012).

The $p16^{INK4a}$ Gene

One of the most important pathways affected in NPC is the *INK4a/ARF* pathway. The *INK4a/ARF* locus encodes two cell cycle regulatory proteins, $p16^{INK4a}$ and $p14^{ARF}$, which share an exon using different reading frames. $p16^{INK4a}$ and $p14^{ARF}$ act through the Rb-CDK4 and *p53* pathways.

$p16^{INK4a}$ is a cyclin-dependant protein kinase 4 (CDK4), which inhibits the ability of CDK4 to interact with cyclin D1. Loss of $p16^{INK4a}$ function would be expected to lead to uncontrolled cell growth. In NPC, loss of *p16*^{INK4a} is mainly caused by aberrant promoter methylation, whereas deletion and mutation of this gene locus are infrequently seen (Lo et al. 1995). CpG island promoter methylation of *p16*^{INK4a} has been reported in 22–65 % of primary NPC but not in biopsies of normal nasopharynx (Lo et al. 1996; Ayadi et al. 2008; Challouf et al. 2012). These data suggest that *p16*^{INK4a} methylation may be a potential biomarker for NPC diagnosis. Furthermore, Chang et al. (2003) have observed moderate methylation rate for *p16*^{INK4a} (20 %) in body fluids from NPC patients. They suggested that *p16*^{INK4a} methylation detection in body fluids may have a potential application in noninvasive screening of NPC.

The *p14*^{ARF} Gene

The main known function of *p14*^{ARF} is to prevent the p53 degradation through its binding to MDM-2 which induces cell cycle arrest. Compared to *p16*^{INK4a} methylation, *p14*^{ARF} promoter methylation has been observed less frequently in NPC (18 %) (Kwong et al. 2002). It has been speculated that epigenetic inactivation of the *p14*^{ARF} gene may interfere with the p53 network in a subset of NPC tumors. Due to its low frequency of methylation in tumors, *p14*^{ARF} needs to be further tested for a potential biomarker for NPC.

The *p15* ^{INK4B} Gene

The *p15* ^{INK4B} gene is also an inhibitor of cyclin-dependent kinase 4, which is an important mediator of cell cycle control, especially in a pathway stimulated by the transforming growth factor β (TGF β) (Hannon and Beach 1994). The *p15* ^{INK4B} gene has been reported to be inactivated by promoter hypermethylation in 21 % of primary NPCs (Kwong et al. 2002), which implied that *p15*^{INK4B} gene promoter methylation may play a role in NPC tumorigenesis.

The Death-Associated Protein Kinase (*DAP-Kinase*) Gene

Death-associated protein, also known as *DAP-kinase*, is a Ca^{2+}-/calmodulin-dependent cytoskeletal-associated protein kinase, with an apoptosis-inducing function (Cohen et al. 1997). *DAP-kinase* expression may affect apoptosis and contributes to immortalization. It is an essential mediator involved in the IFN-γ-induced programmed cell death in HeLa cells. *DAP-kinase* is also involved in tumor necrosis factor-α (TNF-α)- and Fas-induced apoptosis (Cohen et al. 1999).

Hypermethylation of *DAP-kinase* promoter has been initially demonstrated in human neoplasm-derived cell lines (Kissil et al. 1997). Subsequently, several types of cancers including NPC have also reported a repression in *DAP-kinase* expression (Kong et al. 2006; Fendri et al. 2009; Kwong et al. 2002; Challouf et al. 2012). Accordingly, high methylation frequencies have been shown in NPC for *DAP-kinase* ranging from 47 % to 88 % (Fendri et al. 2009; Challouf et al. 2012). Wong et al. (2002) have found that hypermethylation of *DAP-kinase* promoter occurs in early-stage NPC carcinogenesis. Moreover, Tong et al. (2002) have observed a significant frequency of *DAP-kinase* promoter methylation (50 %) in brushing samples from NPC patients. Taken together, these data suggest that *DAP-kinase* gene methylation may be an ideal biomarker candidate for the early detection of NPC. Similarly, Wong et al. (2002) have found a high frequency of hypermethylated *DAP-kinase* promoter in the plasma of NPC patients and suggested that *DAP-kinase* may be one of the potentially useful genes in the clinical monitoring of residual or recurrent disease after treatment in NPC.

The O^6-*Methylguanine-DNA Methyltransferase* (*MGMT*) Gene

O^6-methylguanine-DNA methyltransferase (MGMT) is an important DNA repair with the highest activity in the liver. MGMT protects cells from DNA damage caused by mutagenic and cytotoxic agents leading to alkylation at O^6-guanine (Pegg 1990). Loss or reduced *MGMT* expression due to CpG island methylation occurs in several kinds of human cancers (Esteller et al. 1999). In NPC, aberrant promoter methylation for *MGMT* has been reported with frequencies ranging from 5.5 % to 15 % in primary tumor samples (Challouf et al. 2012; Kwong et al. 2002). Interestingly, Kwong et al. (2002) have reported that *MGMT* methylation may be correlated with the aggressiveness of tumor such as the development of metastasis (Kwong et al. 2002). However, in the study performed by Challouf et al. (2012), the authors did not find any significant relations between the *MGMT* methylation status and clinical characteristics of NPC. These observations need, however, to be confirmed by a larger study with more NPC patients.

The Glutathione S-Transferase P1 (*GSTP1*) Gene

The detoxifying glutathione S-transferase P1 (*GSTP1*) gene protects cells from cytotoxic and carcinogenic agents by conjugation with glutathione (Daniel 1993). Many tumor types including prostate cancer, breast cancers, and cholangiocarcinomas showed *GSTP1* promoter hypermethylation (Esteller et al. 1998). In NPC, methylation of *GSTP1* gene occurred less frequently in only 19 % of cases (Challouf et al. 2012). Kwong et al. (2002) have not, however, detected methylation of *GSTP1* in primary tumor samples. Based on its low frequency of methylation in tumor tissues, the value of *GSTP1* as a potential biomarker for NPC carcinogenesis seems to be limited.

The High-in-Normal-1 (*HIN-1*) Gene

High in normal-1 (*HIN-1*) is a putative cytokine gene located at 5q35-tel. *HIN-1* plays a role in the regulation of epithelial cell proliferation, differentiation, or morphogenesis. The expression of *HIN-1* is significantly downregulated in human breast cancer and its preinvasive lesions. Loss of *HIN-1* expression is caused by DNA methylation of the promoter region (Krop et al. 2001). Methylation of *HIN-1* has been also reported in NPC. Wong et al. (2003b) found *HIN-1* hypermethylation in all NPC cell lines (100 %) and in 77 % of primary NPC. Accordingly, it seems that transcriptional silencing of *HIN-1* pathway might be involved in NPC tumorigenesis. Wong et al. reported also high frequency of methylation in early stages (I and II) of NPC and suggested that methylation of *HIN-1* might be an early event in NPC development (Wong et al. 2003). Moreover, they also detected methylated *HIN-1* promoter in 46 % (12 of 26) of nasopharyngeal swabs, 19 % (5 of 26) of throat-rinsing fluids, 18 % (2 of 11) of plasmas, and 46 % (5 of 11) of buffy coats of peripheral blood of the NPC patients, but it was not detectable in all normal controls. The authors have suggested that detection of methylated promoter DNA in nasopharyngeal swab, throat-rinsing fluid, and peripheral blood might be potentially useful as tumor marker for early detection and for screening of NPC.

Tissue Inhibitor of Metalloproteinase-3 (*TIMP-3*) Gene

The TIMP family has four protein members: *TIMP-1*, *TIMP-2*, *TIMP-3*, and *TIMP-4*. *TIMP-3* is a non-soluble protein that combines with the extracellular matrix. The function of *TIMP-3* is the inhibition of tumor necrosis factor-α (TNF-α)-converting enzymes and the induction of programmed cell death through the stable cell surface TNF-α receptor (Mannello and Gazzanelli 2001). Reduced expression of *TIMP-3* by promoter hypermethylation has been reported in several types of tumors. Furthermore, many authors suggest that hypermethylation of *TIMP-3* occurs in the early stages and tends to accumulate with the multistep tumor progression. In NPC, *TIMP-3* is less frequently methylated. Indeed, Challouf et al. (2012) found that in 19 % of NPC cases, the *TIMP-3* gene 5′ CpG islands exhibited aberrant methylation. Contrary to other cancers, in NPC, promoter hypermethylation of *TIMP-3* is only detectable in tumor tissue and not in adjacent non-tumor tissue. As a diagnostic biomarker, the value of *TIMP-3* may be limited due to its low frequency of methylation in NPC.

Leucyl-tRNA Synthetase 2, Mitochondrial (*LARS2*) Gene

Leucyl-tRNA synthetase 2, mitochondrial (*LARS2*) gene is located at 3p21.3. It encodes the precursor of mitochondrial leucyl-tRNA synthetase which catalyzes the charging of $tRNA^{Leu(UUR)}$ with leucine, an essential step in protein synthesis. *LARS2* performs essential roles in protein synthesis within the mitochondria and is indirectly required for mitochondrial genome maintenance. Promoter hypermethylation of *LARS2* has been found in 64 % of NPC samples and in only 12.5 % of non-tumor samples (chronic nasopharyngitis) (Zhou et al. 2009). This data indicates that DNA methylation in the promoter region of *LARS2* appears to occur at early stages of carcinogenesis and may serve as targets for the development of a novel screening test for cancer (Zhou et al. 2009).

The Deleted in Liver Cancer-1 (*DLC-1*) Gene

The deleted in liver cancer-1 (*DLC-1*) was first isolated from human hepatocellular carcinoma. The *DLC-1* gene, located at the human chromosome region 8p22, behaves like a tumor-suppressor gene. *DLC-1* shares high sequence similarity with Rho family proteins which play essential roles in regulating diverse biological functions, including cytoskeletal organization, cell adhesion, and cell cycle progression (Etienne-Manneville and Hall 2002). The *DLC-1* gene has been frequently methylated in diverse tumors and cell lines (Wong et al. 2003; Kim et al. 2003). Methylation of the *DLC-1* gene is also a common event in NPC (Peng et al. 2006; Seng et al. 2007; Feng et al. 2013). Indeed, 80–89 % of primary NPCs have showed methylation in *DLC-1* promoter (Peng et al. 2006; Seng et al. 2007), which strongly suggested that hypermethylation in the *DLC-1* promoter might perform an important role in the transcriptional silencing of the gene and NPC carcinogenesis. Moreover, based on its high frequency of methylation in tumors, *DLC-1* may be a good biomarker candidate for NPC diagnosis.

Tissue Factor Pathway Inhibitor-2 (*TFPI-2*) Gene

Tissue factor pathway inhibitor-2 (*TFPI-2*) is located on chromosome 7q22 and functions as a protease inhibitor. *TFPI-2* acts in the maintenance of the stability of the tumor environment and inhibits the growth of neoplasms. *TFPI-2* is a candidate TSG with important roles in carcinogenesis and metastasis in human cancers. Transcriptional silencing by promoter hypermethylation of *TFPI-2* has been observed in some human cancers including NPC (Wong et al. 2007; Wang et al. 2010). Using methylation-specific PCR and bisulfate genomic sequencing, Wang et al. (2010) found that *TFPI-2* was aberrantly methylated in 88.6 % (62/70) of NPC primary tumors, but not in normal nasopharyngeal epithelia. The authors suggested that epigenetic inactivation of *TFPI-2* by promoter hypermethylation is common and can be a specific marker for the diagnosis of NPC.

The Tumor Suppressor in Lung Cancer 1 (*TSLC1*) Gene

The tumor suppressor in lung cancer 1 (*TSLC1*) is reported to be a putative TSG on 11q23. The *TSLC1* gene encodes an immunoglobulin superfamily cell adhesion molecule (IgCAM), which is a membrane protein involved in cell–cell interactions (Masuda et al. 2002). Promoter methylation and loss of expression of the *TSLC1* gene have been reported in 20–60 % of cancers from the esophagus, stomach, pancreas, nasopharynx, breast, lung, liver, and uterine cervix, as well as meningiomas (Murakami 2005). Moreover, clinicopathological analyses have revealed that the inactivation of *TSLC1* is likely to be involved in the biological aggressiveness of tumors, including invasion or metastasis (Murakami 2005). Loss of *TSLC1* gene expression by promoter hypermethylation has been also found in 34.2–68 % of primary NPC (Hui et al. 2003; Zhou et al. 2005). No aberrant promoter methylation was, however, found in any of the investigated normal nasopharyngeal epithelia (Hui et al. 2003; Zhou et al. 2005). Lung et al. (2004) reported that the *TSLC1* promoter region is hypermethylated in all NPC cell lines and re-expression of the gene occurs in HONE1 cells after 5-aza-2′-deoxycytidine treatment. Results from fine deletion mapping in 11q22–23 regions and the high inactivation rate of *TSLC1* gave sufficient evidence to consider *TSLC1* as a potential biomarker strongly implicated in NPC development (Lung et al. 2004; Hui et al. 2003).

The Human Disabled-2 (*DAB2*) Gene

Human disabled-2 (*DAB2*) plays an important regulatory role in cellular differentiation. *DAB2* functions also as a negative regulator of canonical Wnt signaling by stabilized beta-catenin degradation complex (Hocevar et al. 2003). Downregulation of *DAB2* has been reported in several cancer types. Although some studies have suggested that DNA methylation of *DAB2* is infrequent, Tong et al. (2010) found promoter methylation of *DAB2* in 65.2 % (30/46) of primary NPC. Being high methylated, Tong et al. (2010) hypothesized that *DAB2* might be a tumor-suppressor gene strongly implicated in NPC carcinogenesis.

The Deleted in Lung and Esophageal Cancer 1 (*DLEC1*) Gene

Deleted in lung and esophageal cancer 1 (*DLEC1*) is located at 3p22.2. *DLEC1* is identified as a candidate tumor-suppressor gene in lung, esophageal, and renal cancers. Downregulation by promoter methylation of *DLEC1* has been reported in various types of tumors. In NPC, hypermethylation of the promoter of *DLEC1* has been observed in 71–86 % of cases (Kwong et al. 2007; Ayadi et al. 2008). Methylation of *DLEC1* promoter has been also detected in NPC cell lines and xenografts but not in normal nasopharyngeal epithelial cells. Moreover, it has been demonstrated that treatment of NPC cell lines with demethylating agent or histone deacetylase inhibitor reversed the methylation and restored *DLEC1* expression. Re-expression of *DLEC1* suppressed the growth and reduced the invasiveness of NPC cells. Taken together, these data strongly suggest that silencing of *DLEC1* expression by promoter hypermethylation can be a biomarker for NPC diagnosis or prevention.

The *BLU* Gene

The *BLU* gene is a candidate tumor-suppressor gene, located at the commonly deleted region 3p21.3. *BLU* gene is an E2F-regulated, stress-responsive gene (Qiu et al. 2004). *BLU* gene is inactivated by both epigenetic and genetic mechanisms in carcinomas (Qiu et al. 2004; Agathanggelou et al. 2003). In NPC, methylation-specific PCR analysis revealed that the *BLU* promoter was highly methylated in 34–74 % of primary NPC (Ayadi et al. 2008; Liu et al. 2003) and in 80 % of nasopharyngeal tumor cell lines (Agathanggelou et al. 2003) but not detected in normal nasopharyngeal tissues. The high incidence of *BLU* alterations suggests that it may be one of the critical tumor-suppressor genes on chromosome 3p21.3 involved in the development of NPC.

The Epithelial (E)-Cadherin (*CDH1*) Gene

Cadherins are a family of transmembrane glycoproteins, which mediates Ca^{2+}-dependent intercellular adhesion. Epithelial (E)-cadherin (*CDH1*) is an important member of this family, which is expressed predominantly on the surface of epithelial cells. The *CDH1* gene acts as an invasion-/metastasis-suppressor gene (Van Roy and Berx 2008). *CDH1* has also a role in organogenesis and morphogenesis (Takeichi 1991). In humans, the *CDH1* gene is considered a tumor suppressor and is located on chromosome 16q22.1. *CDH1* is frequently inactivated by genetic alterations, such as loss of heterozygosity (LOH) and mutations, and also by epigenetic changes (Strathdee 2002). In NPC, hypermethylation of *CDH1* was found in 11–79 % of patient samples (Challouf et al. 2012; Ayadi et al. 2008). It is noteworthy that hypermethylation of *CDH1* was more frequently detected in advanced stages compared to those in early stages of NPC (Niemhom et al. 2008) and was tightly associated with tumor invasion and lymph node metastasis (Li et al. 2004; Ayadi et al. 2008). These data suggested that *CDH1* methylation might be a useful biomarker to assess progression and for the identification of the aggressive NPC. Interestingly, several studies have reported a relation between downregulation of *CDH1* expression and the presence of EBV, the principal etiological factor, in NPC (Krishna et al. 2005; Niemhom et al. 2008). Ran et al. (2011) found high methylation frequency of *CDH1* in NPC clinical specimens (65 %) and in peripheral blood (45 %) of NPC patients and suggest the potential clinical application of *CDH1* as an early diagnostic or predictive marker.

The Stratifin (SFN/14-3-3 Sigma) Gene

The p53-regulated gene *14-3-3 sigma* is a putative tumor-suppressor gene involved in cell cycle regulation and apoptosis following DNA damage. *14-3-3 sigma* undergoes frequent epigenetic silencing in several types of cancer, including carcinoma of the breast, prostate, and skin, suggesting that the loss of *14-3-3 sigma* expression may be causally involved in tumor progression (Lodygin and Hermeking 2005). Similarly, *14-3-3 sigma* promoter methylation occurred at a higher frequency in NPC, 84 % compared to adjacent noncancerous nasopharyngeal epithelial tissue. In addition, Yi et al. (2009) showed a significant correlation between DNA methylation of the *14-3-3 sigma* gene and advanced clinical stage, lymph node involvement, and distant metastasis in NPC.

Summary and Future Perspectives

Aberrant methylation of tumor-related genes is a common event in NPC. Methylation of genes occurs not only in advanced tumor stages, but it is a frequent and early event. Moreover, the frequency of aberrant promoter methylation increases during the progression from precancerous lesion to NPC. Promoter methylation of different kinds of tumor-suppressor genes including *RASSF1A*, *RARbβ-2*, *p16*, or *DAP-kinase* has been demonstrated in body fluids from patients with NPC. Therefore, epigenetic changes in preneoplastic or early neoplastic stages may serve as indicator or "biomarker" for screening of individuals with an increased risk for NPC.

Potential Application to Prognosis and Other Diseases or Conditions

It was demonstrated that re-expression of tumor-suppressor genes that are epigenetically silenced is possible by using demethylating and histone-modifying agents. In the next years, this might be a possible therapeutic approach, but the used therapeutic agents that influence DNA hypermethylation are toxic and lead to genome-wide alteration of the methylation pattern with the possibility of activating oncogenes or imprinted genes. Another possible aspect of chemotherapy might be to modulate the epigenetically involved pathways by using small molecules that are more specific. But further investigations in clinical trials are needed to prove and integrate epigenetic pathway-modulating agents.

Summary Points

- Nasopharyngeal carcinoma (NPC) is a highly invasive and metastatic malignant tumor with remarkable geographic distribution.
- The undifferentiated carcinoma is the major histopathological type of NPC.
- A number of etiological environmental factors, especially the Epstein–Barr virus, along with genetic/host factors might be responsible for the causation of NPC.
- NPC exhibits numerous genetic abnormalities, namely, chromosomal deletions, gene amplifications, and mutations.
- The methylation of DNA is an important epigenetic modification in NPC mediated by three well definite DNA methyltransferases (DNMT), DNMT1, DNMT3a, and DMNT3b.
- NPCs have shown aberrant methylation at CpG islands in a growing list of genes, those belonging to different pathways in cells.
- Promoter methylation of different kinds of tumor-suppressor genes including *RASSF1A*, *p16*, and *DAP-kinase* has been demonstrated in body fluids from patients with NPC and then may serve as biomarker for screening of individuals with an increased risk for NPC.

References

Agathanggelou A, Dallol A, Zöchbauer-Müller S, et al. Epigenetic inactivation of the candidate 3p21.3 suppressor gene BLU in human cancers. Oncogene. 2003;22:1580–8.

Ayadi W, Karray-Hakim H, Khabir A, et al. Aberrant methylation of p16, DLEC1, BLU and E cadherin gene promoters in nasopharyngeal carcinoma biopsies from Tunisian patients. Anticancer Res. 2008;28:2161–7.

Bei JX, Jia WH, Zeng YX. Familial and large-scale case-control studies identify genes associated with nasopharyngeal carcinoma. Semin Cancer Biol. 2012;22:96–106.

Challouf S, Ziadi S, Zaghdoudi R, et al. Patterns of aberrant DNA hypermethylation in nasopharyngeal carcinoma in Tunisian patients. Clin Chim Acta. 2012;413:795–802.

Chan JKC, Pilch BZ, Kuo TT, et al. Tumors of the nasopharynx. In: Barnes L, Eveson JW, Reichart P, Sidransky D, editors. World Health Organization classification of tumors. Pathology and genetics of head and neck tumours. Lyon: IARC Press; 2005. p. 83–97.

Chan KC, Hung EC, Woo JK, et al. Early detection of nasopharyngeal carcinoma by plasma Epstein-Barr virus DNA analysis in a surveillance program. Cancer. 2013;119:1838–44.

Chang ET, Adami HO. The enigmatic epidemiology of nasopharyngeal carcinoma. Cancer Epidemiol Biomarkers Prev. 2006;15:1765–77.

Chang HW, Chan A, Kwong DL, et al. Evaluation of hypermethylated tumor suppressor genes as tumor markers in mouth and throat rinsing fluid, nasopharyngeal swab and peripheral blood of nasopharyngeal carcinoma patient. Int J Cancer. 2003;105:851–5.

Chen J, Fu L, Zhang LY, et al. Tumor suppressor genes on frequently deleted chromosome 3p in nasopharyngeal carcinoma. Chin J Cancer. 2012;31:215–22.

Chow LS, Lo KW, Kwong J, et al. RASSF1A is a target tumor suppressor from 3p21.3 in nasopharyngeal carcinoma. Int J Cancer. 2004;109:839–47.

Cohen O, Feinstein E, Kimchi A. DAP-kinase is a Ca^{2+}/calmodulin-dependent, cytoskeletal-associated protein kinase, with cell death-inducing functions that depend on its catalytic activity. EMBO J. 1997;16:998–1008.

Cohen O, Inbal B, Kissil JL, et al. DAP-kinase participates in TNF-alpha- and Fas-induced apoptosis and its function requires the death domain. J Cell Biol. 1999;146:141–8.

Cottrell SE. Molecular diagnostic applications of DNA methylation technology. Clin Biochem. 2004;37:595–604.

Dammann R, Schagdarsurengin U, Seidel C, et al. The tumor suppressor RASSF1A in human carcinogenesis: an update. Histol Histopathol. 2005;20:645–63.

Daniel V. Glutathione S-transferases: gene structure and regulation of expression. Crit Rev Biochem Mol Biol. 1993;28:173–207.

Donninger H, Vos MD, Clark GJ. The RASSF1A tumor suppressor. J Cell Sci. 2007;120:3163–72.

Esteller M. CpG island hypermethylation and tumor suppressor genes: a booming present, a brighter future. Oncogene. 2002;21:5427–40.

Esteller M, Corn PG, Urena JM, et al. Inactivation of glutathione S-transferase P1 gene by promoter hypermethylation in human neoplasia. Cancer Res. 1998;58:4515–18.

Esteller M, Hamilton SR, Burger PC, et al. Inactivation of the DNA repair gene O^6-methylguanine-DNA methyltransferase by promoter hypermethylation is a common event in primary human neoplasia. Cancer Res. 1999;59:793–7.

Etienne-Manneville S, Hall A. Rho GTPases in cell biology. Nature. 2002;420:629–35.

Fendri A, Masmoudi A, Khabir A, et al. Inactivation of RASSF1A, RARbeta2 and DAP-kinase by promoter methylation correlates with lymph node metastasis in nasopharyngeal carcinoma. Cancer Biol Ther. 2009;8:444–51.

Feng X, Ren C, Zhou W, et al. Promoter hypermethylation along with LOH, but not mutation, contributes to inactivation of DLC-1 in nasopharyngeal carcinoma. Mol Carcinog. 2013;12:53.

Frappier L. Role of EBNA1 in NPC tumourigenesis. Semin Cancer Biol. 2012;22:154–61.

Han BL, Xu XY, Zhang CZ, et al. Systematic review on Epstein-Barr virus (EBV) DNA in diagnosis of nasopharyngeal carcinoma in Asian populations. Asian Pac J Cancer Prev. 2012;13:2577–81.

Hannon GJ, Beach D. p15INK4B is a potential effector of TGF-beta-induced cell cycle arrest. Nature. 1994;371:257–61.

Hocevar BA, Mou F, Rennolds JL, et al. Regulation of the Wnt signaling pathway by disabled-2 (Dab2). EMBO J. 2003;22:3084–94.

Hui AB, Lo KW, Kwong J, et al. Epigenetic inactivation of TSLC1 gene in nasopharyngeal carcinoma. Mol Carcinog. 2003;38:170–8.

Jia WH, Luo XY, Feng BJ, et al. Traditional Cantonese diet and nasopharyngeal carcinoma risk: a large-scale case-control study in Guangdong, China. BMC Cancer. 2010;10:446.

Kim TY, Jong HS, Song SH, et al. Transcriptional silencing of the DLC-1 tumor suppressor gene by epigenetic mechanism in gastric cancer cells. Oncogene. 2003;22:3943–51.

Kissil JL, Feinstein E, Cohen O, et al. DAP-kinase loss of expression in various carcinoma and B-cell lymphoma cell lines: possible implications for role as tumor suppressor gene. Oncogene. 1997;15:403–7.

Kong WJ, Zhang S, Guo CK, et al. Effect of methylation-associated silencing of the death-associated protein kinase gene on nasopharyngeal carcinoma. Anticancer Drugs. 2006;17:251–9.

Krishna SM, Kattoor J, Balaram P. Down regulation of adhesion protein E-cadherin in Epstein-Barr virus infected nasopharyngeal carcinomas. Cancer Biomark. 2005;1:271–7.

Krop IE, Sgroi D, Porter DA, et al. HIN-1, a putative cytokine highly expressed in normal but not cancerous mammary epithelial cells. Proc Natl Acad Sci U S A. 2001;98:9796–801.

Kwong J, Lo KW, To KF, et al. Promoter hypermethylation of multiple genes in nasopharyngeal carcinoma. Clin Cancer Res. 2002;8:131–7.

Kwong J, Chow LS, Wong AY, et al. Epigenetic inactivation of the deleted in lung and esophageal cancer 1 gene in nasopharyngeal carcinoma. Genes Chromosomes Cancer. 2007;46:171–80.

Li Z, Ren Y, Lin SX, et al. Association of E-cadherin and beta-catenin with metastasis in nasopharyngeal carcinoma. Chin Med J (Engl). 2004;117:1232–9.

Li X, Wang E, Zhao YD, et al. Chromosomal imbalances in nasopharyngeal carcinoma: a meta-analysis of comparative genomic hybridization results. J Transl Med. 2006;4:4.
Li X, Fasano R, Wang E, Marincola FM, et al. HLA associations with nasopharyngeal carcinoma. Curr Mol Med. 2009;9:751–65.
Liu XQ, Chen HK, Zhang XS, et al. Alterations of BLU, a candidate tumor suppressor gene on chromosome 3p21.3, in human nasopharyngeal carcinoma. Int J Cancer. 2003;106:60–5.
Lo KW, Huang DP, Lau KM. p16 gene alterations in nasopharyngeal carcinoma. Cancer Res. 1995;55:2039–43.
Lo KW, Cheung ST, Leung SF, et al. Hypermethylation of the p16 gene in nasopharyngeal carcinoma. Cancer Res. 1996;56:2721–5.
Lo KW, Kwong J, Hui AB, et al. High frequency of promoter hypermethylation of RASSF1A in nasopharyngeal carcinoma. Cancer Res. 2001;61:3877–81.
Lodygin D, Hermeking H. The role of epigenetic inactivation of 14-3-3sigma in human cancer. Cell Res. 2005;15:237–46.
Lung HL, Cheng Y, Kumaran MK, et al. Fine mapping of the 11q22-23 tumor suppressive region and involvement of TSLC1 in nasopharyngeal carcinoma. Int J Cancer. 2004;112:628–35.
Mannello F, Gazzanelli G. Tissue inhibitors of metalloproteinases and programmed cell death: conundrums, controversies and potential implications. Apoptosis. 2001;6:479–82.
Mark M, Ghyselinck NB, Chambon P. Function of retinoid nuclear receptors: lessons from genetic and pharmacological dissections of the retinoic acid signaling pathway during mouse embryogenesis. Annu Rev Pharmacol Toxicol. 2006;46:451–80.
Masuda M, Yageta M, Fukuhara H, et al. The tumor suppressor protein TSLC1 is involved in cell-cell adhesion. J Biol Chem. 2002;277:31014–19.
Murakami Y. Involvement of a cell adhesion molecule, TSLC1/IGSF4, in human oncogenesis. Cancer Sci. 2005;96:543–52.
Niemhom S, Kitazawa S, Kitazawa R, et al. Hypermethylation of epithelial-cadherin gene promoter is associated with Epstein-Barr virus in nasopharyngeal carcinoma. Cancer Detect Prev. 2008;32:127–34.
Parkin DM, Bray F, Ferlay J, Pisani P. Global cancer statistics, 2002. CA Cancer J Clin. 2005;55:74–108.
Pegg AE. Mammalian O^6-alkylguanine-DNA alkyltransferase: regulation and importance in response to alkylating carcinogenic and therapeutic agents. Cancer Res. 1990;50:6119–29.
Peng D, Ren CP, Yi HM, et al. Genetic and epigenetic alterations of DLC-1, a candidate tumor suppressor gene, in nasopharyngeal carcinoma. Acta Biochim Biophys Sin (Shanghai). 2006;38:349–55.
Polesel J, Serraino D, Negri E, et al. Consumption of fruit, vegetables, and other food groups and the risk of nasopharyngeal carcinoma. Cancer Causes Control. 2013;24:1157–65.
Qiu GH, Tan LK, Loh KS, et al. The candidate tumor suppressor gene BLU, located at the commonly deleted region 3p21.3, is an E2F-regulated, stress-responsive gene and inactivated by both epigenetic and genetic mechanisms in nasopharyngeal carcinoma. Oncogene. 2004;23:4793–806.
Ran Y, Wu S, You Y. Demethylation of E-cadherin gene in nasopharyngeal carcinoma could serve as a potential therapeutic strategy. J Biochem. 2011;149:49–54.
Robertson KD. DNA methylation and human disease. Nat Rev Genet. 2005;6:597–610.
Seng TJ, Low JS, Li H, et al. The major 8p22 tumor suppressor DLC1 is frequently silenced by methylation in both endemic and sporadic nasopharyngeal, esophageal, and cervical carcinomas, and inhibits tumor cell colony formation. Oncogene. 2007;26:934–44.
Simons MJ, Chao SM, Wee GD, et al. Nasopharyngeal carcinoma and histocompatibility antigens. In: de The G, Ito Y, editors. Nasopharyngeal carcinoma: etiology and control, IARC scientific publication N°20. Lyon: IARC; 1978. p. 271.
Strathdee G. Epigenetic versus genetic alterations in the inactivation of E-cadherin. Semin Cancer Biol. 2002;12:373–9.

Takeichi M. Cadherin cell adhesion receptors as a morphogenetic regulator. Science. 1991;251:1451–5.

Tong JH, Tsang RK, Lo KA, et al. Quantitative Epstein-Barr virus DNA analysis and detection of gene promoter hypermethylation in nasopharyngeal (NP) brushing samples from patients with NP carcinoma. Clin Cancer Res. 2002;8:2612–19.

Tong JH, Ng DC, Chau SL, et al. Putative tumour-suppressor gene DAB2 is frequently down regulated by promoter hypermethylation in nasopharyngeal carcinoma. BMC Cancer. 2010;10:253.

Van der Weyden L, Adams DJ. The Ras-association domain family (RASSF) members and their role in human tumourigenesis. Biochim Biophys Acta. 2007;1776:58–85.

Van Roy F, Berx G. The cell-cell adhesion molecule E-cadherin. Cell Mol Life Sci. 2008;65:3756–88.

Wang S, Xiao X, Zhou X, et al. TFPI-2 is a putative tumor suppressor gene frequently inactivated by promoter hypermethylation in nasopharyngeal carcinoma. BMC Cancer. 2010;10:617.

Wei KR, Xu Y, Liu J, et al. Histopathological classification of nasopharyngeal carcinoma. Asian Pac J Cancer Prev. 2011;12:1141–1147.

Wong TS, Chang HW, Tang KC, et al. High frequency of promoter hypermethylation of the death-associated protein-kinase gene in nasopharyngeal carcinoma and its detection in the peripheral blood of patients. Clin Cancer Res. 2002;8:433–7.

Wong CM, Lee JM, Ching YP, et al. Genetic and epigenetic alterations of DLC-1 gene in hepatocellular carcinoma. Cancer Res. 2003a;63:7646–51.

Wong TS, Kwong DL, Sham JS, et al. Promoter hypermethylation of high-in-normal 1 gene in primary nasopharyngeal carcinoma. Clin Cancer Res. 2003b;9:3042–6.

Wong CM, Ng YL, Lee JM, et al. Tissue factor pathway inhibitor-2 as a frequently silenced tumor suppressor gene in hepatocellular carcinoma. Hepatology. 2007;45:1129–38.

Xu FH, Xiong D, Xu YF, et al. An epidemiological and molecular study of the relationship between smoking, risk of nasopharyngeal carcinoma, and Epstein-Barr virus activation. J Natl Cancer Inst. 2012;104:1396–410.

Yi B, Tan SX, Tang CE, et al. Inactivation of 14-3-3 sigma by promoter methylation correlates with metastasis in nasopharyngeal carcinoma. J Cell Biochem. 2009;106:858–66.

Zhang Z, Sun D, Van do N, et al. Inactivation of RASSF2A by promoter methylation correlates with lymph node metastasis in nasopharyngeal carcinoma. Int J Cancer. 2007;120:32–8.

Zhou L, Jiang W, Ren C, et al. Frequent hypermethylation of RASSF1A and TSLC1, and high viral load of Epstein-Barr virus DNA in nasopharyngeal carcinoma and matched tumor-adjacent tissues. Neoplasia. 2005;7:809–15.

Zhou W, Feng X, Li H, et al. Inactivation of LARS2, located at the commonly deleted region 3p21.3, by both epigenetic and genetic mechanisms in nasopharyngeal carcinoma. Acta Biochim Biophys Sin (Shanghai). 2009;41:54–62.

Whole Blood Transcriptome and Other Biomarkers in Nasopharyngeal Cancer

38

Chun Ren Lim, Michelle Mei Lin Lee, Samuel Chao,
Adel Zaatar, and Choong Chin Liew

Contents

Chun Ren Lim and Michelle Lee contributed equally to this manuscript

C.R. Lim • M.M.L. Lee
GeneNews (Malaysia) Limited, Georgetown, Penang, Malaysia
e-mail: cr_lim@hotmail.com; mlee@genenewsdiagnostics.com

S. Chao
GeneNews Limited, Markham, ON, Canada
e-mail: schao@genenews.com

A. Zaatar
Gleneagles Medical Centre, Penang, Malaysia
e-mail: zaatar@streamyx.com

C.C. Liew (✉)
GeneNews Diagnostics, Kuala Lumpur, Malaysia
e-mail: cliew@genenews.com

V.R. Preedy, V.B. Patel (eds.), *Biomarkers in Cancer, Biomarkers in Disease: Methods, Discoveries and Applications*,
DOI 10.1007/978-94-007-7681-4_3

Abstract

Nasopharyngeal carcinoma is often diagnosed only after the disease has reached late stages and the prognosis is poor. However, when detected early, the disease is highly survivable. This review surveys molecular biomarker studies that aim to identify early, presymptomatic disease, to predict response to treatment, to indicate prognosis, to identify tumor stage, and to monitor disease progression. Blood transcriptomic studies represent a new frontier in the molecular diagnostics of nasopharyngeal carcinoma.

List of Abbreviations

AUC	Area Under the Curve
BCR	B-cell Receptor
CR	Complete Response to Treatment
CT	Computed Tomography
DNA	Deoxyribonucleic Acid
EBV	Epstein-Barr Virus
EGFR1	Epidermal Growth Factor Receptor 1
ELISA	Enzyme-Linked Immunosorbent Assay
GWAS	Genome-Wide Association Study
HLA	Human Leukocyte Antigen
IgA	Immunoglobulin A
IgG	Immunoglobulin G
MHC	Major Histocompatibility Complex
miRNA	MicroRNA
MRI	Magnetic Resonance Imaging
mRNA	Messenger RNA
NPC	Nasopharyngeal Carcinoma
PCR	Polymerase Chain Reaction
PR	Partial Response to Treatment
RNA	Ribonucleic Acid
ROC	Receiver Operating Characteristic Curve
SELDI-TOF-MS	Surface-Enhanced Laser Desorption and Ionization-Time-of-Flight Mass Spectrometry
SNP	Single Nucleotide Polymorphism
TNF	Tumor Necrosis Factor
TNFR	Tumor Necrosis Factor Receptor
TSG	Tumor Suppressor Gene
VCA	Viral Capsid Antigen

Key Facts

Key Facts of Nasopharyngeal Carcinoma (NPC)

- NPC is a cancer arising in the nasopharyngeal epithelial lining, where the back of the nose meets the throat.
- NPC is a carcinoma predominantly found in southern China, Southeast Asia, and North Africa.
- Southern China has the highest incidence of NPC worldwide; in Hong Kong, for example, NPC affects approximately 20–30 per 100,000 men and 15–20 per 100,000 women.
- NPC is caused by a number of factors including EBV infection, genetic susceptibility, ethnic background, and environmental carcinogens.
- The diagnosis of NPC is usually done by computed tomography (CT), magnetic resonance imaging (MRI), and nasopharyngoscopy.
- Symptoms of NPC are nonspecific, and most NPC cases present at late stages, limiting the patient's chance for full recovery.
- Survival rates are high, between 80 % and 95 %, if NPC is detected in the early stages (stages I and II).
- The standard treatment options for NPC are radiotherapy, chemotherapy, and surgery.

Key Facts of Epstein-Barr Virus (EBV)

- Epstein-Barr virus (EBV), a virus from the herpes family, is also known as human herpesvirus 4 (HHV-4).
- EBV is divided into two major types, EBV type 1 and EBV type 2. Both subtypes have different EBNA-3 genes and differ in their transformation capabilities and reactivation abilities.
- EBV is associated with several diseases and cancers, such as Hodgkin's lymphoma, Burkitt's lymphoma, nasopharyngeal carcinoma, and conditions associated with human immunodeficiency virus (HIV).
- EBV is able to affect a number of different cell types (viral tropism) such as B-cells, epithelial cells, T-cells, and smooth muscle cells.
- Most people become infected with EBV and gain adaptive immunity. EBV infects B-cells in the immune system, and once EBV infection is brought under control, it will be present in an individual's B-cells for life.
- EBV has two independent systems for replicating their genomes. The first system employs an active or "lytic" DNA replication system similar to other viruses in the herpesvirus family. The second system is EBV's own system of replication that operates during latent stages of infection to allow circular EBV genomes to be duplicated during cell division.

Key Facts of the Sentinel Principle®

- The Sentinel Principle® was developed by the cofounder and Chief Scientist of GeneNews Limited, Professor C.C. Liew.
- The Sentinel Principle® aims to identify biomarkers of body state using blood transcriptome.
- A biomarker is a measurable molecular, biochemical, or cellular characteristic that indicates the presence or state of a disease.
- Biomarkers are also used to predict the risk of an individual having a specific disease, predict the outcome of a disease, monitor the effects of treatments or disease recurrence, and provide information on accidental exposure to a potential environmental hazard.
- As blood circulates in the body, there are interactions between blood cells and the body's cells. Subtle changes in blood RNA reflect a disease or injury anywhere in the body. Disease-specific blood RNA biomarkers can be developed by measuring and identifying these subtle changes (Fig. 1).
- Blood RNA biomarkers can be a convenient, minimally invasive alternative to tissue biopsy for determining the diagnosis and prognosis of diseases.

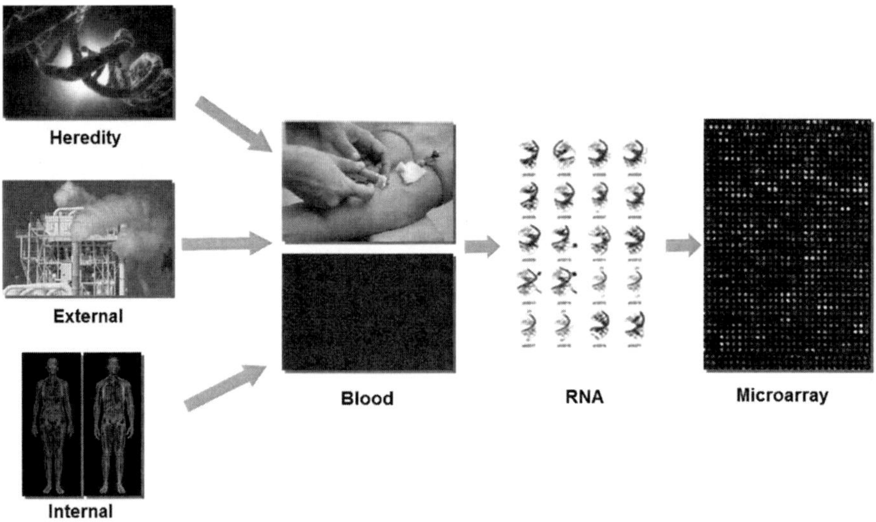

Fig. 1 The Sentinel Principle®. Many factors, including injury or disease, cause subtle changes in gene expression in the blood. The Sentinel Principle® uses the basis that these changes can reflect the body's current state of health to identify blood RNA biomarkers

Definitions of Words and Terms

Transcriptome A collection of all RNA/transcript molecules (mRNA, rRNA, tRNA, noncoding RNA) in a given cell. RNA molecules are called transcripts because they are transcribed from DNA that contains the instructions to perform a particular function.

Pharmacogenomics Many genes affect a person's response to a drug, due to genetic variations. Pharmacogenomics is a branch of science that studies the entire genetic makeup of a person and how it may affect drug response.

CpG Site A section of DNA where a cytosine (C) nucleotide occurs next to a guanine (G) nucleotide, separated by one phosphate (p) in the linear DNA sequence.

DNA Methylation The process of adding a methyl group to the cytosine or adenine DNA nucleotides, usually occurring at CpG sites. DNA methylation alters gene expression without changing the genetic sequence.

Polymorphism The occurrence of two or more different types or characteristics in organisms of the same species. The differences are caused by a sequence variant that is present in a particular population.

Apoptosis Programmed cell death.

Prognosis The predicted likelihood of a patient's recovery from a disease.

Oncogene A gene that promotes uncontrolled cell growth, which may develop into cancer.

Tumor Suppressor Gene (TSG) A tumor suppressor gene is the opposite of an oncogene. It is a cell growth regulating gene. In its normal form, a TSG inhibits the growth of tumors. However, when mutated, cells grow uncontrolled and may progress to cancer.

Genome-Wide Association Study (GWAS) A study that rapidly scans markers across the complete genome of a large population of people to find common genetic variations associated with a particular disease or trait.

Angiogenesis The process of creating new blood vessels. The formation of new tissues requires angiogenesis.

Sentinel Principle® A novel approach, first proposed by Professor C. C. Liew, to identify biomarkers using blood. The Sentinel Principle® is based on the scientific observation that circulating blood reflects, in a detectable way, what is occurring throughout the body.

Introduction

Nasopharyngeal carcinoma (NPC) is a cancer arising in the nasopharyngeal epithelial lining, where the back of the nose meets the throat. NPC is a major carcinoma in southern China (e.g., in Guangdong and Hong Kong), Southeast Asia, and North Africa. The highest incidence worldwide occurs in southeast China; in Hong Kong, for example, NPC affects approximately 20–30 per 100,000 men and 15–20 per 100,000 women (Ferlay et al. 2010). In Malaysia, NPC is the third most common cancer in men (after colon cancer and lung cancer), with an incidence of per 100,000 in Chinese males in Malaysia (National Cancer Registry 2006).

NPC is closely associated with the Epstein-Barr virus (EBV), which infects epithelial cells of the nasopharynx. EBV is a herpesvirus that is transmitted by saliva and carried by 90 % of the population worldwide (Wei and Sham 2005). Genetic susceptibility, ethnic background, and environmental carcinogens are known to play important roles in the etiology of NPC. Consumption of salted fish containing nitrosamines is also a well-established etiological factor for NPC in adults (Chang and Adami 2006).

Because the nasopharynx is difficult to access and because early NPC has minimal or nonspecific symptoms, NPC diagnosis is often only carried out when the disease has reached late stages. The symptoms of NPC include neck mass, nasal and aural dysfunction, and headaches. The usual metastatic sites are the bone and lung.

Primary NPC is very sensitive to radiotherapy and chemotherapy. Earlier stages I and II NPC are readily treated, and patients have excellent survival rates of 80–95 % with radiotherapy alone (Caponigro et al. 2010). Patients with NPC at stages III and IV have reported 3-year survival rates of 70–80 % with chemoradiotherapy (Wee et al. 2005; Al-Sarraf et al. 1998). Relapse, however, is common, and the prognosis for recurrent disease is poor, with a median survival time of less than 1 year (Caponigro et al. 2010). Diagnosis of NPC is by computed tomography (CT), magnetic resonance imaging (MRI) scan of the head and neck, and nasopharyngoscopy to locate the primary tumor. A biopsy of enlarged lymph nodes or the primary tumor is then performed to confirm the diagnosis. There are three types of NPC: undifferentiated carcinoma, keratinizing squamous cell carcinoma, and nonkeratinizing differentiated carcinoma.

Biomarkers for early stage NPC would provide a useful adjunct to current diagnostic methods. Such biomarkers could help improve the prognosis for patients with NPC by providing early disease detection and treatment guidance. A convenient, cost-effective screening technology for the disease would benefit the population at risk for developing NPC and stimulate NPC prevention awareness, especially in high-risk areas, such as in southern China, Southeast Asia, and North Africa. Advances in genetics, genomics, proteomics, and bioinformatics have led to the identification of many potential biomarkers for NPC in recent years. In this chapter we review biomarkers for NPC, with particular emphasis on the use of the whole blood transcriptome.

DNA Biomarkers

More than 90 % of the world's adult population is infected with EBV (Wee et al. 2005; Maeda et al. 2009). In most cases, the virus remains latent in lymphocytes; however, once active, EBV may lead to EBV-related diseases such as nasopharyngeal cancer, Hodgkin's disease, and certain lymphomas. EBV DNA can be detected in tissues from tumors of most patients with NPC. EBV DNA from NPC tumors can also be detected in patient plasma and serum, which enables the use of EBV DNA as a potential diagnostic biomarker.

Quantitative plasma EBV DNA, detected using polymerase chain reaction (PCR), is a relatively inexpensive, noninvasive, and convenient test and has long been accepted as a prognostic marker for NPC. EBV DNA is currently used for tumor growth staging, prediction of prognosis, and posttreatment monitoring. More recently, EBV DNA has been assessed as a screening tool for NPC (Chan et al. 2013; Lo et al. 1999; Le et al. 2005, 2013).

Highly significant differences have been found when EBV DNA levels are measured in NPC and non-NPC groups. Using a real-time PCR, Lo and colleagues found EBV DNA in the plasma of 96 % of NPC patients and only 7 % of healthy controls (Lo et al. 1999). EBV DNA concentration can also be linearly correlated with NPC tumor load, providing information on disease staging (Lo et al. 1999). Primer/probe sets used for real-time quantitative PCR are commonly from the *Bam*HI-W region, which occurs 8–11 times in the EBV genome (Lo et al. 1999; Le et al. 2013). Other single-copy EBV genes used include Epstein-Barr nuclear antigen-1 (EBNA-1), latent membrane protein 2 (LMP2), and DNA polymerase alpha catalytic subunit A (POL1) (Le et al. 2005). Different laboratories, however, have not been able to reproduce similar sensitivity and specificity values for the quantitative plasma/serum EBV DNA test. One possible reason for this failure is that DNA may be liberated during blood clotting, suggesting that important information may be lost if serum DNA is used (Lo et al. 1999). EBV DNA can also be detected in other EBV-linked diseases, reducing the specificity to NPC of the EBV DNA test.

Many studies have also investigated single nucleotide polymorphisms (SNPs) as inherited susceptibility biomarkers for NPC. An SNP, the most common type of genetic variation, is a DNA sequence variation of a single nucleotide. Although most SNPs are common and harmless, some SNPs are located within a gene or a gene's regulatory region, which may cause gene expression to be affected, leading to disease.

Three recent genome-wide association studies (GWASs) have investigated genetic polymorphisms and NPC risk (Bei et al. 2010; Tse et al. 2009; Ng et al. 2009). All of these studies report that genes associated with NPC are located within the major histocompatibility complex (MHC) region on chromosome 6p21. This region includes human leukocyte antigen (HLA) genes, many of which are immune-related genes that differentiate foreign, possibly harmful peptides from the body's own peptides. A number of investigators since the 1970s have suggested that HLA genes, which are categorized into class I, class II, and class III, are associated with the etiology of NPC. The largest GWAS-NPC study to date, reported by Bei and colleagues, used more than 400,000 autosomal SNPs in 1,583 NPC cases and 1,894 controls in the discovery phase (Bei et al. 2010). All of the subjects were of southern Chinese descent, from China and Singapore. The study identified seven SNPs that were significant: rs2860580, rs2894207, and rs28421666, corresponding to the HLA-A, HLA-B/C, and HLA-DQ/DR loci on chromosome 6p21; rs9510787 and rs1572072, corresponding to the TNFRSF19 locus; rs6774494 (MDS1-EVI1); and rs1412829 (CDNK2A/2B) (Bei et al. 2010). The HLA-A*1101 allele was found to have a strong association with a reduced risk for NPC, as reported in other studies (Bei et al. 2010; Tse et al. 2009; Hildesheim et al. 2002). Both TNFRSF19 and MDS1-EVI1 are linked to pathways involved in EBV-related NPC tumorigenesis (Bei et al. 2010). The CDKN2A/CDKN2B gene cluster is deleted in about 40 % of primary NPC tumors, which suggests that these genes may function as tumor suppressor genes for NPC (Bei et al. 2010).

A much smaller GWAS carried out in Taiwan confirmed previous findings on the association of HLA genes with NPC (Tse et al. 2009). This study also reported an association with NPC of two additional genes, gamma-aminobutyric acid B receptor 1 (GABBR1) and HLA complex group 9 (HCG9). Another recent small GWAS from Malaysia (111 NPC cases and 260 controls, all of Chinese descent) reported an association between integrin alpha 9 (ITGA9) and NPC (Ng et al. 2009). Of note, Bei and colleagues in the large study reported above did not observe any association with NPC within the ITGA9 locus (Bei et al. 2010).

Consumption of salted fish containing nitrosamines is one of the factors identified in the etiology of NPC (Chang and Adami 2006). A study by Tiwawech et al. (2006) suggests that polymorphisms of the nitrosamine metabolizing gene, human cytochrome P450 2A6 (CYP2A6), may serve as molecular biomarkers for NPC in high-risk populations whose diet is high in salted fish. CYP2A6 is also known to play a role in the metabolism of nicotine in tobacco smoke (Tiwawech et al. 2006). Six genotypes of the CYP2A6 were identified to have significantly different frequencies in NPC patients as compared with healthy controls (Tiwawech et al. 2006). These results suggest that CYP2A6 polymorphisms may be associated with NPC susceptibility. An increased risk of NPC was also reported in association with a variant form of another cytochrome P450 gene, cytochrome P450, family 2, subfamily E, polypeptide 1 (CYP2E1) (Hildesheim et al. 1995, 1997). Similar to CYP2A6, CYP2E1 is also a nitrosamine metabolizing gene.

A major problem with GWAS is the lack of studies with a large enough sample size for adequate power. GWAS of the same disease or disorder frequently shows inconsistent results, most likely because of small sample sizes of less than a thousand. In addition, GWAS in NPC often do not involve non-Chinese subjects. In order to overcome these problems, pooled or joint studies are usually required.

Methylation (Epigenetics)

DNA methylation is an epigenetic alteration that does not involve the changes of the nucleotide sequence characteristic of genetic mutation. In DNA methylation, a methyl group is added to the cytosine or adenine DNA nucleotides by enzymatic transfer, stably altering gene expression in cells. DNA methylation occurs either as hypermethylation (an increase in methylation of cytosine or adenine nucleotides in DNA relative to their normal counterparts) or hypomethylation (a decrease in methylation of cytosine or adenine nucleotides in DNA relative to their normal counterparts). Methylation often occurs at the CpG island site, so named because it is a short region of high guanine-cytosine (G-C) content and is usually not methylated. The transfer of the methyl group in DNA methylation is performed by DNA methyltransferases. In mammals, DNA methyltransferases mainly target CpG sites, but DNA methylation can still occur at other parts of the DNA (Robertson 2005). DNA methylation of certain genes and sites has been linked to carcinogenesis and to nonmalignant diseases, such as Beckwith-Wiedemann syndrome, Angelman syndrome, and fragile X syndrome (Ambinder et al. 1999).

A CpG island site on a tumor suppressor gene (TSG) that is usually hypomethylated can become hypermethylated and will silence this TSG, thereby preventing transcription of the gene and promoting tumor growth and cancer. Conversely, a usually hypermethylated repeat-rich heterochromatin can become hypomethylated, leading to genomic instability, a characteristic that is often observed in tumor cells (Ambinder et al. 1999). For example, a frequent genomic instability in tumors involves the rearrangement of the large block of pericentromeric heterochromatin on chromosome 1 (Ambinder et al. 1999). In both instances, hypermethylation and hypomethylation may lead to the onset of cancer.

In NPC, CpG island site methylation is known to promote tumorigenesis by inducing the silencing of TSGs and EBV immunodominant antigens, such as EBNA2, EBNA3A, EBNA3B, and EBNA3c, and also suppressing the oncoprotein LMP1 (latent membrane protein 1), which is involved in EBV latency (Laird 2003). Kwong and colleagues analyzed abnormal promoter hypermethylation in CpG sites of eight known cancer-related genes: Ras association domain family 1A (RASSF1A), retinoic acid receptor β-2 (RARβ2), death-associated protein kinase (DAP-kinase), cyclin-dependent kinase inhibitor 2A (CDKN2A/p16), cyclin-dependent kinase inhibitor 2B (CDKN2B/p15), product of CDKN2A beta transcript (ARF/p14), O^6-methylguanine-DNA methyltransferase (MGMT), and glutathione S-transferase pi 1 (GSTP1) (Kwong et al. 2002). Some of the genes had promoter hypermethylation in high proportions of NPC samples, including 84 % of RASSF1A, 80 % of RARβ2, 76 % of DAP-kinase, and 46 % of p16 (Kwong et al. 2002). None of the CpG sites of these genes were methylated in the controls. Epigenetic changes caused by DNA methylation may influence their related cellular pathways, including the Ras signaling pathway, the retinoid signaling pathway, the metastasis-related process, cell cycle, p53 network, and DNA repair in NPC (Kwong et al. 2002). This finding suggests that these genes may be involved in NPC tumorigenesis and that they could possibly be used as targets for NPC biomarkers. Methylation of some of these genes is also linked to other cancers, such as RASSF1A in lung and breast cancers and the tumor suppressor CDKN2A/p16 in melanoma and pancreatic adenocarcinoma (Dammann et al. 2001; Agathanggelou et al. 2001; Kamb et al. 1994; Caldas et al. 1994).

Epigenetic alterations other than DNA methylation that may be linked to cancer include histone modification and chromatin remodeling. The silencing in NPC cells of the osteoprotegerin (OPG) gene, a member of the tumor necrosis factor receptor (TNFR) superfamily, was proven to be caused by both DNA methylation and histone modifications (Lu et al. 2009). Epigenetic alterations such as these often silence tumor suppressor genes, leading to tumor development.

It is possible to compare amounts of DNA methylation with absolute reference points, such as completely unmethylated or completely methylated DNA (Robertson 2005). Such DNA methylation profiling of particular regions, such as CpG sites, can identify useful molecular biomarkers for NPC. DNA methylation tests have been used to screen for diseases. These include the blood-based DNA screening test for colorectal cancer ColoVantage, which detects methylated septin 9 (SEPT9), and the methylation analysis of the promoter region of the small nuclear ribonucleoprotein polypeptide N gene (SNRPN) for Angelman syndrome (Quest 2013; White et al. 2006). There is as yet no known DNA methylation test for NPC.

MicroRNAs

MicroRNAs (miRNAs) are a class of short (20–22 nucleotides), noncoding ribonucleic acids (RNAs). miRNAs form imperfect pairing with messenger RNAs (mRNAs), affecting the regulation of their expression. miRNAs play important roles in many biological processes posttranscriptionally, including cell development, differentiation, proliferation, and apoptosis (Ambros 2004). Approximately 50 % of miRNAs are located in cancer-associated genome regions and have been linked to the onset of cancer and reported as potential cancer biomarkers (Calin and Croce 2006; Iorio et al. 2005; Murakami et al. 2006).

The location of miRNAs is found to affect function. miRNAs in sections of chromosomes that are deleted in cancers usually function as tumor suppressors, whereas those in genomic regions amplified in cancers function as oncogenes and block apoptosis (Calin and Croce 2006). In NPC tissues, miRNAs are expressed differently than they are expressed in normal epithelial tissue and function as oncogenes to promote an aggressive tumor phenotype. The miRNA *mir-29c* targets mRNAs that are usually translated into proteins linked to cell migration and metastasis (Sengupta et al. 2008). mir-29c has been found to be downregulated in NPC, leading to an increase in those proteins that may cause NPC cells to proliferate and spread (Sengupta et al. 2008). Other potential miRNA biomarkers for NPC include miR-17-92 cluster, miR-155, miR-301, miR-219, miR-34 family, miR-143, and miR-145 (Calin and Croce 2006; Chen et al. 2009). These miRNAs were reported either to downregulate TSGs or to cause an overexpression of oncogenes, which will lead to low apoptosis, high tumor cell proliferation, and even metastasis. A recent study reported that a signature of five miRNAs (miRNAs not disclosed) is able to stratify the scores of an individual's risk of NPC and to provide prognostic information (Liu et al. 2012). However, the clinical utility of the signature remains unclear, as miRNA biomarkers for NPC have not yet been introduced onto the market.

miRNA biomarkers have been reported for a number of diseases, including lung cancer, and for several clinical applications, such as to identify the primary origin of cancers with uncertain or unknown origins (Rosetta Genomics 2013).

Proteins

Advances in proteomics using surface-enhanced laser desorption and ionization-time-of-flight mass spectrometry (SELDI-TOF-MS), also known as protein chip profiling, allow for high-throughput and rapid analysis of a large number of proteins in a single study. Protein expression reflects the current biological state of the body; thus, proteins have been intensively studied as a potential source of diagnostic biomarkers. An increased understanding of the structure and function of the proteins involved in pathogenesis will also help develop potential disease treatments.

Potential protein biomarkers for the diagnosis and posttreatment surveillance of NPC include annexin A1, stathmin, amyloid A, fibronectin, Mac-2 Bp, PAI-1, ceruloplasmin, cytokeratin 19 (CK19), Erb3-binding protein (EBP1), and Rho GDP dissociation inhibitor beta (Rho-GDI-2) (Wu et al. 2005; Doustjalali et al. 2006; Li et al. 2008; Cho et al. 2004). Some proteins, however, such as stathmin and annexin A1, are not specific to NPC, which limits their utility as biomarkers. Currently, many putative protein biomarkers for NPC have been reported only by single laboratories, and studies have not been repeated.

NPC patients have higher levels of serum EBV antibodies than do healthy individuals, and circulating EBV antibodies are currently used as NPC tumor markers. Immunoglobulin A (IgA) serology for the EBV viral capsid antigen (VCA) is measured by enzyme-linked immunosorbent assay (ELISA) (Chan et al. 2013; Cho et al. 2004). The sensitivity of the IgA-VCA test is 89 %, but the test has a high false-positive rate of more than 50 % (Tsang et al. 2004). A recent study found that plasma EBV DNA analysis was more sensitive than IgA-VCA analysis in detecting early NPC (Chan et al. 2013). Thus, it may be beneficial to combine several tests for NPC screening. Based on a multi-analyte profiling study using Luminex's xMAP Technology, Gu and colleagues found that IgA and immunoglobulin G (IgG) antibodies against the protein gp78 (tumor autocrine motility factor receptor) have the ability to differentiate NPC from healthy controls (Gu et al. 2009). A SELDI-TOF-MS study, with a sample size of 168 patients, also identified a protein diagnostic pattern consisting of four peaks that is able to distinguish NPC from non-NPC, with a sensitivity and specificity of more than 90 % (Wei et al. 2008).

Messenger RNA (mRNA)

Transcriptomics, or gene expression profiling, studies all transcripts in a particular cell at a particular time. Recent advances in microarray technologies, RNA-seq, high-throughput real-time PCR, and bioinformatics have provided researchers with the opportunity to measure the expression levels of large numbers of genes, simultaneously. Unlike genetic DNA testing, which involves both coding and noncoding materials (which may introduce false information into the results), mRNA markers involve mainly a protein-coding material and are not affected by noncoding "noise." mRNA biomarkers are dynamic, providing information as to the current state of the health and disease of the body, rather than being limited to indicating a predisposition for inherited disease. Today, most mRNA biomarkers are obtained from biopsy tissue, although the use of blood is becoming increasingly common.

Fendri et al. reported the potential use as a prognostic NPC biomarker of B-cell leukemia/lymphoma 2 (BCL2) mRNA, isolated from NPC tissues (Fendri et al. 2010). The BCL2 family of proteins are key regulators that control apoptosis. BCL2 is a proto-oncogene that prevents cell death leading to carcinogenesis (Katsumata et al. 1992). A few studies have also suggested that increased BCL2 and BCL2-like 12 (BCL2L12) mRNA levels may be able to predict treatment response in several cancers, including lung cancer and breast cancer (Fendri et al. 2011; Reed 2003; Thomodaki and Scorilas 2006).

Another study reported that high expression levels of matrix metalloproteinase 9 (MMP9) mRNA may be an unfavorable prognostic factor for patients with NPC (Liu et al. 2010). The authors suggest that MMP9 degrades the extracellular matrix, inducing angiogenesis and enhancing local cell invasion and metastasis (Liu et al. 2010). The overall survival time of NPC patients is inversely correlated to MMP9 expression values (Liu et al. 2010). Overexpression of MMP9 has also been linked to other invasive and metastatic cancers, including breast cancer, colorectal cancer, and gastric carcinoma (Provatopoulou et al. 2009; Bendaraf et al. 2010; Zhao et al. 2008). Other mRNA biomarkers for NPC that have been reported include latent membrane protein LMP1, EBV latent membrane protein LMP2A, and EBV oncogene BARF1 (Kong et al. 2010; Stevens et al. 2006).

Blood Transcriptome

Blood circulates throughout the entire body, and bioinformation regarding the current state of health or disease of an organism is conveyed in the blood through interactions between circulating blood cells and the body's cells, tissues, and organs.

According to the Sentinel Principle®, blood cells act as "sentinels" that can indicate the status of health or disease anywhere in the body (Liew 1999). Furthermore, since blood samples can be obtained readily and with little discomfort to patients, biomarkers derived from blood RNA provide an alternative to tissue biopsy for the diagnosis and prognosis of disease.

Thus, the gene expression pattern of the blood cells is a valuable resource for biomarker identification and pharmacogenomics. With the completion of the full human genome sequence, many groups have utilized whole genome information and technologies developed to profile the whole blood transcriptome. Expression profiling in peripheral blood cells is able to assess environmental exposures or evaluate the host response to different forms of environmental exposures (Lampe et al. 2004). Peripheral blood cells display disease-specific gene expression signatures that could be correlated to clinically relevant patient subgroups, for example, response to treatment and prognosis in hematologic malignancies (Ebert and Golub 2004). Blood mRNA expression profiles can also identify a variety of non-hematologic disorders, such as heart failure (Van Buren et al. 2011), cancer (Marshall et al. 2010; Osman et al. 2006; Liong et al. 2012; Twine et al. 2003; Baine et al. 2011), inflammatory bowel disease (Burakoff et al. 2010, 2011), psychiatric disorders (Tsuang et al. 2005; Glatt et al. 2005, 2011; Kong et al. 2012), and autoimmune diseases (Maas et al. 2002; Aune et al. 2003). In these studies, blood cells are not necessarily involved in pathogenesis but rather signal disease changes.

The Sentinel Principle® approach has been applied in NPC. In 2012, Zaatar et al. reported the first study to develop a blood transcriptomic pharmacogenomics approach to guide treatment for NPC (Zaatar et al. 2012). The methodology of the study is summarized in Fig. 2. In this study, RNA isolated from peripheral whole blood samples was used to identify a blood-based gene expression signature that differentiated NPC from other medical conditions and from healthy controls, as well as to identify a biomarker signature that correlates with NPC patient response to treatment. A blood-based gene expression signature for early stage cancer could form the basis of a clinically useful blood test for the early diagnosis and screening of NPC. Treatment regimens can also be planned as the gene expression signature distinguishes NPC patients who are more likely to experience complete response to treatment from those who can expect partial response to treatment.

In the study, Affymetrix U133 Plus 2.0 GeneChip oligonucleotide arrays (Affymetrix, California, USA) were used to analyze 66 NPC samples and 33 healthy controls. Another 447 expression profiles of samples with other cancers and diseases were included to ensure that the gene signature obtained was specific to NPC alone. These included bladder cancer, breast cancer, prostate cancer, Crohn's disease, cardiovascular disease, and several other cancers and diseases. Using a multivariate logistic regression analysis, 121 candidates of gene combinations that were able to differentiate NPC samples from controls and other diseases were shortlisted. Only the most discriminative gene combinations were retained.

The final gene panel identified was able to distinguish NPC from non-NPC and consisted of three primary genes – low-density lipoprotein receptor adaptor protein 1 (LDLRAP1), PHD finger protein 20 (PHF20), and cisplatin resistant-associated

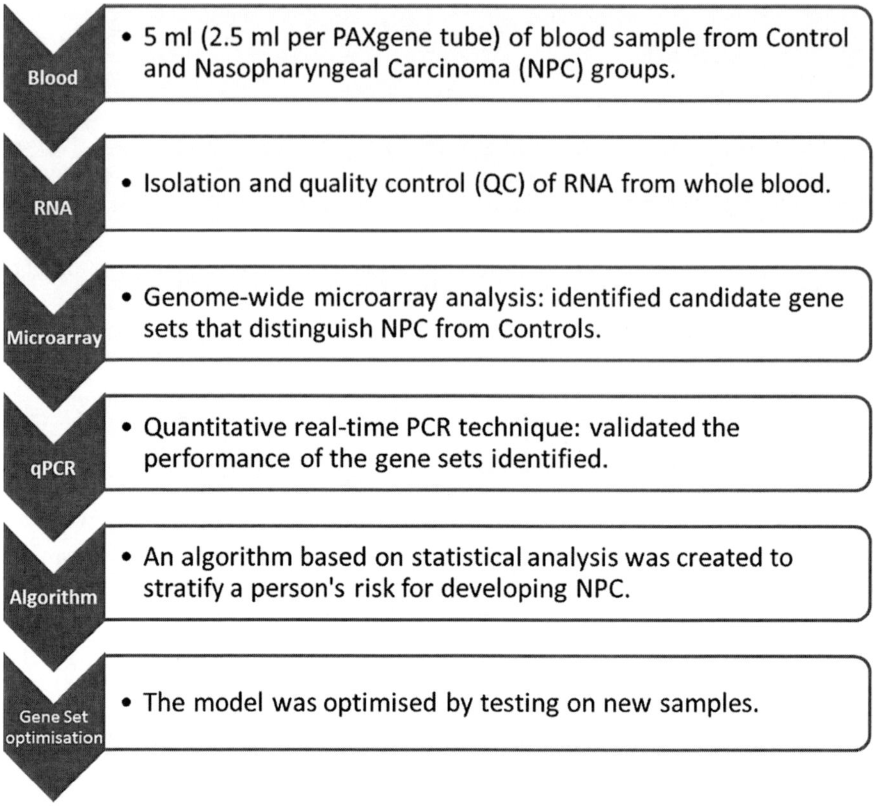

Fig. 2 The methodology of developing blood transcriptome nasopharyngeal carcinoma biomarkers based on the Sentinel Principle®. RNA was isolated from whole blood. Microarray gene profiling data was analyzed to identify candidate genes that distinguish NPC from controls. This was followed by qPCR validation of microarray data. When an algorithm was created, the model was optimized by testing on new independent RNA samples

overexpressed protein (LUC7L3, also known as CROP) – and their associated suppressor genes, enhancer of zeste homologue 1 (Drosophila) (EZH1), interferon-induced protein 35 (IFI35), and ubiquinol-cytochrome c reductase hinge protein (UQCRH). The cluster diagram in Fig. 3 is based on a combination of these three primary genes with three secondary suppressor genes and shows that, to a large extent, the NPC samples stand apart from the controls, which are dispersed throughout the group of samples with other diseases (Zaatar et al. 2012). This final gene panel was tested using a quantitative real-time PCR, and it has been confirmed that the panel maintained a high level of discrimination between NPC and controls with a 95 % confidence interval for an ROC AUC of 0.75–0.93.

Follow-up information 1–3 years posttreatment was obtained for 28 of the NPC cases and was used in the analysis to predict treatment response. CT scan was used

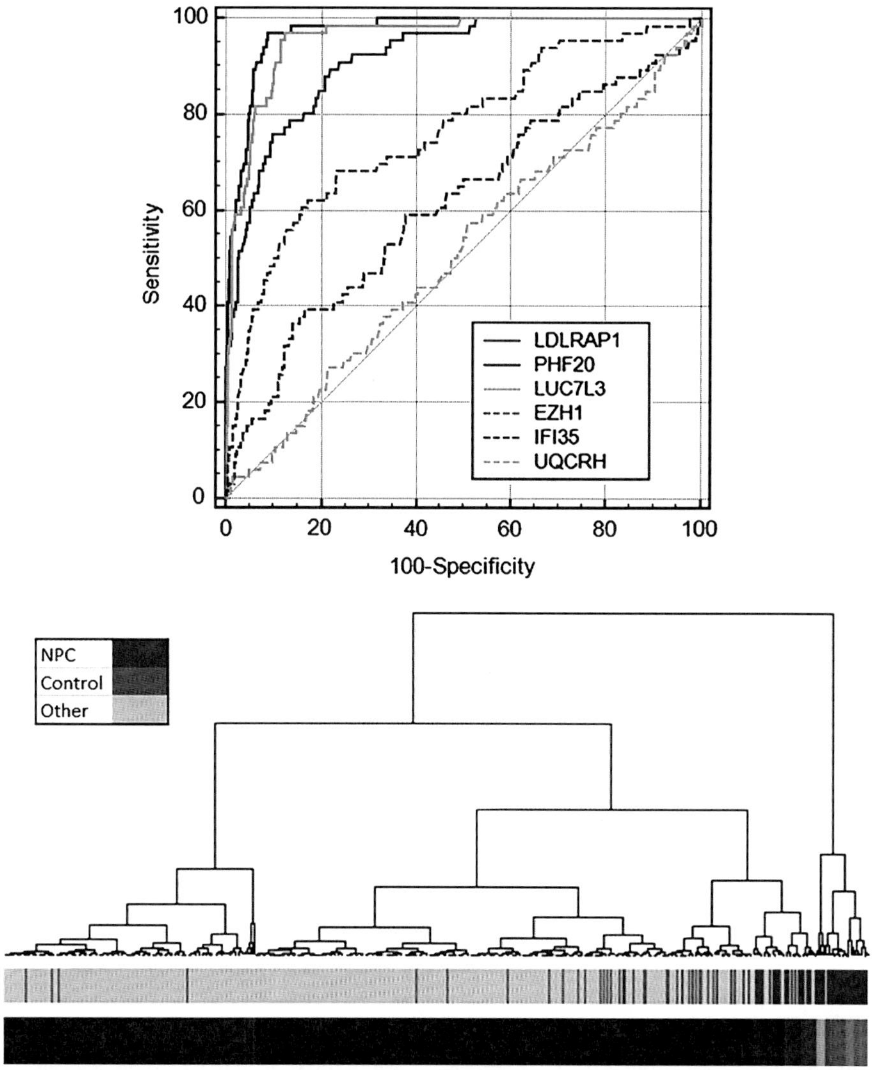

Pair	Prim.	AUC	SE	95% CI	Sec.	AUC	SE	95% CI
1	LDLRAP1	0.92	0.0130	0.89 to 0.94	EZH1	0.77	0.0354	0.73 to 0.80
2	PHF20	0.97	0.0065	0.95 to 0.98	IFI35	0.61	0.0388	0.57 to 0.65
3	LUC7L3	0.96	0.0083	0.94 to 0.97	UQCRH	0.51	0.0381	0.47 to 0.55

Fig. 3 ROCs of probes that contribute to differentiation of nasopharyngeal carcinoma from other conditions. Combination of six genes with three genes appearing most frequently in all top-performing combinations: LDLRAP1, PHF20, and LUC7L3. The additional three secondary genes, EZH1, IFI35, and UQCRH, have little NPC discrimination (ROC AUC, 0.51–0.77) but help suppress confounding factors. ROC AUC for each gene is listed in the table. Dendrogram of the six-gene combination showing control samples dispersed throughout the "other" sample group with a separate cluster consisting mainly of NPC samples on the right. The heat map and clustering are based on results of twofold cross validation iterated 1,000 times

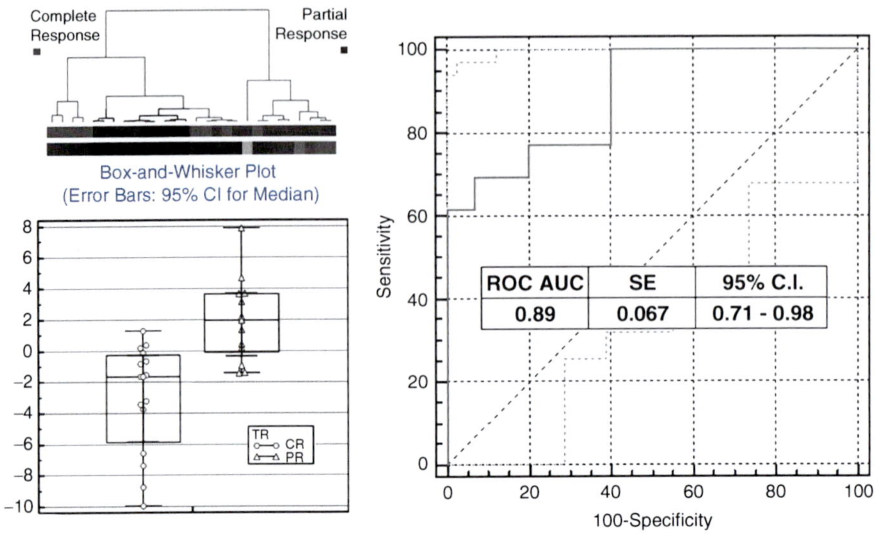

Fig. 4 Box-and-whisker median plot, hierarchical clustering results, and ROC of complete response (*CR*) and partial response (*PR*) samples. The box-and-whisker median (error bars, 95 % CI for medians) plot for distribution of complete response (*CR*) and partial response (*PR*) for pair FOXP1 and STX16, showing good differentiation between the groups. The dendrogram represents the hierarchical clustering results of pre-intervention NPC samples. The boxes directly below the dendrogram represent samples that show complete response (*CR*) to treatment and partial response (*PR*) to treatment, denoted in *light grey* and *black*, respectively. We found two major clusters in the samples; the cluster on the right consists of 8 of 13 (62 %) PR samples (*black*), and the cluster on the left consists of 14 of 15 (93 %) CR samples (*light grey*). The dot plot, heat map, and clustering are based on results of threefold cross validation iterated 1,000 times. The AUC for the single pair equation is 0.89, with a standard error of 0.067

to classify these samples into a complete response to treatment, in which no evidence of disease was present after treatment, and partial response to treatment, in which there was residual disease or metastasis. Gene pairs identified had ROC AUCs of up to 0.94. The most frequent genes in an analysis of the best-performing 6-gene combinations were forkhead box P1 (FOXP1), EGF-like module-containing mucin-like hormone receptor-like 2 (EMR2), syntaxin 16 (STX16), and *N*-acetylglucosamine-1-phosphate transferase (GNPTAB) (Fig. 4; Zaatar et al. 2012).

In these results, the performance of single gene pair, FOXP1-STX16, could be further enhanced with other gene combinations. As shown in Fig. 5, the segregation of complete response and partial response samples was better when three pairs of genes were used together (Fig. 5b) than when one pair of genes was used (Fig. 5a). When three 3-pair genes were used (Fig. 5c), only one complete response was found in the cluster of partial response samples. However, the improvement in segregating complete response and partial response samples was limited, although 18 genes were employed.

The relationship among the biomarkers was studied and plotted onto a network (Fig. 6). All the biomarkers but one (IFI35) were found to be related to cell

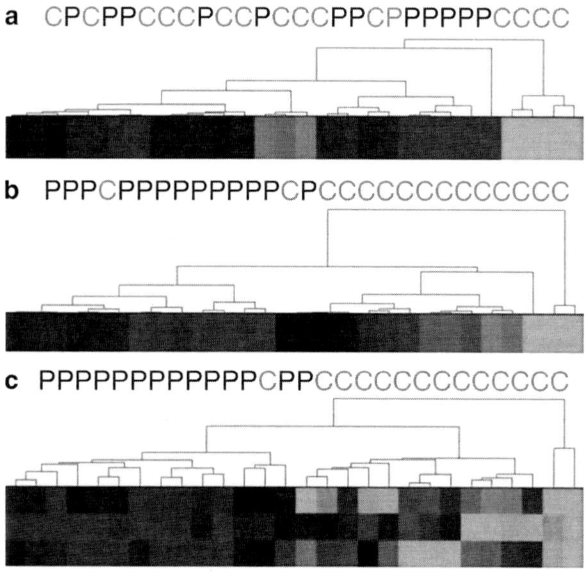

Fig. 5 Hierarchical clustering results using single gene-pair combination (*A*), one 3-pair gene combination (*B*), and three 3-pair gene combinations (*C*). Complete (*C*) and partial (*P*) response samples were shown on top of each clustering result. The distance was calculated using Euclidean, and the clustering method used was UPGMA average linkage

functions, mainly apoptosis and cell growth. Notably, LUC7L3 and LDLRAP1 interact with BCL2, which plays an important role in promoting apoptosis and inhibiting cell growth (Thalasila et al. 2003; Feinman et al. 1999; Vaux et al. 1988). Conversely, PHF20 is a negative regulator of apoptosis and interacts with tumor necrosis factor (TNF) to promote cell growth (Vincenz and Dixit 1996). It is possible that the apoptosis pathway governed by these three primary genes, LDLRAP1, PHF20, and LUC7L3, could be dysregulated in NPC patients, resulting in expression patterns that are different from those of control and non-NPC disease samples. The other secondary genes EZH1, IFI35, and UQCRH are housekeeping genes. It is interesting that UQCRH, which is responsible for releasing cytochrome c from mitochondria, enhances the apoptosis pathway, whereas EZH1 is a general transcription factor promoting apoptosis (Okazaki et al. 1998; Ezhkova et al. 2011). IFI35, also known as IFP35, is an interferon-inducible protein that is involved in protein degradation mediated by proteasome (Chen et al. 2000).

The candidate genes in this study were also located in the B-cell receptor (BCR) and epidermal growth factor receptor 1 (EGFR1) pathways. The BCR pathway responds to specific antigens and is important for antibody production and immune responses (Kurosaki et al. 2010). Changes in the expression of genes in this pathway may cause alterations in signal transmission within the cell, which can result in changes in B-cell production, cell growth, and cell division. EBV replicates in B-cells and epithelial cells and reportedly contributes to NPC tumorigenesis. The finding of gene expression pathways in the BCR pathway of NPC could improve our understanding of NPC treatment response as well as EBV replication and NPC tumor formation.

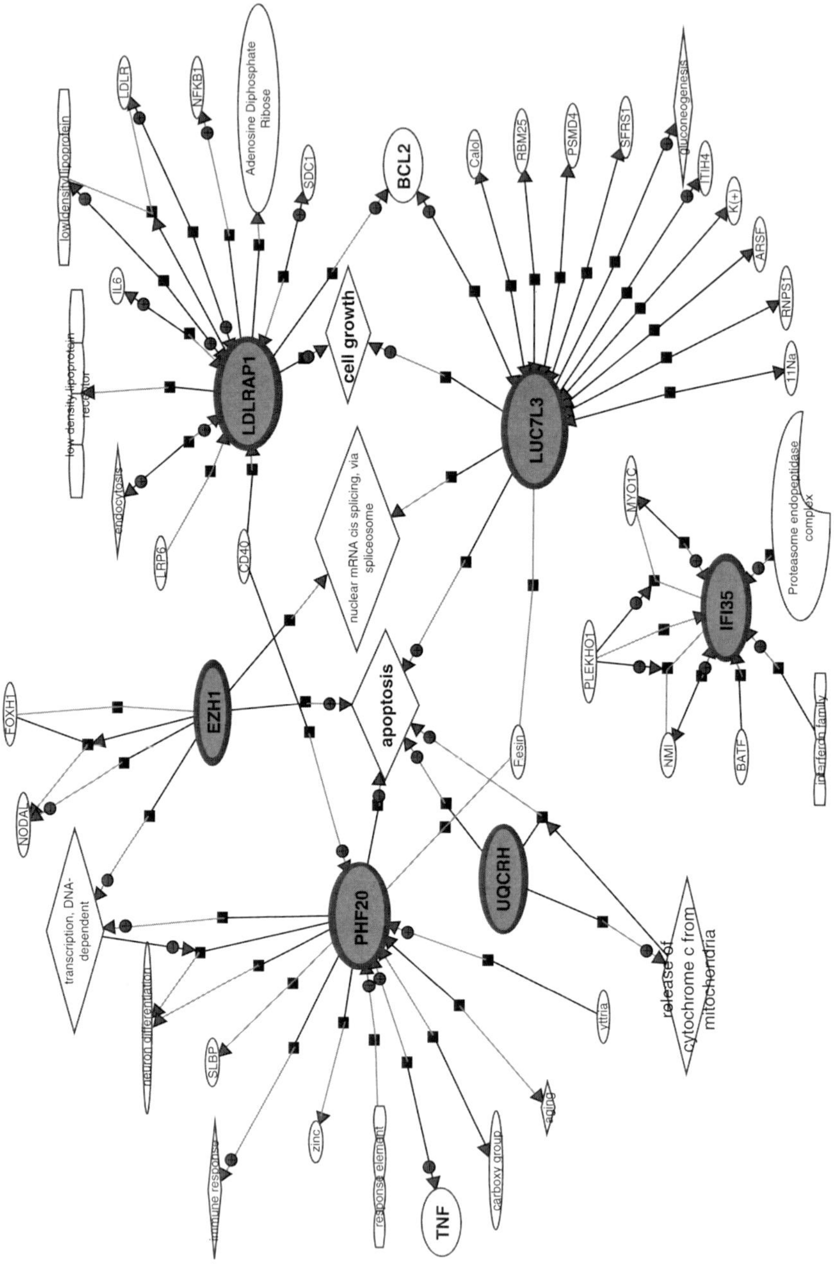

Fig. 6 (continued)

The blood-based gene signature identified in this study may be used to indicate the presence of cancer at presymptomatic, earlier stages, when NPC can be treated with less toxicity and long-term patient survival can be improved. The study also reported genes that are able to distinguish NPC patients more likely to attain complete response to radiation and chemotherapy regiments from patients who can only expect partial response to treatment. Treatment regimens can thus be tailored accordingly. Information on response to treatment may also encourage patient compliance in the presence of treatment side effects.

Potential Applications to Prognosis, Other Diseases, or Conditions

NPC is most often diagnosed only when the disease has reached late stages and the prognosis is poor. However, when detected early, NPC is highly sensitive to radiation and chemotherapy, and stages I and II of NPC can be treated with high survival rates. Thus, the goal of many NPC molecular biomarker studies is to identify early, presymptomatic disease. Biomarkers have also been reported to predict response to treatment, to indicate prognosis, to identify tumor stage, and to monitor disease progression. Biomarker studies may also help to shed light on the pathogenesis of NPC. The findings of NPC biomarker studies may also find application in other head and neck cancers.

The development of optimal NPC biomarkers for clinical use is an important goal. NPC is a complex disease, and the integration of many different platforms and types of studies (such as transcriptomics, proteomics, and bioinformatics) would help us better understand the disease, find and validate optimal biomarkers for NPC, and also develop targeted therapies. A blood-based biomarker test for NPC would be extremely useful as a simple, noninvasive, cost-effective test that would improve screening compliance, reduce NPC, and save lives.

Summary Points

- Molecular biomarkers for the early detection of NPC are important because the disease is not easily diagnosed, although it is readily treated, with high survival rates, if found early.
- This chapter reviews biomarkers for NPC including DNA biomarkers, methylation biomarkers, microRNA biomarkers, protein biomarkers, mRNA biomarkers, and blood transcriptomic biomarkers.

Fig. 6 A gene network illustrating three primary genes, LDLRAP1, PHF20, and LUC7L3, three secondary genes, and other major genes, such as BCL2 and TNF, which interact with the biomarkers. The major cellular aspect of the network is related to apoptosis and cell growth (shown in *diamond rectangles*)

- Molecular biomarkers can be used in the diagnosis of NPC, prognosis of NPC, and management of NPC using chemotherapy or other therapies.
- Biomarkers reported for NPC include quantitative EBV DNA (DNA), CYP2A6 (DNA), Cpg site methylation (methylation), mir-29c (miRNA), annexin A1 (protein), EBV antibodies (protein), BCL2 (mRNA), MMP9 (mRNA), and a six-gene panel consisting of LDLRAP1, PHF20, LUC7L3, EZH1, IFI35, and UQCRH (mRNA).
- Zaatar et al. was the first to report a whole blood transcriptomic study for the discrimination of NPC from controls and other diseases, as well as for the prediction of treatment response in NPC (Zaatar et al. 2012).
- The six genes reported by Zaatar et al. are involved in cellular function, mainly in apoptosis and cell growth; the genes are also involved in BCR and EGFR1 pathways, giving us a better understanding of NPC tumor formation and treatment response (Zaatar et al. 2012).
- A noninvasive blood-based test for NPC would have clinical potential for early diagnosis and screening of NPC, encourage patients to follow treatment schedules, and help doctors plan patient treatments.

References

Agathanggelou A, Honorio S, Macartney DP, Martinex A, Dallol A, Rader J, Fullwood P, Chauhan A, Walker R, Shaw JA, Hosoe S, Lerman MI, Minna JD, Maher ER, Latif F. Methylation associated inactivation of RASSF1A from region 3p21.3 in lung, breast, and ovarian tumours. Oncogene. 2001;20:1509–18.

Al-Sarraf M, LeBlanc M, Giri PG, Fu KK, Cooper J, Vuong T, Forastiere AA, Adams G, Sakr WA, Schuller DE, Ensley JF. Chemoradiotherapy in patients with advanced nasopharyngeal cancer: phase III randomized intergroup study 0099. J Clin Oncol. 1998;16:1310–7.

Ambinder RF, Robertson KD, Tao Q. DNA methylation and the Epstein-Barr virus. Semin Cancer Biol. 1999;9:369–75.

Ambros V. The functions of animal microRNAs. Nature. 2004;431:350–5.

Aune TM, Maas K, Moore JH, Olsen NJ. Gene expression profiles in human autoimmune disease. Curr Pharm Des. 2003;9:1905–17.

Baine MJ, Chakraborty S, Smith LM, Mallya K, Sasson AR, Brand RE, Batra SK, et al. Transcriptional profiling of peripheral blood mononuclear cells in pancreatic cancer patients identifies novel genes with potential diagnostic utility. PLoS One. 2011;6:e17014.

Bei JX, Li Y, Jia WH, Feng BJ, Zhou G, Chen LZ, Feng QS, Low HQ, Zhang H, He F, Tai ES, Kang T, Liu ET, Liu J, Zeng YX. A genome-wide association study of nasopharyngeal carcinoma identifies three new susceptibility loci. Nat Genet. 2010;42:599–603.

Bendaraf R, Buhmeida A, Hilska M, Laato M, Syrjanen S, Syrjanen K, Collan Y, Pyrohonen S. MMP-9 (gelatinase B) expression is associated with disease-free survival and disease-specific survival in colorectal cancer patients. Cancer Invest. 2010;28:38–43.

Burakoff R, Hande S, Ma J, Banks PA, Friedman S, Makrauer F, Liew CC. Differential regulation of peripheral leukocyte genes in patients with active Crohn's disease and Crohn's disease in remission. J Clin Gastroenterol. 2010;44:120–6.

Burakoff R, Chao S, Perencevich M, Ying J, Friedman S, Makrauer F, Odze R, Khurana H, Liew CC. Blood-based biomarkers can differentiate ulcerative colitis from Crohn's disease and noninflammatory diarrhea. Inflamm Bowel Dis. 2011;17:1719–25.

Caldas C, Hahn SA, da Costa LT, Redston MS, Schutte M, Seymour AB, Weinstein CL, Hruban RH, Yeo CJ, Kern SE. Frequent somatic mutations and homozygous deletions of the p16 (MTS1) gene in pancreatic adenocarcinoma. Nat Genet. 1994;9:27–32.

Calin GA, Croce CM. MicroRNA signatures in human cancers. Nat Rev Cancer. 2006;6:857–66.

Caponigro F, Longo F, Ionna F, Perri F. Treatment approaches to nasopharyngeal carcinoma: a review. Anticancer Drugs. 2010;21:471–7.

Chan KCA, Hung ECW, Woo JKS, Chan PKS, Leung SF, Lai FPT, Cheng ASM, Yeung SW, Chan YW, Tsui TKC, Kwok JSS, King AD, Chan ATC, van Hasselt AC, Lo YMD. Early detection of nasopharyngeal carcinoma by plasma Epstein-Barr virus DNA analysis in a surveillance program. Cancer. 2013;119:1834–44.

Chang ET, Adami HO. The enigmatic epidemiology of nasopharyngeal carcinoma. Cancer Epidemiol Biomarkers Prev. 2006;15:1765–77.

Chen J, Shpall RL, Meyerdierks A, Hagemeier M, Böttger EC, Naumovski L. Interferon-inducible Myc/STAT-interacting protein Nmi associates with IFP 35 into a high molecular mass complex and inhibits proteasome-mediated degradation of IFP 35. J Biol Chem. 2000;275:36278–84.

Chen HC, Chen GH, Chen YH, Liao WL, Liu CY, Chang KP, Chang YS, Chen SJ. microRNA deregulation and pathway alterations in nasopharyngeal carcinoma. Br J Cancer. 2009;100:1002–11.

Cho WC, Yip TT, Yip C, Yip V, Thulasiraman V, Ngan RK, Yip TT, Lau WH, Au JS, Law SC, Cheng WW, Ma VW, Lim CK. Identification of serum amyloid a protein as a potentially useful biomarker to monitor relapse of nasopharyngeal cancer by serum proteomic profiling. Clin Cancer Res. 2004;10:43–52.

Dammann R, Yang G, Pfeifer G. Hypermethylation of the CpG island of Ras association domain family 1A (RASSF1A), a putative tumor suppressor gene from the 3p21.3 locus, occurs in a large percentage of human breast cancers. Cancer Res. 2001;61:3105–9.

Doustjalali SR, Yusof R, Govindasamy GK, Bustam AZ, Pillay B, Hashim OH. Patients with nasopharyngeal carcinoma demonstrate enhanced serum and tissue ceruloplasmin expression. J Med Invest. 2006;53:20–8.

Ebert BL, Golub TR. Genomic approaches to hematologic malignancies. Blood. 2004;104:923–32.

Ezhkova E, Lien WH, Stokes N, Pasolli HA, Silva JM, Fuchs E. EZH1 and EZH2 cogovern histone H3K27 trimethylation and are essential for hair follicle homeostasis and wound repair. Genes Dev. 2011;25:485–98.

Feinman R, Koury J, Thames M, Barlogie B, Epstein J, Siegel DS. Role of NF-kappaB in the rescue of multiple myeloma cells from glucocorticoid-induced apoptosis by bcl-2. Blood. 1999;93:3044–52.

Fendri A, Kontos CK, Khabir A, Mokdad-Gargouri R, Ardavanis A, Scorilas A. Quantitative analysis of BLC2 mRNA expression in nasopharyngeal carcinoma: an unfavorable and independent prognostic factor. Tumor Biol. 2010;31:391–9.

Fendri A, Kontos CK, Khabir A, Mokdad-Gargouri R, Scorilas A. BCL2L12 is a novel biomarker for the prediction of short-term relapse in nasopharyngeal carcinoma. Mol Med. 2011;17:163–71.

Ferlay J, Parkin DM, Curado MP, Bray F, Edwards B, Shin HR, Forman D. Cancer incidence in five continents, volumes I to IX: IARC cancer base no 9, Lyon: International Agency for Research on Cancer; 2010. http://ci5.iarc.fr. Accessed 27 May 2013.

Glatt SJ, Everall IP, Kremen WS, Corbeil J, Sásik R, Khanlou N, Han M, Liew CC, Tsuang MT. Comparative gene expression analysis of blood and brain provides concurrent validation of SELENBP1 up-regulation in schizophrenia. Proc Natl Acad Sci U S A. 2005;102:15533–8.

Glatt SJ, Stone WS, Nossova N, Liew CC, Seidman LJ, Tsuang MT. Similarities and differences in peripheral blood gene-expression signatures of individuals with schizophrenia and their first-degree biological relatives. Am J Med Genet B Neuropsychiatr Genet. 2011;156B:869–87.

Gu AD, Lu LX, Xie YB, Chen LZ, Feng QS, Kang T, Jia WH, Zeng YX. Clinical values of multiple Epstein-Barr virus (EBV) serological biomarkers detected by xMAP technology. J Transl Med. 2009;7:73.

Hildesheim A, Chen CJ, Caporaso NE, Cheng YJ, Hoover RN, Hsu MM, Levine PH, Chen IH, Chen JY, Yang CS. Cytochrome P4502E1 genetic polymorphisms and risk of nasopharyngeal carcinoma: results from a case–control study conducted in Taiwan. Cancer Epidemiol Biomarkers Prev. 1995;4:607–10.

Hildesheim A, Anderson LM, Chen CJ, Cheng YK, Brinton LA, Daly AK, Reed CD, Chen IH, Caporaso NE, Hsu MM, Chen JY, Idle JR, Hoover RN, Yang CS, Chhabra SK. CYP2E1 genetic polymorphisms and risk of nasopharyngeal carcinoma in Taiwan. J Natl Cancer Inst. 1997;89:1207–12.

Hildesheim A, Apple RJ, Chen C, Wang SS, Cheng YK, Klitz W, Mack SJ, Chen IH, Hsu MM, Yang CS, Brinton LA, Levine PH, Erlich HA. Association of HLA class I and II alleles and extended haplotypes with nasopharyngeal carcinoma in Taiwan. J Natl Cancer Inst. 2002;94:1780–9.

Iorio MV, Ferracin M, Liu CG, Veronesse A, Spizzo R, Sabbioni S, Magri E, Pedriali M, Fabbri M, Campiglio M, Menard S, Palazzo JP, Rosenberg A, Musiani P, Volinia S, Nenci I, Calin GA, Querzoli P, Negrini M, Croce CM. microRNA gene expression deregulation in human breast cancer. Cancer Res. 2005;65:7065–70.

Kamb A, Shattuck-Eidens D, Eeles R, Liu Q, Gruis NA, Ding W, Hussey C, Tran T, Miki Y, Feldhaus W, McClure M, Aitken JF, Anderson DE, Bergman W, Frants R, Goldgar DE, Green A, MacLennan R, Martin NG, Meyer LJ, Youl P, Zone JJ, Skolnick MH, Cannon-Albright LA. Analysis of the p16 gene (CDKN2) as a candidate for the chromosome 9p melanoma susceptibility locus. Nat Genet. 1994;8:22–6.

Katsumata M, Siegel RM, Louie DC, Miyashita T, Tsujimoto Y, Nowell PC, Greene MI, Reed JC. Differential effects of bcl-2 on t and b cells in transgenic mice. Proc Natl Acad Sci U S A. 1992;89:11376–80.

Kong QL, Hu LJ, Cao JY, Huang YJ, Xu LH, Liang Y, Xiong D, Guan S, Guo BH, Mai HQ, Chen QY, Zhang X, Li MZ, Shao JY, Qian CN, Xia YF, Song LB, Zeng YX, Zeng MS. Epstein-Barr virus-encoded LMP2A induces an epithelial-mesenchymal transition and increases the number of side population stem-like cancer cells in nasopharyngeal carcinoma. PLoS Pathog. 2010;6: e1000940.

Kong SW, Collins CD, Shimizu-Motohashi Y, Holm I, Campbell MG, Lee IH, Brewster SJ, Hanson E, Harris HK, Lowe KR, Saada A, Mora A, Madison K, Hundley R, Egan J, McCarthy J, Eran A, Galdzicki M, Rappaport L, Kunkel LM, Kohane IS. Characteristics and predictive value of blood transcriptome signature in males with autism spectrum disorders. PLoS One. 2012;7:e49475.

Kurosaki T, Shinohara H, Baba Y. B cell signaling and fate decision. Annu Rev Immunol. 2010;28:21–55.

Kwong J, Lo KW, To KF, Teo PML, Johnson PJ, Huang DP. Promoter hypermethylation of multiple genes in nasopharyngeal carcinoma. Clin Cancer Res. 2002;8:131–7.

Laird PW. The power and the promise of DNA methylation markers. Nat Rev Cancer. 2003;4:253–66.

Lampe JW, Stepaniants SB, Mao M, Radich JP, Dai H, Linsley PS, Friend SH, Potter JD. Signatures of environmental exposures using peripheral leukocyte gene expression: tobacco smoke. Cancer Epidemiol Biomarkers Prev. 2004;13:445–53.

Le QT, Jones CD, Yau TK, Shirazi HA, Wong PH, Thomas EN, Patterson BK, Lee AWM, Zehnder JL. A comparison study of different PCR assays in measuring circulating plasma Epstein-Barr virus DNA levels in patients with nasopharyngeal carcinoma. Clin Cancer Res. 2005;11:5700–7.

Le QT, Zhang Q, Cao H, Cheng AJ, Pinsky BA, Hong RL, Chang JT, Wang CW, Tsao KC, Lo YMD, Lee N, Ang KK, Chan ATC, Chan KCA. An international collaboration to harmonize the quantitative plasma Epstein-Barr virus DNA assay for future biomarker-guided trials in nasopharyngeal carcinoma. Clin Cancer Res. 2013;19:2208–15.

Li F, Guan Y, Chen Z. Proteomics in nasopharyngeal carcinoma. Cell Mol Life Sci. 2008;65:1007–12.

Liew CC. Method for the detection of gene transcripts in blood and uses thereof. U.S. patent application no 2002000268730; 1999.

Liong ML, Lim CR, Yang H, Chao S, Bong CW, Leong WS, Das PK, Loh CS, Lau BE, Yu CG, Ooi EJJ, Nam RK, Allen PD, Steele GS, Wassman K, Richie JP, Liew CC. Blood-based biomarkers of aggressive prostate cancer. PLoS One. 2012;7:e45802.

Liu Z, Li L, Yang Z, Luo W, Yang H, Yao K, Wu B, Fang W. Increased expression of MMP9 is correlated with poor prognosis of nasopharyngeal carcinoma. BMC Cancer. 2010;10:270.

Liu N, Chen NY, Cui RX, Li WF, Li Y, Wei RR, Zhang MY, Sun Y, Huang BJ, Chen M, He QN, Jiang N, Chen L, Cho WCS, Yun JP, Zeng J, Liu LZ, Li L, Guo Y, Wang HY, Ma J, et al. Prognostic value of a microRNA signature in nasopharyngeal carcinoma: a microRNA expression analysis. Lancet Oncol. 2012;13:633–41.

Lo YMD, Chan LYS, Lo KW, Leung SF, Zhang J, Chan ATC, Lee JCK, Hjelm M, Johnson PJ, Huang DP. Quantitative analysis of cell-free Epstein-Barr virus DNA in plasma of patients with nasopharyngeal carcinoma. Canc Res. 1999;59:1188–91.

Lu TY, Kao CF, Lin CT, Huang DY, Chiu CY, Huang YS, Wu HC. DNA methylation and histone modification regulate silencing of OPG during tumor progression. J Cell Biochem. 2009;108:315–25.

Maas K, Chan S, Parker J, Slater A, Moore J, Olsen N, Aune TM. Cutting edge: molecular portrait of human autoimmune disease. J Immunol. 2002;169:5–9.

Maeda E, Akahane M, Kiryu S, Kato N, Yoshikawa T, Hayashi N, Aoki S, Minami M, Uozaki H, Fukayama M, Ohtomo K. Spectrum of Epstein-Barr virus-related diseases: a pictorial review. Jpn J Radiol. 2009;27:4–19.

Marshall KW, Mohr S, Khettabi FE, Nossova N, Chao S, Bao W, Ma J, Li XJ, Liew CC. A blood-based biomarker panel for stratifying current risk for colorectal cancer. Int J Cancer. 2010;126:1177–86.

Murakami Y, Yasuda T, Saigo K, Urashima T, Toyoda H, Okanoue T, Shimotohno K. Comprehensive analysis of microRNA expression patterns in hepatocellular carcinoma and non-tumorous tissues. Oncogene. 2006;25:2537–45.

National Cancer Registry, Ministry of Health Malaysia. Malaysia cancer statistics: data and figures peninsular Malaysia. Kuala Lumpur: National Cancer Registry, Ministry of Health Malaysia; 2006. http://www.makna.org.my/PDF/MalaysiaCancerStatistics.pdf. Accessed 1 Aug 2013. ISBN 978-983-3433-51-3.

Ng CC, Yew PY, Puah SM, Krishnan G, Yap LF, Teo SH, Lim PVH, Govindraju S, Ratnevelu K, Sam CK, Takahashi A, Kubo M, Kamatani N, Nakamura Y, Mushiroda T. A genome-wide association study identifies ITGA9 conferring risk of nasopharyngeal carcinoma. J Hum Genet. 2009;54:392–7.

Okazaki M, Ishibashi Y, Asoh S, Ohta S. Overexpressed mitochondrial hinge protein, a cytochrome c-binding protein, accelerates apoptosis by enhancing the release of cytochrome c from mitochondria. Biochem Biophys Res Commun. 1998;243:131–6.

Osman I, Bajorin DF, Sun TT, Zhong H, Douglas D, Scattergood J, Zheng R, Han M, Marshall KW, Liew CC. Novel blood biomarkers of human urinary bladder cancer. Clin Cancer Res. 2006;12:3374–80.

Provatopoulou X, Gounaris A, Kalogera E, Zagouri F, Flessas I, Goussestis E, Nonni A, Papassotoriou I, Zografos G. Circulating levels of matrix metalloproteinase-9 (MMP-9), neutrophil gelatinase-associated lipocalin (NGAL) and their complex MMP-9/NGAL in breast cancer disease. BMC Cancer. 2009;9:390.

Quest Diagnostics. About ColoVantage®. 2013. Available from: http://www.questdiagnostics.com/home/physicians/testing-services/by-test-name/colovantage/about. Accessed 1 Aug 2013.

Reed JC. Apoptosis-targeted therapies for cancer. Cancer Cell. 2003;3:17–22.

Robertson K. DNA methylation and human disease. Nat Rev Genet. 2005;6:597–610.

Rosetta Genomics: Testing Services. Philadelphia; 2013. Available from: http://www.rosettagenomics.com/testing-services. Accessed 1 Aug 2013.

Sengupta S, den Boon JA, Chen IH, Newton MA, Stanhope SA, Cheng YJ, Chen CJ, Hildesheim A, Sugden B, Ahlquist P. microRNA 29c is down-regulated in nasopharyngeal carcinomas, up-regulating mRNAs encoding extracellular matrix proteins. Proc Natl Acad Sci U S A. 2008;105:5874–8.

Stevens SJ, Verjukilen SA, Hariwiyanto B, Harijadi, Paramita DK, Fachiroh J, Adham M, Tan IB, Haryana SM, Middeldorp JM. Noninvasive diagnosis of nasopharyngeal carcinoma: nasopharyngeal brushings reveal high Epstein-Barr virus DNA load and carcinoma-specific viral BARF1 mRNA. Int J Cancer. 2006;119:608–14.

Thalasila A, Poplin E, Shih J, Dvorzhinski D, Capanna T, Doyle-Lindrud S, Beers S, Goodin S, Rubin E, DiPaola RS. A phase I trial of weekly paclitaxel, 13-cis-retinoic acid, and interferon alpha in patients with prostate cancer and other advanced malignancies. Cancer Chemother Pharmacol. 2003;52:119–24.

Thomodaki H, Scorilas A. Bcl2 family of apoptosis-related genes: functions and clinical implications in cancer. Crit Rev Clin Lab Sci. 2006;43:1–67.

Tiwawech D, Srivatanakul P, Karalak A, Ishida T. Cytochrome P450 2A6 polymorphism in nasopharyngeal carcinoma. Cancer Lett. 2006;241:135–41.

Tsang RK, Vlantis AC, Ho RW, Tam JS, To KF, van Hasselt CA. Sensitivity and specificity of Epstein-Barr virus IGA titer in the diagnosis of nasopharyngeal carcinoma: a three-year institutional review. Head Neck. 2004;26:598–602.

Tse KP, Su WH, Chang KP, Tsang NM, Yu CJ, Tang P, See LC, Hsueh C, Yang ML, Hao SP, Li HY, Wang MH, Liao LP, Chen LC, Lin SR, Jorgensen TJ, Chang YS, Shugart YY. Genome-wide association study reveals multiple nasopharyngeal carcinoma-associated loci within the HLA region at chromosome 6p21.3. Am J Hum Genet. 2009;85:194–203.

Tsuang MT, Nossova N, Yager T, Tsuang MM, Guo SC, Shyu KG, Glatt SJ, Liew CC. Assessing the validity of blood-based gene expression profiles for the classification of schizophrenia and bipolar disorder: a preliminary report. Am J Med Genet B Neuropsychiatr Genet. 2005;133B:1–5.

Twine NC, Stover JA, Marshall B, Dukart G, Hidalgo M, Stadler W, Logan T, Dutcher J, Hudes G, Dorner AJ, Slonim DK, Trepicchio WL, Burczynski ME. Disease-associated expression profiles in peripheral blood mononuclear cells from patients with advanced renal cell carcinoma. Cancer Res. 2003;63:6069–75.

Van Buren P, Ma J, Chao S, Mueller E, Schneider DJ, Liew CC. Blood gene expression signatures associate with heart failure outcomes. Physiol Genomics. 2011;43:392–7.

Vaux DL, Cory S, Adams JM. Bcl-2 gene promotes haemopoietic cell survival and cooperates with c-myc to immortalize pre-B cells. Nature. 1988;335:440–2.

Vincenz C, Dixit VM. 14-3-3 proteins associate with A20 in an isoform-specific manner and function both as chaperone and adapter molecules. J Biol Chem. 1996;271:20029–34.

Wee J, Tan EH, Tai BC, Wong HB, Leong SS, Tan T, Chua ET, Yang E, Lee KM, Fong KW, Tan HS, Lee KS, Loong S, Sethi V, Chua EJ, Machin D. Randomized trial of radiotherapy versus concurrent chemoradiotherapy followed by adjuvant radiotherapy in patients with American Joint Committee on Cancer/International Union against Cancer Stage III and IV nasopharyngeal cancer of the endemic variety. J Clin Oncol. 2005;23:6730–8.

Wei WI, Sham JST. Nasopharyngeal carcinoma. Lancet. 2005;365:2041–54.

Wei YS, Zheng YH, Liang WB, Zhang JZ, Yang ZH, Lv ML, Jia J, Zhang L. Identification of serum biomarkers for nasopharyngeal carcinoma by proteomic analysis. Cancer. 2008;112:544–51.

White HE, Durston VJ, Harvery JF, Cross NCP. Quantitative analysis of SRNPN gene methylation by pyrosequencing as a diagnostic test for Prader-Willi syndrome and Angelman syndrome. Clin Chem. 2006;52:1005–13.

Wu CC, Chien KY, Tsang NM, Chang KP, Hao SP, Tsao CH, Chang YS, Yu JS. Cancer cell secreted proteomes as a basis for searching potential tumor markers: nasopharyngeal carcinoma as a model. Proteomics. 2005;5:3173–82.

Zaatar AM, Lim CR, Bong CW, Lee MML, Ooi JJ, Suria D, Raman R, Chao S, Yang H, Neoh SB, Liew CC. Whole blood transcriptome correlates with treatment response in nasopharyngeal carcinoma. J Exp Clin Cancer Res. 2012;31:76.

Zhao ZS, Wang YY, Ye ZY, Tao HQ. Prognostic value of tumor-related molecular expression in gastric carcinoma. Pathol Oncol Res. 2008;15:589–96.

Biomarkers in Nasopharyngeal Carcinoma and Ionizing Radiation

39

Thian-Sze Wong, Wei Gao, and Jimmy Yu-Wai Chan

Contents

T.-S. Wong (✉) • W. Gao
Department of Surgery, Queen Mary Hospital, The University of Hong Kong, Pokfulam, Hong Kong
e-mail: thiansze@gmail.com; thiansze@graduate.hku.hk

J.Y.-W. Chan
Department of Surgery, Queen Mary Hospital, The University of Hong Kong, Hong Kong, Hong Kong
e-mail: chanjyw@gmail.com

V.R. Preedy, V.B. Patel (eds.), *Biomarkers in Cancer, Biomarkers in Disease: Methods, Discoveries and Applications*,
DOI 10.1007/978-94-007-7681-4_39

Abstract

Cancer of the nasopharynx is an epithelial cancer developed in the retro-nasal area in the nasal cavity. Nasopharyngeal carcinoma (NPC) is prevalent in the endemic regions including Southern China and Southeast Asia. The primary tumor of NPC is small and usually causes no symptoms. Patients often present with bilateral glands enlargement and local/regional lymph node metastasis leading to poor prognosis and local control rate. Therefore, there is a desperate need to develop early diagnosis method to improve the treatment outcome. Detection of EBV-derived biomarkers in tissues and EBV DNA in the peripheral blood of NPC patients opens up the possibility to monitor the disease using molecular markers with high sensitivity. Among the biomarkers in tissue, in situ hybridization for EBER remains to be the most efficient and reliable way because EBER is the most abundantly expressed viral transcript. In addition to diagnosis value, EBER, EBNA1, and LMP1 levels in tissue after radiation therapy could serve as biomarkers to evaluate response to radiotherapy. In light of the detection of EBV DNA in plasma, serum, nasal brush, and saliva, EBV DNA is particularly useful for periodic monitoring of NPC patients. A systematic review has revealed that circulating EBV DNA could be applied as noninvasive diagnostic biomarker for NPC. Moreover, the close association of circulating EBV DNA with the clinical outcomes of treatment provided new tool to predict the treatment outcome. Nevertheless, circulating EBV DNA was not detectable in all the undifferentiated NPC patients, and EBV latent infection was not associated with WHO-1 NPC, which limits the utility of EBV DNA. Further studies are warranted to identify complementary biomarkers originating from the human cancer cells to overcome the limitation of EBV-based biomarkers in NPC screening and monitoring treatment outcome.

List of Abbreviations

CT	Computerized Tomography
EA	Early Antigen
EBER	Epstein–Barr-Encoded RNA
EBNA	Epstein–Barr Nuclear Antigen
EBV	Epstein–Barr Virus
IARC	International Agency for Research on Cancer
IM	Infectious Mononucleosis
LMP	Latent Membrane Protein
MHC	Major Histocompatibility Complex
MRI	Magnetic Resonance Imaging
NPC	Nasopharyngeal Carcinoma
VCA	Viral Capsid Antigen
WHO	World Health Organization

Key Facts

Key Facts of NPC

High incidence occurs in Southeastern Asia including Southeastern China, Thailand, Malaysia, and Indonesia.
It is predominant in male patients.
Most symptoms of NPC are vague and nonspecific at the early stages.
By the time of diagnosis, the patients are usually at the advanced stages.
Radiotherapy is recommended for the mainstay treatment regime as the cancer cells demonstrated high sensitivity to radiation.
Cisplatin-based concurrent chemoradiotherapy is recommended for advanced disease.
NPC in the endemic areas is characterized by its consistent association with the EBV.

Key Facts of EBV

It is a double-stranded DNA virus and was first identified in Burkitt's lymphoma cells in 1964.
It belongs to the herpes family and is one of the most common viruses in human.
EBV is capable of selecting two different lifestyles including latent replication and lytic replication.
Since it exerts causal roles in human malignancies, it is classified as group I carcinogen.
The closed association between EBV and NPC was observed, and EBV could serve as a biomarker for diagnosis and monitoring of NPC.
In addition to NPC, EBV was associated with a wide variety of human malignancies such as Hodgkin's disease, non-Hodgkin's lymphoma, and gastric adenocarcinoma.

Definition of Words and Terms

NPC NPC is an epithelial cancer occurring in the retro-nasal area in the nasal cavity, which is predominant in male patients and prevalent in Southeastern Asia.

EBV EBV is a double-stranded DNA virus and belongs to the herpes family, which exerts causal roles in human malignancies such as NPC, Hodgkin's disease, non-Hodgkin's lymphoma, and gastric adenocarcinoma.

Lifestyles of EBV EBV is capable of selecting two different lifestyles including latent replication or lytic replication, and induction of lytic form of EBV infection results in destruction of malignancies with latently infected EBV.

Latent phase of EBV The EBV genomic DNA presents as a closed circular plasmid and is replicated only once during S phase. Viral DNA maintenance requires oriP cis element, EBNA1 protein, and chromosomal initiation factors.

Lytic phase of EBV Lytic phase is a viral productive cycle in which multiple rounds of replication occur. Two key EBV immediate early lytic genes, BZLF1 and BRLF1, activate lytic replication.

Epstein–Barr-encoded RNA They are noncoding RNA transcripts which exhibited the highest abundance among viral transcripts; thus, they represent the most efficient and reliable method to detect EBV in biopsy samples.

Epstein–Barr nuclear antigen 1 It is a DNA-binding protein and acts as transcription activator to enhance EBV gene expression. It is essential for maintaining EBV genome in host cells by protecting the virus from being recognized by the immune system.

Latent membrane protein 1 It is an integral membrane protein associated with advanced and metastatic disease. It contributes to aggressive phenotype in NPC and is a promising therapeutic target for NPC treatment.

Introduction

Cancer of the nasopharynx is an epithelial cancer developed in the retro-nasal area in the nasal cavity. It was first documented and reported by Regaud and Schmincke separately in 1921 (Regaud 1921; Schmincke 1921). Nasopharyngeal carcinoma (NPC) is frequently confined at the mucosal lining of the fossa of Rosenmuller (pharyngeal recess), posteromedial to the medial crura of the Eustachian tube opening in the nasopharynx (Sham et al. 1990). Due to the small volume and peculiar anatomical structure of nasal cavity (with curved surface), comprehensive inspection of the nasal epithelium by visual means to locate the primary tumor is difficult (Loh et al. 1991). The tumor could spread in different directions (e.g., submucosally) making it difficult to be detected by endoscopy. NPC is highly proliferative and infiltrating and could result in the obstruction of larynx and pharynx. Due to the close proximity of nasopharynx to the skull base, skull base erosion with intracranial extension and/or involvement of the cranial nerve is also common (Roh 2004). NPC is also known as lymphoepithelioma as the primary tumor is infiltrated with abundant leukocyte (majority T lymphocytes). The infiltrating lymphocytes could be found in together with other immune cells such as eosinophils, dendritic cells, and macrophages at the periphery or inside the tumor mass (Jayasurya et al. 2000). It is suspected that the infiltrating immune cells interact with the cancer cells intimately allowing the tumor to escape from immune evasion (Yip et al. 2009). The primary tumor is small and usually causes no symptoms. Patients often present with bilateral glands enlargement and local/

regional lymph node metastasis. Other symptoms include cranial nerve palsies, diplopia, headache, hearing loss, numbness, otitis media, and trismus (Wei and Sham 2005). If the tumor mass is large, it will lead to epistaxis, nasal obstruction, and discharge. Most symptoms are vague and nonspecific at the early stages. By the time of diagnosis, the patients are usually at the advanced stages leading to poor prognosis and local control rate. Hence, there is a desperate need to develop early diagnosis method to improve the treatment outcome.

Clinical Inspection and Radiation Treatment of Undifferentiated NPC

Endoscopy and endoscopic biopsy is the routine procedure for NPC screening (Sham et al. 1989). Computerized tomography (CT) scans and magnetic resonance imaging (MRI) of the skull base will also be used to localize the extent of tumor in the head and neck regions (Brennan 2006). For histological assessment, biopsy is collected at the suspicious site with aid of fiber optic nasopharyngoscope and local anesthesia. Routine and frequent monitoring of the nasopharynx with endoscopic examination is useful to monitor the disease. However, due to the workload and expenses, continuous monitoring of the high-risk group is practically difficult. For histological presentation, cancer cells will have an increase in nuclear size with prominent nucleoli (Pathmanathan et al. 1995). In addition, loss of nuclear polarity and an increased in nuclei to cytoplasm ratio are commonly observed in the epithelial layers (Pathmanathan et al. 1995). For severe dysplasia, the biopsy is characterized with hypercellularity and an increased thickness of the mucosal epithelium, with the preexisting epithelial cells replaced by abnormal cells throughout most of the epithelium (Pathmanathan et al. 1995). For undifferentiated NPC, radiotherapy is recommended for the mainstay treatment regime as the cancer cells demonstrate high sensitivity to radiation with over 90 % locoregional control rate (Lee et al. 2012). Concurrent chemoradiotherapy (radiation treatment together with the use of chemotherapeutic agents such as cisplatin and fluorouracil) is recommended for advanced disease as the chemotherapeutic agents could control the distant metastasis (Lu et al. 2009; Wee et al. 2005).

The use of Molecular Markers in NPC Diagnosis

NPC in the endemic areas is characterized by its consistent association with the human herpesvirus 4, Epstein–Barr virus (EBV). In 1970, zur Hausen et al. observed that EBV virus DNA was harbored in the biopsies collected from the NPC patients but was absent in other tumor cells. At that point, the host cells of EBV remained controversial as it could possibly be derived from the anaplastic cells or from the lymphoid tissues (zur Hausen et al. 1970). Later, the presence of EBV in the tumor cells was confirmed, and many attempts have been made to employ EBV as a form of molecular marker in NPC detection. EBV is a double-stranded DNA virus, and the genome was protected within the toroid-shaped protein core and a lipid envelope with virus-encoded glycoprotein spikes (Young and Rickinson 2004). According to the International Agency for Research on Cancer (IARC), EBV is classified as group I carcinogen affirming that EBV has a causal role in human malignancies. The virus was first identified in Burkitt's lymphoma cells in 1964 using electronic microscope and is now known to be associated with other human malignancies including Hodgkin's disease, non-Hodgkin's lymphoma, infectious mononucleosis (IM), lymphoepithelioma-like carcinoma, oral leukoplakia and chronic interstitial pneumonitis in AIDS patients, posttransplant lymphoproliferative disease, gastric adenocarcinoma, as well as nasopharyngeal carcinoma.

To date, it is recognized that the virus was present in virtually all the WHO-2 and WHO-3 NPC cells (Sam et al. 1993). For WHO-1 keratinizing NPC, the causal role of EBV remains unresolved as the virus could only be found in a few numbers of patients. In undifferentiated NPC, the carcinogenic role of EBV in the cancer development is much more established. In the epithelial cells, EBV undergoes two phases of life cycle: the latent infection phase and lytic infection phase. At lytic phase, the virus will express specific proteins including early antigen and viral capsid antigen. The immune response of the host cells will induce elevated antibody titers. In latent infection phase, the EBV will express different proteins including Epstein–Barr nuclear antigens (EBNAs), membrane proteins (LMP1, LMP2A, and LMP2B), and nonpolyadenylated nuclear RNAs (EBERs) in their host cells (Fig. 1) (Kieff 1996). In NPC cells, expressions of EBER, EBNA1, LMP2A, and LMP2B are predominant (Raab-Traub 2002). Rowe et al. characterized the latency phase by

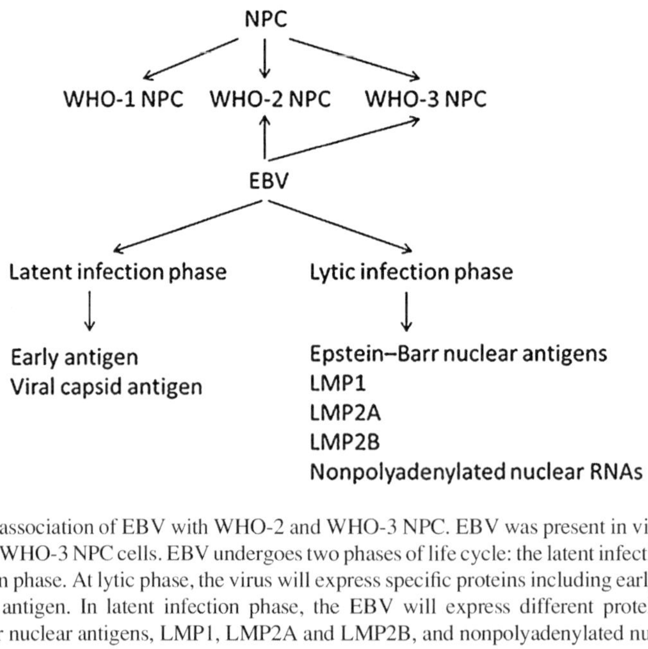

Fig. 1 The association of EBV with WHO-2 and WHO-3 NPC. EBV was present in virtually all the WHO-2 and WHO-3 NPC cells. EBV undergoes two phases of life cycle: the latent infection phase and lytic infection phase. At lytic phase, the virus will express specific proteins including early antigen and viral capsid antigen. In latent infection phase, the EBV will express different proteins including Epstein–Barr nuclear antigens, LMP1, LMP2A and LMP2B, and nonpolyadenylated nuclear RNAs

Table 1 EBV-related biomarkers in NPC

	Type	Detection method	Source of samples
EBER	Noncoding RNA	In situ hybridization	Tissue
EBNA1	Protein	Immunohistochemical staining	Tissue
LMP1	Protein	Immunohistochemical staining	Tissue
EBV DNA	DNA	qPCR	Tissue, blood, saliva
Antibody against EBV antigen	Protein	ELISA	Blood

EBER, EBNA1, LMP1, EBV DNA, and EBV antigens could serve as biomarkers for the diagnosis and prognosis of NPC. EBER, Epstein–Barr-encoded RNA; EBNA1, Epstein–Barr nuclear antigen 1; and LMP1, latent membrane protein 1

the expression patterns of gene products derived from the viral genome (Rowe et al. 1987). For NPC, expression of EBNA1, LMP1, LMP2, EBER, BARTs, and BARF1 in the neoplastic cells was considered as type II latency (Rowe et al. 1987; Fåhraeus et al. 1988; Shibata and Weiss 1992; Gulley and Tang 2008). EBER, EBNA1, LMP1, EBV DNA, and EBV antigens could serve as biomarkers for the diagnosis and prognosis of NPC (Table 1).

Epstein–Barr-Encoded RNA (EBER) 1 and 2 (GenBank Accession Numbers AB065135 and AB065136)

To locate the EBV genome in the biopsy samples, in situ hybridization for EBER remains to be the most efficient and reliable way because EBERs are the most abundantly expressed viral transcripts in the WHO-3 NPC cells and Asian/Chinese ethnicity (Table 2) (Shi et al. 2002). EBERs are thought to be noncoding RNA transcripts (do not code for any protein) as they are nonpolyadenylated (Gulley and Tang 2008). At present, no protein product of EBER is discovered, and the functions of EBER remain unclear. In NPC cells, EBER is transcribed by RNA polymerase III. EBER expression is tumor specific. EBER signals could be detected in the nucleus of the carcinoma cells and are absent in the adjacent normal surface epithelium or the benign stromal cells (Gulley 2001). It is estimated that there are about 1 million copies of EBER transcripts in the nuclei of the latently infected cell (Clemens 1993; Gulley 2001). EBERs are considered as RNA markers for the latently infected cells and are stable in paraffin-embedded tissue sections (Fan et al. 2006). EBER could be detected in all the EBV-associated malignancies except oral hairy leukoplakia (Gilligan et al. 1990). The majority of nasopharyngeal carcinoma patients initially present with enlarged lymph nodes containing metastatic undifferentiated carcinoma of unknown primary. At this circumstance, detection of EBER expression will be useful in identifying the squamous cell-positive lymph node with the squamous cell originating from the NPC (Gulley 2001). As EBER is used as

Table 2 Comparison of diagnostic values of EBV-related biomarkers in NPC

	Abundance	Mode of expression	Samples	Comparison with other biomarkers
EBER	1 million copies per cell	Tumor specific	Paraffin-embedded tissue	The most efficient and reliable way
EBNA1	Not determined	Tumor specific	Paraffin-embedded tissue	High sensitivity and specificity
LMP1	Not determined	Tumor specific	Paraffin-embedded tissue	Low sensitivity
EBV DNA	6,200 copies/mL plasma	Tumor specific	Plasma, serum, nasal brush, saliva	High sensitivity and specificity
Antibody against EBV antigen	Not determined	Not specific to NPC	Blood	Low sensitivity and specificity

EBERs were the most efficient and reliable biomarkers in tissue due to their highest abundance. The diagnosis value of circulating EBV DNA as a noninvasive biomarker for NPC has been demonstrated by a systematic review. EBER, Epstein–Barr-encoded RNA; EBNA1, Epstein–Barr nuclear antigen 1; and LMP1, latent membrane protein 1

Table 3 Prognostic values of EBV-related biomarkers in NPC

	Prognostic values	Samples
EBER	Patients with EBER-positive NPC had a better survival rate after radiation treatment	Paraffin-embedded tissue
EBNA1	High EBNA1 expression in the nasal swab obtained from NPC patients after radiation therapy is a prognostic factor for early and local recurrence	Paraffin-embedded tissue
LMP1	Detection of LMP1 expression in the nasopharyngeal biopsies obtained from postradiation treatment patients could also be regarded as an indicator of early local recurrence	Paraffin-embedded tissue
EBV DNA	The circulating EBV DNA level is a prognostic factor for NPC patients subjected to radiotherapy and is closely associated with the progression-free and overall survival	Plasma, serum, saliva
Antibody against EBV antigen	Measuring the changes in antibody level is only useful in a subset of patients with recurrence or metastases after radiotherapy	Blood

Given the detection of EBV DNA in plasma, serum, and saliva, EBV DNA is particularly useful for periodic monitoring of NPC patients. EBER, Epstein–Barr-encoded RNA; EBNA1, Epstein–Barr nuclear antigen 1; and LMP1, latent membrane protein 1

an indication of NPC cells, in situ hybridization of EBER has been used to monitor NPC patients prospectively after external radiotherapy and is used as a marker for monitoring treatment efficacy (Nicholls et al. 1996). Generally, patients with EBER-positive NPC had a better survival rate after radiation treatment as EBV-positive NPC had a good response rate to radiotherapy (Table 3) (Yip et al. 2006). However, at present, the underlying mechanisms remain poorly understood.

EBNA1 (Epstein–Barr Nuclear Antigen 1, GenBank Accession Number CAD53427)

EBNA1 is a DNA-binding protein and is expressed in all the EBV-associated cancers (Levitskaya et al. 1995; Westhoff Smith and Sugden 2013). It is also expressed in all the EBV-infected NPC cells (Gulley 2001). EBNA1 functions as transcription activator in enhancing EBV gene expression and is essential in maintaining the latently infected status and EBV genome in the host cells (Table 4) (Westhoff Smith and Sugden 2013). The expression level of EBNA1 is closely correlated with the tumor burden (Kottaridis et al. 1996). In addition, EBNA1 expression is essential for the persistent infection of EBV in the host cells as it could prevent the presentation of viral antigen on major histocompatibility complex (MHC) class I molecules and protect the virus from being recognized by the immune cells such as cytotoxic T lymphocyte (Levitskaya et al. 1995). Immunohistochemical staining for EBNA1 protein could be used in screening biopsies obtained from the nasal cavity and regional metastatic lymph node (Table 2). The EBNA transcript could be used as a molecular marker in screening the nasopharyngeal swabs obtained from the NPC patients. Together with the transcript of another EBV gene, LMP1, a sensitivity of 91.4 % (64/70) and a specificity of 98.3 % (348/354) could be reached (Hao et al. 2004). High EBNA1 expression in the nasal swab obtained from NPC patients after radiation therapy is a prognostic factor for early and local recurrence (Table 3) (Hao et al. 2004). EBNA staining is also useful in detecting the cancer cells from the fine-needle aspirate of the regional metastatic lymph node using exfoliative cytologic analysis (Chan and Huang 1990).

Latent Membrane Protein 1 (GenBank Accession Number X58140)

LMP1 is characterized by its transforming properties in the cell lines model (Wang et al. 1985; Kaye et al. 1993). Inhibiting LMP1 expression can trigger cell cycle arrest in NPC cells and could enhance the susceptibility to chemotherapeutic agent

Table 4 Biological functions of EBV-related biomarkers in NPC

	Biological functions	Mechanisms
EBER	No protein product of EBER is discovered, and the functions of EBER remain unclear	Unclear
EBNA1	EBNA1 functions in enhancing EBV gene expression and is essential in maintaining the latently infected status and EBV genome in the host cells	Functions as transcription activator
LMP1	LMP1-expressing NPC cells are phenotypically aggressive	Regulates cell cycle and apoptosis

Targeting LMP1 expression is a promising therapeutic strategy for NPC treatment as expression inhibition of LMP1 could increase the radiation sensitivity of the EBV-infected cells. EBER, Epstein–Barr-encoded RNA; EBNA1, Epstein–Barr nuclear antigen 1; and LMP1, latent membrane protein 1

(Mei et al. 2007). Structurally, LMP1 is a constitutively active homologue of TNFR CD40 receptor. Thus, it will have similar functions in the expressing cells leading to the activation of antiapoptotic genes (Dawson et al. 2012). LMP1-expressing NPC cells are phenotypically aggressive (Table 4) (Busson et al. 2004). Statistical evidence suggested that expression of LMP1 is closely linked to the advanced disease (Zhao et al. 2012). Cases with LMP1 expression exhibited higher cumulative metastatic rates than those without LMP1 expression (Zhao et al. 2012). However, in terms of diagnostic value, LMP1 is not sensitive in comparison with other EBV markers (Table 2). LMP1 is expressed in 50–80 % NPC samples (Zhao et al. 2012). In comparison with EBNA1, LMP1 is less sensitive in detecting the cancer cells in the nasal swabs (Hao et al. 2004). Samples without LMP1 staining may still have strong EBER expression suggesting that LMP1 is not expressed universally in all the EBV-infected cells (Gulley 2001). Targeting LMP1 expression however is a promising therapeutic strategy for NPC treatment as expression inhibition of LMP1 could increase the radiation sensitivity of the EBV-infected cells (Abdulkarim et al. 2003). Detection of LMP1 expression in the nasopharyngeal biopsies obtained from postradiation treatment patients could also be regarded as an indicator of early local recurrence (Table 3) (Hao et al. 2004).

EBV DNA and Viral Load

EBV is a DNA virus (genome size: 173-kb DNA), and the DNA is detected in the nucleus of all the undifferentiated NPC cells (Gulley 2001). The use of in situ hybridization in localizing the tumor cells in the biopsy is not recommended as ERER will offer better sensitivity as a matter of fact that EBER has a higher copy number in the NPC cells (Gulley 2001). EBV DNA could be detected in the peripheral blood of NPC patients with high sensitivity and specificity (Chan and Lo 2002). In a study measuring the plasma EBV DNA concentration, high circulating EBV DNA concentration was detected in patients with primary NPC (6,200 copies/mL), local recurrent NPC (9,200 copies/mL), and distant metastatic NPC (2,050 copies/mL) (Shao et al. 2004a). Circulating EBV DNA may be useful in continuous monitoring of the high-risk group for the development of sporadic disease (Chan et al. 2013). In the NPC tissues, the EBV DNA level is positively correlated with the ERER1-positivie cells and the staging of the tumor patients suggesting that it is correlated with the tumor load (Shao et al. 2004b). Han et al. performed a systematic review on the diagnostic value of circulating EBV DNA in NPC diagnosis. A total of 1,492 NPC and 2,641 controls are used in generating the pooled diagnostic value. The pooled sensitivity and specificity were 0.73 (0.71–0.75) and 0.89 (0.88–0.90) (Table 2). Plasma EBV DNA, in general, had a better detection sensitivity and specificity in comparison with the serum EBV DNA (Han et al. 2012).

The circulating EBV DNA level is a prognostic factor for NPC patients subjected to radiotherapy and is closely associated with the progression-free and overall survival (Table 3) (Chan et al. 2002). Plasma EBV DNA will rise during the first week post-radiotherapy. The increase is suggested to be caused by the release of EBV DNA from the radiation-induced chronic cell death (Lo et al. 2000). Afterwards, the circulating EBV DNA level will drop significantly with a median half-life of 3.8 days (Lo et al. 2000). In locally recurrent NPC patients treated with nasopharyngectomy (in which the tumor is removed by surgical means immediately), the half-life of circulating EBV is much shorter (i.e., 139 min) after the removal of tumor (To et al. 2003). After 1 week post-radiotherapy, plasma DNA will become undetectable in all the NPC patients (Shao et al. 2004a). It is suggested that the circulating EBV DNA level is an indicator of residual tumor load of the NPC patients (Chan et al. 2002). EBV will shed its virion from the oral mucosa into the saliva of the host (Gulley 2001). It was discovered that EBV DNA could also be detected in the saliva of 80 % primary NPC patients before treatment (Pow et al. 2011). Saliva EBV DNA level was higher in advanced NPC patients, and the level dropped significantly after treatment suggesting that saliva EBV DNA is a candidate indicator of tumor burden (Pow et al. 2011).

Antibody Against EBV Antigen

Peptide-based anti-EBV antibody ELISA has been recommended for use in NPC detection and monitoring the treatment efficacy (Zeng 1985). This is because persistent high anti-EBV antibody against the EBV lytic phase protein is present in the NPC patients (Chien et al. 2001). It is suggested that reactivation of EBV replication at the mucosal layer of head and neck region precedes the development of NPC leading to the production of antibody responses by the hosts' immune system (Henle and Henle 1976). A broad spectrum of anti-EBV antibody is suggested to be useful for NPC detection. Examples included anti-early antigen (EA) IgA, antiviral capsid antigen (VCA) IgA, anti-EBNA1 IgA, and EBV DNase-specific neutralizing antibody. However, the detection sensitivity is highly varying with different antibody titers, and the detection rate could range from 20 % to 100 % (Chang et al. 2013). One major problem of using ELISA is that the antibody could also be detected in normal individuals and non-NPC tumors, including liver, brain, lung, and bone metastases (Table 2) (Shao et al. 2004a). For anti-VCA IgA, anti-EBNA1 IgA, and EBV DNase-specific neutralizing antibody, it could also be detected in 18 % normal individuals (Pickard et al. 2004). About 50 % of the unaffected high-risk individuals from families in which two or more individuals were affected with NPC had high anti-EBV antibody titer (Pickard et al. 2004). In a continuous follow-up and surveillance program with 1,318 volunteers involved in anti-VCA IgA and circulating EBV DNA screening, combination of the two markers could only identify three patients with NPC at the beginning of the program, among which only one patient was serology positive (Chan et al. 2013). EBV antibody titer in combination with other EBV markers could offer a better performance than being used alone (Adham et al. 2013). For monitoring the patients after radiotherapy, the EBV serology has limited value because of the fact that it will remain high in particular patients and in the group with clinical remission

(Shao et al. 2004a). The use of EBV serology may have some value in confirming the clinical remission after radiotherapy (de Vathaire et al. 1988). Measuring the changes in antibody level is only useful in a subset of patients with recurrence or metastases after radiotherapy (Table 3) (Shimakage et al. 1987).

Conclusion

Detection of EBV-derived biomarkers in tissues and EBV DNA in the peripheral blood of NPC patients opens up the possibility to monitor the disease using molecular markers with high sensitivity (Liu et al. 2011). For periodic monitoring of NPC patients, EBV DNA is particularly useful as it could be done on different samples (such as plasma, serum, nasal brush, and saliva) obtained by noninvasive means. The samples could be collected from the patients periodically for continuous monitoring of the pathophysiological changes (Yang et al. 2006). The close association of circulating EBV DNA with the clinical outcomes of treatment provided new tool to predict the treatment outcome. However, the utility of EBV DNA has its limitation as the circulating DNA is not detectable in all the undifferentiated NPC patients in the endemic area (Shotelersuk et al. 2000). In addition, for WHO-1 NPC, which is not associated with EBV latent infection, the use of ERER staining and EBV DNA is not applicable. At present, most of the biomarkers examined for NPC diagnosis are derived from the EBV virus, and little is known about the suitability using somatic biomarkers originating from the cancer cell. Further studies are warranted to identify complementary biomarkers to overcome the limitation of EBV-based biomarkers in NPC screening and monitoring treatment outcome.

Potential Application to Prognosis, Other Diseases, or Conditions

Besides NPC, EBV was also associated with Burkitt's lymphoma and Hodgkin's lymphoma (Table 5) (Kutok and Wang 2006). EBV infection played a crucial role in the development of Burkitt's lymphoma. EBNA1 regulated the cell growth by

Table 5 The association of EBV with Burkitt's lymphoma and Hodgkin's lymphoma

	Diagnosis	Functional roles
Burkitt's lymphoma	EBV infection was only found in 15–30 % cases	EBNA1 regulated the cell growth by inhibiting apoptosis
Hodgkin's lymphoma	EBV infection was only found in about 40 % cases	LMP1 activated NFκB expression, resulting in the accumulation of genetic events that contribute to the initiation and progression of Hodgkin's lymphoma

In light of that EBV infection was only found in 15–30 % Burkitt's lymphoma cases and approximately 40 % of Hodgkin's lymphoma cases, EBV could not serve as a satisfactory diagnostic biomarker in these diseases. EBNA1, Epstein–Barr nuclear antigen 1; LMP1, latent membrane protein 1 inhibiting apoptosis in Burkitt's lymphoma cells. When EBV infected Hodgkin's lymphoma, EBER, EBNA1, LMP1, and LMP2A were expressed. LMP1 activated NFκB expression, resulting in the accumulation of genetic events that contribute to the initiation and progression of Hodgkin's lymphoma. In light of that EBV infection was only found in 15–30 % Burkitt's lymphoma cases and approximately 40 % of Hodgkin's lymphoma cases, EBV could not serve as a satisfactory diagnostic biomarker in these diseases.

Summary points

- EBER, EBNA1, and LMP1 can be applied for diagnosis of NPC and evaluation of the treatment effects of radiotherapy.
- EBERs were the most efficient and reliable biomarkers in tissue due to their highest abundance.
- The combination of EBNA1 and LMP1 resulted in an elevated sensitivity and specificity in screening the nasopharyngeal swabs obtained from the NPC patients.
- Given the detection of EBV DNA in plasma, serum, nasal brush, and saliva, EBV DNA is particularly useful for periodic monitoring of NPC patients.
- The diagnosis value of circulating EBV DNA as a noninvasive biomarker for NPC has been demonstrated by a systematic review.
- The circulating EBV DNA level is a prognostic factor for NPC patients subjected to radiotherapy and is closely associated with the progression-free and overall survival.
- Circulating EBV DNA is not applicable for all the NPC patients; therefore, biomarkers originating from the human cancer cells are required to circumvent the limitation of EBV-based biomarkers in NPC screening and treatment outcome monitoring.

References

Abdulkarim B, Sabri S, Zelenika D, et al. Antiviral agent cidofovir decreases Epstein-Barr virus (EBV) oncoproteins and enhances the radiosensitivity in EBV-related malignancies. Oncogene. 2003;22:2260–71.

Adham M, Greijer AE, Verkuijlen SA, et al. Epstein-Barr virus DNA load in nasopharyngeal brushings and whole blood in nasopharyngeal carcinoma patients before and after treatment. Clin Cancer Res. 2013;19:2175–86.

Brennan B. Nasopharyngeal carcinoma. Orphanet J Rare Dis. 2006;1:23.

Busson P, Keryer C, Ooka T, et al. EBV-associated nasopharyngeal carcinomas: from epidemiology to virus-targeting strategies. Trends Microbiol. 2004;12:356–60.

Chan MK, Huang DP. The value of cytologic examination for nasopharyngeal carcinoma. Ear Nose Throat J. 1990;69:268–71.

Chan KC, Lo YM. Circulating EBV DNA as a tumor marker for nasopharyngeal carcinoma. Semin Cancer Biol. 2002;12:489–96.

Chan AT, Lo YM, Zee B, et al. Plasma Epstein-Barr virus DNA and residual disease after radiotherapy for undifferentiated nasopharyngeal carcinoma. J Natl Cancer Inst. 2002;94:1614–19.

Chan KC, Hung EC, Woo JK, et al. Early detection of nasopharyngeal carcinoma by plasma Epstein-Barr virus DNA analysis in a surveillance program. Cancer. 2013;119:1838–44.

Chang C, Middeldorp J, Yu KJ, et al. Characterization of ELISA detection of broad-spectrum anti-Epstein-Barr virus antibodies associated with nasopharyngeal carcinoma. J Med Virol. 2013;85:524–9.

Chien YC, Chen JY, Liu MY, et al. Serologic markers of Epstein-Barr virus infection and nasopharyngeal carcinoma in Taiwanese men. N Engl J Med. 2001;345:1877–82.

Clemens MJ. The small RNAs of Epstein-Barr virus. Mol Biol Rep. 1993;17:81–92.

Dawson CW, Port RJ, Young LS. The role of the EBV-encoded latent membrane proteins LMP1 and LMP2 in the pathogenesis of nasopharyngeal carcinoma (NPC). Semin Cancer Biol. 2012;22:144–53.

de Vathaire F, Sancho-Garnier H, de Thé H, et al. Prognostic value of EBV markers in the clinical management of nasopharyngeal carcinoma (NPC): a multicenter follow-up study. Int J Cancer. 1988;42:176–81.

Fåhraeus R, Fu HL, Ernberg I, et al. Expression of Epstein-Barr virus-encoded proteins in nasopharyngeal carcinoma. Int J Cancer. 1988;42:329–38.

Fan SQ, Ma J, Zhou J, Xiong W, et al. Differential expression of Epstein-Barr virus-encoded RNA and several tumor-related genes in various types of nasopharyngeal epithelial lesions and nasopharyngeal carcinoma using tissue microarray analysis. Hum Pathol. 2006;37: 593–605.

Gilligan K, Rajadurai P, Resnick L, et al. Epstein-Barr virus small nuclear RNAs are not expressed in permissively infected cells in AIDS-associated leukoplakia. Proc Natl Acad Sci U S A. 1990;87:8790–4.

Gulley ML. Molecular diagnosis of Epstein-Barr virus-related diseases. J Mol Diagn. 2001;3:1–10.

Gulley ML, Tang W. Laboratory assays for Epstein-Barr virus-related disease. J Mol Diagn. 2008;10:279–92.

Han BL, Xu XY, Zhang CZ, et al. Systematic review on Epstein-Barr virus (EBV) DNA in diagnosis of nasopharyngeal carcinoma in Asian populations. Asian Pac J Cancer Prev. 2012;13:2577–81.

Hao SP, Tsang NM, Chang KP. Monitoring tumor recurrence with nasopharyngeal swab and latent membrane protein-1 and epstein-barr nuclear antigen-1 gene detection in treated patients with nasopharyngeal carcinoma. Laryngoscope. 2004;114:2027–30.

Henle G, Henle W. Epstein-Barr virus-specific IgA serum antibodies as an outstanding feature of nasopharyngeal carcinoma. Int J Cancer. 1976;17:1–7.

Jayasurya A, Bay BH, Yap WM, et al. Lymphocytic infiltration in undifferentiated nasopharyngeal cancer. Arch Otolaryngol Head Neck Surg. 2000;126:1329–32.

Kaye KM, Izumi KM, Kieff E. Epstein-Barr virus latent membrane protein 1 is essential for B-lymphocyte growth transformation. Proc Natl Acad Sci U S A. 1993;90:9150–4.

Kieff E. Epstein-Barr virus and its replication. In: Fields B, Knipes D, Howley PM, et al., editors. Fields virology. 3rd ed. Philadelphia: Lippincott-Raven; 1996. p. 2343–95.

Kottaridis SD, Panotopoulou E, Diamantis I, et al. Nasopharyngeal carcinoma: Epstein-Barr Virus significance. Anticancer Res. 1996;16:785–9.

Kutok JL, Wang F. Spectrum of Epstein-Barr virus-associated diseases. Annu Rev Pathol. 2006;1:375–404.

Lee AW, Lin JC, Ng WT. Current management of nasopharyngeal cancer. Semin Radiat Oncol. 2012;22:233–44.

Levitskaya J, Coram M, Levitsky V, et al. Inhibition of antigen processing by the internal repeat region of the Epstein-Barr virus nuclear antigen-1. Nature. 1995;375:685–8.

Liu Y, Fang Z, Liu L, et al. Detection of Epstein-Barr virus DNA in serum or plasma for nasopharyngeal cancer: a meta-analysis. Genet Test Mol Biomarkers. 2011;15:495–502.

Lo YM, Leung SF, Chan LY, et al. Kinetics of plasma Epstein-Barr virus DNA during radiation therapy for nasopharyngeal carcinoma. Cancer Res. 2000;60:2351–5.

Loh LE, Chee TS, John AB. The anatomy of the Fossa of Rosenmuller – its possible influence on the detection of occult nasopharyngeal carcinoma. Singapore Med J. 1991;32:154–5.

Lu H, Peng L, Yuan X, et al. Concurrent chemoradiotherapy in locally advanced nasopharyngeal carcinoma: a treatment paradigm also applicable to patients in Southeast Asia. Cancer Treat Rev. 2009;35:345–53.

Mei YP, Zhou JM, Wang Y, et al. Silencing of LMP1 induces cell cycle arrest and enhances chemosensitivity through inhibition of AKT signaling pathway in EBV-positive nasopharyngeal carcinoma cells. Cell Cycle. 2007;6:1379–85.

Nicholls JM, Chua D, Chiu PM, et al. The detection of clinically occult nasopharyngeal carcinoma in patients following radiotherapy – an analysis of 69 patients. J Laryngol Otol. 1996;110:496–9.

Pathmanathan R, Prasad U, Sadler R, et al. Clonal proliferations of cells infected with Epstein-Barr virus in preinvasive lesions related to nasopharyngeal carcinoma. N Engl J Med. 1995;333:693–8.

Pickard A, Chen CJ, Diehl SR, et al. Epstein-Barr virus seroreactivity among unaffected individuals within high-risk nasopharyngeal carcinoma families in Taiwan. Int J Cancer. 2004;111:117–23.

Pow EH, Law MY, Tsang PC, et al. Salivary Epstein-Barr virus DNA level in patients with nasopharyngeal carcinoma following radiotherapy. Oral Oncol. 2011;47:879–82.

Raab-Traub N. Epstein-Barr virus in the pathogenesis of NPC. Semin Cancer Biol. 2002;12:431–41.

Regaud C. Lympho-epitheliome de l'hypopharynx traité par la roentgenthérapie. Bull Soc Franc Otorhinolaryngol. 1921;34:209–14.

Roh JL. Transpalatal endoscopic resection of residual nasopharyngeal carcinoma after sequential chemoradiotherapy. J Laryngol Otol. 2004;118:951–4.

Rowe M, Rowe DT, Gregory CD, et al. Differences in B cell growth phenotype reflect novel patterns of Epstein-Barr virus latent gene expression in Burkitt's lymphoma cells. EMBO J. 1987;6:2743–51.

Sam CK, Brooks LA, Niedobitek G, et al. Analysis of Epstein-Barr virus infection in nasopharyngeal biopsies from a group at high risk of nasopharyngeal carcinoma. Int J Cancer. 1993;53:957–62.

Schmincke A. Über lymphoepitheliale Geschwülste. Beitr Pathol Anat. 1921;68:161–70.

Sham JS, Wei WI, Kwan WH, et al. Fiberoptic endoscopic examination and biopsy in determining the extent of nasopharyngeal carcinoma. Cancer. 1989;64:1838–42.

Sham JS, Wei WI, Zong YS, et al. Detection of subclinical nasopharyngeal carcinoma by fibreoptic endoscopy and multiple biopsy. Lancet. 1990;335:371–4.

Shao JY, Li YH, Gao HY, et al. Comparison of plasma Epstein-Barr virus (EBV) DNA levels and serum EBV immunoglobulin A/virus capsid antigen antibody titers in patients with nasopharyngeal carcinoma. Cancer. 2004a;100:1162–70.

Shao JY, Zhang Y, Li YH, et al. Comparison of Epstein-Barr virus DNA level in plasma, peripheral blood cell and tumor tissue in nasopharyngeal carcinoma. Anticancer Res. 2004b;24:4059–66.

Shi W, Pataki I, MacMillan C, et al. Molecular pathology parameters in human nasopharyngeal carcinoma. Cancer. 2002;94:1997–2006.

Shibata D, Weiss LM. Epstein-Barr virus-associated gastric adenocarcinoma. Am J Pathol. 1992;140:769–74.

Shimakage M, Ikegami N, Chatani M, et al. Serological follow-up study on the antibody levels to Epstein-Barr virus-determined nuclear antigen (EBNA) patients with nasopharyngeal carcinoma (NPC) after radiation therapy. Biken J. 1987;30:45–51.

Shotelersuk K, Khorprasert C, Sakdikul S, et al. Epstein-Barr virus DNA in serum/plasma as a tumor marker for nasopharyngeal cancer. Clin Cancer Res. 2000;6:1046–51.

To EW, Chan KC, Leung SF, et al. Rapid clearance of plasma Epstein-Barr virus DNA after surgical treatment of nasopharyngeal carcinoma. Clin Cancer Res. 2003;9:3254–9.

Wang D, Liebowitz D, Kieff E. An EBV membrane protein expressed in immortalized lymphocytes transforms established rodent cells. Cell. 1985;43:831–40.

Wee J, Tan EH, Tai BC, et al. Randomized trial of radiotherapy versus concurrent chemoradiotherapy followed by adjuvant chemotherapy in patients with American Joint Committee on Cancer/International Union against cancer stage III and IV nasopharyngeal cancer of the endemic variety. J Clin Oncol. 2005;23:6730–8.

Wei WI, Sham JS. Nasopharyngeal carcinoma. Lancet. 2005;365:2041–54.

Westhoff Smith D, Sugden B. Potential cellular functions of Epstein-Barr Nuclear Antigen 1 (EBNA1) of Epstein-Barr Virus. Viruses. 2013;5:226–40.

Yang X, Goldstein AM, Chen CJ, et al. Distribution of Epstein-Barr viral load in serum of individuals from nasopharyngeal carcinoma high-risk families in Taiwan. Int J Cancer. 2006;118:780–4.

Yip KW, Shi W, Pintilie M, et al. Prognostic significance of the Epstein-Barr virus, p53, Bcl-2, and survivin in nasopharyngeal cancer. Clin Cancer Res. 2006;12:5726–32.

Yip WK, Abdullah MA, Yusoff SM, Seow HF. Increase in tumour-infiltrating lymphocytes with regulatory T cell immunophenotypes and reduced zeta-chain expression in nasopharyngeal carcinoma patients. Clin Exp Immunol. 2009;155:412–22.

Young LS, Rickinson AB. Epstein-Barr virus: 40 years on. Nat Rev Cancer. 2004;4:757–68.

Zeng Y. Seroepidemiological studies on nasopharyngeal carcinoma in China. Adv Cancer Res. 1985;44:121–38.

Zhao Y, Wang Y, Zeng S, et al. LMP1 expression is positively associated with metastasis of nasopharyngeal carcinoma: evidence from a meta-analysis. J Clin Pathol. 2012;65:41–5.

zur Hausen H, Schulte-Holthausen H, Klein G, et al. EBV DNA in biopsies of Burkitt tumours and anaplastic carcinomas of the nasopharynx. Nature. 1970;228:1056–8.

Molecular Biomarkers of Laryngeal Cancer 40

Christos K. Kontos, Panagiotis G. Adamopoulos, and
Andreas Scorilas

Contents

C.K. Kontos • P.G. Adamopoulos • A. Scorilas (✉)
Department of Biochemistry and Molecular Biology, Faculty of Biology, School of Science, University of Athens, Athens, Greece
e-mail: chkontos@biol.uoa.gr; padamopoulos@biol.uoa.gr; ascorilas@biol.uoa.gr

V.R. Preedy, V.B. Patel (eds.), *Biomarkers in Cancer, Biomarkers in Disease: Methods, Discoveries and Applications*,
DOI 10.1007/978-94-007-7681-4_33

Abstract

Laryngeal cancer represents the second most common type of head and neck cancer, with approximately 12,000 new laryngeal squamous cell carcinoma cases being yearly diagnosed only in the USA. Despite the fact that the survival rates of laryngeal cancer patients have improved, owing to the more effective treatment than in the past decades, the prognosis of patients with metastatic laryngeal cancer remains poor, even for those treated with both radiotherapy and chemotherapy. Therefore, the relapse rates of laryngeal cancer patients are still very high, compared to patients suffering from other types of cancer. Laryngeal cancer is often diagnosed at an advanced stage, mostly due to the fact that this cancer causes nonspecific symptoms and hence to a delayed start of treatment after the true onset of the disease. To date, several genes have been studied for their diagnostic and/or prognostic potential in laryngeal cancer. Moreover, quantification of RNA or protein products of some genes could be used for the monitoring of laryngeal cancer treatment efficacy. As tumor biomarkers are considered as very important in the personalized medicine era that has just emerged, this chapter summarizes the current knowledge regarding molecular biomarkers in this disease.

List of Abbreviations

ARCON	Accelerated Radiotherapy with Carbogen (98 % O_2, 2 % CO_2) and Nicotinamide
CA9	Carbonic Anhydrase IX
CCNA2	Cyclin A2
CCNB1	Cyclin B1
CCND1	Cyclin D1
CCND3	Cyclin D3
CCNE1	Cyclin E1
CDH1	Cadherin 1, Type 1
CDK4	Cyclin-Dependent Kinase 4
CDKN1A	Cyclin-Dependent Kinase Inhibitor 1A
CDKN1B	Cyclin-Dependent Kinase Inhibitor 1B
CDKN2A	Cyclin-Dependent Kinase Inhibitor 2A
CDKN2B	Cyclin-Dependent Kinase Inhibitor 2B
COX2	Cyclooxygenase 2
CST3	Cystatin C
CSTA	Cystatin A
CSTB	Cystatin B
CTSB	Cathepsin B
CTSD	Cathepsin D
DDC	*L*-DOPA Decarboxylase
DFS	Disease-Free Survival
ECAD	E-cadherin

EGFR	Epidermal Growth Factor Receptor
ELISA	Enzyme-Linked Immunosorbent Assay
FFPE	Formalin Fixed, Paraffin Embedded
FLT1	fms-Related Tyrosine Kinase 1
FLT4	fms-Related Tyrosine Kinase 4
HOTAIR	HOX Transcript Antisense RNA
HOXC	Homeobox C
IHC	Immunohistochemistry
KDR	Kinase Insert Domain Receptor
KLK11	Kallikrein-Related Peptidase 11
lncRNA	Long Noncoding RNA
LSCC	Laryngeal Squamous Cell Carcinoma
MFS	Metastasis-Free Survival
miRNA	microRNA
MKI67	Marker of Proliferation Ki-67
OPN	Osteopontin
OS	Overall Survival
PARK7	Parkinson Protein 7
PCNA	Proliferating Cell Nuclear Antigen
PFS	Progression-Free Survival
PGF	Placental Growth Factor
PTEN	Phosphatase and tensin homolog
PTGS2	Prostaglandin-Endoperoxide Synthase 2
qRT-PCR	Quantitative Real-Time Polymerase Chain Reaction
rRNA	Ribosomal RNA
SPP1	Secreted Phosphoprotein 1
TERT	Telomerase Reverse Transcriptase
TNM	Tumor Extent, Nodes, and Metastases
TP53	Tumor Protein p53
VEGF	Vascular Endothelial Growth Factor
VEGFA	Vascular Endothelial Growth Factor A
VEGFB	Vascular Endothelial Growth Factor B
VEGFC	Vascular Endothelial Growth Factor C
VEGFD	Vascular Endothelial Growth Factor D
VEGFR1	Vascular Endothelial Growth Factor Receptor 1
VEGFR3	Vascular Endothelial Growth Factor Receptor 3

Key Facts of Laryngeal Cancer

- The larynx is a part of the throat, extends from the tip of the epiglottis to the inferior border of the cricoid cartilage, and comprises the supraglottis, glottis, and subglottis.

- Laryngeal squamous cell carcinoma is the most common malignancy of the head and neck region and can arise in any part of the larynx.
- The most common symptoms of laryngeal cancer include hoarseness, a lump in the neck (because of enlarged lymph nodes), ear pain, and difficulty in swallowing.
- Laryngeal tumors may spread by direct extension to adjacent tissues and by metastasis to the regional cervical lymph nodes or, even more distantly (e.g., to the lung), through the blood and lymph vessels.
- Second primary tumors are additional primary malignant neoplasms that are distinctly separate from the index tumor; they can be diagnosed either at the same time or up to 6 months after the initial diagnosis.
- There are different types of treatment for laryngeal cancer patients, the most common being radiation therapy, surgery, and chemotherapy.
- Recurrent laryngeal cancer is a cancer that has relapsed after it has been treated. Laryngeal cancer recurrence is most likely to occur in the first 3 years after treatment for primary laryngeal cancer, in the larynx or in other parts of the body.

Definitions of Words and Terms

Supraglottis The upper part of the larynx above the vocal cords, including the epiglottis.

Glottis The middle part of the larynx containing the vocal cords.

Laryngeal Squamous Cell Carcinoma An uncontrolled growth of abnormal reserve cells that replaced injured or damaged cells in laryngeal epithelia.

Locoregional Restricted to a localized area of the body.

Histological Grade A measure of loss of differentiation occurring in cancer cells, based on the similarity of the tumor to the tissue of origin.

TNM Staging System The most detailed classification of tumors, comprising the tumor extent, the nodal status, and the presence (or absence) of distant metastases.

Radiotherapy Treatment with irradiation of the malignant tumor.

Disease-Free Survival The time interval after primary treatment for a cancer ending with the disappearance of cancer signs and symptoms, until diagnosis of tumor recurrence (locoregional or systemic), last contact with the patient, or end of follow-up.

Metastasis-Free Survival The time interval after primary treatment for a cancer ending with the disappearance of cancer signs and symptoms until the detection of distant metastases originating from the initial tumor, last contact with the patient, or end of follow-up.

Overall Survival The time interval after primary treatment for a cancer until patient's death from the specific disease, last contact with the patient, or end of follow-up.

Introduction

Head and neck carcinomas constitute the sixth most commonly diagnosed cancer worldwide, and the vast majority of them belong in the category of squamous cell carcinoma (SCC) (Chin et al. 2006). This type of carcinoma originates from squamous cells lining the moist, mucosal surfaces inside the mouth, the nose, and the throat. Head and neck SCC holds a remarkable position among causes leading to death. SCC can arise in the nasal cavity, paranasal sinuses, nasopharynx, hypolarynx, larynx, trachea, oral cavity, oropharynx, salivary glands, and ears (Argiris et al. 2008). The second most common type of head and neck cancer is laryngeal cancer. New cases of laryngeal cancer diagnosed in the USA every year are estimated at 12,000. The incidence of laryngeal cancer is much higher in men than in women, especially for those found between 60 and 70 years old (Ferlay et al. 2010). Among the causative risk factors of this malignancy, tobacco use and alcohol consumption are considered to be heavily involved in the carcinogenesis of the larynx (Argiris et al. 2008).

The implication of a wide gamut of molecules in laryngeal cancer and their fundamental role in this malignancy has been widely investigated, so far (Table 1). Dysregulation of the expression of several genes is associated with many hallmarks of cancer, including uncontrolled cell proliferation, defective apoptosis, attenuation or complete loss of cell differentiation, epithelial–mesenchymal transition, metastasis, and angiogenesis. Moreover, the potential of such molecules as molecular biomarkers for prognosis or monitoring of treatment efficacy in laryngeal cancer patients has already been demonstrated. Specific molecular biomarkers are of high importance in the personalized medicine era that has just emerged (Table 2). Therefore, immunohistochemical detection and/or mRNA expression profiling of promising molecular biomarkers will contribute to the generation of novel screening tests with high sensitivity and specificity, as well as tailor-made therapies against laryngeal cancer. Furthermore, selective targeting of interactions between specific molecules participating in key biochemical pathways could dramatically impede tumor progression and, hence, elongate the survival of laryngeal cancer patients.

Table 1 Molecular biomarkers of laryngeal cancer and their functions.

Gene symbol (and aliases)	Name	Function
BAX	BCL2-associated X protein	Promotion of apoptosis
BCL2	B-cell lymphoma 2	Inhibition of apoptosis
BCL2L1 (BCLX)	BCL2-like 1	Promotion or inhibition of apoptosis (depending on the protein isoform)
BCL2L12	BCL2-like 12	Promotion or inhibition of apoptosis (depending on the protein isoform)
CA9	Carbonic anhydrase IX	Catalysis of the reversible hydration of carbon dioxide
CCNA2	Cyclin A2	Cell cycle control
CCNB1	Cyclin B1	
CCND1	Cyclin D1	
CCND3	Cyclin D3	
CCNE1	Cyclin E1	
CD44	CD44 molecule	Regulation of cell–cell and cell–matrix interactions
CDH1 (ECAD)	E-cadherin	Ca^{2+}-dependent cell–cell adhesion
CDK4	Cyclin-dependent kinase 4	Promotion of the cell cycle
CDKN1A (p21, CIP1, WAF1)	Cyclin-dependent kinase inhibitor 1A	Inhibition of the enzymatic activity of cyclin-dependent kinases
CDKN1B (p27, KIP1)	Cyclin-dependent kinase inhibitor 1B	
CDKN2A (p21, p16, p14, INK4A, ARF)	Cyclin-dependent kinase inhibitor 2A	
CDKN2B (p15 and INK4B)	Cyclin-dependent kinase inhibitor 2B	
CSTA	Cystatin A (stefin A)	Inhibition of the activity of cathepsins
CTSB	Cathepsin B	Lysosomal cysteine and aspartyl proteases of lysosomes
CTSD	Cathepsin D	
DDC	*L*-DOPA decarboxylase	Catalysis of the synthesis of dopamine and serotonin
EGFR	Epidermal growth factor receptor	Receptor tyrosine kinase activity (multiple functions)
ERBB2 (HER2)	v-erb-b2 avian erythroblastic leukemia viral oncogene homologue 2	
ERBB3 (HER3)	v-erb-b2 avian erythroblastic leukemia viral oncogene homologue 3	
ERBB4 (HER4)	v-erb-b2 avian erythroblastic leukemia viral oncogene homologue 4	

(*continued*)

Table 1 (continued)

Gene symbol (and aliases)	Name	Function
FLT1 (VEGFR1)	fms-related tyrosine kinase 1	Receptor tyrosine kinase activity (angiogenesis)
FLT4 (VEGFR3)	fms-related tyrosine kinase 1	
HOTAIR	HOX transcript antisense RNA	Retargeting of chromatin-remodeling complexes
KLK11	Kallikrein-related peptidase 11	Trypsin-like serine protease
miR-155	microRNA-155	Posttranscriptional regulation of protein-coding gene expression
miR-455-5p	microRNA-455-5p	
miR-196a	microRNA-196a	
MKI67	Marker of proliferation Ki-67	Participation in rRNA synthesis and cellular proliferation
PARK7 (DJ1)	Parkinson protein 7	Peptidase C56 family member
PCNA	Proliferating cell nuclear antigen	Cofactor of DNA polymerase delta
PTGS2 (COX2)	Prostaglandin-endoperoxide synthase 2	Catalysis of the biosynthesis of prostaglandin
SPP1 (OPN)	Secreted phosphoprotein 1	Cell adhesion molecule and cytokine
TERT	Telomerase reverse transcriptase	Protein component of telomerase (a ribonucleoprotein polymerase that maintains telomere ends)
TP53	Tumor suppressor protein p53	Cell cycle arrest, induction of apoptosis, senescence, DNA repair
VEGFA	Vascular endothelial growth factor A	Angiogenesis
VEGFC	Vascular endothelial growth factor C	

This table exhibits the gene symbols, names, and function of the molecules that could serve as molecular biomarkers on laryngeal cancer, as presented in this chapter. Gene symbols are listed alphabetically

Tumor Protein p53 (TP53)

The tumor protein p53 (*TP53*) gene encodes a tumor-suppressor protein regulating the expression of many genes in response to diverse cellular stresses, thus having multiple functions, including the induction of cell cycle arrest, apoptosis, senescence, and DNA repair (Fig. 1). Although several studies during the last two decades have sought to shed light on the potential associations of p53 expression with distinct tumor clinicopathological features and its putative prognostic value in LSCC, established prognostic factors, results are still inconclusive, mostly due to variations in the selection of LSCC patients included in each study. Moreover, there

Table 2 Clinical significance of molecular biomarkers of laryngeal cancer.

Gene	Type of molecule	Expression in cancerous *vs.* noncancerous specimens	Association with clinicopathological variables	Prognostic value	References
BAX	Protein	Downregulated		Independent favorable predictor of OS	(Nix et al. 2005)
BCL2	Protein	Upregulated		Predictor of radiotherapy failure	(Condon et al. 2002)
				Not significant	(Ogawa et al. 2003)
BCL2L1 ($BCLX_L$)	Protein	Upregulated		Independent unfavorable predictor of OS	(Nix et al. 2005)
BCL2L12	mRNA	Downregulated	Associated with TNM stage		(Geomela et al. 2013)
CA9	Protein			Unfavorable predictor of MFS and OS	(Rademakers et al. 2013)
CCNA2	Protein		Associated with locoregional recurrence	Unfavorable predictor of DFS and OS	(Saarilahti et al. 2003)
CCNB1	Protein		Associated with tumor site, tumor extent, and clinical stage	Unfavorable predictor of DFS and OS	(Dong et al. 2002)
CCND1	Gene	Amplified	Associated with positive nodal status		(Bellacosa et al. 1996; Jares et al. 1994)
	mRNA	Upregulated	Associated with advanced local invasion and stage IV carcinomas		
	Protein		Associated with tumor site, tumor extent, and clinical stage	Unfavorable predictor of DFS and OS	(Dong et al. 2001)
CCND3	Protein	Upregulated		Independent unfavorable predictor of DFS and OS	(Pruneri et al. 2005)
CCNE1	Protein	Upregulated	Associated with tumor site, tumor extent, and clinical stage	Unfavorable predictor of DFS and OS	(Dong et al. 2001; Dong et al. 2000)

CD44v6	Protein		Associated with severe tumor invasion and positive nodal status	Unfavorable predictor of DFS	(Staibano et al. 2007; Zhao et al. 2008)
CDH1 (ECAD)	Protein	Downregulated	Associated with histological grade of tumor cells, high tumor extent, and positive nodal status	Independent predictor of nodal metastases	(Franchi et al. 1996; Rodrigo et al. 2002)
CDK4	Protein			Unfavorable predictor of OS	(Dong et al. 2001)
CDKN1A	Protein		Inversely associated with histological grade and nodal status	Independent favorable predictor of OS	(Pruneri et al. 1999) (Chernock et al. 2013)
CDKN1B	Protein		Inversely associated with high tumor extent and clinical stage	Independent favorable predictor of DFS and OS	(Pruneri et al. 1999)
CDKN2A	Gene	Deleted		Unfavorable predictor of PFS and OS	(Swellam et al. 2008)
CDKN2B	Gene	Deleted		Unfavorable predictor of PFS and OS	(Swellam et al. 2008)
CSTA	Protein		Inversely associated with lymphatic metastasis, LSCC recurrence, and patients' survival rate		(Li et al. 2011)
CTSB	Protein		Associated with migration, invasion, and proliferation of tumor cells	Not significant	(Li et al. 2011)
CTSD	Protein		Associated with lymph node metastasis in the region of the neck	Independent unfavorable predictor of MFS and OS	(Maurizi et al. 1996a)
DDC	mRNA	Upregulated	Inversely associated with TNM stage	Favorable predictor of DFS and OS	(Geomela et al. 2012; Patsis et al. 2012a)
EGFR	Protein	Upregulated	Associated with high tumor histological grade	Independent unfavorable predictor of DFS and OS	(Maurizi et al. 1996b; Maurizi et al. 1992)
ERBB2	Protein			Independent predictor of chemoradiotherapy failure; favorable predictor of DFS	(Almadori et al. 2010; Ganly et al. 2007)

(continued)

Table 2 (continued)

Gene	Type of molecule	Expression in cancerous *vs.* noncancerous specimens	Association with clinicopathological variables	Prognostic value	References
ERBB3	Protein			Favorable predictor of DFS	(Almadori et al. 2010)
ERBB4	Protein			Favorable predictor of DFS	(Almadori et al. 2010)
FLT1	Protein	Upregulated	Associated with tumor extent	Independent unfavorable predictor of DFS	(Pentheroudakis et al. 2012)
FLT4	Protein			Unfavorable predictor of OS	(Pentheroudakis et al. 2012)
HOTAIR	lncRNA	Upregulated	Associated with tumor histological grade and positive nodal status	Independent unfavorable predictor of OS	(Li et al. 2013)
KLK11	mRNA	Downregulated	Inversely associated with TNM stage	Independent favorable predictor of OS	(Patsis et al. 2012b)
miR-155	miRNA	Upregulated	Associated with the progression of the disease and histological grade		(Zhao et al. 2013)
miR-455-5p	miRNA	Upregulated (in the blood plasma)	Associated with the progression of the disease and histological grade		(Saito et al. 2013)
miR-196a	miRNA	Upregulated (in the blood plasma)	Associated with the progression of the disease and histological grade		(Saito et al. 2013)
MKI67 (Ki-67)	Protein		Associated with high tumor histological grade	Predictor of occult neck metastases	(Franchi et al. 1996; Liu et al. 2003; Saarilahti et al. 2003)
PARK7	Protein	Upregulated	Associated with tumor extent, positive nodal status, and cancer cell proliferation and invasiveness	Unfavorable predictor of DFS; independent unfavorable predictor of OS	(Zhu et al. 2012; Zhu et al. 2010)
PCNA	Protein		Associated with high histological grade, lymphatic and vascular invasion, depth of tumor margins, neck metastasis, and locoregional recurrence	Predictor of occult neck metastases, unfavorable predictor of DFS and OS	(Franchi et al. 1996; Liu et al. 2003; Sarac et al. 1998)

PTGS2	Protein		Inversely associated with histological grade	Independent unfavorable predictor of DFS and OS	(Ranelletti et al. 2001)
SPP1	Protein	Upregulated	Associated with high tumor histological grade, positive nodal status, degree of dysplasia, tumor invasion, and presence of distant metastases	Unfavorable predictor of DFS	(Celetti et al. 2005; Lu et al. 2011; Staibano et al. 2007)
TERT	mRNA			Unfavorable predictor of OS	(Eissa et al. 2005)
	Protein (activity)			Unfavorable predictor of DFS and OS	(Swellam et al. 2008)
TP53 (p53)	Protein	Upregulated		Unfavorable predictor of DFS and OS	(Hirvikoski et al. 1997; Jin et al. 1998; Narayana et al. 2000; Nathan et al. 2000; Osman et al. 2002)
				Favorable predictor of DFS and OS	(Hirvikoski et al. 1997)
				Not significant	(Kokoska et al. 1996; Nadal et al. 1995; Narayana et al. 1998; Tan and Ogden 1997; Tomasino et al. 1994)
VEGFA	mRNA	Upregulated	Associated with tumor extent	Independent unfavorable predictor of DFS	(Pentheroudakis et al. 2012)
	Protein		Associated with high histological grade	Unfavorable predictor of DFS and OS	(Parikh et al. 2007; Pentheroudakis et al. 2012)
		Upregulated (in the blood serum)	Associated with tumor size, high histological grade, and positive nodal status	Independent unfavorable predictor of DFS	(Sullu et al. 2010; Teknos et al. 2002)
VEGFC	Protein	Upregulated		Independent unfavorable predictor of DFS	(Hinojar-Gutierrez et al. 2007)

This table provides an overview of the molecular biomarkers of laryngeal cancer, their association with the clinicopathological features of laryngeal tumors, and their clinical value. Moreover, it presents briefly the differences observed in the expression levels of these molecules between laryngeal tumors and noncancerous laryngeal tissue specimens. Gene symbols are listed alphabetically

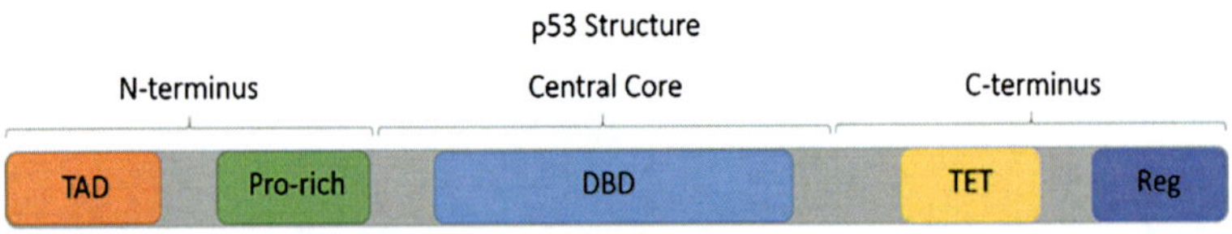

Fig. 1 Schematic representation of the p53 structure. The p53 protein comprises three functional domains, namely, an N-terminal activation domain, a DNA-binding domain (*DBD*), and a C-terminal domain. The N-terminal domain includes a transactivation subdomain (*TAD*) and a proline-rich region. The central DBD binds specific DNA sequences and constitutes a hot spot mutation region. The C-terminal includes a region that performs a regulatory function (Reg domain) containing residues that undergo posttranslational modifications including phosphorylation and acetylation, as well as a tetramerization domain (*TET*) facilitating the oligomerization of p53

has been much controversy about the ability of p53 to predict radiotherapy failure and locoregional recurrence of the tumor.

p53 overexpression is, most likely, unrelated to the biological aggressiveness of laryngeal tumors. Hence, no significant associations have been found between p53 expression status and tumor extent, histological grade, nodal status, or clinical stage of LSCC patients (Dolcetti et al. 1992; Jin et al. 1998; Nadal et al. 1995; Narayana et al. 1998). It has been suggested that aberrant p53 expression is an early event in the process of laryngeal carcinogenesis leading finally to LSCC (Dolcetti et al. 1992; Tomasino et al. 1994), or that it may also play its own role in the early steps of the malignant transformation of the laryngeal mucosa. However, it seems that p53 immunopositivity is not associated with further progression of the disease (Nadal et al. 1995). Regarding the prognostic power of immunohistochemically assessed p53 expression, a number of studies converge at its significance regarding both disease-free survival (DFS) (Hirvikoski et al. 1997; Jin et al. 1998; Narayana et al. 2000; Nathan et al. 2000) and overall survival (OS) (Hirvikoski et al. 1997; Osman et al. 2002) of LSCC patients, treated either with curative radiotherapy (at an early stage) or with surgical resection of the tumor (at an advanced stage). Nonetheless, there is a discrepancy among these studies, as the study of Hirvikoski et al. is the only one to suggest a favorable prognostic role for p53 overexpression in LSCC (Hirvikoski et al. 1997). Furthermore, the utility of intense p53 immunostaining as a prognostic indicator has been questioned, as several other scientific works demonstrated that p53 expression is not predictive of tumor recurrence or radiotherapy failure in LSCC (Kokoska et al. 1996; Nadal et al. 1995; Narayana et al. 1998; Tan and Ogden 1997; Tomasino et al. 1994). In more detail, nuclear accumulation of p53 could not predict tumor recurrence in patients with early-stage glottic LSCC treated with radiotherapy (Kokoska et al. 1996; Narayana et al. 1998) nor in patients with other types of LSCC (Ogawa et al. 2003; Tan and Ogden 1997). Besides that, p53 overexpression failed to predict the DFS and OS of advanced-stage LSCC patients who underwent radical surgical resection of their tumors (Nadal et al. 1995; Tomasino et al. 1994). Taking all the aforementioned data into consideration, it seems that large meta-analyses of

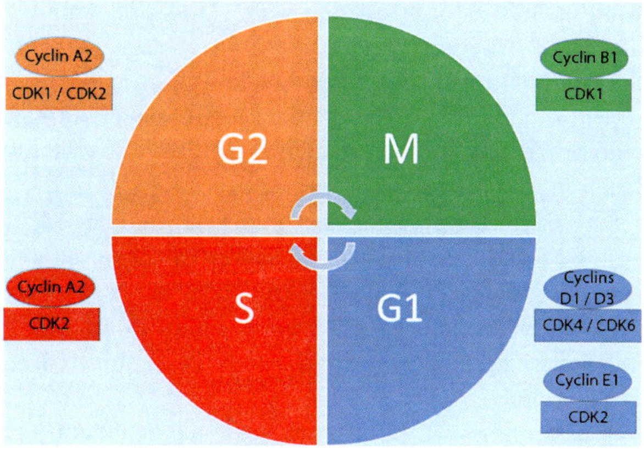

Fig. 2 Schematic representation of some CDKs involved in cell cycle progression

LSCC patient data are needed to determine the prognostic importance of p53 for specific subgroups of patients undergoing specific treatments.

Cyclins, Cyclin-Dependent Kinases, and Their Inhibitors

Cyclins belong to a highly conserved family, whose members control the progression of cells through the cell cycle by forming complexes with and activating cyclin-dependent kinases. Their protein levels are characterized by a dramatic periodicity through the cell cycle (Fig. 2). The cyclins that have mostly been studied in LSCC are cyclin A2 (CCNA2; in the past, known as cyclin A), cyclin B1 (CCNB1), cyclin D1 (CCND1), cyclin D3 (CCND3), and cyclin E1 (CCNE1; in the past, known as cyclin E).

CCNB1, CCND1, and CCNE1 expression was significantly associated with the tumor site, tumor extent, and clinical stage. In particular, CCNB1, CCND1, and CCNE1 overexpression was more common among tumors of the supraglottic larynx, of high extent (T3 or T4), and advanced clinical stage (III or IV) (Dong et al. 2000, 2001, 2002; Pignataro et al. 1998). CCND1 and CCNE1 immunopositivity was also related to the presence of metastases in patients' regional lymph nodes (Dong et al. 2000, 2001; Pignataro et al. 1998). Moreover, high cyclin E expression was more frequently observed in poorly differentiated LSCC than in well- or moderately differentiated malignant neoplasms (Dong et al. 2000). In addition to CCND1 protein overexpression, mRNA overexpression of this gene was noticed in a considerable percentage of LSCC specimens and was significantly associated with advanced local invasion and stage IV carcinomas. In many cases, elevated *CCND1* mRNA levels could be attributed to *CCND1* gene amplification, which was related to positive nodal status, as well (Jares et al. 1994).

The prognostic value of cyclins in LSCC has been well documented so far. CCNA2 overexpression, detected by immunohistochemistry (IHC), was associated with locoregional recurrence, as patients with CCNA2-positive laryngeal tumors were at a 40 % risk of locoregional relapse within a 5-year period from LSCC diagnosis, whereas patients with CCNA2-negative LSCC had an 18 % risk of locoregional recurrence. Strong CCNA2 immunostaining was also an unfavorable prognosticator of DFS and OS in LSCC patients treated with surgery and postoperative radiotherapy (Saarilahti et al. 2003). Furthermore, high CCNB1 immunoreactivity was an unfavorable – albeit not independent – prognostic factor in LSCC (Dong et al. 2002). The most important indicators of poor prognosis, in terms of both DFS and OS, were CCND1 and CCNE1 immunopositivities (Dong et al. 2000, 2001; Pignataro et al. 1998; Pruneri et al. 1999). Besides these cyclins, *CCND3* overexpression and *CCND1* gene amplification were demonstrated to constitute independent predictors of high death risk in this malignancy (Bellacosa et al. 1996; Pruneri et al. 2005).

Co-staining of LSCC tissue specimens with anti-CCND1 and anti-CCND3 was an even more powerful prognosis predictor. Hence, patients with CCND1+/CCND3+ tumors were more prone to succumbing than the rest of patients, whereas patients with CCND1-/CCND3- LSCC exhibited the most prolonged survival. CCND1-/CCND3+ or CCND1+/CCND3- had an intermediate prognosis (Pruneri et al. 2005). Moreover, immunohistochemical assessment of CCND1 and its enzymatic partner, CDK4, revealed that co-overexpression of CCND1 and CDK4 was a strong prognostic factor of poor patient outcome (Dong et al. 2001). Combined CCND1 and CDK4 immunopositivities as well as CCNE1 overexpression retained their unfavorable prognostic value also in the subgroup of early-stage (I or II) LSCC cases (Dong et al. 2000, 2001). Therefore, it is evident that evaluation of expression of cyclins could assist the clinical management of LSCC patients by selecting patients with poor prognosis and/or those who should be treated with more aggressive therapies.

The enzymatic activity of activated cyclin-dependent kinases can be blocked by specific inhibitors, usually during the G1 phase of the cell cycle or in response to signals originating from the environment or from damaged DNA. The most prominent examples of such inhibitory molecules are cyclin-dependent kinase inhibitor 1A (CDKN1A; also known as p21, CIP1, and WAF1), cyclin-dependent kinase inhibitor 1B (CDKN1B; also known as p27 and KIP1), cyclin-dependent kinase inhibitor 2A (CDKN2A; also known as p21, p16, p14, INK4A, and ARF), and cyclin-dependent kinase inhibitor 2B (CDKN2B; also known as p15 and INK4B).

Significant associations were noticed between the immunohistochemically detected expression of both *CDKN1A* and *CDKN1B* genes and clinicopathological features of malignant laryngeal tumors. Low CDKN1A expression was associated with poor tumor differentiation and positive nodal status of LSCC patients, while weak CDKN1B expression was related to high tumor extent and advanced clinical stage (Pruneri et al. 1999). In accordance with these findings, LSCC patients with CDKN1A-positive tumors had better OS rates than those with CDKN1A-negative tumors (Chernock et al. 2013). CDKN1B immunopositivity constitutes another independent favorable prognosticator in LSCC, predicting longer DFS and OS intervals (Pruneri et al. 1999). On the contrary, patients with CDKN1B-negative laryngeal tumors that were simultaneously CCND3 positive (CDKN1B-/CCND3+)

had a very poor prognosis, with regard to both DFS and OS (Pruneri et al. 1999). Similarly, in basaloid LSCC (a rare and aggressive variant of laryngeal cancer), negative CDKN1B immunostaining was linked to high tumor aggressiveness and predicted poor patient outcome (Salerno et al. 2006). Furthermore, genomic deletions of *CDKN2A* and/or *CDKN2B* were associated with worse progression-free survival (PFS) and OS of LSCC patients (Swellam et al. 2008). In summary, loss of expression of each aforementioned cyclin-dependent kinase inhibitor is an adverse prognostic factor in LSCC.

Marker of Proliferation Ki-67 (MKI67)

Marker of proliferation Ki-67 (MKI67) is a nuclear protein, associated with ribosomal RNA (rRNA) synthesis and cellular proliferation. Intense nuclear MKI67 staining was related to poor histologic differentiation. Although MKI67 expression was not an independent prognosticator, malignant laryngeal tumors with high MKI67 expression recurred locoregionally more frequently when treated with split-course radiotherapy than when treated with a continuous course of therapy, while the presence of a planned split did not influence the frequency of locoregional recurrences when MKI67 expression was lower (Saarilahti et al. 2003). Another study demonstrated that MKI67 protein levels are higher in laryngeal tumors accompanied by metastases in the regional lymph nodes than in the LSCC of node-negative patients (Franchi et al. 1996). Furthermore, strong MKI67 expression is a reliable predictor of the existence of occult neck metastases in LSCC (Franchi et al. 1996; Liu et al. 2003). Thus, immunohistochemical detection of MKI67 could distinguish patients who are more likely to benefit from elective neck dissection.

Proliferating Cell Nuclear Antigen (PCNA)

Proliferating cell nuclear antigen (PCNA) is a cofactor of DNA polymerase delta, localized in the cell nucleus. Quantification of PCNA expression (PCNA index) on histological sections from paraffin-embedded biopsies by using monoclonal antibodies reveals the rate of tumor cell proliferation. In LSCC, the PCNA index is associated with histological grade, lymphatic and vascular invasion, depth of tumor margins, neck metastasis, and locoregional recurrence (Sarac et al. 1998). Laryngeal tumors having metastasized in the regional lymph nodes present higher PCNA levels than tumors of the node-negative patients (Franchi et al. 1996). Additionally, the PCNA index values of patients with occult metastasis were significantly higher than those of patient without metastases (Sarac et al. 1998). In accordance with these findings, it has been suggested that PCNA immunostaining in preoperative biopsies could be used for the prediction of occult neck metastases (Franchi et al. 1996; Liu et al. 2003; Sarac et al. 1998). PCNA expression possesses also an important prognostic value, as it is related to patients' DFS (Dong et al. 2000;

Sarac et al. 1998) and OS (Dong et al. 2000). Furthermore, T1N0M0 glottic cancer patients with low intratumoral PCNA expression should receive treatment regimens other than radiotherapy (Munck-Wikland et al. 1993). Interestingly, patients with malignant laryngeal neoplasms overexpressing both PCNA and CCNE1 had the poorest prognosis, when compared to all other LSCC cases (Dong et al. 2000). Therefore, it is evident that immunohistochemical determination of PCNA expression in LSCC could assist in the decision-making for treatment and assessment of prognosis.

BCL2 Family Members

BCL2 family members are key regulators of apoptosis. They are distinguished into antiapoptotic (e.g., *BCL2*) and proapoptotic members (e.g., *BAX*), while some BCL2 family genes are considered as double-edged swords (e.g., *BCLX*, *BCL2L12*) as they encode both antiapoptotic and proapoptotic isoforms. Immunohistochemical examination of LSCC specimens revealed that BCL2 protein expression is associated with the supraglottic location of the tumor, positive regional lymph nodes, and advanced clinical stage of the disease (Pruneri et al. 1998). On the other hand, data regarding the clinical value of BCL2 protein overexpression as a predictor of tumor resistance to radiotherapy – the therapy of choice against early-stage laryngeal tumors – are contradictory. In more detail, two previous studies have shown that high BCL2 protein levels, either alone (Condon et al. 2002) or combined with $BCLX_L$ immunopositivity, and loss of BAX expression (Nix et al. 2005) predict radiotherapy failure in LSCC, therefore also suggesting that radioresistance is due to the inhibition of apoptosis; still, Ogawa et al. argued that BCL2 protein expression assessed by IHC does not have any predictive value, despite its strong association with recurrent LSCC treated by radiotherapy (Ogawa et al. 2003). Furthermore, *BCL2L12* mRNA expression, quantified with the use of SYBR Green-based, quantitative real-time polymerase chain reaction (qRT-PCR), was shown to be lower in laryngeal tumors of advanced TNM stage than in early-stage malignant neoplasms of the larynx (Geomela et al. 2013).

Epidermal Growth Factor Receptor (EGFR) Family Members

The epidermal growth factor receptor (EGFR) is a transmembrane receptor with tyrosine kinase activity, regulating the activation of several important signaling pathways (Fig. 3). Using IHC, EGFR was shown to be overexpressed in LSCC, compared to normal mucosa (Maurizi et al. 1992; Scambia et al. 1991), and to diagnose second primary tumors; thus, EGFR expression could be used to identify LSCC patients with an increased risk of locoregional recurrence (Farhadieh et al. 2009). Moreover, EGFR levels were higher in poorly differentiated laryngeal tumors than in well- or moderately differentiated malignant neoplasms (Maurizi et al. 1992; Scambia et al. 1991). Regarding its prognostic significance in LSCC,

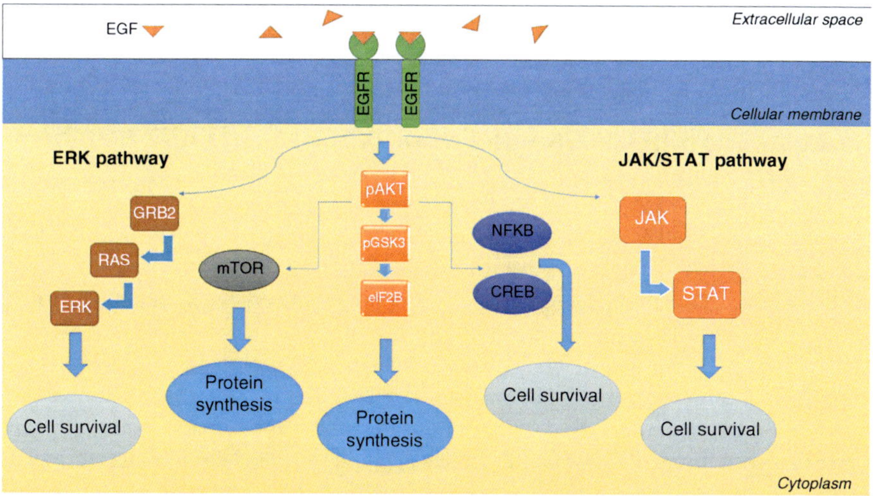

Fig. 3 Activation of the EGF receptor results in autophosphorylation of key tyrosine residues; EGFR acts then as a scaffold to bind different signaling protein molecules, thus leading to the activation of downstream signaling cascades. These pathways act cooperatively to promote cell survival

Cox univariate regression analysis demonstrated that EGFR expression, used as a continuous variable, was associated with the risk of regional metastatic recurrence. As a consequence, a positive EGFR status at the time of diagnosis is indicative of high patient susceptibility to neck node metastases and could be exploited for better decision regarding LSCC patient treatment (Almadori et al. 1999). A positive EGFR expression status ($\geq$20 fmol/mg of protein) predicts a short-term relapse and poor OS, independently of other important clinicopathological parameters, such as the depth of tumor invasion, involvement of regional lymph nodes, histological grade, tumor site, and patient age (Maurizi et al. 1992, 1996b). According to Pivot et al., EGFR determination seems to be a very strong prognosticator especially for LSCC patients treated by induction chemotherapy followed by exclusive radiotherapy (Pivot et al. 2005).

The prognostic significance of EGFR expression can be strengthened by the co-assessment of the expression of the rest of EGFR family members, namely, ERBB2 (HER2), ERBB3 (HER3), and ERBB4 (HER4). In more detail, among the patients bearing laryngeal tumors strongly expressing EGFR, those with tumors co-expressing ERBB2, ERBB3, and ERBB4 are at lower risk of regional relapse and death than those with tumors displaying a negative ERBB2/ERBB3/ERBB4 expression status (Almadori et al. 2010). Moreover, ERBB2 expression, assessed by IHC, was shown to constitute an independent predictor of locoregional recurrence in laryngopharyngeal cancer patients treated with chemoradiotherapy (Ganly et al. 2007).

Besides its emerging prognostic value, EGFR expression could be regarded as a predictive biomarker for the selection of patients who would benefit from accelerated radiotherapy with carbogen (98 % O_2; 2 % CO_2) and nicotinamide (ARCON), a treatment strategy with which high locoregional control rates are achieved, in particular for oropharynx and larynx tumors presenting low EGFR expression (Nijkamp et al. 2013).

Vascular Endothelial Growth Factor (VEGF) Subfamily Members and Their Receptors

The members of the vascular endothelial growth factor (VEGF) subfamily – namely, VEGFA, VEGFB, VEGFC, VEGFD, and placental growth factor (PGF) – constitute pivotal angiogenic effectors produced by tumor and stromal cells. Some small isoforms of the VEGF subfamily members are secreted proteins and act as diffusible agents, whereas the larger ones remain cell associated. They act by binding their receptors such as FLT1, KDR, and FLT4, which subsequently dimerize and become activated through transphosphorylation to promote angiogenesis. The formation of new blood vessels, which supports tumor growth and is considered to be a hallmark of tumor progression, is active in localized LSCC (Pentheroudakis et al. 2012). In fact, soluble VEGFA levels measured in serum using a commercially available enzyme-linked immunosorbent assay (ELISA) were significantly higher in patients with advanced laryngeal carcinoma than in healthy controls (Teknos et al. 2002). Total VEGFA expression was shown to be significantly related to tumor size, histological grade, and nodal status of LSCC patients (Sullu et al. 2010).

Regarding the prognostic significance of VEGFA, its elevated pretreatment levels in patient serum tended to indicate a more aggressive disease phenotype and a worse outcome (Teknos et al. 2002). Moreover, quantification of *VEGFA* and *FLT1* (*VEGFR1*) mRNA levels using qRT-PCR revealed an association of enhanced transcription of both genes with high tumor extent (T3 and T4) as well as their unfavorable independent prognostic value with regard to DFS (Pentheroudakis et al. 2012). High VEGFC expression detected by IHC is also an independent predictive factor of cervical lymph node relapse and short DFS in laryngopharyngeal carcinoma patients with negative regional lymph nodes at the time of surgery (Hinojar-Gutierrez et al. 2007). In addition, VEGFA immunopositivity was associated with high histological grade (Pentheroudakis et al. 2012) and predicted poor OS, independently of patient age, gender, and tumor extent (Parikh et al. 2007), similarly to high *VEGFC* and *FLT1* mRNA expression. FLT4 (VEGFR3) is another unfavorable prognosticator of OS, though not independent of the classical clinicopathological parameters of LSCC (Pentheroudakis et al. 2012).

Secreted Phosphoprotein 1 (SPP1) and Its Receptor (CD44v6)

Secreted phosphoprotein 1 (SPP1), also known as osteopontin (OPN), is a highly acidic Ca^{2+}-binding glycosylated phosphoprotein that can function either as a cell adhesion molecule or as cytokine, binding to its receptor, CD44v6.

SPP1 expression does not differ between hyperplastic and normal laryngeal tissue specimens (Staibano et al. 2007), but is significantly elevated in LSCC samples, in comparison with its expression in matched normal laryngeal mucosa carcinomas, both at the mRNA (Celetti et al. 2005) and protein levels (Celetti et al. 2005; Staibano et al. 2007). *SPP1* seems to be linked to the progression of LSCC, as its protein levels increase in parallel with the loss of differentiation of the cancerous laryngeal tissue. SPP1 expression, detected using IHC on tissue microarrays, is also higher in patients with positive lymph nodes than in those without any metastases (Lu et al. 2011). Besides its association with the histological grade and the positive nodal status of LSCC patients (Celetti et al. 2005), SPP1 immunopositivity is also related to the degree of dysplasia (Staibano et al. 2007), tumor invasion, and presence of distant metastases (Celetti et al. 2005). In accordance with all these findings, high SPP1 expression predicts poor DFS (Staibano et al. 2007).

The CD44v6 is a protein isoform of CD44, a cell surface glycoprotein that is implicated in the regulation of cell–cell and cell–matrix interactions, cell migration, tumor growth, and progression. Immunohistochemical detection of CD44v6 expression in formalin-fixed, paraffin-embedded LSCC biopsies showed that a positive CD44v6 status is associated with severe tumor invasion and positive regional lymph nodes. Additionally, it has been suggested that strong CD44v6 immunostaining in negative surgical margins could predict short DFS interval in LSCC patients (Staibano et al. 2007; Zhao et al. 2008). The predictive role of total CD44 expression with regard to locoregional recurrence has recently been highlighted by another study, in which mRNA and protein expression of this gene correlated with the probability of recurrence after radiotherapy for early-stage LSCC patients (de Jong et al. 2010).

Cathepsins and Their Endogenous Inhibitors

Cathepsins B (CTSB) and D (CTSD) are lysosomal cysteine and aspartyl proteases, respectively, distributed in almost all mammalian cells. They become activated at the low pH found in lysosomes and are heavily involved in mammalian cellular turnover. The activity of cathepsins is regulated by endogenous inhibitors, namely, cystatin A (stefin A, CSTA), cystatin B (stefin A, CSTB), and cystatin C (CST3). CSTA protein expression has been proposed as a potential diagnostic biomarker of laryngeal cancer. Immunohistochemical staining of laryngeal cancerous tissue specimens demonstrated that CSTA protein expression was inversely associated with lymphatic metastasis, LSCC recurrence, and patients' survival rate (Li et al. 2011). Lymph node metastasis in the region of the neck was also associated with CTSD protein levels (Maurizi et al. 1996a). Moreover, CSTA upregulation along with CTSB downregulation impeded in vitro the migration, invasion, and proliferation of laryngeal cancer cells. However, CTSB expression – evaluated using IHC – does not possess prognostic value in LSCC (Li et al. 2011). On the other hand, CTSD expression, determined using a solid-phase two-site

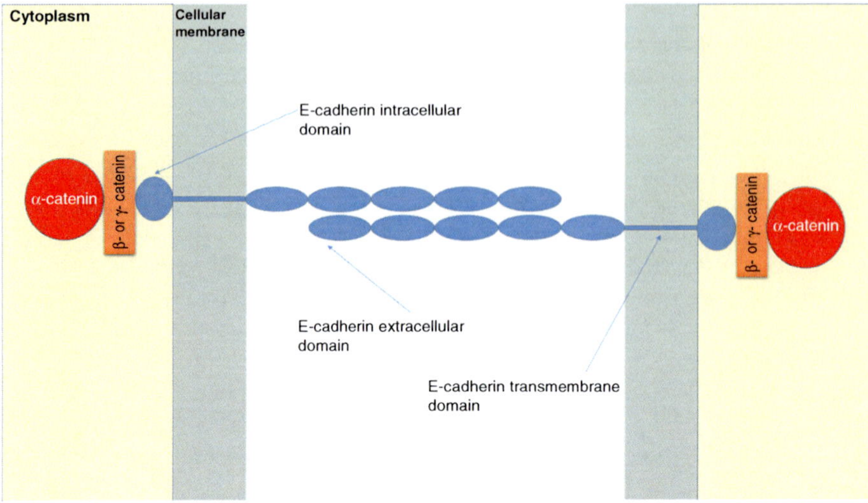

Fig. 4 E-cadherin is a transmembrane protein expressed in epithelial cells, with adhesion and signaling roles. Its extracellular domains interact in a Ca^{2+}-dependent manner to form E-cadherin homodimers between adjacent cells. The intracellular domain of E-cadherin interacts with the actin cytoskeleton via α-catenin and either β- or γ-catenin. Cadherin–catenin complexes constitute the adherens junction

immunoradiometric assay, is an independent factor for reliable prediction of short metastasis-free survival (MFS) interval and poor OS (Maurizi et al. 1996a).

E-Cadherin (ECAD; Cadherin 1, Type 1; CDH1)

E-cadherin (ECAD; officially known as cadherin 1, type 1; CDH1) is a Ca^{2+}-dependent cell–cell adhesion glycoprotein and the mostly studied member of the cadherin superfamily. Loss of E-cadherin function or expression accounts for defective cellular adhesion (Fig. 4) and increased cell motility and proliferation and is heavily implicated in cancer progression, invasion, and metastasis. As might be expected, E-cadherin constitutes a marker of epithelial–mesenchymal transition, a process leading to the acquisition of stemness by epithelial tumor cells of the head and neck (Zhang et al. 2012). Diminished E-cadherin immunopositivity in supraglottic LSCC is associated with poor differentiation of the tumor cells and high tumor extent as well as with the presence of nodal metastases. Most importantly, loss of E-cadherin expression is an independent predictor of the presence of nodal metastases in supraglottic LSCC patients (Rodrigo et al. 2002). Hence, IHC-based determination of E-cadherin expression could be applied for the identification of LSCC patients with clinically negative lymph nodes who are at considerable risk for occult metastases and who might benefit from prophylactic lymphadenectomy in the neck region (Franchi et al. 1996; Rodrigo et al. 2002).

Prostaglandin-Endoperoxide Synthase 2 (PTGS2)

Prostaglandin-endoperoxide synthase 2 (PTGS2), also known as cyclooxygenase 2 (COX2), is one the two isozymes that catalyze the biosynthesis of prostaglandin. PTGS2 regulates angiogenesis in endothelial cells and acts both as a dioxygenase and as a peroxidase. Its expression is triggered by EGFR signaling in normal human keratinocytes as well as in squamous carcinoma cells. The PTGS2 protein is overexpressed in less aggressive, low-grade LSCC specimens, whereas its expression is downregulated or even lost in tumors with poor differentiation, as shown by means of IHC and Western blot (Ranelletti et al. 2001). In pretreatment laryngeal biopsies from early-stage LSCC patients who were next subjected to single-modality radiotherapy, intense PTGS2 immunostaining was more frequent among tumors that proved to be radioresistant than among radiosensitive ones. The accuracy of prediction of radiotherapy failure in LSCC patients was 67 % (Nix et al. 2004). Moreover, loss of PTGS2 expression seems to constitute an unfavorable prognosticator in this malignancy, as it predicts a significantly higher risk for relapse and death, independently from other prognostic clinicopathological factors (Ranelletti et al. 2001). On the contrary, IHC conducted on pretreatment biopsies of patients with early-stage glottic cancer treated by radiotherapy demonstrated that PTGS2 overexpression was associated with poor OS and an increased risk of developing second primary tumors during the early follow-up period (Sackett et al. 2008).

Carbonic Anhydrase IX (CA9)

Carbonic anhydrase IX (CA9) is a transmembrane zinc metalloenzyme catalyzing the reversible hydration of carbon dioxide. It participates in various biological processes, including respiration, calcification, acid–base balance, and bone resorption, and may also be involved in cell proliferation and transformation. IHC for CA9 performed on formalin-fixed, paraffin-embedded (FFPE) samples obtained before any treatment from glottic LSCC patients who were subsequently treated with radiotherapy showed that CA9 overexpression predicts an increased risk for locoregional recurrence (Schrijvers et al. 2008). Nevertheless, a very recent study showed clearly that CA9 does not possess any prognostic significance in early-stage glottic LSCC patients who are treated with radiotherapy (Douglas et al. 2013). On the other hand, patients with advanced LSCC showing a perinecrotic CA9-immunostaining pattern had a significantly worse locoregional control as well as poor MFS and OS, in contrast with those bearing tumors with a diffuse CA9 pattern. Besides that, the same patients did not benefit from ARCON treatment, whereas MFS intervals of ARCON-treated patients with low intratumoral CA9 expression were prolonged (Rademakers et al. 2013). Therefore, further studies are needed for the better determination of the prognostic potential of this hypoxia factor in LSCC.

Parkinson Protein 7 (PARK7)

Parkinson protein 7 (PARK7; also known as DJ1), a member of the peptidase C56 family of proteins, is another potential biomarker in glottic and supraglottic LSCC. PARK7 overexpression, assessed by IHC, is more frequent in glottic and supraglottic LSCC than in its adjacent noncancerous counterparts. Furthermore, PARK7 immunopositivity was associated with the histopathologically assessed primary tumor extent and the postsurgically defined TNM stage of malignant glottic and supraglottic tumors (Zhu et al. 2010, 2012). In supraglottic LSCC, high PARK7 staining intensity was also associated with the presence of nodal metastases. This significant association could be attributed to the fact that PARK7 downregulates phosphatase and tensin homolog (PTEN), thus inducing laryngeal cancer cell proliferation and invasiveness (Zhu et al. 2012). More importantly, high PARK7 protein expression predicted poor outcome in glottic and supraglottic LSCC, independently of clinicopathological parameters (Zhu et al. 2010, 2012).

Telomerase Reverse Transcriptase (TERT)

Telomerase reverse transcriptase (TERT) is the protein component of telomerase, a ribonucleoprotein polymerase that preserves telomere ends by addition of the telomere repeat TTAGGG. This immortalizing enzyme, which also consists of an RNA component serving as a template for the telomere repeat, is heavily implicated in carcinogenesis. It has been proposed that *TERT* mRNA quantification using qRT-PCR could be applied for the molecular reevaluation of the safety margin for conservational laryngeal surgery. High *TERT* mRNA level at the laryngeal tumor edge is a significant unfavorable prognosticator in LSCC, predicting poor patient outcome (Eissa et al. 2005). Additionally, LSCC patients bearing tumors with high telomerase activity were shown to have significantly lower DFS rates than those having tumors with low telomerase activity (Swellam et al. 2008). Hence, quantification of *TERT* mRNA expression and determination of telomerase activity in LSCC might assist in better assessment of prognosis and subsequent classification of patients for treatment.

L-DOPA Decarboxylase (DDC)

L-DOPA decarboxylase (DDC) is a pyridoxal-phosphate-dependent enzyme catalyzing the synthesis of dopamine and serotonin. Analysis of *DDC* mRNA expression in primary LSCC specimens and adjacent noncancerous laryngeal tissues using qRT-PCR uncovered its significant prevalence in the malignant tumors of the larynx (Geomela et al. 2012; Patsis et al. 2012a). Moreover, receiver operating characteristic analysis showed that *DDC* mRNA expression possesses a significant diagnostic potential and suggested its further evaluation in larger cohorts of samples (Patsis et al. 2012a). *DDC* mRNA levels are inversely associated with progression of LSCC, as tumors of early TNM stage display higher *DDC* mRNA expression than advanced-stage tumors (Geomela et al. 2012; Patsis et al. 2012a). *DDC* mRNA positivity has recently been described as a novel molecular prognostic biomarker in LSCC, predicting longer DFS and OS (Patsis et al. 2012a).

Kallikrein-Related Peptidase 11 (KLK11)

Kallikrein-related peptidase 11 (KLK11) is a trypsin-like serine protease belonging to the family of the tissue kallikrein and kallikrein-related peptidases. *KLK11* mRNA expression, as assessed by qRT-PCR, was significantly lower in laryngeal cancerous specimens of primary or recurrent origin, in comparison with their nonmalignant counterparts. Furthermore, TNM stage I and II carcinomas of the larynx were more frequently *KLK11* positive, in contrast with TNM stage III or IV tumors. Patients bearing *KLK11*-positive laryngeal tumors had higher OS probabilities than those with *KLK11*-negative malignant neoplasms. Therefore, *KLK11* appears to be a promising diagnostic and/or independent prognostic biomarker in LSCC (Patsis et al. 2012b).

microRNAs (miRNAs)

microRNAs (miRNAs) are small noncoding RNA molecules of approximately 19–25 nucleotides that posttranscriptionally regulate protein-coding gene expression. miRNAs usually – albeit not exclusively – bind to the 3′ untranslated region of target mRNAs, leading to mRNA degradation and/or translational repression (Ambros 2004). In addition to the fact that these small regulatory RNAs are heavily involved in carcinogenesis, they constitute emerging biomarkers in cancer as they are stable RNA molecules than can be accurately quantified in FFPE samples and blood plasma of patients, as well.

To date, there are only a few studies investigating the diagnostic, prognostic, and predictive potential of miRNAs in LSCC. Using high-throughput qRT-PCR, Ayaz et al. have recently discovered a panel of 26 miRNAs that are differentially expressed (fold change >2) in the plasma of LSCC patients, compared to the control cohort. Out of these 26 RNA molecules, 16 miRNAs were significantly upregulated and 10 miRNAs were significantly downregulated in the plasma of LSCC patients. Interestingly, the same study demonstrated that 17 miRNAs are present exclusively in the patients' plasma (Ayaz et al. 2013). Therefore, this LSCC-specific signature of miRNAs detected in plasma could serve as noninvasive biomarkers for this malignancy. Furthermore, three miRNAs – namely, miR-155 (Zhao et al. 2013), miR-455-5p, and miR-196a (Saito et al. 2013) – were found to be aberrantly expressed in LSCC tissues. Overexpression of these three miRNAs appeared to be associated with the progression of the disease. In more detail, miR-455-5p and miR-196a levels were higher in dysplasias than in normal tissues or benign tumors of the larynx and even higher in LSCC. Besides that, miR-196a and miR-155 expression was more elevated in T3 and T4 tumors than in low invasion LSCC (T1 and T2 for miR-196a, only T2 for miR-155) (Saito et al. 2013; Zhao et al. 2013). miR-155 overexpression was also associated with histological grade, being more profound in high-grade LSCC (Zhao et al. 2013). Several miRNAs among those which are differentially expressed in LSCC patients could be combined in multiparametric panels of biomarkers with diagnostic purposes.

HOX Transcript Antisense RNA (*HOTAIR*)

HOX transcript antisense RNA (*HOTAIR*) is a long noncoding RNA (lncRNA) generated by a gene located in the homeobox C (*HOXC*) gene cluster on chromosome 12 and is co-expressed with *HOXC* genes. *HOTAIR* interacts with both polycomb repressive complex 2 and lysine-specific demethylase 1 to retarget chromatin-remodeling complexes. This intergenic lncRNA is heavily implicated in human malignancies and its clinical significance in solid tumors has just emerged. *HOTAIR* expression has recently been linked to the progression and prognosis of LSCC. *HOTAIR* levels were significantly elevated in LSCC tissue specimens compared to their adjacent noncancerous counterparts, as shown using qRT-PCR. Furthermore, *HOTAIR* overexpression was observed in laryngeal tumors with poor histological differentiation or, to a large extent, in tumors resected from patients with positive regional lymph nodes and/or those at an advanced clinical stage. Thus, high *HOTAIR* expression was shown to constitute an independent indicator of unfavorable prognosis in LSCC (Li et al. 2013).

Conclusion

The clinical value of the aforementioned molecules as putative diagnostic, prognostic, and treatment-response biomarkers in laryngeal cancer has been widely investigated during the last two decades. The elucidation of the biochemical pathways involved in laryngeal carcinogenesis, tumor progression, and metastasis, taking also into account the heterogeneity of laryngeal tumors, would absolutely assist the discovery of novel candidate biomarkers in laryngeal cancer. Moreover, some of the molecular biomarkers presented in this chapter may also have prognostic value in specific laryngeal cancer subtypes. The frequently observed dysregulation of protein and/or mRNA expression in malignant laryngeal tumors compared to benign tumors, dysplasias, or normal specimens originating from the larynx implies that some of these potential biomarkers merit further validation in independent and larger cohorts of laryngeal cancer patients.

Summary Points

- The tumor protein p53 has been extensively studied so far as a potential molecular biomarker in LSCC. Although the *TP53* gene is overexpressed in malignant laryngeal tumors, this overexpression does not seem to be associated with important clinicopathological features. Moreover, data about the potential prognostic significance of immunohistochemically detected p53 expression in laryngeal cancer are conflicting.
- High protein expression levels of several cyclins, a group of important cell cycle regulators which determine the activity of cyclin-dependent kinases, predict short-term relapse and poor overall survival in LSCC. On the other hand, expression of major cyclin-dependent kinase inhibitors is a favorable prognosticator in this malignancy.
- Marker of proliferation Ki-67 could serve as a biomarker for the selection of these LSCC patients who are more likely to benefit from elective neck dissection, as its expression constitutes a reliable predictor of the existence of occult neck metastases.
- PCNA expression is associated with tumor histological grade, lymphatic and vascular invasion, depth of tumor margins, neck metastasis, and locoregional recurrence of laryngeal cancer. Its assessment in preoperative biopsies could be applied for the prediction of occult neck metastases.
- Co-expression of the antiapoptotic BCL2 and $BCLX_L$ proteins along with reduced expression of the proapoptotic BAX protein predicts radiotherapy failure in LSCC and suggests that inhibition of apoptosis accounts for radioresistance.
- EGFR expression appears a very reliable prognosticator, especially for LSCC patients treated by induction chemotherapy followed by exclusive radiotherapy. The prognostic value of EGFR expression can be strengthened by immunohistochemical co-assessment of the expression of ERBB2 (HER2), ERBB3 (HER3), and ERBB4 (HER4).
- The quantification of *VEGFA* and *FLT1* (*VEGFR1*) mRNA expression levels using qRT-PCR uncovered the unfavorable prognostic value of these two key players of angiogenesis, with regard to the DFS of laryngeal cancer patients. This prognostic significance is independent from the prognostic factors that are currently used in clinical practice.
- The expression of cathepsin D, quantified using a solid-phase two-site immunoradiometric assay, is a strong independent predictor of short MFS interval and poor OS.
- Positive immunostaining against E-cadherin could be used for the selection of those LSCC patients with clinically negative lymph nodes who are at risk for occult metastases and who might benefit from prophylactic lymphadenectomy in the neck region.
- Noncoding RNAs, including miRNAs (e.g., miR-155, miR-455-5p, and miR-196a) and lncRNAs (e.g., HOTAIR), are emerging biomarkers in laryngeal cancer. miRNAs that are differentially expressed in LSCC patients could be

exploited by multiparametric panels of biomarkers for the early detection of laryngeal cancer. Furthermore, *HOTAIR* expression has recently been linked to the progression and prognosis of this malignancy.

References

Almadori G, Cadoni G, Galli J, et al. Epidermal growth factor receptor expression in primary laryngeal cancer: an independent prognostic factor of neck node relapse. Int J Cancer. 1999;84:188–91.

Almadori G, Bussu F, Gessi M, et al. Prognostic significance and clinical relevance of the expression of the HER family of type I receptor tyrosine kinases in human laryngeal squamous cell carcinoma. Eur J Cancer. 2010;46:1144–52.

Ambros V. The functions of animal microRNAs. Nature. 2004;431:350–5.

Argiris A, Karamouzis MV, Raben D, Ferris RL. Head and neck cancer. Lancet. 2008;371:1695–709.

Ayaz L, Gorur A, Yaroglu HY, Ozcan C, Tamer L. Differential expression of microRNAs in plasma of patients with laryngeal squamous cell carcinoma: potential early-detection markers for laryngeal squamous cell carcinoma. J Cancer Res Clin Oncol. 2013;139:1499–506.

Bellacosa A, Almadori G, Cavallo S, et al. Cyclin D1 gene amplification in human laryngeal squamous cell carcinomas: prognostic significance and clinical implications. Clin Cancer Res. 1996;2:175–80.

Celetti A, Testa D, Staibano S, et al. Overexpression of the cytokine osteopontin identifies aggressive laryngeal squamous cell carcinomas and enhances carcinoma cell proliferation and invasiveness. Clin Cancer Res. 2005;11:8019–27.

Chernock RD, Wang X, Gao G, et al. Detection and significance of human papillomavirus, CDKN2A(p16) and CDKN1A(p21) expression in squamous cell carcinoma of the larynx. Mod Pathol. 2013;26:223–31.

Chin D, Boyle GM, Porceddu S, Theile DR, Parsons PG, Coman WB. Head and neck cancer: past, present and future. Expert Rev Anticancer Ther. 2006;6:1111–8.

Condon LT, Ashman JN, Ell SR, Stafford ND, Greenman J, Cawkwell L. Overexpression of Bcl-2 in squamous cell carcinoma of the larynx: a marker of radioresistance. Int J Cancer. 2002;100:472–5.

de Jong MC, Pramana J, van der Wal JE, et al. CD44 expression predicts local recurrence after radiotherapy in larynx cancer. Clin Cancer Res. 2010;16:5329–38.

Dolcetti R, Doglioni C, Maestro R, et al. p53 over-expression is an early event in the development of human squamous-cell carcinoma of the larynx: genetic and prognostic implications. Int J Cancer. 1992;52:178–82.

Dong Y, Sui L, Tai Y, Sugimoto K, Hirao T, Tokuda M. Prognostic significance of cyclin E overexpression in laryngeal squamous cell carcinomas. Clin Cancer Res. 2000;6:4253–8.

Dong Y, Sui L, Sugimoto K, Tai Y, Tokuda M. Cyclin D1-CDK4 complex, a possible critical factor for cell proliferation and prognosis in laryngeal squamous cell carcinomas. Int J Cancer. 2001;95:209–15.

Dong Y, Sui L, Watanabe Y, Sugimoto K, Tokuda M. Clinical relevance of cyclin B1 overexpression in laryngeal squamous cell carcinoma. Cancer Lett. 2002;177:13–9.

Douglas CM, Bernstein JM, Ormston VE, et al. Lack of prognostic effect of carbonic anhydrase-9, hypoxia inducible factor-1alpha and bcl-2 in 286 patients with early squamous cell carcinoma of the glottic larynx treated with radiotherapy. Clin Oncol (R Coll Radiol). 2013;25:59–65.

Eissa S, Kenawy G, Moteleb FA, El-Makhzangyc AN, Nassar M. Real-time PCR hTERT mRNA pattern in tumor core, edge, resection margin, and lymph nodes in laryngeal tumors: relation to proliferative index and impact on prognosis. Clin Biochem. 2005;38:873–8.

Farhadieh RD, Salardini A, Rees CG, Russell PJ, Yang JL, Smee R. Protein expression of epidermal growth factor receptor in laryngeal squamous cell carcinoma index tumors correlates with diagnosis of second primary tumors of the upper aero-digestive tract. Ann Surg Oncol. 2009;16:2888–94.

Ferlay J, Shin HR, Bray F, Forman D, Mathers C, Parkin DM. Estimates of worldwide burden of cancer in 2008: GLOBOCAN 2008. Int J Cancer. 2010;127:2893–917.

Franchi A, Gallo O, Boddi V, Santucci M. Prediction of occult neck metastases in laryngeal carcinoma: role of proliferating cell nuclear antigen, MIB-1, and E-cadherin immunohistochemical determination. Clin Cancer Res. 1996;2:1801–8.

Ganly I, Talbot S, Carlson D, et al. Identification of angiogenesis/metastases genes predicting chemoradiotherapy response in patients with laryngopharyngeal carcinoma. J Clin Oncol. 2007;25:1369–76.

Geomela PA, Kontos CK, Yiotakis I, Fragoulis EG, Scorilas A. L-DOPA decarboxylase mRNA expression is associated with tumor stage and size in head and neck squamous cell carcinoma: a retrospective cohort study. BMC Cancer. 2012;12:484.

Geomela PA, Kontos CK, Yiotakis I, Scorilas A. Quantitative expression analysis of the apoptosis-related gene, BCL2L12, in head and neck squamous cell carcinoma. J Oral Pathol Med. 2013;42:154–61.

Hinojar-Gutierrez A, Fernandez-Contreras ME, Gonzalez-Gonzalez R, et al. Intratumoral lymphatic vessels and VEGF-C expression are predictive factors of lymph node relapse in T1-T4 N0 laryngopharyngeal squamous cell carcinoma. Ann Surg Oncol. 2007;14:248–57.

Hirvikoski P, Kumpulainen E, Virtaniemi J, et al. p53 expression and cell proliferation as prognostic factors in laryngeal squamous cell carcinoma. J Clin Oncol. 1997;15:3111–20.

Jares P, Fernandez PL, Campo E, et al. PRAD-1/cyclin D1 gene amplification correlates with messenger RNA overexpression and tumor progression in human laryngeal carcinomas. Cancer Res. 1994;54:4813–7.

Jin YT, Kayser S, Kemp BL, et al. The prognostic significance of the biomarkers p21WAF1/CIP1, p53, and bcl-2 in laryngeal squamous cell carcinoma. Cancer. 1998;82:2159–65.

Kokoska MS, Piccirillo JF, el-Mofty SK, Emami B, Haughey BH, Schoinick SB. Prognostic significance of clinical factors and p53 expression in patients with glottic carcinoma treated with radiation therapy. Cancer. 1996;78:1693–700.

Li C, Chen L, Wang J, et al. Expression and clinical significance of cathepsin B and stefin A in laryngeal cancer. Oncol Rep. 2011;26:869–75.

Li D, Feng J, Wu T, et al. Long intergenic noncoding RNA HOTAIR is overexpressed and regulates PTEN methylation in laryngeal squamous cell carcinoma. Am J Pathol. 2013;182:64–70.

Liu M, Lawson G, Delos M, et al. Predictive value of the fraction of cancer cells immunolabeled for proliferating cell nuclear antigen or Ki67 in biopsies of head and neck carcinomas to identify lymph node metastasis: comparison with clinical and radiologic examinations. Head Neck. 2003;25:280–8.

Lu JG, Li Y, Li L, Kan X. Overexpression of osteopontin and integrin alphav in laryngeal and hypopharyngeal carcinomas associated with differentiation and metastasis. J Cancer Res Clin Oncol. 2011;137:1613–8.

Maurizi M, Scambia G, Benedetti Panici P, et al. EGF receptor expression in primary laryngeal cancer: correlation with clinico-pathological features and prognostic significance. Int J Cancer. 1992;52:862–6.

Maurizi M, Almadori G, Cadoni G, et al. Cathepsin D concentration in primary laryngeal cancer: correlation with clinico-pathological parameters, EGFR status and prognosis. Int J Cancer. 1996a;69:105–9.

Maurizi M, Almadori G, Ferrandina G, et al. Prognostic significance of epidermal growth factor receptor in laryngeal squamous cell carcinoma. Br J Cancer. 1996b;74:1253–7.

Munck-Wikland E, Fernberg JO, Kuylenstierna R, Lindholm J, Auer G. Proliferating cell nuclear antigen (PCNA) expression and nuclear DNA content in predicting recurrence after radiotherapy of early glottic cancer. Eur J Cancer B Oral Oncol. 1993;29b:75–9.

Nadal A, Campo E, Pinto J, et al. p53 expression in normal, dysplastic, and neoplastic laryngeal epithelium. Absence of a correlation with prognostic factors. J Pathol. 1995;175: 181–8.

Narayana A, Vaughan AT, Gunaratne S, Kathuria S, Walter SA, Reddy SP. Is p53 an independent prognostic factor in patients with laryngeal carcinoma? Cancer. 1998;82:286–91.

Narayana A, Vaughan AT, Kathuria S, Fisher SG, Walter SA, Reddy SP. P53 overexpression is associated with bulky tumor and poor local control in T1 glottic cancer. Int J Radiat Oncol Biol Phys. 2000;46:21–6.

Nathan CO, Sanders K, Abreo FW, Nassar R, Glass J. Correlation of p53 and the proto-oncogene eIF4E in larynx cancers: prognostic implications. Cancer Res. 2000;60:3599–604.

Nijkamp MM, Span PN, Terhaard CH, et al. Epidermal growth factor receptor expression in laryngeal cancer predicts the effect of hypoxia modification as an additive to accelerated radiotherapy in a randomised controlled trial. Eur J Cancer. 2013;49:3202–9.

Nix P, Lind M, Greenman J, Stafford N, Cawkwell L. Expression of Cox-2 protein in radioresistant laryngeal cancer. Ann Oncol. 2004;15:797–801.

Nix P, Cawkwell L, Patmore H, Greenman J, Stafford N. Bcl-2 expression predicts radiotherapy failure in laryngeal cancer. Br J Cancer. 2005;92:2185–9.

Ogawa T, Shiga K, Tateda M, et al. Protein expression of p53 and Bcl-2 has a strong correlation with radiation resistance of laryngeal squamous cell carcinoma but does not predict the radiation failure before treatment. Oncol Rep. 2003;10:1461–6.

Osman I, Sherman E, Singh B, et al. Alteration of p53 pathway in squamous cell carcinoma of the head and neck: impact on treatment outcome in patients treated with larynx preservation intent. J Clin Oncol. 2002;20:2980–7.

Parikh RR, Yang Q, Haffty BG. Prognostic significance of vascular endothelial growth factor protein levels in T1-2 N0 laryngeal cancer treated with primary radiation therapy. Cancer. 2007;109:566–73.

Patsis C, Glyka V, Yiotakis I, Fragoulis EG, Scorilas A. l-DOPA Decarboxylase (DDC) expression status as a novel molecular tumor marker for diagnostic and prognostic purposes in laryngeal cancer. Transl Oncol. 2012a;5:288–96.

Patsis C, Yiotakis I, Scorilas A. Diagnostic and prognostic significance of human kallikrein 11 (KLK11) mRNA expression levels in patients with laryngeal cancer. Clin Biochem. 2012b;45:623–30.

Pentheroudakis G, Nicolaou I, Kotoula V, et al. Prognostic utility of angiogenesis and hypoxia effectors in patients with operable squamous cell cancer of the larynx. Oral Oncol. 2012;48:709–16.

Pignataro L, Pruneri G, Carboni N, et al. Clinical relevance of cyclin D1 protein overexpression in laryngeal squamous cell carcinoma. J Clin Oncol. 1998;16:3069–77.

Pivot X, Magne N, Guardiola E, et al. Prognostic impact of the epidermal growth factor receptor levels for patients with larynx and hypopharynx cancer. Oral Oncol. 2005;41:320–7.

Pruneri G, Pignataro L, Carboni N, et al. Clinical relevance of p53 and bcl-2 protein over-expression in laryngeal squamous-cell carcinoma. Int J Cancer. 1998;79:263–8.

Pruneri G, Pignataro L, Carboni N, et al. Clinical relevance of expression of the CIP/KIP cell-cycle inhibitors p21 and p27 in laryngeal cancer. J Clin Oncol. 1999;17:3150–9.

Pruneri G, Pignataro L, Valentini S, et al. Cyclin D3 immunoreactivity is an independent predictor of survival in laryngeal squamous cell carcinoma. Clin Cancer Res. 2005;11:242–8.

Rademakers SE, Hoogsteen IJ, Rijken PF, et al. Pattern of CAIX expression is prognostic for outcome and predicts response to ARCON in patients with laryngeal cancer treated in a phase III randomized trial. Radiother Oncol. 2013;108:517–22.

Ranelletti FO, Almadori G, Rocca B, et al. Prognostic significance of cyclooxygenase-2 in laryngeal squamous cell carcinoma. Int J Cancer. 2001;95:343–9.

Rodrigo JP, Dominguez F, Alvarez C, Manrique C, Herrero A, Suarez C. Expression of E-cadherin in squamous cell carcinomas of the supraglottic larynx with correlations to clinicopathological features. Eur J Cancer. 2002;38:1059–64.

Saarilahti K, Kajanti M, Kouri M, Aaltonen LM, Franssila K, Joensuu H. Cyclin A and Ki-67 expression as predictors for locoregional recurrence and outcome in laryngeal cancer patients treated with surgery and postoperative radiotherapy. Int J Radiat Oncol Biol Phys. 2003;57:986–95.

Sackett MK, Bairati I, Meyer F, et al. Prognostic significance of cyclooxygenase-2 overexpression in glottic cancer. Clin Cancer Res. 2008;14:67–73.

Saito K, Inagaki K, Kamimoto T, et al. MicroRNA-196a is a putative diagnostic biomarker and therapeutic target for laryngeal cancer. PLoS One. 2013;8:e71480.

Salerno G, Di Vizio D, Staibano S, et al. Prognostic value of p27Kip1 expression in basaloid squamous cell carcinoma of the larynx. BMC Cancer. 2006;6:146.

Sarac S, Ayhan A, Hosal AS, Kaya S. Prognostic significance of PCNA expression in laryngeal cancer. Arch Otolaryngol Head Neck Surg. 1998;124:1321–4.

Scambia G, Panici PB, Battaglia F, et al. Receptors for epidermal growth factor and steroid hormones in primary laryngeal tumors. Cancer. 1991;67:1347–51.

Schrijvers ML, van der Laan BF, de Bock GH, et al. Overexpression of intrinsic hypoxia markers HIF1alpha and CA-IX predict for local recurrence in stage T1-T2 glottic laryngeal carcinoma treated with radiotherapy. Int J Radiat Oncol Biol Phys. 2008;72:161–9.

Staibano S, Merolla F, Testa D, et al. OPN/CD44v6 overexpression in laryngeal dysplasia and correlation with clinical outcome. Br J Cancer. 2007;97:1545–51.

Sullu Y, Gun S, Atmaca S, Karagoz F, Kandemir B. Poor prognostic clinicopathologic features correlate with VEGF expression but not with PTEN expression in squamous cell carcinoma of the larynx. Diagn Pathol. 2010;5:35.

Swellam M, El-Arab LR, Adly A. Prognostic value of cell-cycle regulators and cellular biomarkers in laryngeal squamous cell carcinoma. Clin Biochem. 2008;41:1059–66.

Tan LK, Ogden GR. p53 over-expression in laryngeal carcinoma is not predictive of response to radiotherapy. Oral Oncol. 1997;33:177–81.

Teknos TN, Cox C, Yoo S, et al. Elevated serum vascular endothelial growth factor and decreased survival in advanced laryngeal carcinoma. Head Neck. 2002;24:1004–11.

Tomasino R, Morello V, Bazan V, et al. P53 expression in stage iii-iv squamous-cell carcinoma of the larynx – an immunohistochemical study related to clinicopathological, flow-cytometric DNA analysis and prognosis. Int J Oncol. 1994;5:495–500.

Zhang Z, Filho MS, Nor JE. The biology of head and neck cancer stem cells. Oral Oncol. 2012;48:1–9.

Zhao H, Ren J, Zhuo X, Ye H, Zou J, Liu S. Prognostic significance of Survivin and CD44v6 in laryngeal cancer surgical margins. J Cancer Res Clin Oncol. 2008;134:1051–8.

Zhao XD, Zhang W, Liang HJ, Ji WY. Overexpression of miR −155 promotes proliferation and invasion of human laryngeal squamous cell carcinoma via targeting SOCS1 and STAT3. PLoS One. 2013;8:e56395.

Zhu XL, Wang ZF, Lei WB, Zhuang HW, Jiang HY, Wen WP. DJ-1: a novel independent prognostic marker for survival in glottic squamous cell carcinoma. Cancer Sci. 2010;101:1320–5.

Zhu XL, Wang ZF, Lei WB, et al. Tumorigenesis role and clinical significance of DJ-1, a negative regulator of PTEN, in supraglottic squamous cell carcinoma. J Exp Clin Cancer Res. 2012;31:94.

Nuclear BMI-1 as a Biomarker in Laryngeal Cancer

41

Eugenia Allegra and Serena Trapasso

Contents

Abstract

The main cause of treatment failure and death in laryngeal squamous cell carcinoma is metastasis to the regional lymph nodes. The current clinical staging criteria fail to differentiate patients with occult metastasis from patients without metastasis. Identifying molecular markers of the disease might improve our understanding of the molecular mechanisms underlying the pathogenesis and development of laryngeal carcinoma and may help improve clinical staging and treatment.

Emerging studies show BMI1 has an important function as a biomarker of cancer stem cells (CSCs), which are cells with self-renewal characteristics and capable of initiation, progression, invasion, metastasis, tumor recurrence, and resistance to chemotherapy and radiotherapy. There are increasing studies that consider the role of CSCs in head and neck cancers and the potential result of this knowledge on clinical-surgical outcome. A promising intracellular marker of

E. Allegra (✉) • S. Trapasso
Otolaryngology-Head and Neck Surgery, Department of Medical and Surgical Sciences, University Magna Graecia of Catanzaro, Catanzaro, Italy
e-mail: eualle@unicz.it; dr.serena.trapasso@gmail.com

V.R. Preedy, V.B. Patel (eds.), *Biomarkers in Cancer, Biomarkers in Disease: Methods, Discoveries and Applications*,
DOI 10.1007/978-94-007-7681-4_15

CSCs in head and neck cancer is the oncoprotein BMI1, with specific data about its prognostic value based on the specific location. More precisely, the nuclear expression of BMI1 in patients with laryngeal carcinoma seems to correlate with lymph node metastasis.

List of Abbreviations

BMI1	B-Cell-Specific moloney Murine Leukemia Virus Integration site 1
BTRC	Beta-Transducin Repeat Containing
cBMI1	Cytoplasmatic B-Cell-Specific Moloney Murine Leukemia Virus Integration Site 1
CSCs	Cancer Stem Cells
EMT	Epithelial-Mesenchymal Transition
HTH	Helix-Turn-Helix
LSCC	Laryngeal Squamous Cell Carcinoma
nBMI1	Nuclear B-Cell-Specific Moloney Murine Leukemia Virus Integration Site 1
PcG	Polycomb Group
PRC1	Polycomb-Repressive Complex 1
PRC2	Polycomb-Repressive Complex 2
PSC	Posterior Sex Control
RF	Ring Finger
TERT	Telomerase Reverse Transcriptase

Key Facts

(A) The prognosis for laryngeal squamous cell carcinoma (LSCC) has not shown any improvement in the last 30 years because of inadequate prognostic stratification.

(B) In LSCC, the evidence seems to indicate that BMI1 overexpression correlates with a greater capacity of cell proliferation and tumor progression, and more importantly, BMI1 suppresses the sensitivity of laryngeal tumor cells to radiotherapy with negative prognostic significance.

(C) The high expression of BMI1 in laryngeal tumors seems to correlate more prominently with a poor prognosis because of higher capacity of metastasis (locoregional and distant) and resistance to radiochemotherapy treatments.

(D) The expression of nuclear BMI1 (nBMI1) (immunohistochemical determination) correlates significantly with the pN status of the primary tumors, while the high cytoplasmatic BMI1 (cBMI1) expression correlates significantly with distant metastasis.

(E) The expression of BMI1 in patients with laryngeal carcinoma seems to be a potential marker of tumor aggressiveness.

Definition of Words and Terms

Laryngeal Cancer Tumors of the larynx are common in southern Europe. The crucial factor in laryngeal carcinogenesis is tobacco, often associated with alcohol abuse. Even some occupational exposures appear to be indicted in the appearance of these tumors. Despite some early signs, a large number of laryngeal tumors, in particular supraglottic, are diagnosed at a relatively advanced stage of disease. The evaluation of the extension is based on the endoscopic evaluation and on diagnostic imaging quality sections. There are multiple surgical techniques that allow partial and radical excision of adapting to all kinds of local extension. The endoscopic laser surgery has gained a place in the treatment of laryngeal tumors. The transcutaneous radiotherapy is an alternative for tumors very limited and vegetating; its place in the treatment of more advanced forms has evolved with the emergence of new methods and techniques with the combination of chemotherapy, especially in laryngeal preservation strategies. Healing depends on the location and extent of the tumor and the general condition of health. Overall, the 5-year survival from diagnosis is approximately 60 %, ranging between 90 % and 95 % in patients with limited tumors, and it is 19 % in patients with metastatic disease.

Cancer Stem Cells Many studies in recent years have shown that some forms of cancer are characterized by the presence of specific cells with stem-like properties, also called cancer stem cells (CSCs). These cells are considered the cells "that start" the tumor, and they probably are responsible for the recurrence of the tumor. CSCs have the ability to self-renew, the potential to give rise to one or more cell types within the tumor, and the ability to drive, in a continuous manner, the proliferation of malignant cells. Many studies have described the tumorigenic potential of CSCs with formulation of the cancer stem cell (CSC) hypothesis, according to which, to support the tumor growth and cause relapses, it would be a restricted cell population.

Introduction

BMI1 (B-cell-specific Moloney murine leukemia virus integration site 1) is a member of polycomb-repressive complex 1 (PRC1), which maintains chromatin silencing (Gil et al. 2005). Emerging studies show BMI1 has an important function as a biomarker of cancer stem cells (CSCs), which are tumor cells responsible for the origin, progression, metastasis, and cancer resistance to chemotherapy and radiotherapy (Trapasso and Allegra 2012). The main characteristics of CSCs are the ability of self-renewal, duplication, differentiation, tumorigenesis, and influence on cell homeostatic control (tumoral and peritumoral – creation of the "niche" and maintaining the so-called side population); they would determine the biological behavior of the tumor, propensity to relapse/recurrence, and metastasis (Allegra et al. 2013). Moreover, CSCs would possess transmembrane transporters involved in resistance to chemotherapy (by transporting the chemotherapy out of the cell and preventing the therapeutic action), and they have developed repair mechanisms for oxidative stress with ineffectiveness of radian treatments (Allegra et al. 2006).

The early identification of the pool of CSCs by the use of specific markers may constitute as an effective method for early detection, and the identification of antigenic markers revealing metastatic ability and resistance to chemoradiotherapy could be useful for the prognostic framework (Allegra et al. 2012a, b).

Increasing evidence suggests that the polycomb group (PcG) proteins play a major role in the initiation, progression, and recurrence of cancer. The PcG proteins are chromatin modifiers involved in the maintenance of embryonic and adult stem cells and cancer formation (Valk-Lingbeek et al. 2004). PcG proteins are multimeric transcriptional repressor complexes including polycomb-repressive complex 1 (PRC1) and polycomb-repressive complex 2 (PRC2). PcG proteins can occupy the promoters of developmental regulators, and silencing of these genes confers stemness in a PcG-dependent manner (Gil et al. 2005). In addition, deregulation of PcG gene expression leads to cell proliferation and tumor progression (Satijn and Otte 1999).

BMI1 (B-Cell-Specific Moloney Murine Leukemia Virus Integration Site 1)

The BMI1 gene, a member of the PcG proteins, was first isolated as an oncogene that cooperates with c-myc in the oncogenesis of murine lymphomas (Haupt et al. 1991). BMI1 was shown to be necessary to maintain normal and leukemic hematopoietic stem cells and was essential in the lineage specification and multipotency of hematopoietic stem and progenitor cells (Lessar and Sauvageau 2003). It functions as a transcriptional repressor through chromatin modification and plays a role in axial patterning, cell cycle regulation, hematopoiesis, and senescence (Jacobs et al. 1999a, b).

Through chromatin and histone modifications, BMI1 controls the cell cycle and self-renewal of tissue stem cells: it influences the central tumor suppressors Rb and p53 by suppressing the *INK4a* locus, which encodes the tumor suppressors p16 and $p14^{ARF}$ (Pardal et al. 2005; Itahana et al. 2003) (Fig. 1).

BMI1 is an intracellular oncoprotein with an N-terminal ring-finger (RF) domain, required for the activation of telomerase reverse transcriptase (TERT) transcription and immortalization of epithelial cells; a functional recognition motif for the F box protein BTRC (beta-transducin repeat containing), which regulates ubiquitination and proteasome-mediated degradation of various proteins; a C-terminal HTH (helix-turn-helix) domain, also required for the activation of TERT transcription and immortalization of epithelial cells; two highly conserved BMI1-binding motifs, which were required for BMI1-mediated CDKN2A promoter

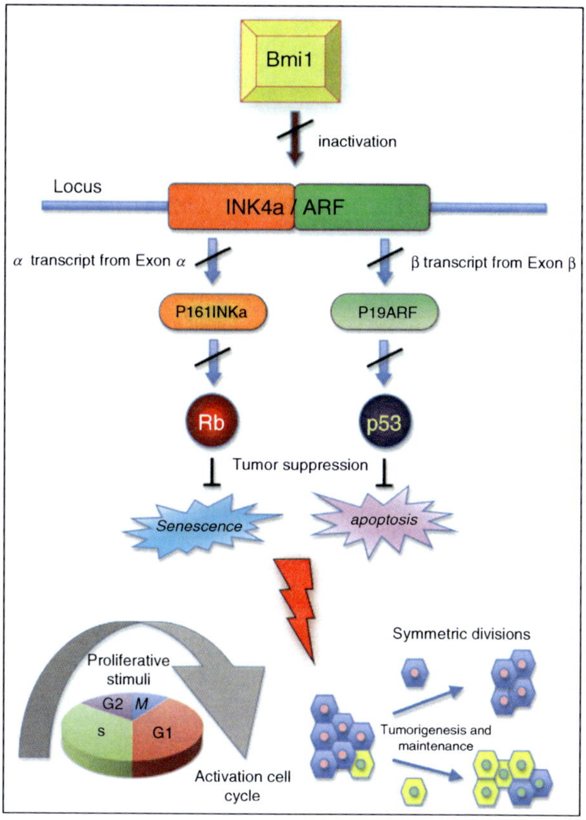

Fig. 1 Schematic representation of the consequences of BMI1 dysregulation for cell cycle activation and tumorigenesis (From Allegra E, Trapasso S, Pisani D, Puzzo L. The Role of BMI1 as a Biomarker of Cancer Stem Cells in Head and Neck Cancer: A Review. Oncology. 2014;86:199–205, with permission)

regulation; and a domain of homology to *Drosophila* posterior sex control (PSC) (Meng et al. 2010; Sahasrabuddhe et al. 2011).

Principal functions of BMI1 are as follows:

1. Senescence regulator, involved in maintaining the transcriptionally repressive state of genes
2. Essential role for the generation of self-renewing adult hematopoietic stem cells and in the maintenance and expansion of immature granule cell precursors
3. Incorporates DMAP1 in polycomb gene silencing
4. Cooperates with FOXG1 to maintain neural stem cell self-renewal (Fasano et al. 2009)
5. Necessary for optimal proliferation of CD8-positive T cells (Heffner and Fearon 2007)
6. Activating NFKappaB through stimulation of IKappaB phosphorylation

BMI1 has important connections with the transcription factor c-myc, which affects cell proliferation and apoptosis: both BMI1 and c-myc are capable of immortalizing certain cells in vitro, and these factors converge on the same pathways as c-myc signaling can influence BMI1 activity and vice versa (Sahasrabuddhe et al. 2011). C-myc is also assumed to participate in oral carcinogenesis, and downregulation of c-myc mRNA has even been associated with poor prognosis (Häyry et al. 2010).

BMI1 also cooperates with Snail, a zinc-finger transcription factor essential for epithelial-mesenchymal transition (EMT) because it downregulates the expression of cell adhesion and basement membrane proteins, most importantly cadherins (Kang et al. 2007). Snail expression in the invasive tumor front seems to correlate with lymph node metastases and with the clinicopathological tumor stage (Koehn et al. 2008).

BMI1 is regulated by TWIST1 in a direct manner, with functional interdependence, and it is involved in promoting EMT and in the tumor-initiating capability of head and neck cancer cells (Yang et al. 2010a).

Thus, BMI1 plays an essential role in maintaining the self-renewal of normal and malignant stem cells (Liu et al. 2006). Meanwhile, aberrant BMI1 expression has been associated with many solid malignancies (Lu et al. 2012; Saeki et al. 2009; Yang et al. 2010b; Qin et al. 2009; Song et al. 2006; Vrzalikova et al. 2008). Chen et al. reported a higher expression of BMI1 in laryngeal carcinomas (Chen et al. 2011b). As already mentioned, BMI1 has also been reported to be overexpressed in cell immortalization and in EMT of cancer cells (Wu and Yang 2011).

Currently, researchers continue to study, but with conflicting results at times, the biological characterization of the oncoprotein BMI1, with others, as a marker of CSCs; however, there are still certain data about their clinical applicability (Allegra et al. 2014).

Clinical Studies and Potential Applications to Prognosis

Currently, there are few studies about the expression of oncoprotein BMI1 in head and neck cancer.

The prognosis for laryngeal squamous cell carcinoma (LSCC) has not shown any improvement in the last 30 years because of inadequate prognostic stratification. In LSCC, the evidence seems to indicate that BMI1 overexpression correlates with a greater capacity of cell proliferation and tumor progression, and more importantly, BMI1 suppresses the sensitivity of laryngeal tumor cells to radiotherapy with negative prognostic significance (Allegra et al. 2014). Chen et al. have confirmed with other studies that BMI1 correlates with laryngeal carcinoma and with the maintenance of the proliferative capacity of laryngeal CSCs (Chen et al. 2011a). The high expression of BMI1 in laryngeal tumors seems to correlate more prominently with a poor prognosis because of higher capacity of metastasis (locoregional and distant) and resistance to radiochemotherapy treatments (Allegra et al. 2014).

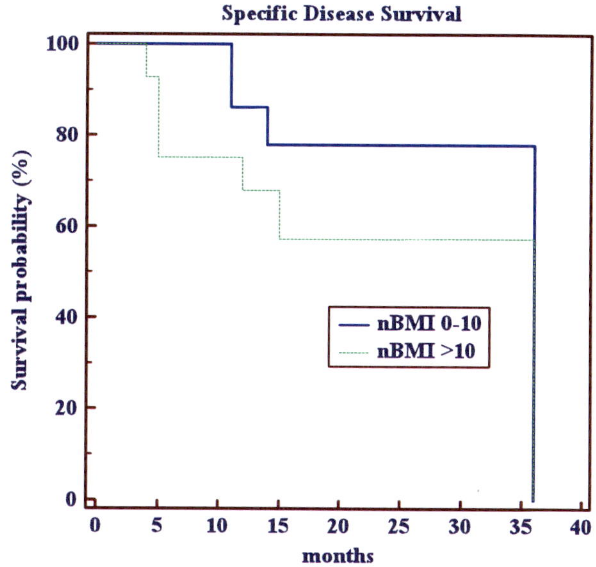

Fig. 2 The 3-year specific survival in the cohort of patients expressing negative or low level of nBMI compared to patients with high expression of nBMI ($p = 0.058$) (From Allegra E, Puzzo L, Zuccalà V, Trapasso S, Vasquez E, Garozzo A, Caltabiano R. Nuclear BMI1 expression in laryngeal carcinoma correlates with lymph node pathological status. World J Surg Oncol 2012;10:206, with permission)

In fact, lymph node metastasis represents the most adverse clinical prognostic factor; it decreases the overall survival approximately 50 %. Actually, neck treatment, performed considering primary tumor localization and T and N classification, has improved regional control and time even if clinical determination of lymph node metastasis made by palpation and CT and MRI imaging reveals a sensitivity ranging 38–78 % for occult metastatic lymph node (Sten et al. 1991; Yucel et al. 1997) and the probability of metastatic lymph nodes in patients classified as N0 ranging 7–37 % (Kirchner and Carter 2004). Immunohistochemical and molecular prognostic markers should be useful to identify at diagnosis patients with occult metastasis to improve the modality of treatment (Almadori et al. 2005). The metastatic potential identified by BMI1 has been recognized in previous studies, with significant results for clinical outcome; in fact, in laryngeal cancers, it was demonstrated that BMI1 expression, in the absence of p16 expression, seems to characterize a subset of patients with a high risk of developing lymph node metastasis. More precisely, the expression of nuclear BMI1 (nBMI1) (immunohistochemical determination) correlates significantly with the pN status of the primary tumors, while high cytoplasmatic BMI1 (cBMI1) expression correlates significantly with distant metastasis (Allegra et al. 2012b, 2013). The expression of BMI1 in patients with laryngeal carcinoma seems to be a potential marker of tumor aggressiveness (Allegra et al. 2014). A high nBMI1 expression may detect lymph node metastasis at diagnosis and can be useful in a subset of patients with to decide on neck treatment (Fig. 2).

However, further and larger studies are needed to confirm these results.

Summary Points

1. BMI1 (B-cell-specific Moloney murine leukemia virus integration site 1) is a member of polycomb-repressive complex 1 (PRC1), which maintains chromatin silencing.
2. BMI1 functions as a transcriptional repressor through chromatin modification and plays a role in axial patterning, cell cycle regulation, hematopoiesis, and senescence.
3. BMI1 has an important function as a biomarker of cancer stem cells (CSCs), which are cells with self-renewal characteristics and capable of initiation, progression, invasion, metastasis, tumor recurrence, and resistance to chemotherapy and radiotherapy.
4. BMI1 plays an essential role in maintaining the self-renewal of normal and malignant stem cells. Meanwhile, aberrant BMI1 expression has been associated with many solid malignancies.
5. The high expression of BMI1 in laryngeal tumors seems to correlate more prominently with a poor prognosis because of higher capacity of metastasis (locoregional and distant) and resistance to radiochemotherapy treatments.
6. The expression of nuclear BMI1 (nBMI1) (immunohistochemical determination) correlates significantly with the pN status of the primary tumors.
7. High cytoplasmatic BMI1 (cBMI1) expression (immunohistochemical determination) correlates significantly with distant metastasis.
8. The expression of BMI1 in patients with laryngeal carcinoma seems to be a potential marker of tumor aggressiveness.

References

Allegra E, Trapasso S. Cancer stem cells in head and neck cancer. Onco Targets Ther. 2012;5:375–83.

Allegra E, Garozzo A, Lombardo N, et al. Mutations and polymorphisms in mitochondrial DNA in head and neck cancer cell lines. Acta Otorhinolaryngol Ital. 2006;26:185–90.

Allegra E, Trapasso S, Sacco A, et al. ELISA detection of salivary levels of Cd44sol as a diagnostic test for laryngeal carcinomas. J Cancer Sci Ther. 2012a;4:330–4.

Allegra E, Puzzo L, Zuccalà V, et al. Nuclear BMI1 expression in laryngeal carcinoma correlates with lymph node pathological status. World J Surg Oncol. 2012b;10:206.

Allegra E, Caltabiano R, Amorosi A, et al. Expression of BMI1 and p16 in laryngeal squamous cell carcinoma. Head Neck. 2013;35(6):847–51.

Allegra E, Trapasso S, Pisani D, et al. The role of BMI1 as a biomarker of cancer stem cells in head and neck cancer: a review. Oncology. 2014;86:199–205.

Almadori G, Bussu F, Cadoni G, et al. Molecular markers in laryngeal squamous carcinoma: towards an integrated clinicobiological approach. Rev Eur J Cancer. 2005;41(5):683–93.

Chen H, Zhou L, Dou T, et al. BMI1's maintenance of the proliferative capacity of laryngeal cancer stem cells. Head Neck. 2011a;33(8):1115–25.

Chen H, Zhou L, Wan G, et al. BMI1 promotes the progression of laryngeal squamous cell carcinoma. Oral Oncol. 2011b;47(6):472–81.

Chiu RJ, Myer EN, Johnson JT. Efficacy of routine neck dissection in the management of supraglottic cancer. Otolaryngol Head Neck Surg. 2004;131:485–8.

Fasano CA, Phoenix TN, Kokovay E, et al. BMI1 cooperates with Foxg1 to maintain neural stem cell self-renewal in the forebrain. Genes Dev. 2009;23(5):561–74.

Gil J, Bernard D, Peters G. Role of polycomb group proteins in stem cell self-renewal and cancer. DNA Cell Biol. 2005;24:117–25.

Haupt Y, Alexander WS, Barri G, et al. Novel zinc finger gene implicated as myc collaborator by retrovirally accelerated lymphomagenesis in Emu-myc transgenic mice. Cell. 1991;65(5): 753–63.

Häyry V, Mäkinen LK, Atula T, et al. BMI1 expression predicts prognosis in squamous cell carcinoma of the tongue. Br J Cancer. 2010;102(5):892–7.

Heffner M, Fearon DT. Loss of T cell receptor-induced BMI1 in the KLRG1(+) senescent CD8(+) T lymphocyte. Proc Natl Acad Sci U S A. 2007;104(33):13414–9.

Itahana K, Zou Y, Itahana Y, et al. Control of the replicative life span of human fibroblasts by p16 and the polycomb protein BMI1. Mol Cell Biol. 2003;23(1):389–401.

Jacobs JJ, Kieboom K, Marino S, DePinho RA, van Lohuizen M. The oncogene and polycomb-group gene BMI1 regulates cell proliferation and senescence through the ink4a locus. Nature. 1999a;397(6715):164–8.

Jacobs JJ, Scheijen B, Voncken JW, et al. BMI1 collaborates with c-Myc in tumorigenesis by inhibiting c-Myc-induced apoptosis via INK4a/ARF. Genes Dev. 1999b;13(20):2678–90.

Kang MK, Kim RH, Kim SJ, et al. Elevated BMI1 expression is associated with dysplastic cell transformation during oral carcinogenesis and is required for cancer cell replication and survival. Br J Cancer. 2007;96(1):126–33.

Kirchner JA, Carter D. Pathology of the larynx. In: Mills SE, editor. Sternberg's diagnostic surgical pathology, vol. 2. 4th ed. Noida: Gopson Papers; 2004. p. 1007–32.

Koehn J, Krapfenbauer K, Huber S, et al. Potential involvement of MYC- and p53-related pathways in tumorigenesis in human oral squamous cell carcinoma revealed by proteomic analysis. J Proteome Res. 2008;7(9):3818–29.

Lessar J, Sauvageau G. BMI1 determines the proliferative capacity of normal and leukaemic stem cells. Nature. 2003;423:255–60.

Liu S, Dontu G, Mantle ID, et al. Hedgehog signaling and BMI1 regulate self-renewal of normal and malignant human mammary stem cells. Cancer Res. 2006;66:6063–71.

Lu H, Sun HZ, Li H, et al. The clinicopathological significance of BMI1 expression in pathogenesis and progression of gastric carcinomas. Asian Pac J Cancer Prev. 2012;13(7):3437–41.

Meng S, Luo M, Sun H, et al. Identification and characterization of BMI1-responding element within the human p16 promoter. J Biol Chem. 2010;285(43):33219–29.

Pardal R, Molofsky AV, He S, et al. Stem cell self-renewal and cancer cell proliferation are regulated by common networks that balance the activation of proto-oncogenes and tumor suppressors. Cold Spring Harb Symp Quant Biol. 2005;70:177–85.

Qin ZK, Yang JA, Ye YL, Zhang X, Xu LH, Zhou FJ, Han H, Liu ZW, Song LB, Zeng MS. Expression of BMI1 is a prognostic marker in bladder cancer. BMC Cancer. 2009;9:61.

Saeki M, Kobayashi D, Tsuji N, et al. Diagnostic importance of overexpression of BMI1 mRNA in early breast cancers. Int J Oncol. 2009;35:511–5.

Sahasrabuddhe AA, Dimri M, Bommi PV, et al. βTrCP regulates BMI1 protein turnover via ubiquitination and degradation. Cell Cycle. 2011;10(8):1322–30.

Satijn DP, Otte AP. RING1 interacts with multiple polycomb-group proteins and displays tumorigenic activity. Mol Cell Biol. 1999;19(1):57–68.

Song L, Zeng MS, Liao WT, et al. BMI1 is a novel molecular marker of nasopharyngeal carcinoma progression and immortalizes primary human nasopharyngeal epithelial cells. Cancer Res. 2006;66:6225–32.

Sten WB, Silver CE, Zeifer BA, et al. Computed tomography of the clinically negative neck. Head Neck. 1991;13:73–5.

Trapasso S, Allegra E. Role of CD44 as a marker of cancer stem cells in head and neck cancer. Biologics. 2012;6:379–83.

Valk-Lingbeek ME, Bruggeman SW, van Lohuizen M. Stem cells and cancer: the polycomb connection. Cell. 2004;118:409–18.

Vrzalikova K, Skarda J, Ehrmann J, et al. Prognostic value of BMI1 oncoprotein expression in NSCLC patients: a tissue microarray study. J Cancer Res Clin Oncol. 2008;134:1037–42.

Wu KJ, Yang MH. Epithelial-mesenchymal transition and cancer stemness: the Twist1-BMI1 connection. Biosci Rep. 2011;31(6):449–55.

Yang MH, Hsu DS, Wang HW, et al. BMI1 is essential in Twist1-induced epithelial-mesenchymal transition. Nat Cell Biol. 2010a;12(10):982–92.

Yang G, He WP, Cai MY, et al. Intensive expression of BMI1 is a new independent predictor of poor outcome in patients with ovarian carcinoma. BMC Cancer. 2010b;10:33.

Yucel T, Saatci I, Sennaroglu L, et al. MR imaging in squamous carcinoma of the head and neck with no palpable lymph nodes. Acta Radiol. 1997;38:810–4.

Part VIII

Leukaemia and Hodgkin Lymphoma

Immunophenotyping as Biomarker Platform in Acute Leukemia

42

Ying Li, Christopher M. Carter, Samer Z. Al-Quran, and Robert W. Allan

Contents

Abstract

In the past two decades, scientific advances have yielded new insights into the genetic and biological features of acute leukemia. Despite these advances, the mortality rate of patients with acute leukemia is still high. Over the same time period, flow cytometric immunophenotyping has become a major tool in current clinical practice for the diagnosis and classification of acute leukemia and the detection of residual leukemic cells after chemotherapy. However, the identification of patients with a high risk of relapse following therapy through the detection of leukemic minimal residual disease (MRD) remains a major challenge since it is difficult to identify small numbers of residual leukemic blasts in a background of nonmalignant regenerating bone marrow cells. The detection of

Y. Li (✉) • C.M. Carter • S.Z. Al-Quran • R.W. Allan
Department of Pathology, Immunology and Laboratory Medicine, University of Florida, Gainesville, FL, USA
e-mail: liying@pathology.ufl.edu; ccarter2@pathology.ufl.edu; alqurs@pathology.ufl.edu; allar@pathology.ufl.edu

V.R. Preedy, V.B. Patel (eds.), *Biomarkers in Cancer, Biomarkers in Disease: Methods, Discoveries and Applications*,
DOI 10.1007/978-94-007-7681-4_7

leukemic blasts rests on the identification of characteristic immunophenotypic aberrancies by flow cytometry that allow discrimination from normal hematopoietic cells. Unfortunately, the immunophenotype of leukemic blasts often closely resembles their normal counterparts in regenerating bone marrows after cytotoxic chemotherapy which makes definitive assessment of leukemic MRD difficult. Emerging molecular analyses such as mRNA profiling by DNA microarray and proteomic analysis by mass spectrometry have been employed to identify new biomarkers of leukemic MRD. Despite these advanced methods, few new biomarkers of leukemic blasts are available clinically which hinders the assessment of leukemic MRD. One way to overcome this barrier is to develop new molecular probes and to discover new biomarkers, which can be used in flow cytometric analysis to distinguish leukemia cells from their normal counterparts.

List of Abbreviations

AML	Acute Myeloid Leukemia
B-ALL	B-Cell Acute Lymphoblastic Leukemia
FISH	Fluorescence In Situ Hybridization
FLT3-ITD	FMS-Like Tyrosine Kinase 3-Internal Tandem Duplication
MRD	Minimal Residual Disease
NPM1	Nucleophosmin 1
PCR	Polymerase Chain Reaction
PTK-7	Protein Tyrosine Kinase-7
SELEX	Systematic Evolution of Ligands by Exponential Enrichment
T-ALL	T-Cell Acute Lymphoblastic Leukemia

Key Facts of Acute Leukemia

- Acute leukemia is a disease of immature hematopoietic cells such as myeloblasts and lymphoblasts.
- Acute leukemia typically presents with decreased numbers of mature blood elements (e.g., anemia, thrombocytopenia, leukopenia, or pancytopenia).
- Bone marrow examination is the usual method for determining the degree of leukemic involvement and the affected cell lineage (e.g., myeloblastic, lymphoblastic, monocytic, promyelocytic, etc.).
- The bone marrow evaluation may include a bone marrow biopsy requiring decalcification and fixation prior to examination, a bone marrow biopsy "touch preparation," a bone marrow aspirate with smear preparation, or, more typically, a combination of the three methods.
- Bone marrow examination typically shows increased bone marrow cellularity with increased numbers of leukemic blasts.

- Leukemic blasts may be present in the blood, but are not always present or a necessity for diagnosis.
- With rare exception, the diagnosis of acute leukemia requires the presence of 20 % or greater leukemic blasts in the bone marrow or blood.
- Proper identification of the leukemic subtype and prognostic factors guides a selection of the appropriate treatment regimen and is essential to determine the likelihood of remission/relapse.
- Adjunct studies, including evaluation of surface and cytoplasmic antigens via flow cytometry, immunohistochemistry, and cytochemistry and evaluation for recurrent chromosomal translocations/abnormalities via cytogenetic karyotyping and FISH, are often necessary to precisely identify the leukemic subtype.
- Acute leukemia treatment consists of chemotherapy and potential bone marrow stem cell transplant depending on the leukemic subtype, prognostic factors, and clinical status.

Definitions of Words and Terms

Aptamer Aptamers are target-specific single-stranded RNA or DNA fragments produced from repetitive binding, extraction, and amplification of what is initially a randomly generated pool of RNA or DNA fragments. In contrast to an antigen-specific antibody, aptamers do not require a living source/laboratory animal to generate the antigen-specific product and can be used to identify an unknown target molecule in a significantly more rapid time frame (1–2 weeks).

Cluster analysis A method of data analysis where data with similarities in selected data subsets is grouped or clustered, optimally resulting in greater separation between the data clusters than between individual data points for a given value.

Flow cytometry A high-throughput, high-sensitivity laser-based method for sorting and evaluating cellular physical properties via light scatter and immunophenotypes via the binding of antigen-specific antibodies conjugated to fluorochromes.

Immunophenotyping Immunophenotyping is the identification of the cytoplasmic and surface antigens (i.e., phenotype) of a target, typically a cell, through the binding of antigen-specific antibodies that are typically conjugated to a secondary molecule, which exhibit different traits (e.g., color change, fluorescence, radioactivity, etc.) depending on the detection method.

Minimal residual disease (MRD) The presence of rare residual or persistent leukemic blasts, historically stated as <5 %, during or following the conclusion of a chemotherapeutic regimen. The residual leukemic blasts are presumed to be the source of relapsed and chemoresistant leukemia following therapy.

Introduction

Acute leukemia is a group of heterogeneous hematologic malignancies arising from hematopoietic stem cells, which typically presents with decreased numbers of mature blood elements (e.g., anemia, thrombocytopenia, leukopenia, or pancytopenia) (O'Donnell et al. 2012). Historically, acute leukemia has been classified into the major categories of acute myeloid leukemia (AML), B-cell acute lymphoblastic leukemia (B-ALL), and T-cell acute lymphoblastic leukemia (T-ALL) according to the FAB (French-American-British) system that was based on morphology and cytochemistry. With few exceptions, such as the favorable survival of acute promyelocytic leukemia (APL), we have not yet succeeded in translating our scientific discoveries into more effective treatments for the majority of patients with acute myeloid leukemia (AML). Most patients will die from their disease. While therapeutic intensification, improved supportive care, and bone marrow transplantation have led to gradual improvements of outcome in children and younger adults with AML, the overall survival rate of AML approaches 50 % (Middeke et al. 2012). In older individuals (>55–60 years) and in patients with therapy-related AML or AML with a prior myelodysplastic syndrome, which often possess unfavorable cytogenetic features (e.g., complex karyotypes, partial deletions, or loss of chromosome 5 and/or 7), the outlook is more dismal with overall survival rates of 10–15 % (Estey 2013). In acute lymphoblastic leukemia (ALL), the majority of which are of B-cell lineage and afford a better prognosis compared to T-ALL, a complete remission rate of 80–85 % can be achieved with contemporary intensive therapy (Khaled et al. 2012; Mathisen et al. 2013).

The Advantage of Immunophenotyping and Common Biomarkers Used for Clinical Flow Cytometry

During the 1990s, flow cytometry became widely used in clinical laboratories for immunophenotyping leukocytes. The majority of the biomarkers expressed by leukemic cells were measured by three or four color flow cytometry, although a few lineage biomarkers could also be determined by immunohistochemical or cytochemical techniques. There is a general misconception that there are many leukemia-specific antibodies or biomarkers available for detecting leukemic blasts by immunophenotyping. In fact, the surface biomarkers currently used for phenotyping AML are adopted from the advancement of immunology research in the last several decades, and thus they are not specific to leukemic cells. Table 1 lists common markers used in the majority of clinical flow cytometry laboratories, and most, if not all, of the listed antigens were discovered more than two decades ago. At the time of a new leukemia diagnosis, leukemic cells (i.e., blasts) are identified by their sheer number, and these markers are applied in daily clinical practice to classify leukemia into myeloid or lymphoid lineages. However, when very few leukemic cells remain in regenerating bone marrow after chemotherapy, the detection sensitivity of flow cytometric immunophenotyping may vary significantly.

Table 1 Common markers used in the majority of clinical flow cytometry laboratories

Antigens	Normal cellular expression
CD1a	Subsets of thymic T cells and Langerhans cells
CD2	Thymic immature T cells and mature T cells
CD3	Thymic immature T cells and mature T cells
CD4	Subsets of mature and immature T cells
CD5	Thymic immature T cells and mature T cells
CD7	Subsets of mature and immature T cells
CD8	Subsets of mature and immature T cells
CD9	Immature B cells
CD10	Immature B cells, germinal center B cells, and subsets of granulocytes
CD11b	Monocytes and subsets of granulocytes
CD11c	Monocytes, subsets of granulocytes, and T cells
CD13	Early CD34-positive bone marrow precursors and subsets of granulocytes and monocytes
CD14	Mature monocytes
CD15	Granulocytes in all maturational stages and early immature monocytes
CD16	Mature granulocytes and NK cells
CD19	Mature and immature B cells and plasma cells, but it is often lost in myeloma cells
CD20	Mature B cells
CD22	Mature and immature B cells and basophils
CD23	Subsets of mature B cells
CD33	Early CD34-postive bone marrow precursors, granulocytes, and monocytes
CD34	Early precursors of B, T, and myeloid lineages
CD38	Immature B, T, or myeloid precursors and subsets of mature B or T cells, granulocytes, and monocytes
CD45	All type of normal leukocytes, but it may be lost in B-ALL or myeloma cells
CD56	T/NK and NK cells including subsets of large granular lymphocytes
CD57	T/NK and NK cells including subsets of large granular lymphocytes
CD64	Mature and immature monocytes and immature granulocytes
CD71	Nucleated red cells of all maturational stages
CD117	Early precursors of granulocytic or erythroid lineages
CD123	Plasmacytoid dendritic cells and basophils
HLA-DR	Early myeloid precursors and mature and immature monocytes and B cells
Glycophorin A	Red cells and late stages of nucleated red cells during maturation

In 1997, the *US-Canadian Consensus Recommendations on the Immunophenotypic Analysis of Hematologic Neoplasia by Flow Cytometry: Data Analysis and Interpretation* was published in order to establish criteria for flow cytometric analysis in the diagnosis and/or classification of malignant hematological disorders (Borowitz et al. 1997). The publication has served as a general guideline for clinical laboratories for more than a decade and emphasizes that the leukemic cell phenotype should be described based on the physical characteristics of the cell (size, cytoplasmic complexity) as determined by light scatter characteristics as well as the presence and intensity of expression of various antigens. Upon completion, an interpretation can then be rendered based on the overall phenotypic pattern seen. The necessity of evaluating both antigenic presence and expression intensity is due to two factors: (1) leukemic cells may express the same antigens as normal bone marrow cells, but at different levels; and (2) the absence of leukemia-specific biomarkers. The 2006 Bethesda International Consensus Recommendations on the Immunophenotypic Analysis of Hematolymphoid Neoplasia further provided the guidelines for flow cytometry immunophenotyping, including indication, reagent or panel selection, and training and education of laboratory professionals (Davis et al. 2007; Greig et al. 2007; Wood et al. 2007).

In 2001, the WHO classification of acute leukemia was introduced, which required that the diagnosis of both adult and pediatric acute leukemia must be based on a combination of morphologic examination, immunophenotypic analysis by flow cytometry, and cytogenetic karyotyping or molecular analysis of prognostically relevant genetic abnormalities. The inclusion of the final criterion was based on the knowledge that the morphologic and immunophenotypic features used previously cannot reliably predict patient outcome or the complex molecular abnormalities underlying these neoplastic processes. However, flow cytometry is still one of the preferred platforms for clinical testing of AML because of the following advantages as compared to molecular assays: (1) It allows for the selection of very small subsets of neoplastic cells (<0.01 %) from background normal cells if adequate biomarkers are available. (2) In the majority of clinical laboratories in Western countries, it can simultaneously evaluate four or more biomarker signals. (3) With adequate biomarkers, flow cytometry-based immunophenotyping assays have significantly less false-positive results than molecular assays. Due to unnecessary treatment and the associated comorbidity/mortality, false-positive results are much more detrimental than false-negative results during the evaluation for residual disease following acute leukemia therapy.

Using Immunophenotyping for Detection of MRD in Acute Leukemia

The detection of MRD in acute leukemia plays an important role in the evaluation of therapy efficacy and identification of early relapse. Currently, identifying patients with MRD who remain at a high risk for relapse following therapy remains a major challenge (Paietta 2012). Due to the difficulty of distinguishing between leukemic blasts and normal recovering blasts, the post-therapy evaluation of remission in acute leukemia has traditionally permitted the presence of 5 % or less leukemic blasts in the bone marrow, and this cutoff value is still used in daily clinical practice. Therefore, more sensitive techniques are required to detect post-therapy malignant cells in lower frequencies, and both molecular methods (e.g., PCR, fluorescence in situ hybridization, FISH) and flow cytometric analysis have been employed. If the leukemic cells have chromosomal abnormalities that can be monitored via FISH, the detection sensitivity is approximately 1–2 % leukemic cells. The detection of MRD by PCR techniques is relatively sensitive (sensitivity: 10^{-4} to 10^{-6}) for lymphoid-associated (B- or T-cell) leukemias; however, it requires knowledge of the patient-specific clonal junctional region sequences of rearranged immunoglobulin or T-cell receptor genes by DNA sequencing (van der Velden et al. 2003). Overall, analysis via molecular methods is useful in less than 30 % of patients with AML. In fact, many AML and some ALL blasts are karyotypically normal and/or do not express leukemic fusion transcripts or other traceable molecular markers identifiable by most molecular methods. Other methods which may identify an abnormality, such as mRNA-DNA microarray studies, are applicable in specimens containing almost exclusively tumor cells, but the DNA microarray-based profiling technique does not function well for detection of residual leukemia in post-therapy specimens with low tumor burden and thus cannot detect MRD. Therefore, immunophenotypic analysis of leukemic cells by flow cytometry still has a pivotal role to play in the diagnosis and classification of acute leukemia before therapy and detection of MRD after therapy. In addition, the turnaround time of immunophenotyping by flow cytometry (2–3 h) is significantly shorter than that of many molecular methods requiring DNA extraction, PCR amplification, and final separation of PCR products (days).

Phenotypical Identification of Leukemic Cells Is Based on Aberrant Antigen Expression and/or Aberrant Patterns of Antigen Expression

Due to the lack of specific biomarkers, much of the knowledge regarding leukemic immunophenotypes has developed from the study of normal hematopoietic cells and their immunophenotypic patterns. By comparison with the immunophenotypes of normal hematopoietic cells, the leukemic cells can immunophenotypically be determined even when mixed in with their normal counterparts. In this way, the antigens expressed by both leukemic and normal cells may still be used for detection:

1. Immunophenotype of B cells in human bone marrow: The B-cell maturation process occurs in the bone marrow, and B cells can be subdivided into at least three subgroups. (1) The earliest immature B-cell precursors express CD34 and CD19, bright levels of CD10 and CD38, and dim intensity CD45 and CD22 without CD20. (2) While still immature, the second group of B-cell precursors loses expression CD34 and maintains expression of CD10 while gradually gaining expression of CD20. This is accompanied by a simultaneous increase in expression of CD19, CD22, and CD45 (Fig. 1a, b). (3) The third group of B cells represents naïve B cells with mature B-cell expression levels of CD20 and CD45. At the same time, the expression of CD10 and CD38 is decreased compared to the immature B-cell precursors, such that the naïve B cells are CD10 negative. The naïve B cells may regain expression of CD10 when they migrate into germinal centers under the stimulation of antigens.

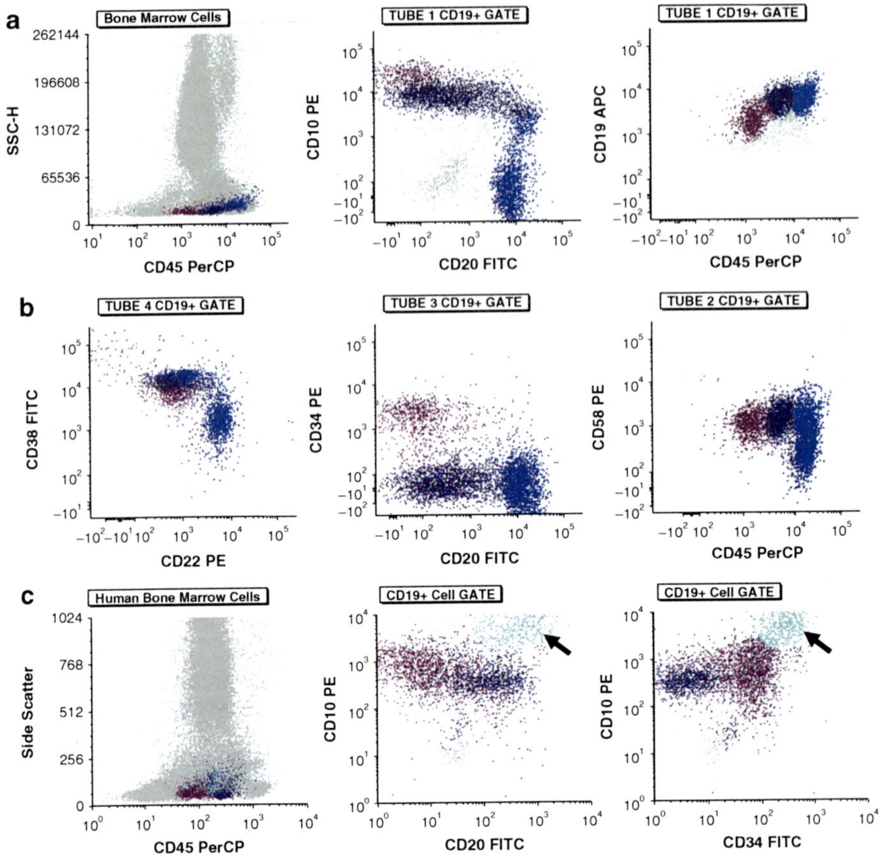

Fig. 1 Antigen expression patterns of normal B cells during maturation and an example of detecting B-ALL MRD by comparing patterns of antigen expression. *Panels **a*** and ***b*** show the phenotypic changes of precursor B cells during their normal maturation. The nonmalignant B-cell precursors are separated according to CD34, CD10, and CD20 expression into the early stage (*purple*), mid stage (*navy*), and naïve B-cell (*blue*) maturational groups. *Panel **c*** illustrates an example of B-ALL cells (0.6 %) that are detected by their higher levels of expression of CD10 and CD34 with discordant levels of CD20

2. Immunophenotype of T cells in human thymus: Unlike B-cell maturation, the very early stem cells of the T-cell lineage are thought to originate in bone marrow before migrating into thymus, and they are not detectable in bone marrow samples by routine clinical flow cytometry immunophenotyping. Clinically, the majority of T-ALL originate from the thymus, and therefore understanding the immunophenotypic changes during thymic T-cell maturation is essential for immunophenotyping T-ALL. The earliest T-cell precursors are few in number even in nonneoplastic thymus, and they are best characterized by their expression of CD34, PTK7, and dim CD1a (Fig. 2a, b). At this stage, the T-cell precursors do not express surface CD3, CD4, or CD8. As these immature

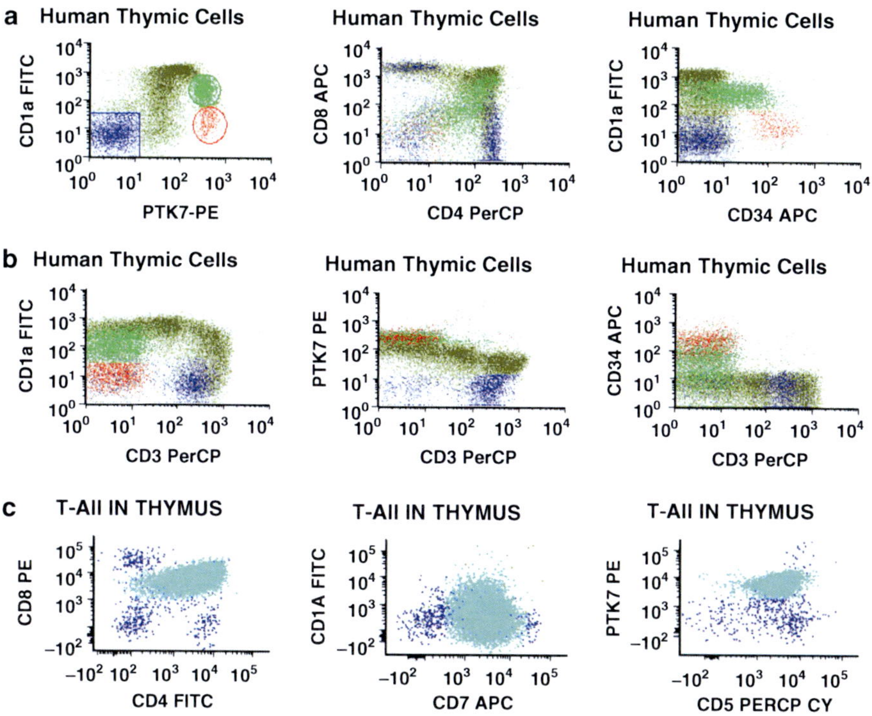

Fig. 2 Immunophenotyping immature thymic T cells. PTK7 expression in nonmalignant immature thymic T cells and T-ALL cells. (**a**) The nonmalignant thymic T cells are separated according to CD1a and PTK7 levels into early stage (*red*), mid stage (*green*), late stage (*olive*), and mature T cells (*blue*). The expression of CD4, CD8, and CD34 of T cells each stage is also shown. (**b**) The temporal relationship is demonstrated between the expression levels of CD3, CD1a, PTK7, and CD34. (**c**) The immunophenotype of a representative case of T-ALL cells (*cyan*) arising in thymus is shown (Jiang et al. Leukemia Res. 2002;36(11):1347–53. © 2002 Elsevier)

T cells mature, CD34 expression is diminished, and they gradually gain expression of CD1a, and CD3, while remaining negative for CD4 and CD8. They then transition from CD4-/CD8- "double-negative" immature T cells to CD4+/CD8+ "double-positive" immature T cells and lose expression of CD1a. Eventually, the majority will then become either CD4- or CD8-positive mature T cells (Fig. 2). However, T-ALL arising in the thymus lost the temporal relationship of PTK7, CD1a, or T-cell antigen expression as seen in normal maturing thymic T cells (Fig. 2c).

3. Immunophenotype of myeloid cells in human bone marrow: The immunophenotypes of myeloid cells during maturation are much more complicated to understand than those of B or T cells in that megakaryocytes, erythrocytes, and all subsets of leukocytes originate from myeloid stem cells. Generally, immunophenotyping by flow cytometry is applied best to leukocytes and, to a lesser extent, erythroid precursors. The relative immunophenotypic limitations

of erythroid precursors are secondary to inadequate markers capable of characterizing the phenotypic changes in erythroid neoplasia. In addition, flow cytometric analysis cannot be routinely used for phenotyping megakaryocytes; however, it can be useful when leukemia blasts show feature of megakaryocytic differentiation. It is well known that the early myeloid stem cells are present as a CD34-positive/CD38 dim positive population, which usually represents <0.1 % of the bone marrow cells. This population may become prominent in regenerating bone marrow or in subsets of myelodysplastic syndrome and acute leukemia. The majority of CD34-positive myeloid precursors have relatively bright CD38 and CD117 (Fig. 3a, b). As these CD34-positive cells differentiate toward granulocytes and monocytes, they gradually gain intensity of CD13, CD33, and HLA-DR (dotted arrows in Fig. 3). Eventually, the granulocytic precursors will increase the expression of CD15 (and CD11b in later stage) while losing HLA-DR expression, but monocytic precursors will retain HLA-DR expression while gaining expression of CD64, CD11b, and finally CD14.

The data used in Figs. 1c, 3c, 4, and 8, respectively, come from clinical cases in which residual leukemic cells were detected according to their immunophenotypes. Leukemic cells can be identified through two strategies:

1. Aberrant antigen expression, which occurs when abnormal cells express antigens that their normal counterparts do not, such as CD56 expression on CD34+ residual AML cells in Fig. 3c. However, leukemic cells with aberrant antigens as illustrated in Fig. 3c are only present in minor subsets of AML, B-ALL, or T-ALL cases. The majority of acute leukemia cases do not have identifiable aberrant antigen expression.
2. Aberrant patterns of normal antigen expression, which refers to quantitative differences in the expression intensity of multiple antigens as compared to normal counterpart cells ("temporal relation changes"), for example, B-ALL blasts with brighter than normal CD10 and CD34 expression illustrated in Fig. 1c and AML blasts with dimmer HLA-DR and brighter CD33 than normal myeloblasts in Fig. 4.

As illustrated in Fig. 1a, b, normal maturing B-cell lymphoblasts have tightly regulated expression of CD10, CD19, CD20, CD22, CD38, and CD34 in human bone marrow. By comparison, B-ALL blasts often lose one or more of these antigens or have a combination of lost antigen expression with concomitant increased expression of one or more other antigens. The leukemic cells in Fig. 1c have increased expression levels of CD10 and CD34, allowing the identification of small numbers of leukemic cells (0.6 %) from background normal immature B cells in the same bone marrow specimen. The example illustrated in Fig. 4 is a more difficult case involving AML. Similar to normal lymphoblasts, normal myeloblasts also have tightly regulated expression of subsets of antigens. In this example, the typical maturational expression of CD33 and HLA-DR in normal human bone

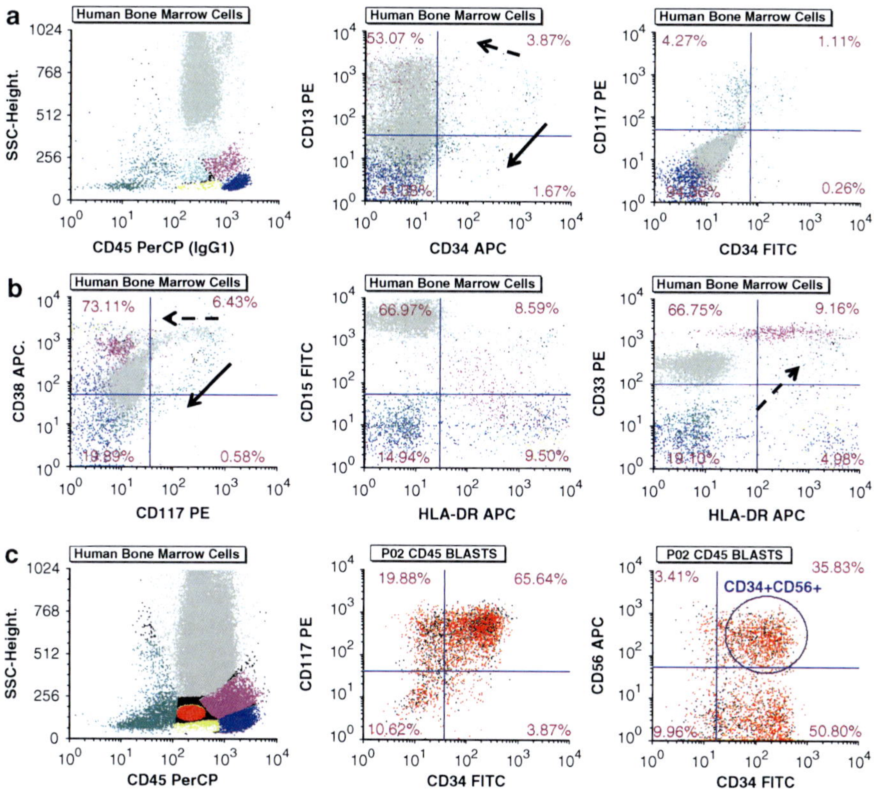

Fig. 3 An example of normal myeloid maturation and detection of AML MRD through aberrant CD56 expression on myeloblasts. *Panels **a*** and ***b*** illustrate the phenotypic changes of leukocytes in human bone marrow during their differentiation, and C shows an AML case with aberrant expression of CD56. The CD34-positive cells in the CD13-CD34 color dot plot (**a**) have two directions, differentiating toward granulocytes while gaining high levels of CD13 (*dotted arrow*) or differentiating toward erythrocytes while losing CD13 (*solid arrow*). The CD34-/CD117-positive cells in the CD38-CD117 color dot plot (*panel **b***) also have two directions, differentiating toward granulocytes or monocytes while maintaining their levels of CD38 (*dotted arrow* in *panel **b***) or differentiating toward erythrocytes while losing CD38 (*solid arrow* in *panel **b***). The AML cells at the time of diagnosis showed coexpression of CD45, CD34, and aberrant CD56. Therefore, aberrant CD56 expression on CD34-positive leukemia cells can be used to detect residual leukemia. Approximately 40 % of the CD34-positive cells expressed CD56 (in *panel **c***), which represented 2–3 % of the total leukocytes. The patient presented with recurrent AML several months later

marrow myeloblasts follows the dotted line in Fig. 4e. While the leukemic blasts, the normal myeloblasts, and other normal bone marrow cells express CD33 and HLA-DR, the temporal relation of CD33 and HLA-DR expression has changed on the AML blasts, indicated by the solid lines in Fig. 4b, e. This phenomenon has not been observed in non-leukemic human bone marrow cells in our experienced laboratory.

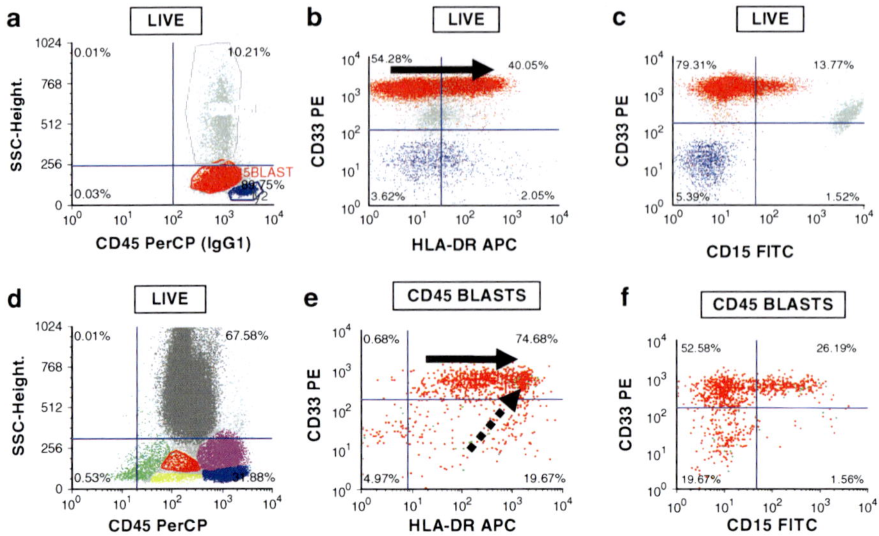

Fig. 4 An example of using aberrant patterns of surface antigen expression to detect AML MRD. The AML leukemic cells at the diagnosis (*red* in *plots* ***a***, ***b***, *and* ***c***) and following therapy (*red* in *plots* ***d***, ***e***, and ***f***) show coexpression of HLA-DR, CD33, and dim CD15. Although HLA-DR, CD33, and CD15 are expressed by leukemia blasts as well as normal bone marrow cells, the aberrant expression patterns (*solid lines* in ***b*** and ***e***) formed by the CD33 and HLA-DR are quite different from the pattern of normal early precursors in human bone marrow (the *dotted line* in ***e***). In addition, the majority of the gated cells (*red dots* under the *solid line* in ***e***) are not monocytes because they lack expression of CD64 and CD14 (not shown here), and they are not early granulocytes because of the relatively bright HLA-DR and very dim CD15 expression. Therefore, one can conclude that AML MRD is present (*red dots* under the *solid line* in ***e***). The patient presented with recurrent AML with a similar immunophenotype several months later

Despite the absence of temporal relation changes in normal human bone marrow cells, and the diagnostic power their identification provides, the analysis of aberrant patterns of antigen expression is significantly more complex than the relatively simple identification of aberrant antigens. The source of the diagnostic degree of difficulty is multifactorial and dependent on the divergence of the leukemic cells from the normal maturation pattern, the proportion of normal background counterparts to the leukemic cells, and the presence of additional cell types and nonviable components that occur temporally in the bone marrow following therapy. For example, in the majority of cases, B-ALL cells often demonstrate markedly different phenotypic patterns than those of normal immature B cells (hematogones), and in these instances, the leukemic cells can be detected even when comprising less than 0.01 % of the total cells. Similarly, the detection of residual T-ALL is also feasible in the majority of clinical flow cytometry laboratories due to the relative absence of immature T cells in human bone marrow and relative abundance of well-studied T-cell lineage antigens, though the sensitivity for detecting T-ALL would be lower than B-ALL.

However, it is much more difficult to use the currently available biomarkers to detect MRD in AML given that AMLs are a heterogeneous group of acute leukemia arising from myeloid stem cells, which unlike immature lymphoblasts differentiate into significantly more diverse mature cell populations. A more fundamental complication is the immunophenotypic resemblance (with available biomarkers) between the leukemic blasts of MRD and their normal counterparts in regenerating human bone marrow after therapy. Published studies report that it is possible to detect AML MRD down to 0.1 % (Kern et al. 2008). However, the detection limit often depends on whether tumor cells express distinct molecular or cytogenetic markers and the types of cases used as negative controls. In clinical practice, cases containing large numbers of regenerating bone marrow cells often result in higher background "noise" with the expected shift in the lower limit of detection. It has also been reported that immunophenotyping and WT1-RNA quantification showed a comparable capacity in terms of technical performance and clinical significance to identify high-risk patients who eventually relapsed. Recently, the integration of Wilms' tumor gene 1 (WT1) and flow cytometry immunophenotyping results has been shown to improve minimal residual disease stratification in acute myeloid leukemia (Marani et al. 2013).

Additional difficulty arises when one considers the intrinsic antigenic variability hematopoietic cells normally demonstrate in the setting of other disease processes. For example, inflammation caused by patient comorbidities, such as autoimmune diseases or infections, can induce certain changes in antigen expression of hematopoietic cells. In addition, medications, in particular hematopoietic growth factors such as GM-CSF, nutritional deficiencies, and unintended toxic effects of ingested or administered substances, can affect the maturation and differentiation of hematopoietic cells with subtle alterations in the patterns of antigen expression. Even when ignoring the presence of preexisting conditions, most, if not all, acute leukemia patients are treated with a battery of supplementary medications, and a true interpretation necessitates correlation of the observed immunophenotypic information with morphological findings and other clinical laboratory findings. For instance, the quantitation of CD34-positive blasts may not always reflect the "true" bone marrow status due to sampling errors or localized leukemia cells after therapy, but the diagnostic accuracy is greatly enhanced when interpreted in combination with CD34 immunohistochemistry performed on the bone marrow biopsy which allows assessment of the quantity and topographical (clustered vs. dispersed) distribution of blasts. Increased bone marrow blasts with an abnormal immunophenotype following growth factor administration (G-CSF) are another common example of an iatrogenic intervention altering the normal immunophenotype of hematopoietic cells. As should now be evident, the lack of a clear consensus on how to interpret flow cytometric immunophenotypic data in these various clinical scenarios makes interpretation of the various aberrancies challenging. In many regards, this is similar to the assessment of subtle morphologic changes by a pathologist in the interpretation of a bone marrow specimen; prior working experience and clinical judgment are important.

Development of Biomarkers for Acute Leukemia

As previously stated, many leukemic cells demonstrate sufficient immunophenotypic similarity to normal early precursor cells in regenerative bone marrow that the detection by flow cytometry of residual low percentage involvement by leukemia cells becomes very difficult. One of the key deficiencies is the lack of sufficiently specific biomarkers for leukemic cells. In fact, the efficacy of flow cytometric analysis is still limited by the available biomarkers/probes, particularly when six to twelve-color flow cytometry is utilized in clinical laboratories. The inconsistency in AML MRD detection hinders the design of new clinical protocols or treatment strategies to treat patients who truly have AML MRD with a presumed higher risk of leukemia relapse. As a result, the development of new molecular panels that can distinguish leukemia cells from their normal counterparts is consistently sought after, as they will have a major impact on the detection of residual acute leukemia.

Unlike the primarily immunohistochemistry-based solid tumor immunophenotyping of recent years, flow cytometry-based immunophenotyping has been applied to clinical practice for more than two decades. However, despite such experience, there are few published studies dedicated to the development of biomarkers for immunophenotyping acute leukemia (Hofmann et al. 2010). As molecular biology and microarray-based profiling have advanced, many molecular markers have been studied or characterized as components of acute leukemia pathogenesis, predictive of chemotherapeutic response, or as prognostic markers for acute leukemia patients after chemotherapy (e.g., FLT3 internal tandem duplication (FLT3-ITD), nucleophosmin mutation (NPM1)) (Murati et al. 2012; Rau and Brown 2009). Since most of these molecular markers are intracellular components related to cell growth, aging, or apoptosis, they cannot be detected through immunophenotyping reliably.

The most recent and promising studies dedicated to the development of new molecular probes and biomarkers for hematopoietic tumors were performed with aptamer nucleotides (Gold et al. 2010). Molecular aptamers consist of single-stranded DNA or RNA that can recognize target proteins, peptides, and other small molecules (Ellington and Conrad 1995; Gold et al. 2002). Aptamers are selected from libraries of random sequences of synthetic DNA or RNA by repetitive binding to the target molecules, a process called SELEX (systematic evolution of ligands by exponential enrichment) (Gold 1995; Vant-Hull et al. 2000). Through this iterative in vitro selection process, single-stranded oligonucleotide aptamers with high specificity and affinity to their targets can be obtained (Fig. 5). The dissociation constants of aptamers to targets can be well below 10^{-8} M, and aptamers can typically discriminate between protein targets that are highly homologous or differ by only a few amino acids (Conrad et al. 1994; Hirao et al. 1998). The basis for this target protein recognition is the tertiary structure formed by the single-stranded oligonucleotide molecules (Kelly et al. 1996).

The identification of surface protein biomarkers is a difficult process. This is in part due to the fact that only limited numbers of molecules are present on individual cells for the majority of surface proteins, and thus it often takes a large numbers of

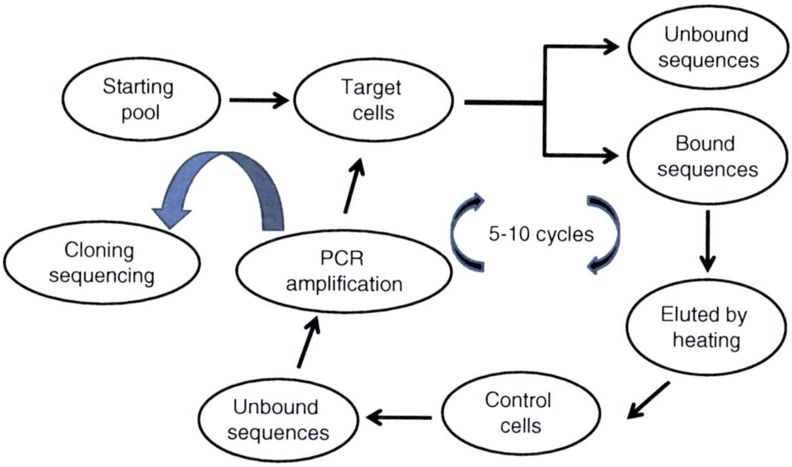

Fig. 5 Schematic presentation of cell SELEX. Aptamer DNA library contains a central randomized sequence of 40–50 nucleotides flanked by PCR primer binding sites at each end. For each selection, more than 10^{14} unique sequences are used, and they are exposed to the target cells (positive selection). The molecules with weak or no affinity for the target cells will remain free in solution, while those that can recognize cell surface molecules will bind to the cells. The bound molecules are eluted by heating and then mixed with negative control cells (negative selection). The unbound DNA will be collected and amplified by PCR amplification. The amplified DNAs are used for the next round of selection. The negative selection step is designed to select aptamers that can recognize markers differentially expressed on target cells. The selection process is monitored by flow cytometry analysis of FITC-labeled DNA sequences bound to cells. The final selected sequences are cloned into plasmid vectors to identify their sequences

cells ($>1 \times 10^8$ cells) to enrich for the target proteins. In addition, adequately solubilizing membrane proteins are often technically difficult, and hydrophobic peptides are often difficult to recover during purification steps such as high-performance liquid chromatography (HPLC). During the past decade, mass spectrometry (MS) in combination with several separation techniques, such as two-dimensional gel electrophoresis (2DGE) or multidimensional liquid chromatography, has become a key tool for protein analysis and proteomic studies. However, one group of proteins that is often underrepresented in proteome analysis is membrane proteins (Santoni et al. 2000). Compared with proteomic studies, the cell-SELEX method is designed to target cell surface proteins, and it is much easier to develop an assay for surface proteins than for intracellular proteins. While it seems that oligonucleotide aptamers offer many advantages, there are problems associated with their application that still need to be explored. As aptamers are single-stranded DNA oligonucleotides, they are sensitive to nuclease digestion unless modified. In addition, the aptamer binding affinity may be more sensitive to environmental changes when compared to antibodies.

While aptamers have demonstrated some in vitro applications, an active area of research is the application of aptamers for in vivo diagnostics or in vivo imaging. In addition to their discriminating and targeting capacities, aptamers have other characteristics that give them promising potential for use as imaging agents in diagnostic procedures. For instance, unlike proteins, aptamers are generated by chemical synthesis, which easily enables a wide range of site-specific modifications, such as tagging with fluorescent dyes, radionucleotides, and biotin, or conjugation to cytotoxic agents (Barbas et al. 2010; Cerchia et al. 2009; Chu et al. 2006). In addition, many synthetic modifications to the phosphate backbone or sugar moiety have been developed to increase the resistance of aptamers to nucleases (Wang and Li 2011), enabling their use in biological fluids. Moreover, oligonucleotide aptamers have not yet shown any toxicity or immunogenicity after testing in several mammalian species, theoretically allowing for repeated administration to the same patient for therapy or diagnostic imaging (de Francis et al. 2009).

The cell-SELEX method has been applied to live leukemia cells (Sefah et al. 2009; Shangguan et al. 2006). The core-binding domains of aptamers typically range from 25 to 60 nucleotides in length, and Fig. 5 illustrates the basic principle of the cell-SELEX process. In this setting, the live leukemic cells and their full repertoire of surface antigens are used as targets to select aptamers that can recognize the patient-specific leukemic cells. The cell-SELEX method uses a single-stranded DNA library containing greater than 10^{14} unique sequences, and the target cells are exposed to the full library of nucleotide sequences. The library sequences with weak or no affinity for the target cells will remain free in solution, while those that recognize surface proteins or other moieties will bind to the cells. The target-bound molecules, containing the highest affinity aptamers, are eluted from the cells by heating and then amplified by PCR amplification. If necessary or desired, a negative selection step can be added to enhance selection of aptamers that recognize a specific cell subtype. After repetitive binding and amplification of these oligonucleotides to the target molecules and control cells, a group of cell-specific aptamers is developed that can differentially recognize target and control cells without ever knowing which target molecules are present on the cell surface (Fig. 6). Individual sequences in the mixture are then cloned into plasmid vectors, and their nucleotide sequences are determined.

The selected aptamers can easily be conjugated with fluorophores for flow cytometric and imaging analysis to study patterns of cell surface protein expression in clinical specimens. In addition, if one of the aptamer probes detects a protein of interest, the specific aptamer probe can then be used to enrich and purify the target protein. For example, a DNA aptamer (Sgc-8) demonstrated high affinity for a T-ALL cell line (CEM) and then was used to phenotype leukemic cells in clinical specimens by flow cytometry (Shangguan et al. 2007). With streptavidin magnetic beads, the biotinylated Sgc-8 aptamer was used to enrich its target protein, which was then later identified as the PTK7 protein (Shangguan et al. 2008). PTK7 is a tyrosine kinase-like molecule that was known to be involved in solid tissue malignancies, but had not been previously evaluated during the thymic T-cell maturation process or on T-ALL blasts. Because the PTK7-specific Sgc-8 aptamer was developed via selection for a T-cell lymphoblastic leukemia (T-ALL) cell line, anti-PTK-7 antibody was used to phenotype the thymic T-cell maturation process (Fig. 2) and later to detect T-ALL MRD in human bone marrow specimens (Figs. 7 and 8)

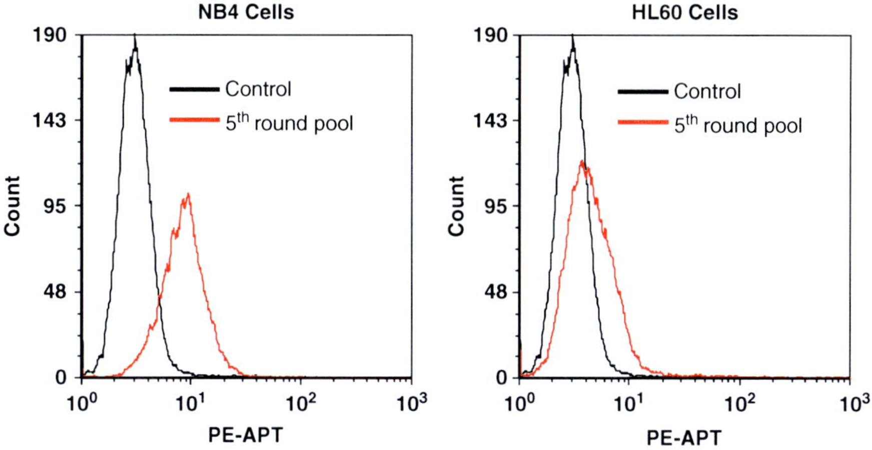

Fig. 6 Flow cytometry assay for monitoring enrichment of the specific aptamer pool against NB4 leukemia cells. After five rounds of selection processes, the phycoerythrin-labeled selected aptamer pool (PE-APT) showed significant increases in fluorescence intensity on target NB4 cells, but it produced minimal change in fluorescence intensity on HL60 cells (negative control). These results indicate that the aptamers recognizing target NB4 cells were enriched preferentially

(Jiang et al. 2012). Therefore, these studies demonstrated that cell-SELEX process can be a useful technique for identification of novel surface markers, and PTK7 may be a useful biomarker for detecting residual T-ALL blasts in combination with the other available T markers. Several other proteins identified through aptamer probes include pigpen from the rat endothelial cell line YPEN-1 (Blank et al. 2001), tenascin-C of U251 glioblastoma cells (Daniels et al. 2003), and immunoglobulin mu heavy chain in Burkitt lymphoma cells (Mallikaratchy et al. 2011). In summary, aptamer technology has shown the potential to identify new biomarkers of leukemic cells and then to use them as novel molecular probes for detecting small numbers of leukemia cells in clinical specimens.

An Alternative Approach for Immunophenotype Data Analysis Needed

Traditionally, flow cytometric data are analyzed by manually gating cells to display discrete populations in concert with the knowledge of general leukocyte classification. In recent years, efforts have been made to develop computational models that may identify cell populations in flow cytometric data, which have shown variable levels of success (Aghaeepour et al. 2013;Lo et al. 2009). Automation in flow cytometry gating will certainly help further the flow cytometric analysis, but work remains in the identification of accurate antigen expression patterns. Most flow cytometry laboratories typically use at least 20–30 markers for immunophenotypic analysis, but the total number of markers is still insufficient to evaluate all cases due

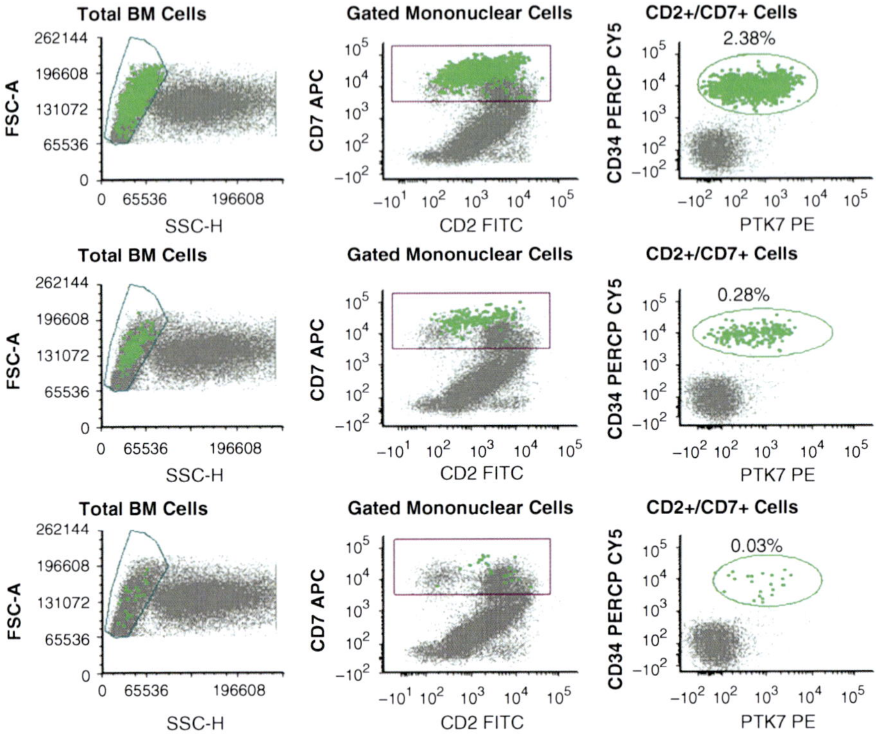

Fig. 7 **Detection of T-ALL cells spiked into normal bone marrow cells**. T-ALL cells were mixed into normal human bone marrow cells to final concentrations of 3 %, 0.3 %, and 0.03 %. T-ALL cells (*green*) can be identified from the background normal cells by sequential gating on mononuclear cells, T cells, and CD34+/PTK7+ cells (Jiang et al. Leukemia Res. 2002;36 (11):1347–53. © 2002 Elsevier)

to the different patterns of antigen expression inherent to leukemic cells. In addition, clinical specimens contain many different subtypes of normal bone marrow cells at different maturational stages. As a result, we are often unable to identify all of the aberrant expression patterns and to then link them to specific diseases or disease processes through direct observation. In order to resolve the issue, cluster analysis has been applied to flow cytometric data and the problem of immunophenotyping (Fiser et al. 2012), and studies have shown a potential role for cluster analysis as an aid in the identification of different antigen expression patterns.

Summary Points

- Acute leukemia is a phenotypically and genetically heterogeneous group.
- Immunophenotyping, particularly through flow cytometric analysis, still plays a critical role in the diagnosis of acute leukemia and detection of MRD after chemotherapy.

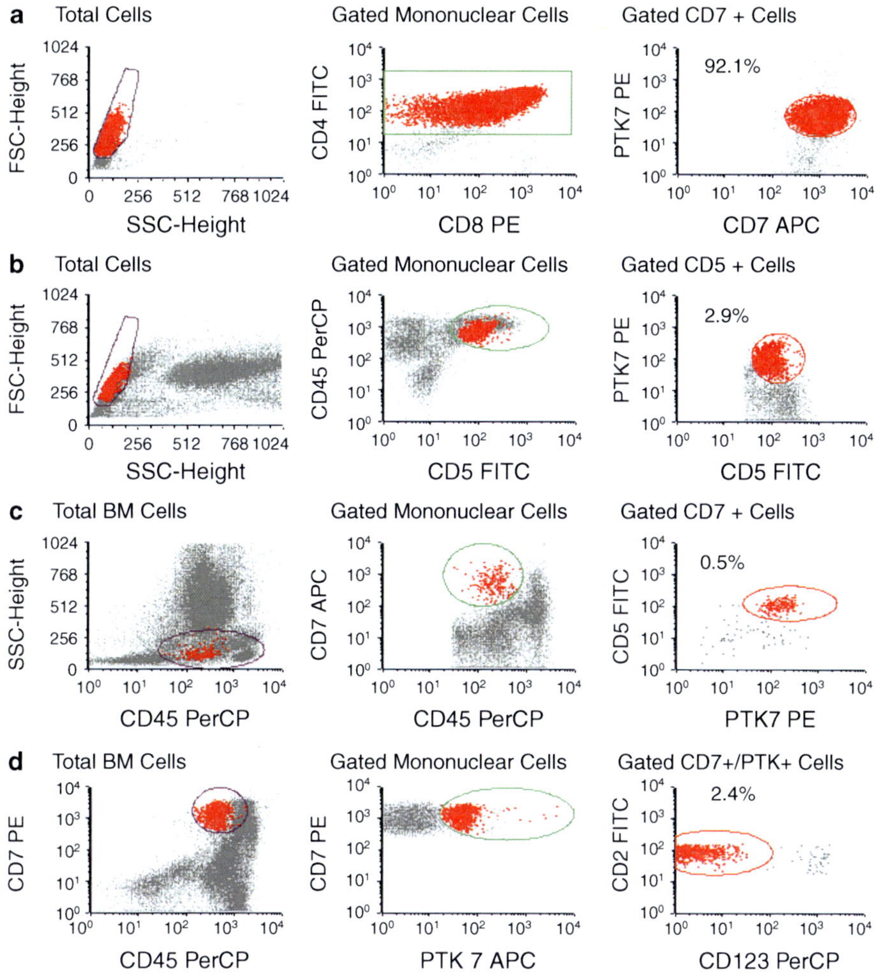

Fig. 8 Examples utilizing PTK7 and other available surface markers for residual T-ALL detection. T-ALL cells in all of the color dot plots are identified and shown as *red dots*. (**a**) and (**b**) show a representative case of T-ALL, (**a**) before therapy and (**b**) after therapy. (**c** and **d**) Show residual T-ALL cell detection in the bone marrow specimens of two other representative cases. Because the expression of T-cell antigens differs in individual T-ALL cases, different immunophenotypic panels and gating strategies are necessary to detect the residual T-ALL cells. CD123 was used to exclude PTK7+ dendritic cells (Jiang et al. Leukemia Res. 2002;36(11):1347–53. © 2002 Elsevier)

- Phenotypic identification of leukemic cells is based on aberrant antigen expression and/or aberrant patterns of antigen expression.
- In spite of the intensive research aimed at discovering novel biomarkers, only a few biomarkers have been introduced into clinical practice in recent years that can reliably be interpreted as aberrant or can create aberrant expression patterns to aid leukemic cell detection.

- The efficacy of flow cytometry and molecular analysis is still limited by inadequate quantity or insufficiently specific biomarkers.
- Further development of tools, such as automation, may aid the detection of differential biomarker expression patterns produced by tumor and normal cells that can be perceived through direct observation alone.
- The development of new molecular probes, new biomarker discovery, and subsequent testing panels for clinical specimens will ultimately be most beneficial to clinical laboratories and eventually lead to improvement in therapeutic outcomes for acute leukemia.

References

Aghaeepour N, Finak G, Hoos H, Mosmann TR, Brinkman R, Gottardo R, Scheuermann RH. Critical assessment of automated flow cytometry data analysis techniques. Nat Methods. 2013;10(3):228–38 (Available from: PM: 23396282).

Barbas AS, Mi J, Clary BM, White RR. Aptamer applications for targeted cancer therapy. Future Oncol. 2010;6(7):1117–26 (Available from: PM: 20624124).

Blank M, Weinschenk T, Priemer M, Schluesener H. Systematic evolution of a DNA aptamer binding to rat brain tumor microvessels. selective targeting of endothelial regulatory protein pigpen. J Biol Chem. 2001;276(19):16464–8 (Available from: PM:11279054).

Borowitz MJ, Bray R, Gascoyne R, Melnick S, Parker JW, Picker L, Stetler-Stevenson M. U.S.-Canadian Consensus recommendations on the immunophenotypic analysis of hematologic neoplasia by flow cytometry: data analysis and interpretation. Cytometry. 1997;30(5): 236–44 (Available from: PM:9383097).

Cerchia L, Giangrande PH, McNamara JO, de Franciscis V. Cell-specific aptamers for targeted therapies. Methods Mol Biol. 2009;535:59–78 (Available from: PM:19377980).

Chu TC, Marks III JW, Lavery LA, Faulkner S, Rosenblum MG, Ellington AD, Levy M. Aptamer: toxin conjugates that specifically target prostate tumor cells. Cancer Res. 2006;66(12):5989–92 (Available from: PM:16778167).

Conrad R, Keranen LM, Ellington AD, Newton AC. Isozyme-specific inhibition of protein kinase C by RNA aptamers. J Biol Chem. 1994;269(51):32051–4 (Available from: PM:7528207).

Daniels DA, Chen H, Hicke BJ, Swiderek KM, Gold L. A tenascin-C aptamer identified by tumor cell SELEX: systematic evolution of ligands by exponential enrichment. Proc Natl Acad Sci U S A. 2003;100(26):15416–21 (Available from: PM:14676325).

Davis BH, Holden JT, Bene MC, Borowitz MJ, Braylan RC, Cornfield D, Gorczyca W, Lee R, Maiese R, Orfao A, Wells D, Wood BL, Stetler-Stevenson M. 2006 Bethesda International Consensus recommendations on the flow cytometric immunophenotypic analysis of hematolymphoid neoplasia: medical indications. Cytometry B Clin Cytom. 2007;72 Suppl 1: S5–13 (Available from: PM:17803188).

de Francis V, Esposito CL, Catuogno S, Cellai L, Cerchia L. Aptamers as innovative diagnostic and therapeutic agents in the central nervous system. CNS Neurol Disord Drug Targets. 2009;8(5):393–401 (Available from: PM:19702567).

Ellington AD, Conrad R. Aptamers as potential nucleic acid pharmaceuticals. Biotechnol Annu Rev. 1995;1:185–214 (Available from: PM:9704089).

Estey EH. Acute myeloid leukemia: 2013 update on risk-stratification and management. Am J Hematol. 2013;88(4):318–27 (Available from: PM:23526416).

Fiser K, Sieger T, Schumich A, Wood B, Irving J, Mejstrikova E, Dworzak MN. Detection and monitoring of normal and leukemic cell populations with hierarchical clustering of flow cytometry data. Cytometry A. 2012;81(1):25–34 (Available from: PM:21990127).

Gold L. The SELEX process: a surprising source of therapeutic and diagnostic compounds. Harvey Lect. 1995;91:47–57 (Available from: PM:9127985).

Gold L, Brody E, Heilig J, Singer B. One, two, infinity: genomes filled with aptamers. Chem Biol. 2002;9(12):1259–64 (Available from: PM:12498875).

Gold L, Ayers D, Bertino J, Bock C, Bock A, Brody EN, Carter J, Dalby AB, Eaton BE, Fitzwater T, Flather D, Forbes A, Foreman T, Fowler C, Gawande B, Goss M, Gunn M, Gupta S, Halladay D, Heil J, Heilig J, Hicke B, Husar G, Janjic N, Jarvis T, Jennings S, Katilius E, Keeney TR, Kim N, Koch TH, Kraemer S, Kroiss L, Le N, Levine D, Lindsey W, Lollo B, Mayfield W, Mehan M, Mehler R, Nelson SK, Nelson M, Nieuwlandt D, Nikrad M, Ochsner U, Ostroff RM, Otis M, Parker T, Pietrasiewicz S, Resnicow DI, Rohloff J, Sanders G, Sattin S, Schneider D, Singer B, Stanton M, Sterkel A, Stewart A, Stratford S, Vaught JD, Vrkljan M, Walker JJ, Watrobka M, Waugh S, Weiss A, Wilcox SK, Wolfson A, Wolk SK, Zhang C, Zichi D. Aptamer-based multiplexed proteomic technology for biomarker discovery. PLoS One. 2010;5(12):e15004 (Available from: PM:21165148).

Greig B, Oldaker T, Warzynski M, Wood B. 2006 Bethesda International Consensus recommendations on the immunophenotypic analysis of hematolymphoid neoplasia by flow cytometry: recommendations for training and education to perform clinical flow cytometry. Cytometry B Clin Cytom. 2007;72 Suppl 1:S23–33 (Available from: PM:17803190).

Hirao I, Spingola M, Peabody D, Ellington AD. The limits of specificity: an experimental analysis with RNA aptamers to MS2 coat protein variants. Mol Divers. 1998;4(2):75–89 (Available from: PM:10425631).

Hofmann A, Gerrits B, Schmidt A, Bock T, Bausch-Fluck D, Aebersold R, Wollscheid B. Proteomic cell surface phenotyping of differentiating acute myeloid leukemia cells. Blood. 2010;116(13):e26–34 (Available from: PM:20570859).

Jiang G, Zhang M, Yue B, Yang M, Carter C, Al-Quran SZ, Li B, Li Y. PTK7: a new biomarker for immunophenotypic characterization of maturing T cells and T cell acute lymphoblastic leukemia. Leuk Res. 2012;36(11):1347–53 (Available from: PM:22898210).

Kelly JA, Feigon J, Yeates TO. Reconciliation of the X-ray and NMR structures of the thrombin-binding aptamer d(GGTTGGTGTGGTTGG). J Mol Biol. 1996;256(3):417–22 (Available from: PM:8604127).

Kern W, Haferlach C, Haferlach T, Schnittger S. Monitoring of minimal residual disease in acute myeloid leukemia. Cancer. 2008;112(1):4–16 (Available from: PM:18000811).

Khaled SK, Thomas SH, Forman SJ. Allogeneic hematopoietic cell transplantation for acute lymphoblastic leukemia in adults. Curr Opin Oncol. 2012;24(2):182–90 (Available from: PM:22234252).

Lo K, Hahne F, Brinkman RR, Gottardo R. Flowclust: a bioconductor package for automated gating of flow cytometry data. BMC Bioinform. 2009;10:145 (Available from: PM:19442304).

Mallikaratchy PR, Ruggiero A, Gardner JR, Kuryavyi V, Maguire WF, Heaney ML, McDevitt MR, Patel DJ, Scheinberg DA. A multivalent DNA aptamer specific for the B-cell receptor on human lymphoma and leukemia. Nucleic Acids Res. 2011;39(6):2458–69 (Available from: PM:21030439).

Marani C, Clavio M, Grasso R, Colombo N, Guolo F, Kunkl A, Ballerini F, Giannoni L, Ghiggi C, Fugazza G, Ravetti JL, Gobbi M, Miglino M. Integrating post induction WT1 quantification and flow-cytometry results improves minimal residual disease stratification in acute myeloid leukemia. Leuk Res. 2013;37(12):1606–11 (Available from: PM: 23891447).

Mathisen MS, Kantarjian H, Thomas D, O'Brien S, Jabbour E. Acute lymphoblastic leukemia in adults: encouraging developments on the way to higher cure rates. Leuk Lymphoma. 2013;54(12):2592–600 (Available from: PM:23547835).

Middeke JM, Beelen D, Stadler M, Gohring G, Schlegelberger B, Baurmann H, Bug G, Bellos F, Mohr B, Buchholz S, Schwerdtfeger R, Martin H, Hegenbart U, Ehninger G, Bornhauser M, Schetelig J. Outcome of high-risk acute myeloid leukemia after allogeneic hematopoietic cell transplantation: negative impact of abnl(17p) and –5/5q-. Blood. 2012;120(12):2521–8 (Available from: PM:22855604).

Murati A, Brecqueville M, Devillier R, Mozziconacci MJ, Gelsi-Boyer V, Birnbaum D. Myeloid malignancies: mutations, models and management. BMC Cancer. 2012;12:304 (Available from: PM: 22823977).

O'Donnell MR, Abboud CN, Altman J, Appelbaum FR, Arber DA, Attar E, Borate U, Coutre SE, Damon LE, Goorha S, Lancet J, Maness LJ, Marcucci G, Millenson MM, Moore JO, Ravandi F, Shami PJ, Smith BD, Stone RM, Strickland SA, Tallman MS, Wang ES, Naganuma M, Gregory KM. Acute myeloid leukemia. J Natl Compr Canc Netw. 2012;10(8):984–1021 (Available from: PM: 22878824).

Paietta E. Minimal residual disease in acute myeloid leukemia: coming of age. Hematology Am Soc Hematol Educ Program. 2012;2012:35–42 (Available from: PM: 23233558).

Rau R, Brown P. Nucleophosmin (NPM1) mutations in adult and childhood acute myeloid leukaemia: towards definition of a new leukaemia entity. Hematol Oncol. 2009;27(4):171–81 (Available from: PM: 19569254).

Santoni V, Kieffer S, Desclaux D, Masson F, Rabilloud T. Membrane proteomics: use of additive main effects with multiplicative interaction model to classify plasma membrane proteins according to their solubility and electrophoretic properties. Electrophoresis. 2000;21(16): 3329–44 (Available from: PM: 11079553).

Sefah K, Tang ZW, Shangguan DH, Chen H, Lopez-Colon D, Li Y, Parekh P, Martin J, Meng L, Phillips JA, Kim YM, Tan WH. Molecular recognition of acute myeloid leukemia using aptamers. Leukemia. 2009;23(2):235–44 (Available from: PM:19151784).

Shangguan D, Li Y, Tang Z, Cao ZC, Chen HW, Mallikaratchy P, Sefah K, Yang CJ, Tan W. Aptamers evolved from live cells as effective molecular probes for cancer study. Proc Natl Acad Sci U S A. 2006;103(32):11838–43 (Available from: PM:16873550).

Shangguan D, Cao ZC, Li Y, Tan W. Aptamers evolved from cultured cancer cells reveal molecular differences of cancer cells in patient samples. Clin Chem. 2007;53(6):1153–5 (Available from: PM:17463173).

Shangguan D, Cao Z, Meng L, Mallikaratchy P, Sefah K, Wang H, Li Y, Tan W. Cell-specific aptamer probes for membrane protein elucidation in cancer cells. J Proteome Res. 2008;7(5):2133–9 (Available from: PM:18363322).

van der Velden VH, Hochhaus A, Cazzaniga G, Szczepanski T, Gabert J, van Dongen JJ. Detection of minimal residual disease in hematologic malignancies by real-time quantitative PCR: principles, approaches, and laboratory aspects. Leukemia. 2003;17(6):1013–34 (Available from: PM:12764363).

Vant-Hull B, Gold L, Zichi DA. Theoretical principles of in vitro selection using combinatorial nucleic acid libraries. Curr Protoc Nucleic Acid Chem. 2000; Chapter 9, Unit available from: PM:18428805.

Wang J, Li G. Aptamers against cell surface receptors: selection, modification and application. Curr Med Chem. 2011;18(27):4107–16 (Available from: PM:21838694).

Wood BL, Arroz M, Barnett D, DiGiuseppe J, Greig B, Kussick SJ, Oldaker T, Shenkin M, Stone E, Wallace P. 2006 Bethesda International Consensus recommendations on the immunophenotypic analysis of hematolymphoid neoplasia by flow cytometry: optimal reagents and reporting for the flow cytometric diagnosis of hematopoietic neoplasia. Cytometry B Clin Cytom. 2007;72 Suppl 1:S14–22 (Available from: PM:17803189).

Serum CD163 and TARC as Circulating Biomarkers in Hodgkin Lymphoma

43

Kimberley Jones, Louise Seymour, and Maher K. Gandhi

Contents

Abstract

Although the long-term disease control of classical Hodgkin lymphoma (cHL) is relatively high, significant treatment-related morbidities are common. These include secondary cancers, cardiopulmonary complications, stroke, peripheral neuropathy, and infertility. In the 20 % of patients who do not respond to first-line agents, prolonged exposure to suboptimal therapy can induce chemoresistance. Patients with a rapid response may be overtreated and might benefit from a truncated treatment regimen. Accurate risk stratification is needed

K. Jones • L. Seymour • M.K. Gandhi (✉)
University of Queensland Diamantina Institute, Translational Research Institute, Brisbane, QLD, Australia
e-mail: kimberley.jones@uq.edu.au; l.seymour@uq.edu.au; m.gandhi@uq.edu.au

V.R. Preedy, V.B. Patel (eds.), *Biomarkers in Cancer, Biomarkers in Disease: Methods, Discoveries and Applications*,
DOI 10.1007/978-94-007-7681-4_5

in order to optimally treat cHL. However, this requires defined predictive and treatment response markers. Existing clinical parameters have limited prognostic value prior to therapy, and the only established marker of value once treatment has commenced is 18-fluorodeoxyglucose positron emission tomography (FDG-PET) combined with computerized tomography (CT). Although PET/CT is currently the most important tool used, interpretation is imperfect with low false-negative rates countered by high false positives. Furthermore, PET/CT is unavailable in many rural or underprivileged centers and, even in the most advantaged centers, is impractical for frequent testing. In order to risk-stratify patients once therapy has commenced, clinicians need an accurate marker of treatment response that can be performed throughout the therapy, prior to each follow-up visit. This chapter focuses on two newly identified serum disease response biomarkers, CD163 and TARC, for cHL that have the potential to greatly assist clinical decision making and aid interpretation of PET/CT.

List of Abbreviations

cDNA	Complementary DNA
cHL	Classical Hodgkin Lymphoma
CR	Complete Remission
CT	Computerized Tomography
CTL	Cytotoxic T Lymphocyte
DSS	Disease-Specific Survival
EBNA	Epstein-Barr Virus Nucleic Acid
EBV	Epstein-Barr Virus
EFS	Event-Free Survival
EIA	Enzyme Immunoassay
ELISA	Enzyme-Linked Immunosorbent Assay
ESR	Erythrocyte Sedimentation Rate
FACS	Fluorescence-Activated Cell Sorter
FDG	18-Fluorodeoxyglucose
FFS	Failure-Free Survival
FFTF	Freedom from First-Line Treatment Failure
GHSG	German Hodgkin Study Group
HL	Hodgkin Lymphoma
HRS	Hodgkin and Reed-Sternberg
IHC	Immunohistochemistry
IM	Infectious Mononucleosis
IPS	International Prognostic Score
ISH	In Situ Hybridization
LD	Lymphocyte Depleted
LDH	Lactate Dehydrogenase
LMP	Latent Membrane Protein
LP	Lymphocyte Predominant
LR	Lymphocyte Rich

MC	Mixed Cellularity
NLPHL	Nodular Lymphocyte-predominant HL
NS	Nodular Sclerosis
OS	Overall Survival
PBMC	Peripheral Blood Mononuclear Cell
PET	Positron Emission Tomography
PFS	Progression-Free Survival
PR	Partial Remission
PTLD	Posttransplant Lymphoproliferative Disorder
qRT-PCR	Quantitative Real-Time *Polymerase Chain Reaction*
ROC	Receiver Operating Characteristic
sCD163	Serum CD163
sTARC	Serum TARC
TAMs	Tumor-Associated Macrophages
TARC	Thymus and Activation-Related Chemokine
TILs	Tumor-Infiltrating Lymphocytes
WHO	World Health Organization

Key Facts

- cHL is the commonest lymphoma in young adults.
- Treatment-related complications including secondary cancers, cardiopulmonary complications, stroke, peripheral neuropathy, and infertility frequently occur in patients with cHL.
- Prognostic and disease response biomarkers are needed in order to accurately risk-stratify and optimally treat cHL.
- PET/CT is the only validated biomarker that reflects disease response during and post-therapy; however, it is impractical for frequent testing and unavailable in many centers, and cross-center standardization is still required.
- Blood-based biomarkers are practical for frequent testing and may be measured by common laboratory techniques.

Definitions of Words and Terms

Classical Hodgkin Lymphoma (cHL) The commonest lymphoma in young adults. It is characterized by the presence of malignant Hodgkin and Reed-Sternberg cells and a cure rate of >80 %.

Nodular Lymphocyte-Predominant Hodgkin Lymphoma (NLPHL) Is a rare lymphoma and a different disease entity to cHL. Hodgkin and Reed-Sternberg cells are not present in NLPHL.

Disease response biomarkers Biological markers of disease during and following therapy.

Prognostic biomarkers Biological markers of disease prior to therapy that predicts response to treatment and survival.

Positron Emission Tomography (PET) Is a mode of radiological imaging using radioactively labeled 18-fluorodeoxyglucose to visualize cellular glucose uptake in the body.

Computerized Tomography (CT) An imaging method that uses x-rays to create cross-sectional views of the body.

ELISA The enzyme-linked immunosorbent assay is used to detect and quantify proteins in solution.

Risk-stratified therapy Using prognosis and response to therapy to determine the type, intensity, and duration of treatment.

CD163 Is a scavenger receptor for the hemoglobin-haptoglobin complex and is expressed on M2-type immunosuppressive macrophages.

Thymus and Activation-Related Chemokine (TARC) Is a chemokine expressed in the thymus and by HRS cells. TARC binds the chemokine receptor CCR4, expressed by Th2 T cells.

Introduction

Cancer biomarkers enable patients to have risk-stratified therapy. Specifically, patients with poor prognosis disease should have more aggressive therapy than those with good prognosis. This forms the basis for risk-adapted therapy. Historically, cancer-specific clinical scoring systems are used, but these fail to take into account the disease biology. More recently, rapidity of response to therapy has been used to guide subsequent therapy. Although this chapter discusses the serum protein biomarkers CD163 and TARC in the context of classical Hodgkin lymphoma (cHL), its lessons are applicable to other cancers. Intuitively, the blood would be expected to at least in part reflect a lymphoid malignancy, yet currently there are no circulating cell-free (cf) biomarkers in HL. Blood biomarkers might be *prognostic* (i.e., serve as an early predictor of refractory disease or future relapse) and/or be markers of *disease response*. The latter enable clinicians to monitor their patient's progress. Validated prognostic and/or disease response blood biomarkers will assist the clinical decision paradigm, to identify those that could be spared excessive treatment, and those where change in therapy should be expedited.

Classical Hodgkin Lymphoma

Epidemiology, Classification, and Diagnosis of HL

Classical HL (cHL) has an incidence in developed countries of three cases per 100,000 and is the commonest lymphoma in young adults (Kuppers 2009). Current treatment strategies for cHL involve chemotherapy and radiotherapy. At present, a long-term disease control of cHL is relatively high (Evens et al. 2008) with greater than 80 % cure rates of newly diagnosed patients under the age of 60 (Diehl et al. 2004). However, if patients do relapse, survival rates are a lot lower. Furthermore, treatment-related morbidity and mortality are frequent in long-term survivors (Diehl et al. 2004; Gandhi et al. 2004). cHL has two peak ages of incidence in developed countries. The first peak is in young adulthood, around the third decade, and the second peak is in old age. In developing countries, there is an additional peak of incidence in children, primarily male children (Caporaso et al. 2009).

HL is divided into two entities: cHL which accounts for 95 % of cases and the rarer nodular lymphocyte-predominant HL (NLPHL). cHL is further divided into four histological subtypes: lymphocyte rich (LR), lymphocyte depleted (LD), mixed cellularity (MC), and nodular sclerosis (NS) which accounts for the majority of cases (Pileri et al. 2002). Histological classification is made according to the World Health Organization (WHO) classification of leukemia and lymphoma (Swerdlow et al. 2008).

The hallmark of cHL is the presence of multinucleated giant Hodgkin and Reed-Sternberg (HRS) cells within an inflammatory microenvironment. The HRS cells are generally CD30+ with a large proportion also CD15+ (Swerdlow et al. 2008). NLPHL is considered a distinct pathologic entity and lacks the typical HRS cells. The malignant cells in NLPHL are large, generally mononuclear, and referred to as lymphocyte-predominant (LP) cells. Unlike HRS cells, LP cells are often CD20 + CD30-. Furthermore, approximately 40 % of cHL cases are Epstein-Barr virus (EBV) associated where the virus resides in the malignant HRS cells and is clonal. In contrast, NLPHL is not an EBV-associated disease (Swerdlow et al. 2008).

The cause of cHL is largely unknown, although the frequent presence of EBV suggests that the virus contributes, but is not pivotal, to pathogenesis (Herbst et al. 1991; Jarrett et al. 1991; Pallesen et al. 1991). EBV-associated cHL rises to greater than 95 % in immunocompromised patients, further implicating both the immune system and EBV in the pathogenesis of this disorder (Gandhi et al. 2004).

The diagnosis of cHL is made by tumor biopsy and requires the histological identification of HRS cells. Importantly, HRS cells only comprise 1–5 % of the diseased node. Hence, histopathological diagnosis can be difficult, and the importance of obtaining an excision biopsy (rather than a core or fine-needle aspirate) cannot be overemphasized. The majority of the diseased tissue is composed of nonneoplastic cells, including macrophages, T cells, B cells, neutrophils, eosinophils, fibroblasts, plasma cells, and mast cells. These tumor-infiltrating lymphocytes (TILs) and tumor-associated macrophages (TAMs) are critical to the biology of the disease, aiding the survival of HRS cells through immune evasion mechanisms and survival signals. HRS cells are thought to actively define the tumor microenvironment via the secretion of numerous cytokines and chemokines that limit cytotoxic T-cell (CTL) activity and promote a type 2 helper T-cell (Th2) and regulatory T-cell environment. Examples include the secretion of IL-10, IL-7, TGF-β, galectin-1, CCL5, CCL22, and thymus and activation-related chemokine (TARC/CCL17) (Fischer et al. 2003). Furthermore, HRS cells express PDL-1, the ligand for PD-1, which induces T-cell exhaustion further restricting immunity in the tumor microenvironment (Yamamoto et al. 2008).

Staging, Prognostication, and Risk-Adapted Treatment Strategies

Once a diagnosis has been established, staging and risk stratification need to occur prior to determining a therapy regimen. The Ann Arbor staging system (with Cotswold modification) is commonly employed. This classification is based on the involvement of lymph nodes on one or both sides of the diaphragm, the number of involved sites, the presence or absence of bulky disease, whether there is contiguous or noncontiguous extranodal disease, and the presence of B symptoms (fever, night sweats, and weight loss). PET/CT is also commonly employed in the staging of patients.

There are several clinical algorithms to prognosticate patients. These include the German Hodgkin Study Group (GHSG) system for early stage (Tubiana et al. 1989; Diehl et al. 2003) and the International Prognostic Score (IPS) for advanced stage (Hasenclever and Diehl 1998). However, these are relatively crude and involve the extent of disease, patient fitness, and surrogates of disease biology such as anemia, lymphocyte count, and erythrocyte sedimentation rate (ESR).

As the long-term disease control of advanced-stage HL is becoming the norm, the emerging issue is to minimize treatment-related complications such as secondary cancer, cardiopulmonary complications, stroke, and infertility (Evens et al. 2008). The intention is to optimize therapy by more accurately identifying patients for risk-stratified therapy. Those with a rapid response to initial treatment have the best outcomes and may benefit from truncated ("de-escalated") treatment regimens to reduce toxicity and minimize late effects of treatment. Paradoxically, there remains a significant minority with refractory disease. In these patients, prolonged exposure to first-line agents can induce chemoresistance and unnecessary toxicity, and alternate rescue strategies should be instituted early. A risk-adapted treatment approach is currently based on limited or advanced stage, presence or absence of poor prognostic features, bulky disease (commonly defined as $\geq$10 cm in diameter or one third the cardiothoracic diameter), and constitutional symptoms. Patients with a positive PET at the end of treatment have a significantly higher recurrence rate than those with a negative PET (Jerusalem et al. 1999; Zinzani et al. 1999). Data to date indicates that interim PET (after two cycles) appears to predict PFS and overall survival (OS) (Hutchings et al. 2005, 2006; Gallamini et al. 2007). The utility of PET to adapt therapy during the course of treatment (PET-directed therapy) is currently being investigated in large prospective cohorts. However, should these studies indicate that interim PET/CT is beneficial, outstanding issues still remain. PET/CT is impractical for frequent testing and unavailable in many centers, and cross-center standardization is still required. A blood-based disease response biomarker measured by simple laboratory techniques would be highly advantageous both when PET/CT is and is not available.

There are no readily accessible, rapid biomarkers capable of accurate risk stratification routinely measured for cHL.

Biomarkers in cHL

Prognostic biomarkers for cHL can be divided into those that risk-stratify patients pre-therapy and those that reflect disease response throughout therapy. These are not mutually exclusive, however, of the known prognostic biomarkers for cHL (Table 1); little is known of their usefulness once therapy has commenced. Indeed, several pre-therapy prognostic biomarkers are routinely measured for staging, yet there is no disease response biomarker routinely monitored for cHL. Despite treatment response being the single most important prognostic factor, the majority of biomarker studies for cHL are not designed to investigate disease response. Instead, the focus has been on prognostic markers in cHL tissue biopsies. Although tissue biomarkers may be useful prior to therapy, it is an impractical source for repeated measures to monitor disease response. Nevertheless, markers elevated in cHL tumor tissues may also be elevated in blood. Blood, in contrast to tissue, is an ideal specimen for disease response monitoring. Indeed, numerous studies have looked for prognostic markers in pre-therapy serum or plasma; however, few studies have used serial monitoring to evaluate disease response.

The high composition of nonmalignant cells within cHL tumors complicates the possible sources of biomarkers. Evidence suggests that both tumor-infiltrating cells and HRS cells have high glucose uptake; thus, PET avidity likely reflects both the malignant and nonmalignant components of the tumor (Shim et al. 2009). It is yet to be determined whether disease response will be best reflected by an HRS-specific marker or a tumor microenvironment-specific marker or the combination of both.

Tissue Biomarkers

Several overexpressed markers have been identified from HRS cells, HRS cell lines, or cHL primary biopsy tissue. From the latter, markers are either overexpressed in HRS cells or in the nonmalignant tumor infiltrate. In HRS cells, increased expression of IL-6 (Reynolds et al. 2002), topoisomerase IIalpha (Doussis-Anagnostopoulou et al. 2008), and CSF1R (Steidl et al. 2012) and decreased expression of HLA class II (Diepstra et al. 2007) have all been associated with poor outcome. In older patients with cHL (>50 years), the expression of EBV-encoded small RNAs (EBER) in HRS cells has been associated with poor

Table 1 Prognostic and disease response markers for cHL

Marker	Source	Method	Outcome
Prognostic markers (prior to therapy)			
Granzyme B + CD8+	**Tissue** (microenvironment: activated T cells)	IHC	**Elevated levels (≥15 %) with unfavorable prognosis** (Oudejans et al. 1997; ten Berge et al. 2001; Alvaro-Naranjo et al. 2005)
CD4 + CD25 + FOXP3+	**Tissue** (microenvironment: regulatory T cells)	IHC	**Elevated levels with favorable prognosis:** ***prolonged EFS and DFS*** (Alvaro et al. 2005; Tzankov et al. 2008)
CD20+	**Tissue** (microenvironment: benign B cells)	IHC	**Elevated levels with favorable prognosis:** ***prolonged EFS*** (Chetaille et al. 2009; Steidl et al. 2010)
CD68 + CD163+	**Tissue** (microenvironment: M2 macrophages)	IHC	**Elevated levels with unfavorable prognosis:** ***poor EFS, DSS, and OS*** (Kamper et al. 2011a; Yoon et al. 2012)
Galectin-1	**Tissue** (microenvironment and HRS cells)	IHC	**Elevated levels with unfavorable prognosis:** ***poor EFS and OS*** (Kamper et al. 2011b)
	Serum (microenvironment and HRS cells)	ELISA	**Levels correlate with tumor burden and clinical features in newly diagnosed cHL** (Ouyang et al. 2013)
HRS-specific IL-6	**Tissue** (HRS cells)	IHC	**Expression by HRS cells with unfavorable prognosis:** ***failure to achieve CR*** (Reynolds et al. 2002)
IL-6	**Serum** (microenvironment and HRS)		**Detectable IL-6 (≥22 pg/mL) with unfavorable prognosis:** ***reduced median survival*** (Kurzrock et al. 1993)
Topoisomerase IIα	**Tissue** (HRS cells)	IHC	**Elevated levels with unfavorable prognosis:** ***inferior FFS*** (Doussis-Anagnostopoulou et al. 2008)
CSF1-R expression	**Tissue** (HRS cells)	mRNA ISH	**Elevated levels with unfavorable prognosis:** ***Inferior PFS and OS*** (Steidl et al. 2012)
EBV-DNA	**Plasma** (HRS cells)	qRT-PCR	**Elevated levels with unfavorable prognosis:** ***inferior EFS*** (Kanakry et al. 2013)
TARC	**Serum** (HRS cells)	ELISA	**Elevated levels correlate with stage, bulk, and metabolic tumor volume** (Plattel et al. 2012)
CD30	**Serum** (HRS cells)	ELISA	**Detectable sCD30 (≥5U/mL) with unfavorable prognosis:** ***increased progressive disease*** **and** ***reduced rates of CR*** (Gause et al. 1991, 1992; Christiansen et al. 1995)

(continued)

Table 1 (continued)

Marker	Source	Method	Outcome
IL-2R (CD25)	**Serum** (microenvironment and HRS cells)	ELISA	**Reduced levels with favorable prognosis:** ***Excellent EFS*** (Gause et al. 1992)
			Elevated levels with unfavorable prognosis: ***poor EFS and OS*** (Christiansen et al. 1995)
ICAM-1	**Serum** (microenvironment)	ELISA	**Elevated levels associate with unfavorable prognosis:** ***inferior DFS and OS*** (Christiansen et al. 1995)
VCAM-1	**Serum** (microenvironment)	EIA	**Elevated levels associate with unfavorable prognosis:** ***inferior DFS and OS*** (Christiansen et al. 1998)
Disease response markers (during and/ or post-therapy)			
FDG avidity	**Patient imaging** (microenvironment and HRS cells)	PET/CT	**Elevated levels with disease, normalize in remission** (Hutchings et al. 2006; Gallamini et al. 2007; Meignan et al. 2010; Gallamini and Kostakoglu 2012)
IL-6	**Serum** (microenvironment)	ELISA	**Elevated levels with disease, normalize in remission** (Seymour et al. 1997)
TARC	**Serum** (HRS cells)	ELISA	**Elevated levels with disease, normalize in remission** (Plattel et al. 2012; Jones et al. 2013)
CD163	**Serum** (microenvironment)	ELISA	**Elevated levels with disease, normalize in remission** (Jones et al. 2013)

CR complete remission, *CT* computerized tomography, *DFS* disease-free survival, *DSS* disease-specific survival, *EFS* event-free survival, *EIA* enzyme immunoassay, *ELISA* enzyme-linked immunosorbent assay, *FFS* failure-free survival, *GHSG* German Hodgkin Study Group, *HRS* Hodgkin and Reed-Sternberg, *IHC* immunohistochemistry, *ISH* in situ hybridization, *PET* positron emission tomography, *PFS* progression-free survival, *OS* overall survival, *qRT-PCR* quantitative real-time polymerase chain reaction

failure-free survival (FFS) (Diepstra et al. 2009). The expression of the EBV latent membrane protein 1 (LMP1) in HRS cells has been associated with favorable outcomes in young adults and early-stage disease (Glavina-Durdov et al. 2001), while a subsequent study found that LMP1 expression negatively impacted overall survival (OS) in specific subgroups (Claviez et al. 2005). However, a recently published meta-analysis of numerous previously published studies concluded that LMP1 expression was not associated with survival in HL (Mao et al. 2013). Galectin-1 is highly expressed by both HRS cells and cells of the tumor microenvironment (TAMs and endothelial cells); however, only increased expression in the tumor microenvironment was associated with poor event-free survival (EFS) (Kamper et al. 2011b).

Within the tumor microenvironment, T cells, B cells, and macrophages have all been associated with outcome. Two studies reported by Meijer and colleagues found that increased numbers of activated T cells (granzyme $B^{+}CD8^{+}$) in tissue biopsies were associated with unfavorable outcomes (Oudejans et al. 1997; ten Berge et al. 2001). This was validated by a number of subsequent studies which also identified T-cell subsets associated with prognosis including FOXP3+ Treg cells being correlated with prolonged event-free and disease-free survival (Alvaro et al. 2005; Alvaro-Naranjo et al. 2005; Tzankov et al. 2008). In addition, an increased number of benign CD20+ B cells in the tumor microenvironment are associated with favorable outcomes in cHL (Chetaille et al. 2009; Steidl et al. 2010). More recently, tumor-associated macrophages (TAMs) have been shown to have prognostic potential in cHL with increased expression of the M2-type immunosuppressive macrophage markers CD68 and CD163 being significant, independent predictors of inferior failure-free survival and overall survival (Steidl et al. 2010; Kamper et al. 2011a; Yoon et al. 2012). Although reports have challenged these findings, elevated levels of the macrophage markers CD68 and CD163 were confirmed in the disease nodes of cHL (Azambuja et al. 2012; Sanchez-Espiridion et al. 2012). Building on these previous studies, Greaves et al. recently showed that increased CD20 and FOXP3 expressions both conferred superior OS and that increased CD68 expression conferred inferior freedom from first-line treatment failure (FFTF) and overall survival (Greaves et al. 2013). Studies comparing CD163 and CD68 immunohistochemistry staining found CD68 to be less specific for the monocyte/macrophage lineage and to have higher nonspecific background staining in primary cHL biopsies, suggesting CD163 may be a better M2 macrophage marker in cHL (Harris et al. 2012).

Blood Biomarkers

Circulating Cell-Free EBV-DNA

One of the best-studied disease response biomarker for cHL is cell-free (serum or plasma) EBV-DNA. Although this HRS-specific marker is only applicable to 40 % of patients, it has been well-established that, in these patients, plasma EBV-DNA is elevated prior to therapy and remains elevated in refractory/relapsed disease but returns to normal levels in remission (Drouet et al. 1999; Gallagher et al. 1999; Wagner et al. 2001; Gandhi et al. 2006; Hohaus et al. 2011; Spacek et al. 2011; Jones et al. 2012). A recent study of a large cHL cohort demonstrated that pre-therapy levels of plasma EBV-DNA also have value as a prognostic marker prior to therapy (Kanakry et al. 2013). Elevated pre-therapy EBV-DNA levels predicted inferior EFS independent of the known poor prognostic factors in the IPS and that plasma EBV-DNA positivity at 6 months post-therapy is associated with poor outcomes. Thus, compounding evidence over the past two decades strongly indicates that EBV-DNA has potential as a robust biomarker for pre-therapy prognostication and as a post-therapy disease response biomarker for EBV^{+}cHL. Importantly, data indicates that EBV-DNA may have limited value as an interim treatment disease response marker, becoming negative early during therapy in both complete and partial responders (Jones et al. 2012). Although methods for quantifying circulating EBV-DNA are yet to be standardized, qRT-PCR is the most widely used technique with the Namalwa cell line used as the commonest standard. It has also been demonstrated that amplification of single- versus multiple-copy EBV-gene targets is equivalent and that cell-free sources serum and plasma are also equivalent but not interchangeable (Jones et al. 2012).

Circulating Cell-Free Protein Biomarkers

Cross talk between HRS cells and the surrounding milieu is mediated by chemokines and cytokines and is critical to HL pathogenesis (Skinnider and Mak 2002). These soluble chemokines and cytokines are an important source of potential biomarkers and can be divided into those that are specific to the HRS cells (tumor specific) and those that originate from the benign infiltrate (tumor associated). Soluble markers originating from HRS cells hold the promise of high specificity, whereas markers from the microenvironment may be more sensitive owing to their relative abundance. Importantly, tumor specificity is not absolute and is more likely a spectrum. Other factors influencing circulating protein levels include relative abundance within expressing cells and ability for the protein to be released into the circulation.

Serum levels of IL-10 (Vassilakopoulos et al. 2001), IL-6 (Seymour et al. 1997), CD30 (Gause et al. 1991, 1992; Christiansen et al. 1995), IL-2R (Gause et al. 1992; Christiansen et al. 1995), ICAM-1 (Christiansen et al. 1995), VCAM-1 (Christiansen et al. 1998), and thymus and activation-related chemokine (TARC) (Weihrauch et al. 2005; Niens et al. 2008) are all elevated in cHL patients prior to therapy and have been associated with survival. A recent study of 60 cHL patients with serial samples throughout therapy found that serum TARC levels reflected disease response in both early- and advanced-stage cHL and in relapsed disease (Plattel et al. 2012). In cHL, HRS cells are known to have elevated levels of TARC (van den Berg et al. 1999; Peh et al. 2001).

Serum CD163 and TARC as Biomarkers for cHL

A recently published prospective multicenter observational study of 47 patients with HL (43 cHL and 4 NLPHL) reports an analysis of the HRS-specific protein TARC and the tumor microenvironment-specific M2-type immunosuppressive macrophage marker CD163 serum levels at five timepoints prior to, during, and post-therapy (Jones et al. 2013). Results were compared to healthy donors and to disease response as determined by radiological assessment. Tissue CD163 immunohistochemistry was correlated to matched serum samples.

Methods and Sample Preparation

Blood was collected from patients at defined timepoints – pre-therapy, immediately pre-second and pre-third cycles of therapy, and 1 month and 6 months post-therapy – as well as from healthy donors. Serum tubes were spun at 3,000 rpm for 10 min. Serum was removed, aliquoted, and stored at −80 °C until thawed in batches. CD163 and TARC were quantified in serum samples using the Quantikine® Human CD163 ELISA kit (R&D Systems) and the RayBio® Human TARC ELISA kit (RayBiotech) as per manufacturer's instructions. A 1:20 dilution was used for sCD163.

Primary tumor biopsies were obtained for the majority of patients, and tissue CD163 expression was quantified by immunohistochemistry. $CD163^{+}$ monocytes were also quantified in the blood of a subset of patients and healthy controls, and the effect of monocyte depletion on T-cell proliferation was investigated.

Analysis and Interpretation

sTARC and sCD163 Levels in Pre-therapy cHL, Complete Remission, and Healthy Donors

By ELISAs, both sTARC and sCD163 reflected disease response in complete responders (sCD163, AUC 0.7333, $P = 0.001$, 95 % C.I. 0.6072–0.8594; TARC, AUC 0.8793, $P < 0.0001$, 95 % C.I. 0.7492–0.9613; Fig. 1). Cutoff levels were defined by two criteria: a value greater than the healthy participant mean plus one standard deviation and a value with greater than 80 % sensitivity and specificity from the receiver operating characteristic (ROC) curve analysis of pre-therapy versus healthy participant values. A cutoff level of 500 ng/ml for sCD163 resulted in 86 % sensitivity and 81 % specificity differentiating pre-therapy from healthy controls and 62 % sensitivity and 75 % specificity distinguishing pre-therapy from complete remission (CR) 6 months post-therapy. For sTARC, the cutoff value was defined as 300 pg/ml with 90 % sensitivity and 86 % specificity for pre-therapy versus healthy donors and 70 % sensitivity and 84 % specificity for pre-therapy versus CR 6 months post-therapy.

Value of sTARC and sCD163 Levels as an Interim Therapy Biomarker

Importantly, the kinetics of the two biomarkers were strikingly different. sCD163 levels gradually declined throughout therapy, while sTARC rapidly dropped to normal levels prior to second therapy (Fig. 2). Notably, sTARC and EBV-DNA (both HRS-specific markers) had the same kinetic profile, dropping to normal levels after one treatment even in patients that responded slowly to therapy (by radiological assessment). Accordingly, sCD163 interim values, and not sTARC, reflected interim therapy response. For sCD163 levels, there was no significant difference between pre-therapy samples and those in partial remission (PR) at the interim timepoint. However, there was a significant difference for sCD163 between pre-therapy and those in CR at the interim timepoint ($P = 0.0152$). In contrast, there was a significant difference between pre-therapy sTARC levels and both PR and CR samples at the interim timepoint ($P = 0.0001$ for both). In addition, the kinetics of the biomarker (stratified by CR/PR) at the

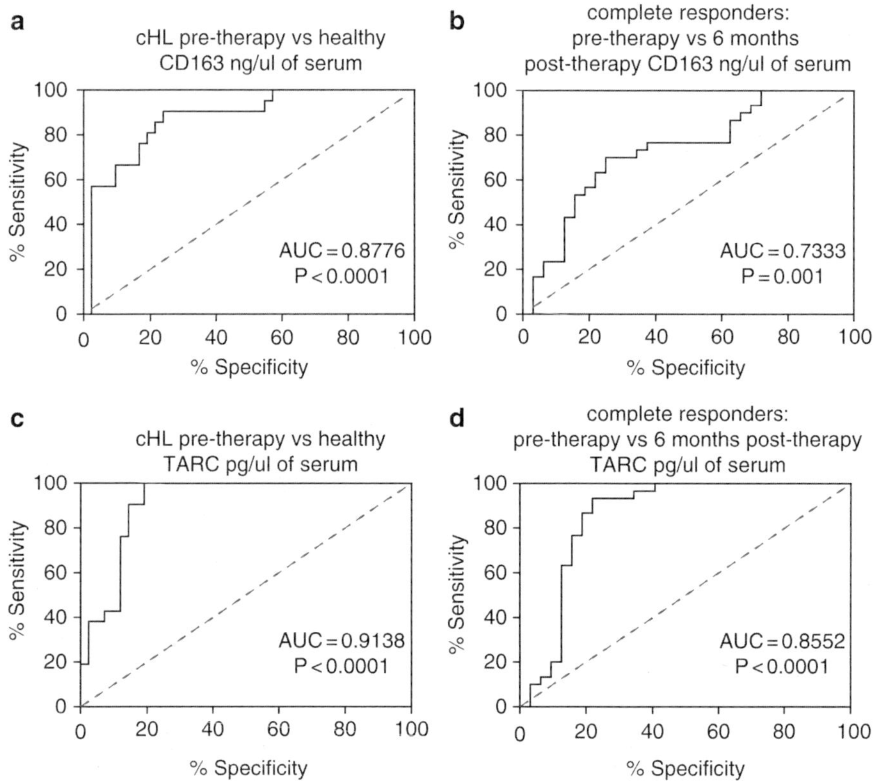

Fig. 1 Sensitivity and specificity of sCD163 and sTARC as biomarkers in cHL (Taken with permission from Jones et al. (2013)). (**a–d**) Receiver operating characteristic (*ROC*) plots demonstrate high sensitivity and specificity of (**a**) sCD163 pre-therapy cHL versus healthy participant, (**b**) sCD163 pre-therapy cHL versus CR 6 months post-therapy, (**c**) sTARC pre-therapy cHL versus healthy participants, and (**d**) sTARC pre-therapy cHL versus CR 6 months post-therapy. *AUC* area under the curve

interim timepoint was evaluated for associations with outcome once chemotherapy was completed. All patients in CR at the interim timepoint maintained ongoing CR at 1 and 6 months post-therapy. Interestingly, of those PR patients below the sCD163 threshold at the interim timepoint, all achieved and maintained ongoing CR, while four of the eight patients above the sCD163 threshold went on to have refractory/relapsed disease. However, for sTARC, of the four patients below the sTARC threshold at the interim therapy timepoint, two remained in ongoing CR, whereas one had refractory disease and one relapsed by 6 months post-therapy. Similarly, two of the nine patients above the sTARC threshold had relapsed disease by 6 months post-therapy.

Thus, the results suggest that a marker of tumor infiltrate (sCD163) and not HRS cells (sTARC) may more accurately reflect interim therapy tumor bulk. The rapid

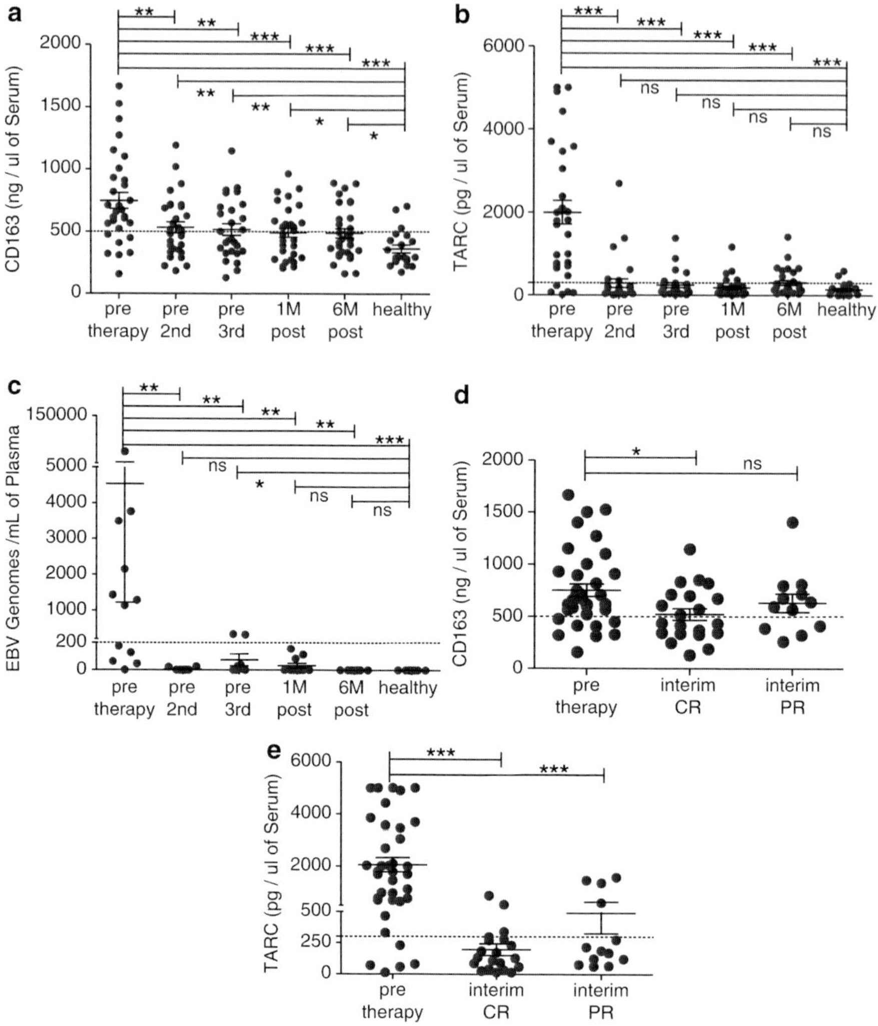

Fig. 2 sCD163 and sTARC as biomarkers in cHL (Taken with permission from Jones et al. (2013)). (**a–c**) Comparison of sCD163, sTARC, and plasma EBV-DNA levels in cHL patients with CR by 1 month post-therapy and who remained in CR at 6 months post-therapy. (**a**) sCD163 levels, (**b**) sTARC levels, and (**c**) plasma EBV-DNA levels. (**d, e**) Comparison of interim therapy treatment response. cHL patients, restricted to those with paired interim samples that matched interim radiological assessment. (**d**) sCD163 levels show a significant difference between paired pre-therapy and CR interim therapy ($P = 0.0152$), while no significant difference was seen between paired pre-therapy and PR interim therapy ($P =$ NS). (**e**) sTARC levels show a significant difference between paired pre-therapy versus CR interim therapy ($P = 0.0001$) and paired pre-therapy versus PR interim therapy ($P = 0.0001$). *Error bars* represent mean with SEM. $***P < 0.001$, $**P < 0.01$, $*P < 0.05$, NS $= P > 0.05$

decline of HRS-specific markers (sTARC and EBV-DNA) may be due to the low numbers of HRS cells such that reduction after just one cycle is sufficient to make sTARC and EBV-DNA equivalent to threshold values. Indeed, sTARC pre-therapy levels were 300-fold lower than sCD163 levels. Alternatively, it is possible that HRS cells are preferentially chemosensitive compared to the tumor microenvironment (or at least TAMs); however, there is currently no evidence to support this. One way to address this would be to biopsy the diseased lymph node following the first cycle of therapy. However, such an invasive procedure would present regulatory challenges and may not give a definitive answer as a single biopsy may not be a representative of the entire tumor. An accurate animal model reflecting both HRS cells and the tumor microenvironment is needed and would be invaluable for future cHL research.

Value of sTARC and sCD163 Levels as Markers of Refractory/Relapsed Disease

Although the results clearly demonstrate that both sTARC and sCD163 are sensitive and specific markers of disease resolution post-therapy, the data of post-therapy levels in refractory or relapsed disease is less definitive. Out of the entire cohort, five patients had either refractory or relapsed disease post-therapy. As such, this study was underpowered to make any definitive conclusions. Of these five patients, one patient had refractory disease at 1 month post-therapy (Fig. 3a), one patient had resolution of disease at the interim timepoint but elapsed at 1 month post-therapy (Fig. 3b), and three patients relapsed after 1 month post-therapy (Fig. 3c–e). The time course of sCD163 and sTARC is shown in Fig. 3, in association with the tumor burden. All five patients had elevated sTARC levels pre-therapy, and all but one had elevated sCD163 levels pre-therapy. Two patients had low-volume relapsed/refractory disease, and neither marker was elevated at the corresponding timepoint. In contrast, three patients had extensive relapsed/refractory disease, and sTARC was well above threshold at the time of refractory/relapsed disease in all three. In one of these cases, sCD163 was also elevated at the time of refractory/relapsed disease, while in two of these cases, sCD163 was not (although in one of these patients sCD163 was also not elevated pre-therapy). Further work is required to confirm the role of sTARC and sCD163 as biomarkers for refractory/relapsed disease.

Potential Applications to Prognosis, Other Diseases, or Conditions

Association of sTARC and sCD163 with Other Known Prognosticators

Pre-therapy levels of sCD163, but not sTARC, were associated with "B" symptoms, stage, and low lymphocyte count ($P = 0.0351$, $P = 0.0328$, and $P = 0.0297$, respectively). In addition, sCD163 levels strongly correlated with plasma

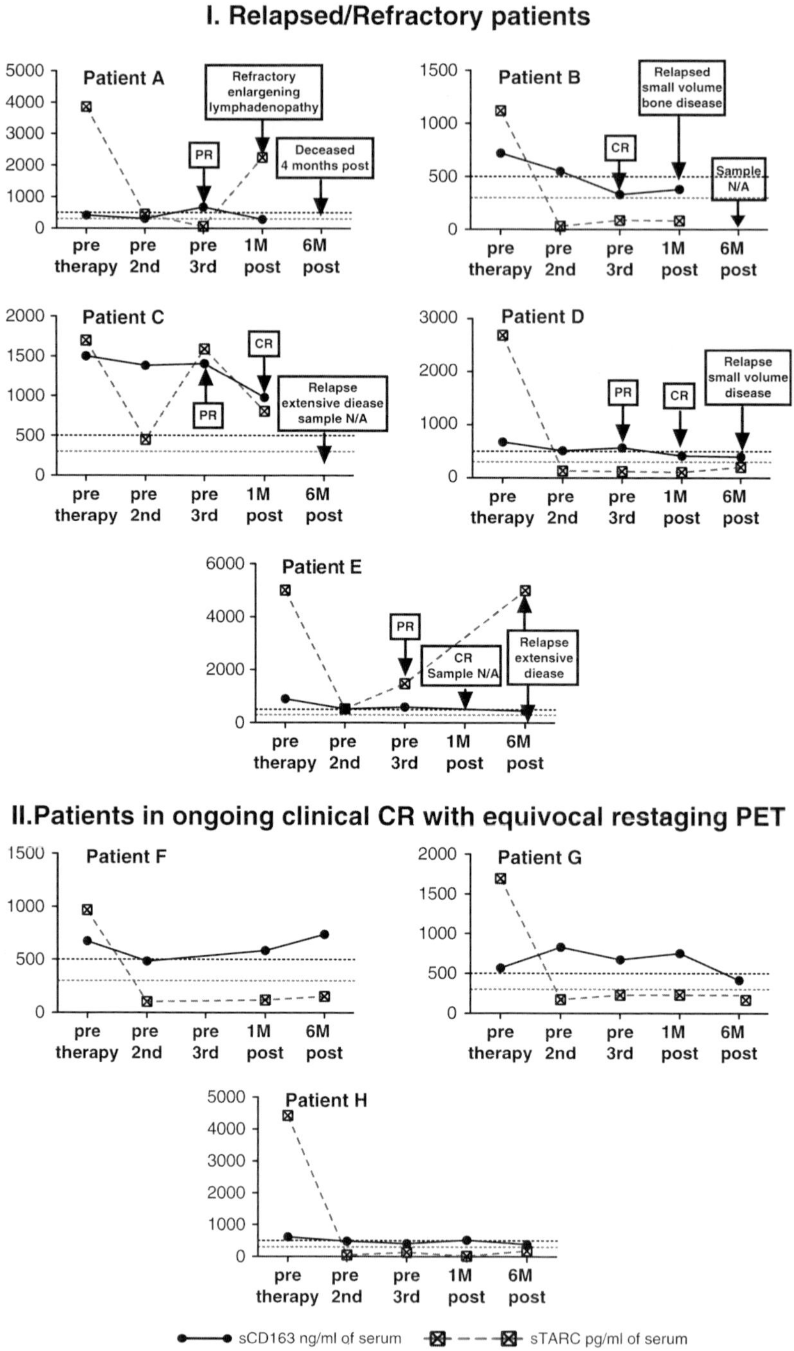

Fig. 3 Kinetics of serum CD163 and TARC in relapsed/refractory cHL and in patients in ongoing CR with equivocal restaging PET (Taken with permission from Jones et al. (2013)).

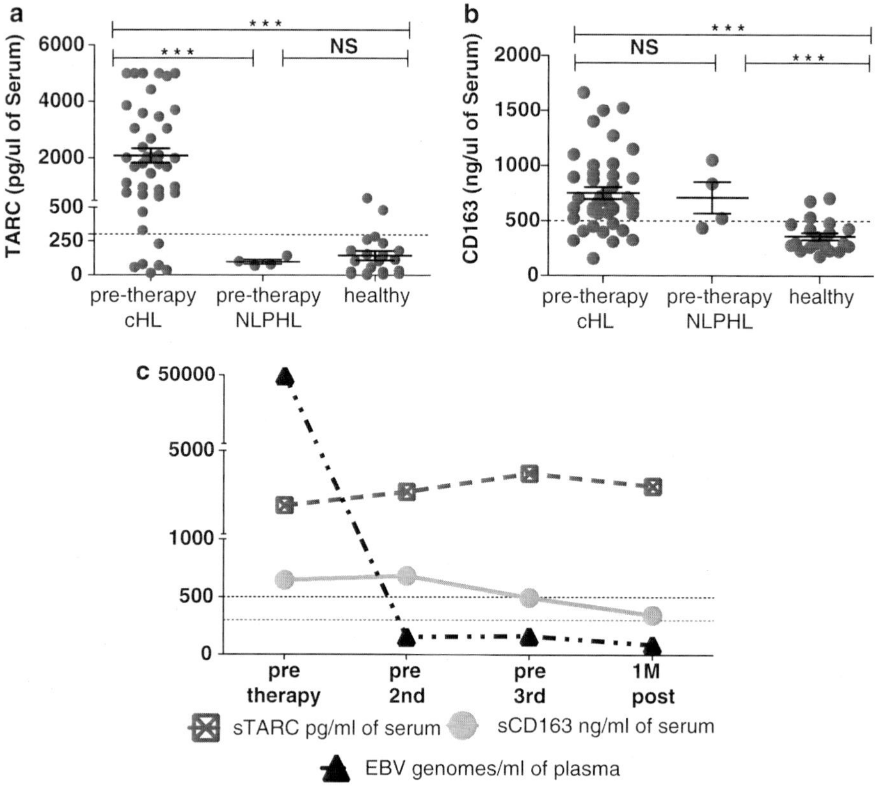

Fig. 4 **Serum CD163 and TARC in other diseases** (Figure not previously published). (**a**, **b**) Comparison of pre-therapy serum CD163 and TARC in NLPHL. *Error bars* represent mean with SEM. (**a**) sCD163: cHL pre-therapy versus NLPHL pre-therapy ($P =$ NS), cHL pre-therapy versus healthy participants ($P < 0.0001$), and NLPHL versus healthy participants ($P = 0.001$). (**b**) sTARC: cHL pre-therapy versus NLPHL pre-therapy ($P < 0.0001$), cHL pre-therapy versus healthy participants ($P < 0.0001$), and NLPHL versus healthy participants ($P =$ NS). (**c**) cHL patient with severe atopic dermatitis that persisted throughout therapy. sTARC, sCD163, and plasma EBV-DNA levels are shown. This patient achieved radiological PR at the interim timepoint and CR at the end of therapy. $***P < 0.001$, $**P < 0.01$, $*P < 0.05$, NS = $P > 0.05$

EBV-DNA ($r = 0.791$, $P = 0.001$). Given that tissue CD163 may be an independent predictor of inferior failure-free survival and overall survival, tissue CD163 in pre-therapy diagnostic tissue biopsies was compared with sCD163 and results demonstrated that tissue CD163 modestly correlated to matching pre-therapy

Fig. 3 (continued) The *dashed gray lines* represent sTARC and the solid black lines sCD163. The *dotted gray* and *black lines* are the sTARC and sCD163 thresholds, respectively. The *arrows* represent the timing of the radiological assessment. Limited small volume disease was defined as disease confined to a single site and ≤2 cm. Patients *A–E* had refractory or relapsed disease as indicated. Patients *F–H* had persistent clinical CR despite low-grade PET avidity of uncertain significance at restaging

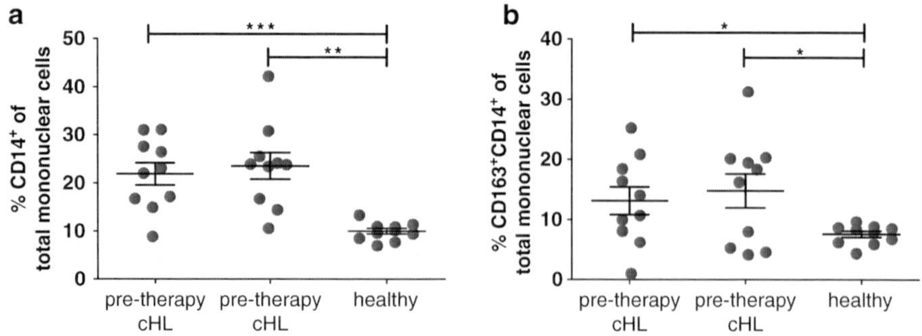

Fig. 5 Comparison of total circulating CD163$^+$CD14$^+$ monocytes in cHL patients versus healthy participants (Taken with permission from Jones et al. (2013)). *Error bars* represent mean with SEM. (**a**) Percentage of monocytes (defined as CD14+) within the total population of viable mononuclear cells (pre-therapy cHL versus healthy $P = 0.0006$, post-therapy cHL versus healthy $P = 0.0010$). (**b**) Percentage of CD163+ monocytes within the total population of viable mononuclear cells (pre-therapy cHL versus healthy $P = 0.0437$, post-therapy cHL versus healthy $P = 0.0332$). $^{***}P < 0.001$, $^{**}P < 0.01$, $^{*}P < 0.05$, NS = $P > 0.05$

sCD163 levels ($r = 0.4005$, $P = 0.0256$) and associated with IPS ($P = 0.0332$) and the presence of early- or advanced-stage disease ($P = 0.0025$).

sCD163, sTARC, and NLPHL

TARC is expressed by the HRS cells of cHL, as well as the thymus, subsets of dendritic cells, endothelial cells, and activated peripheral blood mononuclear cells (van den Berg et al. 1999; Shimada et al. 2004). HRS cells are not present in NLPHL, and TARC is not expressed by primary NLPHL tissues (van den Berg et al. 1999; Peh et al. 2001). Consistent with this, sTARC was not elevated in pre-therapy NLPHL patients compared to healthy participants and was significantly lower than pre-therapy cHL ($P < 0.0001$, Fig. 4a), indicating that sTARC might be highly specific for cHL. In contrast, sCD163 levels were elevated in pre-therapy NLPHL patients compared to healthy participants ($P = 0.001$, Fig. 4b) at a similar level compared to pre-therapy cHL samples. Thus, sCD163 is not specific to cHL, and further investigation into the use of sCD163 as a disease response biomarker for NLPHL is warranted.

sCD163, sTARC, and Allergic Disease

Although sTARC was specific for cHL and not NLPHL, sTARC is known to be elevated in a range of allergic disease such as atopic dermatitis (Hijnen et al. 2004; Shimada et al. 2004). A patient with stage IV_B EBV-related nodular sclerosing cHL was excluded from analysis based on a history of long standing methotrexate therapy for severe atopic dermatitis. The dermatitis remained poorly controlled for the duration of the study. Despite the patient achieving radiological PR at the interim timepoint and CR at the end of therapy, sTARC was grossly elevated at all

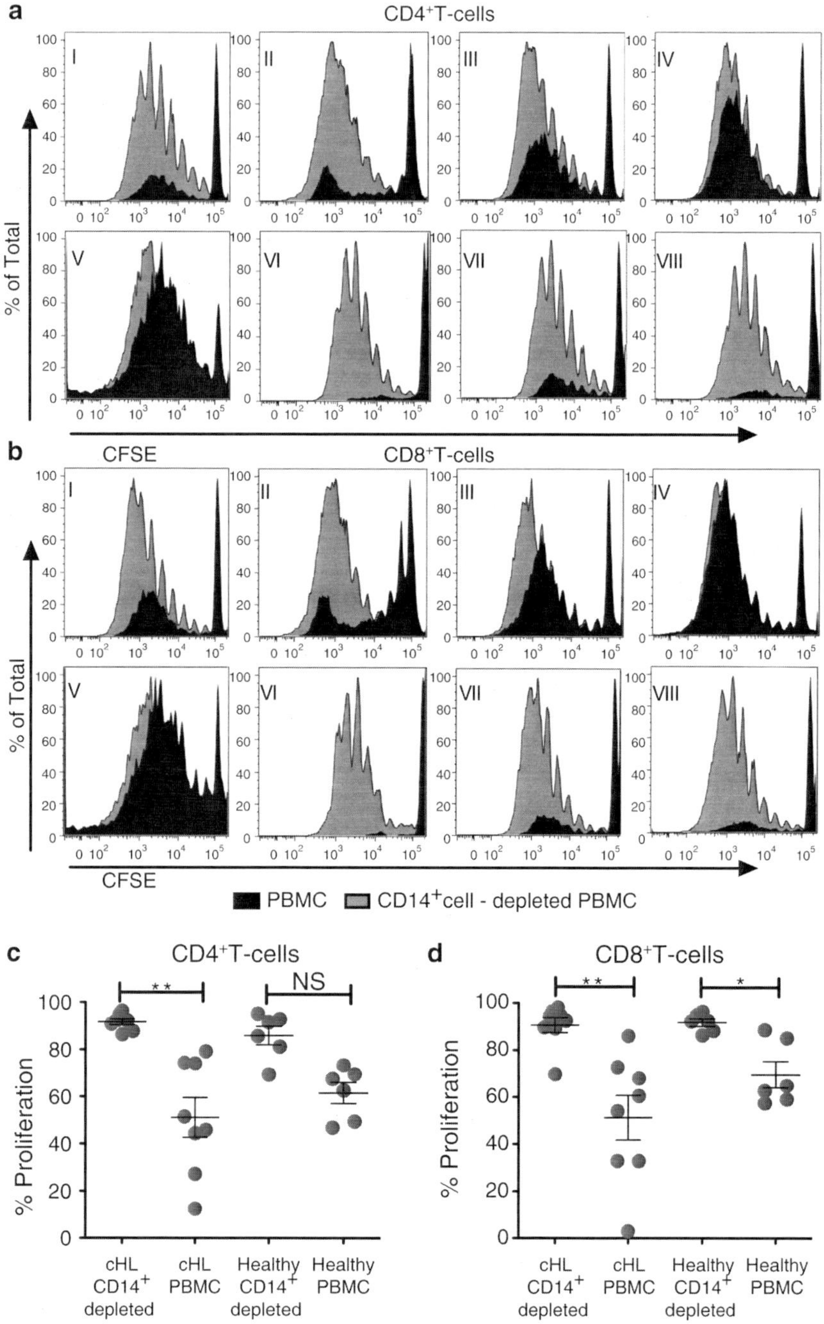

Fig. 6 Monocyte depletion enhances T-cell proliferation in cHL patients (Taken with permission from Jones et al. (2013)). *Histograms* show (**a**) CD4$^+$ and (**b**) CD8$^+$ T-cell proliferation from eight cHL patients (labeled *I–VIII*). T-cell proliferation from CD14$^+$ cell-depleted PBMC in

timepoints with the mean over 10× the defined threshold value (mean 3,163 pg/ml, range 2,383–3,920 pg/ml) (Fig. 4c). These results demonstrate that concurrent allergic disease can greatly affect sTARC, rendering interpretation of disease response from sTARC levels impossible. In contrast, this patient's sCD163 and EBV-DNA levels reflected cHL disease throughout therapy.

Specificity of sTARC and sCD163

CD163+ monocytes were elevated in the peripheral blood of cHL patients ($P = 0.0437$) compared to healthy donors, implicating circulating "shed" CD163 as only partially tumor derived (Fig. 5). Interestingly, monocyte depletion markedly enhanced both CD4+ and CD8+ T-cell proliferation in cHL patients (both $P < 0.01$), suggesting monocyte-mediated immunosuppression may occur in cHL and offer a potential explanation for the association with sCD163 levels and lymphopenia (Fig. 6).

Thus, elevated sCD163 levels are not specific to cHL and may not be entirely tumor derived; however, sCD163 levels were not influenced by concurrent allergic disease. On the other hand, elevated sTARC levels are specific to cHL versus NLPHL and are likely to be mostly HRS cell derived in the absence of additional disease but in the presence of concurrent allergic dermatitis; sTARC levels can be greatly affected.

Conclusions and Future Challenges

The histological uniqueness of cHL, in which the microenvironment comprises 95 % of the diseased node, provides a unique opportunity to study the relative role of tumor-specific and tumor-associated biomarkers. Serum CD163 and TARC reflect different components of the diseased HL lymph node, namely, the tumor microenvironment and the tumor cell. Assaying both sequentially provides complimentary information that potentially will assist clinicians in prognosis, disease response assessment (both when PET/CT is and is not available), and surveillance as an early marker of relapse. The data presented is from an observational cHL study, in which neither therapy nor timing/nature of radiological monitoring was mandated. Definitive validation is required and can only be achieved through the use of large international, uniformly treated cohorts, ideally with data on their association with quantitative tumor burden assessment by PET/CT.

Fig. 6 (continued) gray and from nondepleted PBMC in *black*. (**c**) $CD4^+$ and (**d**) $CD8^+$ T-cell proliferation from cHL patient and healthy participant $CD14^+$ cell-depleted PBMC and nondepleted PBMC represented as total percent proliferation above background. *Error bars* represent mean with SEM. ***$P < 0.001$, **$P < 0.01$, *$P < 0.05$, NS = $P > 0.05$

Summary Points

- Serum CD163 and TARC are promising disease response biomarkers in classical Hodgkin lymphoma.
- Serum CD163 reflects the (benign) tumor microenvironment, and serum TARC is a biomarker of the (malignant) Hodgkin and Reed-Sternberg cell.
- Serum CD163 and TARC have distinct kinetics during therapy, with CD163 levels best reflecting interim therapy response.
- Serum CD163, but not TARC, may be of value as a disease response biomarker for NLPHL.
- Pre-therapy serum CD163 levels associated with lymphopenia and IPS.

References

Alvaro T, Lejeune M, et al. Outcome in Hodgkin's lymphoma can be predicted from the presence of accompanying cytotoxic and regulatory T cells. Clin Cancer Res. 2005;11(4):1467–73.

Alvaro-Naranjo T, Lejeune M, et al. Tumor-infiltrating cells as a prognostic factor in Hodgkin's lymphoma: a quantitative tissue microarray study in a large retrospective cohort of 267 patients. Leuk Lymphoma. 2005;46(11):1581–91.

Azambuja D, Natkunam Y, et al. Lack of association of tumor-associated macrophages with clinical outcome in patients with classical Hodgkin's lymphoma. Ann Oncol. 2012;23(3):736–42.

Caporaso NE, Goldin LR, et al. Current insight on trends, causes, and mechanisms of Hodgkin's lymphoma. Cancer J. 2009;15(2):117–23.

Chetaille B, Bertucci F, et al. Molecular profiling of classical Hodgkin lymphoma tissues uncovers variations in the tumor microenvironment and correlations with EBV infection and outcome. Blood. 2009;113(12):2765–3775.

Christiansen I, Enblad G, et al. Soluble ICAM-1 in Hodgkin's disease: a promising independent predictive marker for survival. Leuk Lymphoma. 1995;19(3–4):243–51.

Christiansen I, Sundstrom C, et al. Soluble vascular cell adhesion molecule-1 (sVCAM-1) is an independent prognostic marker in Hodgkin's disease. Br J Haematol. 1998;102(3):701–9.

Claviez A, Tiemann M, et al. Impact of latent Epstein-Barr virus infection on outcome in children and adolescents with Hodgkin's lymphoma. J Clin Oncol. 2005;23(18):4048–56.

Diehl V, Stein H, et al. Hodgkin's lymphoma: biology and treatment strategies for primary, relapsed disease. Hematology Am Soc Hematol Educ Program. 2003:225–47.

Diehl V, Thomas RK, et al. Part II: Hodgkin's lymphoma–diagnosis and treatment. Lancet Oncol. 2004;5(1):19–26.

Diepstra A, van Imhoff GW, et al. HLA class II expression by Hodgkin Reed-Sternberg cells is an independent prognostic factor in classical Hodgkin's lymphoma. J Clin Oncol. 2007; 25(21):3101–8.

Diepstra A, van Imhoff GW, et al. Latent Epstein-Barr virus infection of tumor cells in classical Hodgkin's lymphoma predicts adverse outcome in older adult patients. J Clin Oncol. 2009; 27(23):3815–21.

Doussis-Anagnostopoulou IA, Vassilakopoulos TP, et al. Topoisomerase IIalpha expression as an independent prognostic factor in Hodgkin's lymphoma. Clin Cancer Res. 2008;14(6):1759–66.

Drouet E, Brousset P, et al. High Epstein-Barr virus serum load and elevated titers of anti-ZEBRA antibodies in patients with EBV-harboring tumor cells of Hodgkin's disease. J Med Virol. 1999;57(4):383–9.

Evens AM, Hutchings M, et al. Treatment of Hodgkin lymphoma: the past, present, and future. Nat Clin Pract Oncol. 2008;5(9):543–56.

Fischer M, Juremalm M, et al. Expression of CCL5/RANTES by Hodgkin and Reed-Sternberg cells and its possible role in the recruitment of mast cells into lymphomatous tissue. Int J Cancer. 2003;107(2):197–201.

Gallagher A, Armstrong AA, et al. Detection of Epstein-Barr virus (EBV) genomes in the serum of patients with EBV-associated Hodgkin's disease. Int J Cancer. 1999;84(4):442–8.

Gallamini A, Kostakoglu L. Interim FDG-PET in Hodgkin lymphoma: a compass for a safe navigation in clinical trials? Blood. 2012;120(25):4913–20.

Gallamini A, Hutchings M, et al. Early interim 2-[18F]fluoro-2-deoxy-D-glucose positron emission tomography is prognostically superior to international prognostic score in advanced-stage Hodgkin's lymphoma: a report from a joint Italian-Danish study. J Clin Oncol. 2007; 25(24):3746–52.

Gandhi MK, Tellam JT, et al. Epstein-Barr virus-associated Hodgkin's lymphoma. Br J Haematol. 2004;125(3):267–81.

Gandhi MK, Lambley E, et al. Plasma Epstein-Barr virus (EBV) DNA is a biomarker for EBV-positive Hodgkin's lymphoma. Clin Cancer Res. 2006;12(2):460–4.

Gause A, Pohl C, et al. Clinical significance of soluble CD30 antigen in the sera of patients with untreated Hodgkin's disease. Blood. 1991;77(9):1983–8.

Gause A, Jung W, et al. Soluble CD8, CD25 and CD30 antigens as prognostic markers in patients with untreated Hodgkin's lymphoma. Ann Oncol. 1992;3 Suppl 4:49–52.

Glavina-Durdov M, Jakic-Razumovic J, et al. Assessment of the prognostic impact of the Epstein-Barr virus-encoded latent membrane protein-1 expression in Hodgkin's disease. Br J Cancer. 2001;84(9):1227–34.

Greaves P, Clear A, et al. Expression of FOXP3, CD68, and CD20 at diagnosis in the microenvironment of classical Hodgkin lymphoma is predictive of outcome. J Clin Oncol. 2013; 31(2):256–62.

Harris JA, Jain S, et al. CD163 versus CD68 in tumor associated macrophages of classical Hodgkin lymphoma. Diagn Pathol. 2012;7:12.

Hasenclever D, Diehl V. A prognostic score for advanced Hodgkin's disease. International Prognostic Factors Project on Advanced Hodgkin's Disease. N Engl J Med. 1998;339 (21):1506–14.

Herbst H, Dallenbach F, et al. Epstein-Barr virus latent membrane protein expression in Hodgkin and Reed-Sternberg cells. Proc Natl Acad Sci U S A. 1991;88(11):4766–70.

Hijnen D, De Bruin-Weller M, et al. Serum thymus and activation-regulated chemokine (TARC) and cutaneous T cell- attracting chemokine (CTACK) levels in allergic diseases: TARC and CTACK are disease-specific markers for atopic dermatitis. J Allergy Clin Immunol. 2004; 113(2):334–40.

Hohaus S, Santangelo R, et al. The viral load of Epstein-Barr virus (EBV) DNA in peripheral blood predicts for biological and clinical characteristics in Hodgkin lymphoma. Clin Cancer Res. 2011;17(9):2885–92.

Hutchings M, Mikhaeel NG, et al. Prognostic value of interim FDG-PET after two or three cycles of chemotherapy in Hodgkin lymphoma. Ann Oncol. 2005;16(7):1160–8.

Hutchings M, Loft A, et al. FDG-PET after two cycles of chemotherapy predicts treatment failure and progression-free survival in Hodgkin lymphoma. Blood. 2006;107(1):52–9.

Jarrett RF, Gallagher A, et al. Detection of Epstein-Barr virus genomes in Hodgkin's disease: relation to age. J Clin Pathol. 1991;44(10):844–8.

Jerusalem G, Beguin Y, et al. Whole-body positron emission tomography using 18F-fluorodeoxyglucose for posttreatment evaluation in Hodgkin's disease and non-Hodgkin's lymphoma has higher diagnostic and prognostic value than classical computed tomography scan imaging. Blood. 1999;94(2):429–33.

Jones K, Nourse JP, et al. Tumor-specific but not nonspecific cell-free circulating DNA can be used to monitor disease response in lymphoma. Am J Hematol. 2012;87(3):258–65.

Jones K, Vari F, et al. Serum CD163 and TARC as disease response biomarkers in classical Hodgkin lymphoma. Clin Cancer Res. 2013;19(3):731–42.

Kamper P, Bendix K, et al. Tumor-infiltrating macrophages correlate with adverse prognosis and Epstein-Barr virus status in classical Hodgkin's lymphoma. Haematologica. 2011a;96(2): 269–76.

Kamper P, Ludvigsen M, et al. Proteomic analysis identifies galectin-1 as a predictive biomarker for relapsed/refractory disease in classical Hodgkin lymphoma. Blood. 2011b;117(24): 6638–49.

Kanakry JA, Li H, et al. Plasma Epstein-Barr virus DNA predicts outcome in advanced Hodgkin lymphoma: correlative analysis from a large North American cooperative group trial. Blood. 2013;121(18):3547–53.

Kuppers R. The biology of Hodgkin's lymphoma. Nat Rev Cancer. 2009;9(1):15–27.

Kurzrock R, Redman J, et al. Serum interleukin 6 levels are elevated in lymphoma patients and correlate with survival in advanced Hodgkin's disease and with B symptoms. Cancer Res. 1993;53(9):2118–22.

Mao Y, Lu MP, et al. Prognostic significance of EBV latent membrane protein 1 expression in lymphomas: evidence from 15 studies. PLoS One. 2013;8(4):e60313.

Meignan M, Gallamini A, et al. Report on the Second International Workshop on interim positron emission tomography in lymphoma held in Menton, France, 8–9 April 2010. Leuk Lymphoma. 2010;51(12):2171–80.

Niens M, Visser L, et al. Serum chemokine levels in Hodgkin lymphoma patients: highly increased levels of CCL17 and CCL22. Br J Haematol. 2008;140(5):527–36.

Oudejans JJ, Jiwa NM, et al. Activated cytotoxic T cells as prognostic marker in Hodgkin's disease. Blood. 1997;89(4):1376–82.

Ouyang J, Plutschow A, et al. Galectin-1 serum levels reflect tumor burden and adverse clinical features in classical Hodgkin lymphoma. Blood. 2013;121(17):3431–3.

Pallesen G, Hamilton-Dutoit SJ, et al. Expression of Epstein-Barr virus latent gene products in tumour cells of Hodgkin's disease. Lancet. 1991;337(8737):320–2.

Peh SC, Kim LH, et al. TARC, a CC chemokine, is frequently expressed in classic Hodgkin's lymphoma but not in NLP Hodgkin's lymphoma, T-cell-rich B-cell lymphoma, and most cases of anaplastic large cell lymphoma. Am J Surg Pathol. 2001;25(7):925–9.

Pileri SA, Ascani S, et al. Hodgkin's lymphoma: the pathologist's viewpoint. J Clin Pathol. 2002;55(3):162–76.

Plattel WJ, van den Berg A, et al. Plasma thymus and activation-regulated chemokine as an early response marker in classical Hodgkin's lymphoma. Haematologica. 2012;97(3):410–5.

Reynolds GM, Billingham LJ, et al. Interleukin 6 expression by Hodgkin/Reed-Sternberg cells is associated with the presence of 'B' symptoms and failure to achieve complete remission in patients with advanced Hodgkin's disease. Br J Haematol. 2002;118(1):195–201.

Sanchez-Espiridion B, Martin-Moreno AM, et al. Immunohistochemical markers for tumor associated macrophages and survival in advanced classical Hodgkin lymphoma. Haematologica. 2012;97(7):1080–4.

Seymour JF, Talpaz M, et al. Clinical correlates of elevated serum levels of interleukin 6 in patients with untreated Hodgkin's disease. Am J Med. 1997;102(1):21–8.

Shim HK, Lee WW, et al. Relationship between FDG uptake and expressions of glucose transporter type 1, type 3, and hexokinase-II in Reed-Sternberg cells of Hodgkin lymphoma. Oncol Res. 2009;17(7):331–7.

Shimada Y, Takehara K, et al. Both Th2 and Th1 chemokines (TARC/CCL17, MDC/CCL22, and Mig/CXCL9) are elevated in sera from patients with atopic dermatitis. J Dermatol Sci. 2004;34(3):201–8.

Skinnider BF, Mak TW. The role of cytokines in classical Hodgkin lymphoma. Blood. 2002;99(12):4283–97.

Spacek M, Hubacek P, et al. Plasma EBV-DNA monitoring in Epstein-Barr virus-positive Hodgkin lymphoma patients. Acta Pathol Microbiol Immunol Scand. 2011;119(1):10–6.

Steidl C, Lee T, et al. Tumor-associated macrophages and survival in classic Hodgkin's lymphoma. N Engl J Med. 2010;362(10):875–85.

Steidl C, Diepstra A, et al. Gene expression profiling of microdissected Hodgkin Reed-Sternberg cells correlates with treatment outcome in classical Hodgkin lymphoma. Blood. 2012;120(17): 3530–40.

Swerdlow SH, Campo E, et al. WHO Classification of Tumours of Haematopoietic and Lymphoid Tissues. 4th ed. Lyon, France: IARC Press; 2008.

ten Berge RL, Oudejans JJ, et al. Percentage of activated cytotoxic T-lymphocytes in anaplastic large cell lymphoma and Hodgkin's disease: an independent biological prognostic marker. Leukemia. 2001;15(3):458–64.

Tubiana M, Henry-Amar M, et al. Toward comprehensive management tailored to prognostic factors of patients with clinical stages I and II in Hodgkin's disease. The EORTC Lymphoma Group controlled clinical trials: 1964–1987. Blood. 1989;73(1):47–56.

Tzankov A, Meier C, et al. Correlation of high numbers of intratumoral FOXP3+ regulatory T cells with improved survival in germinal center-like diffuse large B-cell lymphoma, follicular lymphoma and classical Hodgkin's lymphoma. Haematologica. 2008;93(2):193–200.

van den Berg A, Visser L, et al. High expression of the CC chemokine TARC in Reed-Sternberg cells. A possible explanation for the characteristic T-cell infiltrate in Hodgkin's lymphoma. Am J Pathol. 1999;154(6):1685–91.

Vassilakopoulos TP, Nadali G, et al. Serum interleukin-10 levels are an independent prognostic factor for patients with Hodgkin's lymphoma. Haematologica. 2001;86(3):274–81.

Wagner HJ, Schlager F, et al. Detection of Epstein-Barr virus DNA in peripheral blood of paediatric patients with Hodgkin's disease by real-time polymerase chain reaction. Eur J Cancer. 2001;37(15):1853–7.

Weihrauch MR, Manzke O, et al. Elevated serum levels of CC thymus and activation-related chemokine (TARC) in primary Hodgkin's disease: potential for a prognostic factor. Cancer Res. 2005;65(13):5516–9.

Yamamoto R, Nishikori M, et al. PD-1-PD-1 ligand interaction contributes to immunosuppressive microenvironment of Hodgkin lymphoma. Blood. 2008;111(6):3220–4.

Yoon DH, Koh YW, et al. CD68 and CD163 as prognostic factors for Korean patients with Hodgkin lymphoma. Eur J Haematol. 2012;88(4):292–305.

Zinzani PL, Magagnoli M, et al. The role of positron emission tomography (PET) in the management of lymphoma patients. Ann Oncol. 1999;10(10):1181–4.

Part IX

Further Knowledge

Biomarkers in Health and Disease: Cancer Further Knowledge

44

Rajkumar Rajendram, Roshanna Rajendram, Vinood B. Patel, and Victor R. Preedy

Contents

R. Rajendram (✉)
Department of General Medicine and Intensive Care, John Radcliffe Hospital, Oxford, UK

Diabetes and Nutritional Sciences Research Division, School of Medicine, King's College London, London, UK
e-mail: rajkumarrajendram@doctors.org.uk; rajkumarrajendram@hotmail.com

R. Rajendram
School of Medicine, University of Birmingham, Edgbaston, Birmingham, UK

V.B. Patel
Department of Biomedical Sciences, Faculty of Science and Technology, University of Westminster, London, UK
e-mail: v.b.patel@westminster.ac.uk

V.R. Preedy
Department of Nutrition and Dietetics, Division of Diabetes and Nutritional Sciences, Faculty of Life Sciences and Medicine, King's College London, London, UK
e-mail: victor.preedy@kcl.ac.uk

V.R. Preedy, V.B. Patel (eds.), *Biomarkers in Cancer, Biomarkers in Disease: Methods, Discoveries and Applications*,
DOI 10.1007/978-94-007-7681-4_47

Abstract

A cancer biomarker is a substance that indicates the presence of cancer. It could be secreted by a tumor or result from a specific response to the cancer. Genetic, epigenetic, proteomic, glycomic, and imaging biomarkers can be used for cancer diagnosis, prognosis, and epidemiology. This chapter outlines the sources of the most up-to-date information on the regulatory bodies, journals on biomarkers, journals on cancer, professional bodies, books, emerging techniques and platforms, and websites that are relevant to an evidence-based use of biomarkers in health and disease.

Introduction

A cancer develops when cells reproduce uncontrollably. These cancer cells destroy the surrounding tissue and can spread to other organs (metastasize). There are over 200 different types of cancer, each of which can cause a multitude of symptoms and each has its own methods of diagnosis and treatment.

Biomarkers have significant scientific and clinical value in oncology. In 2001 a consensus panel defined biomarkers as "characteristics that are objectively measured and evaluated as indicators of normal biological processes, pathogenic processes, or pharmacologic responses to a therapeutic intervention or other health care intervention" (Atkinson et al. 2001).

A cancer biomarker is a substance that indicates the presence of cancer. It could be secreted by a tumor or result from a specific response to the cancer. Genetic, epigenetic, proteomic, glycomic, and imaging biomarkers can be used for cancer diagnosis, prognosis, and epidemiology. Ideally, such biomarkers can be assayed in noninvasively collected biofluids like blood or serum (Atkinson et al. 2001).

Biomarkers can be used to diagnose cancers at an early stage, suggest the likely outcome (prognosis) in the absence of treatment, and predict the likely response to treatment. Thus there are three main uses for biomarkers in oncology:

Diagnosis
Prognosis
Prediction

While challenges exist in translating research on novel biomarkers into clinical practice, several biomarkers are currently used routinely by oncologists (doctors who specialize in the management of patients with cancer). These include AFP (liver cancer), BCR-ABL (chronic myeloid leukemia), BRCA1/BRCA2 (breast/ovarian cancer), CEA (colorectal cancer), HER-2 (breast cancer), and PSA (prostate-specific antigen) (prostate cancer).

Table 1 This table lists the regulatory bodies and organizations involved with various aspects of biomarkers

Regulatory bodies and organizations	
Biomarkers Consortium	www.biomarkersconsortium.org
Biomarker, Imaging and Quality of Life Studies Funding Program, National Cancer Institute, USA	www.cancer.gov/aboutnci/organization/ccct/funding/BIQSFP
Biomarker Qualification Program US Food and Drug Administration	www.fda.gov/Drugs/DevelopmentApprovalProcess/DrugDevelopmentToolsQualificationProgram/ucm284076.htm
Cancer Australia	www.canceraustralia.gov.au
Cancer Diagnosis Program, National Cancer Institute, USA	www.cancerdiagnosis.nci.nih.gov
Cancer Institute New South Wales	www.cancerinstitute.org.au
Clinical Proteomic Technologies for Cancer Initiative 2006–2011, National Cancer Institute, USA	www.proteomics.cancer.gov/programs/completed/cptac
Early Detection Research Network, National Cancer Institute, USA	www.edrn.nci.nih.gov
European Medicines Agency	www.ema.europa.eu/ema/index.jsp?curl=pages/special_topics/general/general_content_000349.jsp
Medicines and Healthcare products Regulatory Agency (MHRA)	www.mhra.gov.uk
National Cancer Institute	www.cancer.gov
Oncologic Drugs Advisory Committee of the US Food and Drug Administration	www.fda.gov/AdvisoryCommittees/CommitteesMeetingMaterials/Drugs/OncologicDrugsAdvisoryCommittee

Table 2 Journals publishing original research and review articles related to biomarkers

Journals on biomarkers or on the applications and use of biomarkers	
Biomarkers	www.informahealthcare.com/bmk
Biomarkers in Medicine	www.futuremedicine.com/loi/bmm
Journal of Biomarkers	www.hindawi.com/journals/jbm
Journal of Molecular Biomarkers & Diagnosis	www.omicsonline.org/molecular-biomarkers-diagnosis.php
Molecular and Cellular Proteomics	www.mcponline.org
Nature Medicine	www.nature.com/nm
New England Journal of Medicine	www.nejm.org

Several potentially relevant cancer biomarkers have been discovered through omic technologies such as genomics and proteomics. The use of emerging high-throughput technologies to integrate biomarkers into clinical practice will allow "personalization" of disease management in the future.

Table 3 This table lists the journals publishing original research and review articles related to cancer

Journals on cancer or covering material on cancer	
Annals of Oncology	www.annonc.oxfordjournals.org
British Journal of Cancer	www.nature.com/bjc
BMC Cancer	www.biomedcentral.com/bmccancer
Blood	www.bloodjournal.hematologylibrary.org
Cancer Epidemiology, Biomarkers & Prevention	www.cebp.aacrjournals.org
Clinical Cancer Research	www.clincancerres.aacrjournals.org
Cancer Cell	www.cell.com/cancer-cell/home
Cancer Discovery	www.cancerdiscovery.aacrjournals.org
Cancer Research	www.cancerres.aacrjournals.org
Journal of Clinical Oncology	www.jco.ascopubs.org
Journal of National Cancer Institute	www.jnci.oxfordjournals.org
Lancet Oncology	www.thelancet.com/journals/lanonc/issue/current
Leukemia	www.nature.com/leu/index.html

Examples of the definitions, measurement, and applications of biomarkers can be found in this book and also via the recommended resources in the tables below.

Tables 1–7 list the most up-to-date information on the regulatory bodies (Table 1), journals on biomarkers (Table 2), journals on cancer (Table 3), professional bodies (Table 4), books (Table 5), emerging techniques and platforms (Table 6), and websites (Table 7) that are relevant to an evidence-based use of biomarkers in health and disease.

Summary Points

- Biomarkers have significant clinical value in modern medicine.
- Biomarkers can be used in screening for cancer.
- Biomarkers can be used in staging of cancer, in grading, and to direct initial therapy after diagnosis.
- Biomarkers can be used to screen for cancer recurrence, monitor the response to treatment, and guide the choice of further treatments.
- This chapter lists the most up-to-date resources on the regulatory bodies, journals, books, professional bodies, and websites that are relevant to an evidence-based approach to the use of biomarkers.

Table 4 This table lists the professional societies involved with biomarkers and/or cancer

Professional societies	
American Association for Cancer Research	www.aacr.org
American Cancer Society	www.cancer.org
American Society of Clinical Oncology	www.asco.org
Biomed Central (BMC) Biomarkers Research	www.biomarkerres.org
European Association for Cancer Research	www.eacr.org
European Organisation for Research and Treatment of Cancer (EORTC)	www.eortc.org
Korean Breast Cancer Society	www.kbcs.or.kr
Korean Cancer Association	www.cancer.or.kr
International Clinical Cytometry Society	www.cytometry.org/web/index.php
National Cancer Institute (NCI) and National Human Genome Research Institute (NHGRI)	

Table 5 This table lists books on cancer and/or biomarkers

Relevant books
Oxford Textbook of Oncology. Souhami RL, Tannock I, Hohenberger P, Horiet JC (editors). Oxford University Press, 2001, Oxford, UK
Cancer: Principles and Practice of Oncology. De Vita VT, Lawrence TS, Rosenberg SA. Lippincott Williams & Wilkins, 2011, Philadelphia, USA
Abeloff's Clinical Oncology. Niederhuber JE, Armitage JO, Doroshow JH, Kastan MB, Tepper JE. Saunders, 2013, USA
The Aptamer Handbook: Functional Oligonucleotides and Their Applications. Klussmann S (editor). Wiley-VCH, 2006, Weinheim
Aptamers in Bioanalysis. Mascini M. Wiley-Interscience, 2009, New Jersey, USA
Cancer Medicine. Hong WK, Bast RC Jr., Hait WN, Kufe DW, Pollock RE, Weichselbaum, JF, Holland EF III. American Association for Cancer Research December, 2009, Philadelphia, USA

Table 6 This table lists some emerging source and resource platforms in biomarker discovery and application

Sources and resources for emerging techniques and platforms	
Archemix	www.archemix.com
Biobanking and Biomolecular Resources Research Infrastructure	www.bbmri.eu
Cancer Genome Atlas	www.cancergenome.nih.gov
Cancer Human Biobank (caHUB)	www.cancer.gov/aboutnci/recovery/recoveryfunding/cahub
European Human Tumor Frozen Tissue Bank	www.tubafrost.org
Lucerna, Inc	www.lucernatechnologies.com/About-Us-17.html
OTC Biotech	www.otcbiotech.com/
University of Zurich Progenetix database	www.progenetix.org/cgi-bin/pgHome.cgi

Table 7 This table lists some internet resources on biomarkers

Relevant internet resources	
Adjuvant online	www.adjuvantonline.com
American Association for Cancer Research	www.aacr.org
American Cancer Society	www.cancer.org
American Society of Clinical Oncology	www.asco.org
Biomed Central (BMC) Biomarkers	www.biomarkerres.org
European Association for Cancer Research	www.eacr.org
European Organisation for Research and Treatment of Cancer (EORTC)	www.eortc.org
ISCIII	www.cnio.es
Gene Card	www.genecards.org
NCBI	www.ncbi.nlm.nih.gov
National Cancer Institute	www.cancer.gov
NCCN	www.nccn.org
Oncomine	www.oncomine.org
Telomerase Database	www.telomerase.asu.edu/
World Health Organization	www.who.int/mediacentre/factsheets/fs297/en/index.html

Acknowledgement We would like to thank the following authors for contributing to the development of this resource (Carnero A, Clarke S, De Rossi A, Diakos C, Noh D-Y, Schraml PH, Takenaka S, Wonshik H, Yi L).

References

Atkinson AJ, Colburn WA, DeGruttola VG, DeMets DL, Downing GJ, Hoth DF, Oates JA, Peck CC, Schooley RT, Spilker BA, Woodcock J, Zeger SL. NCI-FDA Biomarkers Definitions Working Group; Biomarkers and surrogate endpoints: preferred definitions and conceptual framework. Clin Pharmacol Ther. 2001;69:89–95.

Index

V.R. Preedy, V.B. Patel (eds.), *Biomarkers in Cancer, Biomarkers in Disease: Methods, Discoveries and Applications*,
DOI 10.1007/978-94-007-7681-4

MIX
Papier aus verantwortungsvollen Quellen
Paper from responsible sources
FSC® C105338

Printed by Books on Demand, Germany